WITHDRAWN
FROM LIBRARY

BRITISH MEDICAL ASSOCIATION

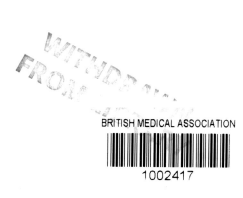

1002417

DIAGNOSTIC PATHOLOGY

Endocrine

SECOND EDITION

NOSÉ

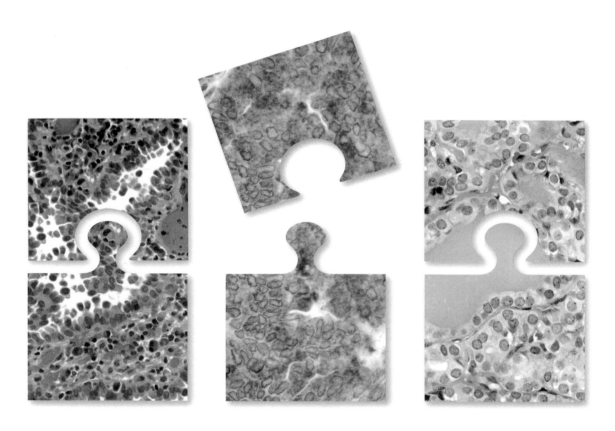

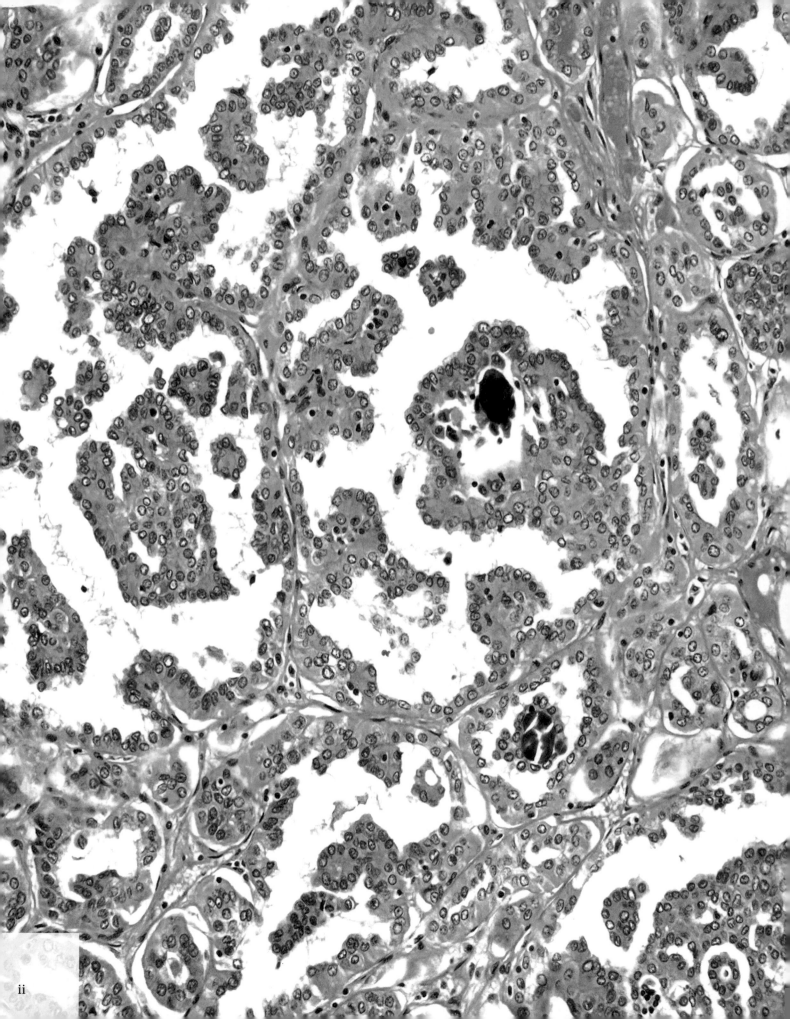

DIAGNOSTIC PATHOLOGY

Endocrine

SECOND EDITION

Vania Nosé, MD, PhD

Associate Chief of Pathology
Director of Anatomic and Molecular Pathology
Massachusetts General Hospital
Professor of Pathology
Harvard Medical School
Boston, Massachusetts

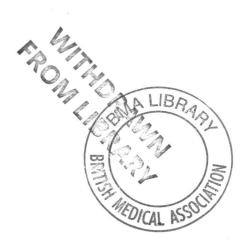
WITHDRAWN FROM LIBRARY
BMA LIBRARY
BRITISH MEDICAL ASSOCIATION

ELSEVIER

1600 John F. Kennedy Blvd.
Ste 1800
Philadelphia, PA 19103-2899

DIAGNOSTIC PATHOLOGY: ENDOCRINE, SECOND EDITION

ISBN: 978-0-323-52480-3

Copyright © 2018 by Elsevier. All rights reserved.

No part of this publication may be reproduced or transmitted in any form or by any means, electronic or mechanical, including photocopying, recording, or any information storage and retrieval system, without permission in writing from the publisher. Details on how to seek permission, further information about the Publisher's permissions policies and our arrangements with organizations such as the Copyright Clearance Center and the Copyright Licensing Agency, can be found at our website: www.elsevier.com/permissions.

This book and the individual contributions contained in it are protected under copyright by the Publisher (other than as may be noted herein).

Notices

Knowledge and best practice in this field are constantly changing. As new research and experience broaden our understanding, changes in research methods, professional practices, or medical treatment may become necessary.

Practitioners and researchers must always rely on their own experience and knowledge in evaluating and using any information, methods, compounds, or experiments described herein. In using such information or methods they should be mindful of their own safety and the safety of others, including parties for whom they have a professional responsibility.

With respect to any drug or pharmaceutical products identified, readers are advised to check the most current information provided (i) on procedures featured or (ii) by the manufacturer of each product to be administered, to verify the recommended dose or formula, the method and duration of administration, and contraindications. It is the responsibility of practitioners, relying on their own experience and knowledge of their patients, to make diagnoses, to determine dosages and the best treatment for each individual patient, and to take all appropriate safety precautions.

To the fullest extent of the law, neither the Publisher nor the authors, contributors, or editors, assume any liability for any injury and/or damage to persons or property as a matter of products liability, negligence or otherwise, or from any use or operation of any methods, products, instructions, or ideas contained in the material herein.

Publisher Cataloging-in-Publication Data

Names: Nosé, Vania.
Title: Diagnostic pathology. Endocrine / [edited by] Vania Nosé.
Other titles: Endocrine.
Description: Second edition. | Salt Lake City, UT : Elsevier, Inc., [2018] | Includes bibliographical references and index.
Identifiers: ISBN 978-0-323-52480-3
Subjects: LCSH: Endocrine glands--Diseases--Diagnosis--Handbooks, manuals, etc. | Endocrine glands--Tumors--Handbooks, manuals, etc. | Pathology, Surgical--Handbooks, manuals, etc. | MESH: Endocrine System Diseases--pathology--Atlases. | Endocrine System Diseases--diagnosis--Atlases.
Classification: LCC RC280.E55 N67 2018 | NLM WK 17 | DDC 616.4--dc23

International Standard Book Number: 978-0-323-52480-3

Cover Designer: Tom M. Olson, BA

Printed in Canada by Friesens, Altona, Manitoba, Canada

Last digit is the print number: 9 8 7 6 5 4 3 2 1

 Working together to grow libraries in developing countries

www.elsevier.com • www.bookaid.org

Dedication

To my wonderful sons and best friends, Gustave, Erick, and Philip, and to their wives, Carla, Suzana, and Bianca, and to my future grandchildren (no pressure!), for making my life so lovely, happy, interesting, and complete.

To my dearest parents, Dalva and Antonio, for their amazing life example, invaluable guidance, and support.

To my adored brothers, Dalton and Walton, and their lovely families, for their tremendous support and invaluable friendship.

To the contributing authors of this book, for their contributions, wonderful work, and extreme dedication to this project.

To my mentors in endocrine pathology, Drs. Shields Warren, William A. Meissner, and Merle A. Legg: it was a real honor and a privilege to train with such legends, and for their guidance shaping my career since.

To my residents and fellows, who make endocrine pathology more exciting.

To Lisa Gervais and the Elsevier group, for their extraordinary work in making this book a reality.

VN

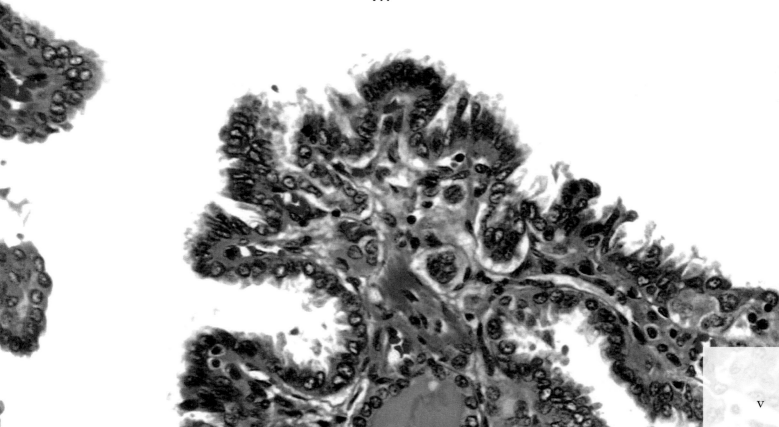

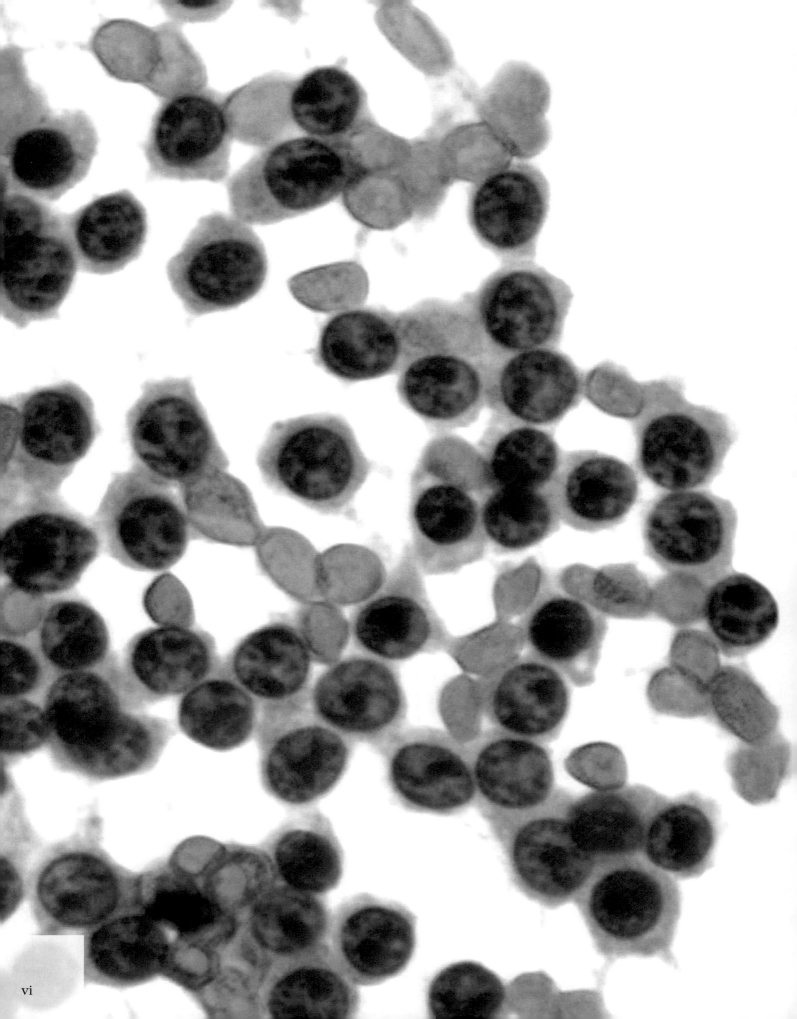

Contributing Authors

Carla Martins Alberti, MD
Department of Cardiology
Hospital Beneficência Portuguesa de São Paulo
São Paulo, Brazil

Lori A. Erickson, MD
Professor of Pathology
Mayo Clinic
Rochester, Minnesota

Nada A. Farhat, MD, MA, MPH
Attending Pathologist and
Assistant Professor of Pathology
New York Eye and Ear Infirmary of Mount Sinai
Icahn School of Medicine
New York, New York

Julie Guilmette, MD
Endocrine/Head and Neck Pathology Fellow
Massachusetts General Hospital
Boston, Massachusetts

Suzana Leite, MD
Department of Ophthalmic Plastic Surgery
Eye Clinic
São Paulo, Brazil

M. Beatriz S. Lopes, MD, PhD
Professor of Pathology and Neurological Surgery
University of Virginia School of Medicine
University of Virginia Health System
Charlottesville, Virginia

Michelle Menon Miyake, MD
Otolaryngologist and Head and Neck Surgeon
Department of Otolaryngology
Santa Casa de Misericórdia de São Paulo
São Paulo, Brazil

Peter M. Sadow, MD, PhD
Associate Professor of Pathology
Harvard Medical School
Director, Head and Neck Pathology
Massachusetts General Hospital
Pathologist
Massachusetts Eye and Ear
Boston, Massachusetts

Dipti P. Sajed, MD, PhD
Assistant Professor of Pathology
UCLA David Geffen School of Medicine
Los Angeles, California

Martin Taylor, MD, PhD
Chief Resident, Anatomic Pathology
Massachusetts General Hospital and
Harvard Medical School
Boston, Massachusetts

Arthur S. Tischler, MD
Professor of Pathology
Tufts University School of Medicine
Tufts Medical Center
Boston, Massachusetts

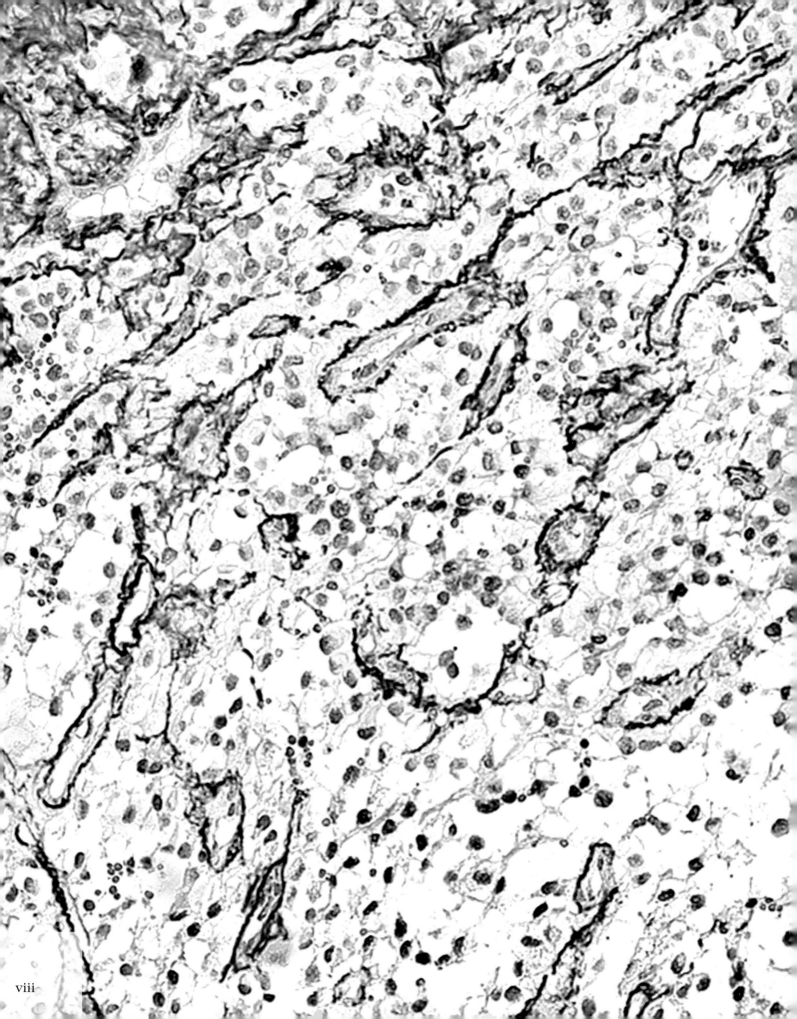

Preface

Our goal for this book is to offer comprehensive and updated information on the latest developments in endocrine pathology, presented in an easy and intuitive format. We hope that students, residents, fellows, and practicing pathologists and endocrinologists will find it useful for improving their skillset and aiding in the diagnosis of distinct endocrine lesions and tumors.

Diagnostic Pathology: Endocrine, second edition conveys intensive insight on conditions of the pituitary, thyroid, parathyroid, adrenal gland, neuroendocrine pancreas, and neuroendocrine skin. The classic and newly described inherited tumor syndromes and paraneoplastic syndromes are also presented.

New entities were added to the second edition, including noninvasive follicular neoplasm with papillary-like nuclear features (NIFTP), IgG4-related thyroid diseases, DICER1 syndrome, and multiple neoplasia type 4 (MEN4). This new edition is also completely updated according to the new 2017 WHO Classification of Tumors of Endocrine Organs.

The relevant characteristics of 128 diagnoses are discussed, including key factors such as clinical presentation, pathogenesis, molecular findings, electron microscopy, and immunohistochemical features, to name a few.

The user-friendly outline format highlights pertinent information for easy review and quick reference. Tables are included when relevant. Each entity is richly illustrated; there are more than 2,400 illustrations, micrographs, gross photographs, and other images in the book.

Contributions from renowned pathologists and physicians in their subspecialties have allowed us to present not only common/classic endocrine diagnoses, but also newly recognized diseases and unusual cases. Moreover, the Expert Consult™ eBook version included with the purchase of the print book will allow us to update this volume periodically.

We hope that the second edition of *Diagnostic Pathology: Endocrine* will be an informative, enlightening, and beneficial resource for pathologists, pathologists in training, endocrinologists, endocrine surgeons, and all healthcare professionals with an interest in endocrine diseases.

Vania Nosé, MD, PhD

Associate Chief of Pathology
Director of Anatomic and Molecular Pathology
Massachusetts General Hospital
Professor of Pathology
Harvard Medical School
Boston, Massachusetts

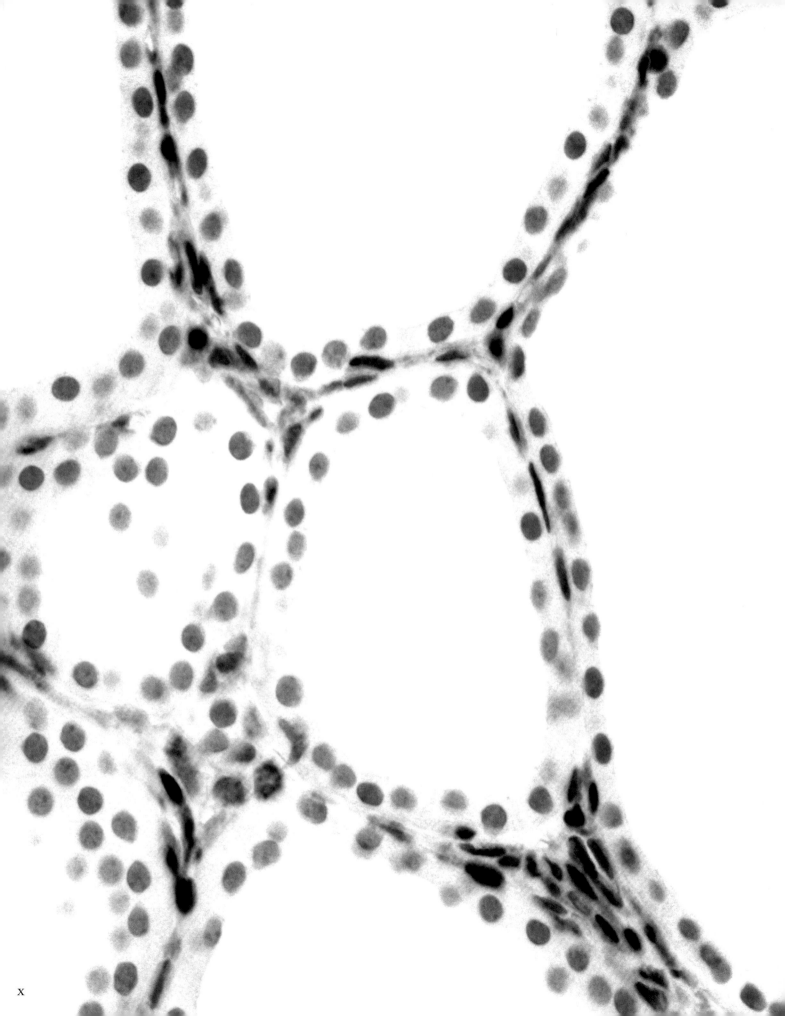

Acknowledgments

Lead Editor

Lisa A. Gervais, BS

Text Editors

Arthur G. Gelsinger, MA
Rebecca L. Bluth, BA
Nina I. Bennett, BA
Terry W. Ferrell, MS
Matt W. Hoecherl, BS
Megg Morin, BA

Image Editors

Jeffrey J. Marmorstone, BS
Lisa A. M. Steadman, BS

Illustrations

Richard Coombs, MS
Lane R. Bennion, MS
Laura C. Wissler, MA

Art Direction and Design

Tom M. Olson, BA
Laura C. Wissler, MA

Production Coordinators

Angela M. G. Terry, BA
Emily C. Fassett, BA

ELSEVIER

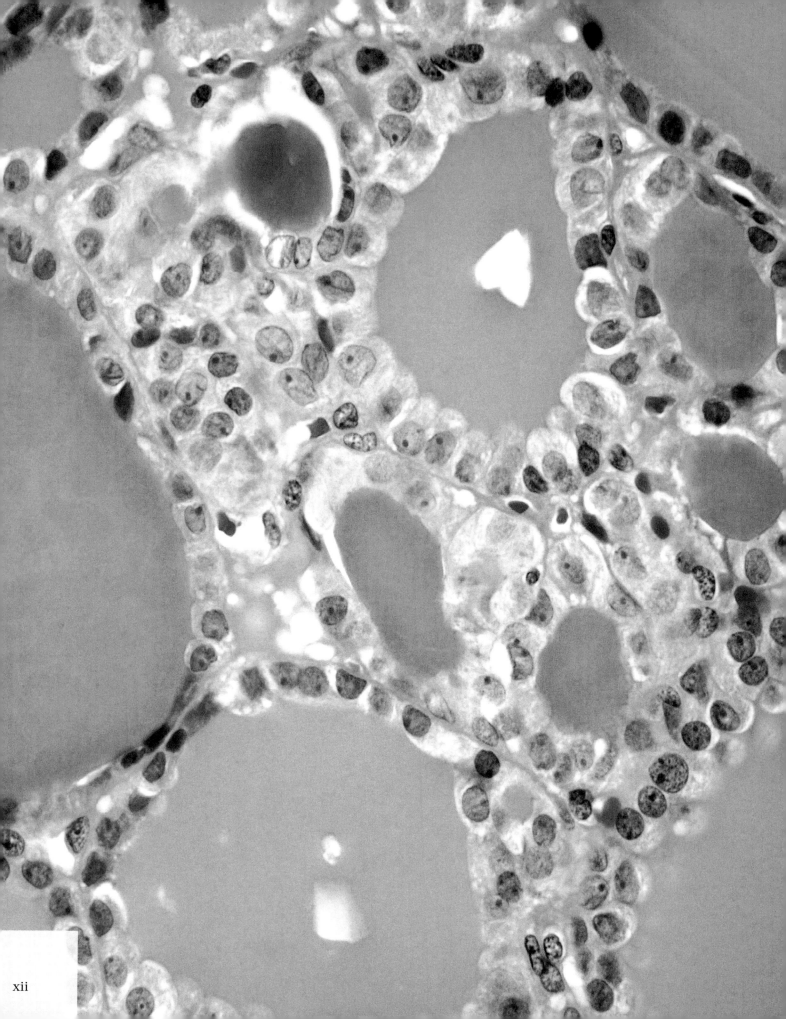

Sections

SECTION 1:
Thyroid

SECTION 2:
Parathyroid Gland

SECTION 3:
Adrenal Glands

SECTION 4:
Pituitary Gland

SECTION 5:
Endocrine Pancreas

SECTION 6:
Endocrine Skin

SECTION 7:
Inherited Tumor Syndromes

SECTION 8:
Paraneoplastic Syndromes

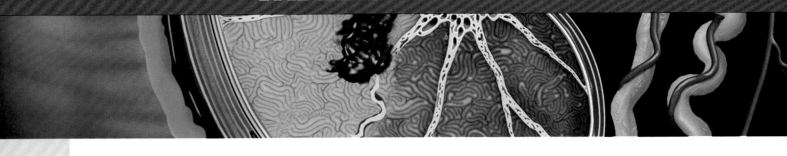

TABLE OF CONTENTS

TABLE OF CONTENTS

TABLE OF CONTENTS

DIAGNOSTIC PATHOLOGY

Endocrine

SECOND EDITION

NOSÉ

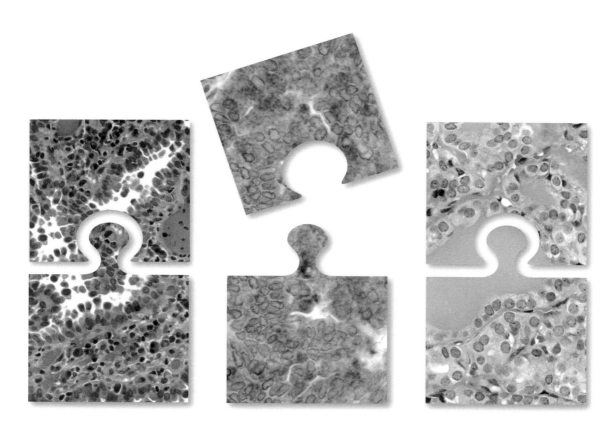

SECTION 1
Thyroid

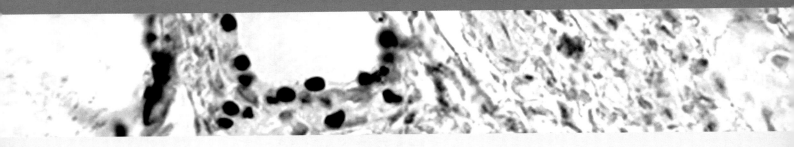

Nonneoplastic

Neoplastic

Molecular Pathology of Thyroid Neoplasms

Protocol for Examination of Specimens From Patients With Carcinoma of Thyroid Gland

Thyroglossal Duct Cyst

ETIOLOGY/PATHOGENESIS

- Derived from thyroglossal duct, which is connection between median anlage, foramen cecum, and descended thyroid gland
- Thyroglossal duct cyst (TGDC) is result of persistence of thyroglossal duct

CLINICAL ISSUES

- Fistulas may develop secondary to infection and may drain into skin or pharynx
- Papillary thyroid carcinoma may arise in TGDC

IMAGING

- Ultrasound and CT scan
  - Shows cyst intimately associated with hyoid bone with fluid density

CYTOPATHOLOGY

- Ciliated respiratory-type cells &/or squamous cells
- Mature lymphocytes

MACROSCOPIC

- Cysts vary greatly in size
  - 1- to 4-cm in diameter
- Usually contains clear fluid
- Smooth-walled cystic structure

MICROSCOPIC

- Midline location and distinct lining with lymphoid follicles
  - Helpful establishing diagnosis
- Cyst lined by respiratory epithelium
- Cyst wall may contain thyroid follicles

TOP DIFFERENTIAL DIAGNOSES

- Branchial cleft cyst and other benign embryologic abnormalities
- Cystic degeneration of colloid nodule in multinodular hyperplasia
- Lymphatic malformation
- Abscess

(Left) Sagittal oblique graphic shows the course of a thyroglossal duct cyst from the foramen cecum ➡ to the thyroid bed. Note the close relationship to the midportion of the hyoid bone. The cyst can occur anywhere along this tract. (Right) Thyroglossal duct cyst shows ciliated respiratory-type epithelium lining cells ➡ in juxtaposition to scattered thyroid follicles. The cyst fluid is usually clear, fibrinous, and acellular.

Graphic of Thyroglossal Duct and Cyst

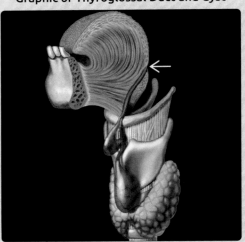

Thyroglossal Duct Cyst

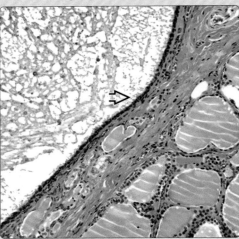

(Left) The high-power view highlights the cyst wall lined by a cylindrical, ciliated-type respiratory epithelium and a submucosa with lymphocytic infiltration. (Right) Histologic sections of a thyroglossal duct cyst shows both respiratory-type epithelium ➡ and an adjacent epithelium with squamous metaplasia ➡. Note a lymphoid follicle in the cyst wall ➡, a characteristic feature of thyroglossal duct cysts.

High Power of Thyroglossal Duct Cyst

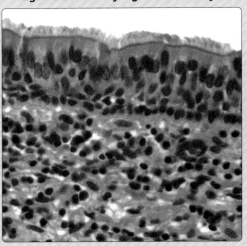

Cyst Wall of Thyroglossal Duct Cyst

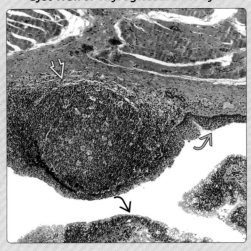

TERMINOLOGY

Abbreviations

- Thyroglossal duct cyst (TGDC)

Definitions

- Developmental anomaly derived from persistence of thyroglossal duct
  - Leading to development of cysts and fistulas

ETIOLOGY/PATHOGENESIS

Developmental Anomaly

- Derived from thyroglossal duct, which is connection between median anlage, foramen cecum, and descended thyroid gland
  - TGDC is result of persistence of thyroglossal duct
- Knowledge of typical course of thyroid primordium during embryologic development is essential to understand variant locations along this path where thyroid tissue can be found
- Migration of thyroid primordium begins at foramen cecum at base of tongue and then loops around hyoid bone anteriorly and inferiorly and descends anteriorly to thyrohyoid membrane into orthotopic location in infrahyoid portion of neck
- Thyroid ectopia is categorized into 1 of 4 typical locations with respect to this embryologic course
  - Base of tongue
  - Adjacent to hyoid bone
  - Midline infrahyoid portion of neck
  - Rarely in lateral part of neck

CLINICAL ISSUES

Epidemiology

- Incidence
  - No predisposition for male or female gender
  - Usually presents before 4th decade of life
  - 685 patients were recently described (344 males; 341 females)
    - Age at presentation was bimodal (1st and 5th decades) and ranged from 0.8-87.0 years (mean: 31.3 years)
    - Males predominate in children (150:111); females in adults (230:194)

Presentation

- Most frequently present with mobile midline neck mass in infrahyoid location
- Located at or below level of hyoid bone in anterior midline of neck
- Usually between 1-4 cm in diameter
  - Average cyst size: 2.4 cm
  - Pediatric patients have smaller cysts (mean: 2.1 cm) than adults (mean: 2.8 cm)
- Fistulas may develop secondary to infection and may drain into skin or pharynx
- Radiological studies demonstrate midline cystic area
  - Expansion or destruction of cartilaginous structure of hyoid may occur

Treatment

- Surgery
  - Necessary to avoid potential complications of fistulas
    - In rare instances, TGDCs can rupture and lead to life-threatening complications

Prognosis

- Cancer has been reported in TGDCs
  - Most common is papillary thyroid carcinoma
    - Occurs in 3.2% of all TGDCs in series of 685 cases
      - 22 patients (17 females, 5 males)
      - Aged 12-64 years (mean: 39.9 years; median: 39.0 years)
    - Typical cytologic and morphologic features of papillary thyroid carcinoma in context of cyst
    - Papillary thyroid carcinoma in TGDC is more common in women than men, tends to have classic morphologic features of papillary carcinoma, and carries similar prognosis
    - All of tumors are classic PTC, showing sclerotic and infiltrative pattern
  - Other malignancies
    - Adenosquamous cell carcinoma arising in TGDC
- Infection, rupture
  - May lead to life-threatening complications if not treated early
- Recurrence after surgery: 10%

IMAGING

CT Findings

- Imaging characteristics of TGDC as simple cyst and of ectopic thyroid tissue as hyperattenuating soft tissue mass at CT
- From retrospective study of all CT and MR imaging studies obtained in head and neck region
  - From over 60,00 CT and MR images, 69 cases (0.1%) had TGDCs
  - Ages ranged from 3 days to 17 years old,with the mean age at 5 years
  - Locations varied with majority at base of tongue (83%) followed by hyoid (13%) then infrahyoid straps (4%)
  - Sizes ranged from 2-28 mm with average size at 8 mm

MACROSCOPIC

General Features

- 1- to 4-cm cyst; usually contains clear fluid
- Smooth-walled cystic structure
  - May contain brown fluid
  - When infected, may contain purulent material
- Fistulas may occur secondary to inflammation and infection
  - May open into pharynx or skin
  - May have drainage

MICROSCOPIC

Histologic Features

- Cysts are usually lined by ciliated respiratory-type epithelium
  - ~ 38% are lined by respiratory epithelium alone
  - ~ 10% are lined by squamous epithelium alone

- o ~ 50% are lined by both respiratory and squamous epithelium
- Cyst wall contains lymphoid aggregates and lymphoid follicles
- Squamous metaplasia may be present
  - o Occurs in setting of chronic inflammation within TGDC
    - – Squamous cell carcinoma subtypes may rarely occur in setting of TGDC
- Granulation tissue and loss of epithelium may be seen after inflammation and infection
  - o It may be associated with skin fistula in ~ 10% of cases
- Cyst wall may contain thyroid follicles
  - o ~ 70% TGDC has associated thyroid gland tissue present within cyst wall
- Papillary thyroid carcinoma was identified in 22 patients (3.2%) in series of 685 cases
- Xanthogranulomatous inflammation with accumulation of foamy histiocytes, multinucleated giant cells (Touton type), cholesterol clefts, and chronic inflammatory cells may occur

Cytologic Features

- Squamous or respiratory cells
  - o Inflammatory cells usually composed of mature lymphocytes

DIFFERENTIAL DIAGNOSIS

Neoplastic vs. Nonneoplastic

- Carcinoma, lymphoma
  - o Metastatic cystic papillary thyroid carcinoma may be difficult to distinguish from papillary thyroid carcinoma occurring within TGDC
    - – Presence of respiratory or squamous epithelium as well as anatomic location helps in differentiation
  - o Squamous cell carcinoma
- Other benign cysts
  - o Epidermoid cysts may be present in thyroid gland
    - – Lined by squamous epithelium
      - □ They may be filled with keratin
      - □ Does not contain lymphoid follicles in wall
  - o Branchial cleft cyst and other benign embryologic abnormalities
  - o Cystic degeneration of colloid nodule in multinodular hyperplasia
  - o Lymphatic malformation
  - o Abscess
  - o Saccular cyst
  - o Relationship of mass to landmarks as
    - – Foramen cecum, hyoid bone, strap muscles, thyrohyoid membrane, and thyroid cartilage
    - – May help differentiate TGDC and ectopic thyroid tissue from other anterior neck masses when embryologic thyroid course is considered

DIAGNOSTIC CHECKLIST

Pathologic Interpretation Pearls

- Look for respiratory epithelium as well as gross features
- Squamous metaplasia occurs in setting of chronic inflammation within TGDC
- Be wary of carcinomas found incidentally within TGDCs excised without clinical suspicion of cancer

SELECTED REFERENCES

1. Bakkar S et al: The extent of surgery in thyroglossal cyst carcinoma. Langenbecks Arch Surg. 402(5):799-804, 2016
2. O'Neil LM et al: Wide anterior neck dissection for management of recurrent thyroglossal duct cysts in adults. J Laryngol Otol. 130 Suppl 4:S41-4, 2016
3. Shemen L et al: Imaging characteristics and findings in thyroglossal duct cancer and concurrent thyroid cancer. BMJ Case Rep. 2016, 2016
4. Thompson LD et al: Thyroglossal duct cyst carcinomas: a clinicopathologic series of 22 cases with staging recommendations. Head Neck Pathol. 11(2):175-185, 2016
5. Thompson LD et al: A clinicopathologic series of 685 thyroglossal duct remnant cysts. Head Neck Pathol. 10(4):465-474, 2016
6. Zizic M et al: Upper neck papillary thyroid cancer (UPTC): A new proposed term for the composite of thyroglossal duct cyst-associated papillary thyroid cancer, pyramidal lobe papillary thyroid cancer, and Delphian node papillary thyroid cancer metastasis. Laryngoscope. 126(7):1709-14, 2016
7. Baglam T et al: Does papillary carcinoma of thyroglossal duct cyst develop de novo? Case Rep Otolaryngol. 2015:382760, 2015
8. Taskin OC et al: Thyroglossal duct cyst associated with xanthogranulomatous inflammation. Head Neck Pathol. 9(4):530-3, 2015
9. Rohof D et al: Recurrences after thyroglossal duct cyst surgery: results in 207 consecutive cases and review of the literature. Head Neck. 37(12):1699-704, 2014
10. Rossi ED et al: Thyroglossal duct cyst cancer most likely arises from a thyroid gland remnant. Virchows Arch. 465(1):67-72, 2014
11. Zander DA et al: Imaging of ectopic thyroid tissue and thyroglossal duct cysts. Radiographics. 34(1):37-50, 2014
12. Wilsher MJ: IgG4 related disease of the thyroglossal duct. Pathology. 45(6):618-22, 2013
13. Yamada S et al: Papillary carcinoma arising in thyroglossal duct cyst in the lateral neck. Pathol Res Pract. 209(10):674-8, 2013
14. Altay C et al: CT and MRI findings of developmental abnormalities and ectopia varieties of the thyroid gland. Diagn Interv Radiol. 18(4):335-43, 2012
15. Kinoshita N et al: Adenosquamous carcinoma arising in a thyroglossal duct cyst: report of a case. Surg Today. 41(4):533-6, 2011
16. Rosenberg TL et al: Evaluating the adult patient with a neck mass. Med Clin North Am. 94(5):1017-29, 2010
17. Ozolek JA: Selective pathologies of the head and neck in children: a developmental perspective. Adv Anat Pathol. 16(5):332-58, 2009
18. Turkyilmaz Z et al: Congenital neck masses in children and their embryologic and clinical features. B-ENT. 4(1):7-18, 2008
19. Mussak EN et al: Surgical and medical management of midline ectopic thyroid. Otolaryngol Head Neck Surg. 136(6):870-2, 2007
20. Falvo L et al: Papillary thyroid carcinoma in thyroglossal duct cyst: case reports and literature review. Int Surg. 91(3):141-6, 2006
21. Foley DS et al: Thyroglossal duct and other congenital midline cervical anomalies. Semin Pediatr Surg. 15(2):70-5, 2006
22. Magro G et al: [Unusual non-neoplastic lesions in the "surgical pathology" of the thyroid.] Pathologica. 98(2):119-38, 2006
23. Niedziela M: Pathogenesis, diagnosis and management of thyroid nodules in children. Endocr Relat Cancer. 13(2):427-53, 2006
24. Sauvageau A et al: Fatal asphyxia by a thyroglossal duct cyst in an adult. J Clin Forensic Med. 13(6-8):349-52, 2006
25. Burnell I et al: Mucin-secreting papillary adenocarcinoma of the hyoid bone: a unique case. J Laryngol Otol. 119(6):498-502, 2005
26. Tarnaris A et al: Lymphoma mimicking a thyroglossal duct cyst in an adolescent. J Laryngol Otol. 119(3):216-8, 2005

CT of Thyroglossal Duct Cyst

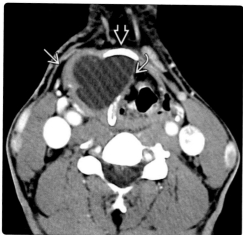

Cyst Wall of Thyroglossal Duct Cyst

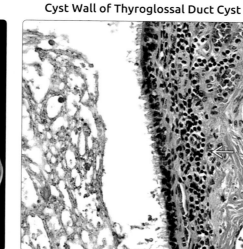

(Left) *Axial CECT shows a thyroglossal duct cyst at the level of the hyoid bone embedded in strap muscles* ➡. *The cyst abuts the hyoid bone* ➡ *and impinges on the preepiglottic space* ➡. (Right) *Thyroglossal duct cyst shows a cyst lined by a ciliated epithelium-lined wall with lymphoplasmacytic infiltration* ➡ *in the submucosa. Note dilated vessels in the wall and an amorphous material in the lumen.*

Papillary Thyroid Carcinoma Arising Within Thyroglossal Duct Cyst

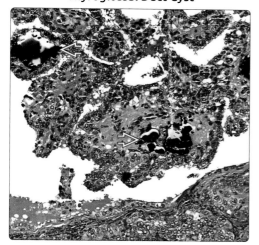

Papillary Thyroid Carcinoma Within Thyroglossal Duct Cyst

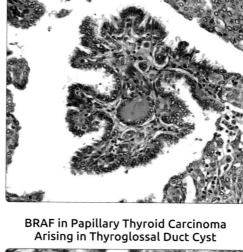

(Left) *Microphotograph shows a papillary thyroid carcinoma that arose in a thyroglossal duct cyst with the typical nuclear features of papillary carcinoma and with the presence of psammoma bodies* ➡. (Right) *Histological section shows a papillary thyroid carcinoma, classic variant, arising within a thyroglossal duct cyst. The papillary architecture and the nuclear features are characteristic of papillary carcinoma.*

Immunohistochemistry for TTF-1 in Thyroglossal Duct Cyst With Carcinoma

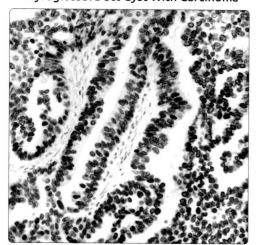

BRAF in Papillary Thyroid Carcinoma Arising in Thyroglossal Duct Cyst

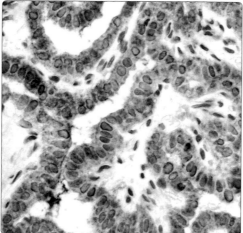

(Left) *Thyroglossal duct cyst is shown with areas of papillary thyroid carcinoma. These areas show TTF-1 immunostain positivity in this papillary thyroid carcinoma. These tumors have a similar immunophenotype as the tumors from thyroid origin.* (Right) *BRAF immunostain shows immunopositivity in the cytoplasm of the tumor cells of this papillary thyroid carcinoma arising within a thyroglossal duct cyst. The BRAF immunopositivity correlates with the BRAF V600 mutation.*

Ectopic Thyroid

TERMINOLOGY

- Thyroid tissue may be located in abnormal location along thyroglossal duct tract or at another site

ETIOLOGY/PATHOGENESIS

- Ectopic thyroid is result of improper descent of thyroid along its natural course during embryogenesis along thyroid anlage tract

CLINICAL ISSUES

- Ectopic thyroid tissue is one of most common anomalies occurring during histogenesis of thyroid gland
- Ectopic thyroid may be only thyroid tissue in some patients, so surgeons need to be wary of accidental removal of ectopic gland
- May be present in lingual, sublingual, suprathyroidal, or intrathymic location
- Lingual thyroid results from developmental abnormality due to failure to descend to its pretracheal position

○ Ectopic lingual thyroid tissue is rarely associated with obstructive oropharyngeal symptoms due to progressive enlargement

- Ectopic thyroid has been reported in variety of nontraditional places, including pericardium, heart, chest wall, vagina, inguinal region, and porta hepatis
- Normal-appearing thyroid tissue may be found in lymph nodes
- Ectopic tissue may also be found within striated muscles and fibroadipose tissues of central neck

MICROSCOPIC

- Normal thyroid tissue
- Subject to same diseases of thyroid as inflammation, hyperplasia, and tumors
- Most malignancies are histologically classified as papillary thyroid carcinomas
- As in many cases, ectopic thyroid gland may be only functioning thyroid tissue

Embryological Descent of Thyroid Gland

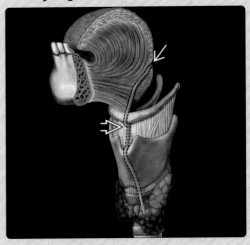

(Left) The path of descent ⇨ of the thyroid gland from the foramen cecum ⇨ to the normal location in the neck can be arrested. An ectopic thyroid can be found anywhere on this path. Lingual thyroid involves the tongue base. (Right) Ectopic thyroid gland is present within lingual tissue. Note the skeletal muscle ⇨ interspersed between the collagen fibers ⇨ and thyroid follicles ⇨.

Thyroid Tissue Within Tongue

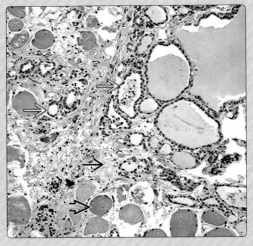

Lingual Thyroid

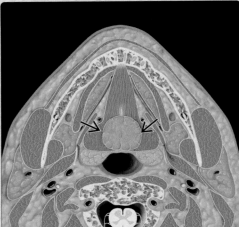

(Left) Axial graphic depicts a lingual thyroid focus ⇨ in the posterior midline of the tongue, just deep to the location of the foramen cecum. (Right) Aberrant ectopic thyroid is composed by normal-appearing thyroid follicles composed by follicular cells with regular nuclei. The follicles usually contain colloid.

Normal Thyroid Follicles

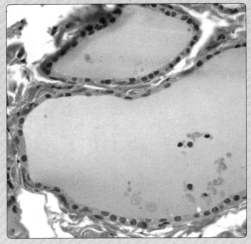

TERMINOLOGY

Synonyms

- Heterotopia
  - Presence of otherwise normal-appearing tissue in abnormal location
- Aberrant rest
- Choristoma

Definitions

- Thyroid tissue may be located in abnormal location along thyroglossal duct tract or at another site
- Thyroid tissue located in abnormal location
  - Most common occurrence is base of tongue: Lingual thyroid
  - Sublingual
  - Suprahyoid
  - Pericardium
  - Chest wall
  - Mediastinum
  - Other locations
    - Trachea and larynx
    - Adrenal
    - Gallbladder
    - Porta hepatis
    - Inguinal region
- Normal-appearing thyroid tissue may be found in lymph nodes
  - This most likely represents metastatic papillary thyroid carcinoma to lymph nodes
    - Especially if thyroid tissue is present within nodes lateral to jugular vein
  - Some believe this may represent ectopic thyroid tissue
- Ectopic tissue may also be found within striated muscles and fibroadipose tissues of central neck
  - Result of developmental defect arising from close association of thyroid and neck tissues during development
  - May be found in perithyroidal soft tissue of neck
  - Needs to be differentiated from detachment of thyroid tissue from large multinodular hyperplasia

ETIOLOGY/PATHOGENESIS

Developmental Anomaly

- Presence of thyroid tissue outside gland
  - Aberrant thyroid rests: Ectopic thyroid tissue
  - Thyroid tissue as component of teratoma

Embryology

- Result of improper descent of thyroid along its natural course during embryogenesis
  - Lingual thyroid tissue results from failure of medial anlage to descend from pharynx
    - So it remains at base of tongue

CLINICAL ISSUES

Epidemiology

- Incidence
  - Excluding thyroglossal duct cysts, it is extremely rare to find heterotopic thyroid tissue

- Few reports of familial ectopic thyroid tissue
  - Ectopic thyroid tissue is one of most common anomalies occurring during histogenesis of thyroid gland

Presentation

- May be present in lingual, sublingual, suprathyroidal, or intrathymic location
- Ectopic thyroid has been reported in variety of nontraditional places, including pericardium, heart, chest wall, vagina, inguinal region, and porta hepatis
- Lingual thyroid results from developmental abnormality due to failure to descend to its pretracheal position
  - Ectopic lingual thyroid tissue is rarely associated with obstructive oropharyngeal symptoms due to progressive enlargement
  - Lingual thyroid data
    - 29 patients with lingual thyroid were reported in series
    - 83% were female; age at diagnosis ranged from 2 weeks to 68 years
    - Almost 1/3 of patients were symptomatic
    - Most common symptoms: Cough and hoarseness
    - Incidental finding in 9 patients (31%)
    - 72% of patients developed hypothyroidism
- Papillary thyroid carcinoma in thyroglossal duct cysts and in ectopic thyroid tissue occurs at younger age
  - More aggressive features at presentation
  - Concomitant cancer in thyroid and lymph node metastases is usually present

Treatment

- Surgical approaches
  - Ectopic thyroid may be only thyroid tissue in some patients, so surgeons need to be wary of accidental removal of ectopic gland
  - Radioiodine therapy with I-131 is effective treatment modality for ablation of ectopic thyroid tissue as alternative to surgery
  - Differentiated thyroid cancer in thyroglossal duct cysts is uncommon
    - Requirement of total thyroidectomy and lymph node dissection is still controversial

Prognosis

- Generally good; however, thyroid carcinoma may arise in ectopic tissue
  - Because of atypical clinical presentation in these instances, diagnosis may be easily missed by clinician

Radiology

- Radioactive iodine tracing may establish diagnosis

IMAGING

General Features

- Presence of encapsulated mass at base of tongue
  - Tc-99m scintigraphy showing isotope uptake of the ectopic thyroid
  - Magnetic resonance imaging T2 FFS MR

MACROSCOPIC

Gross

- Tissue may be distorted; however, cut surface will be purple-red, resembling normal thyroid parenchyma

MICROSCOPIC

Histologic Features

- Like normal thyroid tissue
  - Follicles, solid cell nests, C cells, and colloid
- Ectopic thyroid tissue may also be involved in same processes as normal, orthotopic thyroid gland
- Subject to same diseases of thyroid as inflammation, hyperplasia, and tumors
  - Most malignancies are histologically classified as papillary thyroid carcinomas
- Incidence of malignancy arising in ectopic thyroid is ~ 1%
- As in many cases, ectopic thyroid gland may be only functioning thyroid tissue

ANCILLARY TESTS

Immunohistochemistry

- Tissue will display normal immunoprofile of thyroid tissue
  - TTF-1, pax-8, thyroglobulin, calcitonin in C cells

DIFFERENTIAL DIAGNOSIS

Carcinoma

- Invasive or metastatic
  - Case reports of ectopic thyroid tissue masquerading as metastatic papillary thyroid carcinoma
    - Use morphologic clues to discern from true malignancy, such as desmoplastic response surrounding tissue and cytologic evidence of malignancy
  - If any morphologic signs of malignancy are identified, then diagnosis is papillary thyroid carcinoma until proven otherwise

DIAGNOSTIC CHECKLIST

Pathologic Interpretation Pearls

- Ectopic, histologically normal-appearing thyroid can be present in lymph nodes in H&N region, commonly making diagnosis of metastatic thyroid cancer difficult
  - This may mimic metastatic papillary thyroid carcinoma
  - Index of clinical suspicion of papillary carcinoma should be high if thyroid tissue appears in nodes adjacent to jugular vein
  - Rare finding
- Ectopic thyroid may appear within skeletal muscle adjacent to thyroid
- Recent molecular techniques suggest that ectopic thyroid tissue in tongue and bilateral neck nodes represents normal nonneoplastic thyroid tissue
- Ectopic thyroid tissue is rare but important differential diagnosis when investigating mediastinal lesions
- Struma ovarii
  - Monodermal form of ovarian teratoma, which is mostly composed of thyroid tissue
  - Most are benign; however, small percentage of these cases are malignant (malignant struma ovarii)

SELECTED REFERENCES

1. Carranza Leon BG et al: Lingual thyroid: 35-year experience at a tertiary care referral center. Endocr Pract. 22(3):343-9, 2016
2. Gandhi A et al: Lingual thyroid ectopia: diagnostic SPECT/CT imaging and radioactive iodine treatment. Thyroid. 26(4):573-9, 2016
3. Garcia-Rodriguez L et al: Ectopic thyroid tissue with Hashimoto's thyroiditis. WMJ. 115(1):47-8, 2016
4. Gomez JS et al: Ectopic thyroid tissue simulating metastasis. Ear Nose Throat J. 95(3):100-3, 2016
5. Paragliola RM et al: A rare case of lateral ectopic thyroid. Clin Nucl Med. 41(12):936-937, 2016
6. Raskin A et al: Incidental ectopic thyroid follicular adenoma on myocardial perfusion imaging. J Nucl Cardiol. 23(1):153-4, 2016
7. Santangelo G et al: Prevalence, diagnosis and management of ectopic thyroid glands. Int J Surg. 28 Suppl 1:S1-6, 2016
8. Schneider B et al: Intrapericardial left-sided ectopic thyroid mass supplied by the left circumflex artery. Interact Cardiovasc Thorac Surg. 23(4):671-3, 2016
9. Sturniolo G et al: Thyroid cancer in lingual thyroid and thyroglossal duct cyst. Endocrinol Nutr. 64(1):40-43, 2016
10. Sturniolo G et al: Differentiated thyroid carcinoma in lingual thyroid. Endocrine. 51(1):189-98, 2016
11. Gordini L et al: Tall cell carcinoma arising in a thyroglossal duct cyst: a case report. Ann Med Surg (Lond). 4(2):129-32, 2015
12. Warner E et al: Mucoepidermoid carcinoma in a thyroglossal duct remnant. Int J Surg Case Rep. 13:43-7, 2015
13. Wei S et al: Pathology of thyroglossal duct: an institutional experience. Endocr Pathol. 26(1):75-9, 2015
14. Pellegriti G et al: Thyroid cancer in thyroglossal duct cysts requires a specific approach due to its unpredictable extension. J Clin Endocrinol Metab. 98(2):458-65, 2013
15. Noussios G et al: Ectopic thyroid tissue: anatomical, clinical, and surgical implications of a rare entity. Eur J Endocrinol. 165(3):375-82, 2011
16. Chowhan AK et al: Cervical ectopic thymus masquerading as metastatic thyroid papillary carcinoma. Malays J Pathol. 32(1):65-8, 2010
17. Li J et al: WNT5A antagonizes WNT/β-catenin signaling and is frequently silenced by promoter CpG methylation in esophageal squamous cell carcinoma. Cancer Biol Ther. 10(6):617-24, 2010
18. Adotey JM: Papillary adenocarcinoma of thyroid in a patient with right submandibular mass--a rare case of 'lateral aberrant thyroid'. Niger J Clin Pract. 12(3):333-4, 2009
19. Uludag M et al: Ectopic mediastinal thyroid tissue: cervical or mediastinum originated? BMJ Case Rep. 2009, 2009
20. Hernandez-Cassis C et al: A six-year-old boy with a suspicious thyroid nodule: intrathyroidal thymic tissue. Thyroid. 18(3):377-80, 2008
21. Hardy RG et al: Snail family transcription factors are implicated in thyroid carcinogenesis. Am J Pathol. 171(3):1037-46, 2007
22. Schmidt J et al: BRAF in papillary thyroid carcinoma of ovary (struma ovarii). Am J Surg Pathol. 31(9):1337-43, 2007
23. Giusan AO et al: [Aberrant goiter of the root of the tongue.] Vestn Otorinolaringol. (1):65, 2006
24. Kalaany NY et al: LXRs regulate the balance between fat storage and oxidation. Cell Metab. 1(4):231-44, 2005

Thyroglossal Duct

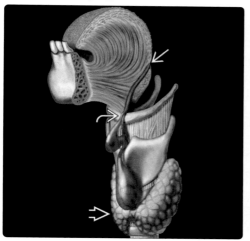

Aberrant Thyroid Tissue Locations

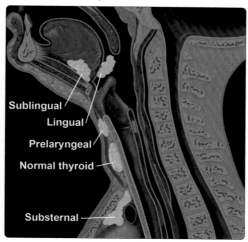

Sublingual
Lingual
Prelaryngeal
Normal thyroid
Substernal

(Left) *Sagittal oblique graphic shows the potential sites of a thyroglossal duct cyst or ectopic thyroid tissue from the foramen cecum ➡ to the thyroid bed ➡. Note the close relationship of the midportion of the hyoid bone ➡ to this pathway. A cyst can occur anywhere along this tract.* (Right) *Thyroid tissue may be located in abnormal locations along thyroglossal duct tract or at other sites. Lingual thyroid results from complete arrest of the descent of the medial thyroid anlage.*

Ectopic Midline Neck Thyroid

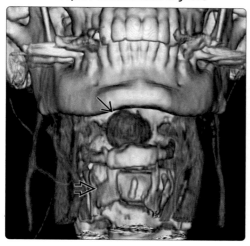

Mediastinal Goiter

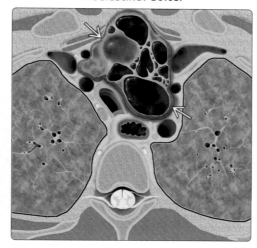

(Left) *Anterior 3D MR shows absence of thyroid tissue in the thyroid bed ➡ and a well-circumscribed ectopic thyroid ➡ in the midline along the path of the thyroglossal duct tract.* (Right) *Ectopic thyroid tissue can be seen in the pericardium and anterior mediastinum. Ectopic tissue may have the usual changes as the topic thyroid as multinodular hyperplasia ➡ (as depicted here) thyroiditis and carcinoma.*

Ectopic Thyroid With Normal Architecture

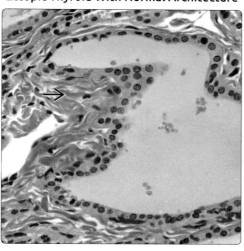

Thyroid Within Adipose Tissue

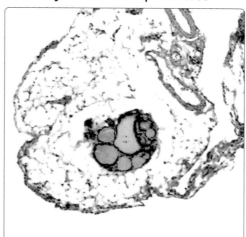

(Left) *Ectopic thyroid gland present within ectopic locations has the same morphological features as the topic thyroid tissue. Note the thyroid follicles interspersed between the collagen fibers ➡.* (Right) *Ectopic thyroid tissue is present within adipose tissue in strumosis. The thyroid tissue has its normal architecture and it is usually benign.*

KEY FACTS

TERMINOLOGY

- Cell type within thyroid gland, remnant of ultimobranchial apparatus, associated with development of thyroid C cells (CCs)

ETIOLOGY/PATHOGENESIS

- Thought to represent ultimobranchial body rests

CLINICAL ISSUES

- May mimic squamous metaplasia, which is seen in many other thyroid conditions
- SCNs were usually composed of mixture of main cells (MCs) and CCs

MICROSCOPIC

- Well-demarcated small cellular nests present in interfollicular distribution
- Consist of polygonal to oval cells with oval nuclei and granular chromatin
- Nuclear grooves may be present

  - Mimicking papillary thyroid carcinoma
- Lesions may have cysts in up to 60% of nests
- Distinct eosinophilic basement membrane
- Calcitonin-producing CCs are associated with SCNs

ANCILLARY TESTS

- Solid cell nests (SCNs) are positive for p63, p40, low-molecular-weight keratins, CEA
- CD5(+) intraepithelial lymphocytes
- SCNs are negative for TTF-1, HBME-1, and thyroglobulin
- No somatic *BRAF* mutation was found in any of SCNs
- No *RET* rearrangement

TOP DIFFERENTIAL DIAGNOSES

- Squamous metaplasia
- Papillary thyroid microcarcinoma
- Squamous cell carcinoma
- Inclusions within thyroid
- Squamous morules

SCN With Solid and Cystic Components

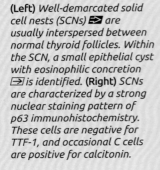

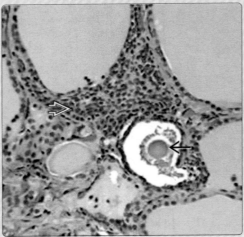

(Left) *Well-demarcated solid cell nests (SCNs)* ➡ *are usually interspersed between normal thyroid follicles. Within the SCN, a small epithelial cyst with eosinophilic concretion* ➥ *is identified.* (Right) *SCNs are characterized by a strong nuclear staining pattern of p63 immunohistochemistry. These cells are negative for TTF-1, and occasional C cells are positive for calcitonin.*

P63 is Strongly Positive in SCN

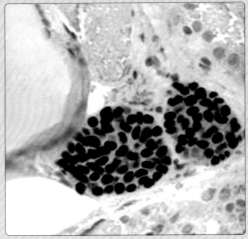

Hyperplastic SCNs

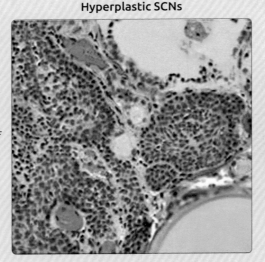

(Left) *SCNs may have a lobulated appearance and may be hypercellular, hyperplastic, and associated with C cells.* (Right) *Immunopositivity for carcinoembryonic antigen* ➡ *in SCNs is shown. p63, CD5, and CEA staining provides a much more sensitive means of detecting SCNs than staining for other markers.*

CEA Immunoreactivity in SCNs

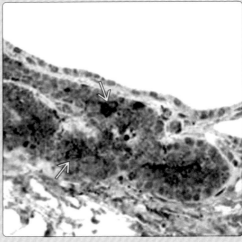

TERMINOLOGY

Abbreviations

- Solid cell nest (SCN)

Definitions

- Cell type within thyroid gland, remnant of ultimobranchial apparatus, associated with development of thyroid C cells (CCs)
  - Located in posterolateral or posteromedial portion of lateral midlobes of thyroid

ETIOLOGY/PATHOGENESIS

Pathogenesis

- Thought to represent ultimobranchial body rests
  - Derived from endoderm
- May be derived from branchial pouch remnants

Possible Relation to Carcinogenesis

- SCNs have been examined as precursor lesions to thyroid carcinoma
  - Studies suggesting intrathyroid thymic carcinoma (CASTLE) may originate from SCNs
- Intrathyroid thymic carcinoma (CASTLE) may arise from branchial pouch remnants, thyroid SCNs
  - Similar immunophenotype
    - Focal squamous differentiation resembling Hassall corpuscles
    - Immunopositivity for
      - CD5
      - CD117
      - High-molecular-weight cytokeratin
      - Cytokeratin
      - p63
      - Carcinoembryonic antigen
      - Epithelial membrane antigen
      - p40
    - Negativity for
      - TTF-1
      - pax-8
      - Thyroglobulin
      - HBME-1
      - Calcitonin
      - PTH
  - *BRAF* mutations in SCN hyperplasia have been investigated as a possible precursor to *BRAF* (+) papillary thyroid carcinoma

CLINICAL ISSUES

Presentation

- Found in 3% of routinely examined thyroid glands
  - Has been found in up to 61% of glands in some studies
    - May mimic squamous metaplasia, which is seen in many other thyroid conditions
  - Has been found in cases of struma ovarii and branchial-like cysts of thyroid
- SCNs were usually composed of mixture of main cells (MCs) and CCs
- Thyroid-type SCNs has been reported associated with struma ovarii

MICROSCOPIC

Histologic Features

- Well-demarcated cellular nests with interfollicular distribution
- SCNs of thyroid are single or multiple foci of solid &/or cystic clusters of squamoid MCs with minor proportion of CCs
- Consists of polygonal to oval to spindle cells with elongated nuclei and granular chromatin
  - Nuclear grooves may be present
    - This may mimic papillary thyroid carcinoma
  - Some cells may have clear cytoplasm and round nuclei
  - Usually < 0.1 mm in diameter
  - Presence of intraepithelial lymphocytes
- Lesions may have cysts in up to 60% of nests
  - Larger cysts may resemble branchial cleft cysts
- Distinct eosinophilic basement membrane
- Cytological mimicry of papillary thyroid carcinoma most frequently occurs in setting of thyroiditis, such as Hashimoto thyroiditis and Graves disease

ANCILLARY TESTS

Cytology

- Rarely observed on cytology

Immunohistochemistry

- SCNs are positive for p63
  - p63, p53-homolog nuclear transcription factor, is consistently expressed in basal/stem cells of several multilayered epithelia
  - It is reliable immunohistochemical marker of SCN
  - Strong nuclear signal is observed in SCN
    - Important to know that p63 will not help in differentiation from squamous metaplasia
- SCNs are positive for low-molecular-weight keratin, CK5, CK5/6
- Intraepithelial lymphocytes are CD5(+)
- SCNs are negative for
  - TTF-1
  - pax-8
  - HBME-1
  - Thyroglobulin
  - Calcitonin
  - Parathormone
    - May assist in distinguishing from papillary thyroid carcinoma when nuclear grooves and atypia are present
- In oncocytic SCNs, 80% of MCs showed oncocytic cytoplasm
  - These oncocytic SCNs have positivity for cytokeratin 19, p63, p40, galectin-3, and HBME-1
  - Negativity for thyroglobulin, TTF-1, pax-8, Oct-4, and α-fetoprotein in oncocytic SCNs
- Some SCN express focally calcitonin, chromogranin, synaptophysin, neuron-specific enolase, and carcinoembryonic antigen
  - These stains will help identify thyroid CCs that are usually present within nests

Genetic Testing

- No somatic *BRAF* mutation was found in any of SCNs

- o *BRAF* mutation in SCN hyperplasia has been suggested to be precursor lesion to papillary thyroid carcinoma
- No *RET* rearrangement
- No germinal mutation of GRIM-19 was detected in one study

Electron Microscopy

- Desmosomes, intermediate filaments, and intraluminal cytoplasmic projections

DIFFERENTIAL DIAGNOSIS

Squamous Metaplasia

- Multifocal, shows keratinization
- In setting of chronic thyroid inflammation
- Immunohistochemistry may help
  - o p63 is positive in both SCNs and squamous metaplasia

Papillary Thyroid Microcarcinoma

- Enlarged cells with overlapping nuclei, nuclear grooves, irregular nuclear membranes
- Some features may mimic SCNs
- Best differentiated by the immunoprofile
- Positive for TTF-1, pax-8, HBME-1, and thyroglobulin

Squamous Cell Carcinoma

- Primary thyroid carcinoma or metastatic carcinoma to thyroid
- Nuclear atypia, keratinization, and mitosis favor diagnosis of squamous cell carcinoma rather than SCNs

Inclusions Within Thyroid

- Intrathyroid thymic tissue
  - o These may be in close association with SCNs
  - o They may also contain scattered calcitonin-producing CCs
- Intrathyroid parathyroid tissue
- Salivary gland tissue

Squamous Morules

- Squamous morules may be present as part of papillary thyroid carcinoma, diffuse sclerosing variant
- Squamous morules are part of cribriform morular variant of papillary thyroid carcinoma
- Squamous morules usually have concentric arrangement
- Squamous morules have similar immunophenotype as SCNs
  - o Immunopositivity for CK5/6, p63, p40
  - o However, these are negative for CEA
- These usually don't have cystic changes or intraepithelial lymphocytes

DIAGNOSTIC CHECKLIST

Pathologic Interpretation Pearls

- Differentiation from papillary thyroid carcinoma
  - o Use immunohistochemistry
- Differentiation from squamous metaplasia
  - o Important as squamous metaplasia is commonly seen in several other thyroid conditions

SELECTED REFERENCES

1. Vázquez-Román V et al: Immunohistochemical profiling of the ultimobranchial remnants in the rat postnatal thyroid gland. J Morphol. 278(8):1114-1124, 2017
2. Handra-Luca A: Thyroid solid cell nests: usefulness of cytokeratin 5/6?: cytokeratin 5/6 in thyroid cell nests. Endocr Pathol. 27(1):83-5, 2016
3. Manzoni M et al: Thyreoglossal duct cyst with evidence of solid cell nests and atypical thyroid follicles. Endocr Pathol. 27(2):175-7, 2016
4. Manzoni M et al: Solid cell nests of the thyroid gland: morphological, immunohistochemical and genetic features. Histopathology. 68(6):866-74, 2016
5. Yerly S et al: A carcinoma showing thymus-like elements of the thyroid arising in close association with solid cell nests: evidence for a precursor lesion? Thyroid. 23(4):511-6, 2013
6. Bellevicine C et al: Ultimobranchial body remnants (solid cell nests) as a pitfall in thyroid pathology. J Clin Endocrinol Metab. 97(7):2209-10, 2012
7. Cameselle-Teijeiro J et al: Absence of the BRAF and the GRIM-19 mutations in oncocytic (Hürthle cell) solid cell nests of the thyroid. Am J Clin Pathol. 137(4):612-8, 2012
8. Eloy C et al: Tumor-in-tumor of the thyroid with basaloid differentiation: a lesion with a solid cell nest neoplastic component? Int J Surg Pathol. 19(2):276-80, 2011
9. Ríos Moreno MJ et al: Inmunohistochemical profile of solid cell nest of thyroid gland. Endocr Pathol. 22(1):35-9, 2011
10. Seethala RR et al: Solid cell nests, papillary thyroid microcarcinoma, and HBME1. Am J Clin Pathol. 134(1):169-70, 2010
11. Asioli S et al: Solid cell nests in Hashimoto's thyroiditis sharing features with papillary thyroid microcarcinoma. Endocr Pathol. 20(4):197-203, 2009
12. Cameselle-Teijeiro J et al: BRAF mutation in solid cell nest hyperplasia associated with papillary thyroid carcinoma. A precursor lesion? Hum Pathol. 40(7):1029-35, 2009
13. Cameselle-Teijeiro J et al: Thyroid-type solid cell nests in struma ovarii. Int J Surg Pathol. 19(5):627-31, 2009
14. Yamazaki M et al: Carcinoma showing thymus-like differentiation (CASTLE) with neuroendocrine differentiation. Pathol Int. 58(12):775-9, 2008
15. Kuhn E et al: Images in pathology. solid and cystic cell nests. Int J Surg Pathol. 14(3):223, 2006
16. Michal M et al: Branchial-like cysts of the thyroid associated with solid cell nests. Pathol Int. 56(3):150-3, 2006
17. Reimann JD et al: Carcinoma showing thymus-like differentiation of the thyroid (CASTLE): a comparative study: evidence of thymic differentiation and solid cell nest origin. Am J Surg Pathol. 30(8):994-1001, 2006
18. Ryska A et al: Massive squamous metaplasia of the thyroid gland– report of three cases. Pathol Res Pract. 202(2):99-106, 2006

SCNs: Peripheral Location

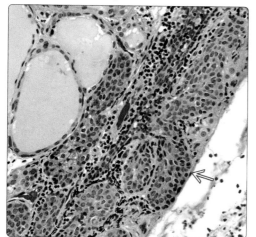

Large Solid Cell Nests

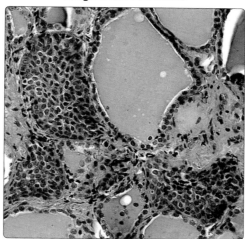

(Left) *This SCN is located at the periphery* ➡ *of the thyroid with only a thin perithyroid tissue over it. The SCNs are usually located in the posterolateral or posteromedial portion of the lateral midlobes of the thyroid.* (Right) *SCNs of the thyroid are ultimobranchial body remnants. SCNs are composed of main cells and C cells. It has been suggested that main cells might be pluripotent cells contributing to the histogenesis of C cells and follicular cells as well as to the formation of certain thyroid tumors.*

Solid and Cystic SCN

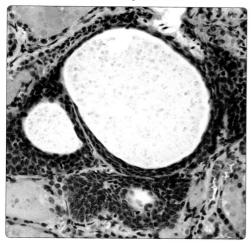

Intraepithelial Lymphocytes

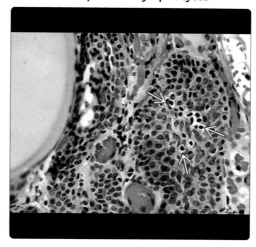

(Left) *SCNs of the thyroid are composed of main cells and C cells and can present as a solid mass, cystic mass, or mixed solid-cystic mass within thyroid follicles.* (Right) *SCNs form an aggregate of epithelioid cells that characteristically have intraepithelial lymphocytes* ➡. *These lymphocytes are CD5(+).*

Cystic SCN

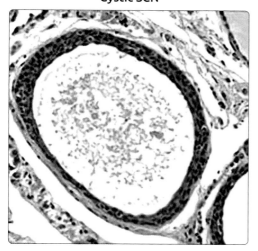

CK5/6 in SCNs and Squamous Morules

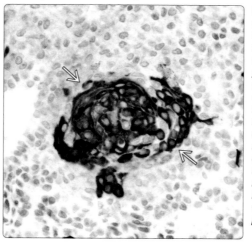

(Left) *SCN can be cystically changed and contained a small amount of mucus-type material. These are labyrinth-like cystic structures lined by a few layers of benign-appearing squamoid main cells and filled by mucinous material.* (Right) *Squamous morules may be present in association with the cribriform morular thyroid carcinoma or as a component of papillary thyroid carcinoma. These morules may mimic SCNs and have the same immunoprofile with positivity for CK5/6* ➡, *p63, and p40.*

TERMINOLOGY

- Acute inflammation of thyroid gland with destruction of thyroid follicles with polymorphonuclear leukocyte infiltration

ETIOLOGY/PATHOGENESIS

- May be caused by several different organisms, including bacteria, mycobacteria, fungi, and viruses

CLINICAL ISSUES

- Associated with systemic infection
- Thyroid gland is relatively resistant to infections, making infectious thyroiditis rare occurrence
- Protective mechanisms
  - Rich blood supply
  - Rich lymphatic drainage
  - High glandular iodine content: May act as bactericidal agent
    - Anatomic separation from other neck structures by facial planes
- Most common predisposing factors for thyroid infections are preexisting thyroid conditions
- Tends to develop in immunocompromised or malnourished patients
  - Immunocompetent patients have typical signs of infection
- Acute suppurative thyroiditis is uncommon in children

MACROSCOPIC

- Abscess formation may be appreciable on gross exam as identified by histology

MICROSCOPIC

- Typical histologic evidence of acute infection is present
  - Focal to diffuse acute inflammatory cell infiltration
  - Destruction of follicular cells
- Mycobacterial organisms or fungi may evoke granulomatous response

Acute Inflammation Within Thyroid

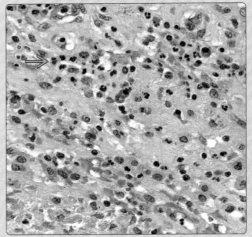

Acute Thyroiditis in Resolution

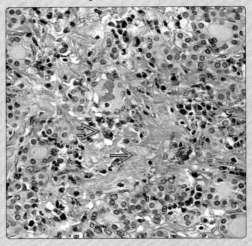

(Left) High-power microphotograph shows polymorphonuclear cells ➡ within the thyroid parenchyma with destroyed follicles in the setting of acute thyroiditis. This is typical of acute thyroiditis caused by bacteria. (Right) Resolving acute thyroiditis with reparative fibrosis ➡ and hemosiderin deposition ➡ is shown. The acute inflammatory infiltrate is absent. Instead, there is a lymphoplasmacytic infiltrate around the thyroid follicles.

Acute Granulomatous Thyroiditis

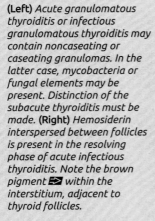
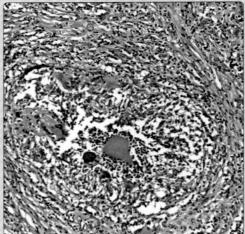

Resolving Thyroiditis

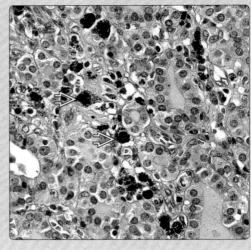

(Left) Acute granulomatous thyroiditis or infectious granulomatous thyroiditis may contain noncaseating or caseating granulomas. In the latter case, mycobacteria or fungal elements may be present. Distinction of the subacute thyroiditis must be made. (Right) Hemosiderin interspersed between follicles is present in the resolving phase of acute infectious thyroiditis. Note the brown pigment ➡ within the interstitium, adjacent to thyroid follicles.

TERMINOLOGY

Synonyms

- Infectious thyroiditis
- Acute suppurative thyroiditis

Definitions

- Acute inflammation of thyroid gland with polymorphonuclear leukocyte infiltration

ETIOLOGY/PATHOGENESIS

Infectious Agents

- May be caused by several different organisms
- Acute bacterial thyroiditis is most common cause of infectious thyroiditis
  - Bacteria
    - *Streptococcus haemolyticus, Staphylococcus aureus, Pneumococcus, Actinomyces*
    - *E. coli*
      - Rare case of acute suppurative thyroiditis caused by *Escherichia coli* secondary to urinary tract infection
    - Variety of anaerobes in children
- Fungi infection is 2nd most common cause of thyroiditis
  - *Aspergillus* species is most common fungal infection in thyroid
    - *Aspergillus* is most common fungal cause of suppurative thyroiditis
    - Most patients with *Aspergillus* thyroiditis have disseminated infection, primarily with lung compromise
  - *Candida* species, *Histoplasma*, *Cryptococcus*, *Pneumocystis* species, *Nocardia*, and *Coccidioides*
- Mycobacterial infection
  - Infrequent
  - *Mycobacterium tuberculosis*: Presents as disseminated tuberculosis
  - *M. avium-intracellulare*: In patients with AIDS
- Virus
  - Cytomegalovirus
    - Usually in immunosuppressed patients
  - Rubella
- Other agents
  - *Echinococcus granulosus, Strongyloides stercoralis, Taenia solium*

CLINICAL ISSUES

Epidemiology

- Incidence
  - Rare
    - Acute suppurative thyroiditis is rare disorder
      - Only 500 cases have been reported in literature to date
  - No age or sex predisposition
  - Thyroid gland is relatively resistant to infections, making infectious thyroiditis rare occurrence
    - Protective mechanisms
      - Rich blood supply
      - Rich lymphatic drainage
      - High glandular iodine content: May act as bactericidal agent
      - Anatomic separation from other neck structures by facial planes
  - Tends to develop in immunocompromised or malnourished patients
    - Frequently associated with concomitant infections
  - Most common predisposing factors for thyroid infections are preexisting thyroid conditions
    - Multinodular goiter
    - Hashimoto thyroiditis
    - Thyroid carcinoma
    - Riedel thyroiditis: Report of 1 case associated with acute suppurative thyroiditis
- Modes of infection
  - Spread from primary focus via bloodstream
  - Direct spread from adjoining neck structures
  - After surgery
  - Neck trauma

Presentation

- Especially common in setting of neck trauma
- Acute suppurative thyroiditis is uncommon in children
  - Usually presents subacutely following upper respiratory tract infection
  - Usually caused by *Streptococcus* species
- Immunocompetent patients have typical signs of infection
  - Physical exam may show fever, variable enlargement of thyroid, as well as tenderness to palpation
    - Thyroid gland is warm to palpation
    - Swelling and pain in neck region
  - Hypothyroidism or hyperthyroidism may occur
    - Most patients are euthyroid
  - Local mechanical compression leading to dysphagia and dysphonia
- Also associated with upper respiratory infection, otitis media, infected thyroglossal duct cyst, tonsillitis
- Fungal organisms may also be causative agents, such as *Aspergillus*, *Cryptococcus*, *Candida*, and *Coccidioides*
- Viral agents, such as rubella and cytomegalovirus, may occur, particularly in immunosuppressed patients
  - Extremely rare
- Microbial studies can help identify organism

Treatment

- Surgical approaches
  - Only when life-threatening situations involving compromise of airway or spread to adjacent tissues
- Drugs
  - Antibiotics can be used in milder cases

Prognosis

- Responsive to treatment
- Patients completely recover

IMAGING

General Features

- Thyroid ultrasound usually reveals well-defined hypoechogenic clusters in both lobes
- May present with fluid-filled masses and cavities

- Computed tomography may better evaluate presence of abscess and allow better distinctions between diagnostic possibilities

MACROSCOPIC

General Features

- Focal or diffuse enlargement
  - Thyroid can appear normal
- Abscess formation may be appreciable on gross exam as identified by histology
- Areas of necrosis may be seen

MICROSCOPIC

Histologic Features

- Acute thyroiditis, acute phase: Acute suppurative inflammation
  - Typical histologic evidence of acute infection is present
    - Focal to diffuse acute inflammatory cell infiltration with destruction of follicular cells
    - Areas of abscess may be present
    - Necrosis, fibrin, and nuclear debris may be present
      - Necrotic foci associated with microabscesses
  - Thick colloid globules and multinucleated giant cells are frequent findings
  - Calcification could be due to dystrophic changes in old colloid cyst
  - Follicular cells may have some atypical features, such as
    - Nuclear overlapping and pleomorphism, coarse chromatin, and nuclear irregularities
- Granulomatous inflammation
  - Classic caseating granulomas may be present
  - Associated with mycobacterial infection
    - Causes granulomatous thyroiditis: Epithelioid and mostly noncaseating granulomas
  - Some granulomatous inflammation associated with fungal infections
- Mycobacterial organisms will evoke granulomatous response
  - Not to be confused with other granulomatous thyroid diseases
- Immunocompromised patients may not develop appropriate granulomatous response to mycobacterial or fungal organisms
- Resolving infection will show fibrosis, chronic inflammation, and hemosiderin deposition
- Special stains for acid-fast bacilli, fungi, virus, and bacteria may be helpful in identifying causative agent
  - Acid-fast bacilli stain
  - Cytomegalovirus immunohistochemistry
  - Methenamine silver stains

Cytologic Features

- Smears from thyroid aspirates are predominated by sheets of polymorphonuclear cells
  - Neutrophils are present
- Microorganisms may be present

DIFFERENTIAL DIAGNOSIS

Subacute Thyroiditis

- Subacute granulomatous thyroiditis or de Quervain thyroiditis
  - Due to systemic viral infection epidemics
    - Mumps
    - Coxsackie adenovirus
    - Measles
    - Influenza viruses
- Granulomas have multinucleated giant cells, lymphocytes, plasma cells, histiocytes, areas of acute inflammation, and variable degree of fibrosis
- Differentiate with physical exam and clinical and laboratory findings

Ischemic Necrosis

- Ischemic necrosis will have necrosis and vascular changes

Hemorrhagic Cyst

- Lack of predominant acute inflammatory cells

Other Thyroiditis

- Differentiate with physical exam and clinical and laboratory findings

Thyroid Tumors

- Thyroid lymphoma
  - Be careful not to miss hematolymphoid malignancy
- Anaplastic thyroid carcinoma

DIAGNOSTIC CHECKLIST

Pathologic Interpretation Pearls

- Treatment is directly dependent on proper identification of offending organism
  - Consultation with microbiology is important as well as review of patient's clinical history
  - Prompt treatment and early detection is key for good prognosis
- Look for typical signs of acute inflammation
  - Gross and microscopic findings

SELECTED REFERENCES

1. Sen S et al: Acute suppurative thyroiditis secondary to urinary tract infection by E. coli: a rare clinical scenario. BMJ Case Rep. 2016
2. Koirala KP et al: Treatment of acute painful thyroiditis with low dose prednisolone: a study on patients from Western Nepal. J Clin Diagn Res. 9(9):MC01-3, 2015
3. Samanta S: Unusual cytomorphology of acute suppurative thyroiditis. J Cytol. 32(1):25-7, 2015
4. Marui S et al: Suppurative thyroiditis due to aspergillosis: a case report. J Med Case Rep. 8:379, 2014
5. Hong JT et al: Case of concurrent Riedel's thyroiditis, acute suppurative thyroiditis, and micropapillary carcinoma. Korean J Intern Med. 28(2):236-41, 2013
6. Valina S et al: [Abscess formation after puncture of a thyroid cyst - a case report.] Zentralbl Chir. 138 Suppl 2:e108-9, 2013
7. Wongphyat O et al: Acute suppurative thyroiditis in young children. J Paediatr Child Health. 48(3):E116-8, 2012
8. Ikuyama S: [Acute suppurative thyroiditis.] Nihon Rinsho. Suppl 1:412-4, 2006

Destruction of Follicles by Inflammation

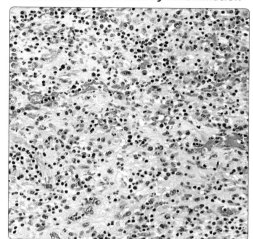

Acute Thyroiditis

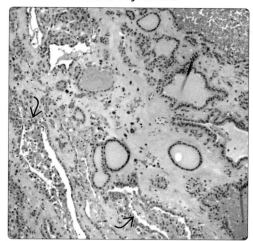

(Left) *Acute thyroiditis may be suppurative or nonsuppurative with numerous neutrophils and destruction of the thyroid parenchyma.* (Right) *Residual thyroid follicles are shown in a background of acute inflammatory exudate with neutrophils. Some follicles have been destroyed by the inflammatory process and some have histiocytic infiltrate* ⤴.

Necrosis

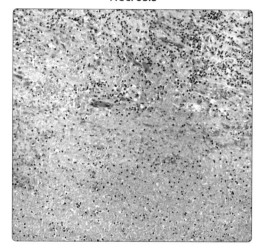

Necrosis in Acute Thyroiditis

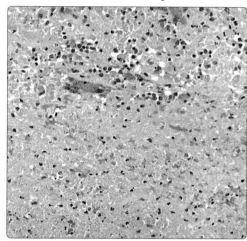

(Left) *Infiltration with neutrophils, areas with microabscesses, extensive necrosis, and thyroid follicle destruction are usually present multifocally.* (Right) *Foci of necrosis may be present throughout the thyroid. Special stains are very helpful for identifying the etiologic microorganisms.*

Resolving Acute Thyroiditis

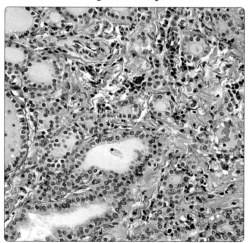

Subacute Thyroiditis

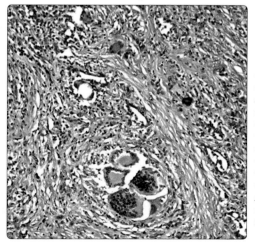

(Left) *Resolving acute thyroiditis is characterized by early fibrosis, hemosiderin deposition between follicles, and lymphoplasmacytic infiltrate. Note the brown pigment adjacent to thyroid follicles.* (Right) *The granulomas have multinucleated giant cells, lymphocytes, plasma cells, histiocytes, areas of acute inflammation, and variable degrees of fibrosis. Subacute thyroiditis shows microabscess formation and should not to be confused with acute granulomatous thyroiditis.*

TERMINOLOGY

- Granulomatous inflammatory condition of thyroid typically following viral infection

ETIOLOGY/PATHOGENESIS

- Known to occur as sequela of viral infections

CLINICAL ISSUES

- Accounts for < 3% of all thyroid diseases
- Female predisposition 3-6x that of males
- Gland is enlarged, tender, and hard to palpation
- Initial hyperthyroid phase
- Subsequent hypothyroid phase
- Most patients with granulomatous thyroiditis have complete resolution within period of months

MICROSCOPIC

- Histologic features change throughout progression of disease

- Early disease shows destruction of follicular epithelial cells
  - Areas of acute inflammation with focal abscess formation
- Late disease phase
  - Polymorphonuclear leukocytes are replaced by chronic inflammatory infiltrate
    - Multinucleated giant cells, lymphocytes, plasma cells, histiocytes
  - Early fibrosis may be present
- Resolution phase shows fibrosis with regenerating follicles

TOP DIFFERENTIAL DIAGNOSES

- Mycobacterial thyroiditis
- Fungal thyroiditis
- Sarcoidosis
- Minocycline-related thyroiditis
- Lymphocytic thyroiditis
- Neoplastic process

Characteristic Cut Surface

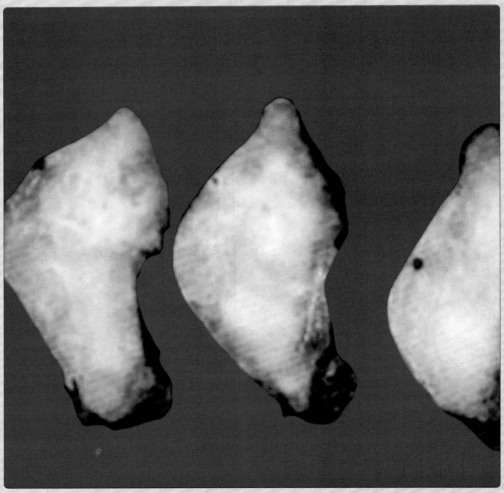

Gross cut surface of granulomatous thyroiditis shows parenchyma with vague nodularity, variably sized nodules, and a fibrotic, white-tan appearance. The entire thyroid is involved.

TERMINOLOGY

Abbreviations

- Granulomatous thyroiditis (GT)

Synonyms

- Subacute thyroiditis
- Nonsuppurative thyroiditis
- Giant cell thyroiditis
- Pseudotuberculous thyroiditis
- de Quervain thyroiditis

Definitions

- Granulomatous inflammatory condition of thyroid typically following viral infection

ETIOLOGY/PATHOGENESIS

Infectious Agents

- Known to occur as sequela of systemic viral infections
  - Mechanism is not fully elucidated
  - Many cases are known to arise in patients with initial upper respiratory infections with prodromal symptoms
  - Most frequently occurs in summer months
  - Circulating antibodies to various viruses, including
    - Measles, influenza, adenovirus, Epstein-Barr virus, coxsackievirus, influenza viruses, measles, mumps
    - Primary HIV infection
    - New cases H1N1-related have been documented

Autoimmunity

- Thyroid antibodies are present in some patients with GT
  - Typically disappear after resolution of disease
    - May suggest transient state of autoimmunity within thyroid
- Presence of antithyroid antibodies may be related to reaction against transiently elevated antigens from follicular destruction as opposed to true autoimmune state

Genetic

- Association between GT and HLA-BW35

CLINICAL ISSUES

Epidemiology

- Incidence
  - Accounts for < 3% of all thyroid diseases
- Age
  - Most common in 2nd-5th decades
    - Uncommon in children and elderly
- Sex
  - Female predisposition 3-6x that of males

Presentation

- Subacute thyroiditis is most common cause of thyroid pain
- Clinical presentation
  - Pain, which is presenting symptom in > 90% of cases
    - Aggravated by swallowing or head movement
  - General symptoms
    - May include malaise, fatigue, fever, chills, weight loss, anorexia, and myalgias
    - Fever of unknown origin is sometimes diagnostic dilemma for clinicians
      - Endocrine causes reported in literature include subacute thyroiditis, thyrotoxicosis, adrenal insufficiency, and pheochromocytoma
      - Among these, subacute thyroiditis is often overlooked as it can occasionally lack typical symptoms
  - Symptoms
    - ~ 50% of patients with subacute thyroiditis have initial thyrotoxic phase
      - Due to unregulated release of preformed thyroid hormone from damaged thyroid follicular cells
  - Physical examination
    - Gland is enlarged, tender, and hard upon palpation
    - Enlargement is usually symmetrical but may be asymmetrical
    - Thyroid gland can be enlarged up to 3-4x its normal size
      - Extremely large or grossly nodular goiter is not characteristic of subacute thyroiditis
      - This should raise possibility of alternate diagnoses
- Clinically, 3 phases of disease are recognized
  - Hyperthyroid phase: Increased serum T3 and T4 associated with low radioactive iodine uptake
  - Hypothyroid phase with proportion of gland destroyed
  - Recovery phase: Euthyroid phase

Laboratory Tests

- Initial hyperthyroid phase
  - Result of damage to thyroid follicular cells
    - Elevation of serum T3, T4, and thyroglobulin levels
- Subsequent hypothyroid phase
  - Result of progressive destruction of gland with depletion of hormone production and iodine uptake
    - Will generally last few months, after which most patients recover

Treatment

- Drugs
  - Corticosteroids are primary method of treatment with excellent results in most patients
    - Patients typically receive short course of tapered steroids
  - NSAIDs are used to treat pain

Prognosis

- Most patients have complete resolution within period of months and are sequelae free
  - Hypothyroidism may persist in 5-15% of patients
    - Hormone replacement therapy is required

IMAGING

Ultrasonographic Findings

- Hypoechogenicity within involved thyroid gland
  - Characteristic sonographic finding of subacute thyroiditis: Heterogeneous, poorly defined hypoechoic area within thyroid gland

Radioisotope Scan

- Patchy, irregular, or absent iodine uptake
  - PET/US fusion technique may help in small and uncertain findings

MACROSCOPIC

General Features

- Thyroid gland is asymmetrically enlarged, firm to hard and tan-white in appearance
  - Gland may have nodules of varying size and shape
  - Nodules may be present throughout parenchyma

MICROSCOPIC

Histologic Features

- Include multinucleated giant cells, lymphocytes, plasma cells, histiocytes
  - Areas of acute inflammation and variable degrees of fibrosis
  - Will change over progression of disease
- Early disease phase
  - Destruction of follicular epithelial cells with extravasation and depletion of colloid
    - Colloid may be found within inflammatory infiltrate
  - Infiltration of follicles by inflammatory infiltrate consisting of polymorphonuclear leukocytes
    - Lymphocytes, histiocytes, and giant cells may be seen
  - Microabscesses may be present
- Late disease phase
  - Polymorphonuclear leukocytes are replaced by chronic inflammatory infiltrate
  - Histiocytes, giant cells, and plasma cells are present
  - Inflammatory cells replace follicular epithelial cells
  - Fibrosis is present between follicles and lobules
- Regenerative phase
  - Normal follicles reappear with varying, but mostly minimal, degrees of residual fibrosis

ANCILLARY TESTS

Cytology

- Follicular cells admixed with inflammatory cells
  - Neutrophils, lymphocytes, histiocytes, multinucleated giant cells (up to 50 nuclei per cell), and foamy histiocytes
- Cytology will change with disease progression
  - Early disease will show acute inflammatory cells with microabscesses
  - Later-phase disease will show mixed inflammatory infiltrate with giant cells, histiocytes, and follicular cells with degenerative changes
  - Aspirates may be acellular with advanced fibrosis

DIFFERENTIAL DIAGNOSIS

Infectious

- Mycobacterial thyroiditis
  - Presence of necrosis within granulomas should warrant investigation of mycobacterial etiologies
  - GT will not have necrotizing granulomas
- Fungal thyroiditis
  - Occasionally, granulomatous inflammation occurs with fungal reaction

Other Thyroiditides

- Hashimoto disease
- Graves disease
- Radioactive iodine administration
- Amiodarone-induced thyroiditis
- Contrast dye-induced thyroiditis
- Acute suppurative thyroiditis
- Amyloid goiter
- Sarcoidosis
  - Noncaseating granulomas
  - Look for extrathyroid manifestations to rule in/out sarcoidosis
    - Elevated calcium in patients with sarcoidosis
  - Treatment and resolution with corticosteroids may make this difficult diagnosis
    - Close clinical follow-up is vital if sarcoidosis is suspected
- Lymphocytic (Hashimoto) thyroiditis
  - Squamous metaplasia, prominent lymphoid aggregates, other typical histologic signs of Hashimoto thyroiditis
- Postoperative necrotizing granulomas
- Granulomatous vasculitis
- Palpation thyroiditis

Neoplastic

- Nodularity may give physicians clinical impression of neoplastic process
  - Histologic distinction from neoplastic disease is fairly straightforward

Conditions Associated With Granulomas in Thyroid

- Mycobacterial and fungal infections
- Sarcoidosis
- Minocycline granulomatous thyroiditis
  - Thyroid disease in patients treated with minocycline for acne associated with autoimmune thyroiditis and granulomas
- Foreign body reaction
- Postoperative necrotizing granulomas
- Postbiopsy granulomas to cholesterol clefts
- Palpation thyroiditis

DIAGNOSTIC CHECKLIST

Clinically Relevant Pathologic Features

- Symptom time frame
  - Rapid progression after viral prodromal phase with swift resolution of symptoms
- Treatment and prognosis
  - Corticosteroids are 1st-line treatment
  - Prognosis is excellent

Pathologic Interpretation Pearls

- Histologic picture varies with progression of disease
  - Early disease shows destruction of follicular epithelial cells
  - Later disease shows chronic inflammatory changes
  - Resolution phase shows fibrosis with regenerating follicles

SELECTED REFERENCES

1. Bahowairath FA et al: Lesson of the month 1: Subacute thyroiditis: a rare cause of fever of unknown origin. Clin Med (Lond). 17(1):86-87, 2017

Granulomatous Thyroiditis

	Early Phase	Late Phase	Regenerative Phase
Cytology	Acute inflammatory cells, microabscesses	Mixed inflammatory population with giant cell formation	May be normal or may be acellular if gland has extensive fibrosis
Morphology	Predominantly acute inflammatory cells	Acute inflammatory cells are replaced by chronic inflammation	
	Destruction of follicular cells with extravasation of colloidal material, which may be found within inflammatory infiltrate	Histocytes, giant cells, lymphocytes, and plasma cells are present	
	Microabscess formation	Follicular epithelium is replaced by inflammatory cells	
	Fibrosis is absent	Fibrosis is present between follicles	

2. Altay FA et al: Subacute thyroiditis following seasonal influenza vaccination. Hum Vaccin Immunother. 12(4):1033-4, 2016

3. Fang F et al: Concurrent onset of subacute thyroiditis and Graves disease. Am J Med Sci. 352(2):224-6, 2016

4. Jonas C et al: Painful thyroid nodule, a misleading presentation of subacute thyroiditis. Acta Chir Belg. 116(5):301-304, 2016

5. Lee YJ et al: Sonographic characteristics and interval changes of subacute thyroiditis. J Ultrasound Med. 35(8):1653-9, 2016

6. Mo Z et al: Acute transverse myelitis and subacute thyroiditis associated with dengue viral infection: a case report and literature review. Exp Ther Med. 12(4):2331-2335, 2016

7. Rosa M: Cytologic features of subacute granulomatous thyroiditis can mimic malignancy in liquid-based preparations. Diagn Cytopathol. 44(8):682-4, 2016

8. Sheraz F et al: Dengue fever presenting atypically with viral conjunctivitis and subacute thyroiditis. J Coll Physicians Surg Pak. 26(6):S33-4, 2016

9. Hallengren B et al: Presence of thyroid-stimulating hormone receptor antibodies in a patient with subacute thyroiditis followed by hypothyroidism and later Graves' disease with ophthalmopathy: a case report. Eur Thyroid J. 4(3):197-200, 2015

10. Mazza E et al: Thyroidectomy for painful thyroiditis resistant to steroid treatment: three new cases with review of the literature. Case Rep Endocrinol. 2015:138327, 2015

11. Abo Salook M et al: IgG4-related thyroiditis: a case report and review of literature. Endocrinol Diabetes Metab Case Rep. 2014:140037, 2014

12. Alfadda AA et al: Subacute thyroiditis: clinical presentation and long term outcome. Int J Endocrinol. 2014:794943, 2014

13. Freesmeyer M et al: Diagnosis of de quervain's subacute thyroiditis via sensor-navigated 124Iodine PET/ultrasound (124I-PET/US) fusion. Endocrine. 49(1):293-5, 2014

14. Michas G et al: De Quervain thyroiditis in the course of H1N1 influenza infection. Hippokratia. 18(1):86-7, 2014

15. Cappelli C et al: Ultrasound findings of subacute thyroiditis: a single institution retrospective review. Acta Radiol. 55(4):429-33, 2013

16. Schenke S et al: Thyroiditis de Quervain. are there predictive factors for long-term hormone-replacement? Nuklearmedizin. 52(4):137-40, 2013

17. Frates MC et al: Subacute granulomatous (de Quervain) thyroiditis: grayscale and color Doppler sonographic characteristics. J Ultrasound Med. 32(3):505-11, 2013

18. Calvi L et al: Acute thyrotoxicosis secondary to destructive thyroiditis associated with cardiac catheterization contrast dye. Thyroid. 21(4):443-9, 2011

19. Mordes DA et al: Cytopathology of subacute thyroiditis. Diagn Cytopathol. 40(5):433-4, 2012

20. Samuels MH: Subacute, silent, and postpartum thyroiditis. Med Clin North Am. 96(2):223-33, 2012

21. Carlé A et al: Epidemiology of subtypes of hyperthyroidism in Denmark: a population-based study. Eur J Éndocrinol. 164(5):801-9, 2011

22. Engkakul P et al: de Quervain thyroiditis in a young boy following hand-foot-mouth disease. Eur J Pediatr. 170(4):527-9, 2011

23. Engkakul P et al: Eponym: de Quervain thyroiditis. Eur J Pediatr. 170(4):427-31, 2011

24. Horai Y et al: A case of Takayasu's arteritis associated with human leukocyte antigen A24 and B52 following resolution of ulcerative colitis and subacute thyroiditis. Intern Med. 50(2):151-4, 2011

25. Janssen OE: Atypical presentation of subacute thyroiditis. Dtsch Med Wochenschr. 136(11):519-22, 2011

26. Lee JI et al: Diagnostic value of a chimeric TSH receptor (Mc4)-based bioassay for Graves' disease. Korean J Intern Med. 26(2):179-86, 2011

27. Ruchala M et al: Sonoelastography in de Quervain thyroiditis. J Clin Endocrinol Metab. 96(2):289-90, 2011

28. Sharma M et al: Hyperthyroidism. Med Sci Monit. 17(4):RA85-91, 2011

29. Xie P et al: Real-time ultrasound elastography in the diagnosis and differential diagnosis of subacute thyroiditis. J Clin Ultrasound. 39(8):435-40, 2011

30. Akahori H et al: Graves' disease associated with infectious mononucleosis due to primary Epstein-Barr virus infection: report of 3 cases. Intern Med. 49(23):2599-603, 2010

31. Chang T et al: Hashimoto encephalopathy: clinical and MRI improvement following high-dose corticosteroid therapy. Neurologist. 16(6):394-6, 2010

32. Dimos G et al: Subacute thyroiditis in the course of novel H1N1 influenza infection. Endocrine. 37(3):440-1, 2010

33. Espinoza PG et al: A comparison between two imaging techniques for the diagnosis of subacute thyroiditis (de Quervain thyroiditis): brief communication. Clin Nucl Med. 35(11):862-4, 2010

34. Karkare M: Subacute thyroiditis following ginger (Zingiber officinale) consumption. Int J Ayurveda Res. 1(2):134, 2010

35. Levenson JN et al: Discordance between cytologic results in multiple thyroid nodules within the same patient. Acta Cytol. 54(5):673-8, 2010

36. Girgis CM et al: Subacute thyroiditis following the H1N1 vaccine. J Endocrinol Invest. 33(7):506, 2010

37. Rao NL et al: Salivary C-reactive protein in Hashimoto's thyroiditis and subacute thyroiditis. Int J Inflam. 2010:514659, 2010

38. Richard J et al: Sweet's syndrome and subacute thyroiditis: an unrecognized association? Thyroid. 20(12):1425-6, 2010

Early Phase of de Quervain Thyroiditis

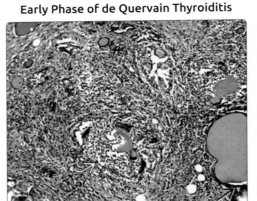

Residual Thyroid Follicles

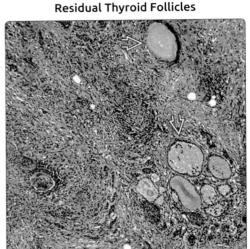

(Left) *Low-power view of a thyroid with subacute de Quervain thyroiditis shows the variable appearance of the lesions. Areas of granulomatous inflammation* ➡ *are adjacent to focal areas with fibrosis and to areas of noninvolved parenchyma* ➡. **(Right)** *Residual thyroid follicles* ➡ *can be identified in this section, adjacent to inflammation, early fibrosis, and noncaseating granulomas. Fibrotic background with granulomas is characteristic of later phase granulomatous thyroiditis.*

Microabscess Formation in Early Phase

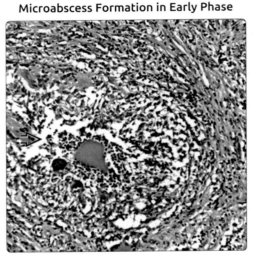

Subacute Thyroiditis

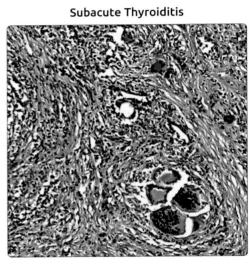

(Left) *Granulomatous thyroiditis in the acute phase shows giant cells with microabscess* ➡ *formation surrounded by early fibrosis; however, fibrosis is not as striking as is seen in the later phase of the disease.* **(Right)** *Acute inflammation within the parenchyma is present surrounding extensive giant cell granulomatous formation. There is more fibrosis and giant cell formation than in the immediate acute phase. This may represent the interphase between early- and late-phase disease.*

Fibrotic Phase

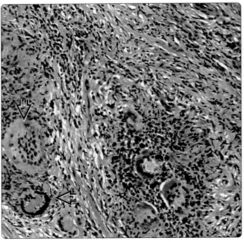

Giant Cell Granuloma

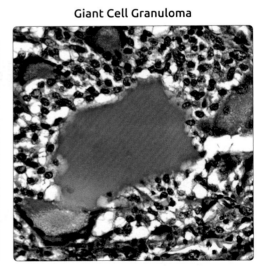

(Left) *Fibrotic background with noncaseating granulomas is characteristic of the later phase of granulomatous thyroiditis. Note the numerous nuclei* ➡ *present in the giant cell.* **(Right)** *Higher power image of a granuloma with giant cell formation and mixed inflammatory component formed by lymphocytes, plasma cells, histiocytes, and neutrophils is shown. In the acute phase, there is microabscess formation. In the later phase, the follicular epithelium disappears, and there is mixed inflammatory infiltrate.*

Giant Cells in Late Fibrotic Phase

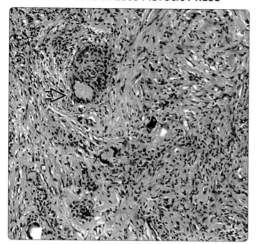

Giant Cells Forming Granuloma

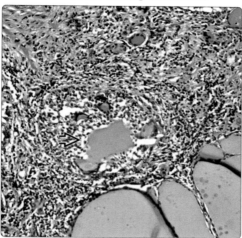

(Left) *Scattered multinucleated giant cells* ⇒ *are present within a background of extensive fibrosis, characteristic of late-phase granulomatous thyroiditis. In this phase, lymphocytes and plasma cells predominate the inflammatory cell infiltrate.* (Right) *Prominent multinucleated giant cells are present in the area of disrupted follicles and surrounding colloid* ⇒. *Note the inflammatory infiltration and an adjacent preserved thyroid follicle.*

Granulomatous Thyroiditis

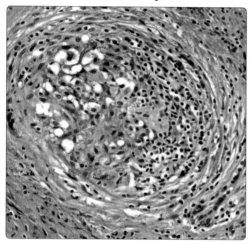

Minocycline Black Thyroid

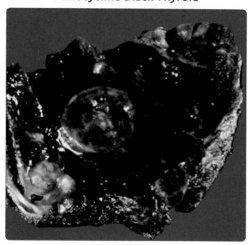

(Left) *H&E shows an area with a well-formed granuloma composed by a mixed population of histiocytes and inflammatory cells, surrounded by fibrous tissue.* (Right) *This gross cut surface of a thyroid from a patient treated with minocycline shows a dark brown to black appearance with a well-circumscribed adenomatous nodule. This gross appearance is different from the typical subacute thyroiditis which shows a vague nodularity and a fibrotic, white-tan appearance.*

Minocycline Granuloma

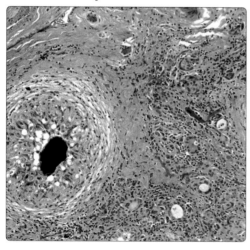

Minocycline Thyroiditis

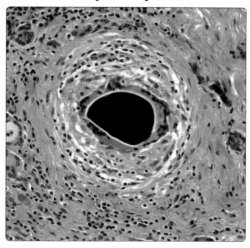

(Left) *The differential diagnosis of subacute thyroiditis should include minocycline-associated thyroiditis. In this thyroid, the giant cell granulomas are surrounding black colloid.* (Right) *High-power view of granulomatous thyroiditis due to prior minocycline treatment is shown. This condition is within the differential diagnosis of granulomatous de Quervain thyroiditis. The black pigment within giant cells is characteristic.*

Palpation Thyroiditis

TERMINOLOGY

- Palpation thyroiditis (PT) is iatrogenic condition caused by vigorous palpation of thyroid gland

ETIOLOGY/PATHOGENESIS

- Similar histologic findings were reproduced in study involving rigorous palpation of animal thyroid glands for 3 days
- Palpation of thyroid gland may impair physical integrity of follicular basement membrane
  - It reflects release of preformed hormone from damaged follicular cells
  - With consequent development of inflammatory response

CLINICAL ISSUES

- Self-limiting entity of little clinical significance other than its propensity to mimic other disease processes

- Majority of patients are asymptomatic; however, clinically significant thyrotoxicosis occurs in minority

IMAGING

- Technetium-99m scintigraphy scan may show radiotracer uptake focally or diffusely decreased throughout both lobes of thyroid gland

MICROSCOPIC

- Folliculitis with mixed inflammatory infiltrate consisting of histiocytes, lymphocytes, and multinucleated giant cells
  - With multifocal foreign body giant cell reaction to colloid
- Inflammatory response is usually seen within follicles to extravasated colloid
- Loss of follicular epithelial cells

ANCILLARY TESTS

- CD68, CD163, and lysozyme positive

Giant Cell Reaction

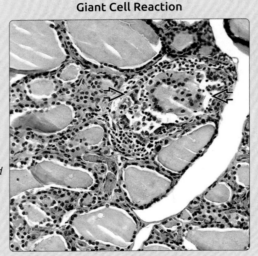

Extravasated Colloid

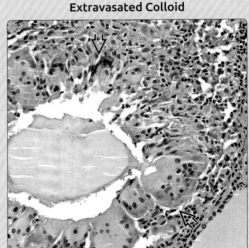

(Left) Giant cell granulomatous formation ⇥ is identified within an area of a ruptured follicle in palpation thyroiditis in response to extravasated colloid. Note the lack of follicular cells. *(Right)* High-power view shows a prominent, histiocytic, inflammatory, and foreign body-type giant cell ⇥ reaction to extravasated colloid from a ruptured thyroid follicle.

Residual Colloid Within Granuloma

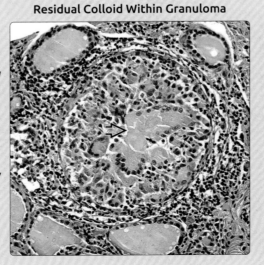

Giant Cells and Histiocytes

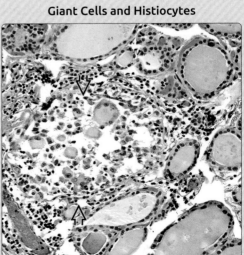

(Left) Giant cell formation surrounded by chronic inflammatory infiltrate is usually present in palpation thyroiditis. Residual colloid ⇥ can be identified in the center of this inflammatory reaction. *(Right)* Ruptured thyroid follicle ⇥ in palpation thyroiditis shows giant cells and histiocytes in a granulomatous reaction adjacent to and surrounded by normal follicles.

TERMINOLOGY

Abbreviations

- Palpation thyroiditis (PT)

Synonyms

- Multifocal granulomatous folliculitis
- Martial arts thyroiditis

Definitions

- Iatrogenic condition caused by vigorous palpation of thyroid gland

ETIOLOGY/PATHOGENESIS

Historical Perspective

- Condition was observed in 83% of surgically removed thyroid glands with nodularity as compared to glands examined at autopsy (10-40%) at Mayo Clinic
  - Authors concluded that condition was caused by preoperative injury or rupture
    - Similar histologic findings were reproduced in study involving rigorous palpation of animal thyroid glands for 3 days

CLINICAL ISSUES

Laboratory Tests

- Patients with PT have been found to have normal laboratory findings
  - This is in contrast to post-FNA patients who have occasionally been found to have elevated serum thyroglobulin levels
  - Despite this, there is case report of subsequent atrial fibrillation after PT
- Rare reports of thyrotoxicosis resulting from PT
  - Occur due to mechanical damage of thyroid follicles by vigorous palpation

Prognosis

- PT is self-limiting entity of little clinical significance other than its propensity to mimic other disease processes
  - Diagnosis is usually not rendered in routinely examined thyroid glands
    - No treatment is indicated

MACROSCOPIC

General Features

- Gross areas of hemorrhage may be present

MICROSCOPIC

Histologic Features

- Folliculitis with mixed inflammatory infiltrate consisting of histiocytes, lymphocytes, and multinucleated giant cells
  - Inflammatory response is usually seen within follicles to extravasated colloid
    - May be adjacent to ruptured follicles
  - Loss of follicular epithelial cells
  - Necrosis is seldom found
    - If necrosis is found, consider other etiologies

Cytologic Features

- Nonacute inflammatory cells and giant cell formation

ANCILLARY TESTS

Immunohistochemistry

- CD68, CD163, and lysozyme positive

Special Stains

- PAS stain may be helpful in identifying residual colloid within giant cell formation

DIFFERENTIAL DIAGNOSIS

Sarcoidosis and Other Granulomatous Processes

- Sarcoidosis
  - Will have interstitial granulomas
- Infectious processes
  - Such entities will usually produce caseating granulomas
- Subacute thyroiditis
  - Will have acute inflammatory cells

C-Cell Hyperplasia

- Chromogranin and calcitonin positive by immunohistochemistry

DIAGNOSTIC CHECKLIST

Pathologic Interpretation Pearls

- Foreign body-type reaction within follicles or adjacent to ruptured follicles
  - Be mindful of other processes that may produce granulomas
- Normal laboratory findings
  - Sarcoidosis will frequently have elevated calcium
- Absence of necrosis
  - Necrosis is usually not present in PT
    - This finding warrants investigation of other possible etiologies

SELECTED REFERENCES

1. Madill EM et al: Palpation thyroiditis following subtotal parathyroidectomy for hyperparathyroidism. Endocrinol Diabetes Metab Case Rep. 2016, 2016
2. Blazak JK et al: Palpation thyroiditis seen on F-18 FDG PET/CT. Clin Nucl Med. 36(3):261-3, 2011
3. Lanas A et al: Frequency of positive anti thyroid peroxidase antibody titers among normal individuals. Rev Med Chil. 138(1):15-21, 2010
4. Tonacchera M et al: Assessment of nodular goitre. Best Pract Res Clin Endocrinol Metab. 24(1):51-61, 2010
5. Nys P et al: Etiologic discussion and clinical relevance of thyroid ultrasonography in subclinical hypothyroidism. a retrospective study in 1845 patients. Ann Endocrinol (Paris). 70(1):59-63, 2009
6. Mai VQ et al: Palpation thyroiditis causing new-onset atrial fibrillation. Thyroid. 18(5):571-3, 2008
7. Uchino S et al: Examination strategy for thyroid nodules. Nihon Rinsho. 65(11):2016-20, 2007
8. Paunkovic J et al: Does autoantibody-negative Graves' disease exist? a second evaluation of the clinical diagnosis. Horm Metab Res. 38(1):53-6, 2006
9. Vitti P et al: Thyroid ultrasound as a predicator of thyroid disease. J Endocrinol Invest. 26(7):686-9, 2003
10. Lawrence W Jr et al: Diagnosis and management of patients with thyroid nodules. J Surg Oncol. 80(3):157-70, 2002
11. Rueda FL et al: Atypical thyroiditis in Huelva, Spain. Endocr Pract. 5(3):109-13, 1999
12. Carney JA et al: Palpation thyroiditis (multifocal granulomatour folliculitis). Am J Clin Pathol. 64(5):639-47, 1975

Riedel Thyroiditis

TERMINOLOGY

- Riedel thyroiditis (RT): Densely sclerotic inflammatory process involving thyroid gland and adjacent tissue
- IgG4-related thyroid disease (IgG4-RTD)

ETIOLOGY/PATHOGENESIS

- Autoimmune basis suggested
- RT considered IgG4-related disease variant
  - Has long association with systemic fibrosclerosing diseases, included within IgG4-related disease spectrum

CLINICAL ISSUES

- Often sudden inflammatory goiter with compressive symptoms and nontender, hard thyroid gland on palpation
- May be associated with retroperitoneal fibrosis or sclerosing mediastinitis

MACROSCOPIC

- Enlargement of gland with extensive fibrosis

- Cut surfaces tan-gray, woody, and without normal apparent lobulation of gland

MICROSCOPIC

- Normal thyroid gland obliterated by dense, sclerotic, keloid-like fibrous tissue
- Extensive inflammatory infiltrate present
- Sclerotic tissue may involve adjacent extrathyroidal soft tissue and parathyroid glands

ANCILLARY TESTS

- > 50 IgG4(+) cells per HPF
- Elevated IgG4 to IgG ratio (> 40%)

TOP DIFFERENTIAL DIAGNOSES

- Fibrous variant of Hashimoto thyroiditis
- Undifferentiated thyroid carcinoma
- Subacute thyroiditis

Differential Diagnosis of Thyroiditis

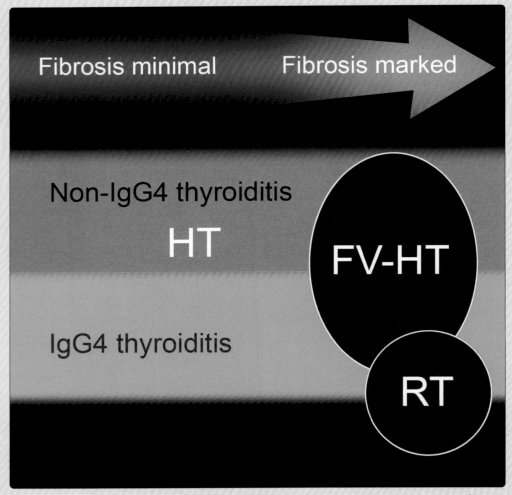

The differential diagnosis of some thyroiditis is based according to the degree of fibrosis, IgG4 immunostaining, and invasive fibrosis beyond the thyroid surface. There is an overlap in histopathological features between IgG4 thyroiditis, fibrosing variant of Hashimoto thyroiditis (FV-HT), and Riedel thyroiditis (RT).

TERMINOLOGY

Abbreviations

- Riedel thyroiditis (RT)

Synonyms

- Riedel struma
- Invasive fibrous thyroiditis
- IgG4-related thyroiditis or IgG4-related thyroid disease
  - RT is member of family of IgG4-related disease

Definitions

- Idiopathic, densely sclerotic process involving thyroid gland and adjacent tissue

ETIOLOGY/PATHOGENESIS

Autoimmune

- Autoimmune basis suggested but not proven
  - Association between RT and Hashimoto thyroiditis also suggests autoimmune process
  - Presence of antithyroid antibodies may be result of release of thyroid antigens into circulation due to destruction of follicles
    - Mechanism in contrast to more active autoimmune thyroiditides, such as Hashimoto and Graves diseases
  - Presence of mononuclear cells and detection of autoantibodies directed against thyroid-specific antigens favors autoimmune pathogenesis
- Possible relation to eosinophilia
  - Recent study of 16 patients with RT showed striking eosinophilia and abundant extracellular deposition of eosinophil-derived protein
  - Additionally, immunofluorescence studies of proteins in human eosinophilic granules show extracellular deposition of major basic protein in RT but not in Hashimoto disease

Systemic Fibrosing Disease/IgG4-Related Systemic Disease

- RT associated with systemic fibrosing disease (inflammatory fibrosclerosis)
- RT, now firmly considered IgG4-related disease variant, has had long association with systemic fibrosclerosing diseases, many of which are now included within IgG4-related disease spectrum
  - Significant proportion of cases of fibrosing Hashimoto thyroiditis, and minority of cases with classic Hashimoto thyroiditis, belong to spectrum of IgG4-related disease
- Recent evidence suggests RT part of IgG4-related systemic disorder
  - RT may coexist with 1 or more anatomic sites of involvement, including
    - Retroperitoneum, retroorbital, sinonasal tract, parotid gland, lacrimal glands, lung, mediastinum, and hepatobiliary tract
  - Supported by fact that RT shows elevated numbers of IgG4-positive plasma cells as well as morphologic features of IgG4-related disease

CLINICAL ISSUES

Epidemiology

- Incidence
  - Extremely rare condition (0.5% of all thyroidectomy cases at Mayo Clinic)
  - Occurs mostly in adults and has female predominance

Presentation

- Often sudden inflammatory goiter with compressive symptoms and nontender, hard thyroid gland on palpation
  - Patients present with stone-hard, painless neck mass frequently associated with dysphagia, dyspnea, and stridor
  - Vocal cord paralysis due to involvement of recurrent laryngeal nerve may occur
  - Frequent involvement of surrounding neck structures, including compression and encasement of carotid artery and internal jugular vein
- May be associated with various inflammatory conditions such as retroperitoneal fibrosis, sclerosing cholangitis, or sclerosing mediastinitis
  - Less frequently associated with mediastinal fibrosis, orbital and lacrimal sclerosis, pituitary or testicular fibrosis

Laboratory Tests

- Laboratory findings may demonstrate elevated antithyroglobulin antibodies and antimicrosomal antibodies
- Thyroid function may be normal, low, or high
  - Hypothyroidism occurs in ~ 30-40% of patients
    - Hypoparathyroidism may occur and can be indication of involvement of parathyroid glands

Treatment

- Surgical approaches
  - Surgical resection may be necessary to preserve tracheal and esophageal functions
    - Resection of uninvolved thyroid not necessary
- Drugs
  - Steroids and tamoxifen to diminish inflammation
  - Patients frequently require thyroid hormone replacement as they are hypothyroid
  - Mycophenolate mofetil has been recently used for systemic fibrosis

Prognosis

- Favorable after surgery

MACROSCOPIC

General Features

- Extensive fibrosis involving thyroid gland
- Cut surfaces are tan-gray, avascular, woody, and without normal apparent lobulation of gland
- Fibrosis frequently extends to adjacent soft tissue

MICROSCOPIC

Histologic Features

- Normal thyroid gland obliterated by dense, sclerotic, keloid-like fibrous tissue

- Thyroid follicles may occasionally be present within fibrotic stroma
- Sclerotic tissue may involve extrathyroidal soft tissue, including muscles, nerves, and adipose tissue and may also involve parathyroid glands
- Occasional giant cells may be present
- Oxyphilic cells not present
  - Presence of these cells suggests diagnosis of chronic lymphocytic thyroiditis or granulomatous inflammation of thyroid
- Inflammatory infiltrate consisting of lymphocytes, plasma cells, a few neutrophils, and eosinophils
- Remnant thyroid follicles may be present, entrapped within dense collagen, with extensive atrophic changes
- Occasionally vasculitis with intimal proliferation and thrombosis
  - Vasculitis may effect entire thickness of vessel
    - May create thrombus-like effect
- Follicular adenoma, adenomatous nodules, and follicular carcinomas have been reported within fibrosis in few select cases
- Histology is gold standard for diagnosis of IgG4-related disease
  - Storiform-type fibrosis and obliterative phlebitis constitute characteristic features of this disease
  - Definitive diagnosis of IgG4-related disease also requires presence of elevated numbers of IgG4-positive plasma cells as well as IgG4 to IgG ratio > 40%

ANCILLARY TESTS

Cytology
- Typically scant colloid indicative of dry tap

Immunohistochemistry
- Recent studies have shown predominance of λ-light chains
- > 50 IgG4-positive cells per HPF

DIFFERENTIAL DIAGNOSIS

Fibrous Variant of Hashimoto Thyroiditis
- Demonstrates smaller gland with some preservation of lobules
- No involvement of adjacent head and neck tissue
- Oxyphilic metaplasia may be present, as opposed to RT

Undifferentiated Thyroid Carcinoma, Paucicellular Variant
- Patients with undifferentiated thyroid carcinoma will also present with thyroid mass that may or may not be painful
  - Occurrence in elderly patients
  - Fatal outcome within months
  - Rapidly growing mass
- Gross exam will demonstrate necrosis and hemorrhage in carcinoma
- Rare variant of anaplastic carcinoma that may histologically resemble RT
  - Microscopic exam may demonstrate more atypia than RT
    - Usually hypocellular foci comprised by atypical spindle cells
  - Acellular fibrous tissue with extensive necrosis and dystrophic calcification

- Presence of lymph node metastases helps in differential diagnosis
- Presence of lymphovascular invasion
- May be extremely difficult to distinguish from RT on small biopsy specimens
- Thyroglobulin and TTF-1 immunohistochemistry usually negative

Subacute Thyroiditis
- Clinical presentation includes neck pain in thyroid region
- Diverse systemic manifestations including fever, chills, weight loss, anorexia, and fatigue
- Early or hyperthyroid phase: Elevated thyroglobulin, T3, and T4, and decreased serum TSH
- Later or hypothyroid phase: Decreased thyroglobulin, T3 and T4, and increased serum TSH
- Granulomatous inflammation of thyroid with distinct histological findings
  - Early phase: Destruction of follicular cells and acute inflammatory infiltrate including microabscesses
  - Later phase: Lymphoplasmacytic infiltrate predominant
  - Regenerative phase: Follicular cell regeneration and minimal residual fibrosis
- Minimal residual fibrosis present in later regenerative phase, but keloid-like fibrosis absent

DIAGNOSTIC CHECKLIST

Pathologic Interpretation Pearls
- Destruction and replacement of thyroid parenchyma by keloid-like dense collagen
- Extension of fibrosis into extrathyroidal soft tissue
- Thyroglobulin and TTF-1 immunohistochemistry may be useful to identify tissue as thyroid tissue

SELECTED REFERENCES

1. Jokisch F et al: A small subgroup of Hashimoto's thyroiditis is associated with IgG4-related disease. Virchows Arch. 468(3):321-7, 2016
2. Stan MN et al: Riedel's thyroiditis association with IgG4-related disease. Clin Endocrinol (Oxf). ePub, 2016
3. Takeshima K et al: Clinicopathological features of Riedel's thyroiditis associated with IgG4-related disease in Japan. Endocr J. 62(8):725-31, 2015
4. Oriot P et al: Fibrosis of the thyroid gland caused by an IgG4-related sclerosing disease: three years of follow-up. Acta Clin Belg. 69(6):446-50, 2014
5. Li Y et al: Distinct histopathological features of Hashimoto's thyroiditis with respect to IgG4-related disease. Mod Pathol. 25(8):1086-97, 2012
6. Pusztaszeri M et al: Riedel's thyroiditis with increased IgG4 plasma cells: evidence for an underlying IgG4-related sclerosing disease? Thyroid. 22(9):964-8, 2012
7. Hennessey JV: Clinical review: Riedel's thyroiditis: a clinical review. J Clin Endocrinol Metab. 96(10):3031-41, 2011
8. Kakudo K et al: Diagnosis of Hashimoto's thyroiditis and IgG4-related sclerosing disease. Pathol Int. 61(4):175-83, 2011
9. Li Y et al: Hashimoto's thyroiditis: old concepts and new insights. Curr Opin Rheumatol. 23(1):102-7, 2011
10. Dahlgren M et al: Riedel's thyroiditis and multifocal fibrosclerosis are part of the IgG4-related systemic disease spectrum. Arthritis Care Res (Hoboken). 62(9):1312-8, 2010
11. Lu L et al: Clinical and pathological features of Riedel's thyroiditis. Chin Med Sci J. 25(3):129-34, 2010
12. McIver B et al: Graves' disease after unilateral Riedel's thyroiditis. J Clin Endocrinol Metab. 95(6):2525-6, 2010
13. Piazza O et al: Riedel's thyroiditis and cerebral venous sinuses thrombosis: a case report. Panminerva Med. 52(4):362-4, 2010
14. Shahi N et al: Riedel's thyroiditis masquerading as anaplastic thyroid carcinoma: a case report. J Med Case Reports. 4:15, 2010
15. Yamamoto M et al: [IgG4-related systemic disease/systemic IgG4-related disease.] Rinsho Byori. 58(5):454-65, 2010

Riedel vs. Fibrous Variant Hashimoto Thyroiditis

	Riedel Thyroiditis	Fibrous Variant Hashimoto
Age	Variable	Elderly
Clinical findings	Nonpainful, enlarging thyroid mass	Painless goiter
Laboratory findings	May have slightly elevated thyroid antibodies	Extremely elevated thyroid antibodies relative to Riedel
Gross findings	Variable size but tends to be smaller than Hashimoto	Larger than Riedel
Extrathyroidal invasion	More likely to have adherence and infiltration of surrounding tissues of head and neck	Confined to thyroid gland
Normal thyroid tissue	Sharply demarcated	Diffuse involvement
Architecture	Near complete loss of lobular architecture with dense fibrosis	Less obliterative fibrotic pattern
Venulitis	Yes	No
Oncocytic (Hürthle) cells	No	Yes
Associated autoimmune disease	Yes	Yes

16. Buła G et al: [Riedel's goitre - rare and difficult to diagnose reason for surgical treatment of goiters.] Endokrynol Pol. 60(6):488-91, 2009
17. Erdoğan MF et al: A case of Riedel's thyroiditis with pleural and pericardial effusions. Endocrine. 35(3):297-301, 2009
18. Kojima M et al: Inflammatory pseudotumor of the thyroid gland showing prominent fibrohistiocytic proliferation. A case report. Endocr Pathol. 20(3):186-90, 2009
19. Brihaye B et al: Diffuse periarterial involvement in systemic fibrosclerosis with Riedel's thyroiditis, sclerosing cholangitis, and retroperitoneal fibrosis. Scand J Rheumatol. 37(6):490-2, 2008
20. Gire J et al: [Orbital pseudotumors and Riedel's thyroiditis: case report.] J Fr Ophtalmol. 31(7):715, 2008
21. Michels JJ et al: [What diagnosis can be made by the pathologist in a case of sclerosing thyroiditis?.] Ann Pathol. 28(4):263-7, 2008
22. Perimenis P et al: [Riedel's thyroiditis: current aspects.] Presse Med. 37(6 Pt 2):1015-21, 2008
23. Won YS et al: A case of Riedel's thyroiditis associated with benign nodule: mimic of anaplastic transformation. Int J Surg. 6(6):e24-7, 2008
24. Cho MH et al: Riedel's thyroiditis in a patient with recurrent subacute thyroiditis: a case report and review of the literature. Endocr J. 54(4):559-62, 2007
25. Zimmermann-Belsing T et al: Riedel's thyroiditis: an autoimmune or primary fibrotic disease? J Intern Med. 235(3):271-4, 1994

(Left) *Keloid-like bands of fibrosis and extensive inflammatory infiltrate replaces the thyroid parenchyma. The keloid-like fibrosis is characteristic of RT/IgG4-related disease.* **(Right)** *Keloid-like bands of fibrosis and extensive lymphoplasmacytic inflammatory infiltrate replaces the thyroid parenchyma. The keloid-like fibrosis is characteristic of RT/IgG4-related disease.*

Extensive Storiform Fibrosis

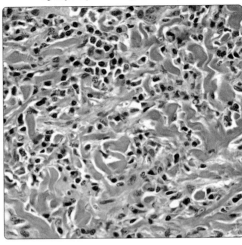

Lymphoplasmacytic Infiltrate

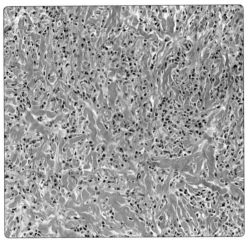

(Left) *High-power view demonstrates diffuse keloid-like fibroblastic proliferation in a paucicellular fashion, almost completely replacing the thyroid parenchyma with scattered atrophic thyroid follicles. Lymphoplasmacytic inflammatory infiltrate is present.* **(Right)** *Thyroid is replaced by cellular fibrous tissue arranged in a storiform pattern with keloid-like appearance intermixed with lymphoplasmacytic infiltrate and plump fibroblasts. There is extensive destruction of the thyroid follicles.*

Keloid-Like Fibrosis

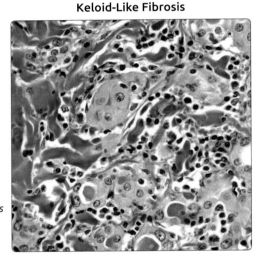

Keloid-Like Fibrosis

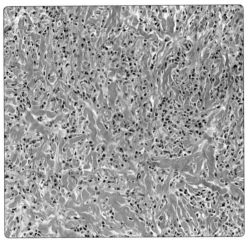

(Left) *H&E shows IgG4-related disease with keloid-like fibroblastic proliferation in a paucicellular fashion, with a prominent lymphoplasmacytic inflammatory infiltrate, completely replacing the thyroid parenchyma.* **(Right)** *IgG4-related systemic disease is now increasingly recognized in multiple organs, including an established thyroid involvement. RT is now included within IgG4-related disease. Elevated numbers of IgG4-positive plasma cells are identified within the lymphoplasmacytic infiltrate.*

Numerous Plasma Cells Within Fibrosis

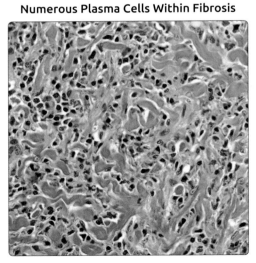

Numerous IgG4-Positive Cells

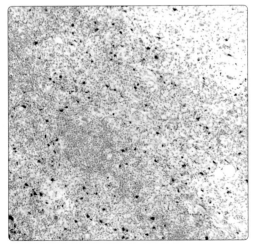

Residual Follicles Within Keloid

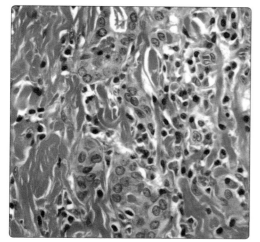

Loss of Thyroid Follicles by Fibrosis

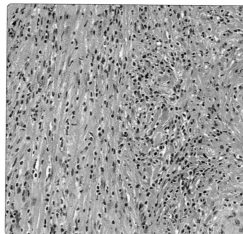

(Left) *H&E shows IgG4-related disease with keloid-like fibroblastic proliferation in a paucicellular fashion, with a prominent lymphoplasmacytic inflammatory infiltrate, replacing the thyroid parenchyma.* **(Right)** *The normal thyroid gland is completely replaced by a dense, keloid-like fibroblastic proliferation, associated with lymphoplasmacytic inflammatory infiltrate. Note the absence of thyroid follicles.*

Early Phase of RT

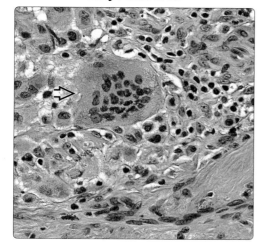

Fibrosis

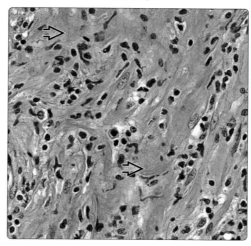

(Left) *Occasional multinucleated giant cells ⊃, associated with destroyed follicular cells, macrophages, lymphocytes, and eosinophils are present in areas of thyroid follicle destruction seen in early phases of RT.* **(Right)** *Keloid-like bands of fibrosis and extensive inflammatory infiltrate replace the thyroid parenchyma. The keloid-like fibrosis is characteristic of RT ⊃.*

Skeletal Muscle Involved by Inflammation

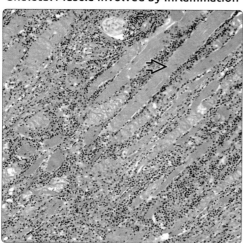

Extrathyroidal Fibrosis

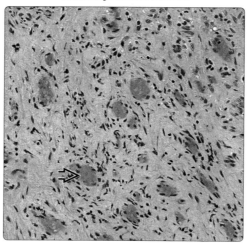

(Left) *The extensive fibrosing process present in RT is not confined to the thyroid and usually involves adjacent skeletal muscle ⊃. Involvement of other extrathyroidal tissues, such as parathyroid, vessels, nerves, and fat may be present.* **(Right)** *High-power view of an extensive fibrosing process shows sclerotic tissue surrounding skeletal muscle bundles ⊃. The inflammatory component present is scarce and includes lymphocytes, plasma cells, and eosinophils.*

TERMINOLOGY

- Autoimmune disease characterized by elevated circulating antiperoxidase and antithyroglobulin antibodies

CLASSIFICATION

- Hashimoto thyroiditis (HT) can be divided into 2 groups: IgG4 thyroiditis [IgG4(+) plasma cell-rich] and non-IgG4 thyroiditis [IgG4(+) plasma cell-poor]
- IgG4-related thyroiditis
- Fibrous variant
- Fibrous atrophy variant
- Juvenile variant
- Cystic variant

CLINICAL ISSUES

- Female predominance 5-7x that of men
- Antithyroid microsomal antibodies present in 95% of cases
- IgG4-related HT has its own clinical, serological, and sonographic features

MACROSCOPIC

- Diffuse symmetric enlargement with bosselated or irregular surfaces and prominent pyramidal lobe
- Usually 2-3x size of normal gland and may weigh up to 200 g

MICROSCOPIC

- Gland showing lymphoplasmacytic infiltrate with prominent germinal centers
- Thyroid follicles are atrophic with fibrotic background
  o Interfollicular fibrosis, interlobular fibrosis, and scar storiform fibrosis
- Squamous metaplasia of follicles may be present

TOP DIFFERENTIAL DIAGNOSES

- Riedel thyroiditis as another candidate for IgG4-related thyroiditis
- Thyroid carcinoma, lymphoma, Graves disease

Imaging Findings

Lobulated Cut Surface

(Left) *Axial CECT shows Hashimoto thyroiditis (HT) as diffuse enlargement of both lobes ➡ and the pyramidal lobe ➡ of the thyroid. Note the absence of adenopathy, thyroid lobe necrosis, and calcifications.* (Right) *Gross cut surface of IgG4 thyroiditis shows well demarcated nodules with sharp border from the surrounding tissue. The surface appearance is ivory-white with extensive lobulations, indicating replacement of the thyroid parenchyma by fibrous tissue and inflammatory infiltrate.*

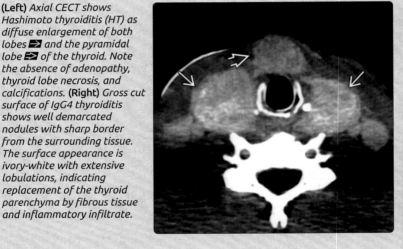

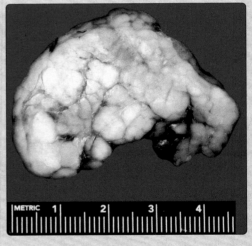

Features of Non-IgG4-Related HT

Features of IgG4-Related HT Thyroiditis

(Left) *This photomicrograph shows prominent lymphoid follicles ➡ within the thyroid parenchyma as well as follicular atrophy ➡, squamous metaplasia ➡, and lymphocytic infiltrate in the thyroid follicles that are devoid of colloid.* (Right) *This H&E highlights the large thick fibrous bands in between the oncocytic cells and abundant plasma cell infiltration in fibrosing variant of HT/IgG4-related disease.*

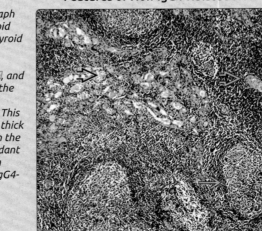

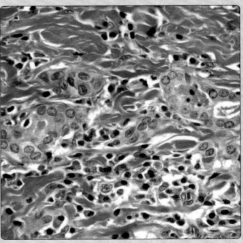

TERMINOLOGY

Abbreviations

- Hashimoto thyroiditis (HT)

Synonyms

- Struma lymphomatosa
- Hashimoto struma
- Lymphadenoid goiter
- IgG4-related thyroiditis

Definitions

- Autoimmune disease characterized by elevated circulating antithyroid peroxidase and antithyroglobulin antibodies
  o Infiltration of thyroid by inflammatory cells
  o Hypothyroidism due to destruction and eventual fibrous replacement of follicular cells

ETIOLOGY/PATHOGENESIS

Pathogenesis

- Activation of CD4(+) helper cells targeted at thyroid antigens
  o Exact mechanism of this pathway has yet to be identified

Infectious

- Potential role as molecular mimicry of infectious agents has been implicated
- Serologic evidence of recent viral and bacterial infections has been reported
  o This link has not been conclusively documented

Autoimmunity

- Possible, as follicular cells in Hashimoto have been shown to demonstrate HLA proteins, which are required for antigen presentation to CD4 helper cells
- Exact antigens causing autoimmunity are unknown
  o Elevated antithyroglobulin and antithyroid microsomal antibodies suggest that these may be involved
- Patients with HT are at greater risk for
  o Type II diabetes mellitus
  o Addison disease
  o Autoimmune oophoritis
  o Hypoparathyroidism
  o Sjögren syndrome
  o Myasthenia gravis
  o Pernicious anemia
  o Thrombocytopenic purpura

IgG4-Related Disease

- IgG4-related thyroiditis has its own clinical, serological, and sonographic features that are distinct from those associated with non-IgG4 thyroiditis
- IgG4-related disease (IgG4-RD) is characterized by elevated serum IgG4 levels, IgG4(+) plasmocytes, and lymphocyte infiltration into multiple organs
- IgG4 thyroiditis is subset of patients with HT who exhibit histopathological features of IgG4-RD
- HT patients with elevated serum IgG4 levels shared clinical features with both IgG4-RD and IgG4 thyroiditis
  o Definitive diagnosis of IgG4-RD also requires presence of elevated numbers of IgG4(+) plasma cells as well as IgG4:IgG ratio > 40%

CLINICAL ISSUES

Presentation

- Female predominance 5-7x that of men
- Mean age is 59 for women and 58 for men
- Rare in children; however, may account for 40% of adolescent goiters
- Compression of trachea of recurrent laryngeal nerve can occur but is rare
- Patients do not frequently report pain but do report uncomfortable tight sensation in neck
- May be associated with IgG4-type diseases (i.e., autoimmune pancreatitis)
- May be associated with other autoimmune diseases (Sjögren, pernicious anemia, chronic active hepatitis)
- Hashimoto encephalopathy
  o Rare disorder characterized by
    - Encephalopathy and CNS dysfunction
    - Elevated antithyroid antibodies
    - Absence of infection or structural abnormalities in CNS
    - Response to treatment with steroids
    - Serum autoantibodies against NH2-terminal of α-enolase may be used as diagnostic biomarker
- IgG4 thyroiditis
  o Distinctive subtype of HT characterized by an increased number of IgG4(+) plasma cells, high serum IgG4 levels, and thyroid storiform fibrosis
    - Thyroid involvement
      □ Younger age group
      □ Lower F:M ratio
      □ Higher levels of thyroid autoantibodies
      □ Diffuse low echogenicity
      □ Rapid progress requiring surgical treatment
      □ More subclinical hypothyroidism
    - Fibrous variant of HT was prior diagnosis in ~ 95% of IgG4-related thyroiditis
    - IgG4-RD of thyroid gland differs from that in other organ systems, exhibiting dense fibrosis without intense eosinophilia or obliterative phlebitis
      □ Obliterative phlebitis is one of characteristic features of IgG4-RD reported in other organs, but this type of vasculitis has not been reported in any variants of HT, including IgG4 thyroiditis

Laboratory Tests

- Antithyroglobulin antibody in > 60% of patients
- Antithyroid microsomal antibodies in 95% of patients

Treatment

- Surgical approaches
  o Necessary with excessive compression or discomfort or under clinical suspicion of possible carcinoma
  o Option for patients who do not respond well to medical treatment of hormonal symptoms
- Drugs
  o T4 (levothyroxine) is treatment of choice for all patients with hypothyroidism (overt or subclinical) as result of hypothyroidism
    - Treatment is usually lifelong

- – Response to T4 therapy will include decrease in levels of thyroid antibodies
  - – Clinicians must be careful of overtreating patients and causing iatrogenic thyrotoxicosis
  - o Immunosuppressive therapy may decrease thyroid antibody levels and diminish thyroid enlargement
    - – However, steroids are contraindicated due to their side effects
  - o Appropriate management of patients who are euthyroid but have enlarged glands remains controversial
    - – T4 administration may result in shrinkage of gland, easing compressive symptoms
    - – Other patients may experience enlargement of gland with treatment
    - – 10-15% of patients may develop hypothyroidism

Prognosis

- Potential complications
  - o Hypothyroidism
  - o Thyroid lymphoma may develop
    - – Usually B-cell phenotype
  - o In pregnant women, most common complication is postpartum thyroiditis
  - o Thyroid carcinoma (papillary or follicular)
- Prognosis is generally good
  - o Most patients are managed favorably with medical or surgical therapy
  - o No increased incidence of medullary thyroid carcinoma

Similarities to Graves Disease

- HT is similar to Graves in number of ways; however, they should be regarded as distinct clinical entities
  - o Conditions may occur concurrently in families or individuals
  - o Lymphocytic infiltration and Ig are found in both conditions
  - o Thymic enlargement
  - o Thyroid antibodies
  - o Graves may precede HT and vice versa

IMAGING

General Features

- Radioiodine not generally useful but may demonstrate increased uptake as compared to subacute thyroiditis
  - o Radioiodine scan can be misleading since it is similar to Graves disease and multinodular goiter
  - o Normal glandular enlargement or diffuse abnormality with heterogeneous hypoechogenicity
  - o T2 MR may demonstrate increased intensity
  - o Heterogeneous echotexture may occur in fibrous variant in concordance with atrophied and fibrotic thyroid gland

MACROSCOPIC

General Features

- Diffuse, symmetric enlargement with bosselated or irregular surfaces and prominent pyramidal lobe
- Usually 2-3x size of normal gland and may weigh up to 200 g
- Sectioning reveals accentuated lobulation with increased fibrosis

- Parenchyma is tan-yellow instead of red-brown due to excess lymphoid tissue
- Inflammation may lead to adherence to adjacent skeletal muscle
- Dominant nodule may be present, making gross assessment between HT and neoplastic processes difficult
- Lymphoepithelial cysts
  - o Part of spectrum of changes associated with HT
  - o Represent secondary changes
  - o Incidental findings
  - o May attain large sizes and present clinically as mass
  - o Can be multifocal and bilateral
  - o Lined by squamous epithelium consisting of multiple layers of cells
  - o Occasionally, columnar epithelium may be present containing goblet cells

MICROSCOPIC

Histologic Features

- Gland showing lymphoplasmacytic infiltrate with prominent germinal centers
- Thyroid follicles are atrophic with fibrotic background
- Squamous metaplasia of follicles may be present
- Metaplastic follicles contain eosinophilic, granular cytoplasm (Hürthle changes)

Histologic Variants of Hashimoto Thyroiditis

- Fibrous variant (non-IgG4 related)
  - o Comprises 10% of cases
  - o Occurs in slightly older population than usual HT
  - o Gland is usually larger and more fibrotic than usual HT
  - o Histology shows preservation of lobulated pattern as opposed to Riedel thyroiditis
    - – Unlike Riedel, fibrosis does not extend beyond gland
  - o Atrophic follicular cells with degenerative changes and broad areas of fibrosis
    - – Fibrosis is acellular, keloid-like with irregular broad bands coursing through remaining thyroid parenchyma
    - – Chronic inflammatory infiltrate is mostly present within fibrous tissue
    - – Exaggerated lobular pattern with lobules separated by cellular storiform-type fibrosis, resembling fibrosis seen in other forms of IgG4-RD
  - o More extensive squamous metaplasia
  - o Hürthle cell changes are present as in usual HT
  - o Etiology unknown; however, it has been suggested that fibrous variant is progression of usual HT
- IgG4-related thyroiditis
  - o Distinctive subtype of HT characterized by increased number of IgG4(+) plasma cells
  - o Higher grade of stromal storiform-type fibrosis, lymphoplasmacytic infiltration, and follicular cell degeneration than non-IgG4 thyroiditis
- Fibrous atrophy variant
  - o Patients present with small atrophic thyroid gland
  - o Thyroid gland is very small and weighs 1-6 g
  - o Histology shows extensive destruction of thyroid parenchyma with minimal preservation of follicles

- o Usually occurs in elderly patients with high titers of antithyroid antibodies
- Juvenile variant
  - o Poorly defined variant of HT described in younger patients
  - o Histology similar to usual HT
  - o Follicular atrophy is uncommon
- Cystic variant
  - o Extremely rare, associated with bronchial cleft-like cysts in patients with HT
  - o Cysts are thought to be derived from developmental rests
  - o Cysts are lined by squamous and columnar epithelium and surrounded by follicular lymphoid tissue and fibrous capsule
  - o Thyroid gland shows marked atrophy, Hürthle cell change, lymphocytic infiltrates, and follicle formation
  - o Minimal fibrosis

ANCILLARY TESTS

Cytology

- Cellular aspirate with Hürthle cells and mixed inflammatory infiltrate
  - o Hürthle cells are larger than follicular cells
  - o Hürthle cells appear as sheets or small groups of cells or as single cells
  - o Lymphocytes are usually abundant
  - o Minimal to absent colloid is present
- Plasma cells, macrophages, and giant cells may also be present
  - o Presence of germinal centers may be suggested on cytologic examination, as tingible body macrophages are usually present
- Fibrous variant
  - o Fine-needle aspiration will be low yield depending on level of fibrosis
  - o Low cellularity specimen can be helpful in suggesting fibrotic process

Immunohistochemistry

- Mixed B- and T-cell markers are present on immunohistochemistry
  - o CD20, CD3, CD45
  - o B cells and plasma cells demonstrate κ and λ light chain staining
  - o IgG, IgM, and IgA heavy chains present
    - IgG κ combination most frequent
- IgG4 and IgG immunostains
  - o Cutoff value of > 20/HPF IgG4(+) plasma cells and > 30% IgG4:IgG ratio

Genetic Testing

- No BRAF point mutation
- No gene rearrangements
  - o However, there are reports of RET rearrangements in absence of morphologic findings of papillary thyroid carcinoma
    - Despite this, it is better not to diagnose papillary thyroid carcinoma without morphologic evidence of said disease

- In general, do not order these molecular tests without clinical suspicion of disease
- Concept of early premalignant transformation has been examined but is yet unproven

Electron Microscopy

- Follicular cells demonstrate typical Hürthle cell changes with enlarged mitochondria and diminished amounts of other organelles, including endoplasmic reticulum and Golgi bodies

DIFFERENTIAL DIAGNOSIS

Neoplastic (Thyroid Carcinoma, Lymphoma)

- Especially difficult to differentiate from carcinoma when adjacent skeletal muscle is involved
  - o Molecular studies can be helpful as well as morphologic evidence of papillary thyroid carcinoma
- Dominant nodule in HT may mimic neoplastic process
- Molecular distinction (absence of BRAF, NRAS, KRAS, HRAS, and RET gene rearrangement) can differentiate dominant nodule in HT from papillary thyroid carcinoma

Other Thyroiditides (Riedel Thyroiditis, Graves Disease)

- Distinction between fibrous variant of HT and Riedel can be difficult, but Riedel will demonstrate more prominent obliteration of follicles
  - o Riedel will frequently have extension to adjacent anatomical structures, whereas fibrous variant of HT will not
  - o Riedel will not have high antibody titers
- Graves disease has less inflammatory infiltrate than HT and rare oncocytic metaplasia

DIAGNOSTIC CHECKLIST

Pathologic Interpretation Pearls

- Thyroid grossly shows diffuse symmetric enlargement with bosselated or irregular surfaces
- Sectioning reveals accentuated lobulation with increased fibrosis
- Gland showing lymphoplasmacytic infiltrate with prominent germinal centers
- Metaplastic follicles contain Hürthle cell changes

SELECTED REFERENCES

1. Dutta D et al: Immunoglobulin G4 related thyroid disorders: diagnostic challenges and clinical outcomes. Endokrynol Pol. 67(5):520-524, 2016
2. Jokisch F et al: A small subgroup of Hashimoto's thyroiditis is associated with IgG4-related disease. Virchows Arch. 468(3):321-7, 2016
3. Kottahachchi D et al: Immunoglobulin G4-related thyroid diseases. Eur Thyroid J. 5(4):231-239, 2016
4. Minamino H et al: A novel immunopathological association of IgG4-RD and vasculitis with Hashimoto's thyroiditis. Endocrinol Diabetes Metab Case Rep. 2016:160004, 2016
5. Stan MN et al: Riedel's thyroiditis association with IgG4-related disease. Clin Endocrinol (Oxf). 86(3):425-430, 2016
6. Deshpande V: IgG4 related disease of the head and neck. Head Neck Pathol. 9(1):24-31, 2015
7. Takeshima K et al: Distribution of serum immunoglobulin G4 levels in Hashimoto's thyroiditis and clinical features of Hashimoto's thyroiditis with elevated serum immunoglobulin G4 levels. Endocr J. 62(8):711-7, 2015
8. Takeshima K et al: Clinicopathological features of Riedel's thyroiditis associated with IgG4-related disease in Japan. Endocr J. 62(8):725-31, 2015
9. Caturegli P et al: Hashimoto thyroiditis: clinical and diagnostic criteria. Autoimmun Rev. 13(4-5):391-7, 2014

Variants of Hashimoto Thyroiditis

	Fibrous/IgG4 Related	Fibrous Atrophy	Juvenile	Cystic
Clinical	10% of Hashimoto thyroiditis (HT) cases	High titers of antithyroid antibodies	Poorly defined	Extremely rare
Age	Elderly	Elderly	Younger	Variable
Gross	Larger, more fibrotic than usual HT	Fibrotic and atrophic, very small gland	Similar to usual HT	Thyroid gland has bronchial cleft-like cysts and less fibrosis than usual HT
Microscopic	Fibrous bands and storiform fibrosis	Fibrous effacement with minimal preservation of follicles	Similar to usual HT	Cysts are lined by squamous and columnar epithelium

Differential Diagnosis

	Hashimoto	Riedel	Graves	Papillary Carcinoma
Etiology	Autoimmune	Undetermined	Autoimmune	Neoplastic
Age	6th decade	Variable	3rd and 4th decades	Variable
Clinical presentation	Painless goiter	Sudden painless goiter	Goiter with associated eye symptoms	Indolent
Hormonal status	Hypothyroid	Euthyroid or hypothyroid	Hyperthyroid	Euthyroid
Gross findings	Diffusely enlarged with bosselations	Variable size	Diffusely enlarged and symmetric	Localized lesion
	Fibrotic parenchyma with somewhat lymphoid appearance	Severely fibrotic parenchyma	Beefy deep red parenchyma	Can show papillary projections, microcalcifications
Microscopic findings	Hürthle cell changes, squamous metaplasia, lymphoid aggregate, and fibrotic background; difficult to differentiate IgG4-related Hashimoto thyroiditis (HT) from Riedel thyroiditis (RT)	Diffusely sclerotic parenchyma with almost complete obliteration of follicles; difficult to differentiate RT from IgG4-related HT	Preservation of normal follicular architecture, hyperplastic features, and histologic evidence of hyperthyroidism	Nuclear inclusions, "Orphan Annie" nuclei, papillary projections, and characteristic nuclear grooves

10. Ehlers M et al: Hashimoto's thyroiditis and papillary thyroid cancer: are they immunologically linked? Trends Endocrinol Metab. 25(12):656-64, 2014

11. Kawashima ST et al: Serum levels of IgG and IgG4 in Hashimoto thyroiditis. Endocrine. 45(2):236-43, 2013

12. Taşli F et al: The role of IgG4 (+) plasma cells in the association of Hashimoto's thyroiditis with papillary carcinoma. APMIS. 122(12):1259-65, 2014

13. Kishitani T et al: [The biomarker and treatment in Hashimoto's encephalopahty.] Nihon Rinsho. 71(5):893-7, 2013

14. Olmez I et al: Diagnostic and therapeutic aspects of Hashimoto's encephalopathy. J Neurol Sci. 331(1-2):67-71, 2013

15. Pocsay G et al: [Hashimoto encephalopathy.] Orv Hetil. 154(33):1312-6, 2013

16. Weetman AP: The immunopathogenesis of chronic autoimmune thyroiditis one century after hashimoto. Eur Thyroid J. 1(4):243-50, 2013

17. Deshpande V et al: Fibrosing variant of Hashimoto thyroiditis is an IgG4 related disease. J Clin Pathol. 65(8):725-8, 2012

18. Itoh M: [Hashimoto's thyroiditis(chronic thyroiditis), IgG4-related thyroiditis.] Nihon Rinsho. 70(11):1938-44, 2012

19. Kakudo K et al: IgG4-related disease of the thyroid glands. Endocr J. 59(4):273-81, 2012

20. Li Y et al: Distinct histopathological features of Hashimoto's thyroiditis with respect to IgG4-related disease. Mod Pathol. 25(8):1086-97, 2012

21. Kakudo K et al: Diagnosis of Hashimoto's thyroiditis and IgG4-related sclerosing disease. Pathol Int. 61(4):175-83, 2011

22. Li Y et al: Hashimoto's thyroiditis: old concepts and new insights. Curr Opin Rheumatol. 23(1):102-7, 2011

23. Anil C et al: Hashimoto's thyroiditis is not associated with increased risk of thyroid cancer in patients with thyroid nodules: a single-center prospective study. Thyroid. 20(6):601-6, 2010

24. Li Y et al: Distinct clinical, serological, and sonographic characteristics of hashimoto's thyroiditis based with and without IgG4-positive plasma cells. J Clin Endocrinol Metab. 95(3):1309-17, 2010

25. Sadow PM et al: Absence of BRAF, NRAS, KRAS, HRAS mutations, and RET/PTC gene rearrangements distinguishes dominant nodules in Hashimoto thyroiditis from papillary thyroid carcinomas. Endocr Pathol. 21(2):73-9, 2010

26. Li Y et al: Immunohistochemistry of IgG4 can help subclassify Hashimoto's autoimmune thyroiditis. Pathol Int. 59(9):636-41, 2009

27. Shih ML et al: Thyroidectomy for Hashimoto's thyroiditis: complications and associated cancers. Thyroid. 18(7):729-34, 2008

28. Caturegli P et al: Autoimmune thyroid diseases. Curr Opin Rheumatol. 19(1):44-8, 2007

29. Sargent R et al: BRAF mutation is unusual in chronic lymphocytic thyroiditis-associated papillary thyroid carcinomas and absent in non-neoplastic nuclear atypia of thyroiditis. Endocr Pathol. 17(3):235-41, 2006

30. Aozasa K et al: [Differential diagnosis of Hashimoto's thyroiditis from thyroidal neoplastic diseases.] Nippon Rinsho. 57(8):1894-8, 1999

CT Findings

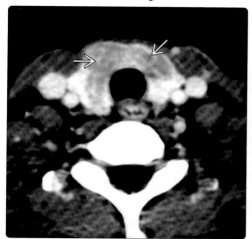

Ultrasound Findings

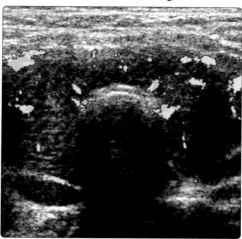

(Left) *Enhanced CT of the thyroid gland in a patient with chronic HT shows fibrous septa* ➡ *within the thyroid gland. The gland is more heterogeneous and smaller than in acute disease. (Courtesy D. Gray, MD.)* (Right) *Color Doppler ultrasound shows diffuse enlargement of the thyroid gland with increased vascularity.*

Characteristic Gross Findings

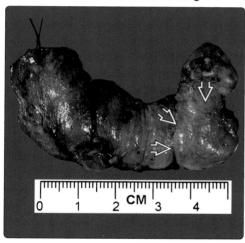

Characteristic Cut Surface

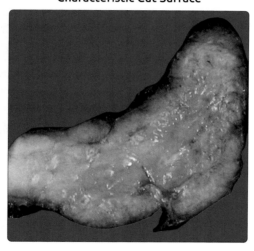

(Left) *Gross photograph shows HT. Note the diffusely enlarged thyroid gland with a bosselated and irregular appearance and a dominant nodule* ➡. *An affected gland is usually 2-3x the size of a normal thyroid gland.* (Right) *The normal brown-red thyroid parenchyma has been replaced by a tan-gray lobulated appearance. The excess lymphoid aggregates and the increased degree of lymphocytic infiltrate in HT is responsible for changes in the gross appearance of the thyroid.*

Pale Tan Cut Surface

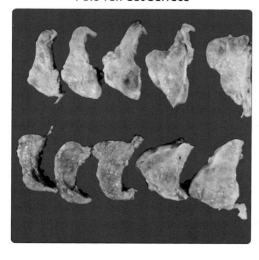

Gross Cut Surface of IgG4 Thyroiditis

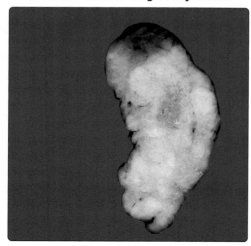

(Left) *Serial section of a thyroid highlights the cut surface appearance of the fibrous variant of HT. The thyroid parenchyma is mostly replaced by fibrous tissue, giving the thyroid a diffuse, tan-white, atrophic appearance.* (Right) *Thyroid gland usually shows diffuse symmetric enlargement without a dominant mass. The cut surface of the thyroid from a patient with IgG4 thyroiditis is usually elastic and soft in consistency and ivory-white in color.*

Microscopic Characteristics

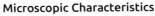

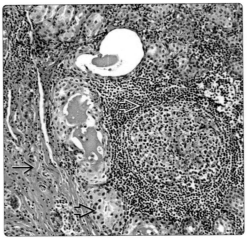

Lymphoid Cells and Follicular Cells

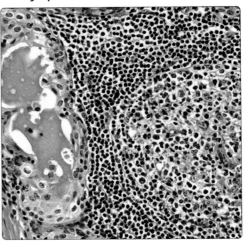

(Left) *H&E highlights focal squamous metaplasia characteristic of HT. Note the juxtaposition of squamous metaplasia* ⇒ *against lymphoid follicles* ⇒, *and a fibrotic background* ⇒, *characteristic of HT.* (Right) *High-power view shows squamous metaplasia of the follicular cells in proximity to reactive lymphoid aggregate with prominent germinal center. There is a mixed inflammatory infiltrate composed predominantly of lymphocytes.*

Squamous Metaplasia

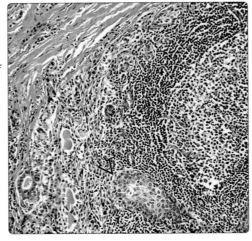

Lymphoid Follicle Formation

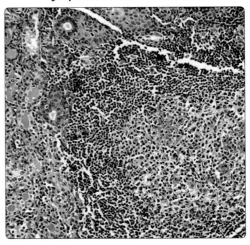

(Left) *H&E illustrates a prominent lymphoid follicle associated with squamous metaplasia* ⇒ *of the follicular cells, in association with thick fibrous bands, characteristic of HT.* (Right) *Prominent lymphoid aggregates with germinal center formation are present within the thyroid parenchyma. The follicles are atrophic, infiltrated by lymphocytes, with oncocytic cell changes and focal squamous metaplasia.*

Dense Lymphoid Infiltrate

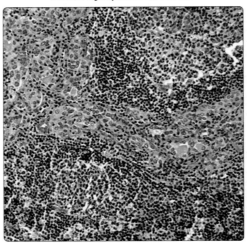

Intraepithelial Lymphocytes

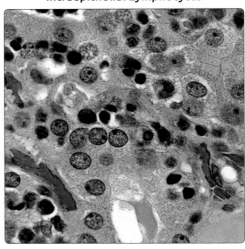

(Left) *Prominent reactive lymphoid aggregates within the thyroid parenchyma are shown. Lymphoid architecture can be so prominent that it may resemble nodal tissue. The differential diagnosis includes lymphoma.* (Right) *High-power H&E of a well-circumscribed dominant nodule in HT highlights numerous intraepithelial lymphocytes and follicles with oncocytic follicular cell cytoplasm with enlarged nuclei.*

Differential Diagnosis of Thyroiditis

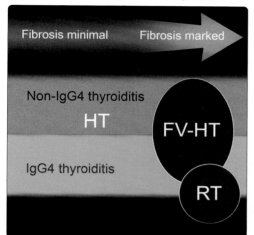

Fibrous Variant of HT

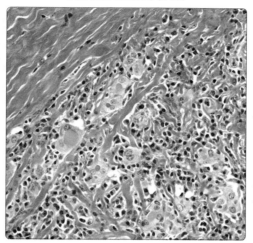

(Left) *There is an overlap in histopathological features between IgG4 thyroiditis, fibrosing variant of Hashimoto thyroiditis (FV-HT), and Riedel thyroiditis (RT). The differential diagnosis is based according to the degree of fibrosis, IgG4 immunostaining, and invasive fibrosis beyond the thyroid surface.* (Right) *Fibrous variant of HT is also now known as part of IgG4 thyroiditis. IgG4 thyroiditis shows a significantly higher grade of lymphoplasmacytic infiltration and stromal keloid-type fibrosis than the non-IgG4 thyroiditis.*

Thick Fibrous Bands

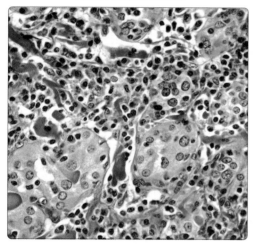

IgG4-Related Thyroiditis

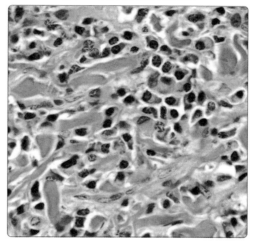

(Left) *There is a predominant plasma cell infiltration in between and within oncocytic cells in HT. The fibrous bands present are thick and in between scattered oncocytic follicular cells.* (Right) *The large, thick, fibrous bands in a storiform arrangement with abundant plasma cell infiltration are seen in the fibrosing variant of HT, IgG4-related disease.*

Thick Fibrosis in IgG4-Related HT

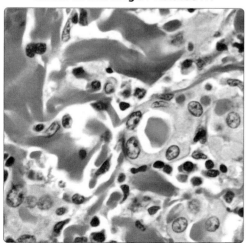

Numerous IgG4(+) Plasma Cells

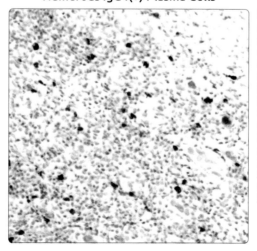

(Left) *Photomicroscopic illustration highlights the marked plasma cell infiltration and thick, fibrous bands in between the oncocytic cells in HT. These features are seen in IgG4-related thyroiditis.* (Right) *Fibrous variant of HT, IgG4-related demonstrates extensive destruction of the thyroid follicles and marked atrophy of the follicular cells. The lymphoplasmacytic inflammatory infiltrate is extensive and with numerous IgG4(+) cells.*

Graves Disease (Diffuse Hyperplasia)

TERMINOLOGY

- Autoimmune disease characterized by diffuse goiter, thyrotoxicosis, infiltrative ophthalmopathy, and occasionally infiltrative dermopathology

CLINICAL ISSUES

- Most common cause of hyperthyroidism in USA
- Most common cause of spontaneous hyperthyroidism in patients < 40 years
- F:M = 8:1
- Diffuse goiter with thyrotoxicosis, eye disease, and possible skin manifestations
- TSH receptor antibody is most specific for Graves disease; however, these may be seen in other thyroiditides such as Hashimoto
- Strongly associated with haplotypes HLA-B8 and HLA-DR3
- Prognosis good with treatment; however, left untreated, patients may develop thyroid storm, which can be deadly

MACROSCOPIC

- Diffuse symmetric enlargement
- Beefy, deep red parenchyma
- Prominent vascular pattern

MICROSCOPIC

- Preserved follicular architecture with prominent stromal vessels and hyperplasia of tall columnar cells in follicle
- Iodine treatment may diminish vascularity of gland, causing involution of follicle, causing follicular cells to be cuboidal rather than columnar

TOP DIFFERENTIAL DIAGNOSES

- Dyshormonogenetic goiter
- Toxic multinodular goiter
- Papillary thyroid carcinoma
- Hashimoto thyroiditis
- Adenomatous nodule

Eye Ophthalmopathy in Graves Disease

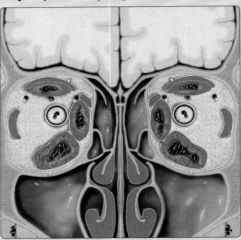

Exophthalmus in Graves Disease

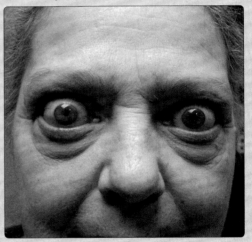

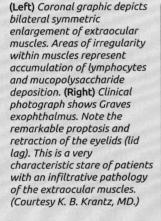

(Left) Coronal graphic depicts bilateral symmetric enlargement of extraocular muscles. Areas of irregularity within muscles represent accumulation of lymphocytes and mucopolysaccharide deposition. (Right) Clinical photograph shows Graves exophthalmus. Note the remarkable proptosis and retraction of the eyelids (lid lag). This is a very characteristic stare of patients with an infiltrative pathology of the extraocular muscles. (Courtesy K. B. Krantz, MD.)

Thyroid Scan

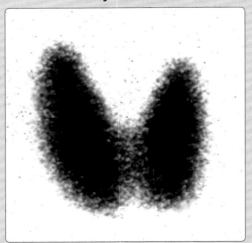

Classical Papillary Hyperplasia

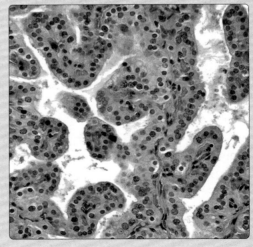

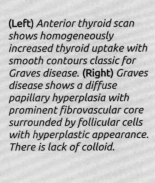

(Left) Anterior thyroid scan shows homogeneously increased thyroid uptake with smooth contours classic for Graves disease. (Right) Graves disease shows a diffuse papillary hyperplasia with prominent fibrovascular core surrounded by follicular cells with hyperplastic appearance. There is lack of colloid.

TERMINOLOGY

Abbreviations
- Graves disease (GD)

Synonyms
- Diffuse hyperplasia
- Diffuse toxic goiter

Definitions
- Autoimmune disease characterized by diffuse goiter, thyrotoxicosis, infiltrative ophthalmopathy, and occasionally infiltrative dermopathology
  - Named after Irish clinician Robert Graves, who described syndrome of cardiac palpitations, thyroid enlargement, and exophthalmos

ETIOLOGY/PATHOGENESIS

Environmental Exposure
- Iodine replacement in previously deficient patients can cause reactive hyperthyroid state and unmask underlying autoimmune process
- Smoking increases risk of Graves 2-3x and is significantly associated with ophthalmopathy

General
- Stronger familial predisposition than Hashimoto (monozygotic twin concordance rate may be as high as 60%)
- Strongly associated with haplotypes HLA-B8 and HLA-DR3
- Hyperthyroidism caused by antibodies
  - Antibodies directed toward extracellular domain of thyroid stimulating hormone receptor (TSHR) on follicular cells
    - Serum of patient with Graves disease has been found to stimulate thyroid activity in animals in controlled experiment
    - These antibodies activate receptor and stimulate hormone synthesis and secretion as well as proliferation of follicular cells
- Possible triggers include infectious etiology as well as physiological and psychological stress
  - Triggered disturbance of immune system confers imbalance that begets autoimmunity
- Role of gonadal steroids has been suggested because of higher incidence in women, particularly in times of hormonal change such as puberty, pregnancy, and menopause
  - 6x increased risk of Graves disease in postpartum women
- In men, Graves disease occurs later in life with more severe symptoms and greater incidence of ophthalmopathy
- Autoimmunity triggered by genetic susceptibility and environmental factors

Ophthalmopathy
- Has not been fully elucidated
- Thought to be related to expression of HLA class II antigens by orbital muscles, to which activated T cells react
- TSH receptor mRNA has been detected in retroorbital fibroblasts

Dermopathy
- Has not been fully elucidated
- Thought to be mechanism involving fibroblasts in skin, similar to that of Graves ophthalmopathy

CLINICAL ISSUES

Epidemiology
- Incidence
  - Most common cause of hyperthyroidism in USA
  - Most common cause of spontaneous hyperthyroidism in patients > 40 years
  - One of most common autoimmune diseases
    - Annual incidence: 20-25 per 100,000
- Age
  - Usually presents in 3rd or 4th decade
- Sex
  - F:M = 8:1

Presentation
- Diffuse goiter with thyrotoxicosis, eye disease, and possible skin manifestations
- Most common symptoms include anxiety, hyperhidrosis, heat intolerance, palpitations, fatigue, tachycardia, muscle wasting, and weight loss
- Patients have goiter, tachycardia, tremors, and warm, moist skin
- Exophthalmos may be present
- Usually presents at later age in men and with more severe symptoms
- Often presents in women undergoing states of hormonal changes such as pregnancy or menopause
- Increased radioiodine uptake on imaging

Laboratory Tests
- Serum antibodies against thyroid peroxidase or microsomal antibodies, thyroglobulin, and TSH receptor
- TSH receptor antibody is most specific for Graves disease; however, these may be seen in other thyroiditides such as Hashimoto
- Strongly associated with haplotypes HLA-B8 and HLA-DR3
- Patients have diminished levels of circulating CD8 T cells

Treatment
- Surgical approaches
  - Thyroidectomy
- Drugs
  - Methimazole, propylthiouracil, carbimazole
    - Inhibit thyroid hormone synthesis through interference with peroxidase-mediated iodination of tyrosine residues
  - Nonradioactive iodine inhibits release of thyroid hormones and peripheral conversion of T4 to T3
    - Additionally, iodine promotes colloid storage, reduces vascularity, and promotes involution of follicles
    - Diminished activity attenuates hyperthyroid symptoms
  - Radiation
    - Radioactive iodine ablation may be used in patients with refractory symptoms or in those whose thyroid function is difficult to manage

– After radioactive ablation, patients need to be supplemented with T4 and followed clinically
  o β-blockers relieve symptoms but do not affect physiology of thyroid gland

Prognosis

- Untreated patients may develop thyroid storm, which can be deadly
  o However, if patients followed, prognosis usually excellent

MACROSCOPIC

General Features

- Diffuse symmetric enlargement with vague nodularity

Size

- 50-150 g

Gross Features

- Prominent vascular pattern
  o Follicular cells may promote vascularity by secreting vascular endothelial growth factor in response to stimulation by TSHR
- Beefy, deep red parenchyma
  o Resembles skeletal muscle
  o Parenchyma has spongy to firm consistency
- Treated Graves disease has less vascularity and lighter pink color than untreated Graves

MICROSCOPIC

Histologic Features

- Preserved follicular architecture with prominent stromal vessels and hyperplasia of tall columnar cells in follicle
  o Tall columnar cells with eosinophilic to amphophilic cytoplasm
  o Nuclei are basally located, round to regular, and with coarse to granular cytoplasm
  o Unlike Hashimoto disease, fibrosis limited and usually absent
    – Fibrosis may be present in treated cases
- Signs of hyperthyroidism in follicle, such as small follicular size and scalloping of colloid
- Papillae with fibrovascular core may be present, mimicking papillary thyroid carcinoma
- Mixed inflammatory infiltrate with lymphocytic infiltrate within stroma surrounding follicles
- Iodine treatment may diminish vascularity of gland, causing involution of follicle, causing follicular cells to be cuboidal rather than columnar
- Radioactive iodine can lead to nuclear pleomorphism, follicular destruction, fibrosis, and oncocytic metaplasia
- Treatment with propylthiouracil can cause hyperplastic changes
- Dendritic cells are increased in number

Ophthalmic Muscles

- Edema, loss of striation, fragmentation of fibers, diffuse lymphocytic infiltration
  o Accumulation of excessive hydrophilic glycosaminoglycans

o Advanced stages will demonstrate atrophy with associated fibrosis

Skin

- Mucopolysaccharides within dermis and thickening of skin (5-10% of Graves patients)

Treatment Effects

- Hyperplastic effects diminished and regressed but still present
- Colloid increased
- Radiative therapy causes follicular atrophy, fibrosis, Hürthle cell changes, nuclear atypia, hyperplastic nodules, and persistence of lymphocytic infiltrate

ANCILLARY TESTS

Cytology

- Low to moderately cellular specimen
- Sheets of follicular cells with peripherally located nuclei and marginal vacuoles adjacent to nuclei
  o Vacuoles clear on Papanicolaou stain, pink on Diff-Quik
  o These cells with marginal vacuolization are called "flame cells"
  o Nuclei contain small nucleoli
- Hürthle cell changes may be present in up to 1/2 of cytologic specimens of patients with Graves disease
- Posttreatment specimens can demonstrate atypia
- Lymphocytes may be present in specimen

Immunohistochemistry

- HLA-DR positive in thyroid cells as well as lymphoid cells
- Hematolymphoid markers demonstrate mixed inflammatory infiltrate
- TTF-1 and thyroglobulin positive

Genetic Testing

- Skewed X chromosome inactivation (XCI)
  o Related to prognosis of GD

Electron Microscopy

- Increased activity of follicular cells and in some cases immune complex deposition within basement membrane

DIFFERENTIAL DIAGNOSIS

Dyshormonogenetic Goiter

- Family history often identified; inherited disorder
- Patients younger than those with Graves disease
- Thyroid diffusely affected with multiple nodules
- Absent, watery colloid
- Marked nuclear atypia

Toxic Multinodular Goiter

- Gross findings demonstrate marked nodularity
- Majority of gland with follicles having abundant colloid
- Patients will be hyperthyroid
  o Characteristic antibody panel of Graves will be absent

Papillary Thyroid Carcinoma

- Graves disease may have papillary structures with fibrovascular cores and psammoma bodies

- Inflammatory response of Graves disease may cause adherence to adjacent skeletal muscle mimicking invasive PTC
- These features can make distinction between Graves disease and papillary carcinoma difficult
- Look closely for nuclear features of papillary thyroid carcinoma in these instances, and always consider clinical history
- Papillary thyroid carcinoma can be found in 1-4% of cases
  o Thyroid nodular lesions in GD patients are highly suspicious for carcinoma
    − Frequently clinically significant tumors
- Incidental thyroid carcinoma in GD patients not uncommon
  o Most of them are microcarcinoma

Hashimoto Thyroiditis

- Distinction from early Hashimoto may be difficult clinically as Hashimoto may present initially with hypothyroid symptoms
- However, Hashimoto will inevitably convert to hypothyroid symptoms
- Autoantibody panel may be similar, but TSH more specific for Graves
- Hashimoto will have more prominent oncocytic metaplasia
- More lymphocytic infiltrate and germinal centers
- Fibrous bands coursing through parenchyma favors diagnosis of Hashimoto over Graves

Adenomatous Nodule

- Clinically resembles multinodular goiter
- Patients are euthyroid
- Nodules of multiple sizes with background of normal-appearing thyroid
- Colloid deposition normal
- Cytologically benign

DIAGNOSTIC CHECKLIST

Pathologic Interpretation Pearls

- Signs of hyperthyroidism in follicle, such as small follicular size and scalloping of colloid during active Graves disease
  o Degree of histologic signs of hyperthyroidism will change with treatment
- Patients with Graves disease generally undergo treatment before thyroidectomy
  o Surgical specimen will almost always have some treatment effect
- Treatment can dramatically change histology of gland; therefore, clinical history essential to signing out cases of suspected Graves disease
  o Histological changes are dependent upon selected treatment modality
    − Radiation, iodine, propylthiouracil
- Be aware of other conditions associated with enlarged thyroid, altered hormone status, and antibodies associated with that condition
  o Hashimoto will be hypothyroid
  o Toxic multinodular goiter will be hyperthyroid
  o Adenomatoid nodules will be euthyroid
- Clinical history is essential in diagnosis
  o Family history, antibodies, hormone status

SELECTED REFERENCES

1. El Hussein S et al: Histologic findings and cytological alterations in thyroid nodules after radioactive iodine treatment for Graves' disease. Int J Surg Pathol. 1066896917693091, 2017
2. Romero-Kusabara IL et al: Distinct inflammatory gene expression in extraocular muscle and fat from patients with Graves' orbitopathy. Eur J Endocrinol. ePub, 2017
3. Smith TJ et al: Graves' disease. N Engl J Med. 376(2):185, 2017
4. Sundaresh V et al: Comparative effectiveness of treatment choices for Graves' hyperthyroidism: A historical cohort study. Thyroid. ePub, 2017
5. Viard J-P et al: Graves' disease. N Engl J Med. 376(2):184-5, 2017
6. Hazen EP et al: Case records of the Massachusetts General Hospital. Case 10-2015. A 15-year-old girl with Graves' disease and psychotic symptoms. N Engl J Med. 372(13):1250-8, 2015
7. Perros P et al: Management of patients with Graves' orbitopathy: initial assessment, management outside specialised centres and referral pathways. Clin Med. 15(2):173-8, 2015
8. Rapoport B et al: Evidence that TSH receptor A-subunit multimers, not monomers, drive antibody affinity maturation in Graves' disease. J Clin Endocrinol Metab. jc20151528, 2015
9. Boutzios G et al: Higher incidence of tall cell variant of papillary thyroid carcinoma in Graves' Disease. Thyroid. 24(2):347-54, 2014
10. Ishido N et al: The relationship between skewed X chromosome inactivation and the prognosis of Graves' and Hashimoto's diseases. Thyroid. ePub, 2014
11. Li Y et al: Increased expression of IL-37 in patients with Graves' disease and its contribution to suppression of proinflammatory cytokines production in peripheral blood mononuclear cells. PLoS One. 9(9):e107183, 2014
12. McCoy AN et al: Rituximab (Rituxan) therapy for severe thyroid-associated ophthalmopathy diminishes IGF-1R(+) T cells. J Clin Endocrinol Metab. 99(7):E1294-9, 2014
13. Nagasaki S et al: Induction of adrenomedullin 2/intermedin expression by thyroid stimulating hormone in thyroid. Mol Cell Endocrinol. 395(1-2):32-40, 2014
14. Wei S et al: Thyroid carcinoma in patients with Graves' disease: an institutional experience. Endocr Pathol. ePub, 2014
15. Ross DS: Radioiodine therapy for hyperthyroidism. N Engl J Med. 364(6):542-50, 2011
16. Domoslawski P et al: Expression of estrogen and progesterone receptors and Ki-67 antigen in Graves' disease and nodular goiter. Folia Histochem Cytobiol. 51(2):135-40, 2013
17. Tortora F et al: Disease activity in Graves' ophthalmopathy: diagnosis with orbital MR imaging and correlation with clinical score. Neuroradiol J. 26(5):555-64, 2013
18. Feldt-Rasmussen U et al: Autoimmunity in differentiated thyroid cancer: significance and related clinical problems. Hormones (Athens). 9(2):109-17, 2010
19. García-Mayor RV et al: Treatment of Graves' hyperthyroidism with thionamides-derived drugs: review. Med Chem. 6(4):239-46, 2010
20. Lytton SD et al: Bioassays for TSH-receptor autoantibodies: an update. Autoimmun Rev. 10(2):116-22, 2010
21. Pezzolla A et al: [Incidental carcinoma in thyroid pathology: our experience and review of the literature.] Ann Ital Chir. 81(3):165-9, 2010
22. Smith TJ: Pathogenesis of Graves' orbitopathy: a 2010 update. J Endocrinol Invest. 33(6):414-21, 2010
23. Tomer Y: Genetic susceptibility to autoimmune thyroid disease: past, present, and future. Thyroid. 20(7):715-25, 2010
24. van Steensel L et al: The orbital fibroblast: a key player and target for therapy in graves' ophthalmopathy. Orbit. 29(4):202-6, 2010
25. Matos K et al: Protein expression of VEGF, IGF-1 and FGF in retroocular connective tissues and clinical correlation in Graves' ophthalmopathy. Arq Bras Oftalmol. 71(4):486-92, 2008
26. Jayaram G et al: Grave's disease. Appearance in cytologic smears from fine needle aspirates of the thyroid gland. Acta Cytol. 33(1):36-40, 1989

Differential Diagnosis

	Graves	Hashimoto	Riedel	Papillary Carcinoma
Etiology	Autoimmune	Autoimmune	Undetermined	Neoplastic
Age	3rd and 4th decade	6th decade	Variable	Variable
Clinical presentation	Goiter with associated eye symptoms	Painless goiter	Sudden painless goiter	Indolent
Hormonal status	Hyperthyroid	Hypothyroid	Euthyroid or hypothyroid	Euthyroid
Gross findings	Diffusely enlarged and symmetric	Diffusely enlarged with bosselations	Variable size	Localized lesion
Characteristic gross findings	Beefy, deep red parenchyma	Fibrotic parenchyma with somewhat lymphoid appearance	Severely fibrotic parenchyma	Can show papillary projections and microcalcifications
Microscopic findings	Preservation of normal follicular architecture, hyperplastic features, histologic evidence of hyperthyroidism	Hürthle cell changes, squamous metaplasia, lymphoid aggregate, and fibrotic background	Diffusely sclerotic parenchyma with almost complete obliteration of follicles	Nuclear inclusions, "Orphan Annie" nuclei, papillary architectures, characteristic nuclear grooves

Treatment Effect and Histological Changes

	Iodine	Radioactive Iodine	Propylthiouracil
Histologic picture	Decreased vascularity and involution of gland	Variable depending on duration but can demonstrate a wide variety of changes leading to difficulty in diagnosis	Leads to decrease in thyroid hormone synthesis
Characteristic findings	Hyperplastic appearance with papillary architecture	Follicular cell destruction, fibrosis, and oncocytic metaplasia can occur	Decrease in colloid may give false impression of hyperplasia
Diagnostic difficulty	Can give impression of hyperplastic nodule of follicular neoplasm	Can mimic Hashimoto, papillary thyroid carcinoma, follicular neoplasm with Hürthle cell changes	Can give impression of hyperplastic nodule or follicular neoplasm

Thyroid Vascularity

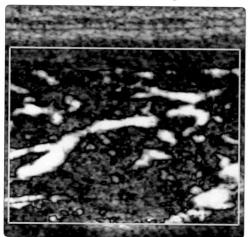

Increased Vascularity

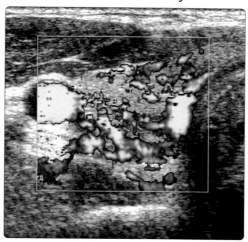

(Left) *Power Doppler US shows marked intrathyroid vascularity in Graves disease. In patients who respond to treatment, such vascularity diminishes. It will increase again in recurrent disease.* (Right) *Power Doppler US shows marked intrathyroid vascularity. Increase in vascularity does not correlate with thyroid function, but it is a reflection of inflammatory activity.*

Ultrasound in Graves Disease

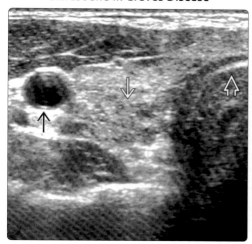

Graves Disease

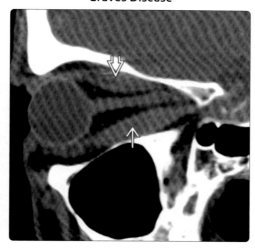

(Left) *Transverse grayscale US of the thyroid in Graves disease shows a hypoechoic, heterogeneous spotty echo pattern ➡. In this patient, the thyroid maintains its normal contour. The trachea ➡ and carotid artery ➡ are shown.* (Right) *Sagittal NECT in a patient with Graves disease and thyroid-associated orbitopathy shows the enlarged muscle bellies of the superior ➡ and inferior ➡ recti. Note the tendinous attachments are spared.*

Papillary Hyperplasia

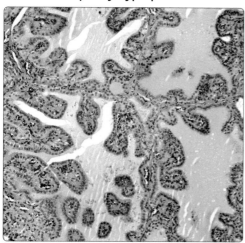

Scalloping of Colloid

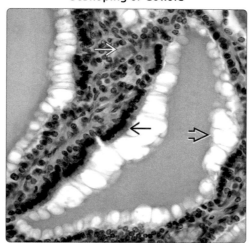

(Left) *Microphotograph of Graves disease shows a papillary follicular architecture and pale colloid. Scalloping of the colloid is less dramatic and sometimes absent in the treated phase.* (Right) *Note the scalloping of the colloid ➡ as well as the columnar shape of the follicular cells ➡. There are fibrovascular structures within the parenchyma ➡.*

(Left) *Section of thyroid with dilated irregular follicles and little colloid, with marked scalloping of colloid, shows extensive papillary hyperplasia. Untreated Graves disease with prominent papillary hyperplasia can be mistaken for papillary thyroid carcinoma.* **(Right)** *Graves disease shows a preserved follicular architecture with dilated follicles and papillary hyperplasia filled with dense colloid. There is extensive scalloping of colloid.*

Marked Hyperplasia

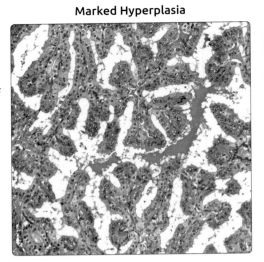

Low-Power Appearance

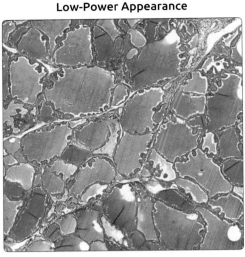

(Left) *High-power microphotograph shows papillary architecture characteristic of Graves disease. Note the more flattened, cuboidal appearance of the follicular cells and pale scalloped colloid.* **(Right)** *Note the scalloping of the colloid ⊟ as well as the columnar shape of the follicular cells. There is a thin, fibrovascular structure within the parenchyma ➡.*

Papillary Hyperplasia

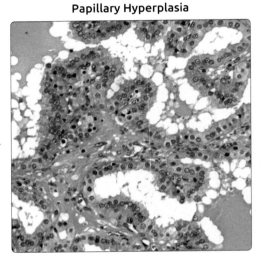

Hyperplastic Changes

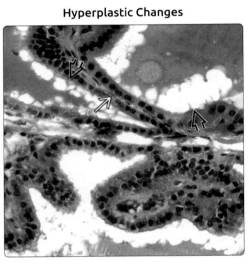

(Left) *Low-power view shows a thyroid with the characteristic architecture seen in untreated Graves disease. Note the irregular follicles (so-called "geographic map") with pale to dark, scalloped colloid.* **(Right)** *This area shows residual papillary hyperplasia, often seen in early treatment with propylthiouracil. The follicular cells are flattened, and the absence of scalloping of the colloid indicates that the patient is no longer hyperthyroid.*

Untreated Graves Disease

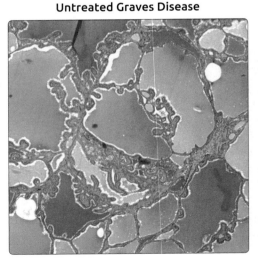

Treatment Effect

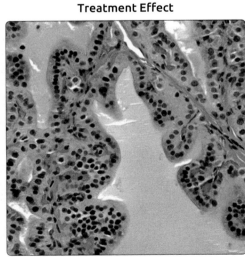

Treatment Effect

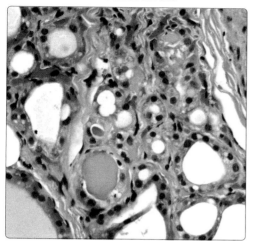

Mild Cellular Pleomorphism

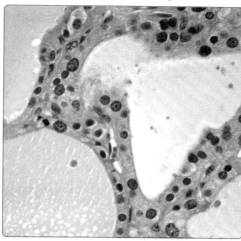

(Left) *The findings in treated Graves disease are those of irregular thyroid follicles with follicular atrophy, surrounded by fibrosis and sclerosis. The follicular cell nuclei show pleomorphism. There is focal lymphocytic infiltrate.* (Right) *High-power view shows a partially treated Graves disease with oncocytic cell change and scattered pleomorphic nuclei. The follicular structure is preserved, and there is no papillary hyperplasia.*

Treated Graves Disease

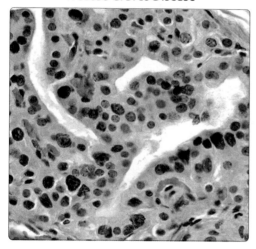

Pleomorphic Nuclei

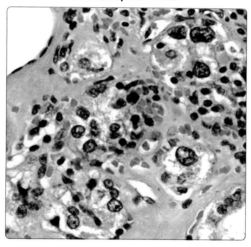

(Left) *Treated Graves disease shows oncocytic cell metaplasia, follicular atrophy, and pleomorphic nuclei, some with nucleoli. There is focal cribriform arrangement.* (Right) *The findings in treated Graves disease are those of irregular thyroid follicles with follicular atrophy, surrounded by fibrosis and sclerosis with pleomorphism of the follicular cell nuclei. There is focal interstitial fibrosis.*

Graves Post Treatment With Radioactive Iodine

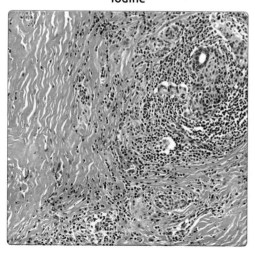

Nuclear Pleomorphism

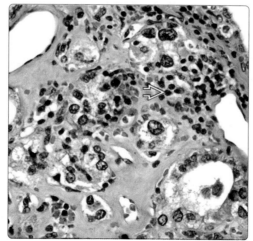

(Left) *Graves disease treated by radioactive iodine therapy creates a diagnostic dilemma, as the distinction between radiation effect, thyroiditis, and a malignant primary thyroid neoplasm can be very challenging.* (Right) *The findings in Graves disease, treated preoperatively, are those of irregular thyroid follicles with follicular atrophy, surrounded by fibrosis and sclerosis. The follicular cells have oxyphilic cytoplasm and the nuclei shows pleomorphism. There is focal lymphocytic infiltrate* ⇒.

Multinodular Thyroid Hyperplasia

TERMINOLOGY

- Benign, nonneoplastic enlargement of thyroid gland

ETIOLOGY/PATHOGENESIS

- Any disruption of normal hypothalamic pituitary axis that results in increase of thyroid stimulating hormone (TSH)
  - Increase in TSH causes increased activity of follicular cells and resulting glandular enlargement
- Lack of iodine may cause increased oxidative damage to follicular cells
  - This in turn damages DNA and may predispose thyroid cells to hyperplasia
- Childhood &/or familial MNGs suggest DICER1 syndrome

CLINICAL ISSUES

- Extremely common finding in surgical pathology
- Symmetric or asymmetric enlargement of thyroid gland on palpation

CYTOPATHOLOGY

- Abundant colloid
- Low cellularity
- Benign nuclear features
  - However, nuclear atypia may be present in some cases

MACROSCOPIC

- Gross enlargement of thyroid gland with distorted outer surface
- 2° degenerative changes, i.e., cystic degeneration, fibrosis, hemorrhage, and calcifications frequently present
- Encapsulated nodules may be present
- Moderate to severe enlargement (sometimes 1,000 g)

MICROSCOPIC

- Multiple variably sized nodules identifiable
- Varying degrees of cellularity and colloid
- Sanderson polsters
- Degenerative changes

CT of Multinodular Hyperplasia

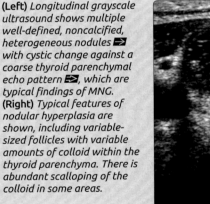

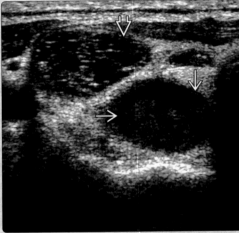

Histological Findings of Multinodular Hyperplasia

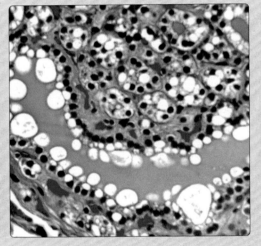

(Left) *Longitudinal grayscale ultrasound shows multiple well-defined, noncalcified, heterogeneous nodules ➡ with cystic change against a coarse thyroid parenchymal echo pattern ➡, which are typical findings of MNG.* (Right) *Typical features of nodular hyperplasia are shown, including variable-sized follicles with variable amounts of colloid within the thyroid parenchyma. There is abundant scalloping of the colloid in some areas.*

CT of Multinodular Hyperplasia

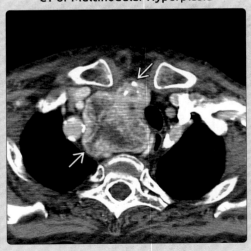

Graphic of Multinodular Hyperplasia

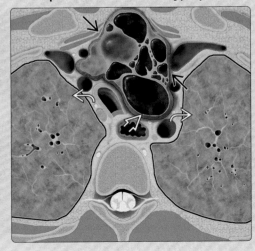

(Left) *Axial CECT reveals substernal extension of MNG ➡ into the superior mediastinum, with compression and displacement of surrounding structures. MNG is the most common cause of a superior mediastinal mass.* (Right) *Graphic depiction of a mediastinal mass shows substernal extension of an MNG. There are characteristic features of MNG, including multiple, well-defined nodules ➡ with cystic changes ➡. This mass is compressing the mediastinal structures and lungs ➡.*

TERMINOLOGY

Abbreviations
- Multinodular hyperplasia (MNH)

Synonyms
- Multinodular goiter (MNG)

Definitions
- Benign, nonneoplastic enlargement of thyroid gland
- Varying degrees of nodularity
- Not associated with hyper-/hypothyroidism

ETIOLOGY/PATHOGENESIS

Environmental Exposure
- Dietary goitrogenic substances and foods
  - Cyanoglucosides
  - Perchlorates
  - Thiocarbamides
  - Aniline derivatives
  - Thiocyanates
  - Cassava
  - Specific plants
- Radiation
  - Can also lead to papillary thyroid carcinoma

Hypothalamic Pituitary Axis Disturbances
- Any disruption of normal hypothalamic pituitary axis that results in increase of thyroid-stimulating hormone (TSH)
  - Increase in TSH causes increased activity of follicular cells and resulting glandular enlargement

Drugs
- Lithium
- Amiodarone
- Aminoglutethimide
- Propylthiouracil, methimazole, perchlorate, thiocyanate
- Sulfonamides, phenylbutazone, and phenindione

Iodine Deficiency
- Historical cause of goiter, as iodine deficiency leads to lack of T3 and T4 and subsequent increase in TSH

Mutagenesis
- Has been suggested that lack of iodine may cause increased oxidative damage to follicular cells
  - This in turn damages DNA and may predispose thyroid cells to hyperplasia
- Genetic and epigenetic events associated with origin and malignant potential of FTH are poorly understood

PTEN-Hamartoma Tumor Syndrome/Cowden Disease
- Autosomal dominant disorder characterized by germline mutation in *PTEN* gene
  - Multiple carcinomas and hamartomas of uterus, breast, and thyroid
- Patients frequently present with multinodular thyroid

DICER1 Syndrome
- Childhood &/or familial MNGs suggest DICER1 syndrome

CLINICAL ISSUES

Epidemiology
- Incidence
  - Extremely common finding in surgical pathology
    - Palpable nodules found in 3-7% of adult population
    - More frequent in women
  - Thyroid cancer in multinodular goiter ~ 5-10%

Presentation
- Physical exam
  - Symmetric or asymmetric enlargement of thyroid gland on palpation
  - Patient may have fullness or discomfort
    - Most noticeable upon swallowing

Treatment
- Surgical approaches
  - Surgery provides permanent cure of excessive nodular hyperplasia
- Drugs
  - Thyroxine
  - Radioactive iodine

Prognosis
- Excellent with appropriate medical intervention

IMAGING

Ultrasonographic Findings
- Most sensitive and cost-effective means of detecting thyroid nodules
  - May reveal nodules too small to be detected clinically
  - Large nodules may protrude into anterior mediastinum
    - May also compress adjacent structures such as trachea, esophagus, or large vessels

MACROSCOPIC

General Features
- Gross enlargement of thyroid gland with distorted outer surface
- Secondary degenerative changes such as cystic degeneration, fibrosis, hemorrhage, and calcifications frequently present
- Encapsulated nodules may be present

Size
- Moderate to severe enlargement (sometimes 1,000 g)

Sections to Be Submitted
- Many sections of nodular areas in relation to normal tissue
  - Areas of degeneration should be sampled
  - Any areas suspicious for neoplastic processes
  - Nonnodular areas should be sampled well, as goitrogenic conditions may have characteristic features in nonnodular areas
    - Dyshormonogenetic goiter

MICROSCOPIC

Histologic Features
- Multiple variably sized nodules identifiable

- o Varying degrees of cellularity and colloid
  - – Enlarged follicles with flattened epithelium
  - – Smaller follicles with taller epithelium
- Sanderson polsters
  - o Papillary-type projections into lumina of follicles
    - – May mimic papillary thyroid carcinoma; however, nuclear features of Sanderson polsters are benign
- Cellular atypia may be present
  - o Oncocytic changes
  - o Nuclear clearing
  - o Signet ring changes
- Variable degree of fibrosis, cystic changes, evidence of hemorrhage, and calcification

ANCILLARY TESTS

Cytology

- Abundant colloid
- Low cellularity
- Degenerative features may be present
- Benign nuclear features

Immunohistochemistry

- Loss of staining for PTEN in thyroid glands with nodular hyperplasia
  - o Suggested as means of detecting patients with Cowden syndrome
- Otherwise, normal immunoprofile of thyroid gland remains intact

Genetic Testing

- May demonstrate genetic abnormalities associated with syndromes that lead to clinical presentations of goiter
  - o Dyshormonogenetic goiter
    - – Genetic disorder that may have mutations in any of number of proteins associated with thyroid hormonogenesis
- PTEN mutation in suspected cases of PTEN-hamartoma tumor syndrome
- Childhood &/or familial MNGs suggest DICER1 syndrome
  - o Particularly when other highly characteristic diseases like CN or lung cysts co-occur
  - o Genetic counseling is strongly recommended before DICER1 mutation analysis
  - o In patients with DICER1 mutations, tumor surveillance critical
    - – Increased risk of multiple tumors, including ovarian tumors and pleuropulmonary blastoma
- Epigenetic analysis shows significant promoter hypermethylation of tumor-suppressor gene *RASSF1A*
  - o Silencing of tumor suppressor *RASSF1A* in subset of MNH

DIFFERENTIAL DIAGNOSIS

Follicular Adenoma

- Generally solitary encapsulated neoplasm
  - o Nodular hyperplasia demonstrates diffuse nodularity of entire gland with less fibrosis and tendency for encapsulated lesions

Papillary Thyroid Carcinoma

- Demonstrates more striking nuclear atypia than that occasionally seen in nodular hyperplasia

- o PTC has characteristic nuclear features (clearing, grooves, pseudoinclusions)
- Sanderson polsters may mimic papillary architecture of carcinoma

Dyshormonogenetic Goiter

- Has nodules with interspersed fibrous banding through parenchyma
  - o Patients have family history of goiter and hypothyroidism
  - o Usual age of presentation is mid teens

Follicular Carcinoma

- Encapsulated follicular neoplasm with capsular &/or vascular invasion

DIAGNOSTIC CHECKLIST

Clinically Relevant Pathologic Features

- Gross appearance
  - o Asymmetric nodular enlargement of thyroid gland
  - o Distorted outer contours
  - o Gland may be extremely enlarged
- Cytoplasmic features
  - o Hürthle cell changes are absent
- Nuclear features
  - o Bland nuclei
  - o Dense chromatin
- Age distribution
  - o Highly variable
- Histologic patterns
  - o Dilated follicles
  - o Multiple nodules of varying sizes
  - o Sanderson polsters
  - o Variable scalloping of colloid within follicles

SELECTED REFERENCES

1. de Kock L et al: Deep sequencing reveals spatially distributed distinct hot spot mutations in DICER1-related multinodular goiter. J Clin Endocrinol Metab. 101(10):3637-3645, 2016
2. Brown TC et al: Frequent silencing of RASSF1A via promoter methylation in follicular thyroid hyperplasia: a potential early epigenetic susceptibility event in thyroid carcinogenesis. JAMA Surg. ePub, 2014
3. Rath SR et al: Multinodular goiter in children: an important pointer to a germline DICER1 mutation. J Clin Endocrinol Metab. 99(6):1947-8, 2014
4. Syrenicz A et al: New insights into the diagnosis of nodular goiter. Thyroid Res. 7:6, 2014
5. Laury AR et al: Thyroid pathology in PTEN-hamartoma tumor syndrome: characteristic findings of a distinct entity. Thyroid. 21(2):135-44, 2011
6. Smith JR et al: Thyroid nodules and cancer in children with PTEN hamartoma tumor syndrome. J Clin Endocrinol Metab. 96(1):34-7, 2011
7. Peteiro-Gonzalez D et al: New insights into thyroglobulin pathophysiology revealed by the study of a family with congenital goiter. J Clin Endocrinol Metab. 95(7):3522-6, 2010
8. Couch RM et al: An autosomal dominant form of adolescent multinodular goiter. Am J Hum Genet. 39(6):811-6, 1986
9. Ramelli F et al: Pathogenesis of thyroid nodules in multinodular goiter. Am J Pathol. 109(2):215-23, 1982

CT of Multinodular Hyperplasia

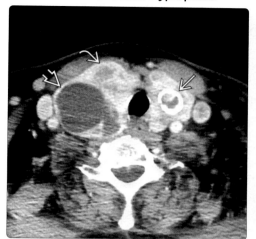

Gross Photograph of Multinodular Hyperplasia

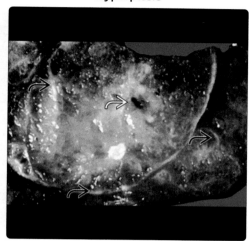

(Left) *Axial CECT reveals the many varied imaging manifestations of MNG. Note the diffusely enlarged thyroid gland with calcified ➡, cystic ➡, and solid ➡ nodular regions.* (Right) *Cut surface of a thyroid with multinodular hyperplasia shows a heterogeneous surface with areas of fibrosis ➡, areas mimicking a pseudocapsule, and areas of degenerative changes ➡.*

Histological Findings

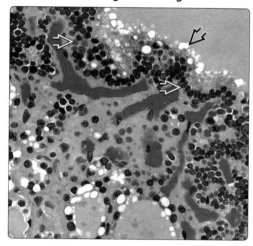

Histological Findings

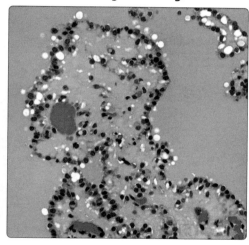

(Left) *High-power photomicrograph of a Sanderson polster ➡ shows nuclei that are round and regular with dense chromatin. The adjacent colloid has minimal scalloping ➡.* (Right) *High-power photomicrograph of a Sanderson polster shows round and regular nuclei with dense chromatin. Papillary protrusions into the lumina of dilated follicles may mimic papillary carcinoma; however, the atypical papillary thyroid carcinoma nuclear features are absent.*

Histological Findings

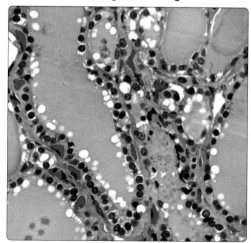

Histological Findings

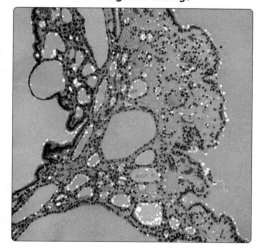

(Left) *High-power photomicrograph shows densely packed follicles with varying amounts of colloid, some with excessive scalloping. This type of histologic pattern may mimic a follicular neoplasm.* (Right) *There is marked variability of follicle size and shape. The colloid also has variable appearance. Focal papillary protrusions into the lumina of dilated follicles are commonly seen and are known as Sanderson polsters.*

Dyshormonogenetic Goiter

TERMINOLOGY

- Familial goiter that develops from defect in metabolism of thyroid hormone secondary to inherited disorder

ETIOLOGY/PATHOGENESIS

- Multiple inherited biochemical defects lead to decreased thyroid hormone synthesis
- Resultant alterations in thyroid gland homeostasis, disturbance of feedback system, and chronic TSH stimulation lead to enlarged thyroid glands or goiters
- Some known gene mutations
  - *DUOX2*
  - *TG*
  - *TPO*

CLINICAL ISSUES

- Prevalence of 1 in 30,000-50,000 live births in Europe and North America

- May be associated with nerve deafness (Pendred syndrome)

MACROSCOPIC

- Thyroid gland is enlarged asymmetrically
- Cut surface is firm and tan with nodules of varying size, which may be up to few centimeters in diameter

MICROSCOPIC

- Solid &/or microfollicular patterns predominating
- Papillary proliferations and insular growth pattern
- Nuclear abnormalities: Enlarged, irregularly shaped, hyperchromatic nuclei and vesicular nuclei
- Colloid is usually absent

ANCILLARY TESTS

- Positive staining for TTF-1 and pax-8
- Negative or focal faint staining for thyroglobulin

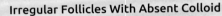

Irregular Follicles With Absent Colloid

Irregular Follicles Devoid of Colloid

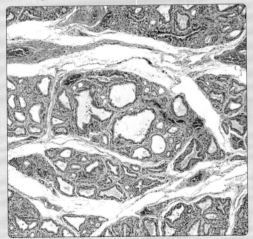

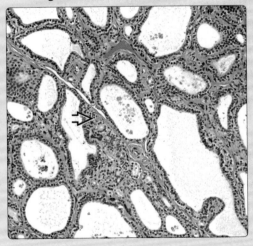

(Left) Low-power view of an area characteristic of a dyshormonogenetic goiter is shown. There are irregular-shaped follicles lacking colloid and surrounded by fibrous bands and dilated lymphatics. (Right) Irregular thyroid follicles with no colloid in a background of fibrosis ⟹ is a characteristic finding in dyshormonogenetic goiter. The cellular nodules exhibiting a variety of architectural appearances, the solid &/or microfollicular patterns, are predominate.

TTF-1 Immunoexpression is Maintained

Absence of Thyroglobulin

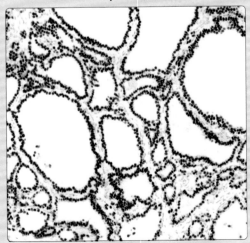

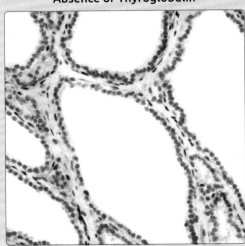

(Left) There is lacking of thyroglobulin expression in a dyshormonogenetic goiter, but there is preservation of TTF-1 immunoexpression. (Right) A dyshormonogenetic goiter is characterized by the lack of thyroglobulin production, as demonstrated in this figure, with follicular cells and lumen contents with no immunoreaction for thyroglobulin.

TERMINOLOGY

Abbreviations

- Dyshormonogenetic goiter (DHG)

Synonyms

- Inherited goiter

Definitions

- DHGs are genetically determined thyroid hyperplasias due to enzyme defects in thyroid-hormone synthesis
- DHG is one of most common causes of hypothyroidism in children and adolescents in iodine nonendemic areas
- Familial goiter that develops from defect in metabolism of thyroid hormone secondary to inherited disorder

ETIOLOGY/PATHOGENESIS

Developmental Anomaly

- Multiple inherited biochemical defects, which lead to decreased thyroid hormone synthesis
  - Resulting alterations in thyroid gland homeostasis, disturbance of feedback system, and chronic TSH stimulation lead to enlarged thyroid gland or goiters

Known Genetic Etiologies

- Deficiencies may be present in multiple steps of thyroid hormone synthesis
  - Thyroglobulin synthesis
  - Iodine transport (into and out of follicular cell)
  - Iodine oxidation
  - Organification of thyroglobulin
  - Coupling and dehalogenation of iodotyrosine compounds
  - Breakdown of thyroglobulin
- *TG*
  - Thyroglobulin (TG) defects due to *TG* gene mutations
  - *TG* gene defects are inherited in autosomal recessive manner
    - Affected individuals are either homozygous or compound heterozygous for mutations
  - This dyshormonogenesis displays wide phenotype variation
- *DUOX2*
  - *Dual oxidase 2 (DUOX2)* mutations are cause of dyshormonogenesis
    - *DUOX2* mutations might be most common cause of
      - Both permanent congenital hypothyroidism and transient hypothyroidism
      - In Japanese series
- *TPO*
  - Thyroid peroxidase (TPO) defects, typically transmitted as autosomal recessive traits, result in hypothyroid goiters with failure to convert iodide into organic iodine
  - TPO is heme binding protein localized on apical membrane of thyrocyte
  - TPO enzymatic activity is essential for thyroid hormonogenesis
  - Inactivating mutations form molecular basis for specific subtype of congenital hypothyroidism
    - Thyroid dyshormonogenesis due to iodide organification defect

- Most common phenotype is total iodide organification defect, with severe and permanent hypothyroidism as consequence
  - c.2268dup mutation in thyroid peroxidase (*TPO*) gene was reported to be founder mutation in Taiwanese patients with dyshormonogenetic congenital hypothyroidism
  - c.2268dup mutation leads to formation of normal and alternatively spliced TPO mRNA transcripts with consequential loss of TPO enzymatic activity
- *NIS*
  - *NIS* gene mutations appears to be most prevalent mutations among Indian children

Pendred Syndrome

- Familial syndrome in which patient has DHG and familial deaf-mutism from sensorineural deafness
- Is autosomal recessive disease classically characterized by DHG
- Pendred syndrome is one cause of congenital hypothyroidism due to thyroid dyshormonogenesis
- Incidence of Pendred syndrome is 7.5-10/100,000 in general population
  - It carries 1 % risk of developing thyroid carcinoma
- Is caused by biallelic mutations (homozygous or compound heterozygous) of *SLC26A4*(PDS) gene
- Mutations in *SLC26A* gene
  - Encoding for pendrin
    - Anion transporter, mostly expressed in thyroid gland, kidney, and inner ear
  - This gene encompasses 21 exons and contains open reading frame of 2,343 base pairs
  - *SLC26A4* gene mutations are associated with broad phenotypic spectrum
    - Including Pendred syndrome
    - Nonsyndromic autosomal recessive hearing loss with enlarged vestibular aqueduct
- Patients with Pendred syndrome have genotypic and phenotypic variability, leading to challenges in definitive diagnosis
  - There is correlation between SLC26A4 genotype and thyroid phenotype
- *TP53* mutation was found in one case of papillary thyroid carcinoma, follicular variant, in patient with Pendred syndrome
  - Evidence support that thyroid carcinomas arising from DHG require additional genetic alteration
    - In addition to purported TSH overstimulation

CLINICAL ISSUES

Epidemiology

- Incidence
  - Prevalence of 1 in 30,000-50,000 live births in Europe and North America
  - 2nd most frequent cause of permanent congenital hypothyroidism after thyroid dysgenesis, including aplastic and hypoplastic thyroid disorders

Site

- Thyroid is diffusely involved, as this is constitutional genetic condition

Presentation

- Goiter is usually not present at birth but appears later in life
  - 75% of goiters develop before 24 years of age (average age 15)
    - Ranges from adults to neonates (only most severe inherited mutations result in infant presentation)
- Patients usually present with clinical evidence of goiter, although sometimes diagnosis is made at autopsy
- May be associated with nerve deafness (Pendred syndrome)
- Slight predilection for female gender
- Family history of hypothyroidism or goiter is reported in roughly 20% of patients

Laboratory Tests

- Laboratory studies demonstrate diminished hormone levels
  - Due to absent or severely decreased thyroid hormone synthesis
    - TSH is increased, illustrating pituitary axis compensation
    - Minimal to absent T4 and T3

Natural History

- Neonatal hypothyroidism will produce cretinism
- Hypothyroidism will progress without proper treatment

Treatment

- Options, risks, complications
  - Treatment can be medical or surgical and is usually based on symptoms
    - Determined on individual basis

Prognosis

- Approach is same as that used for multinodular goiter

MACROSCOPIC

General Features

- Thyroid gland is enlarged asymmetrically

Size

- May weigh up to 600 g

Gross Features

- Thyroid gland is enlarged and multinodular
- Weighing up to 600g
- Areas of cystic change, fibrosis, old and recent hemorrhage may be present
- Cut surface is firm and tan with nodules of varying size, which may be up to few centimeters in diameter

MICROSCOPIC

Histologic Features

- Nodules are hypercellular and often have trabecular pattern with no colloid or rare pale-staining colloid
- Most common alteration is markedly cellular nodules exhibiting variety of architectural appearances
  - Predominantly solid &/or microfollicular patterns
- Prominent papillary hyperplasia may be present in nodules
- Insular growth pattern were also present

- Some authors have described characteristic microcystic pattern in dyshormonogenic goiters with associated thyroglobulin synthetic defect
- Myxoid changes may be seen
- Extensive fibrosis in internodular tissue may simulate true capsular invasion
- Nuclear abnormalities consist of enlarged, irregularly shaped, hyperchromatic and vesicular nuclei
  - Cytologic atypia in DHG may mimic papillary thyroid carcinoma, may be comparable to radiation thyroiditis
- May have focal areas with clear cytoplasmic change
- Colloid is usually absent
  - When present, colloid frequently has pale, washed out appearance

ANCILLARY TESTS

Cytology

- Cytologic examination is not capable of excluding follicular neoplasm
- Cellular aspirate
- Scant colloid
- Prominent atypical nuclei

Immunohistochemistry

- Positive staining for TTF-1 and pax-8
- Negative or focal faint staining for thyroglobulin
- Negative staining for calcitonin

Electron Microscopy

- Ultrastructural studies show cells with abundant mitochondria, rough endoplasmic reticulum with dilated cisternae, and tall follicular cells with numerous microvilli

DIFFERENTIAL DIAGNOSIS

Neoplastic vs. Other Goiters

- 2 most concerning differential diagnoses are thyroid neoplasms and multinodular goiter
- Identification can be extremely difficult
  - Due to propensity of DHG to have
    - Marked hypercellularity
    - Extensive hyperplasia
    - Nuclear pleomorphism
- Some types of iatrogenic goiter

Iatrogenic goiter

- Due to administration of antithyroidal agents
- This is most challenging differential diagnosis
  - Other differential diagnosis below are less challenging

Multinodular Goiter

- May be markedly enlarged as DHG
- More likely to show degenerative changes such as hemorrhage, cystic degeneration, and hemosiderin-laden macrophages
- Toxic multinodular goiter will have elevated T3 and T4 in laboratory studies
- Nontoxic multinodular goiter will have euthyroid laboratory studies
- Thyroglobulin and colloid present within follicles

Adenomatous Nodule

- Asymmetric thyroid enlargement in middle-aged patient
- Does not have cytologic atypia characteristic of DHG
- Abundant colloid
- Degenerative changes such as calcification, hemorrhage, and hemosiderin are present

Radiation Thyroiditis

- Cytologic atypia is present throughout gland as opposed to being mostly limited to areas interspersed between nodules
- Diffusely similar degree of cytologic atypia warrants consideration of radiation thyroiditis
- Patient history of thyroid radiation

Follicular Carcinoma

- Extensive fibrotic background of DHG may mimic capsular invasion seen in follicular carcinoma
  - Follicular carcinoma will have localized lesion with capsular invasion amongst otherwise uninvolved thyroid parenchyma
    - Definitive capsular invasion must be present to correctly diagnose follicular thyroid carcinoma
- Capsule in follicular carcinoma will have vessels
- Key interpretive points include laboratory studies, clinical history, and family history
  - Patients with DHG will have diminished thyroid hormone levels and elevated TSH on laboratory studies

DIAGNOSTIC CHECKLIST

Clinically Relevant Pathologic Features

- Family history of hypothyroidism
- Diminished T3 and T4
- Elevated TSH

Pathologic Interpretation Pearls

- Markedly cellular nodules exhibiting variety of architectural appearances
- Atypical, pleomorphic nuclei
- Diffuse involvement of thyroid
- No or minimal pale colloid

SELECTED REFERENCES

1. Bassot C et al: Mapping pathogenic mutations suggests an innovative structural model for the pendrin (SLC26A4) transmembrane domain. Biochimie. 132:109-120, 2017
2. Noguchi Y et al: A nationwide study on enlargement of the vestibular aqueduct in Japan. Auris Nasus Larynx. 44(1):33-39, 2017
3. Wolf A et al: A novel mutation in SLC26A4 causes nonsyndromic autosomal recessive hearing impairment. Otol Neurotol. 38(2):173-179, 2017
4. Ajiji M et al: Pendred syndrome in a newborn with neck swelling: a case report. J Trop Pediatr. 62(4):338-40, 2016
5. Fu C et al: Mutation screening of the SLC26A4 gene in a cohort of 192 Chinese patients with congenital hypothyroidism. Arch Endocrinol Metab. 60(4):323-7, 2016
6. Gonçalves AC et al: Further characterisation of the recently described SLC26A4 c.918+2T>C mutation and reporting of a novel variant predicted to be damaging. Acta Otorhinolaryngol Ital. 36(3):233-8, 2016
7. Matsuo K et al: High prevalence of DUOX2 mutations in Japanese patients with permanent congenital hypothyroidism or transient hypothyroidism. J Pediatr Endocrinol Metab. 29(7):807-12, 2016
8. Ramesh BG et al: Genotype-phenotype correlations of dyshormonogenetic goiter in children and adolescents from South India. Indian J Endocrinol Metab. 20(6):816-824, 2016
9. Tong GX et al: Targeted next-generation sequencing analysis of a pendred syndrome-associated thyroid carcinoma. Endocr Pathol. 27(1):70-5, 2016
10. Soh LM et al: Evaluation of genotype-phenotype relationships in patients referred for endocrine assessment in suspected Pendred syndrome. Eur J Endocrinol. 172(2):217-26, 2015
11. Lee CC et al: Functional analyses of C.2268dup in thyroid peroxidase gene associated with goitrous congenital hypothyroidism. Biomed Res Int. 2014:370538, 2014
12. Miyagawa M et al: Mutation spectrum and genotype-phenotype correlation of hearing loss patients caused by SLC26A4 mutations in the Japanese: a large cohort study. J Hum Genet. 59(5):262-8, 2014
13. Chertok Shacham E et al: Minimally invasive follicular thyroid carcinoma developed in dyshormonogenetic multinodular goiter due to thyroid peroxidase gene mutation. Thyroid. 22(5):542-6, 2012
14. Narumi S et al: Molecular basis of thyroid dyshormonogenesis: genetic screening in population-based Japanese patients. J Clin Endocrinol Metab. 96(11):E1838-42, 2011
15. Fukata S et al: Diagnosis of iodide transport defect: do we need to measure the saliva/serum radioactive iodide ratio to diagnose iodide transport defect? Thyroid. 20(12):1419-21, 2010
16. Ris-Stalpers C et al: Genetics and phenomics of hypothyroidism and goiter due to TPO mutations. Mol Cell Endocrinol. 322(1-2):38-43, 2010
17. Drut R et al: Papillary carcinoma of the thyroid developed in congenital dyshormonogenetic hypothyroidism without goiter: Diagnosis by FNAB. Diagn Cytopathol. 37(10):707-9, 2009
18. Francois A et al: Fetal treatment for early dyshormonogenetic goiter. Prenat Diagn. 29(5):543-5, 2009
19. Kallel R et al: [Papillary carcinoma arising from dyshormonogenetic goiter.] Ann Endocrinol (Paris). 70(6):485-8, 2009
20. Mayor-Lynn KA et al: Antenatal diagnosis and treatment of a dyshormonogenetic fetal goiter. J Ultrasound Med. 28(1):67-71, 2009
21. Rubio IG et al: Mutations of the thyroglobulin gene and its relevance to thyroid disorders. Curr Opin Endocrinol Diabetes Obes. 16(5):373-8, 2009
22. Banghova K et al: Thyroidectomy in a patient with multinodular dyshormonogenetic goitre--a case of Pendred syndrome confirmed by mutations in the PDS/SLC26A4 gene. J Pediatr Endocrinol Metab. 21(12):1179-84, 2008
23. Banghová K et al: [Pendred syndrome among patients with hypothyroidism: genetic diagnosis, phenotypic variability and occurrence of phenocopies.] Cas Lek Cesk. 147(12):616-22, 2008
24. Chang XY et al: [Dyshormonogenetic goiter: clinicopathologic study of four cases.] Zhonghua Bing Li Xue Za Zhi. 36(1):39-42, 2007
25. Pfarr N et al: Congenital primary hypothyroidism with subsequent adenomatous goiter in a Turkish patient caused by a homozygous 10-bp deletion in the thyroid peroxidase (TPO) gene. Clin Endocrinol (Oxf). 64(5):514-8, 2006
26. Deshpande AH et al: Cytological features of dyshormonogenetic goiter: case report and review of the literature. Diagn Cytopathol. 33(4):252-4, 2005
27. Thompson L: Dyshormonogenetic goiter of the thyroid gland. Ear Nose Throat J. 84(4):200, 2005
28. Karak AK et al: Fine needle aspiration cytology, histology and MIB-1 proliferative index in a case of dyshormonogenetic goitre. Indian J Pathol Microbiol. 44(2):169-72, 2001
29. Pedrinola F et al: Overexpression of epidermal growth factor and epidermal growth factor-receptor mRNAs in dyshormonogenetic goiters. Thyroid. 11(1):15-20, 2001
30. Perrotin F et al: Prenatal diagnosis and early in utero management of fetal dyshormonogenetic goiter. Eur J Obstet Gynecol Reprod Biol. 94(2):309-14, 2001
31. Camargo RY et al: Pathological findings in dyshormonogenetic goiter with defective iodide transport. Endocr Pathol. 9(3):225-233, 1998
32. de Lima MA et al: [Immunohistochemical identification of biochemical defect of dyshormonogenetic goiter.] Rev Hosp Clin Fac Med Sao Paulo. 53(2):86-90, 1998
33. Kavishwar VS et al: Dyshormonogenetic goitre with clear cell change resembling parathyroid adenoma--a case report. Indian J Pathol Microbiol. 41(4):469-71, 1998
34. Medeiros-Neto G et al: Metastatic thyroid carcinoma arising from congenital goiter due to mutation in the thyroperoxidase gene. J Clin Endocrinol Metab. 83(11):4162-6, 1998
35. Ghossein RA et al: Dyshormonogenetic goiter: a clinicopathologic study of 56 cases. Endocr Pathol. 8(4):283-292, 1997
36. Medeiros-Neto G et al: Prenatal diagnosis and treatment of dyshormonogenetic fetal goiter due to defective thyroglobulin synthesis. J Clin Endocrinol Metab. 82(12):4239-42, 1997

(Left) *The nodular formations of a dyshormonogenetic goiter tend to have less severe nuclear atypia than the areas of extranodular parenchyma. The density of the follicles and scarcity of colloid can give the false impression of a follicular neoplasm.* **(Right)** *Characteristic low-power view of a dyshormonogenetic goiter is shown. There is absence of colloid in the lumen of the irregular follicles. There is focal papillae formation and interstitial fibrosis.*

Adenomatous Changes in Dyshormonogenetic Goiter

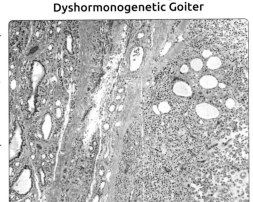

Irregular Follicles Lacking Colloid

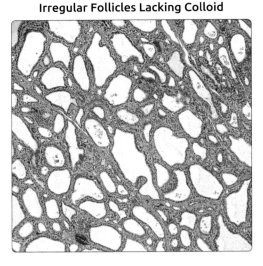

(Left) *Banding fibrosis in the thyroid parenchyma is characteristic of a dyshormonogenetic goiter, usually associated with the highest degree of nuclear atypia. There is a fluffy eosinophilic material in the lumen.* **(Right)** *Small and larger follicles lack colloid, and only a small of pale pink fluffy material is within the follicles. The density of the follicles and scarcity of colloid may give the false impression of a follicular neoplasm.*

Follicular Cells With Nuclear Enlargement

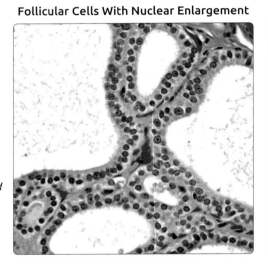

Lack of Colloid

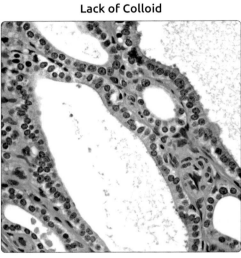

(Left) *Immunohistochemistry for thyroglobulin is completely negative in a dyshormonogenetic goiter. Note the follicular cells and the lumen contents with absence of immunoreaction.* **(Right)** *The follicular cells do not produce thyroglobulin but maintain the immunoexpression of TTF-1 and pax-8. These findings are characteristic of dyshormonogenetic goiter.*

Absence of Thyroglobulin

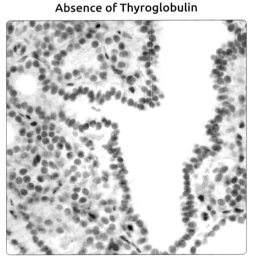

pax-8 Immunopositivity Retained

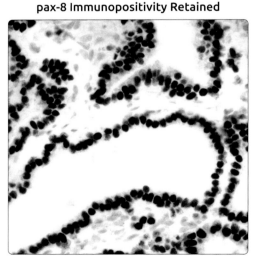

Papillary Proliferations

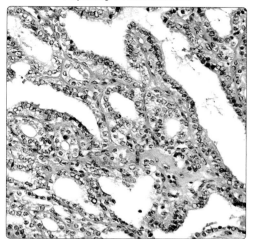

Papillae and Nuclear Pleomorphism

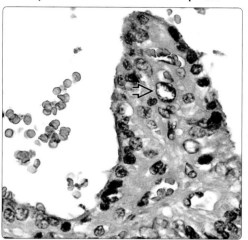

(Left) *Papillae formation is characteristic of a dyshormonogenetic goiter. There are abundant clear nuclei that may mimic papillary thyroid carcinoma. For this reason, clinical history and laboratory studies are necessary.* (Right) *High-power photomicrograph shows papillary hyperplasia with projection of the papillae into the follicular lumen. There is a lack of colloid, and the cells show nuclear membrane irregularities, nuclear atypia, and focally striking nuclear clearing* ⇒.

Papillary Proliferations

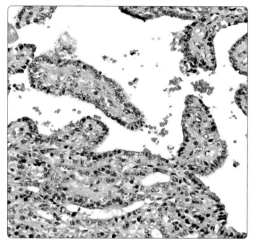

Area With Papillary Hyperplasia

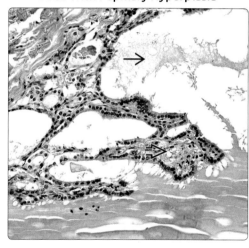

(Left) *Low-power microphotograph shows papillary projections with abundant cytoplasmic clearing. This is a common feature of a dyshormonogenetic goiter. There is no appreciable colloid.* (Right) *Papillary architecture* ⇒ *is frequently observed in a dyshormonogenetic goiter. This may mimic thyroid carcinoma, especially if there is nuclear atypia (not seen here). The pale-staining, watery colloid* ⇒ *is focally present within this field.*

Area With Interstitial Fibrosis

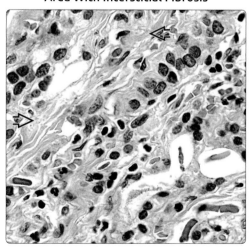

Nuclear Atypia

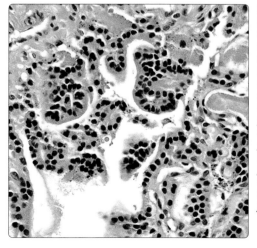

(Left) *Banding fibrosis* ⇒ *in the thyroid parenchyma is characteristic of a dyshormonogenetic goiter, usually associated with the highest degree of nuclear atypia. There is a dense eosinophilic colloid-like material and nuclear pleomorphism.* (Right) *Nuclear atypia may be present within papillary formations. Note the hyperchromatism and pleomorphism of the follicular cells lining the follicles. There is minimal colloid within the follicles.*

Amyloid Goiter

TERMINOLOGY

- Amyloid goiter: Rare condition characterized by clinically detectable enlargement of thyroid gland due to deposition of amyloid
- Systemic amyloidogenic conditions with thyroid involvement include plasma cell dyscrasias, chronic infections, autoimmune conditions, familial Mediterranean fever, and familial amyloid polyneuropathy

ETIOLOGY/PATHOGENESIS

- Amyloid deposition in thyroid can occur as part of
- Primary amyloidosis
  - Defined as not associated with underlying chronic disease
  - Chemical composition: IgG-light chain (κ or λ) origin (AL)
- Secondary amyloidosis
  - Defined as associated with underlying chronic disease
  - Chemical composition: Serum amyloid A

CLINICAL ISSUES

- Painless thyroid mass
- History of persistent hoarseness for several years before presentation with compressive symptoms

MACROSCOPIC

- Thyroid gland usually uniformly and diffusely enlarged
- Gross appearance: Uniform, lobulated, fleshy, tan-yellow thyroid tissue

MICROSCOPIC

- Marked decrease in number of follicles with corresponding increase in adiposity
- Histologic appearance of thyroid predominantly consists of diffuse amyloid deposition surrounding thyroid follicles
- Confirmation of amyloid made by presence of congophilia and apple-green birefringence under polarized-light microscopy

Gross Cut Surface

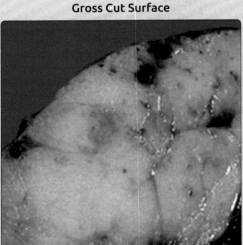

Fibrovascular Core

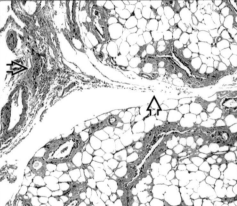
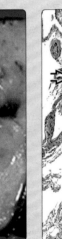

(Left) The thyroid gland in amyloid goiter (AG) is usually uniformly and diffusely enlarged. The cut surface is lobulated and yellow, the color depending on the amount of adipose tissue present. (Right) The characteristic gross findings are correlated with the lobulated microscopic findings. There is a thin fibrovascular core ⊟ separating the thyroid lobules with amyloid and fat deposition with a marked increase in fat content.

Residual Thyroid Follicle

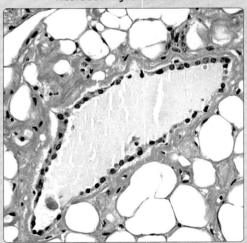

Congophilic Material and Birefringency

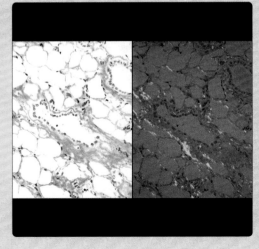

(Left) Diffuse amyloid deposition surrounding thyroid follicles intermixed with mature adipose tissue is shown. The amyloid is evenly distributed around follicles and appears eosinophilic, acellular, and amorphous. (Right) AG is characterized by the presence of amyloid deposition, with destruction of thyroid follicles and adipocytic proliferation. Amyloid is confirmed by the congophilic material and apple-green birefringence under polarized light microscopy.

TERMINOLOGY

Abbreviations
- Amyloid goiter (AG)

Synonyms
- Lipomatous hamartoma

Definitions
- Rare condition characterized by clinically detectable enlargement of thyroid gland due to deposition of amyloid
  - Not associated with neoplasm causing clinically detectable thyroid enlargement (goiter)

ETIOLOGY/PATHOGENESIS

Pathogenesis
- Most amyloid deposits in thyroid are calcitonin-derived and seen in association with medullary thyroid carcinoma
- Amyloid deposition in thyroid can occur as part of
  - Primary amyloidosis
  - Secondary amyloidosis
- **Primary amyloidosis**
  - Defined as not associated with underlying chronic disease
  - Amyloid deposition in variety of viscera, including heart, gastrointestinal tract, tongue
  - Chemical composition: IgG-light chain (κ or λ) origin (AL)
- **Secondary amyloidosis**
  - Defined as associated with underlying chronic disease
  - Amyloid deposition in kidneys, adrenal glands, liver, and spleen
  - Chemical composition: Serum amyloid A (SAA)
  - AG in secondary amyloidosis characterized by deposition of amyloid A protein (AA) in gland, associated with atrophic follicles
- More commonly seen as part of secondary systemic amyloidosis
  - In this setting, amyloid usually found at autopsy rather than resulting in symptomatic mass
- Predisposing disorders associated with secondary systemic amyloidosis with deposition in thyroid include
  - Chronic inflammatory diseases including infections
    - Chronic osteomyelitis
    - Pulmonary tuberculosis
    - Chronic bronchitis with bronchiectasis
    - Chronic peritonitis
  - Rheumatoid arthritis
  - Familial Mediterranean fever
  - Crohn disease
  - Hodgkin disease
  - Extramedullary plasmacytoma (EMP) either as
    - Solitary plasma cell tumor (primary EMP)
    - Manifestation of multiple myeloma (secondary EMP)
- **Classification of amyloidosis**
  - Systemic amyloidosis (primary and secondary)
  - Multiple myeloma-associated amyloidosis
    - Chemical composition: IgG-light chain (κ or λ) origin (AL)
  - Localized or solitary amyloidosis
    - Chemical composition: IgG-light chain (κ or λ) origin (AL)
  - Familial Mediterranean fever
    - Chemical composition: SAA
  - Senile amyloidosis
    - Chemical composition: Transthyretin (TTR; prealbumin)
  - Dialysis-associated amyloidosis
    - Chemical composition: β2-microglobulin (Aβ2M)
  - Systemic amyloidogenic conditions with thyroid involvement include plasma cell dyscrasias, chronic infections, autoimmune conditions, familial Mediterranean fever, and familial amyloid polyneuropathy
    - Few cases of familial amyloid polyneuropathy have demonstrated transthyretin amyloid deposits in thyroid, although goitrous enlargement of thyroid in this condition is rare

CLINICAL ISSUES

Presentation
- Painless mass
- In symptomatic patients, clinical presentation includes nontender thyroid enlargement
  - History of persistent hoarseness for several years before presentation with compressive symptoms
- Some degree of thyroid dysfunction

Laboratory Tests
- Light-chain amyloidosis warrants search for lymphoproliferative disorder
- Calcitonin amyloidosis suggests sporadic medullary thyroid carcinoma or multiple endocrine neoplasia syndrome
- Diagnosis of familial form of amyloidosis in patient warrants increased surveillance in family members

Treatment
- In symptomatic patients, thyroidectomy to alleviate pressure symptoms
- Secondary (AA) amyloidosis may indicate presence of chronic inflammatory condition or infection, and management of underlying disease is optimal course of therapy

MACROSCOPIC

General Features
- Uniform, lobulated, fleshy, white-tan-yellow, enlarged thyroid, from 50-130 g
  - Gross color of thyroid may vary depending on adipose tissue content

MICROSCOPIC

Histologic Features
- Diffuse amyloid deposition and fat infiltration surrounding thyroid follicles
- Follicles lined by cuboidal epithelium, filled with homogeneous pale eosinophilic colloid, and surrounded by fat and wispy, paucicellular deposits of eosinophilic amyloid

- Diffuse deposition of amorphous eosinophilic material between follicles, in interstitium around and within vessels, and between adipocytes
- Areas of mature adipose tissue and focal lymphocytic thyroiditis ± foreign body-type giant cells
  o Although multivacuolated cells resembling lipoblasts are not infrequent, no atypia or hyperchromasia of adipocyte nuclei seen
  o Significant variation in adipocyte size and shape attributable to irregular expansion of intercellular space by amyloid
- Presence of amyloid confirmed by congophilia and apple-green birefringence under polarized-light microscopy
- **Diffuse amyloid deposition surrounding thyroid follicles**
  o Amyloid evenly distributed throughout gland
- **Focal nodular pattern of amyloid deposition**
- Amyloid deposition can be angiocentric, seen around vascular spaces
  o Less often, amyloid within vessel walls
- Residual thyroid follicles vary in appearance
  o Elongated thyroid follicles with normal colloid content
  o Small, slit-like atrophic follicles without colloid
  o Scattered remnant follicular cells may be found
  o Follicular cells may appear normal or flat, single-cell layer
  o Squamous metaplasia may be present

ANCILLARY TESTS

Cytology

- Aspirated material contains
  o Few cells (paucicellular)
  o Small fragments of cyanophilic material (amyloid)
  o Amyloid is congophilic

Histochemistry

- Congo red
  o Reactivity: Positive

Immunohistochemistry

- IHC studies needed for definitive histopathologic classification
  o Subtypes differ in etiology, genetics, and treatment
- No immunoreactivity with calcitonin or thyroglobulin
- Immunohistochemical evaluation may demonstrate presence of AA immunoreactivity

Electron Microscopy

- Nonbranching fibrils varying in size from 50-150 Å in diameter

DIFFERENTIAL DIAGNOSIS

Hyalinizing Trabecular Tumor

- Characterized by
  o Trabecular to organoid (paraganglioma-like) growth
  o Extracellular hyalinization
    – May be prominent and excessive, simulating amyloid
    – May be intratrabecular and extratrabecular
  o Neoplastic cellular proliferation shows
    – Elongated cells with nuclei that display morphologic similarities to papillary carcinoma

  – Cytoplasmic (yellow) inclusions surrounded by clear halo
  o Hyalinization negative for Congo red
    – No birefringence
  o Hyalinization negative for immunoreactivity associated with amyloid goiter
- Characteristic Ki-67/MIB-1 cytoplasmic membranous staining

Adenomatous Nodule With Degenerative Changes

- Degenerative changes seen in adenomatoid nodules may include irregular fibrosis
  o Fibrosis may be intralesional or at periphery
  o Fibrosis negative for Congo red

Medullary Thyroid Carcinoma

- Presence of neuroendocrine neoplastic cellular proliferation
- Immunoreactivity for calcitonin and other neuroendocrine markers
- Amyloid deposition limited to neoplastic proliferative area
  o Not diffuse pattern as seen in amyloid goiter

DIAGNOSTIC CHECKLIST

Pathologic Interpretation Pearls

- Marked decrease in number of follicles with corresponding increase in adiposity and amyloid deposition

SELECTED REFERENCES

1. Oueslati I et al: Amyloid goiter as the first manifestation of systemic amyloidosis. Tunis Med. 94(1):82, 2016
2. Cabrejas Gómez Mdel C et al: Amyloid goiter as an initial manifestation of systemic amyloidosis. Reumatol Clin. 11(6):404-5, 2015
3. Law JH et al: Symptomatic amyloid goiters: report of five cases. Thyroid. 23(11):1490-5, 2013
4. Pinto A et al: Localized amyloid in thyroid: are we missing it? Adv Anat Pathol. 20(1):61-7, 2013
5. Ozdemir D et al: Amyloid goiter and hypopituitarism in a patient with systemic amyloidosis. Amyloid. 18(1):32-4, 2011
6. Yaeger KA et al: Amyloid goiter. Diagn Cytopathol. 38(10):742-3, 2010
7. Abdou AG et al: A case of amyloid goiter associated with intrathyroid parathyroid and lymphoepithelial cyst. Endocr Pathol. 20(4):243-8, 2009
8. Vanguri VK et al: Transthyretin amyloid goiter in a renal allograft recipient. Endocr Pathol. 19(1):66-73, 2008
9. Siddiqui MA et al: Amyloid goiter as a manifestation of primary systemic amyloidosis. Thyroid. 17(1):77-80, 2007
10. Ozdemir BH et al: Diagnosing amyloid goitre with thyroid aspiration biopsy. Cytopathology. 17(5):262-6, 2006
11. Ozdemir BH et al: Amyloid goiter in familial Mediterranean fever (FMF): a clinicopathologic study of 10 cases. Ren Fail. 23(5):659-67, 2001
12. Srivastava A et al: Juvenile rheumatoid arthritis with amyloid goiter: report of a case with review of the literature. Endocr Pathol. 12(4):437-41, 2001
13. Coli A et al: Papillary carcinoma in amyloid goitre. J Exp Clin Cancer Res. 19(3):391-4, 2000
14. D'Antonio A et al: Amyloid goiter: the first evidence in secondary amyloidosis. Report of five cases and review of literature. Adv Clin Path. 4(2):99-106, 2000
15. Villamil CF et al: Amyloid goiter with parathyroid involvement: a case report and review of the literature. Arch Pathol Lab Med. 124(2):281-3, 2000
16. Hamed G et al: Amyloid goiter. A clinicopathologic study of 14 cases and review of the literature. Am J Clin Pathol. 104(3):306-12, 1995
17. Haouet S et al: [Thyrolipoma. A case report and review of the literature.] Arch Anat Cytol Pathol. 38(5-6):230-2, 1990
18. Gnepp DR et al: Fat-containing lesions of the thyroid gland. Am J Surg Pathol. 13(7):605-12, 1989

Yellow Lobulated Cut Surface

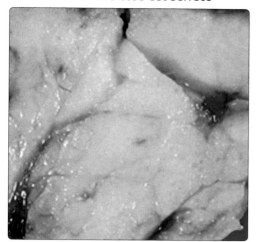

Thin Fibrovascular Core

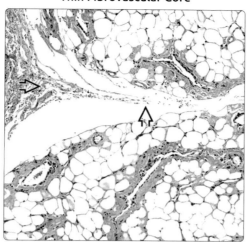

(Left) The thyroid gland is usually uniformly and diffusely enlarged; the cut surface is homogeneously tan/yellow and lobulated with a soft, greasy texture reflecting a marked increase in fat content. (Right) The characteristic gross lobulated appearance correlates with the microscopic findings. There is a thin, fibrovascular band ⇒ separating lobules of atrophic follicles surrounded by amyloid and a variable amount of adipose tissue.

Predominance of Adipocytes

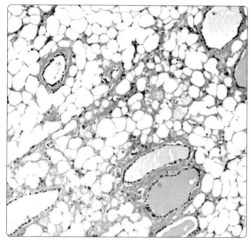

Residual Thyroid Follicle

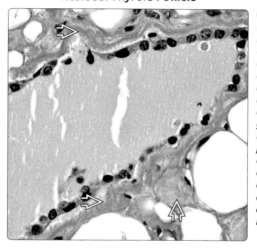

(Left) A marked decrease in the number of follicles is noted, and there is a corresponding increase in adiposity. Thin, fibrous septa are randomly arranged, as are aggregates of eosinophilic amyloid. The amyloid is evenly distributed throughout the gland. (Right) The follicles are lined by cuboidal epithelium filled with homogeneous, pale, eosinophilic colloid. The extracellular amyloid ⇒ deposited around the follicles appears as eosinophilic, acellular, and amorphous material.

Follicular Destruction

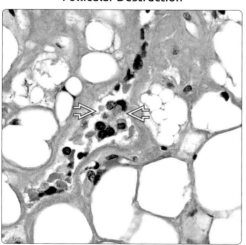

Extensive Deposition of Acellular Material

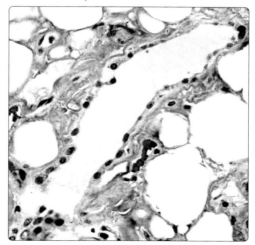

(Left) The thyroid follicles are progressively destroyed and have an atrophic appearance due to the amyloid deposition. This gives a slit-like appearance of the follicle without colloid ⇒. Scattered follicular cell remnants may be seen. The amyloid is intermixed with adipose tissue. (Right) Trichrome stain shows extensive areas of thyroid parenchyma replacement by homogeneous acellular material with scattered capillaries within the amyloid deposition and adipocytes.

Congophilia

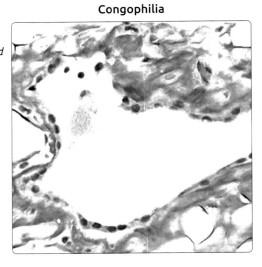

Apple-Green Birefringence

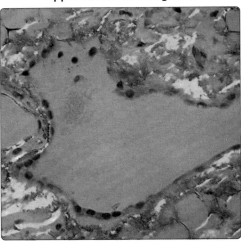

(Left) *Congo red stain highlights the diffuse amyloid deposition surrounding thyroid follicles with the congophilia appearance.* (Right) *The presence of congophilia and apple-green birefringence under polarized light microscopy confirms amyloid deposition.*

Residual Follicles

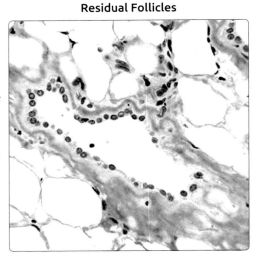

Apple-Green Birefringence

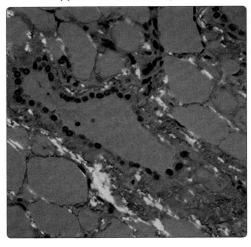

(Left) *The follicles are lined by cuboidal epithelium and are surrounded by adipocytes of variable size and shape, attributable to the irregular expansion of the intercellular space by amyloid. The deposits show bright congophilic staining.* (Right) *Amyloid goiter is characterized by the presence of amyloid deposition, which is confirmed by apple-green birefringence and congophilic material under polarized light microscopy.*

Calcitonin Negativity

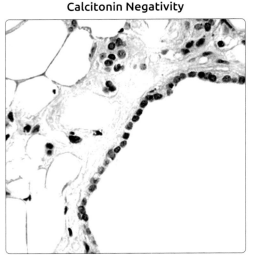

TTF1(+) Residual Follicular Cells

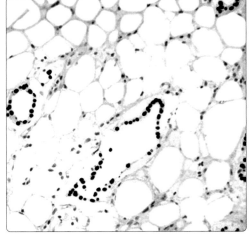

(Left) *Most amyloid deposits seen in thyroid are calcitonin derived; however, calcitonin stain is characteristically negative in cases of amyloid goiter, even with confirmed amyloid deposition.* (Right) *TTF-1 immunostain reveals that the residual follicular cells are still immunoreactive for this antigen. Such reactivity is gradually lost as thyroid follicles are destroyed. The adjacent adipose tissue is negative for this antigen and positive for S100 protein.*

Parathyroid With Amyloid Deposition

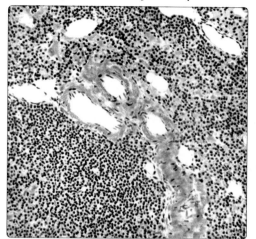

Parathyroid With Amyloid Deposition

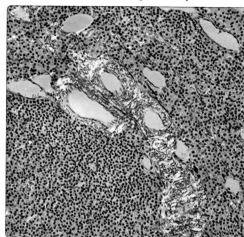

(Left) *Photomicrograph shows a parathyroid gland from a patient with AG. The gland has a chief cell adenoma, and congophilic deposits are present in numerous vessels in the parenchyma but not within the parathyroid adenoma.* (Right) *Photomicrograph shows amyloid deposition in vessels within a parathyroid gland in a patient with AG. The presence of congophilia and apple-green birefringence under polarized light microscopy confirms amyloid deposition.*

Ultrastructural Findings

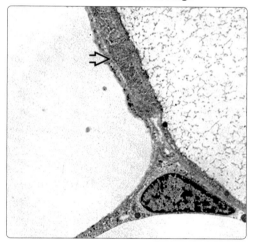

Ultrastructural Findings of Fibrils

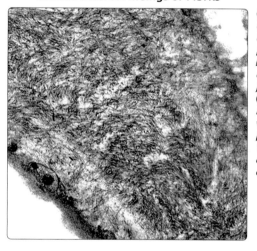

(Left) *Ultrastructural examination of thyroid with amyloid goiter reveals the presence of fibrillary material ⇨ within the adipocytes around residual thyroid follicles and in vessel walls.* (Right) *High-power magnification of an adipocyte within an AG reveals the presence of fibrillary material. The fibrillary material was also arranged around follicles and vessels.*

Ultrastructural Findings Around Cells

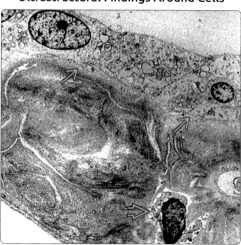

Ultrastructural Findings of Fibrils

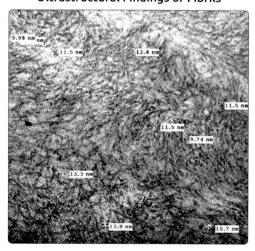

(Left) *The fibrillary material is arranged around follicles and vessels, and amyloid fibrils surround follicular cells ⇨. An endothelial cell is within the amyloid deposition ⇨. The fibrils in the thyroid are short, irregular, and nonbranching.* (Right) *High-power magnification of an AG shows that the fibrils within the thyroid are short, irregular, and nonbranching with a diameter of ~ 10.8 nm.*

ETIOLOGY/PATHOGENESIS

- Result of interventional procedure for diagnostic purposes

CLINICAL ISSUES

- Post-FNA changes (PFNAC) has no clinical significance in itself; however, it has propensity to lead to erroneous diagnoses

MICROSCOPIC

- Reactive histologic features present in thyroid parenchyma
- Acute changes
  - Granulation tissue
  - Fresh hemorrhage
  - Hemosiderin-laden macrophages
- Additional features
  - Nuclear atypia with nuclear membranes irregularities and nuclear clearing
  - Capsular disruption and vascular pseudoinvasion
  - Follicular destruction

- Inflammatory infiltrate
- Chronic changes
  - Squamous and oncocytic metaplasia
  - Pseudoinvasion from capsular disruption
  - Fibrosis
  - Hemosiderin deposition within fibrous tissue
- Reactive spindle cell formation may occur with bland mitosis in reaction to trauma of FNA biopsy

TOP DIFFERENTIAL DIAGNOSES

- Papillary thyroid carcinoma
  - Shows more severe degree of nuclear atypia
- Anaplastic thyroid carcinoma
  - Marked nuclear atypia
  - Invasive growth pattern
- Vascular entities
  - Vascular proliferation at prior FNA site may mimic hemangioma and angiosarcoma

---

(Left) Recent post-FNA site changes in the thyroid gland usually demonstrate abundant hemosiderin deposition, disruption of thyroid follicles, and early fibroblastic proliferation. (Right) FNA site changes from a removal procedure show focal hemosiderin deposition ⊟ within the thyroid parenchyma in a background of extensive reactive fibrosis. There is mild chronic inflammation.

Heavy Hemosiderin Deposition

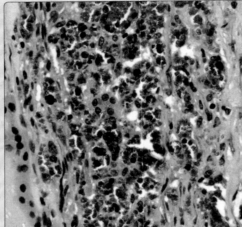

Fibrosis and Hemosiderin Deposition

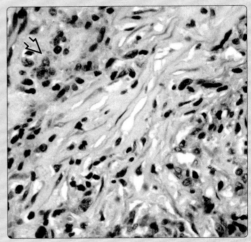

(Left) Hemosiderin deposition within fibrous bands and in the thyroid parenchyma is present after FNA biopsy. There is disruption of the follicular architecture. (Right) Adjacent to fibrosis and hemosiderin deposition, there are characteristic reactive nuclear changes that mimic papillary thyroid carcinoma ⊟. Pseudoinvasion from capsular disruption is another finding that may mimic thyroid carcinoma.

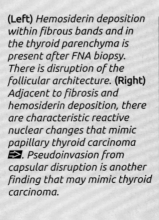

Follicular Thyroid Disruption

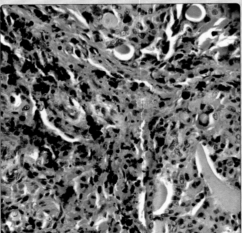

Cellular Atypia at Prior FNA Site

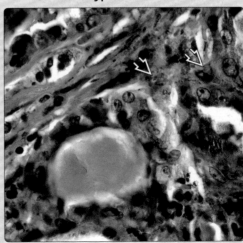

TERMINOLOGY

Abbreviations

- Post-FNA changes (PFNAC)

Synonyms

- FNA site changes
- Worrisome histologic alterations following FNA of thyroid

Definitions

- Changes in normal histology of thyroid gland following FNA
  - Reactive or degenerative

ETIOLOGY/PATHOGENESIS

Iatrogenic

- Result of interventional procedure for diagnostic purposes

CLINICAL ISSUES

Epidemiology

- Incidence
  - Common clinical procedure
- Age
  - No age predilection
- Sex
  - No gender predilection

Presentation

- Patients presenting with nodule frequently undergo FNA biopsy

Prognosis

- PFNAC has no clinical significance in itself; however, it has propensity to lead to erroneous diagnoses
  - May subject patients to unnecessary clinical interventions

Clinical implications

- Most important clinical implications of PFNAC are that they are frequently superimposed in other pathologic entities
  - May make distinction between benign and malignant entities difficult
  - 0.15% FNA have complications

MICROSCOPIC

Histologic Features

- Reactive histologic features present in thyroid parenchyma
  - May be acute or chronic
- Acute changes
  - Granulation tissue
  - Fresh hemorrhage
  - Hemosiderin-laden macrophages
- Additional features
  - Nuclear atypia
    - Mitotic figures may be present
  - Capsular disruption
  - Follicular destruction
    - May mimic thyroiditis
- Chronic changes
  - Infarction
  - Fibrosis

- Squamous and oncocytic metaplasia
- Pseudoinvasion from capsular disruption
  - May mimic thyroid carcinoma
  - Absence of follicular cells within needle tract in addition to other reactive features indicates PFNAC
- Floater cells
  - Cells with reactive atypia may become dislodged into vessels mimicking appearance of vascular invasion

Post-FNA Spindle Cell Proliferation

- Reactive spindle cell formation may occur with bland mitosis in reaction to trauma of FNA biopsy
  - May mimic anaplastic thyroid carcinoma or sarcoma
  - Lesion is well circumscribed and nonencapsulated
  - Nuclear atypia may be present to mild degree

DIFFERENTIAL DIAGNOSIS

Papillary Thyroid Carcinoma

- Shows more severe degree of nuclear atypia
- Classic features of nuclear grooves, clearing, and papillary architecture

Anaplastic Thyroid Carcinoma

- Marked nuclear atypia
- Atypical mitotic figures
- Invasive growth pattern

Vascular Entities

- PFNAC may produce reactive vascular proliferation, which may mimic vascular neoplasms, such as hemangioma and angiosarcoma

DIAGNOSTIC CHECKLIST

Clinically Relevant Pathologic Features

- Regenerative changes, which may mimic atypia

Pathologic Interpretation Pearls

- Localized degenerative changes in patient with neoplasm and known history of FNA should warrant consideration of PFNAC
  - Especially true in borderline-type cases

SELECTED REFERENCES

1. Cappelli C et al: Complications after fine-needle aspiration cytology: a retrospective study of 7449 consecutive thyroid nodules. Br J Oral Maxillofac Surg. 55(3):266-269, 2016
2. Yegen G et al: Not all post-FNA spindle cell proliferations in the thyroid are of myofibroblastic origin: follicular adenoma with spindle cell metaplasia. Endocr Pathol. 26(4):374-6, 2015
3. Nissan A et al: Prospective trial evaluating electrical impedance scanning of thyroid nodules before thyroidectomy: final results. Ann Surg. 247(5):843-53, 2008
4. Baloch ZW et al: Cytologic and architectural mimics of papillary thyroid carcinoma. diagnostic challenges in fine-needle aspiration and surgical pathology specimens. Am J Clin Pathol. 125 Suppl:S135-44, 2006
5. Krishnamurthy S et al: Ultrasound-guided fine-needle aspiration biopsy of the thyroid bed. Cancer. 93(3):199-205, 2001
6. Baloch ZW et al: Post-fine-needle aspiration spindle cell nodules of the thyroid (PSCNT). Am J Clin Pathol. 111(1):70-4, 1999
7. Pinto RG et al: Infarction after fine needle aspiration. a report of four cases. Acta Cytol. 40(4):739-41, 1996

Adenomatous Nodules

TERMINOLOGY

- Thyroid gland enlargement as result of follicular hyperplasia due to impaired thyroid hormone production

ETIOLOGY/PATHOGENESIS

- Endogenous characteristics in addition to genetic and environmental conditions

CLINICAL ISSUES

- Present in < 5% of patients clinically
- Enlarged thyroid, asymmetric in most instances
- Rarely, thyroid gland may be so enlarged that patients become hoarse due to laryngeal nerve compression or experience dysphagia

MACROSCOPIC

- Asymmetrically enlarged gland with multiple nodules of variable size
- Dominant nodule frequently identified
- Thyroid gland distorted by nodular enlargement

- Degenerative cystic changes common
- Can range in size from extremely large to microscopic lesions found incidentally
- Asymmetrically enlarged gland with multiple nodules of variable size

MICROSCOPIC

- Usually microfollicular appearance
- Nodules usually compress surrounding uninvolved thyroid
- Nodules unencapsulated
- Recognized as mimicker of follicular neoplasm on cytology

ANCILLARY TESTS

- Loss of PTEN IHC staining occurs in isolated nodules related to *PTEN* gene mutations/deletions
- PTEN immunoexpression serves as screening molecular correlate to predict for germline *PTEN* mutation in PTEN-hamartoma tumor syndrome

Multinodular Thyroid Cut Surface

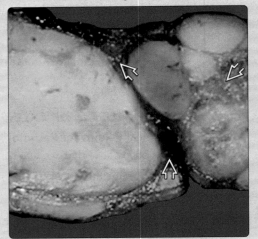

Multiple Adenomatous Nodules

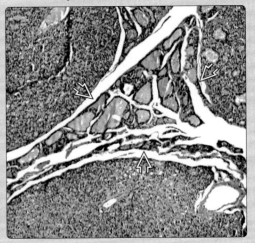

(Left) *Gross photograph of adenomatous nodules (ANs) shows multiple well-circumscribed and unencapsulated nodules compressing the adjacent uninvolved thyroid parenchyma* ➡. (Right) *Microphotograph of multiple adenomatous nodules shows the adjacent compressed normal thyroid parenchyma* ➡. *Note the lack of a fibrous capsule surrounding the ANs.*

Unencapsulated Adenomatous Nodules

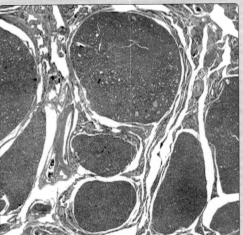

PTEN Immunostaining in Syndromic Adenomatous Nodules

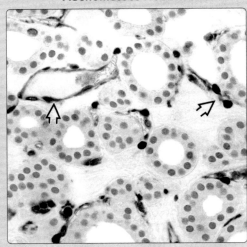

(Left) *Characteristic histology of an AN is shown. There is minimal colloid within the nodule. The lesion is unencapsulated and well circumscribed with abrupt continuity to the normal thyroid parenchyma. (Right) Loss of PTEN immunostaining occurs in isolated nodules related to PTEN gene mutations/deletions in patients with PTEN-hamartoma syndrome. The endothelial cells* ➡ *within the nodules are PTEN(+).*

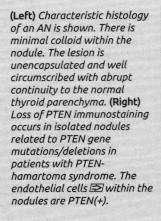

TERMINOLOGY

Abbreviations
- Adenomatous nodule (AN)

Synonyms
- Adenomatous hyperplasia
- Adenomatoid nodule

Definitions
- Thyroid gland enlargement as result of follicular hyperplasia due to impaired thyroid hormone production

ETIOLOGY/PATHOGENESIS

Developmental Anomaly
- As part of inherited tumor syndromes
  - *PTEN*-hamartoma tumor syndrome (Cowden disease; BRRS)
    - Caused by germline mutation of *PTEN* in autosomal dominant fashion
    - Thyroid disease usually diagnosed in young patients
    - May be associated with multiple follicular adenomas and follicular carcinoma
    - Thyroid usually has > 20 adenomatous nodules
  - Carney complex
    - Autosomal dominant disorder caused by mutations in *PRKAR1A* gene in 80% of affected families
    - Amplification of 2p16-23 in patients with *PRKAR1A*-negative Carney complex
      - With activation of protein kinase A pathway
    - Up to 75% of patients present with multiple adenomatous nodules
  - McCune-Albright syndrome
    - Mutation in GNAS
    - Leading to increase in cAMP levels
  - DICER1 syndrome
    - Pleuropulmonary blastoma and dysplasia syndrome associated with multinodular thyroid disease in children
  - Pendred syndrome
    - Autosomal recessive syndrome resulting from mutations in *SLC2*

Environmental Exposure
- Diet
  - Some foods thought to be goitrogenic
    - Raw vegetables, seafood
- Drugs
  - Amiodarone, lithium, methimazole, carbimazole, propylthiouracil, thalidomide, rifampin, carbamazepine, and perchlorate are all examples of drugs associated with adenomatous nodules

In Iodine-Deficient Areas
- Diminished iodine within nodules

Multifactorial
- Endogenous characteristics in addition to genetic and environmental conditions

CLINICAL ISSUES

Epidemiology
- Incidence
  - Present in < 5% of patients clinically
    - Autopsy series show as many as 50% of patients have adenomatous nodules
  - Mostly present in iodine-deficient areas
- Age
  - Peak range: 5th-7th decades
    - Occurs at earlier age when part of inherited syndromes
- Sex
  - F:M = 5-10:1
    - Nodules often detected by clinicians in pregnant patients

Presentation
- Enlarged thyroid, asymmetric in most instances
  - Rarely, thyroid gland may be so enlarged that patients become hoarse due to laryngeal nerve compression or experience dysphagia

Treatment
- Surgical approaches
  - Surgery often performed, as adenomatoid nodules may cause clinicians concern for malignancy
  - Additionally, excessive goiter may cause discomfort

Prognosis
- Excellent: Surgery is curative
  - Patients with thyroidectomy require thyroid hormone replacement therapy

IMAGING

Radiographic Findings
- Diffuse enlargement of thyroid gland with multiple nodules
- CT scan most useful imaging exam as it best assesses airway compromise and substernal extension in severe cases

Ultrasonographic Findings
- Prominent single or multiple nodules
  - May be hypoechoic or hyperechoic

CT Findings
- Multiple solid masses; some may have degenerative changes

Nuclear Medicine Findings
- Heterogeneous radiotracer uptake with nodular, asymmetric image

MACROSCOPIC

General Features
- Asymmetrically enlarged gland with multiple nodules of variable size
  - Dominant nodule frequently identified
  - Thyroid gland distorted by nodular enlargement
- Sectioning demonstrates nodularity and heterogeneity
  - Surrounding parenchyma firm and beefy red
  - Nodules pale tan, and degenerative changes common

- Central scarring
- Hemorrhage
- Fibrous pseudocapsule
- Ossification and calcification
- Marked cystic changes in larger nodules
- Multiple nodules (> 20) in young patients raise suspicion of inherited syndrome

Size

- Can range in size from extremely large to microscopic lesions found incidentally

MICROSCOPIC

Histologic Features

- General features
  - Nodules may compress surrounding uninvolved thyroid parenchyma
  - Nodules unencapsulated
  - Large follicles with abundant colloid
    - Papillary projections may be present mimicking carcinoma
    - Papillae simple, without arborization, and lack complexity as compared to papillary thyroid carcinoma
    - Cells have rounded basally located nuclei with coarse, dense chromatin
    - Cells maintain their polarity
- Areas of increased cellularity present throughout parenchyma
- Sanderson polsters may be present within follicular lumina
- Follicular cells
  - Flattened
  - Cuboidal or columnar
  - Hemosiderin may be present
  - Oncocytic changes may be present
  - Signet ring type vacuoles may be present in cytoplasm
  - Round, uniform, small nuclei
  - Nuclei lack nuclear features of papillary thyroid carcinoma
  - Oncocytic changes may occur
    - Abundant eosinophilic granular cytoplasm
    - Round nuclei with prominent cherry red macronucleoli
- Reactive changes
  - Hemorrhage
    - Hemosiderin-laden macrophages common
  - Cholesterol clefting
  - Fibrosis
  - Granulation tissue
  - Dystrophic calcification
  - Typical post-FNA site changes common as mass-forming lesions frequently undergo fine-needle aspiration biopsy
  - Follicular rupture and subsequent colloidal spill may lead to granuloma formation
    - These areas may appear similar to characteristic granulomas in palpation thyroiditis
- Metaplastic changes common
  - Most frequently osseous metaplasia
  - Cartilage, squamous, and adipose tissue may be present
- Concurrent neoplasms

- Papillary microcarcinoma common

ANCILLARY TESTS

Cytology

- Highly variable colloid
  - May be thin, viscous, scant, abundant, and serous to reddish brown
- Typical characteristics low cellularity
  - Large flat sheets of follicular epithelium in characteristic honeycomb arrangement
    - Monolayer of cells evenly spaced
    - Oncocytic cells may be present
- Nuclei round, small, and contain dense chromatin
- Background of hemosiderin-laden macrophages and foamy histiocytes may be present
  - Multinucleated giant cells may be present
- Has been recognized as common mimicker of follicular neoplasm on cytology

Immunohistochemistry

- Loss of PTEN IHC staining occurs in isolated nodules related to *PTEN* gene mutations/deletions
- Loss of PTEN expression [PTEN(-)] in thyroid nodules, whether in all nodules or in subset of nodules, is both sensitive and specific for these syndromes
- Thyroid follicular cells in background thyroid PTEN(+)
- Endothelial cells within adenomatous nodule show preserved expression of PTEN immunostaining
- PTEN immunoexpression serves as screening molecular correlate to predict for germline *PTEN* mutation in these syndromes

Genetic Testing

- Mutations in thyroglobulin, thyroperoxidase, sodium iodide transporter, and thyroid stimulating hormone receptor (TSHR) may be responsible for development of nodules
- RAS mutation may be present in some adenomatous nodules
- Majority of ANs nodules occur in sporadic setting
  - However, multiple and numerous ANs can be identified in inherited tumor syndromes
- Syndrome mostly associated with numerous AN is PTEN-hamartoma tumor syndrome
- Patients with PTEN-hamartoma tumor syndrome harbor germline inactivating mutations in *PTEN*
  - *PTEN* encodes tumor suppressor protein PTEN (phosphatase and tensin homolog protein)
  - Leading to clonal follicular epithelial proliferations in thyroid gland
  - Recognition of this syndrome is important so that cancer screening and genetic counseling can be initiated
- Other tests may be performed (as *PRKAR1A, GNAS, DICER1*) to identify other syndromes

DIFFERENTIAL DIAGNOSIS

Follicular Adenoma

- Solitary lesion
- Encapsulated
- Less colloid
- Tends to lack degenerative features

Adenomatous Nodules in Familial Syndromes

PTEN-Hamartoma Tumor Syndrome	Carney Complex	McCune-Albright Syndrome	DICER1 Syndrome
Germline inactivating mutations in *PTEN*	Germline mutations in *PRKAR1A* and amplification of 2p16-23	Mosaicism for spontaneous postzygotic mutation in *GNAS*	Mutations in *DICER1*
Encodes tumor suppressor protein PTEN	Leading to activation of protein kinase A pathway	Leading to increase in cAMP levels	Pleuropulmonary blastoma-family tumor predisposition syndrome
Leading to clonal thyroid follicular cell proliferation	Leading to development of benign hyperfunctioning thyroid follicular cell proliferation	With development of hyperthyroidism and follicular cell proliferation	Linked to childhood familial multinodular adenomatous hyperplasia

Dyshormonogenetic Goiter

- May have nodules but develop in characteristic fibrotic background
- Follicles irregularly shaped
- Lack of colloid

Papillary Thyroid Carcinoma

- Characteristic overlapping of tumor cells with marked follicular cell disarray
- Has characteristic nuclear features (clearing, pseudo-inclusions, indentations, nuclear membrane irregularities)
- May have papillary architecture, trabecular architecture, solid architecture
- Molecular and immunohistochemistry may be needed to distinguish difficult cases

Follicular Carcinoma

- Encapsulated
  - Capsule tends to be thick
- Neoplasm demonstrates capsular &/or vascular invasion
- Molecular testing may be necessary in difficult cases
  - However, AN does not have real fibrous capsule

Hyalinizing Trabecular Tumor

- Trabecular growth pattern of medium-sized elongated cells with numerous intranuclear inclusions and PAS(+) basement membrane material

DIAGNOSTIC CHECKLIST

Pathologic Interpretation Pearls

- Unencapsulated nodule with adjacent normal appearing thyroid
  - Microfollicular-patterned nodules
  - Encapsulated lesions should raise concern for other follicular lesions such as adenoma or carcinoma
- Loss of PTEN immunostaining within follicular cells may indicate inherited syndrome

SELECTED REFERENCES

1. Nosé V: Genodermatosis affecting the skin and mucosa of the head and neck: Clinicopathologic, genetic, and molecular aspect–PTEN-hamartoma tumor syndrome/Cowden syndrome. Head Neck Pathol. 10(2):131-8, 2016
2. Cameselle-Teijeiro J et al: Thyroid pathology findings in Cowden syndrome: A clue for the diagnosis of the PTEN hamartoma tumor syndrome. Am J Clin Pathol. 144(2):322-8, 2015
3. Feng X et al: Characteristics of benign and malignant thyroid disease in familial adenomatous polyposis patients and recommendations for disease surveillance. Thyroid. 25(3):325-32, 2015
4. Barletta JA et al: Immunohistochemical staining of thyroidectomy specimens for PTEN can aid in the identification of patients with Cowden syndrome. Am J Surg Pathol. 35(10):1505-11, 2011
5. Laury AR et al: Thyroid pathology in PTEN-hamartoma tumor syndrome: characteristic findings of a distinct entity. Thyroid. 21(2):135-44, 2011
6. Nosé V: Familial thyroid cancer: a review. Mod Pathol. 24 Suppl 2:S19-33, 2011
7. Smith JR et al: Thyroid nodules and cancer in children with PTEN hamartoma tumor syndrome. J Clin Endocrinol Metab. 96(1):34-7, 2011
8. Turanli S et al: Predictors of malignancy in patients with a thyroid nodule that contains Hürthle cells. Otolaryngol Head Neck Surg. 144(4):514-7, 2011
9. Zhang Y et al: Endocrine tumors as part of inherited tumor syndromes. Adv Anat Pathol. 18(3):206-18, 2011
10. Dabelić N et al: Malignancy risk assessment in adenomatoid nodules and suspicious follicular lesions of the thyroid obtained by fine needle aspiration cytology. Coll Antropol. 34(2):349-54, 2010
11. Nosé V: Familial follicular cell tumors: classification and morphological characteristics. Endocr Pathol. 21(4):219-26, 2010
12. Nosé V: Thyroid cancer of follicular cell origin in inherited tumor syndromes. Adv Anat Pathol. 17(6):428-36, 2010
13. Schreiner AM et al: Adenomatoid nodules are the main cause for discrepant histology in 234 thyroid fine-needle aspirates reported as follicular neoplasm. Diagn Cytopathol. Epub ahead of print, 2010
14. Mihai R et al: One in four patients with follicular thyroid cytology (THY3) has a thyroid carcinoma. Thyroid. 19(1):33-7, 2009
15. Nayar R et al: The indeterminate thyroid fine-needle aspiration: experience from an academic center using terminology similar to that proposed in the 2007 National Cancer Institute Thyroid Fine Needle Aspiration State of the Science Conference. Cancer. 117(3):195-202, 2009
16. Nosé V et al: Hyalinizing trabecular tumor of the thyroid: an update. Endocr Pathol. 19(1):1-8, 2008
17. Yassa L et al: Long-term assessment of a multidisciplinary approach to thyroid nodule diagnostic evaluation. Cancer. 111(6):508-16, 2007
18. Deveci MS et al: Fine-needle aspiration of follicular lesions of the thyroid. Diagnosis and follow-Up. Cytojournal. 3:9, 2006
19. Malle D et al: Use of a thin-layer technique in thyroid fine needle aspiration. Acta Cytol. 50(1):23-7, 2006
20. Zagorianakou P et al: The role of fine-needle aspiration biopsy in the management of patients with thyroid nodules. In Vivo. 19(3):605-9, 2005
21. Oertel YC et al: Diagnosis of malignant epithelial thyroid lesions: fine needle aspiration and histopathologic correlation. Ann Diagn Pathol. 2(6):377-400, 1998

(Left) *Axial T1WI MR reveals asymmetric enlargement of the right thyroid lobe with an ill-defined, rounded area of slightly lower intensity* ➡. *Focal hyperintensities* ➡ *are from hemorrhage or calcium.* (Right) *Axial T2WI MR shows uniform hyperintensity of a thyroid nodule* ➡ *that appears more clearly defined and does not extend outside the gland. No neck adenopathy is present.*

Thyroid Nodule

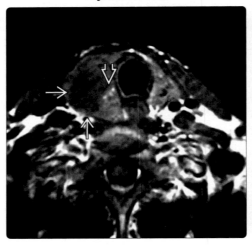

Thyroid Nodule

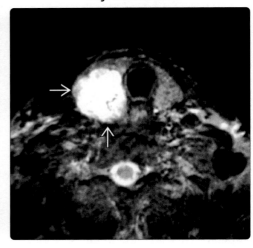

(Left) *Gross photo of a large AN shows central degenerative changes* ➡. *There are multiple smaller ANs* ➡ *and an encapsulated lesion (follicular carcinoma)* ➡. (Right) *Low-power microphotograph of ANs highlights the compression of adjacent thyroid parenchyma. Note that the ANs are unencapsulated and that the adjacent thyroid parenchyma is atrophic.*

Multiple Thyroid Nodules

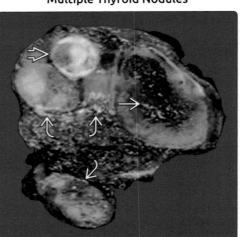

Nodules With Compressed Thyroid Follicles

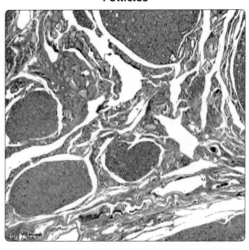

(Left) *Photomicrograph of thyroid in a patient with PTEN-hamartoma tumor syndrome shows multiple ANs and adjacent intervening thyroid parenchyma. There is prominent lymphatic dilatation* ➡ *within the thyroid.* (Right) *ANs have features similar to follicular adenomas, with typical follicular architecture with follicles of various sizes, lined by follicular cells with homogeneous regular nuclei, and with abundant colloid.*

Adenomatous Nodules and Compressed Thyroid Parenchyma

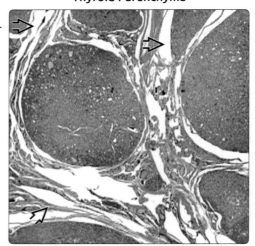

Small Uniform Follicles

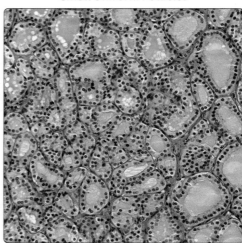

Small Follicles With Uniform Nuclei

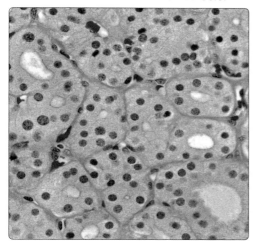

Uniform Follicles and Interstitial Fibrosis

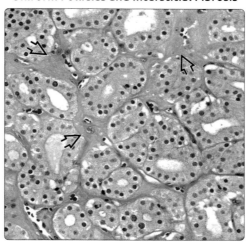

(Left) ANs have similar morphologic findings as follicular adenoma with homogeneous uniform follicles, with pale pink cytoplasm and small round uniform nuclei. However, these nodules are unencapsulated. (Right) ANs have homogeneous, uniformly round follicles, with pale pink cytoplasm and small, round, uniform nuclei. This area of the nodule is centrally located and shows interstitial fibrosis ⊟.

Homogeneous Follicular Appearance

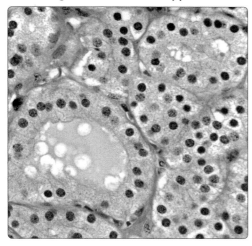

PTEN(-) in Adenomatous Nodules and PTEN(+) in Normal Thyroid

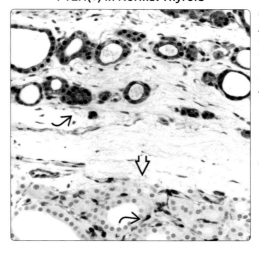

(Left) Thyroid pathology findings suggestive of PTEN-hamartoma tumor syndromes include multiple ANs. These nodules have similar morphologic findings as follicular adenoma with homogeneous follicles. (Right) Loss of PTEN expression in thyroid ANs ⊟, whether in all nodules or in a subset of nodules, is both sensitive and specific for these syndromes. The thyroid follicular cells ⊟ in the background thyroid and endothelial cells within nodule are PTEN(+).

Preservation of PTEN in Adenomatous Nodules

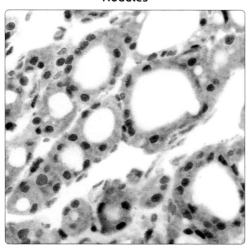

Adenomatous Nodules in Patient With Syndrome

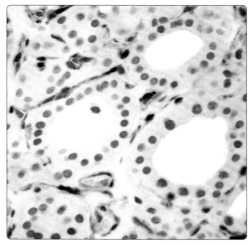

(Left) AN with preservation of PTEN immunoexpression shows nuclear and cytoplasmic staining. (Right) Loss of PTEN expression in thyroid nodules, whether in all nodules or in a subset of nodules, is both sensitive and specific for PTEN-hamartoma syndrome. Note the positivity in endothelial cells.

Pigments and Crystals, Thyroid

TERMINOLOGY

- Deposition of material within thyroid
  - Lipofuscin, calcium oxalate, minocycline, iron

CLINICAL ISSUES

- Tends to occur in older patients when processes conducive to pigments and crystals have had time to manifest themselves within thyroid tissue
- No prognostic implications
- Pigments and crystals are not associated with abnormal laboratory findings clinically significant for thyroid dysfunction
- Pigments and crystals are incidental findings in patients who had their thyroid gland removed for other purposes

MICROSCOPIC

- Iron
  - Hemosiderin can be found within follicular epithelial cells, macrophages, and within stroma

- Special stains for iron may be used to distinguish hemosiderin from other pigments
- Lipofuscin
  - Intracytoplasmic accumulation of granular, light brown pigment
- Minocycline
  - Histology shows granular, black pigment within apical portion of thyroid follicular cells
- Crystals
  - Crystal deposition within thyroid is exclusively found within colloid
  - Crystals are composed of calcium oxalate
- Amiodarone
  - Large involuting follicles with areas of degeneration and destruction of follicles
  - Follicles filled with swollen and foamy cells that may contain fine pigmented material

Black Minocycline Pigment

Crystals Within Colloid

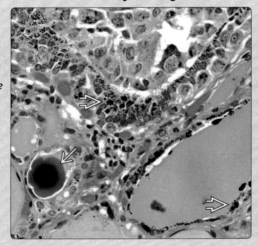
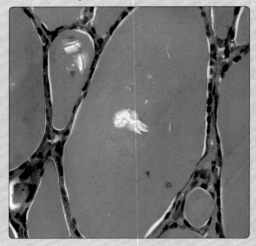

(Left) Intracytoplasmic, granular, black minocycline pigment is present within the follicular epithelial cells ⇒. Pigment also accumulates in the colloid ➡ of the follicular lumen. (Right) Calcium oxalate crystals are present in the colloid and within the follicular lumen.

Hemosiderin

Crystals Under Polarized Light

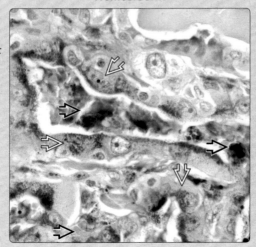
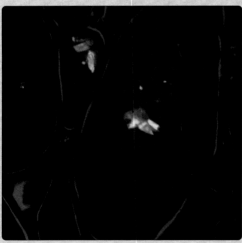

(Left) Hemosiderin pigment is usually present within thyroid parenchyma after fine-needle aspiration biopsy. The pigment is seen in the cytoplasm of follicular cells ➡ and in the macrophages ⇒. (Right) Calcium oxalate crystals within colloid are better identified under polarized microscopy.

TERMINOLOGY

Synonyms

- Black thyroid
  - Name is specifically applied to minocycline-induced discoloration of thyroid gland

Definitions

- Deposition of material within thyroid
  - Lipofuscin
  - Minocycline metabolites
  - Crystals
  - Iron
  - Amiodarone

ETIOLOGY/PATHOGENESIS

Environmental Exposure

- Lipofuscin
  - Product of aging similar to lipofuscin deposition in other organs composed of tryptophan and histidine
  - Lipofuscin is product of oxidation of fatty acids
- Minocycline
  - Commonly administered antibiotic
  - Antibiotic minocycline is tetracycline derivative
  - Prolonged treatment with this drug causes striking black discoloration of thyroid
    - Antibiotic minocycline is virtually pathognomonic for brown-black discoloration of thyroid gland referred to as black thyroid
    - Black thyroid is incidental finding in patients taking drug who undergo thyroid surgery for another indication
  - Can also cause black pigmentation within skin
  - Components of black pigment are not fully understood
    - Thought to result from oxidative degradation of drug
  - Has been investigated as associative condition to papillary thyroid carcinoma
    - Results have been inconclusive
  - Has been associated with hyalinizing trabecular tumor of thyroid, papillary thyroid carcinoma, and other tumors
  - Black thyroid can also be attributable to iodine-containing compound indocyanine green
    - Indocyanine green is cause of black thyroid with histopathological features similar to that induced by minocycline
  - Minocycline pigment is also described in diverse places, as
    - Aorta
    - Atherosclerotic plaques
    - Black bone disease
    - Eye minocycline-induced hyperpigmentation
- Amiodarone
  - Amiodarone is effective cardiac antiarrhythmic drug
  - Long-term, high-dose use of drug is associated with skin discoloration, corneal deposition, and alterations in thyroid hormone levels
  - Amiodarone-induced thyrotoxicosis is due to release of thyroxin as result of thyroid follicle destruction
- Iron
  - Commonly seen in thyroid in areas of hemorrhage in nodular goiter or around previous biopsy site
  - Most frequently result of release of iron from red blood cells
    - Resorption of iron and conversion to hemosiderin by macrophages
  - Disorders of iron metabolism, including cases in which trauma is associated with degeneration and hemorrhage, can lead to iron deposition in thyroid follicular cells
  - Rarely, may be result of hereditary disorders of iron metabolism
    - Hereditary hemochromatosis
- Crystals
  - Most commonly calcium oxalate
    - Associated with renal failure

CLINICAL ISSUES

Epidemiology

- Age
  - Tends to occur in older patients when processes conducive to pigments and crystals have had time to manifest themselves within thyroid tissue
- Sex
  - No predilection for either gender

Presentation

- Incidental finding
  - Pigments and crystals are incidental findings in patients who had their thyroid gland removed for other purposes

Laboratory Tests

- Pigments and crystals are not associated with abnormal laboratory findings clinically significant for thyroid dysfunction

Treatment

- Not necessary

Prognosis

- No prognostic implications

MACROSCOPIC

General Features

- Minocycline
  - Thyroid gland is normal in size and has dark brown to black color and may show only minimal fibrosis
- Amiodarone
  - Diffusely enlarged thyroid

MICROSCOPIC

Histologic Features

- Iron
  - Hemosiderin can be found within follicular epithelial cells, macrophages, and within stroma
  - Hemosiderin has characteristic brown-yellow color
    - Intracytoplasmic and stromal accumulation of granular pigment
  - Special stains for iron may be used to distinguish hemosiderin from other pigments

- o Hemosiderin is usually seen in setting of reorganizing tissue after hemorrhage, prior fine-needle aspiration, or associated with multinodular hyperplasia
- o Location of hemosiderin has been proposed to be possible indication of neoplastic disease
  - Remains controversial
- o Occasionally, increased fibrosis may be present
- Amiodarone
  - o Pathology of amiodarone is characterized by diffusely enlarged hyperplastic gland
  - o On histology, shows large involuting follicles with areas of degeneration and destruction of follicles, which are filled with swollen and foamy cells that may contain fine pigmented material
  - o These degenerated follicles are associated with areas of fibrosis and nonspecific chronic inflammation
- Lipofuscin
  - o As in other organs, lipofuscin may be seen in thyroid follicular cells
  - o Incidental finding in number of thyroid specimens
- Minocycline
  - o Histology shows granular black pigment within apical portion of thyroid follicular cells
  - o Pigment usually localizes within cytoplasm of follicular epithelial cells
  - o Can be seen within colloid as large black depositions
  - o May localize to pathologic or nonpathologic component of resected thyroid gland
  - o Granulomatous reaction to black colloid with numerous histiocytes and giant cells may occur
    - In these cases, findings must be differentiated from subacute granulomatous thyroiditis
- Crystals
  - o Crystal deposition within thyroid is exclusively found within colloid
    - Crystals are composed of calcium oxalate
  - o Calcium oxalate crystals are frequently found in normal thyroid tissue
  - o Readily identified via light microscopy and polarization
  - o Commonly seen in nodular goiters and follicular adenomas
  - o May be seen in association with thyroid malignancies
  - o Not frequently identified in thyroiditis
  - o Anisotropic crystals commonly seen in older patients with normal thyroid glands
  - o Presence of these crystals also help guide pathologist to identification of thyroid origin during frozen section of follicular-patterned lesions
    - Differentiating parathyroid with pseudofollicular architecture from thyroid tissue can be challenging on intraoperative frozen sections
    - Birefringent calcium oxalate crystals are present in colloid of normal thyroid follicles, whereas crystals are rare in parathyroid tissue

DIFFERENTIAL DIAGNOSIS

Melanoma

- Extremely rare but has been known to metastasize to thyroid and may have characteristic melanin pigment

DIAGNOSTIC CHECKLIST

Pathologic Interpretation Pearls

- Iron: Intracytoplasmic and stromal accumulation of granular, yellow-brown pigment
- Minocycline: Granular, black pigment within apical portion of thyroid follicular cells and within colloid
- Lipofuscin: Delicate brown pigment
- Amiodarone: Involuting follicles with foamy cells that may contain finely pigmented material
- Calcium oxalate crystals: Birefringency within colloid

SELECTED REFERENCES

1. Chernock RD et al: Novel cause of 'black thyroid': intraoperative use of indocyanine green. Endocr Pathol. ePub, 2016
2. Nishimoto K et al: A case of minocycline-induced black thyroid associated with papillary carcinoma. Ear Nose Throat J. 95(3):E28-31, 2016
3. Pusztaszeri M: Birefringent crystals in thyroid fine-needle aspiration cytology. Diagn Cytopathol. 44(10):814-5, 2016
4. Bann DV et al: Black thyroid. Ear Nose Throat J. 93(10-11):E54-5, 2014
5. Bosma JW et al: A brown-eyed woman with blue discoloration of the sclera. minocycline-induced hyperpigmentation. Neth J Med. 72(1):33, 37, 2014
6. Wong KS et al: Utility of birefringent crystal identification by polarized light microscopy in distinguishing thyroid from parathyroid tissue on intraoperative frozen sections. Am J Surg Pathol. 38(9):1212-9, 2014
7. Gonzalez-Arriagada WA et al: Facial pigmentation associated with amiodarone. Gen Dent. 61(4):e15-7, 2013
8. Reed DN et al: Minocycline-induced black bone disease encountered during total knee arthroplasty. Orthopedics. 35(5):e737-9, 2012
9. Kandil E et al: Papillary thyroid carcinoma in black thyroids. Head Neck. 33(12):1735-8, 2011
10. Jaffar R et al: Hemosiderin laden macrophages and hemosiderin within follicular cells distinguish benign follicular lesions from follicular neoplasms. Cytojournal. 6:3, 2009
11. Kang SW et al: A case of black thyroid associated with hyalinizing trabecular tumor. Endocr J. 55(6):1109-12, 2008
12. Oertel YC: Black thyroid syndrome. Thyroid. 17(9):905, 2007
13. Sharma V et al: A case of trabecular adenoma of the thyroid with black pigmentation. Thyroid. 17(6):593-4, 2007
14. Raptis L et al: It's all in the face: amiodarone-induced myxedema and skin pigmentation. Eur J Dermatol. 16(5):590-1, 2006
15. Birkedal C et al: Minocycline-induced black thyroid gland: medical curiosity or a marker for papillary cancer? Curr Surg. 58(5):470-1, 2001
16. Bahadir S et al: Amiodarone pigmentation, eye and thyroid alterations. J Eur Acad Dermatol Venereol. 14(3):194-5, 2000
17. Shimizu M et al: Calcium oxalate crystals in thyroid fine needle aspiration cytology. Acta Cytol. 43(4):575-8, 1999
18. Dalefield RR et al: Lipofuscin and abnormalities in colloid in the equine thyroid gland in relation to age. J Comp Pathol. 111(4):389-99, 1994

Findings in Black Thyroid

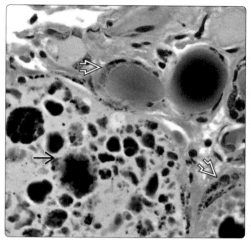

Minocycline Granulomatous Reaction

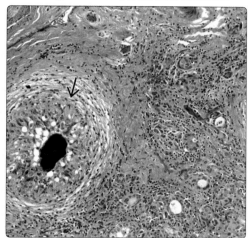

(Left) *Minocycline pigment is present within macrophages in follicular lumen* ➡ *and as granular pigment in the cytoplasm of follicular cells* ➡. **(Right)** *Low-power view of a thyroid of a patient treated with minocycline, showing a giant-cell granulomas with centered the black colloid. This granulomatous inflammation* ➡ *contains giant cells and histiocytes and must be differentiated from subacute granulomatous thyroiditis.*

Giant Cell Granuloma to Minocycline

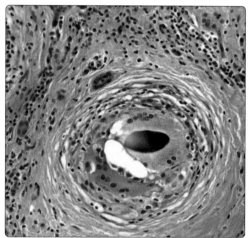

Iron Pigment in Prior FNA Site

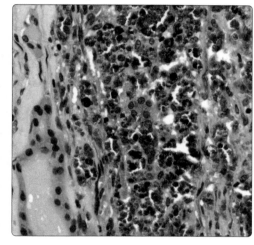

(Left) *Black minocycline pigment is usually seen within colloid and in the apical portion of the follicular cells. In this case, numerous giant-cell granulomas had centered the black colloid.* **(Right)** *Iron pigment is commonly seen in the thyroid in areas of hem-orrhage in a nodular goiter or around a previous biopsy site or trauma.*

Giant Cell

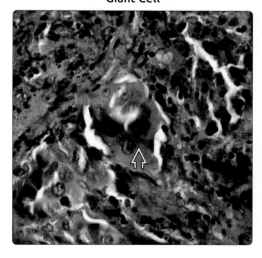

Extensive Hemosiderin Deposition

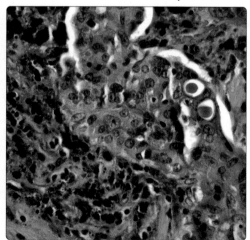

(Left) *Hemosiderin pigment is usually present within thyroid parenchyma after fine-needle aspiration biopsy. A foreign-body giant cell containing granular, golden brown pigment is present* ➡. **(Right)** *Hemosiderin pigment resulted from the release of iron from red blood cells in an area of trauma or rupture of follicles. Resorption of iron and conversion to hemosiderin is done by macrophages.*

TERMINOLOGY

- Tumor of germ cell origin composed of mature or immature tissues derived from all 3 germ cell layers
  - Ectoderm, mesoderm, and endoderm

CLINICAL ISSUES

- Thyroid teratoma has bimodal age distribution
- Neonates and infants: Majority are benign (> 90%)
- Children and adults: ~ 1/2 are malignant
- Patients may present with significant dyspnea, difficulty breathing, and stridor
- Patients diagnosed with thyroid teratomas in newborn period are treated with surgical resection
- If untreated by surgery, neonatal cases will result in death due to severe airway obstruction and mass effect
- In cases of malignant teratoma, chemotherapy may be used ± radiotherapy, although treatment is only palliative

MACROSCOPIC

- Most show smooth and glistening capsule; congested subcapsular vessels or subcapsular hemorrhage may be present
- On cross sections, tumor can have predominantly solid, cystic, or mixed solid-cystic pattern

MICROSCOPIC

- Intimate admixture of thyroid and other tissues with surrounding fibrous pseudocapsule
- Variable amounts of mature and immature tissues from 3 germ cell layers

TOP DIFFERENTIAL DIAGNOSES

- Cervical teratomas
- Cystic hygroma
- Hemangioma
- Small blue round cell tumors

Thyroid Teratoma in Fetus

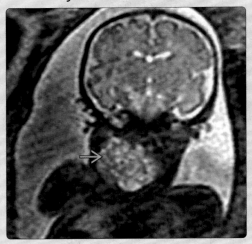

Gross Surface of Thyroid Teratoma

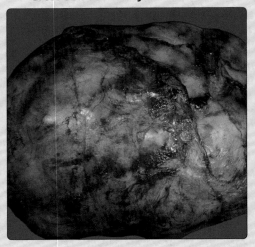

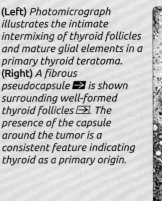

(Left) Magnetic resonance, coronal single shot fast spin echo T2-weighted, shows a heterogeneous cystic and solid mass within the neck ⟹ of a male fetus in uterus during the 3rd trimester. (Right) This gross photograph of a thyroid teratoma removed from a newborn displays a well-circumscribed tumor completely surrounded by a smooth and glistening capsule. This multinodular mass is predominantly solid.

Thyroid Follicles and Glia

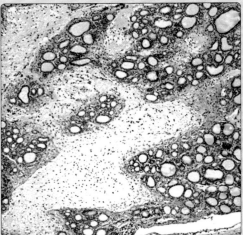

Fibrous Pseudocapsule and Follicles

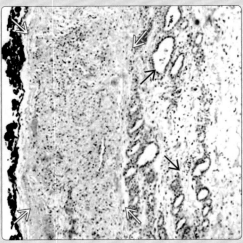

(Left) Photomicrograph illustrates the intimate intermixing of thyroid follicles and mature glial elements in a primary thyroid teratoma. (Right) A fibrous pseudocapsule ⟹ is shown surrounding well-formed thyroid follicles ⟹. The presence of the capsule around the tumor is a consistent feature indicating thyroid as a primary origin.

TERMINOLOGY

Synonyms

- Teratoma of thyroid gland

Definitions

- Tumor of germ cell origin composed of mature or immature tissues derived from all 3 germ cell layers: Ectoderm, mesoderm, and endoderm
  - Ectoderm: Neural tissue, choroid plexus, pigmented cells, skin, hair, etc.
  - Mesoderm: Skeletal muscle, cartilage, bone, fat, connective tissue, etc.
  - Endoderm: GI mucosa, liver, pancreas, urothelium, lung, etc.
- Thyroid teratomas are defined only when following criteria are present
  - Presence of fibrous pseudocapsule
  - Intimate intermingling of thyroid tissue with teratoma
  - Tumor occupies thyroid gland or portion of it
  - Close anatomic relationship between tumor and thyroid gland
  - Direct continuity between tumor and thyroid gland

ETIOLOGY/PATHOGENESIS

Developmental Anomaly

- Arise from misplaced embryonic germ cell rests
  - Embryonic rests from 3 germ cell layers within thyroid continue to develop in new location

CLINICAL ISSUES

Epidemiology

- Incidence
  - Cervical teratomas are very rare, although they are most common neck tumors in newborns and infants
  - Thyroid teratomas are rare: < 0.1 % of all primary thyroid tumors
- Age
  - Occurs in broad age range, from newborn to up 90 yr of age
  - Thyroid teratoma has bimodal age distribution
    - These tumors occur in neonates and infants and in patients > 50 yr
    - Neonates and infants: Majority are benign (> 90%)
    - Children and adults: ~ 1/2 are malignant teratomas
- Sex
  - Equal gender distribution

Presentation

- Commonly presents as large neck mass
  - Tumors in neck occupy thyroid gland area
  - Tumors can be extremely large
- Patients may present with significant shortness of breath, difficulty breathing, and stridor
- Many times diagnosis is made prenatally

Natural History

- If untreated by surgery, neonatal cases will result in death due to severe airway obstruction and mass effect

Treatment

- Options, risks, complications
  - Treatment and outcomes depend on age of patient and tumor size at presentation
- Surgical approaches
  - Patients diagnosed with thyroid teratomas in newborn period should be treated with surgical resection
    - Surgical resection is treatment of choice for neonatal teratoma
    - Surgery must be performed immediately in neonatal patients to avoid complications
  - Surgical excision for benign or immature teratomas is treatment of choice
- Adjuvant therapy
  - In cases of malignant teratoma, chemotherapy may be used ± radiotherapy, although treatment is only palliative

Prognosis

- Prognosis and tumor histology correlates with age at presentation
  - Neonates and infants have benign or immature teratomas
  - Children and adults have preponderance of malignant teratomas
- Neonates and infants with benign, mature, or immature teratomas do not die from disease
  - Death is usually result of local effect and complications of airway obstruction, tracheal compression, or lack of development of neck structures during development
  - Neonatal teratomas must be surgically resected immediately after birth to avoid preoperative morbidity and mortality
  - Case of neonatal thyroid teratoma with immature neuroblastoma-like elements and spread to multiple cervical lymph nodes has been reported
    - After excision of tumor and nodes, baby remained disease free and well for > 5 yr, which reinforces notion that neonatal teratomas tend to have benign course if excised
- Malignant teratomas have clinically aggressive behavior and may invade adjacent structures
  - Local recurrence and metastases to lung occur in < 1/2 of patients
  - Most malignant teratomas have fatal outcome

IMAGING

Ultrasonographic Findings

- Ultrasound is useful diagnostic modality that can provide helpful information as early as in utero
- Heterogeneous thyroid masses containing solid and cystic areas sometimes with fatty or calcific elements

MR Findings

- Multiloculated solid or cystic structure with high signal on T2-weighted images
- Bulk of lesion is usually unilateral extending to midline
- Encapsulation is common

CT Findings

- Well-defined solid and cystic mass that may contain fat nodules
- Distortion and compression of airways and neck structures may be noted

Radiologic Differential Diagnosis

- Cystic hygroma, congenital hemangioma, congenital infantile fibrosarcoma, and rhabdomyosarcoma

MACROSCOPIC

General Features

- Most show smooth and glistening capsule; congested subcapsular vessels or subcapsular hemorrhage may be present
- Multinodular masses or multiloculated cysts are common
- On cross sections, tumor can have predominantly solid, cystic, or mixed solid-cystic pattern
- Most tumors show thyroid and other tissue types intimately intermixed
- Frequently, thyroid is only point of attachment between tumor and normal structures of neck

Sections to Be Submitted

- Sections of thyroid tissue intermixed with other teratoma components
- Sections of periphery to demonstrate surrounding thyroid gland and presence of capsule

Size

- Median reported size is 7 cm (range: 3.5-13.5 cm)

MICROSCOPIC

Histologic Features

- Intimate admixture of thyroid and other tissues with surrounding fibrous pseudocapsule
- In congenital/neonatal thyroid teratomas, immature neuroglial tissue is often identified
- Variable amounts of mature and immature tissues from 3 germ cell layers
- Necrosis and calcification can be present

ANCILLARY TESTS

Cytology

- Cellular specimens may show various tissue components

Immunohistochemistry

- Can be used to help identify tissue types, especially useful for immature components

DIFFERENTIAL DIAGNOSIS

Cervical Teratomas

- Teratomas arising in neck region outside thyroid may have thyroid tissue as component
- Spatial continuity of teratoma with thyroid should be interpreted with caution
- Intimate intermingling of thyroid tissue and other components of tumor and presence of pseudocapsule separating tumor from residual normal thyroid are best indicators of primary thyroid teratoma

Small Blue Round Cell Tumors

- Rhabdomyosarcoma, small cell carcinoma, lymphoma, melanoma, Ewing sarcoma
- Histology, immunohistochemistry, and clinical history are often sufficient to make distinction

Cystic Hygroma

- a.k.a. cavernous lymphangiomas, cystic hygromas are congenital multiloculated lymphatic lesions that can occasionally arise on anterior aspect of neck
- Radiographically, may present as cyst, may show septations, may have infiltrative appearance, and may be uni- or multilocular
- Microscopically, composed of endothelium-lined cystic spaces with scanty stroma

Hemangiomas

- Vascular lesions that appear on ultrasound as homogeneous soft tissue masses and may appear cystic; vascular flow can be demonstrated with Doppler
- Small echogenicities representing calcifications can be present (phleboliths)
- Microscopically, composed of endothelium-lined vascular spaces of variable sizes

DIAGNOSTIC CHECKLIST

Clinically Relevant Pathologic Features

- Age distribution
  - Thyroid teratoma has bimodal age distribution
    - Neonates and infants have benign or immature teratomas
    - Children and adults: ~ 1/2 are malignant teratomas

Pathologic Interpretation Pearls

- Presence of fibrous pseudocapsule: Single most significant criterion to establish diagnosis of primary thyroid teratoma
- Spatial continuity of thyroid and teratoma: Not sufficient and should be regarded as questionable argument in favor of this diagnosis

SELECTED REFERENCES

1. Rabinowits G et al: Successful management of a patient with malignant thyroid teratoma. Thyroid. 27(1):125-128, 2017
2. Alexander VR et al: Head and neck teratomas in children-a series of 23 cases at Great Ormond Street Hospital. Int J Pediatr Otorhinolaryngol. 79(12):2008-14, 2015
3. du Toit J et al: Let's face it - 13 unusual causes of facial masses in children. Insights Imaging. 6(5):519-30, 2015
4. Sheikh F et al: Prenatally diagnosed neck masses: long-term outcomes and quality of life. J Pediatr Surg. 50(7):1210-3, 2015
5. Zielinski R et al: Retrospective chart review of 44 fetuses with cervicofacial tumors in the sonographic assessment. Int J Pediatr Otorhinolaryngol. 79(3):363-8, 2015
6. Corrias A et al: Diagnostic features of thyroid nodules in pediatrics. Arch Pediatr Adolesc Med. 164(8):714-9, 2010
7. Martino F et al: Teratomas of the neck and mediastinum in children. Pediatr Surg Int. 22(8):627-34, 2006
8. Heerema-McKenney A et al: Congenital teratoma: a clinicopathologic study of 22 fetal and neonatal tumors. Am J Surg Pathol. 29(1):29-38, 2005
9. Riedlinger WF et al: Primary thyroid teratomas in children: a report of 11 cases with a proposal of criteria for their diagnosis. Am J Surg Pathol. 29(5):700-6, 2005
10. Thompson LD et al: Primary thyroid teratomas: a clinicopathologic study of 30 cases. Cancer. 88(5):1149-58, 2000
11. Wakhlu A et al: Head and neck teratomas in children. Pediatr Surg Int. 16(5-6):333-7, 2000

Cervical Mass

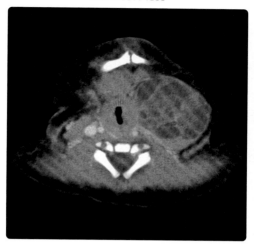

Solid and Cystic Neck Mass

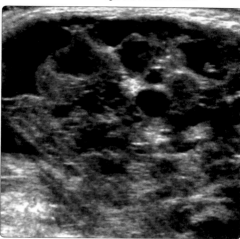

(Left) *Cross-sectional CT imaging reveals cervical mass arising in the central portion of the neck. The mass compresses and causes contralateral deviation of the airways and cervical structures. This lesion has solid and cystic areas.* (Right) *In utero ultrasound of a thyroid teratoma displays the typical appearance of a heterogeneous complex solid and cystic mass. The differential diagnosis includes hemangiomas and cystic hygromas. Doppler imaging can be helpful in establishing the diagnosis.*

Homogeneous Neck Mass

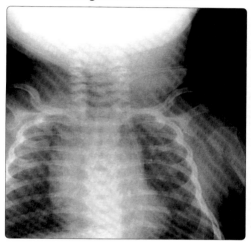

Newborn Baby With Large Neck Mass

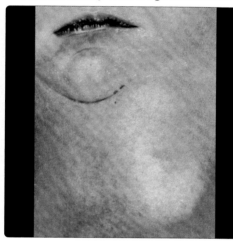

(Left) *Radiograph shows a homogeneous shadow of the neck mass that originates in the central portion of the neck and extends to the left. Distortion of cervical soft tissue structures causing difficulty breathing is a common complication of thyroid teratomas.* (Right) *Clinical photograph shows a cervical mass in a newborn occupying the anterior aspect of the neck and extending to the left. The clinical differential diagnosis for such a lesion includes hemangiomas and cystic hygromas.*

MR of Newborn With Neck Mass

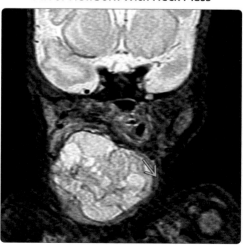

Newborn With Cystic and Solid Neck Mass

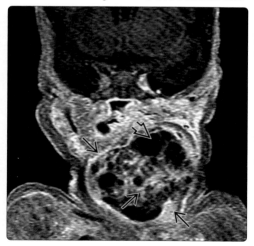

(Left) *Fast spin echo inversion recovery magnetic resonance from the same baby boy in the previous image, now at 1 day of age, demonstrates enlargement of the mass with compression and distortion of the airways ⮕.* (Right) *T1-weighted MR shows cystic ⮕ and solid components ⮕ of a neck mass. The lesion is completely encased by a capsule.*

Gross Appearance at Surgery

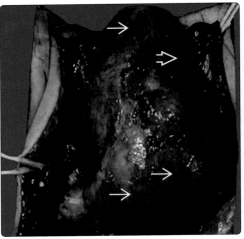

Thin Fibrous Capsule

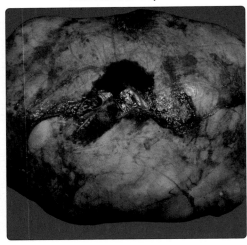

(Left) *This image was obtained from an intraoperative consultation. The picture shows a well-demarcated tumor surrounded by a glistening capsule. Congested capsular vessels* ➡ *and a focus of subcapsular hemorrhage* ⇒ *are noted.* (Right) *A fibrous capsule with congested vasculature and subcapsular hemorrhage is seen. Thorough evaluation of the capsule should be performed to identify adjacent thyroid parenchyma and to rule out invasion.*

Prominent Vessels and Cystic Changes

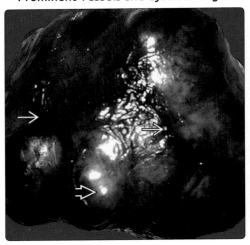

Cut Surface of Thyroid Teratoma

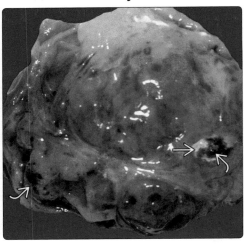

(Left) *Resection specimen in frontal view shows a lobulated tumor completely involved by a thin glistening capsule. Fine congested capsular vessels* ➡ *and bulging fluid-filled cysts are noted* ⇒*.* (Right) *The bisected cut surface of the tumor reveals a variegated and glistening appearance with multiple solid and cystic components. Focal areas of necrosis* ➡*, hemorrhage* ➡*, and pigment deposition are seen.*

Multinodular Appearance

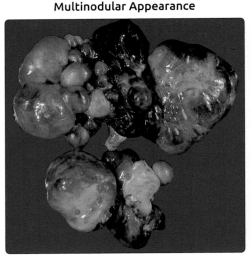

Teratoma Surface With Cysts

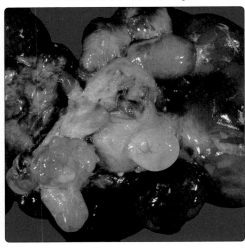

(Left) *Another common gross appearance of thyroid teratomas is shown. This tumor forms heterogeneous multilobular complex masses. Even though it is very irregular in shape, the smooth and glistening capsule is still noticeable throughout the specimen surface.* (Right) *Closer view of the lesion shows encapsulated solid and cystic areas with marked variation in size, color, and cyst contents. No tissue resembling normal thyroid is grossly identifiable.*

Thyroid Follicles, Glia, and Epithelium

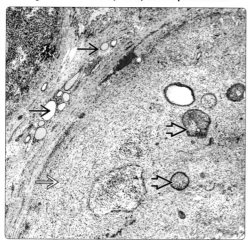

Thyroid Follicles, Neural Tissue, Epithelium

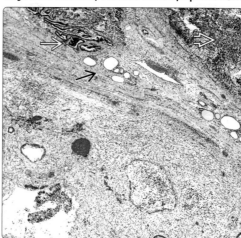

(Left) *Photomicrograph shows the hallmark of teratomas: The intermixing of thyroid follicles ⇒ with elements derived from diverse embryonal layers. Teratoma components identified in this field include mature neuropil ➡, immature neuroglia, and islands of squamous epithelium ⇛.* (Right) *In this H&E, thyroid follicles ⇒ are closely juxtaposed to ciliated epithelium resembling fallopian tube ➡. Immature neural tissue is also noticed in this slide ⇛.*

Mesenchymal and Epithelial Tissues

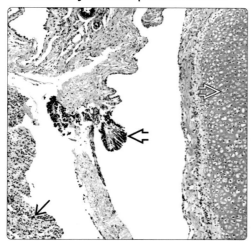

Thyroid Follicles, Adipose Tissue, and Glia

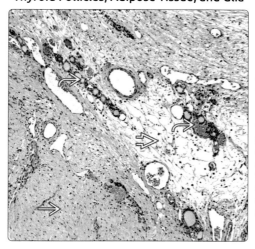

(Left) *This figure illustrates epithelial and mesenchymal-derived tissues found at the center of a teratoma mass. Pigmented epithelium resembling choroid plexus ⇛ and hyalin-type cartilage ⇛ are displayed. Mature-appearing glial elements ⇒ are also present.* (Right) *Low-power view shows thyroid follicles ➡ permeating fibroadipose tissue. Tissue components in this teratoma include adipose tissue ⇛ and neuronal-type tissue ➡ with prominent blood vessels.*

Thyroid Follicles and Epithelium

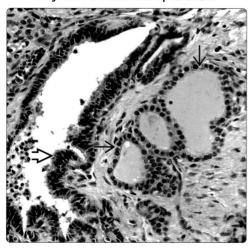

Neuropil Intermixed With Follicles

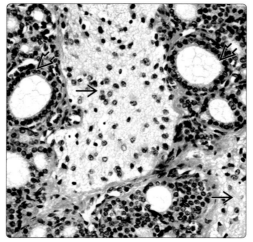

(Left) *High-power magnification shows thyroid follicles with abundant eosinophilic colloid ⇛ adjacent to pseudostratified ciliated cylindrical epithelium ⇛ reminiscent of the cells of the respiratory system.* (Right) *High-power view illustrates the typical intimate intermingling of thyroid follicles ⇛ with tissue elements of the teratoma. In this field, groups of thyroid follicles are permeated by sheets of mature fibrillary neuropil ⇛.*

Follicular Adenoma

TERMINOLOGY

- Follicular adenoma (FA): Benign, encapsulated, noninvasive neoplasm showing evidence of thyroid follicular cell differentiation without nuclear features of papillary thyroid carcinoma

ETIOLOGY/PATHOGENESIS

- After radiation exposure or in iodine-deficient areas
- Inherited tumor syndromes
  - PTEN-hamartoma tumor syndrome (PHTS): Cowden disease and Bannayan-Riley-Ruvalcaba syndrome (BRRS) syndrome
  - Pendred syndrome
  - Carney complex

CLINICAL ISSUES

- Most patients present with solitary nodule
- Multiple adenomatous nodules and adenomas may be part of inherited tumor syndromes

MICROSCOPIC

- Variants
  - Hyperfunctioning (so-called toxic or hot) adenoma
  - FA with papillary hyperplasia
  - Lipoadenoma (so-called adenolipoma)
  - Signet ring cell FA
  - Signet ring cell FA
  - Clear cell FA
  - Spindle cell FA
  - Black FA

TOP DIFFERENTIAL DIAGNOSES

- Follicular carcinoma
- Noninvasive follicular neoplasm with papillary-like nuclear features
- Adenomatous nodules
- Hyalinizing trabecular tumor

Gross Features

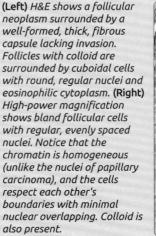

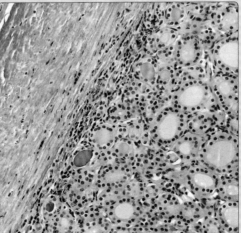

Cut Surface of Large Adenoma

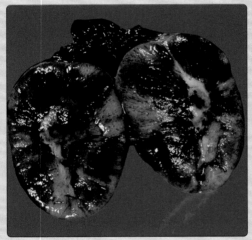

(Left) *Cross section shows a well-circumscribed, encapsulated lesion with a cut surface that is homogeneous and pale compared to normal thyroid tissue. Processing of the specimen to ensure extensive sampling of the tumor capsule throughout the lesion is critical to evaluate capsular &/or vascular invasion.* (Right) *There is a thin, fibrous capsule separating the neoplasm from the surrounding compressed parenchyma. This neoplasm has areas of hemorrhage and central degenerative changes.*

Follicular Adenoma: Thick Fibrous Capsule

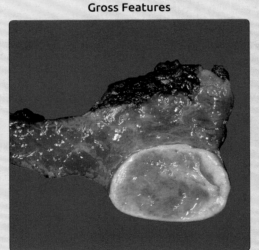

Follicular Adenoma: Morphology

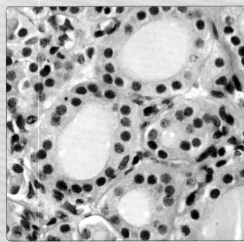

(Left) *H&E shows a follicular neoplasm surrounded by a well-formed, thick, fibrous capsule lacking invasion. Follicles with colloid are surrounded by cuboidal cells with round, regular nuclei and eosinophilic cytoplasm.* (Right) *High-power magnification shows bland follicular cells with regular, evenly spaced nuclei. Notice that the chromatin is homogeneous (unlike the nuclei of papillary carcinoma), and the cells respect each other's boundaries with minimal nuclear overlapping. Colloid is also present.*

TERMINOLOGY

Abbreviations

- Follicular adenoma (FA)

Synonyms

- Follicular thyroid adenoma (FTA)

Definitions

- FA: Benign, encapsulated, noninvasive neoplasm showing evidence of thyroid follicular cell differentiation without nuclear features of papillary thyroid carcinoma

ETIOLOGY/PATHOGENESIS

Environmental Exposure

- Radiation
  - Gamma radiation during childhood
  - FAs may arise < 10 years after exposure
  - May be associated with lymphocytic thyroiditis
  - Associated with other thyroid tumors
  - Age at diagnosis usually 14 years younger than in patients with sporadic tumors
- Iodine deficiency
  - Patients in iodine-deficient areas prone to having multiple adenomas
  - FA may be associated with follicular carcinoma
  - May be associated with nodular hyperplasia

As Part of Inherited Tumor Syndromes

- PTEN-hamartoma tumor syndrome (PHTS): Cowden disease, Bannayan-Riley-Ruvalcaba syndrome
  - Caused by germline mutation of *PTEN* gene in autosomal dominant fashion
  - > 90% of individuals affected by PHTS manifest phenotype by 20 years of age
  - Affected individuals usually develop both benign and malignant tumors of breast, uterus, and thyroid
  - Affected individuals also develop multiple hamartomas of breast, colon, endometrium, and brain and ganglioneuromatous proliferations
  - Thyroid tumors occur at younger age than sporadic tumors
  - May be associated with multiple FAs and follicular carcinomas
  - Often associated with multiple follicular adenomatous nodules
- Pendred syndrome
  - Autosomal recessive syndrome resulting from mutations in *SLC26A4* (PDS) gene that codes for pendrin protein
  - Characterized by bilateral sensorineural deafness, goiter, and hypothyroidism
  - > 100 mutations identified in *SLC26A4* gene; most are family specific
  - Mutations in pendrin lead to impaired iodine transport, which may cause subsequent goiter with possible hypothyroidism
- Carney complex
  - Autosomal dominant disorder caused by mutations in *PRKAR1A* gene in 80% of affected families
  - Defined as cardiac myxomas, multiple endocrine neoplasms, and spotty cutaneous pigmentation

- < 750 cases have been identified as of 2010 (NIH Genetics Home Reference)
- Clinical manifestations can be numerous, and presentation is variable even within same kindred
- Up to 75% of patients present with multiple thyroid nodules, most of which are FA

CLINICAL ISSUES

Epidemiology

- Incidence
  - Most common neoplasm of thyroid
  - Common in areas of endemic goiter and iodine-deficient areas
- Age
  - All ages; most commonly adults 20-50 years
  - Younger age group when part of inherited nonmedullary thyroid tumor syndromes
- Sex
  - More common in females
    - F:M (6:1)

Presentation

- Most patients present with solitary nodule
- Most adenomas lack uptake on iodine scans: "Cold" nodules
- Some adenomas can cause hyperthyroidism, so-called toxic adenomas, and take up iodine on scans
- Multiple adenomatous nodules may be part of inherited tumor syndromes

Treatment

- FTAs adequately treated by simple excision or lobectomy

Prognosis

- Behavior of these tumors is completely benign

IMAGING

Ultrasonographic Findings

- US best modality for initial evaluation of thyroid lesions
- Helpful in separation of single from multiple nodules (adenoma vs. adenomatoid nodules)
- Most FAs are single, solid, homogeneous masses with smooth borders and thin, well-defined, peripheral, echo-poor halo that represents capsule
- Majority of FAs are isoechoic, but they can be hyper- or hypoechoic
- Pattern of peripheral blood vessels extending toward center of lesion is frequently present

MR Findings

- Often used in evaluation of recurrent tumors
- Nodule will appear as iso- or hypointense lesion on T1WI and hyperintense on T2WI with smooth, regular margins
- Compression of adjacent normal gland can be seen

CT Findings

- Appears as solitary hypodense nodule
- Invasion and adenopathy can be evaluated
- Large FAs may show enhancement due to degeneration

MACROSCOPIC

General Features

- Solitary nodule
- Can be multiple when part of genetic syndrome
- Completely surrounded by thin, sharp, fibrous capsule
- Stands out from unaffected gland parenchyma
- Average size: 3 cm; range: 1-10 cm
- Cut surface color ranges from tan-gray to reddish-brown, depending on cellularity and colloid content
- Secondary changes may occur in larger tumors
  o Hemorrhage
  o Degenerative changes
  o Cyst formation
  o Fibrosis and hyalinization

MICROSCOPIC

Histologic Features

- Encapsulated, follicular-patterned neoplasm surrounded by well-defined fibrous capsule
- Variable architecture with different histologic patterns include
  o Normofollicular: Uniform-appearing follicles containing colloid
  o Macrofollicular: Large, colloid-filled follicles
  o Microfollicular: Small follicles lined by flattened epithelial cells (a.k.a. fetal pattern)
  o Trabecular: Cells grouped together forming trabeculae
  o Solid: Cells in sheets
- Tumor architecture and cytologic appearance are very distinct from surrounding thyroid parenchyma
- Colloid usually present within follicular lumen
- Cytoplasm usually pale eosinophilic and can range from clear to oncocytic
- Nuclei basal, evenly spaced, round to oval with homogeneously dark chromatin
- Nucleoli rare, and when present, small and eccentric
- Isolated bizarre nuclei occasionally present
- Mitoses very rare in FAs
- Can present single or multiple combined morphological patterns with no difference in clinical behavior

Cytologic Features

- Cellularity variable
- Rare variants have been reported, including clear cell, signet ring, and oncocytic FAs
- Cells usually bland resembling normal follicular cells, but pleomorphism, if present, does not indicate malignancy
- Nuclear:cytoplasmic ratio variable with clinically hot nodules tending to have more abundant cytoplasm

Histologic Variants

- Hyperfunctioning (so-called toxic or hot) adenoma
- FA with papillary hyperplasia
- Lipoadenoma (so-called adenolipoma)
- FA with bizarre nuclei
- Signet ring cell FA
- Clear cell FA
- Spindle cell FA
- Black FA

ANCILLARY TESTS

Frozen Sections

- Should not be performed on FAs or other encapsulated, follicular-patterned lesions
- Entire capsule should be evaluated to exclude invasion
- Preferable to defer diagnosis of follicular lesions to permanent sections

Immunohistochemistry

- Positive for keratins, TTF-1, pax-8, and thyroglobulin
- Negative for calcitonin, CEA, and neuroendocrine markers synaptophysin, chromogranin, CD56
- In adenomas and adenomatous nodules of PHTS, loss of PTEN immunostaining
- Focal and faint immunoreactivity for galectin-3, HBME-1, and CITED1 very rare
- Panel of markers often positive in PTC and negative in FA (CK19, HBME-1, galectin-3, and MSG1) can assist in evaluation encapsulated lesions with PTC features
  o Strong expression of ≥ 2 of these markers (especially HBME-1) supports diagnosis of PTC; lack of staining of 3 or 4 of markers strongly supports diagnosis of FA
  o CK19 most sensitive marker (up to 96%); HBME-1 most specific (up to 96%)

Genetic Testing

- FAs have monoclonal origin established through detection of oncogenic mutation or cytogenetic abnormalities
- To date, no molecular test has been able to distinguish adenomatous nodules, FA, and carcinoma with 100% sensitivity and specificity
- Clonal cytogenetic aberrations detectable in ~ 1/2 of all FAs
  o Numerical chromosomal changes: Trisomy 7 most common, followed by gains of chromosomes 12 and 5
  o Translocation of 19q13 (ZNF331) and 2p21 (THADA)
- Activating point mutation of NRAS, KRAS, and HRAS present in ~ 30% of FAs
  o RAS mutations play important role in thyroid tumorigenesis
  o RAS mutation significantly associated with larger size and faster tumor growth than those with wild-type RAS
- PAX8/PPRG rearrangements are found in ~ 8% of FAs
- No BRAF V600E mutation or RET/PTC rearrangement in FAs
  o Few cases of FA carrying BRAF K601E reported in literature
- TSHR and GNAS mutations found in most hyperfunctioning FAs
- PIK3CA and PTEN mutations occur in ~ 5% of FAs
- Molecular analyses of miRNAs could be used to improve discrimination of indeterminate fine-needle aspirations (FNAs)

DIFFERENTIAL DIAGNOSIS

Adenomatous Nodules

- Multiple nodules, variable-sized follicles with no capsule
- Well circumscribed but not encapsulated

Hyalinizing Trabecular Tumor

- Rare thyroid neoplasm of follicular cell origin characterized by trabecular growth pattern and prominent intratrabecular and intertrabecular hyalinization
- Encapsulated or well circumscribed
- Medium-sized, elongated cells with finely granular cytoplasm
- Characteristic nuclear features similar to papillary thyroid carcinoma
- PAS(+) basement membrane material
- Diagnosis remains elusive and misleading because of overlapping characteristics with other thyroid tumors
  - Papillary thyroid carcinoma
  - Medullary thyroid carcinoma
  - Newly described noninvasive follicular thyroid neoplasm with papillary-like nuclear features

Noninvasive Follicular Neoplasm With Papillary-Like Nuclear Features

- Encapsulated or well-circumscribed, follicular-patterned neoplasm with PTC nuclear features
  - Including ground-glass nuclei (pale, clear, empty-appearing nuclei), intranuclear pseudoinclusions, nuclear molding, grooves, and overlapping

Follicular Thyroid Carcinoma

- Follicular-patterned neoplasm
- If minimally invasive, surrounded by fibrous capsule, this is characterized by vascular &/or capsular invasion

Parathyroid Adenoma

- Smaller cells in solid or microfollicular pattern
- May be intrathyroidal
- May have follicular pattern

Medullary Thyroid Carcinoma

- Invasive growth
- Cytoplasm is slightly granular
- Nuclei have salt and pepper nuclear chromatin
- May have amyloid deposit
- May have follicular arrangement, difficult to distinguish from follicular neoplasms

DIAGNOSTIC CHECKLIST

Pathologic Interpretation Pearls

- Pathologist's task is to differentiate malignant neoplasms, follicular carcinoma in particular, from numerous morphologic variants of FA
  - Diagnosis of follicular carcinoma rests on demonstration of capsular or vascular invasion
  - Extensive sampling and histological examination of entire tumor capsule essential
  - Topic of what constitutes capsular invasion (invasion into, all the way through, or presence of few follicles within capsule) remains controversial among experts
  - Deeper sectioning of suspicious tumor foci within capsule will often reveal invasion through entire capsule thickness
  - True invading tumor nests should be connected to main tumor mass, as freestanding foci may represent entrapment secondary to previous FNA biopsy
  - Isolated nodules outside capsule that are morphologically similar to tumor can only be considered invasion if direct connection with main mass seen histologically
- Atypical FA
  - Term reserved for encapsulated follicular lesions, which may show spontaneous necrosis, infarction, numerous mitoses, or increased cellularity
  - Atypical adenomas should have no features of papillary tumors and should lack capsular or vascular invasion
  - These tumors have benign clinical behavior

SELECTED REFERENCES

1. LiVolsi VA et al: Non-invasive follicular neoplasm with papillary like nuclear features (NIFTP): If it ain't broke, don't fix it. The cytopathologist's dilemma. Diagn Cytopathol. 45(6):479-480, 2017
2. Lloyd RV et al: WHO Classification olf Tumours of Endocrine Organs. Lyon, France: IARC Press, 2017
3. Macerola E et al: BRAFK601E mutation in a follicular thyroid adenoma. Int J Surg Pathol. 1066896916688083, 2017
4. Rossi ED et al: Cytopathology of follicular cell nodules. Adv Anat Pathol. 24(1):45-55, 2017
5. Saglietti C et al: Hyalinizing trabecular tumour of the thyroid: fine-needle aspiration cytological diagnosis and correlation with histology. J Clin Pathol. ePub, 2017
6. Schopper HK et al: Single thyroid tumour showing multiple differentiated morphological patterns and intramorphological molecular genetic heterogeneity. J Clin Pathol. 70(2):116-119, 2017
7. Xu B et al: Noninvasive follicular thyroid neoplasm with papillary-like nuclear features: Historical context, diagnosis, and future challenges. Endocr Pathol. ePub, 2017
8. Xu B et al: Outcome of large noninvasive follicular thyroid neoplasm with papillary-like nuclear features (NIFTP). Thyroid. ePub, 2017
9. Giordano TJ: Follicular cell thyroid neoplasia: insights from genomics and The Cancer Genome Atlas research network. Curr Opin Oncol. 28(1):1-4, 2016
10. Nikiforov YE et al: Nomenclature revision for encapsulated follicular variant of papillary thyroid carcinoma: A paradigm shift to reduce overtreatment of indolent tumors. JAMA Oncol. ePub, 2016
11. Puzziello A et al: Benign thyroid nodules with RAS mutation grow faster. Clin Endocrinol (Oxf). 84(5):736-40, 2016
12. Tennakoon TM et al: Values of molecular markers in the differential diagnosis of thyroid abnormalities. J Cancer Res Clin Oncol. ePub, 2016
13. Xing M: Clinical utility of RAS mutations in thyroid cancer: a blurred picture now emerging clearer. BMC Med. 14:12, 2016
14. Jin L et al: The diagnostic utility of combination of HMGA2 and IMP3 qRT-PCR testing in thyroid neoplasms. Appl Immunohistochem Mol Morphol. ;23(1):36-43, 2014
15. Maruta J et al: Value of thyroid specific peroxidase and Ki-67 stains in preoperative cytology for thyroid follicular tumors. Diagn Cytopathol. 43(3):202-9, 2014
16. Mathur A et al: Follicular lesions of the thyroid. Surg Clin North Am. 94(3):499-513, 2014
17. Nikiforov YE et al: Highly accurate diagnosis of cancer in thyroid nodules with follicular neoplasm/suspicious for a follicular neoplasm cytology by ThyroSeq v2 next-generation sequencing assay. Cancer. 120(23):3627-34, 2014
18. Petric R et al: Preoperative serum thyroglobulin concentration as a predictive factor of malignancy in small follicular and Hürthle cell neoplasms of the thyroid gland. World J Surg Oncol. 12:282, 2014
19. Roncati L et al: Pre-miR146a expression in follicular carcinomas of the thyroid. Pathologica. 106(2):58-60, 2014
20. Yoon JH et al: Better understanding in the differentiation of thyroid follicular adenoma, follicular carcinoma, and follicular variant of papillary carcinoma: a retrospective study. Int J Endocrinol. 2014:321595, 2014
21. Laury AR et al: Thyroid pathology in PTEN-hamartoma tumor syndrome: characteristic findings of a distinct entity. Thyroid. 21(2):135-44, 2011
22. Stokowy T et al: A two miRNA classifier differentiates follicular thyroid carcinomas from follicular thyroid adenomas. Mol Cell Endocrinol. 399:43-9, 2014
23. Hall JE et al: Thyroid disease associated with Cowden syndrome: a meta-analysis. Head Neck. 35(8):1189-94, 2013
24. Nosé V: Thyroid cancer of follicular cell origin in inherited tumor syndromes. Adv Anat Pathol. 17(6):428-36, 2010
25. Westhoff CC et al: Clear cell follicular adenoma of the thyroid—a challenge in intra-operative diagnostics. Exp Clin Endocrinol Diabetes. 118(1):19-21, 2010

Immunohistochemistry

Antibody	Reactivity	Staining Pattern	Comment
TTF-1	Positive	Nuclear	Strong nuclear staining
Thyroglobulin	Positive	Cytoplasmic	Strong in cytoplasm and luminal borders
pax-8	Positive	Nuclear	
CK-PAN	Positive	Cytoplasmic	
CK8/18/CAM5.2	Positive	Cytoplasmic	
CK19	Positive	Cytoplasmic	Present in ~ 1/2 of adenomas
CEA-M	Negative		
Chromogranin-A	Negative		
Calcitonin	Negative		
Synaptophysin	Negative		
Galectin-3	Negative		Follicular adenomas may have scattered cells weakly positive in < 10% of cases
HBME-1	Negative		Distinguish from papillary carcinoma

26. Osamura RY et al: Current practices in performing frozen sections for thyroid and parathyroid pathology. Virchows Arch. 453(5):433-40, 2008
27. Serra S et al: Controversies in thyroid pathology: the diagnosis of follicular neoplasms. Endocr Pathol. 19(3):156-65, 2008
28. Yeung MJ et al: Management of the solitary thyroid nodule. Oncologist. 13(2):105-12, 2008
29. Baloch ZW et al: Our approach to follicular-patterned lesions of the thyroid. J Clin Pathol. 60(3):244-50, 2007
30. Bertherat J: Carney complex (CNC). Orphanet J Rare Dis. 1:21, 2006
31. Marini F et al: Multiple endocrine neoplasia type 1. Orphanet J Rare Dis. 1:38, 2006
32. Rosai J et al: Pitfalls in thyroid tumour pathology. Histopathology. 49(2):107-20, 2006
33. Scognamiglio T et al: Diagnostic usefulness of HBME1, galectin-3, CK19, and CITED1 and evaluation of their expression in encapsulated lesions with questionable features of papillary thyroid carcinoma. Am J Clin Pathol. 126(5):700-8, 2006
34. LiVolsi VA et al: Use and abuse of frozen section in the diagnosis of follicular thyroid lesions. Endocr Pathol. 16(4):285-93, 2005
35. el-Sahrigy D et al: Signet-ring follicular adenoma of the thyroid diagnosed by fine needle aspiration. report of a case with cytologic description. Acta Cytol. 48(1):87-90, 2004
36. Hirokawa M et al: Observer variation of encapsulated follicular lesions of the thyroid gland. Am J Surg Pathol. 26(11):1508-14, 2002

Follicular Adenoma: CT Scan

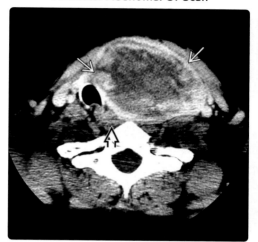

Follicular Adenoma: MR Scan

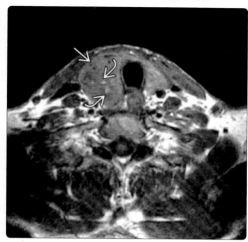

(Left) *Axial CECT through the neck demonstrates a large, heterogeneous mass* ➡️ *in the left thyroid lobe and extending into the superior mediastinum. There is significant mass effect on the larynx, trachea, and esophagus* ➡️, *which are displaced laterally to the right.* (Right) *Axial T1 MR through the neck demonstrates the heterogeneous appearance of a right thyroid mass* ➡️. *The mass is predominantly hypodense but has focal areas of T1 hyperintensity* ➡️.

Gross Features of Large Adenoma

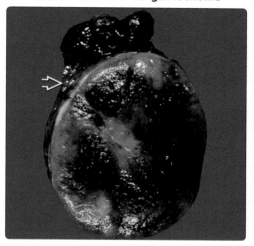

Cut Surface of Thyroid in PHTS

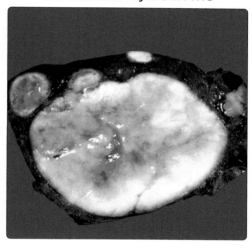

(Left) *Gross cut surface of follicular adenoma is shown. The nodule is well circumscribed and encapsulated. The thick, fibrous capsule* ➡️ *separates the adenoma from the adjacent brown-red compressed thyroid parenchyma, which shows a different gross appearance.* (Right) *Cut surface of a thyroid from a young patient with PTEN-hamartoma tumor syndrome, follicular adenoma, multiple adenomatoid nodules, and hyperplastic nodules is shown.*

Follicular Adenoma: Capsule

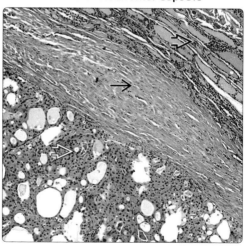

Uniform Thyroid Follicles

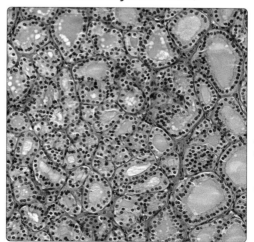

(Left) *Follicular adenoma* ➡️ *is involved by a thick, fibrous capsule* ➡️. *The normal thyroid follicles* ➡️ *surrounding the lesion are often elongated due to compression, and the follicular cells differ from the neoplastic cells.* (Right) *Follicular adenoma shows typical follicular architecture with follicles of various sizes, lined by follicular cells uniformly distributed with homogeneous regular nuclei, and abundant colloid.*

Thyroid With Adenoma

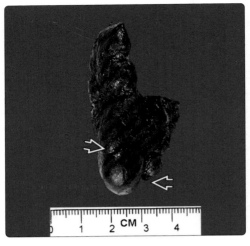

Serial Section of Thyroid Lobe

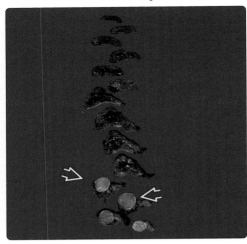

(Left) *External view of a thyroid lobe with a follicular adenoma in the inferior pole is shown. The nodule ⇶ is prominent and protrudes from the surface. The nodule has a smooth surface and is well circumscribed.* (Right) *Gross surface of follicular adenoma is shown. The nodule present in the inferior pole is well circumscribed and encapsulated. The fibrous capsule ⇶ separates the adenoma from the the adjacent brown-red, compressed thyroid parenchyma.*

Microfollicular and Solid Adenoma

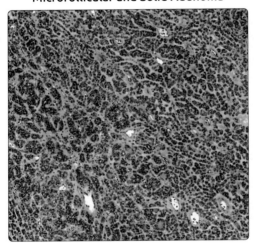

Oncocytic Follicular Thyroid Adenoma

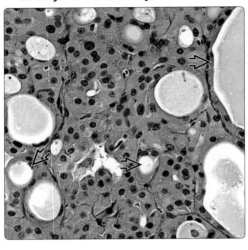

(Left) *Low-power view shows a follicular adenoma with small cell features displaying a mixed pattern of growth, including solid nests, ribbons, and microfollicles. The transition of distinct patterns across the field is also illustrated.* (Right) *Lesion displays follicles formed by somewhat larger cells with abundant eosinophilic cytoplasm and homogeneous nuclei with conspicuous small nucleoli. The size of the follicles varies over a wide range. Colloid can be seen within most follicles ⇨.*

Follicular Adenoma: Signet Ring Cells

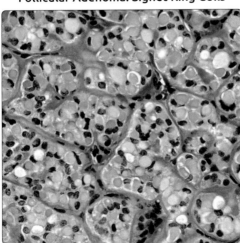

Follicular Adenoma: Hyalinization

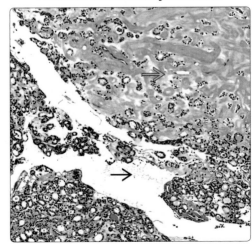

(Left) *Follicular adenoma shows signet ring features in an alveolar pattern. The nests of signet ring cells are separated by thin, fibrous trabeculae with rare follicle spaces showing colloid within the cell cytoplasm.* (Right) *Follicular adenoma shows central degenerative changes. Edema is noted as empty spaces between the follicles ⇨. Prominent hyalinization with small residual follicles is usually present centrally ⇨.*

Characteristic Cellular Features

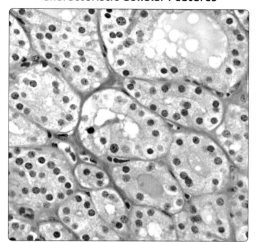

PTEN Immunohistochemistry

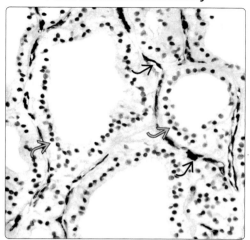

(Left) *H&E shows a follicular adenoma with a normofollicular architecture. The cells are uniformly distributed within the follicles. The nuclei are evenly spaced and round to oval with homogeneous chromatin.* (Right) *Immunohistochemistry for PTEN in a thyroidectomy specimen from a patient with Cowden disease (PHTS) shows loss of staining of the follicular cells ⊿ and preservation of staining of the endothelial cells ⊿.*

Follicular Adenoma: Plasma Cells

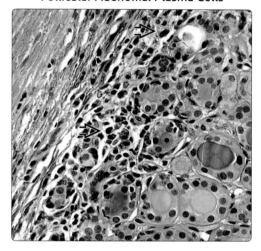

Follicular Adenoma: Surface

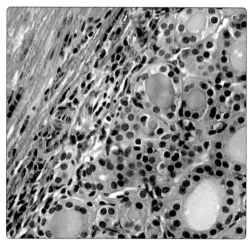

(Left) *This follicular adenoma, surrounded by a thick, fibrous capsule, contains numerous plasma cells ⊿ intermixed with follicles with thick, dark-pink colloid. The cells are uniformly distributed within the follicles, and the nuclei are evenly spaced.* (Right) *Follicular adenoma is surrounded by a thick, fibrous capsule and shows follicular architecture with follicles of various sizes, lined by follicular cells with homogeneous, regular nuclei and pale-pink colloid.*

Follicular Adenoma: Interface

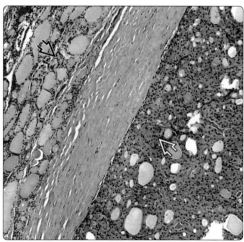

Adenoma With Lipomatous Metaplasia

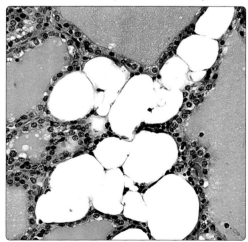

(Left) *A thick, fibrous capsule separates the normal thyroid tissue ⊿ from the follicular adenoma ⊿. Notice the distinct patterns and the sharp demarcation between the lesion and capsule.* (Right) *H&E shows a central portion of a follicular adenoma with focal lipomatous metaplasia. The follicular cells are uniformly distributed within the follicles, around the colloid, and the nuclei are round to oval. The follicular cells are intermixed with adipocytes.*

Noninvasive Follicular Thyroid Neoplasm With Papillary-Like Nuclear Features

TERMINOLOGY

- Noninvasive follicular thyroid neoplasm with papillary-like nuclear features (NIFTP) is noninvasive neoplasm of thyroid follicular cells with follicular growth pattern, and nuclear features of papillary thyroid carcinoma (PTC)
  - NIFTP was introduced to emphasize low biological potential of these tumors
  - Tumors now classified as NIFTP were previously called encapsulated noninvasive follicular variant of PTC

ETIOLOGY/PATHOGENESIS

- Diagnostic Criteria for NIFTP
  - Encapsulation or clear demarcation
  - Follicular growth pattern
  - Nuclear features of PTC, score 2-3
  - No vascular or capsular invasion
  - No tumor necrosis
  - Absence of high mitotic activity
- Exclusion criteria for NIFTP

- "True" papillae
  - Psammoma bodies
  - Infiltrative border
  - Tumor necrosis
  - High mitotic activity
  - Cell morphology characteristic of other variants of PTC
- New proposed terminology, NIFTP, reflects key histopathologic features of this lesion, i.e., lack of invasion, follicular growth pattern, and nuclear features of PTC

CLINICAL ISSUES

- Reclassification of EFVPTC, carcinoma, to NIFTP will encourage risk-adapted management strategy for this tumor
  - It will reduce overtreatment, iatrogenic complications, lessen emotional burden on patients and cost implications
- Prospective studies are needed to validate reported patient outcomes

NIFTP Gross Cut Surface

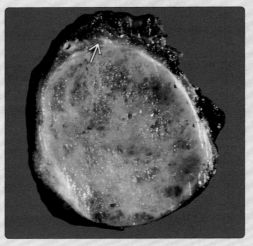

NIFTP Characteristics

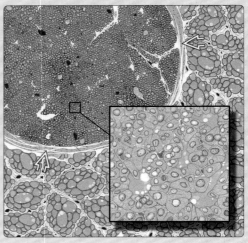

(Left) The gross characteristic features of NIFTP is a well-circumscribed or encapsulated nodule, which is lighter than the adjacent thyroid parenchyma, and compresses the red-brown adjacent thyroid parenchyma ➡. (Right) Well-circumscription, well-demarcation, or encapsulated follicular-patterned neoplasm ➡, with no capsular invasion are some of the criteria for the diagnosis of NIFTP. Nuclear features of papillary thyroid carcinoma (inset) must be present. No papillae should be seen.

PTC-Like Nuclear Features in NIFTP

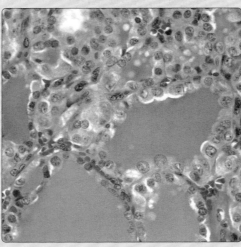

Encapsulated/Well-Circumscribed Tumors

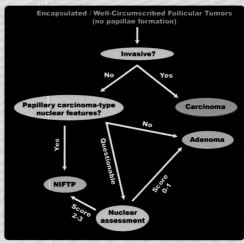

(Left) As with invasive encapsulated tumors and infiltrative tumors, the nuclei show most of the features of those in classic papillary carcinoma except that intranuclear inclusions are rare, and the nuclei often are more rounded than oval. (Right) This diagnostic algorithm for the evaluation of encapsulated follicular-patterned neoplasms uses the evaluation of the capsular invasion and papillary carcinoma-type nuclear features differentiating NIFTP from follicular adenoma and carcinoma.

TERMINOLOGY

Abbreviations

- Noninvasive follicular thyroid neoplasm with papillary-like nuclear features (NIFTP)

Synonyms

- Old terminology:
  - Papillary thyroid carcinoma, follicular variant, encapsulated or well-circumscribed (EFVPTC)
  - Noninvasive follicular variant of papillary thyroid carcinoma (PTC)

Definitions

- Noninvasive follicular thyroid neoplasm with papillary-like nuclear features (NIFTP) is noninvasive neoplasm of thyroid follicular cells with follicular growth pattern, and nuclear features of PTC that has extremely low malignant potential (WHO 2017)
- Recently, tumors classified as NIFTP were formerly classified as noninvasive/encapsulated/well-circumscribed follicular variant of papillary thyroid carcinoma (EFVPTC)
  - EFVPTC has indolent clinical behavior in comparison with other tumors, including invasive follicular variant of PTC
  - Encapsulated PTC, follicular variant without invasion was renamed NIFTP in order to reduce overtreatment of this indolent tumor
- NIFTP reflects key histopathologic features of this lesion, i.e., lack of invasion, follicular growth pattern, and nuclear features of PTC

ETIOLOGY/PATHOGENESIS

New Entity

- Term NIFTP was accepted and new nomenclature was developed
  - Offers designation for lesion before known as noninvasive EFVPTC that would reflect following characteristics
    - Main morphological features are follicular growth pattern and nuclear features of PTC
    - Lack of invasion, which separates this tumor from invasive EFVPTC
    - Clonal origin determined by finding driver mutation, which indicates that lesion is biologically neoplasm
    - Very low risk of adverse outcome as tumor is noninvasive
- New proposed terminology, NIFTP, reflects key histopathologic features of this lesion, i.e., lack of invasion, follicular growth pattern, and nuclear features of PTC
- Molecular analysis performed in this study on limited number of samples confirmed previous observations: Most of these lesions are driven by clonal genetic alterations and are therefore neoplasms rather than hyperplastic proliferations
- When defined with strict histopathologic criteria, these tumors are not expected to show molecular alterations associated with classic PTC, such as BRAF V600E mutations
- Instead, they demonstrate high prevalence of RAS and other mutations, which have been associated with follicular-pattern thyroid tumors, including follicular adenoma (FA), follicular thyroid carcinoma (FTC), and EFVPTC

- Furthermore, tumors analyzed in this study also recapitulate the FA to FTC sequence of progression with capacity for invasion, suggesting that NIFTP likely represents "benign" counterpart or precursor of invasive EFVPTC

Background Information

- Even though all outcomes data pointed to clinically benign behavior, noninvasive encapsulated/well-demarcated FVPTC continued to be overtreated with total thyroidectomy followed by radioactive iodine remnant ablation
- Cancer Genome Atlas research network confirmed all previous molecular studies demonstrating that FVPTC group of tumors, invasive and noninvasive, have RAS-like molecular signature, unlike conventional papillary carcinoma that features BRAF V600E-like profile
- Crisis in overdiagnosis and treatment of encapsulated FVPTC caused working group of Endocrine Pathology Society to critically reexamine this entity
- Reexamination of encapsulated follicular variant of PTC addressed 4 important points
  - Definition of diagnostic histopathologic features of encapsulated FVPTC and correlation with some molecular alterations
  - Follow-up analysis of at least 10 years in many noninvasive cases treated conservatively (surgery alone)
  - Consensus on minimal criteria of nuclear alterations to diagnose FVPTC
    - Using molecular alterations as reference standard, 0- to 3-point scoring scheme based on conventional morphologic criteria has been shown to define what is not PTC
      - Encapsulated noninvasive nodule with nuclear score of 0 to 1 should be diagnosed as FA
  - Consensus terminology: NIFTP
    - Name reflects the clinicopathologic features of lesion

CLINICAL ISSUES

Presentation

- Thyroid nodule

Treatment

- Thyroid lobectomy alone
- Similar to their small counterparts, large (≥ 4 cm) NIFTP appear to have extremely low risk of recurrence
  - Surgical treatment alone, including lobectomy appears to be adequate for large (≥ 4 cm) NIFTP
  - Managing large NIFTP conservatively without radioactive iodine therapy
- When excised lesion is diagnosed as NIFTP, no further surgery is needed
- No postoperative radioactive iodine treatment should be given
- American Thyroid Association (ATA) recommendation on noninvasive/encapsulated/well-circumscribed follicular variant papillary thyroid carcinoma (EFVPTC) without capsular or vascular invasion to NIFTP
  - This is weak recommendation based on moderate-quality evidence

- o Retrospective studies are needed to validate observed patient outcomes (and test performance in predicting thyroid cancer outcomes)
- o Studies are needed to evaluate implications on patients' psychosocial health and economics

Prognosis

- Based on available data, great majority of NIFTPs are of low risk and conservative surgical excision is adequate treatment
- Evidence so far published indicates that those lesions that are adequately examined microscopically do not recur or metastasize

MACROSCOPIC

General Features

- Tumors are well demarcated, well-circumscribed from surrounding thyroid
- Tumor may be encapsulated
- Median tumor size is 2.5 cm (range: 1.0-5.5 cm)

MICROSCOPIC

Histologic Features

- There are diagnostic features that are required for diagnosis of NIFTP (diagnostic inclusion criteria) and exclusion criteria
- **Diagnostic inclusion criteria for NIFTP**
- (1) Encapsulation or circumscription
  - o Thick, thin, or partial capsule or well circumscribed with clear demarcation from adjacent thyroid tissue
- (2) Absence of vascular or capsular invasion
  - o Requires adequate microscopic examination of tumor capsule interface
- (3) Follicular growth pattern with
  - o No papillae
  - o No psammoma bodies
  - o < 30% solid/trabecular/insular growth pattern
  - o Including microfollicular, normofollicular, or macrofollicular architecture with abundant colloid
- (4) Nuclear features of PTC: Score 2-3
  - o **Diagnostic nuclear score**: 3-point scoring scheme
    - Simplified and reproducible criteria for nuclear features for diagnosis of NIFTP in routine pathology practice, 6 main consensus nuclear features were grouped into 3 categories
    - (1) Size and shape (nuclear enlargement/overlapping/crowding, elongation)
    - (2) Nuclear membrane irregularities (irregular contours, grooves, pseudoinclusions)
    - (3) Chromatin characteristics (clearing with margination/glassy nuclei)
    - Each category of nuclear features is assigned score either 0 or 1, with end result of summation nuclear score of 0-3
    - For tumor to be qualified as NIFTP, nuclear features from at least 2 of these 3 categories must be present
    - Score of 0 or 1 was diagnostic of benign nodule and score of 2 or 3 is required for diagnosis of NIFTP
    - Nuclear features may be patchy, focal, or diffuse
    - Sprinkling sign if present, is helpful for diagnosis

- May also include
  - o Dark colloid
  - o Irregularly shaped follicles
  - o Intratumoral fibrosis
  - o Follicles cleft from stroma
  - o Multinucleated giant cells within follicles
- No tumor necrosis
- No high mitotic activity
  - o High mitotic activity defined as at least 3 mitoses per 10 high-power fields (400x)

Cytologic Features

- NIFTP can only be diagnosed in patients who have undergone hemithyroidectomy because final surgical pathology is required to evaluate for vascular or capsular invasion
- Preoperative diagnosis of NIFTP is not possible with our current available modalities
- Cytologic diagnosis of this entity has been studied in retrospective analyses
- ~ 1/2 of NIFTP are cytologically diagnosed as follicular neoplasms
- Distinction between NIFTP and PTC cannot be made on cytological preparations
- Role of preoperative molecular testing is controversial, as it does not replace clinical judgment and findings must be evaluated in individual context
  - o That said, preoperative molecular testing with detection of *RAS*, *PPARG* fusions, *BRAFK601E* or thyroid adenoma-associated (*THADA*) fusions may be helpful, as 80% of NIFTP have these alterations

Exclusion Criteria for NIFTP

- "True" papillae as defined as
  - o Complex, arborizing papillae with fibrovascular cores, lined by cells with nuclear features of PTC
  - o Not associated with fine-needle aspiration area
- Component of solid, trabecular, or insular growth accounting for > 30% of tumor
- High mitotic activity
  - o At least 3 per 10 high-power fields (40x)
- Psammoma bodies
- Infiltrative border
- Tumor necrosis
- Cell morphology characteristic of other variants of PTC
  - o Such as tall cell features, cribriform-morular variant, solid variant
- B*RAFV600E*, *TERT* mutations, and *RET* rearrangements should not be found in NIFTP
- **Reminder**
  - o For diagnosis of NIFTP, as for FA, examination of entire capsule is needed to exclude invasion
  - o Although large nodules can represent NIFTP, tumors over 4 cm should have careful histological assessment of periphery
    - In order to rule out foci of invasion, thereby indicating diagnosis of carcinoma
  - o In cases of fully developed nuclear features of PTC, microscopic examination of entire tumor is required to exclude papillae

Future Directions

- Small NIFTP or micro-NIFTP
  - Original description of NIFTP included only lesions that measured > 1.0 cm
  - Tumors with appropriate histological characteristics that measure < 1.0 cm, and thus would be microcarcinomas, have not been studied in systematic fashion
  - Until additional data are available for these small tumors, it is recommended that they are diagnosed as "follicular variant of papillary thyroid microcarcinoma"
- Multifocal lesions in same gland
  - Some thyroid glands may contain > 1 NIFTP (up to 20%)
  - If so, each needs to be fully examined and diagnosis confirmed
  - Each should carry prognosis of one individual tumor
  - These cases are interesting as they appear to recapitulate "multifocal" classic papillary carcinomas or microcarcinomas
  - Molecular analysis of these unusual multifocal cases should clarify if these NIFTPs are indeed independent clonal proliferations
- NIFTP with oncocytic cytology
  - Presence of foci of or diffuse oncocytic cytology in NIFTP has not been reported
  - As this cytoplasmic change is not uncommon in infiltrative follicular variant of papillary carcinoma, it seems that some NIFTP may show this alteration
    - No data are available on this feature and this awaits further studies

ANCILLARY TESTS

Immunohistochemistry

- HBME-1 does show membrane staining in about 60-70% of these lesions
  - Stain is usual stronger in luminal border
  - Staining may be focal and tends to be concentrated in areas of microfollicular growth
- Special stains for various markers (CK19, galectin-3), as with most papillary carcinomas are not often helpful
- BRAF V600E immunostain is negative

Genetic Testing

- NIFTP share molecular alterations with other follicular-patterned thyroid tumors
  - NIFTPs may harbor mutations in *RAS* in about 30%, and *PPARG* or *THADA* gene fusions
- Rare cases show *BRAF* K601E mutation
- *BRAF* V600E mutations, *TERT* mutations, and *RET* fusions should not be present
- In comparison to invasive lesions, especially those with vascular invasion, NIFTPs cases don't show *TERT* or *p53* mutations

DIFFERENTIAL DIAGNOSIS

Follicular Adenoma

- Lack nuclear features of NIFTP

Papillary Carcinoma, Encapsulated Follicular Variant, With Invasion

- Capsular invasion is noted

Follicular Variant of Papillary Carcinoma, Invasive

- Not encapsulated or well circumscribed, and invasive

Conventional Papillary Thyroid Carcinoma

- Presence of papillae

Solid Variant of Papillary Carcinoma

- Lack follicles

DIAGNOSTIC CHECKLIST

Clinically Relevant Pathologic Features

- Encapsulation or circumscription
- Follicular growth pattern
- Nuclear features of PTC
- No vascular or capsular invasion
- No tumor necrosis
- No increased mitotic index
- No true papillae

Pathologic Interpretation Pearls

- NIFTP was primarily associated with mutations in *RAS*, whereas equal number of IFVPTC cases were associated with *BRAF* V600E or with *RAS* mutations

SELECTED REFERENCES

1. Agrawal N et al: Non-invasive follicular tumor with papillary-like nuclear features (niftp): not a tempest in a teapot. Endocr Pract. ePub, 2017
2. Baloch ZW et al: Managing thyroid tumors diagnosed as non-invasive follicular tumor with papillary like nuclear features (niftp). Endocr Pract. ePub, 2017
3. Brandler TC et al: Can noninvasive follicular thyroid neoplasm with papillary-like nuclear features be distinguished from classic papillary thyroid carcinoma and follicular adenomas by fine-needle aspiration? Cancer. ePub, 2017
4. Cho U et al: Molecular correlates and rate of lymph node metastasis of non-invasive follicular thyroid neoplasm with papillary-like nuclear features and invasive follicular variant papillary thyroid carcinoma: the impact of rigid criteria to distinguish non-invasive follicular thyroid neoplasm with papillary-like nuclear features. Mod Pathol. 30(6):810-825, 2017
5. Giannini R et al: Identification of two distinct molecular subtypes by digital RNA counting of "non-invasive follicular tumour with papillary-like nuclear features (NIFTP)". Thyroid. ePub, 2017
6. Jug R et al: Noninvasive follicular thyroid neoplasm with papillary-like nuclear features: an evidence-based nomenclature change. Patholog Res Int. 2017:1057252, 2017
7. Ohori NP et al: The influence of the noninvasive follicular thyroid neoplasm with papillary-like nuclear features (NIFTP) resection diagnosis on the false-positive thyroid cytology rate relates to quality assurance thresholds and the application of NIFTP criteria. Cancer. ePub, 2017
8. Wong KS et al: The flip side of NIFTP: an increase in rates of unfavorable histologic parameters in the remainder of papillary thyroid carcinomas. Endocr Pathol. ePub, 2017
9. Xu B et al: Evolution of the histologic classification of thyroid neoplasms and its impact on clinical management. Eur J Surg Oncol. ePub, 2017
10. Xu B et al: Noninvasive follicular thyroid neoplasm with papillary-like nuclear features: historical context, diagnosis, and future challenges. Endocr Pathol. ePub, 2017
11. Xu B et al: Outcome of large noninvasive follicular thyroid neoplasm with papillary-like nuclear features (NIFTP). Thyroid. ePub, 2017
12. Haugen BR Md et al: The ATA guidelines on management of thyroid nodules and differentiated thyroid cancer task force review and recommendation on the proposed renaming of eFVPTC without Invasion to NIFTP. Thyroid. ePub, 2017
13. Scharpf J et al: The follicular variant of papillary thyroid cancer and noninvasive follicular thyroid neoplasm with papillary-like nuclear features (NIFTP). Curr Opin Oncol. 29(1):20-24, 2017
14. Paulson VA et al: NIFTP accounts for over half of "carcinomas" harboring RAS Mutations. Thyroid. ePub, 2017
15. Yang GC et al: Sonographic and cytologic differences of NIFTP from infiltrative or invasive encapsulated follicular variant of papillary thyroid carcinoma: a Review of 179 Cases. Diagn Cytopathol. ePub, 2017

Diagnostic Features of NIFTP

Major Features	Minor Features	Features not Present
(1) Encapsulation or well circumscription or clear demarcation of tumor from adjacent thyroid tissue	Dark colloid	True papillae
(2) Absence of invasion	Irregularly shaped follicles	Psammoma bodies
(3) Follicular growth pattern	Multinucleated giant cells within follicles	Cell/morphological characteristics of other variants of papillary thyroid carcinoma
(4) Papillary nuclear features	Sprinkling sign	Tumor necrosis
Enlargement	Follicles cleft from stroma	High mitotic activity
Crowding/overlapping		
Elongation		
Irregular contours		
Grooves		
Pseudoinclusions		
Chromatin clearing		

Noninvasive follicular thyroid neoplasm with papillary-like nuclear features = NIFTP.

Criteria Diagnostic of NIFTP

Characteristics	Diagnostic Findings
Interface	Encapsulation or well circumscribed with clear demarcation from adjacent thyroid
Growth pattern	Follicular growth pattern (Micro-, normo-, or macrofollicular) with
	No Papillae
	No psammoma bodies
	< 30% Solid/trabecular/insular growth patterns
Nuclear score	2-3
Invasion	No capsular or vascular invasion
Necrosis	Absent
Mitosis	No increased mitotic activity (< 3 mitosis per 10 HPF)

Noninvasive follicular thyroid neoplasm with papillary-like nuclear features = NIFTP.

16. Jeon MJ et al: Impact of reclassification on thyroid nodules with architectural atypia: from non-invasive encapsulated follicular variant papillary thyroid carcinomas to non-invasive follicular thyroid neoplasm with papillary-like nuclear features. PLoS One. 11(12):e0167756, 2016
17. Valderrabano P et al: Evaluation of ThyroSeq v2 performance in thyroid nodules with indeterminate cytology. Endocr Relat Cancer. 24(3):127-136, 2017
18. Baloch ZW et al: Noninvasive follicular thyroid neoplasm with papillary-like nuclear features (NIFTP): a changing paradigm in thyroid surgical pathology and implications for thyroid cytopathology. Cancer Cytopathol. 124(9):616-20, 2016
19. Hahn SY et al: Preoperative differentiation between noninvasive follicular thyroid neoplasm with papillary-like nuclear features (NIFTP) and non-NIFTP. Clin Endocrinol (Oxf). ePub, 2016
20. Bizzarro T et al: Young investigator challenge: the morphologic analysis of noninvasive follicular thyroid neoplasm with papillary-like nuclear features on liquid-based cytology: Some insights into their identification. Cancer. 124(10):699-710, 2016
21. Gucer H et al: The value of HBME-1 and claudin-1 expression profile in the distinction of BRAF-like and RAS-like phenotypes in papillary thyroid carcinoma. Endocr Pathol. 27(3):224-32, 2016
22. Zhao L et al: Cytological, molecular, and clinical features of noninvasive follicular thyroid neoplasm with papillary-like nuclear features versus invasive forms of follicular variant of papillary thyroid carcinoma. Cancer. ePub, 2017
23. Jiang XS et al: Young investigator challenge: molecular testing in noninvasive follicular thyroid neoplasm with papillary-like nuclear features. Cancer. 124(12):893-900, 2016
24. Hodak S et al: Changing the cancer diagnosis: the case of follicular variant of papillary thyroid cancer-primum non nocere and nIFTP. Thyroid. 26(7):869-71, 2016
25. Rosario PW et al: Noninvasive follicular thyroid neoplasm with papillary-like nuclear features. Endocr Relat Cancer. 23(12):893-897, 2016
26. Tallini G et al: The history of the follicular variant of papillary thyroid carcinoma. J Clin Endocrinol Metab. jc20162976, 2016
27. Maletta F et al: Cytological features of "non-invasive follicular thyroid neoplasm with papillary-like nuclear features" and their correlation with tumor histology. Hum Pathol. ePub, 2016
28. Strickland KC et al: Preoperative cytologic diagnosis of noninvasive follicular thyroid neoplasm with papillary-like nuclear features: a prospective analysis. Thyroid. 26(10):1466-1471, 2016
29. Nikiforov YE et al: Nomenclature revision for encapsulated follicular variant of papillary thyroid carcinoma: a paradigm shift to reduce overtreatment of indolent tumors. JAMA Oncol. ePub, 2016

Well-Circumscribed Tumor

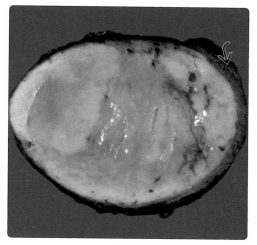

Molecular Findings in Follicular-Patterned Neoplasms

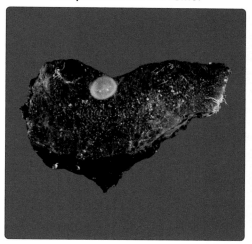

Putative Scheme of Thyroid Carcinogenesis

Growth pattern	Nuclear features of PTC	Main oncogene		
Papillary	Yes	BRAF	Papillary microcarcinoma ⇒	Classic PTC
Follicular	Yes	RAS	NIFTP ⇒	Invasive EFVPTC
Follicular	No	RAS	Follicular adenoma ⇒	Follicular thyroid carcinoma

(Left) *This cut surface photograph demonstrates gross features of a well-circumscribed and nonencapsulated tumor. The nodule is large, solid, and tan and compresses the adjacent thyroid parenchyma ⇒.* **(Right)** *This scheme demonstrates that NIFTP does not demonstrate molecular alterations associated with classic papillary thyroid carcinoma, as BRAF alterations, but shows RAS mutations which have been associated with follicular-patterned neoplasms.*

Encapsulated 0.4-cm Tumor

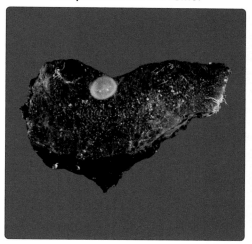

Cytology FNA Flow Chart

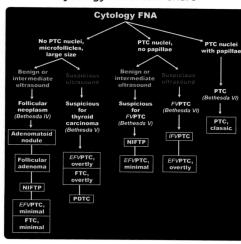

Cytology FNA

- No PTC nuclei, microfollicles, large size
  - Benign or intermediate ultrasound → Follicular neoplasm (Bethesda IV) → Adenomatoid nodule → Follicular adenoma → NIFTP → EFVPTC, minimal → FTC, minimal
  - Suspicious ultrasound → Suspicious for thyroid carcinoma (Bethesda V) → EFVPTC, overtly → FTC, overtly → PDTC
- PTC nuclei, no papillae
  - Benign or intermediate ultrasound → Suspicious for FVPTC (Bethesda V) → NIFTP → EFVPTC, minimal
  - Suspicious ultrasound → FVPTC (Bethesda VI) → IFVPTC → EFVPTC, overtly
- PTC nuclei with papillae → PTC (Bethesda VI) → PTC, classic

(Left) *This cut surface of this encapsulated tumor shows microscopic absence of capsular invasion and nuclear features of papillary carcinoma. As the tumor is < 1.0 cm, the tumor is presently called papillary microcarcinoma, encapsulated follicular variant.* **(Right)** *This cytology fine-needle aspiration flow chart, based on the nuclear features of papillary thyroid carcinoma, helps in evaluation of NIFTP and other thyroid tumors.*

Well-Circumscribed 1.5-cm Nodule

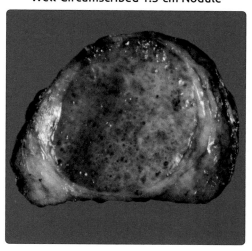

Tumor With Thick Fibrous Capsule

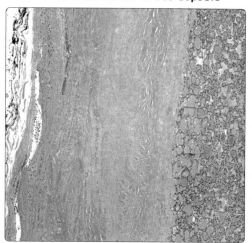

(Left) *This well-circumscribed tumor nodule showed nuclear features of papillary thyroid carcinoma and no invasion into the adjacent thyroid. However, the cells have an oncocytic cytoplasm, and this tumor is not included in the NIFTP category and should be classified as EFVPTC, oncocytic.* **(Right)** *This follicular patterned tumor has a thick fibrous capsule without capsular invasion. To classify a tumor as NIFTP, the tumor should be well-circumscribed or encapsulated, with no capsular invasion.*

Well-Circumscribed Tumor

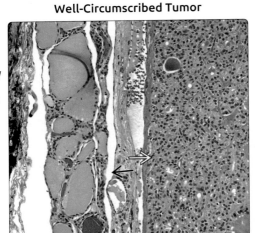

NIFTP Border and Adjacent Thyroid

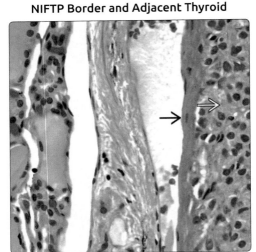

(Left) *Low-power view shows a follicular patterned lesion* ➡, *well demarcated at its periphery, with a distinct border between the tumor and adjacent thyroid* ➡. **(Right)** *This follicular patterned lesion* ➡ *is well demarcated with focal thin fibrous capsule* ➡ *with a distinct border separating the tumor and adjacent thyroid. NIFTP are noninvasive, encapsulated/well-circumscribed follicular cell tumors with papillary thyroid carcinoma-type nuclear features.*

Thick Fibrous Capsule

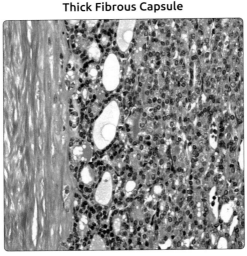

NIFTP Nuclear Features

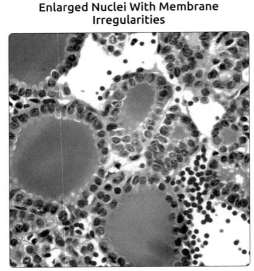

(Left) *PTC-like nuclear features are no longer diagnostic criteria of malignancy, and the invasiveness takes precedence over nuclear features in diagnosis of encapsulated follicular-patterned lesions. For the diagnosis of NIFTP, no capsular invasion should be present.* **(Right)** *This NIFTP shows the characteristic nuclear features: Nuclear overlapping, nuclear membranes irregularities, nuclear grooves, as well as nuclear clearing and thick eosinophilic colloid.*

Follicular-Patterned Neoplasm

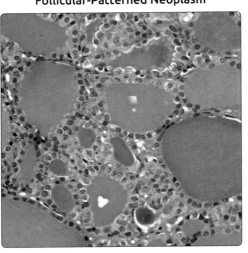

Enlarged Nuclei With Membrane Irregularities

(Left) *Microphotography of a NIFTP showing a follicular-patterned lesion that is well demarcated at its periphery and a mixed pattern consisting of small and medium size follicles with thick eosinophilic colloid. Also, papillae must be absent to classify the tumor as NIFTP.* **(Right)** *High-power view shows follicles lined by cells with atypical nuclei with cytologic features of papillary thyroid carcinoma including cells with enlarged nuclei nuclear grooves and nuclear overlapping.*

Follicular-Patterned Tumor

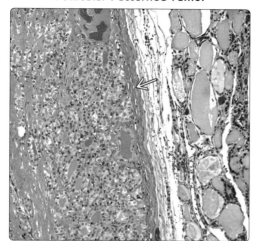

HBME1-Positive Tumor

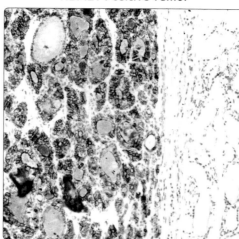

(Left) *This well-circumscribed follicular-patterned neoplasm ➡, has no invasion into adjacent thyroid parenchyma. The lesion is over 1.0 cm and has nuclear features of papillary thyroid carcinoma, and no papillae are present. This tumor meets the criteria for NIFTP.* (Right) *This well-circumscribed follicular-patterned neoplasm has no invasion into adjacent thyroid parenchyma, highlighted by the positive staining for HBME1 in the lesional cells. Note the negative stain in adjacent thyroid.*

PTC-Type Nuclear Features

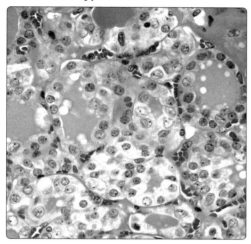

Negativity for BRAF VE1 Antibody

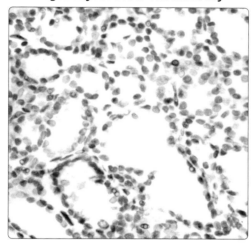

(Left) *This high power view of a NIFTP shows the papillary-like nuclear features including nuclear enlargement, as compared with adjacent normal thyroid parenchyma, overlapping, nuclear membranes irregularities, nuclear grooves, and clearing.* (Right) *Immunohistochemistry performed for BRAF V600E mutation using the mutation-specific BRAF VE1 antibody is characteristically negative in NIFTP.*

HBME1 Membranous Staining

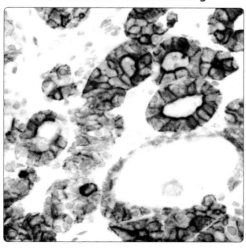

Multifocal Membranous HBME1 Staining

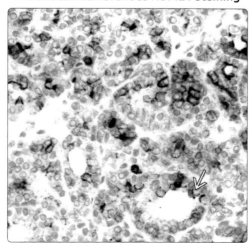

(Left) *The characteristic staining pattern of NIFTP is membranous, patchy, and usually more intense in luminal borders of the follicles.* (Right) *In areas of a microfollicular pattern, the HBME1 immunostain shows focal and patchy membranous staining and focal luminal-pattern staining ➡. This staining pattern is characteristic of these tumors.*

TERMINOLOGY

- Hyalinizing trabecular tumor (HTT): Unique neoplasm of follicular derivation exhibiting prominent trabecular architecture and hyaline appearance

ETIOLOGY/PATHOGENESIS

- Arises in background of lymphocytic thyroiditis; association with papillary thyroid carcinoma or multinodular hyperplasia

CLINICAL ISSUES

- Benign behavior
- Marked female predominance; mean age: 47 years

MACROSCOPIC

- Single, small, solid, well-circumscribed nodule measuring up to 2.5 cm

MICROSCOPIC

- Circumscribed; trabecular; intratrabecular hyalinization

- Trabecular growth pattern of medium-sized, elongated cells with finely granular acidophilic or clear cytoplasm
- Elongated, polygonal and fusiform cells, nuclei with numerous intranuclear grooves and pseudoinclusions

ANCILLARY TESTS

- Characteristic and distinctive cell membrane pattern with Ki-67 (MIB-1)

TOP DIFFERENTIAL DIAGNOSES

- Medullary thyroid carcinoma
- Papillary thyroid carcinoma
- Paraganglioma

DIAGNOSTIC CHECKLIST

- Small, circumscribed nodule
- Trabecular pattern
- Intratrabecular hyalinization
- Numerous intranuclear inclusions

Trabecular Pattern

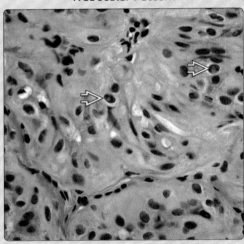

Characteristic Membranous MIB1 Staining

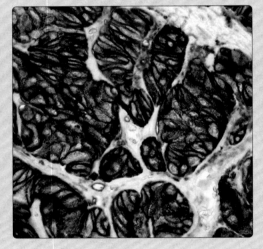

(Left) *H&E of a hyalinizing trabecular tumor (HTT) shows a prominent trabecular-patterned neoplasm with cells with ample eosinophilic cytoplasm and with numerous intranuclear inclusions ➡.* (Right) *Ki-67 (MIB-1) immunostain demonstrates the unique and characteristic membranous pattern of staining. The distinct membranous staining is identified with some Ki-67 antibodies.*

Lymphocytic Thyroiditis

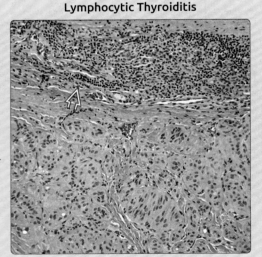

TTF-1 Stain

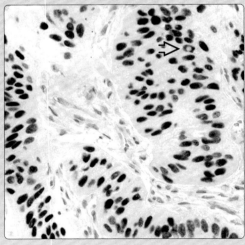

(Left) *Most HTTs are well circumscribed and may have a thin, fibrous capsule separating it from the thyroid, which usually has prominent lymphocytic thyroiditis ➡.* (Right) *TTF-1 highlights the nuclei of most of the neoplastic cells in hyalinizing trabecular tumors and highlights the elongated nuclei, some with intranuclear inclusion ➡.*

TERMINOLOGY

Abbreviations

- Hyalinizing trabecular tumor (HTT)

Synonyms

- Hyalinizing trabecular adenoma (HTA)
  - HTA-like lesion, paraganglioma-like adenoma

Definitions

- Unique neoplasm of follicular derivation exhibiting prominent trabecular architecture and variable intratrabecular hyalinization

ETIOLOGY/PATHOGENESIS

Unknown

- Arises in background of lymphocytic thyroiditis
- May occur following radiation exposure
  - Several reports confirm cases after radiation exposure
- May be present in association with papillary thyroid carcinoma
- May be associated with multinodular hyperplasia

Genetics

- *RET/PTC1* rearrangements have been reported in HTT
- To date, no association of HTT with *RAS* or *BRAF* mutations

CLINICAL ISSUES

Epidemiology

- Incidence
  - Relatively uncommon
- Age
  - Unusual under 30 years
  - Mean: 47 years
- Sex
  - Marked female predominance
    - F:M = 6:1

Presentation

- Single asymptomatic mass
- Abnormal imaging finding

Treatment

- Surgical approaches
  - Thyroid lobectomy
  - Recognition of trabecular pattern in neoplasm of follicular derivation is sufficient for referring patient to surgeon

Prognosis

- Great majority have benign behavior
- Very rarely case report of metastases to local lymph node
- Should be considered neoplasm of extremely low malignant potential

IMAGING

General Features

- Best diagnostic clue
  - Small, well-circumscribed nodule that is solid and cold on ultrasonography and scintigraphy
  - Solid tumors with hypoechogenicity or marked hypoechogenicity

MACROSCOPIC

General Features

- Single, solid, well-circumscribed nodule
- Homogeneous, delicately lobulated cut surface
- Yellow cut surface with white streaks

Size

- Range from small, microscopic tumors to medium-sized nodules measuring up to 2.5 cm

MICROSCOPIC

Histologic Features

- Trabecular growth pattern of medium-sized elongated cells with finely granular acidophilic or clear cytoplasm
- Intratrabecular PAS-positive basement membrane material may resemble amyloid; negative for Congo red
- Absence of follicle formation and absent colloid

Cytologic Features

- Cytologic diagnosis of HTT can be challenging, as these neoplasms share cytomorphological features with other thyroid neoplasms and paraganglioma
- Elongated, polygonal and fusiform cells, nuclei with numerous intranuclear grooves and pseudoinclusions
- Presence of round paranuclear yellow cytoplasmic bodies and rare psammoma bodies

Predominant Pattern/Injury Type

- Circumscribed
  - May be encapsulated
- Solid
  - Trabecular and alveolar growth pattern
  - Intratrabecular hyalinization

Predominant Cell/Compartment Type

- Epithelial
  - Follicular cells

Diagnostic Algorithm for HTT

- Gross
  - Circumscribed or encapsulated nodule up to 2.5 cm
- Architecture
  - Solid, nonpapillary, nonfollicular
- Pattern
  - Trabecular growth pattern with wide or thick trabeculae
- Trabeculae
  - Separated by stroma; some irregular and folded
- Intratrabecular hyalinization
  - PAS-positive material among cells and within trabecula
- Intertrabecular stroma
  - Thin and vascular
- Cellular arrangement
  - Perpendicular to major axis of trabeculae
- Cells
  - Elongated and eosinophilic cytoplasm
  - May contain yellow bodies
- Nuclei

- o Elongated, ground-glass with grooves, intranuclear inclusion
- Immunostains
  - o Ki-67 (MIB-1) membranous and cytoplasmic staining

ANCILLARY TESTS

Cytology

- Cytologic diagnosis of HTT can be challenging
- Characteristic presence of numerous intranuclear inclusions
  - o Mistakenly interpreted as papillary carcinoma because of similar nuclear features
- Key to diagnosis is recognition of hyaline and colloid/amyloid-like material in background of smears
  - o Presence of hyaline material
    - – Key to correct diagnosis is recognition of hyaline and colloid/amyloid-like material in background of smears
    - – Lumpy stromal deposits of basement membrane material
    - – Misinterpreted as medullary thyroid carcinoma because of extracellular matrix
- Elongated tumor cells with abundant eosinophilic cytoplasm

Immunohistochemistry

- Thyroglobulin and TTF-1 positive
- Chromogranin and calcitonin negative
- Characteristic and distinctive cell membrane pattern with Ki-67 (MIB-1)
- May express CK19 and galectin-3

DIFFERENTIAL DIAGNOSIS

Medullary Thyroid Carcinoma

- Amyloid-like amorphous material and elongated cells; expresses neuroendocrine markers and calcitonin

Papillary Thyroid Carcinoma

- Similar cytological features; papillary or follicular structures

Paraganglioma

- Very rare; strikingly similar morphology; expresses neuroendocrine markers

DIAGNOSTIC CHECKLIST

Pathologic Interpretation Pearls

- Small, circumscribed nodule with trabecular pattern, intratrabecular hyalinization, and numerous intranuclear inclusions

SELECTED REFERENCES

1. Yi KI et al: False-positive cytopathology results for papillary thyroid carcinoma: A trap for thyroid surgeons. Clin Otolaryngol. ePub, 2017
2. Jang H et al: Hyalinizing trabecular tumor of the thyroid: diagnosis of a rare tumor using ultrasonography, cytology, and intraoperative frozen sections. Ultrasonography. 35(2):131-9, 2016
3. Bakuła-Zalewska E et al: Hyaline matrix in hyalinizing trabecular tumor: Findings in fine-needle aspiration smears. Diagn Cytopathol. ePub, 2014
4. Chan JK: The wonderful colors of the hematoxylin-eosin stain in diagnostic surgical pathology. Int J Surg Pathol. 22(1):12-32, 2014
5. Choi WJ et al: The ultrasonography features of hyalinizing trabecular tumor of the thyroid gland and the role of fine needle aspiration cytology and core needle biopsy in its diagnosis. Acta Radiol. ePub, 2014
6. Park HS et al: Diagnostic caveats of immunoreactivity for Ki67 and chromogranin A in hyalinizing trabecular tumour of the thyroid. J Clin Pathol. 67(9):835-9, 2014
7. Sung SY et al: Hyalinizing trabecular tumor of thyroid: does frozen section prevent unnecessarily aggressive operation? Six new cases and a literature review. J Chin Med Assoc. 77(11):573-7, 2014
8. Howard BE et al: Hyalinizing trabecular tumor masquerading as papillary thyroid carcinoma on fine-needle aspiration. ORL J Otorhinolaryngol Relat Spec. 75(6):309-13, 2013
9. Lenggenhager D et al: HBME-1 expression in hyalinizing trabecular tumours of the thyroid gland. Histopathology. 62(7):1092-7, 2013
10. Mahajan A et al: Thyroid Bethesda reporting category, 'suspicious for papillary thyroid carcinoma', pitfalls and clues to optimize the use of this category. Cytopathology. 24(2):85-91, 2013
11. Smith NR et al: Hyalinizing trabecular tumour: review and new insights into the molecular biology. J Otolaryngol Head Neck Surg. 41(1):30-4, 2012
12. Arena S et al: Cytological diagnosis difficulties in hyalinizing trabecular adenoma of the thyroid. J Endocrinol Invest. 34(11):887-8, 2011
13. Liu Z et al: Encapsulated follicular thyroid tumor with equivocal nuclear changes, so-called well-differentiated tumor of uncertain malignant potential: a morphological, immunohistochemical, and molecular appraisal. Cancer Sci. 102(1):288-94, 2011
14. Thompson LD: Hyalinizing trabecular adenoma of the thyroid gland. Ear Nose Throat J. 90(9):416-7, 2011
15. Carney JA et al: Hyalinizing trabecular tumors of the thyroid gland are almost all benign. Am J Surg Pathol. 32(12):1877-89, 2008
16. Hyalinizing trabecular tumors of the thyroid gland are almost all benign: Carney JA, Hirokawa M, Lloyd RV, Papotti M, Sebo TJ. Am J Surg Pathol. 32(12):1877-89, 2008
17. Nosé V et al: Hyalinizing trabecular tumor of the thyroid: an update. Endocr Pathol. 19(1):1-8, 2008
18. Volante M et al: A practical diagnostic approach to solid/trabecular nodules in the thyroid. Endocr Pathol. 19(2):75-81, 2008
19. Evenson A et al: Hyalinizing trabecular adenoma–an uncommon thyroid tumor frequently misdiagnosed as papillary or medullary thyroid carcinoma. Am J Surg. 193(6):707-12, 2007
20. Galgano MT et al: Hyalinizing trabecular adenoma of the thyroid revisited: a histologic and immunohistochemical study of thyroid lesions with prominent trabecular architecture and sclerosis. Am J Surg Pathol. 30(10):1269-73, 2006
21. Casey MB et al: Hyalinizing trabecular adenoma of the thyroid gland: cytologic features in 29 cases. Am J Surg Pathol. 28(7):859-67, 2004
22. Lloyd RV: Hyalinizing trabecular tumors of the thyroid: a variant of papillary carcinoma? Adv Anat Pathol. 9(1):7-11, 2002
23. Cheung CC et al: Hyalinizing trabecular tumor of the thyroid: a variant of papillary carcinoma proved by molecular genetics. Am J Surg Pathol. 24(12):1622-6, 2000
24. Hirokawa M et al: Cell membrane and cytoplasmic staining for MIB-1 in hyalinizing trabecular adenoma of the thyroid gland. Am J Surg Pathol. 24(4):575-8, 2000
25. Papotti M et al: RET/PTC activation in hyalinizing trabecular tumors of the thyroid. Am J Surg Pathol. 24(12):1615-21, 2000
26. Katoh R et al: Accumulated basement membrane material in hyalinizing trabecular tumors of the thyroid. Mod Pathol. 12(11):1057-61, 1999
27. Katoh R et al: Hyalinizing trabecular adenoma. A report of three cases with immunohistochemical and ultrastructural studies. Histopathology. 15(3):211-24, 1989
28. Carney JA et al: Hyalinizing trabecular adenoma of the thyroid gland. Am J Surg Pathol. 11(8):583-91, 1987

Interface Between Tumor and Thyroid

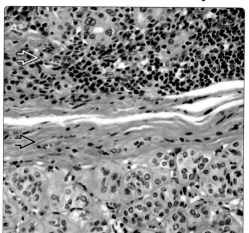

Intranuclear Inclusions

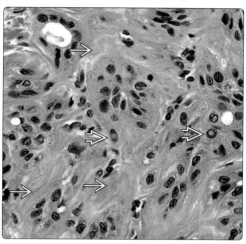

(Left) *Most HTTs are well circumscribed and may have a thin, fibrous capsule ⇒ separating it from the thyroid, usually with lymphocytic thyroiditis ⇒. The tumor is arranged in a nested to trabecular architecture.*
(Right) *The nested to trabecular growth pattern is highlighted by intratrabecular hyalinization ⇒, characteristic of this tumor and distinct from other thyroid tumors with intertrabecular hyalinization. Note the intranuclear inclusions ⇒.*

Intratrabecular Hyalinization

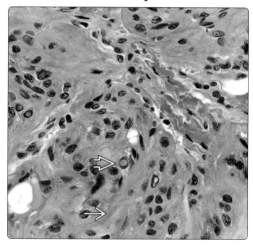

Hyalinization

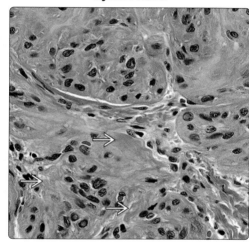

(Left) *H&E of HTT shows a trabecular growth pattern with prominent intratrabecular hyalinization ⇒. The cells are elongated, have irregular nuclei, and some nuclei show characteristic intranuclear pseudoinclusions ⇒. (Right) H&E of HTT shows cells arranged in a nested pattern with areas of prominent hyalinization ⇒. The hyalinization is noted within and between the trabeculae and nests of calls. Numerous intranuclear inclusions are present.*

Elongated Cells by Cytology

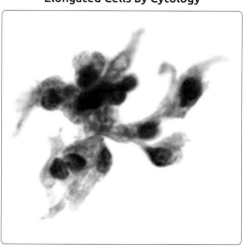

Intranuclear Pseudoinclusion

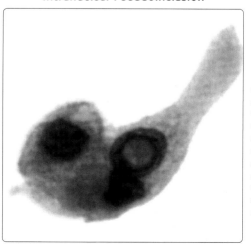

(Left) *HTT cytology shows a characteristic group of elongated tumor cells with abundant cytoplasm (some with intranuclear inclusion). These cells are usually associated with hyalinized material (not shown here). (Right) Cytology of HTT shows characteristic elongated tumor cell with abundant cytoplasm and a large intranuclear inclusion. The tumor cells are usually associated with aggregates of dense, pink, hyalinized material.*

Well-Circumscribed Nodule

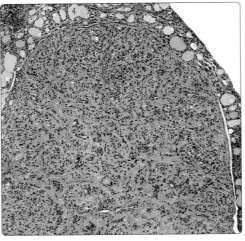

MIB-1 Immunostain

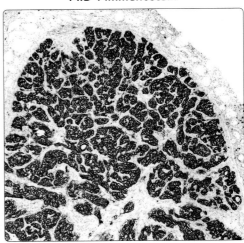

(Left) *H&E shows a well-circumscribed nodule surrounded by a thin, fibrous capsule in a background of lymphocytic thyroiditis. The tumor is arranged in a characteristic trabecular architecture with a prominent intratrabecular hyalinization.* (Right) *Ki-67 (MIB-1) immunostain shows a strong and characteristic membranous staining. This Ki-67 staining is distinct and separates HTTs from all other thyroid tumors.*

Galectin-3 Immunostain

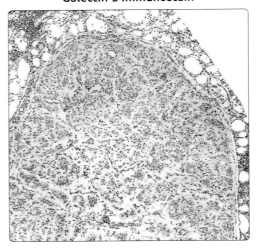

Fibrous Capsule

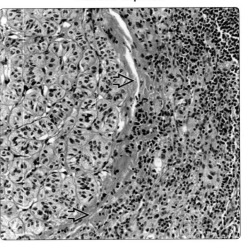

(Left) *Galectin-3 immunostain demonstrates negativity of HTTs with only macrophages demonstrating weak positivity. This is distinct from papillary thyroid carcinomas, which are usually positive.* (Right) *HTT is arranged in a nested architecture. This well-circumscribed tumor stands out from the background of lymphocytic thyroiditis. A thin, fibrous capsule ⊳ surrounds the nodule.*

Characteristic MIB-1 Immunostain

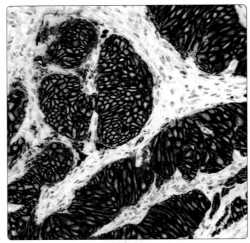

MIB-1 Immunostain in Tumor and Lymphocytes

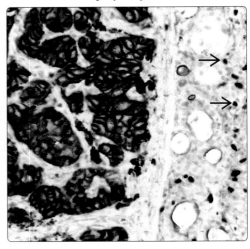

(Left) *Lower power magnification of Ki-67 (MIB-1) immunostain demonstrates characteristic strong membranous and peripheral cytoplasmic staining in tumor cells of HTT.* (Right) *High-power magnification of Ki-67 (MIB-1) immunohistochemical stain shows the characteristic membranous staining pattern of HTT (left portion of image) and the nuclear positivity in lymphocytes in adjacent thyroid ⊳.*

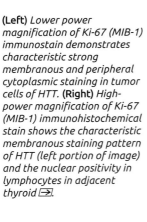

Trabecular Pattern

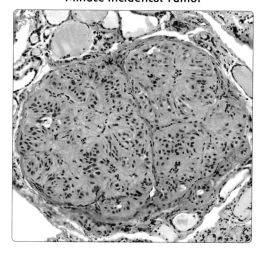

Well-Circumscribed Tumor

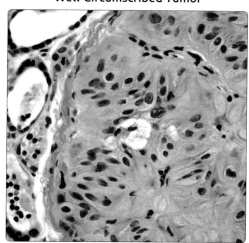

(Left) *H&E shows a trabecular-patterned neoplasm composed of spindle and fusiform cells with abundant eosinophilic cytoplasm and elongated nuclei with occasional intranuclear inclusions.* (Right) *H&E shows nonneoplastic thyroid separated from the tumor by a thin, fibrous pseudocapsule. The tumor cells are elongated with abundant cytoplasm with oval-shaped nuclei with nuclear grooves.*

Minute Incidental Tumor

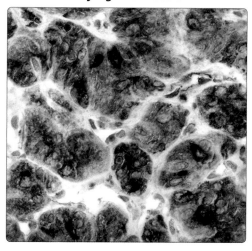

Numerous Nuclear Pseudoinclusions

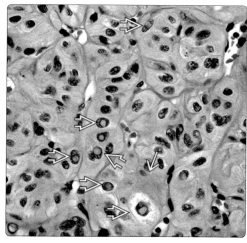

(Left) *H&E shows an HTT found incidentally in the thyroid gland. The tumor is well circumscribed and arranged in a trabecular architecture with intratrabecular hyalinization.* (Right) *H&E shows prominent trabecular-patterned neoplasm with intertrabecular and intratrabecular hyalinization ➡ and numerous intranuclear inclusions ⊟.*

Thyroglobulin Stain

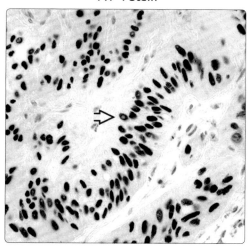

TTF-1 Stain

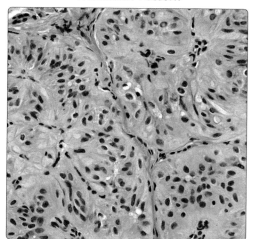

(Left) *Positive thyroglobulin immunostaining in the cytoplasm of the tumor cells is characteristic of these tumors, confirming their follicular cell origin.* (Right) *TTF-1 highlights the nuclei of most of the neoplastic cells in HTTs. TTF-1 staining is strong in the nuclei of HTT cells and highlights the elongated nuclei, some with intranuclear inclusions ⊟.*

TERMINOLOGY

- C-cell hyperplasia (CCH): Increase in C-cell population in thyroid due to reactive/physiologic or neoplastic/primary process
  - For practical purposes, if C cells can be seen on H&E and confirmed by IHC, lesion should be reported as CCH
- **Reactive, Sporadic, or Physiological CCH**
  - Usually difficult to visualize on H&E stains
- **Primary, Hereditary, or Neoplastic CCH**
  - Considered precursor lesion to familial medullary thyroid carcinomas

CLINICAL ISSUES

- **Reactive CCH** unlikely to represent premalignant lesion
- **Neoplastic CCH** is premalignant lesion
- ~ 30% of MTC occur in context of MEN2A and MEN2B or familial MTC
  - Prophylactic thyroidectomy appears to offer best chance of cure to patients with MEN2 and familial MTC

MICROSCOPIC

- Large cell with granular to amphophilic cytoplasm
- Round nuclei, coarse granular or salt and pepper chromatin
- 4 histological patterns
  - **Nodular**: C-cell clusters between or filling thyroid follicle
  - **Diffuse**: Cells scattered between follicles
  - **Solitary**: Single focus of CCH
  - **Multifocal**: Foci of CCH throughout gland

ANCILLARY TESTS

- C cells stain positively for calcitonin, chromogranin, synaptophysin, CRP, and CEA

TOP DIFFERENTIAL DIAGNOSES

- Medullary thyroid microcarcinoma
- Solid cell nests
- Medullary thyroid carcinoma with intrathyroidal spread

Scattered C Cells

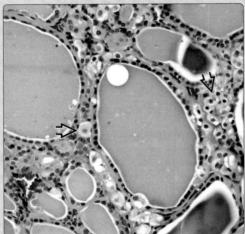

Solid Cell Nests and C Cells

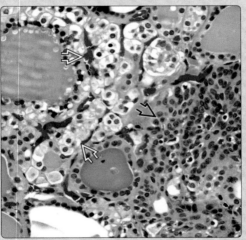

(Left) *Scattered C cells ⇨ can be identified in this field. These cells are within the follicles or in between the follicles and do not form nodules or have a diffuse proliferation pattern.* (Right) *Photomicrograph of thyroid from a patient with MEN2 shows an area of hyperplasia of C cells ⇨ associated with a solid cell nest ⇨. The C-cell proliferation is easily identified by H&E in this syndrome and hardly seen in the thyroid of other syndromes.*

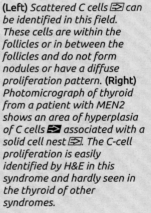

C-Cell Hyperplasia

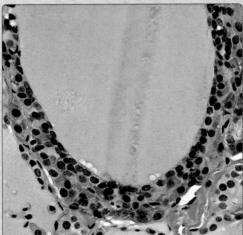

Calcitonin Immunostain

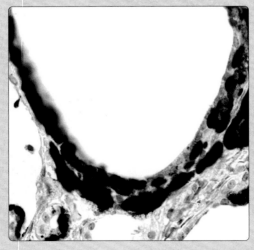

(Left) *The hyperplastic C cells in this photomicrograph surround almost the entire thyroid follicle. The C-cell proliferation has a diffuse pattern and the C cells have an ample blue granular cytoplasm.* (Right) *The thyroid follicular cells are almost completely replaced by an increased number of C cells, highlighted by calcitonin immunostaining. The C cells surround the thyroid follicle in a diffuse pattern.*

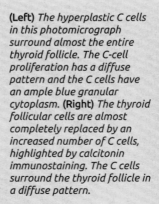

TERMINOLOGY

Abbreviations

- C-cell hyperplasia (CCH)

Synonyms

- C-cell proliferation
- Parafollicular C-cell hyperplasia

Definitions

- Calcitonin-producing C cells are derived from neural crest and descend down into thyroid with ultimobranchial body
  - Habitually associated with ultimobranchial body remnants and solid cell nests
  - C cells are normally found at junction of upper and middle 1/3 of thyroid lobes bilaterally
  - New indications suggest that mouse thyroid C cells are endodermal in origin
- CCH: Increase in C-cell population in thyroid due to reactive/physiologic or neoplastic process
- Proposed diagnostic criteria for diagnosis of CCH include
  - > 50 C cells per low-power field, 100x (WHO 2017)
  - > 50 C cells in 3 low-power fields (100x)
  - > 40 C cells/cm²
  - > 10 cells per cluster
  - For practical purposes, if C cells can be seen on H&E and confirmed by IHC, lesion should be reported as CCH
- **Neoplastic/primary CCH**
  - Considered precursor lesion of familial medullary thyroid carcinomas (MTC)
    - Premalignant lesion; therefore, term hyperplasia is misnomer
  - Caused by mutations in *RET* protooncogene
  - Histopathology
    - Predominantly nodular or mixed nodular/diffuse hyperplasia
    - Usually easy to identify on conventional H&E
    - Cytomorphologically similar to medullary microcarcinomas
    - C-cell quantification not necessary for diagnosis
- **Reactive/physiologic CCH**
  - No clear malignant potential documented
  - Caused by stimuli external to C cell
  - Histopathology
    - Predominantly diffuse
    - Usually difficult to visualize on H&E stains
    - Calcitonin stain improves detection

CLINICAL ISSUES

Presentation

- **Primary, hereditary, or neoplastic CCH**
  - Regarded as precursor of medullary thyroid carcinoma associated with MEN2 syndromes
  - 25-30% occur in context of multiple endocrine neoplasias (MEN2A and MEN2B) or familial MTC
  - Incidence rising due to increase in prophylactic thyroidectomies
    - Patients with family history of MTC and elevated serum calcitonin
    - Carriers of mutations in *RET* gene

- **Reactive, sporadic, or physiological CCH**
  - Most cases sporadic
  - May be associated with
    - Aging
    - Hyperparathyroidism
    - Hypercalcemia
    - Hypergastrinemia
    - Hashimoto thyroiditis
    - PTEN hamartoma tumor syndrome
    - Multinodular goiter
    - Hyperthyroidism
    - Following subtotal thyroidectomy
    - Lymphomas
  - Can be seen in vicinity of large tumors of follicular cell origin

Treatment

- Surgical approaches
  - Prophylactic thyroidectomy appears to offer best chance of cure to patients with MEN2 and familial MTC
  - Thyroidectomy recommended to prevent progression to medullary thyroid microcarcinoma (MMC)
    - Recommended age of prophylactic thyroidectomy depends on *RET* mutation

Prognosis

- **Neoplastic CCH** is premalignant lesion often associated with MMC
  - Generally good prognosis with early detection and thyroidectomy
  - 10-year survival rates of 74-100% reported for MMC
- **Reactive CCH** unlikely to represent premalignant lesion
  - Reports exist of MTC in patients thought to have reactive CCH, but with serum calcitonin > 50 pg/mL

IMAGING

General Features

- Due to diffuse nature or small size, CCH lesions may be easily overlooked on imaging studies

MACROSCOPIC

General Features

- CCH not usually grossly identified
- Associated MMC or MTC may be present as whitish, firm nodules, typically in upper or middle 1/3 of lobe
- In at-risk patients who undergo thyroidectomy, entire gland should be submitted to identify areas of CCH

MICROSCOPIC

Histologic Features

- C-cell hyperplasia appears as multifocal areas of increased numbers of amphophilic large cells replacing follicular epithelium and replacing follicles completely forming nodules
- 4 histological patterns
  - **Nodular**: C-cell clusters between or filling thyroid follicle
  - **Diffuse**: Cells scattered between follicles
  - **Solitary**: Single focus of CCH
  - **Multifocal**: Foci of CCH throughout gland

- **Hereditary, primary, and neoplastic CCH**
  - More likely to be nodular, multifocal, and bilateral
  - Usually detectable on H&E sections
  - Presence of cytological atypia
  - Seen adjacent to MTC
  - Usually bilateral
  - Can be nodular or diffuse
- **Reactive, physiological, and sporadic CCH**
  - Tends to be solitary, diffuse, and unilateral
  - No cytologic atypia, not usually detectable on H&E-stained sections
  - Usually unilateral and diffuse
  - Seen in association with nodular thyroid disease

Cytologic Features

- Round and polygonal cells
- Slightly larger than adjacent follicular cells
- Granular to amphophilic cytoplasm
- Round nuclei, coarse granular or salt-and-pepper chromatin

DIFFERENTIAL DIAGNOSIS

Benign Entities

- Squamous metaplasia, remnants of thymus, solid cell nests, palpation thyroiditis, intrathyroid parathyroid tissue, tangentially cut follicles

Neoplastic Processes

- Intrathyroid spread of MTC, MMC, follicular-derived neoplasms

Medullary Thyroid Microcarcinoma

- < 1 cm
- Can be sporadic or familial
- Incidental finding in patients undergoing thyroidectomies for nodular disease
- Detected by routine calcitonin screening in patients with nodular disease

Medullary Thyroid Carcinoma With Intrathyroidal Spread

- May be seen multifocally in areas where C cells absent
- Present in lymphovascular spaces, most prominent at periphery

Solid Cell Nests

- Can be associated with C cells; finding in normal thyroid
- Positive for p63, CD5, 34bE12, and CEA

Tangentially Cut Follicles

- Smaller cells with small pale cytoplasm
- Absence of immunoexpression of chromogranin, synaptophysin, and calcitonin

Intrathyroid Parathyroid Tissue

- Small round nuclei
- Positive for PTH and negative for calcitonin and TTF-1

Palpation Thyroiditis

- Single or few follicles destroyed
- Presence of histiocytes and giant cells
- Random distribution throughout gland

DIAGNOSTIC CHECKLIST

Pathologic Interpretation Pearls

- Differentiation of nodular CCH from MMC represents challenge
- Demonstration of breach of basement membrane and desmoplasia favor MMC
- One of best ways to distinguish C-cell hyperplasia is by routine histologic examination
  - C-cell hyperplasia associated with familial medullary carcinoma and MEN syndromes is readily observed on routine H&E stains
    - Cells often large and show significant nuclear atypia as well as occasional features of medullary carcinoma
  - Secondary C-cell hyperplasia often only observed by immunohistochemical staining for calcitonin and quantitative analysis

SELECTED REFERENCES

1. Nilsson M et al: On the origin of cells and derivation of thyroid cancer: C cell story revisited. Eur Thyroid J. 5(2):79-93, 2016
2. Johansson E et al: Revising the embryonic origin of thyroid C cells in mice and humans. Development. 142(20):3519-28, 2015
3. Sakorafas GH et al: Incidental thyroid C cell hyperplasia: clinical significance and implications in practice. Oncol Res Treat. 38(5):249-52, 2015
4. Schmid KW: Histopathology of C Cells and Medullary Thyroid Carcinoma. Recent Results Cancer Res. 204:41-60, 2015
5. Synoracki S et al: [Thyroid C cells and their pathology: Part 2: Medullary thyroid carcinoma.] Pathologe. 36(3):254-60, 2015
6. Ting S et al: [Thyroid C cells and their pathology: Part 1: normal C cells, - C cell hyperplasia, - precursor of familial medullary thyroid carcinoma.] Pathologe. 36(3):246-53, 2015
7. Bussolati G: C and APUD cells and endocrine tumours. Pearse's laboratory in the years 1965-1969: a personal recollection. Endocr Pathol. 25(2):133-40, 2014
8. Nakazawa T et al: C-cell-derived calcitonin-free neuroendocrine carcinoma of the thyroid: the diagnostic importance of CGRP immunoreactivity. Int J Surg Pathol. 22(6):530-5, 2014
9. Diazzi C et al: The diagnostic value of calcitonin measurement in wash-out fluid from fine-needle aspiration of thyroid nodules in the diagnosis of medullary thyroid cancer. Endocr Pract. Epub ahead of print, 2013
10. Figlioli G et al: Medullary thyroid carcinoma (MTC) and RET proto-oncogene: mutation spectrum in the familial cases and a meta-analysis of studies on the sporadic form. Mutat Res. 752(1):36-44, 2013
11. Cameselle-Teijeiro J et al: C-cell hyperplasia and papillary thyroid carcinoma. Int J Surg Pathol. 20(6):643-4, 2012
12. Pirola S et al: C-cell hyperplasia in thyroid tissue adjacent to papillary carcinoma. Int J Surg Pathol. 20(1):66-8, 2012
13. Laury AR et al: Thyroid pathology in PTEN-hamartoma tumor syndrome: characteristic findings of a distinct entity. Thyroid. 21(2):135-44, 2011
14. Etit D et al: Histopathologic and clinical features of medullary microcarcinoma and C-cell hyperplasia in prophylactic thyroidectomies for medullary carcinoma: a study of 42 cases. Arch Pathol Lab Med. 132(11):1767-73, 2008
15. Ashworth M: The pathology of preclinical medullary thyroid carcinoma. Endocr Pathol. 15(3):227-31, 2004
16. Guyétant S et al: C-cell hyperplasia and medullary thyroid carcinoma: clinicopathological and genetic correlations in 66 consecutive patients. Mod Pathol. 16(8):756-63, 2003
17. Kaserer K et al: Recommendations for reporting C cell pathology of the thyroid. Wien Klin Wochenschr. 114(7):274-8, 2002
18. Baloch ZW et al: Neuroendocrine tumors of the thyroid gland. Am J Clin Pathol. 115 Suppl:S56-67, 2001
19. Krueger JE et al: Inherited medullary microcarcinoma of the thyroid: a study of 11 cases. Am J Surg Pathol. 24(6):853-8, 2000
20. de Lellis RA et al: The pathobiology of the human calcitonin (C)-cell: a review. Pathol Annu. 16(Pt 2):25-52, 1981

Immunohistochemistry

Antibody	Reactivity	Staining Pattern	Comment
CK-PAN	Positive	Cytoplasmic	
TTF-1	Positive	Nuclear	
pax-8	Positive	Nuclear	
Chromogranin-A	Positive	Cytoplasmic	
Synaptophysin	Positive	Cytoplasmic	
Calcitonin	Positive	Cytoplasmic	Calcitonin gene-related peptide is also positive
ACTH	Positive	Cytoplasmic	ACTH may be present in some cases
Somatostatin	Positive	Cytoplasmic	Somatostatin may be present in few cases
GastrinRP	Positive	Cytoplasmic	Rare cases may express
CEA-M	Positive	Cytoplasmic	
Thyroglobulin	Negative		
Collagen IV	Negative		Used to confirm diagnosis of medullary thyroid microcarcinoma: C cells expanding into interstitium
S100	Negative		Positive in sustentacular cells of intrathyroidal paraganglioma
PTH	Negative		Used to differentiate from intrathyroidal parathyroid tissue
p63	Negative		Used in differential diagnosis of solid cell nests
34bE12	Negative		Used in differential diagnosis of solid cell nests
CD5	Negative		Used in differential diagnosis of solid cell nests

Reactive/Physiologic vs. Neoplastic C-Cell Hyperplasia

Features	Reactive or Physiological C-Cell Hyperplasia	Neoplastic or Primary C-Cell Hyperplasia
Detectable on H&E stains	No	Yes
Cytologic atypia	No	Yes
Seen adjacent to medullary thyroid carcinoma	No	Yes
Bilaterality	No	Yes
Staining with NCAM	No	Yes
Calcitonin reactivity	Yes	Yes
CEA reactivity	No	Yes/no
Chromogranin reactivity	Yes	Yes
Synaptophysin reactivity	Yes	Yes

C Cells Associated With SCNs

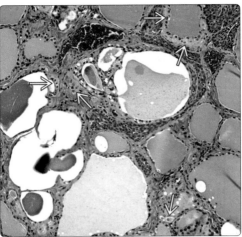

Normal C-Cell Population as Identified by Calcitonin Stain

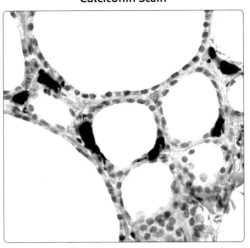

(Left) *The calcitonin-producing C cells are usually associated with ultimobranchial body remnants/solid cell nests (SCNs). Near the SCNs, numerous C cells* ➡ *can be identified by routine stains.* (Right) *Calcitonin stain highlights the normal C-cell distribution within the junction of the upper and middle 1/3 of the thyroid lobes. Normal C-cell population is characterized by < 50 calcitonin-positive cells per low-power field.*

C-Cell Hyperplasia

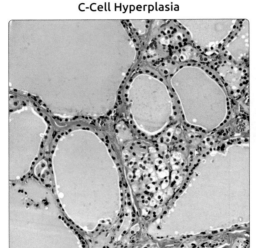

Identification of C Cells

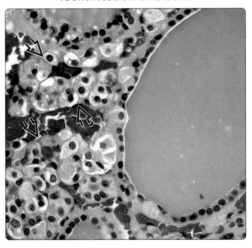

(Left) *An increased number of C cells can be seen adjacent to large thyroid nodules. The reactive C-cell proliferation is usually difficult to identify on H&E.* (Right) *High-power photomicrograph shows a thyroid from a patient with MEN2. The C-cell proliferation* ➡ *is easily identified by H&E. In inherited syndromes, the C-cell hyperplasia usually precedes neoplasia.*

C-Cell Hyperplasia

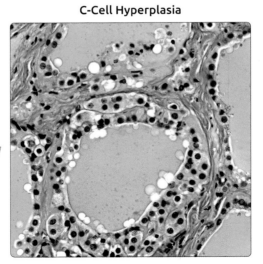

Calcitonin(+) C-Cell Hyperplasia

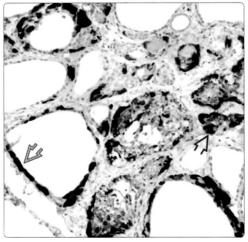

(Left) *C-cell proliferation is easily identified at this magnification. This finding is usually seen in cases of neoplastic C-cell hyperplasia.* (Right) *Calcitonin immunohistochemical stain shows the marked increase in the number of C cells, which are arranged in small clusters in a nodular* ➡ *and diffuse* ➡ *pattern.*

Medullary Microcarcinoma

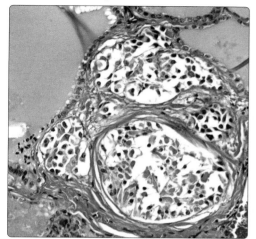

C-Cell Hyperplasia and Microcarcinoma

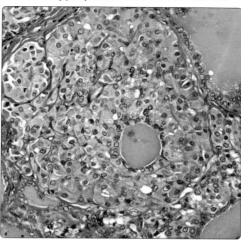

(Left) *Most of the time, the differential diagnosis between C-cell hyperplasia and medullary thyroid microcarcinoma is challenging. The presence of extension of C cells through the basement membranes of expanded C cell-filled follicles into the surrounding thyroid interstitium associated with desmoplasia help in the diagnosis of microcarcinoma.* **(Right)** *Nodular C-cell hyperplasia is a misnomer, as this is considered precursor lesion of familial medullary thyroid carcinomas in MEN2 syndromes.*

C Cells and Solid Cell Nest

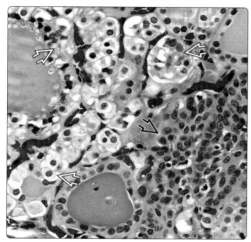

C-Cell Hyperplasia Associated With SCNs

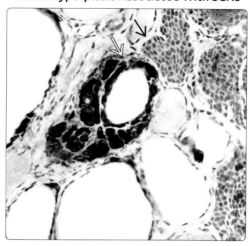

(Left) *The thyroid follicular cells are almost completely replaced by an increased number of C cells ⇒, easily identified by H&E staining. The C cells have ample blue granular cytoplasm. These are adjacent to a solid cell nest ⊟.* **(Right)** *Calcitonin-producing C cells are derived from the neural crest and descend down into the thyroid with the ultimobranchial body/SCNs. C-cell hyperplasia ⇒ can be located near the SCNs ⊟. Note the group of C cells obscuring a follicle.*

Diffuse C-Cell Hyperplasia

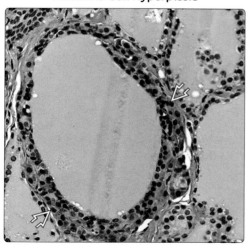

Calcitonin Immunostain

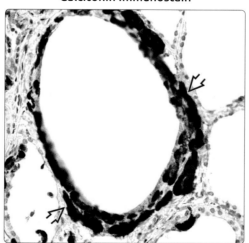

(Left) *The thyroid follicular cells are almost completely replaced by an increased number of C cells ⇒, easily identified by H&E staining. The C cells have ample blue granular cytoplasm.* **(Right)** *C-cell hyperplasia highlighted by calcitonin staining shows the thyroid follicular cells replaced by an increased number of C cells ⊟ that surround the entire follicle.*

Follicular Thyroid Carcinoma

TERMINOLOGY

- Malignant epithelial tumor of thyroid showing evidence of follicular cell differentiation but lacking diagnostic features of papillary thyroid carcinoma

ETIOLOGY/PATHOGENESIS

- Iodine deficiency considered important risk factor for development of follicular adenoma and FTC
- Familial FTC accounts for ~ 5% of FTC in USA

MICROSCOPIC

- Minimally invasive follicular thyroid carcinoma
- Encapsulated angioinvasive follicular thyroid carcinoma
- Widely invasive follicular thyroid carcinoma

ANCILLARY TESTS

- Cytogenetic changes found in ~ 65% of FTC
- Most common somatic mutations in FTC
  - *RAS* point mutations in 30-50% of tumors
  - *PPARG* gene fusions that occur in 20-30% of FTC
- *TERT* promoter mutations found in ~ 20% of FTC
- FTC occurring in familial setting
  - Mutations in *PTEN*, *PRKAR1A*, *WRN*, and *GNAS1*

DIAGNOSTIC CHECKLIST

- Pathologist's most important tasks are:
  - Demonstrate capsular &/or vascular invasion as diagnosis of FTC rests on identifying these
    - **Capsular invasion**: Neoplastic cells penetrate the entire thickness of tumor capsule
    - **Vascular invasion**: Intravascular tumor cells should be adherent to vascular wall, covered by endothelium or in context of thrombus or fibrin
  - Differentiate between FTC and numerous variants of follicular adenoma and other benign or malignant neoplasms
  - Identify pathological characteristics of inherited tumor syndrome: Usually multifocal and bilateral

Capsular Invasion

Lymphovascular Invasion

(Left) *H&E shows the classic mushroom sign, diagnostic of follicular thyroid carcinoma (FTC). The tumor cells ➡ invade across the entire thickness of the fibrous capsule ➡. (Right) H&E illustrates a hallmark in the diagnosis of FTC. Vascular invasion is shown here with tumor cells present within a large capsular blood vessel.*

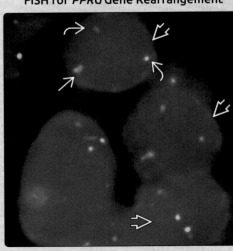

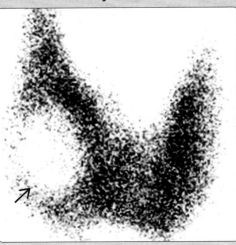

FISH for *PPRG* Gene Rearrangement

Cold Thyroid Nodule

(Left) *Three cells ➡ in this thyroid FNA specimen show typical rearrangements of PPAR-γ seen in some FTC. A FISH break-apart probe was used. Normal chromosomes should have green and red signals next to each other ➡. Rearrangement is shown as separate red and green signals ➡. (Right) Anterior planar I-123 nuclear medicine scan shows a "cold" nodule (differentiated thyroid carcinoma) in the right thyroid lobe ➡. A "cold" nodule has ~ 20% chance of being malignant.*

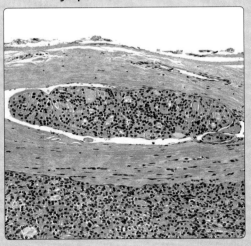

Follicular Thyroid Carcinoma

TERMINOLOGY

Abbreviations
- Follicular thyroid carcinoma (FTC)

Synonyms
- Follicular carcinoma
- Familial nonmedullary thyroid carcinoma
- Familial FTC

Definitions
- FTC: Thyroid malignancy arising from follicular cells in which diagnostic features of papillary thyroid carcinoma are absent
  - Lesions usually encapsulated and show invasive growth
  - Occurs in familial setting

ETIOLOGY/PATHOGENESIS

Environmental Exposure
- Radiation exposure results in 5.2x relative risk for developing FTC
- Iodine deficiency associated with higher risk for development of follicular adenoma and follicular carcinoma

Preexisting Thyroid Disease
- Present in up to 15% of patients with FTC
- Dyshormonogenic goiter with chronic TSH stimulation may predispose to follicular neoplasms
- Associated with other thyroid tumors, mostly follicular adenoma
  - These tumors are identical histologically
  - Follicular adenoma may be precursor to follicular carcinoma
    - Both harbor RAS, PTEN, and PIK3CA mutations
- Lymphocytic thyroiditis and FTC may coexist
- Association between lymphocytic thyroiditis and FTC remains unclear

Inherited Tumor Syndromes
- Accounts for at least 5% of FTC in USA
- **PTEN hamartoma tumor syndrome** (PHTS)
  - Cowden syndrome, Bannayan-Riley-Ruvalcaba syndrome, Proteus syndrome, and Proteus-like syndrome
  - Germline mutation of PTEN gene transmitted in autosomal dominant fashion
  - Individuals may also develop multiple hamartomas of breast, colon, endometrium, brain, and ganglioneuromatous proliferations
    - Trichilemmomas
  - Affected individuals may develop benign and malignant tumors of breast, uterus, and thyroid
    - Breast cancer: Early onset; most women diagnosed between 38-46 years of age
  - May be associated with multiple follicular adenomas and carcinomas of thyroid
    - Thyroid tumors associated with multiple thyroid nodules in young patient
    - FTC major diagnostic criterion for diagnosis of PHTS
- **Carney complex**
  - Autosomal dominant disorder caused by mutations in PRKAR1A
  - Carney complex includes cardiac myxomas, multiple endocrine neoplasms, and spotty cutaneous pigmentation
  - 75% of patients develop multiple thyroid nodules
    - ~ 5% of patients may present with follicular or papillary carcinoma
- **Werner syndrome**
  - Autosomal recessive
  - Caused by mutations in WRN
  - Age-related disorders present early in life, including malignancies
    - Melanoma, soft tissue sarcoma, osteosarcoma
    - Up to 3% of patients will have thyroid disease, usually FTC
- **McCune-Albright syndrome**
  - Patients harbor postzygotic mutations in GNAS1 with mosaic distribution
  - Triad of café au lait skin pigmentation, polyostotic fibrous dysplasia, and hyperfunctioning endocrinopathies
  - Associated with precocious puberty, hyperthyroidism, GH excess, and Cushing syndrome
    - Associated with FTC and papillary thyroid carcinomas
- **Li-Fraumeni syndrome**
  - Caused by germline mutation of TP53
  - Development of diverse sarcomas and carcinomas at young age
  - Unusual thyroid follicular cell tumors with marked nuclear pleomorphism

CLINICAL ISSUES

Epidemiology
- Incidence
  - 6-10% of thyroid malignancies
- Age
  - Inherited syndrome-related FTC affects patients at earlier age than does sporadic FTC
    - Sporadic cases: 5th decade
- Sex
  - More common in women

Presentation
- Painless mass
- Slow growing
- Difficulty swallowing

Prognosis
- 70-80% cure rate if disease confined to thyroid
- 20-30% recurrence when regional lymph node metastases present
- 50-90% of patients who present with distant metastases will die

IMAGING

Ultrasonographic Findings
- In minimally invasive disease, usually well-circumscribed nodule (> 1 cm)
- Cannot distinguish follicular adenoma from FTC

○ Carcinoma usually associated with microcalcifications, hypoechogenicity, irregular margins or absent halo sign, solid aspect, intranodular vascularization, and shape (taller than wide)
- May be helpful in assessing lymph node involvement by thyroid carcinoma

Scintigraphy

- Scan shows "cold" nodule

MACROSCOPIC

General Features

- Round to ovoid encapsulated tumors, tan to light brown
- Usually multiple and bilateral in familial setting
- Minimally invasive tumors: Thick, irregular, fibrous capsule and grossly similar or indistinguishable from follicular adenoma
- Widely invasive carcinomas: Lack of capsule or extensive permeation of capsule

Size

- Round to ovoid encapsulated tumors, 1-10 cm in diameter

MICROSCOPIC

Histologic Features

- Diagnosis of FTC requires demonstration of capsular &/or vascular invasion
- FTC subclassified into 3 groups
  ○ **Minimally invasive**: Capsular invasion only
  ○ **Encapsulated angioinvasive**: Extent of vascular invasion prognostically relevant
  ○ **Widely invasive**: Extensive extension into thyroid and extrathyroidal tissues
- Cytoarchitectural features of FTC similar to those of follicular adenoma
  ○ Trabecular, solid, microfollicular, normofollicular, macrofollicular
  ○ Mixed architectural patterns also occur
- Variants
  ○ Clear cell
  ○ Signet-ring cell type
  ○ Glomeruloid pattern
  ○ Spindle cell type
- FTC lacks nuclear features of PTC
- FTC generally surrounded by thick, irregular, fibrous capsule
- Criteria for capsular invasion
  ○ Tumor bud has invaded beyond outer contour of capsule
  ○ Tumor bud still clothed by thin capsule; however, it has extended through outer capsular surface
  ○ Presence of satellite nodule with cytoarchitectural and cellular features identical to those of tumor cells
  ○ Classic mushroom-like bud that has totally transgressed fibrous capsule
- Criteria for vascular invasion
  ○ Blood vessels should be of larger caliber with identifiable wall the size of a vein, and involved blood vessels must be located within or outside fibrous capsule (i.e., not within tumor)

○ Intravascular polypoid tumor growth must protrude into lumen, be covered by endothelium, and be attached to wall of vessel and associated with thrombus
○ Clusters of epithelial cells floating in vascular lumen and unattached to wall not considered vascular invasion
- Nodal status
  ○ Metastasis present or absent, ipsilateral vs. contralateral, number with metastases, size of largest metastatic deposit
    − Metastases reportedly more frequent in familial cases
- Follicular carcinoma in familial diseases may be incidental finding within thyroid with multiple nodules
  ○ Tumors arise in background of multiple adenomatous nodules, nodular hyperplasia, &/or lymphocytic thyroiditis
  ○ Follicular carcinoma in inherited syndromes tends to be
    − Smaller than sporadic tumors
    − Multiple
    − Bilateral

Categories of Tumor

- Minimally invasive follicular thyroid carcinoma
- Encapsulated angioinvasive follicular thyroid carcinoma
- Widely invasive follicular thyroid carcinoma

ANCILLARY TESTS

Immunohistochemistry

- Expression of lineage-specific antigens: pax-8, TTF-1, thyroglobulin
- Value of any other markers questionable

Genetic Testing

- FTC have significantly higher rate of numerical chromosomal abnormalities and losses and gains of specific chromosomal regions than PTC
- Cytogenetic changes found in ~ 65% of FTC
- Most common somatic mutation in FTC
  ○ *RAS* point mutations in 30-50% of tumors
  ○ *PPARG* gene fusions (*PAX8-PPARG* or *CREB3L2-PPARG*) that occur in 20-30% of FTC
  ○ *TERT* promoter mutations found in ~ 20% of FTC
  ○ *PIK3CA* mutations found in up to 10% of FTC
  ○ Inactivation of *PTEN* found in up to 10% of FTC
- Accumulation of additional mutations, such as *TP53*, may be associated with progression to poorly differentiated carcinomas
- FTC occurring in familial setting
  ○ PTEN-hamartoma tumor syndrome (Cowden disease and other syndromes), Carney complex, Werner syndrome, McCune-Albright syndrome
    − Mutations in *PTEN*, *PRKAR1A*, *WRN*, and *GNAS1*
  ○ Family history of thyroid carcinoma identified in ~ 4% of patients diagnosed with FTC
  ○ **Testing families with history of cancer**
    − Most useful to begin by testing individual with cancer
      □ If multiple affected individuals present within kindred, testing can establish linkage between cancer(s) and mutation

DIFFERENTIAL DIAGNOSIS

Follicular Adenoma

- Encapsulated benign neoplasm with variable architecture and histologic patterns
- Only features to reliably distinguish adenoma from FTC are capsular &/or vascular invasion

Papillary Thyroid Carcinoma, Follicular Variant

- Follicular pattern of growth, can be encapsulated
- Usually shows typical papillary carcinoma features: Ground-glass nuclei, intranuclear pseudoinclusions, nuclear grooves, and overlapping
- Immunohistochemistry for HBME-1, galectin-3, and CK19 may help distinguish follicular variant of PTC from FTC

Noninvasive Follicular Tumor With Papillary-Like Nuclear Features

- Encapsulated or well-circumscribed follicular neoplasm with papillary-like nuclear features
- No capsular or vascular invasion

Adenomatous Nodule

- Frequently multiple, variably sized follicles with no capsule or incomplete capsule
- May have abundant edematous or hyalinized stroma

Hyperplastic Nodules in Hashimoto Thyroiditis

- Diffusely enlarged and firm thyroid
- Lymphocytic infiltration of stroma, formation of large lymphoid follicles
- Thyroid follicles often small and atrophic, lined by Hürthle cells

Hyperplastic Nodules in Dyshormonogenetic Goiter

- Hypercellular nodules with varied appearances commonly solid and microfollicular
- Atypia with bizarre nuclei may be present
- Irregular areas of fibrosis at periphery of nodules may simulate capsular invasion

Hyalinizing Trabecular Tumor

- Trabecular growth pattern with medium-sized, elongated cells with granular cytoplasm
- No follicle formation and absent colloid
- PAS(+) basement membrane material
- Characteristic cytoplasmic and membranous Ki-67/MIB1 staining pattern

Medullary Thyroid Carcinoma: Glandular, Oxyphil, and Hyalinizing, Trabecular

- Invasive growth pattern
- Slightly granular cytoplasm
- Salt and pepper nuclear chromatin
- Calcitonin, CEA, chromogranin, and synaptophysin positivity

Intrathyroid Parathyroid Tumor

- Solitary parathyroid adenomas within thyroid parenchyma may mimic PTC, as they appear as "cold" nodules on imaging studies
- Clinical picture of hyperparathyroidism should raise suspicion
- Histological examination will confirm parathyroid tissue

DIAGNOSTIC CHECKLIST

Pathologic Interpretation Pearls

- Pathologist's most important tasks
  - Demonstrate capsular &/or vascular invasion, as diagnosis of FTC rests on identifying these
  - Differentiate between FTC and numerous variants of follicular adenoma and other benign or malignant neoplasms
  - Identify pathological characteristics of inherited tumor syndrome
    - Thyroid carcinoma in familial setting usually multifocal and bilateral
    - Familial cases usually associated with other thyroid pathology: Adenomatous nodules, multinodular hyperplasia, follicular adenomas, and lymphocytic thyroiditis

SELECTED REFERENCES

1. Glomski K et al: Metastatic follicular thyroid carcinoma and the primary thyroid gross examination: Institutional review of cases from 1990 to 2015. Endocr Pathol. 28(2):177-185, 2017
2. Lang BH et al: The total number of tissue blocks per centimetre of tumor significantly correlated with the risk of distant metastasis in patients with minimally invasive follicular thyroid carcinoma. Endocrine. 55(2):496-502, 2017
3. Vuong HG et al: Pediatric follicular thyroid carcinoma - indolent cancer with low prevalence of RAS mutations and absence of PAX8-PPARG fusion in a Japanese population. Histopathology. ePub, 2017
4. Lee YM et al: Risk factors for distant metastasis in patients with minimally invasive follicular thyroid carcinoma. PLoS One. 11(5):e0155489, 2016
5. Stenson G et al: Minimally invasive follicular thyroid carcinomas: prognostic factors. Endocrine. 53(2):505-11, 2016
6. Mochizuki K et al: Low frequency of PAX8-PPARγ rearrangement in follicular thyroid carcinomas in Japanese patients. Pathol Int. ePub, 2015
7. Ni Y et al: Germline and somatic SDHx alterations in apparently sporadic differentiated thyroid cancer. Endocr Relat Cancer. 22(2):121-30, 2015
8. Duman BB et al: Evaluation of PTEN, PI3K, MTOR, and KRAS expression and their clinical and prognostic relevance to differentiated thyroid carcinoma. Contemp Oncol (Pozn). 18(4):234-40, 2014
9. Kakudo K et al: Prognostic classification of thyroid follicular cell tumors using Ki-67 labeling index: Risk stratification of thyroid follicular cell carcinomas [Review]. Endocr J. ePub, 2014
10. Nikiforov YE et al: Highly accurate diagnosis of cancer in thyroid nodules with follicular neoplasm/suspicious for a follicular neoplasm cytology by ThyroSeq v2 next-generation sequencing assay. Cancer. ePub, 2014
11. Son EJ et al: Familial follicular cell-derived thyroid carcinoma. Front Endocrinol (Lausanne). 3(3):61, 2012
12. Laury AR et al: Thyroid pathology in #I#PTEN#I#-hamartoma tumor syndrome: characteristic findings of a distinct entity. Thyroid. 21(2):135-44, 2011
13. Nosé V: Familial thyroid cancer: a review. Mod Pathol. 24 Suppl 2:S19-33, 2011
14. Paschke R et al: Thyroid nodule guidelines: agreement, disagreement and need for future research. Nat Rev Endocrinol. 7(6):354-61, 2011
15. Zhang Y et al: Endocrine tumors as part of inherited tumor syndromes. Adv Anat Pathol. 18(3):206-18, 2011
16. Nosé V: Thyroid cancer of follicular cell origin in inherited tumor syndromes. Adv Anat Pathol. 17(6):428-36, 2010
17. Dotto J et al: Familial thyroid carcinoma: a diagnostic algorithm. Adv Anat Pathol. 15(6):332-49, 2008
18. Collins MT et al: Thyroid carcinoma in the McCune-Albright syndrome: contributory role of activating Gs alpha mutations. J Clin Endocrinol Metab. 88(9):4413-7, 2003
19. French CA et al: Genetic and biological subgroups of low-stage follicular thyroid cancer. Am J Pathol. 162(4):1053-60, 2003

Differential Diagnosis of Follicular Thyroid Carcinoma

Lesion	Characteristic Findings	Comments
Dominant nodule in nodular hyperplasia	Follicles have different sizes and shapes; colloid ranges from pale to dark red, and these nodules have irregular fibrosis and pseudocapsule	Capsule in follicular carcinoma is thick and surrounds entire nodule; colloid is homogeneous and dark red in follicular carcinoma
Adenomatous nodule	Usually multiple and nonencapsulated	Follicular carcinoma may occur in association with adenomatous nodules
Follicular adenoma	Usually single and surrounded by thin capsule	Fibrous capsule in follicular adenoma is usually thinner than in follicular carcinoma
Noninvasive follicular thyroid neoplasm with papillary-like nuclear features	Encapsulated or well-circumscribed follicular-patterned neoplasm with papillary-like nuclear features	Papillary thyroid carcinoma-like nuclear features
Follicular variant of papillary thyroid carcinoma	Follicular-patterned neoplasm with focal nuclear features of papillary thyroid carcinoma	Usually main differential diagnosis with follicular carcinoma
Poorly differentiated thyroid carcinoma	Pattern of follicular cells usually in solid, trabecular, and insular, and presents with rare follicles	May show apoptosis, necrosis, and high mitotic rate; has higher Ki-67 proliferative index; some positive for p53
Hyalinizing trabecular tumor	Well-circumscribed benign thyroid tumor but lacks fibrous capsule; has trabecular growth pattern and rarely forms follicles	Positive for TTF-1 and thyroglobulin; however, HTT has characteristic membranous staining for Ki-67/MIB1
Medullary thyroid carcinoma, follicular patterned	Tumor cells in medullary thyroid carcinoma have ample eosinophilic granular cytoplasm and salt and pepper nuclei	Both tumors positive for TTF-1; medullary thyroid carcinoma positive for chromogranin, synaptophysin, calcitonin, and CEA

Follicular Thyroid Carcinoma in Familial Setting

Syndrome	Common Clinical Findings	Thyroid Pathology Findings
PTEN hamartoma tumor syndrome	Mucocutaneous lesions, breast carcinoma, endometrial carcinoma, thyroid carcinoma, macrocephaly, gastrointestinal hamartomas, lipomas, and other tumors	Follicular carcinoma associated with multiple adenomatous nodules and multiple follicular adenomas
Carney complex	Myxomas, spotty mucocutaneous pigmentation, psammomatous melanotic schwannoma, breast ductal adenoma, multiple endocrine neoplasms including PPNAD, GH-producing adenoma, thyroid carcinoma	Small percentage (~ 5%) of patients with this syndrome may develop follicular carcinoma, usually associated with other thyroid nodules
Werner syndrome	Bilateral cataracts, characteristic dermatological findings, short stature, osteoporosis, multiple neoplasms at younger age	Small percentage (~ 3%) of patients with this syndrome develop follicular carcinoma
McCune-Albright syndrome	GH excess, Cushing syndrome, precocious puberty	Patients may develop follicular carcinoma and papillary thyroid carcinoma
Li-Fraumeni syndrome	Sarcomas, brain tumor, adrenal cortical carcinoma, breast cancer, other tumors at young age; rarely involves thyroid	Patients develop many thyroid nodules with nuclear pleomorphism and may develop follicular carcinoma

Classification of Follicular Thyroid Carcinoma

Traditional	AFIP 2014	WHO 2017
Minimally invasive	Minimally invasive with capsular invasion	Minimally invasive
Minimally invasive	Minimally invasive with limited vascular invasion (< 4 vessels)	Encapsulated angioinvasive
Minimally invasive	Minimally invasive with extensive vascular invasion (> 4 vessels)	Encapsulated angioinvasive
Widely invasive	Widely invasive	Widely invasive

AFIP = Armed Forces Institute of Pathology; modified from 2017 WHO classification of tumors of endocrine organs.

Ultrasound Findings

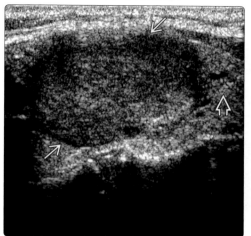

CECT Findings

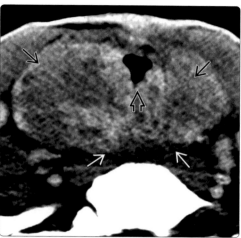

(Left) *Longitudinal grayscale ultrasound shows an ill-defined, solid, hypoechoic thyroid nodule ➡. Ill-defined edges and hypoechogenicity should raise suspicion of malignancy. Normal thyroid echogenicity is seen ➡.* (Right) *Axial CECT shows a large follicular carcinoma with diffuse thyroid involvement ➡, compression of the airway ➡, and extrathyroid spread posteriorly ➡. These features cannot be evaluated by ultrasound.*

Doppler Ultrasound Findings

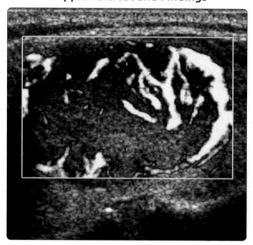

Gross Cut Surface

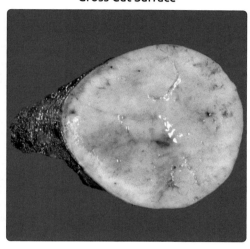

(Left) *Power Doppler ultrasound shows profuse, chaotic intranodular vascularity. FNAC confirmed carcinoma of the thyroid. Such vessels in a thyroid nodule suggest malignancy.* (Right) *Gross photograph shows a minimally invasive follicular carcinoma presenting as a single nodule in a sporadic setting. The tumor is grossly indistinguishable from a follicular adenoma. Thorough examination of the capsule is crucial to identify foci of capsular invasion.*

Multinodular Thyroid

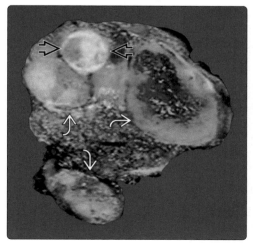

Criteria for Capsular Invasion

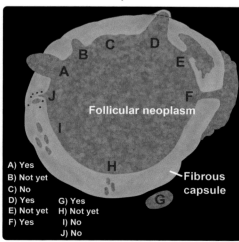

Follicular neoplasm

A) Yes
B) Not yet
C) No
D) Yes
E) Not yet
F) Yes
G) Yes
H) Not yet
I) No
J) No

Fibrous capsule

(Left) *Gross cut surface of a thyroid from a 12-year-old patient with PTEN hamartoma tumor syndrome shows multiple adenomatous nodules ➡ and a follicular carcinoma ➡, confirmed by histopathology.* (Right) *Graphic shows the criteria necessary to interpret and diagnose a follicular neoplasm as follicular carcinoma based on capsular invasion. The follicular neoplasm is surrounded by a thick, fibrous capsule with invasion on A, D, F, and G.*

Overview of Follicular Neoplasm

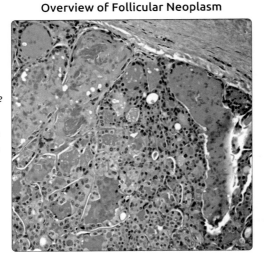

Capsular Invasion

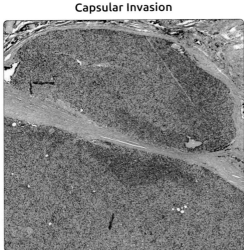

(Left) *Follicular carcinoma demonstrates a thick capsule surrounding the neoplastic follicles. In this area, there is no capsular invasion.* (Right) *Follicular carcinoma with cytologically identical satellite nodules indicates true capsular invasion, even without demonstration of the point of capsular penetration.*

Extension of Tumor Into Thyroid

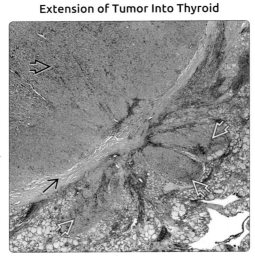

Lymphovascular Invasion

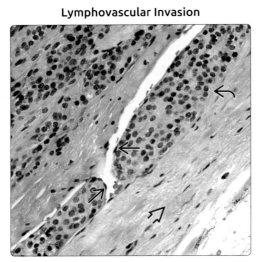

(Left) *H&E of follicular carcinoma ⇒ shows finger-like projections of the tumor ⮕ protruding beyond the capsule ⇥ into the surrounding thyroid parenchyma.* (Right) *High-power view shows 2 groups of tumor cells in a vessel within the tumor capsule ⮕. The tumor cells are attached to the vessel wall ⮕. Endothelial cells can be seen lining both tumor thrombi ⇥.*

Morphological Features

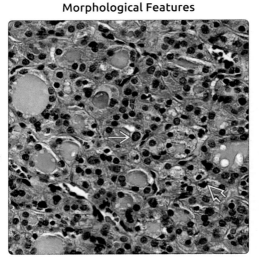

Follicular Cell Atypia

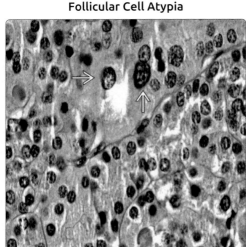

(Left) *Nuclear pleomorphism can be present to various degrees in follicular carcinoma. This case presents microfollicular architecture with a few large, irregular nuclei that may show nucleoli ⮕. Colloid is present throughout the tumor. A mitotic figure is seen ⮕.* (Right) *High-power view of an FTC depicts pleomorphism and cellular atypia. The overall follicular architecture is preserved, but cells with pink granular cytoplasm and irregular large nuclei are present ⮕.*

Vascular Invasion

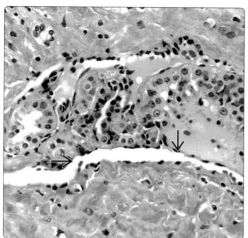

Encapsulated Angioinvasive FTC

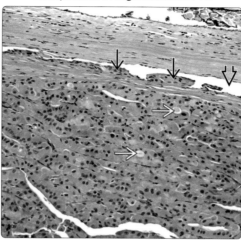

(Left) *In this example of vascular invasion, epithelial tumoral cells are present in the lumen of a vessel within the tumoral capsule. Note that the cluster of tumor cells is lined by endothelium ➡. The neoplastic cells may be associated with a thrombus.* (Right) *Groups of epithelial tumor cells ➡ are attached to the wall of a vascular space ➡ within the tumor capsule. The cells are arranged in a follicular pattern and have abundant eosinophilic cytoplasm. Pools of colloid material can also be seen ➡.*

Capsular Invasion

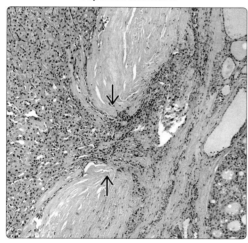

Capsular and Vascular Invasion

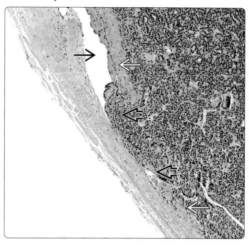

(Left) *Minimally invasive follicular carcinoma shows the point of invasion. There is a tumor capsule invasion ➡ through the entire capsule thickness, invading a large blood vessel along the way.* (Right) *Low-power view depicts a polypoid mass of tumor cells ➡ infiltrating the tumor capsule ➡ and invading a large vascular space ➡. The tumor mass is connected to the intravascular component.*

Vascular Invasion

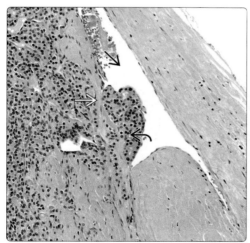

Capsular and Vascular Invasion

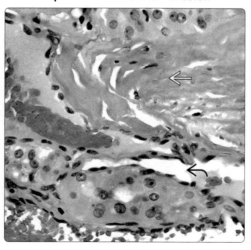

(Left) *Tumor cells are present within a large capsular blood vessel ➡. The cells are attached to the vessel wall ➡. A rim of fibrous capsule is seen between the tumor thrombus and the remainder of the tumoral mass ➡.* (Right) *High-power view of FTC shows the point of invasion where tumor cells penetrate the capsule ➡ and reach a blood vessel ➡.*

Poorly Differentiated Thyroid Carcinoma

TERMINOLOGY

- Follicular cell-derived carcinoma with limited structural follicular or papillary features
- Clinical behavior intermediate between well-differentiated (papillary and follicular) and undifferentiated (anaplastic) carcinomas

ETIOLOGY/PATHOGENESIS

- Iodine deficiency may be contributing environmental factor
- Some tumors are thought to arise from preexisting papillary or follicular carcinomas

CLINICAL ISSUES

- 5-year survival rate: 71%
- Mean: 55-63 years (range: 14-89 years)

MICROSCOPIC

- **Diagnostic criteria**
  - Presence of solid, trabecular, or insular growth pattern
  - Absence of conventional nuclear features of PTC

- Presence of at least 1 of following
  - Convoluted nuclei
  - Mitotic activity ≥ 3/10 HPF
  - Tumor necrosis

ANCILLARY TESTS

- β-catenin and *TP53* mutation
- Poorly differentiated thyroid carcinomas (PDTCs) have mutation load intermediate between that of anaplastic and well-differentiated papillary carcinoma
- Early driver events in thyroid carcinogenesis
  - *HRAS, KRAS,* or *NRAS* mutations, *BRAF* mutation, *ALK* fusions
- Genes that typically occur as late events associated with tumor dedifferentiation
- Activating mutations in *AKT1,* mutations in *TERT, CTNNB1*
- Small number of PDTC shows *RET/TAS2R38* and *NTRK1* rearrangements
- Rearrangements of *RET* and *PAX8/PPARG* less frequent

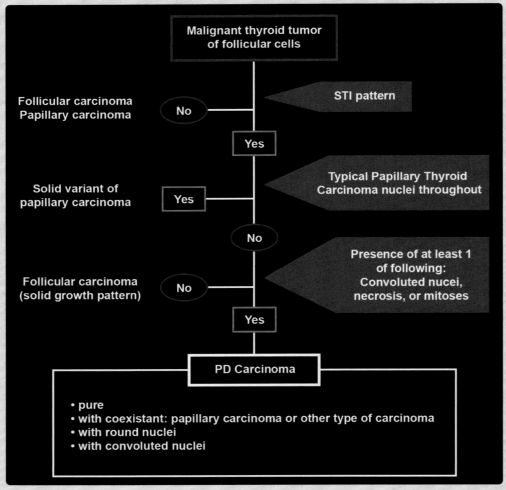

Algorithm for Diagnosis of PDTC Using Turin Consensus Criteria

Malignant thyroid tumor of follicular cells

Follicular carcinoma Papillary carcinoma — No

STI pattern

Yes

Solid variant of papillary carcinoma — Yes

Typical Papillary Thyroid Carcinoma nuclei throughout

No

Follicular carcinoma (solid growth pattern) — No

Presence of at least 1 of following: Convoluted nucei, necrosis, or mitoses

Yes

PD Carcinoma

- pure
- with coexistant: papillary carcinoma or other type of carcinoma
- with round nuclei
- with convoluted nuclei

Algorithmic approach to the histopathological diagnosis of a malignant thyroid tumor with a solid, trabecular, and insular growth pattern (STI) is shown. (Courtesy Volante et al, 2007.)

TERMINOLOGY

Abbreviations

- Poorly differentiated thyroid carcinoma (PDTC)

Synonyms

- Poorly differentiated follicular carcinoma
- Insular carcinoma
- Solid carcinoma
- Trabecular carcinoma

Definitions

- PDTC is follicular cell neoplasm that shows limited evidence of follicular cell differentiation and is morphologically and behaviorally intermediate between differentiated (follicular and papillary) carcinomas and anaplastic thyroid carcinoma (WHO 2017)
- Malignant epithelial thyroid neoplasm showing histological and biological features intermediate between differentiated and anaplastic thyroid carcinoma
  - PDTCs are more aggressive than well-differentiated, but less aggressive than anaplastic, forms
- **Turin diagnostic criteria and algorithm**
  - PDTC was introduced as diagnostic entity in 2004 WHO Classification of Tumours of Endocrine Organs
  - International consensus meeting was held in Turin, Italy in 2006
  - Uniform set of criteria and algorithmic approach for diagnosis of PDTC were put forth in 2007 and further validated in 2010
  - Turin criteria has been shown to reliably diagnose PDTC and stratify patients clinically with prognostic significance
    - Not initially used for oncocytic, poorly differentiated carcinomas
    - Turin criteria now accepted to be applied to oncocytic PDTC
      - Patients with this variant have decreased survival using radioiodine treatment compared to conventional PDTC
      - Patients might be candidates for novel treatment modalities
- Tumor growth pattern alone, as insular, trabecular, or solid, is not defining criteria for PDTC
- Follicular cell carcinoma with limited structural follicular or papillary features
- Presence of necrosis and numerous mitoses are helpful for diagnosis

ETIOLOGY/PATHOGENESIS

Origin

- Unknown etiology
- Iodine deficiency may be contributing environmental factor
  - Given association of PDTC with longstanding nodular hyperplasia
- Some tumors are thought to arise from preexisting papillary or follicular carcinomas
- Some may arise as de novo neoplasms

CLINICAL ISSUES

Epidemiology

- Incidence
  - PDTCs are rare form of thyroid carcinomas
  - As percentage of thyroid cancer cases
    - USA: Rare; 1.8% (Mayo Clinic series)
    - Japan: ~ 0.3%
    - Northern Italy: 6.7% (Turin series)
  - Variations in incidence may be due to histopathological interpretation
- Age
  - Mean: 55-63 years (range: 14-89 years)
- Sex
  - F:M = 1.1-2.1:1.0

Presentation

- No clinical features can accurately diagnose PDTCs
- Solitary, large, cold mass
  - Growth of longstanding nodule
  - New rapidly growing mass
- Locally advanced disease with extrathyroid extension is common at initial presentation
- Distant metastases to lymph nodes, lung, liver, and bone are reported at presentation in ~ 15% of cases

Treatment

- Options, risks, complications
  - Treatment of choice is total thyroidectomy
    - Followed by postoperative radioactive iodine
    - Supplemental thyroxine
  - PDTC is usually resistant to radioactive iodine
  - Usually not responsive to conventional thyroid cancer therapy
  - New target therapy drugs

Prognosis

- Prognostic factors independently associated with survival in PDTC by multivariate analysis
- **Good prognosis**
  - Histological factor
    - Convoluted (papillary carcinoma-like) neoplastic cell nuclei
- **Poor prognosis**
  - **Clinicopathological factors**
    - Age > 45 is associated with worse prognosis and higher risk of death
    - Larger tumors (> 5.0 cm)
    - Presence of extrathyroidal extension (pT4a)
    - Presence of metastatic disease at presentation
      - Local or distant metastases
  - Advanced clinical stage
  - Presence or absence of tumor capsule
  - Presence of capsular invasion
  - **Histopathological factors**
    - Tumor necrosis
    - IMP3 immunoreactivity
    - Oncocytic features
  - Molecular genetic factors
  - RAS gene mutation
  - Downregulation of miR-150

- Intermediate between well- and undifferentiated thyroid carcinoma
  - Death from disease is common
  - Disease course may be long, differing from anaplastic thyroid carcinomas
  - Death may occur after several years
  - 5-year survival rate: 71%
  - 10-year survival rate: 46%

MACROSCOPIC

General Features

- Solid, gray-white mass with pushing borders
- Usually infiltrative but may have thick capsule
- Frequent foci of necrosis and hemorrhage
- Occasional satellite tumor nodules within thyroid parenchyma

Size

- Most tumors are > 3 cm
- Mean tumor size: 5.9 cm (range: 2-13 cm)

MICROSCOPIC

Histologic Features

- Solid, trabecular, or insular growth pattern
  - Insular: Cell nests separated by thin fibrovascular septa
  - Trabecular: Cells arranged in thick ribbons or cords
  - Solid: Patternless arrangement of cells
- Small cells with round to vesicular nuclei with absence of conventional nuclear features of papillary thyroid carcinoma (PTC)
- Presence of at least 1 of following
  - Convoluted nuclei
  - Mitotic activity ≥ 3/10 HPF
  - Tumor necrosis
- Some tumors contain clear or oncocytic cells
- Rare tumors may show rhabdoid features
- Some may have hobnail cells

Associations

- May be associated with follicular carcinoma or papillary carcinoma
  - Presence of associated (separate) papillary carcinoma or convoluted nuclei
  - PDTC portion of tumor cannot have papillary features
- No features of papillary type present
  - Not otherwise specified

Turin Proposal for Diagnosis of Poorly Differentiated Thyroid Carcinoma

- Recommends algorithmic approach to histopathological diagnosis of PDTC
  - Diagnosis of carcinoma of follicular cell derivation by conventional criteria
  - Presence of solid, trabecular, or insular patterns of growth
  - Absence of conventional nuclear features of PTC
  - Presence of at least 1 of following
    - Convoluted nuclei
    - Mitotic activity > 3/10 HPF
    - Tumor necrosis

- Component of follicular or PTC may be present
- Aggressive forms of papillary or follicular thyroid carcinoma should not be included in poorly differentiated category
  - If their distinct features of differentiation are retained throughout tumor
- Component with anaplastic thyroid carcinoma may be identified

ANCILLARY TESTS

Cytology

- Highly cellular
- Small to intermediate-sized, monotonous, noncohesive cells
- Scant colloid, some microfollicles
- Bland nuclei, fine chromatin, small nucleoli
- Sheets of tumor cells with microfollicular, insular, or trabecular pattern
- Necrosis and mitosis are relatively common
- Definitive diagnosis should be made on histology

Immunohistochemistry

- Variably positivity for thyroglobulin
- TTF-1 positive in most nuclei
- pax-8 immunopositivity
- Positivity for cytokeratin
- Cyclin-D1 positive
- p53 immunopositivity in > 1/2 of cases
- Bcl-2 positive > 80% of cases
- IMP3 positive
- Neuroendocrine markers and calcitonin negative
- Ki-67 proliferative index high

Genetic Testing

- PDTCs have mutation load intermediate between that of anaplastic and well-differentiated papillary carcinoma
  - Multiple genetic hits model: Multistep progression from well differentiated to PDTC
- Early driver events in thyroid carcinogenesis
  - HRAS, KRAS, or NRAS mutations in 50%
    - Predominant NRAS mutation
  - BRAF mutation
    - This finding may indicate PDTCs are associated more with papillary carcinoma
  - ALK fusions
- Genes that typically occur as late events associated with tumor dedifferentiation
  - Activating mutations in AKT1 (in 19% of aggressive, radioiodine-refractory PDTCs)
    - Nearly always in combination with BRAF V600E mutation
  - Mutations in TERT are clonal in PDTC and anaplastic thyroid carcinoma
  - Mutation in CTNNB1
  - β-catenin and TP53 mutation
    - Present in poorly differentiated and anaplastic thyroid carcinomas but not in well-differentiated tumors
    - TP53 mutations in 20-30%
    - β-catenin accumulation in nuclei
- Small number of PDTC shows RET/TAS2R38 or NTRK1 rearrangements

- Rearrangement of *RET* (~ 10% of cases) and *PAX8/PPARG* (detected in ~ 5% of cases)

DIFFERENTIAL DIAGNOSIS

Medullary Thyroid Carcinoma

- Growth pattern may include solid, trabecular, or insular
- May have increased mitotic activity and necrosis
- Immunohistochemistry
  - Positivity for neuroendocrine markers, such as chromogranin, synaptophysin, NSE
  - Calcitonin positivity
  - TTF-1 positivity
  - Thyroglobulin negative

Parathyroid Carcinoma

- PTH and chromogranin immunostain

Carcinoma Metastatic to Thyroid Gland

- Immunohistochemistry markers will help in diagnosis

Papillary Thyroid Carcinoma

- Solid, microfollicular, tall cell, and diffuse sclerosing variants
- Diagnosis is based on conventional nuclear features of PTCs
  - Nuclear enlargement
  - Nuclear overlapping/crowding
  - Variation in size and shape
  - Clear to dispersed chromatin
  - Nuclear grooves
  - Nuclear pseudoinclusions
- Growth pattern, mitotic index, and necrosis do not help make distinction
- Immunohistochemistry
  - Diffuse thyroglobulin reactivity
  - TTF-1 strong and diffuse

Follicular or Well-Differentiated Carcinoma

- Absence of PTC nuclear features
- No convoluted nuclei
- Low to nil mitotic activity
- Absence of necrosis
- Encapsulated lesions with capsular &/or vascular invasion

Undifferentiated or Anaplastic Thyroid Carcinoma

- Rapidly enlarging neck or thyroid mass
  - Growth over short period of time
- Highly aggressive tumor
- Poor prognosis with very high mortality rates irrespective of therapy
  - Death within months of diagnosis
  - 5-year survival rate < 14%
  - Median survival rates: 2-6 months
- Pleomorphic neoplasm
- Cell arrangements include solid, trabecular, and insular patterns
  - Growth patterns also include fascicular and storiform
- Markedly atypical cells of various cell types
  - Squamous cell
  - Spindle cell
  - Small cell
  - Rhabdoid cell
  - Giant cell

- Lymphoepithelioma-like
- Paucicellular
- Plasmacytoid
- Irrespective of growth pattern and cell-type neoplastic cellular infiltrate is poorly differentiated
  - No evidence of colloid formation
- Immunohistochemistry
  - Cytokeratin, pax-8, and p53 reactivity are most useful markers
  - Thyroglobulin and TTF-1 reactivity usually absent in majority of cases
  - Chromogranin, synaptophysin, and calcitonin are negative
  - Vimentin reactivity usually present

DIAGNOSTIC CHECKLIST

Clinically Relevant Pathologic Features

- Tumors have widely Invasive pattern
  - Extending to perithyroidal tissue in 60-70% of cases
  - Vascular invasion is seen in 60-90% of cases
  - Distant metastases to lung, bone, and other sites in 40-70% of cases
  - Metastases to lymph nodes in 15-65% of cases
- Association with well-differentiated thyroid carcinomas
  - Follicular thyroid carcinoma
  - PTC

Pathologic Interpretation Pearls

- Follicular cell-derived carcinoma with limited structural follicular or papillary features
- Growth pattern alone not defining criterion for classifying thyroid tumor as poorly differentiated carcinoma
- Even when focal, poorly differentiated component should be mentioned in pathology report

SELECTED REFERENCES

1. Nonaka D: A study of FoxA1 expression in thyroid tumors. Hum Pathol. S0046-8177(17)30164-8, 2017
2. Sasanakietkul T et al: Epigenetic modifications in poorly differentiated and anaplastic thyroid cancer. Mol Cell Endocrinol. ePub, 2017
3. Teng L et al: Hobnail variant of papillary thyroid carcinoma: molecular profiling and comparison to classical papillary thyroid carcinoma, poorly differentiated thyroid carcinoma and anaplastic thyroid carcinoma. Oncotarget. 8(13):22023-22033, 2017
4. Xu B et al: Evolution of the histologic classification of thyroid neoplasms and its impact on clinical management. Eur J Surg Oncol. S0748-7983(17)30478, 2017
5. Yu MG et al: Poorly differentiated thyroid carcinoma: 10-year experience in a Southeast Asian population. Endocrinol Metab (Seoul). 32(2):288-295, 2017
6. Hahn SY et al: Description and comparison of the sonographic characteristics of poorly differentiated thyroid carcinoma and anaplastic thyroid carcinoma. J Ultrasound Med. 35(9):1873-9, 2016
7. Landa I et al: Genomic and transcriptomic hallmarks of poorly differentiated and anaplastic thyroid cancers. J Clin Invest. 126(3):1052-66, 2016
8. Volante M et al: The story of poorly differentiated thyroid carcinoma: from Langhans' description to the Turin proposal via Juan Rosai. Semin Diagn Pathol. 33(5):277-83, 2016
9. Xu B et al: Genomic Landscape of poorly differentiated and anaplastic thyroid carcinoma. Endocr Pathol. 27(3):205-12, 2016
10. Xu B et al: Clinicopathologic features of fatal non-anaplastic follicular cell-derived thyroid carcinomas. Thyroid. 26(11):1588-1597, 2016
11. Sykorova V et al: Search for new genetic biomarkers in poorly differentiated and anaplastic thyroid carcinomas using next generation sequencing. Anticancer Res. 35(4):2029-36, 2015
12. Amacher AM et al: Prevalence of a hobnail pattern in papillary, poorly differentiated, and anaplastic thyroid carcinoma: a possible manifestation of high-grade transformation. Am J Surg Pathol. 39(2):260-5, 2014

13. Arora S et al: Comparing outcomes in poorly-differentiated versus anaplastic thyroid cancers treated with radiation: a surveillance, epidemiology, and end results analysis. J Cancer Res Ther. 10(3):526-30, 2014

14. Asioli S et al: Cell size as a prognostic factor in oncocytic poorly differentiated carcinomas of the thyroid. Hum Pathol. 45(7):1489-95, 2014

15. Burman KD: Is poorly differentiated thyroid cancer poorly characterized? J Clin Endocrinol Metab. 99(4):1167-9, 2014

16. Eloy C et al: Small cell tumors of the thyroid gland: a review. Int J Surg Pathol. 22(3):197-201, 2014

17. Gnemmi V et al: Poorly differentiated thyroid carcinomas: application of the Turin proposal provides prognostic results similar to those from the assessment of high-grade features. Histopathology. 64(2):263-73, 2014

18. Ibrahimpasic T et al: Outcomes in patients with poorly differentiated thyroid carcinoma. J Clin Endocrinol Metab. 99(4):1245-52, 2014

19. Kakudo K et al: Prognostic classification of thyroid follicular cell tumors using Ki-67 labeling index: Risk stratification of thyroid follicular cell carcinomas [Review]. Endocr J. 62(1):1-12. doi: 10.1507/endocrj.EJ14-0293. Epub 2014 Sep 7., 2014

20. Pannone G et al: The role of survivin in thyroid tumors: differences of expression in well-differentiated, non-well-differentiated, and anaplastic thyroid cancers. Thyroid. 24(3):511-9, 2014

21. Patel KN et al: Poorly differentiated thyroid cancer. Curr Opin Otolaryngol Head Neck Surg. 22(2):121-6, 2014

22. Pita JM et al: Cell cycle deregulation and TP53 and RAS mutations are major events in poorly differentiated and undifferentiated thyroid carcinomas. J Clin Endocrinol Metab. 99(3):E497-507, 2014

23. Chernock RD et al: Napsin A expression in anaplastic, poorly differentiated, and micropapillary pattern thyroid carcinomas. Am J Surg Pathol. 37(8):1215-22, 2013

24. Ghossein RA et al: Immunohistochemical detection of mutated BRAF V600E supports the clonal origin of BRAF-induced thyroid cancers along the spectrum of disease progression. J Clin Endocrinol Metab. 98(8):E1414-21, 2013

25. Hannallah J et al: Comprehensive literature review: recent advances in diagnosing and managing patients with poorly differentiated thyroid carcinoma. Int J Endocrinol. 2013:317487, 2013

26. Ibrahimpasic T et al: Poorly differentiated thyroid carcinoma presenting with gross extrathyroidal extension: 1986-2009 Memorial Sloan-Kettering Cancer Center experience. Thyroid. 23(8):997-1002, 2013

27. Landa I et al: Frequent somatic TERT promoter mutations in thyroid cancer: higher prevalence in advanced forms of the disease. J Clin Endocrinol Metab. 98(9):E1562-6, 2013

28. Sadow PM et al: Poorly differentiated thyroid carcinoma: an incubating entity. Front Endocrinol (Lausanne). 3:77, 2012

29. Shaik S et al: SCF(β-TRCP) suppresses angiogenesis and thyroid cancer cell migration by promoting ubiquitination and destruction of VEGF receptor 2. J Exp Med. 209(7):1289-307, 2012

30. Dima M et al: Establishment and characterization of cell lines from a novel mouse model of poorly differentiated thyroid carcinoma: powerful tools for basic and preclinical research. Thyroid. 21(9):1001-7, 2011

31. Fat I et al: Insular variant of poorly differentiated thyroid carcinoma. Endocr Pract. 17(1):115-21, 2011

32. Knauf JA et al: Progression of BRAF-induced thyroid cancer is associated with epithelial-mesenchymal transition requiring concomitant MAP kinase and TGFβ signaling. Oncogene. 30(28):3153-62, 2011

33. Nambiar A et al: The concepts in poorly differentiated carcinoma of the thyroid: a review article. J Surg Oncol. 103(8):818-21, 2011

34. Asioli S et al: Poorly differentiated carcinoma of the thyroid: validation of the Turin proposal and analysis of IMP3 expression. Mod Pathol. 23(9):1269-78, 2010

35. Rivera M et al: Encapsulated thyroid tumors of follicular cell origin with high grade features (high mitotic rate/tumor necrosis): a clinicopathologic and molecular study. Hum Pathol. 41(2):172-80, 2010

36. Rivera M et al: Molecular, morphologic, and outcome analysis of thyroid carcinomas according to degree of extrathyroid extension. Thyroid. 20(10):1085-93, 2010

37. Bongiovanni M et al: Poorly differentiated thyroid carcinoma: a cytologic-histologic review. Adv Anat Pathol. 16(5):283-9, 2009

38. Baloch ZW et al: Unusual tumors of the thyroid gland. Endocrinol Metab Clin North Am. 37(2):297-310, vii, 2008

39. Volante M et al: Poorly differentiated thyroid carcinoma: diagnostic features and controversial issues. Endocr Pathol. 19(3):150-5, 2008

40. Kakudo K et al: [Thyroid carcinoma--differentiated, poorly differentiated and anaplastic carcinoma.] Nippon Rinsho. 65(11):1979-84, 2007

41. Volante M et al: Poorly differentiated thyroid carcinoma: the Turin proposal for the use of uniform diagnostic criteria and an algorithmic diagnostic approach. Am J Surg Pathol. 31(8):1256-64, 2007

42. Albores-Saavedra J et al: Where to set the threshold between well differentiated and poorly differentiated follicular carcinomas of the thyroid. Endocr Pathol. 15(4):297-305, 2004

43. Nikiforov YE: Genetic alterations involved in the transition from well-differentiated to poorly differentiated and anaplastic thyroid carcinomas. Endocr Pathol. 15(4):319-27, 2004

44. Sakamoto A: Definition of poorly differentiated carcinoma of the thyroid: the Japanese experience. Endocr Pathol. 15(4):307-11, 2004

45. Volante M et al: Poorly differentiated carcinomas of the thyroid with trabecular, insular, and solid patterns: a clinicopathologic study of 183 patients. Cancer. 100(5):950-7, 2004

46. Volante M et al: Prognostic factors of clinical interest in poorly differentiated carcinomas of the thyroid. Endocr Pathol. 15(4):313-7, 2004

WHO and Turin Diagnostic Criteria for PDTC

WHO 2004 Diagnostic Criteria	Turin Diagnostic Criteria 2006
Majority of tumor shows solid/trabecular/insular growth pattern	Presence of solid/trabecular/insular growth pattern
Infiltrative pattern of growth	Absence of conventional nuclear features of papillary carcinoma
Presence of necrosis	Presence of at least 1 of following features
Obvious vascular invasion	Convoluted nuclei
	Mitotic activity ≥ 3/10 HPF
	Tumor necrosis

PDTC = poorly differentiated thyroid carcinoma.

Note: WHO 2017 adopts the Turin Diagnostic Criteria.

Genetic Alterations in Well-Differentiated Thyroid Carcinoma (FTC and PTC) and Compared With Those of PDTC and ATC

Tumor Type	TP53	TERT	RAS	BRAF	PIK3CA	PTEN	CTNNB1	EIF1AX	ALK
FTC	0%	10-35%	30-50%	0%	0-10%	0-10%	0%	0%	0%
PTC	0%	5-15%	0-5%	40-80%	0-5%	0-5%	0%	0-5%	0-5%
PDTC	10-35%	20-50%	20-50%	5-15%	0-5%	5-20%	0-5%	5-15%	0-10%
ATC	40-80%	30-75%	10-50%	10-50%	5-25%	10-15%	0-5%	5-15%	0-10%

Well-differentiated thyroid carcinomas: FTC = follicular thyroid carcinoma; PTC = papillary thyroid carcinoma; PDTC = poorly differentiated thyroid carcinoma; ATC = anaplastic thyroid carcinoma.

Estimated published mutation prevalence rates: From 2017 WHO Classification of Tumors of Endocrine Organs.

Immunohistochemistry Table

Antibody	Reactivity	Staining Pattern	Comment
Thyroglobulin	Positive	Cytoplasmic	
TTF-1	Positive	Nuclear	
pax-8	Positive	Nuclear	
AE1/AE3	Positive	Cytoplasmic	
IMP3	Positive	Cytoplasmic	
Cyclin-D1	Positive	Nuclear	
Bcl-2	Positive	Cytoplasmic	Positive in > 80% cases
p53	Positive	Nuclear	Focally positive
BRAF	Positive	Cytoplasmic	BRAF is usually negative in PDTC; positive only when associated with BRAF-positive PTC
p63	Negative		
Chromogranin-A	Negative		
Synaptophysin	Negative		
Calcitonin	Negative		

PDTC = poorly differentiated thyroid carcinoma; PTC = papillary thyroid carcinoma.

(Left) *This poorly differentiated thyroid carcinoma (PDTC) presented as a solid mass with a variegated cut surface showing multiple foci of hemorrhage and necrosis ➡, occupying most of the lobe. A rim of compressed residual normal thyroid ➡ is present.* **(Right)** *PDTCs are usually unencapsulated. The cut surface of this tumor shows a variegated hemorrhagic area ➡ and an area of partially encapsulated neoplasm ➡.*

Gross Cut Surface With Necrosis

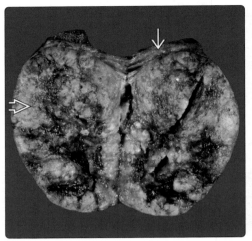

Partially Encapsulated PDTC

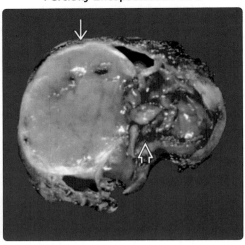

(Left) *PDTC is also characterized by a large trabecular growth pattern with cords of tumor cells forming large ribbons separated by fibrovascular connective tissue. A focus of necrosis ➡ within the trabecula is shown.* **(Right)** *The presence of a mitotic figure ➡ in a background of an otherwise bland homogeneous population of cells growing in a trabecular and focally microfollicular pattern helps make the diagnosis of PDTC. Minimal colloid is present.*

Growth Pattern of PDTC

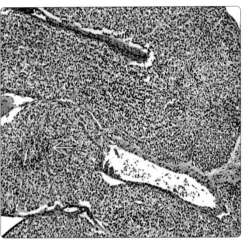

Atypical Mitosis in PDTC

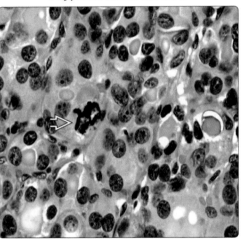

(Left) *PDTC is characterized by a diffuse sheet-like growth pattern ➡ with an occasional microfollicular pattern ➡. In this pattern, the follicles usually lack colloid.* **(Right)** *Large cells with clear cytoplasm and vacuolated nuclei with prominent nucleoli ➡ make up this PDTC. Mitotic figures ➡ and focal apoptosis are also shown.*

Diffuse Growth Pattern

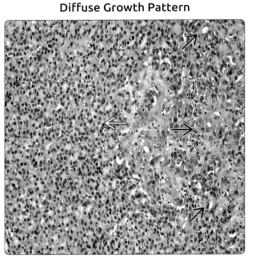

Cytology Aspects

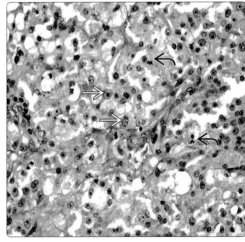

Trabecular Growth Pattern

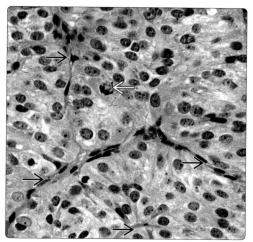

Mitoses

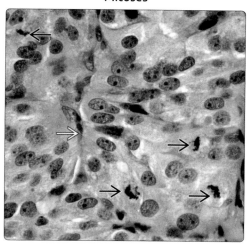

(Left) *High magnification of a trabecular/insular growth-patterned PDTC shows cells with round nuclei arranged in cords and separated by thin fibrovascular septa ➔. A mitotic figure ➔ is also present in the field.* (Right) *High magnification of a PDTC shows a characteristic insular growth pattern with round to oval nuclei, thin fibrovascular septa ➔, and 4 obvious mitoses ➔.*

Unusual Histopathology Pattern

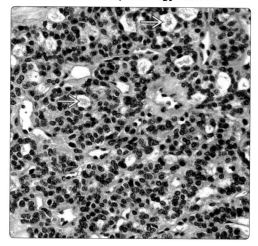

Morphological Features

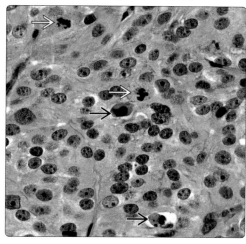

(Left) *A variant of PDTC shows a mixed trabecular and microfollicular pattern. The cells have small homogeneous nuclei and scant cytoplasm. Many of the lumina are filled with blue mucin-like material ➔.* (Right) *This high-magnification micrograph of a PDTC shows small to medium cells with round nuclei and homogeneous chromatin growing in a solid pattern. Scattered mitotic figures ➔ and apoptotic bodies ➔ are often seen and help establish the diagnosis.*

Nuclear Morphology

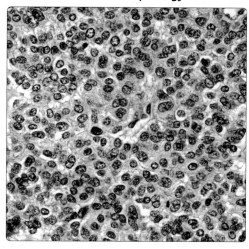

Lymphovascular Invasion

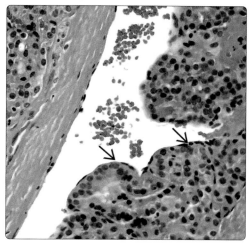

(Left) *In this PDTC, the cells are arranged in a solid growth pattern (sheet-like). Some of the nuclei are convoluted but lack nuclear features of papillary thyroid carcinoma (PTC), such as cleared chromatin and pseudoinclusions.* (Right) *The presence of a lymphovascular invasion can be seen in PDTC, and it is demonstrated here as tumor cells are present inside the vascular space. The PDTC cells are lined by a single layer of endothelial cells ➔.*

Cytology of PDTC

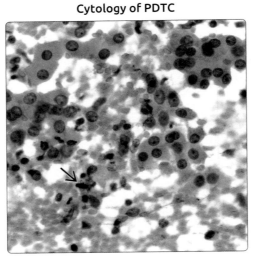

Extensive Necrosis

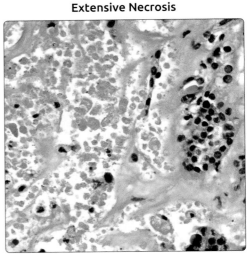

(Left) *PDTC fine-needle aspiration shows a highly cellular specimen with small to medium-sized cells with fine chromatin and scant colloid. Cells may be noncohesive and may form microfollicles. A mitotic figure ⇨ is seen.* **(Right)** *This PDTC shows areas of extensive necrosis. The presence of necrosis, increased mitotic activity, and atypical mitosis are helpful in the diagnosis of PDTC, irrespective of the architectural pattern.*

Minimal Nuclear Pleomorphism

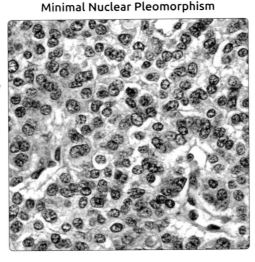

Oncocytic Cells

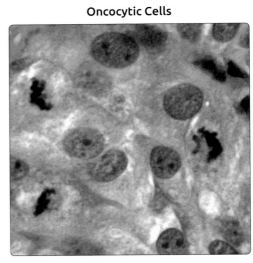

(Left) *High-power view of a PDTC with insular and solid arrangement composed of uniform cells with round hyperchromatic nuclei with minimal nuclear pleomorphism is shown.* **(Right)** *Some PDTCs are composed predominantly of oncocytic cells with mild cellular pleomorphism and nucleoli. In this photomicrography, 3 mitosis are identified. The markedly increased mitotic activity in this case was associated with areas of necrosis.*

PDTC Adjacent to PTC

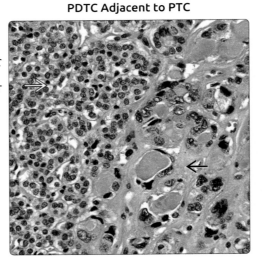

Metastases to Bone

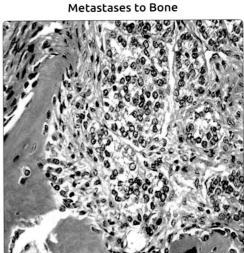

(Left) *The diagnosis of PDTC ⇨ is associated with PTC ⇨ and depends on the exclusion of a separate independent PTC and confirmation that the PDTC cells do not have nuclear features of PTC. The classic PTC nuclear features in this image allow ready distinction of the 2 components.* **(Right)** *Locally advanced disease and distant metastases to lymph nodes, bone, and lung are frequent in PDTC. In this micrograph, an example of metastatic PDTC in bone is shown.*

Cyclin D1 in PDTC

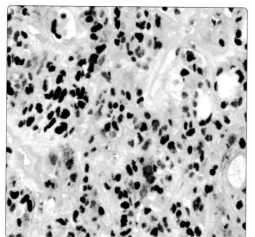

Thyroglobulin Pattern in PDTC

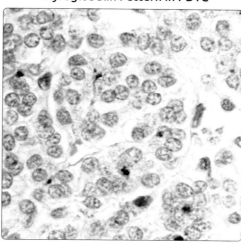

(Left) *Immunohistochemical stain for cyclin-D1 in a case of PDTC shows strong nuclear expression throughout the tumor. Cyclin D1 is usually positive in PDTC and anaplastic thyroid carcinoma. The exact role of cyclin-D1 in the transformation from well-differentiated carcinoma to PDTC remains unknown.*
(Right) *The immunohistochemical staining pattern for thyroglobulin is highly variable in PDTCs. In this example, few scattered cells show weak to moderate focal cytoplasmic positivity.*

HBME-1 Immunostain in PDTC and PTC

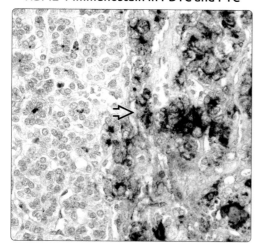

TTF-1 Immunostain in PDTC

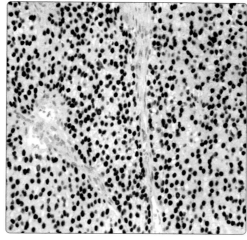

(Left) *HBME-1 immunohistochemical stain in a case of PDTC associated with PTC highlights the positivity of the PTC component ⇉ and negativity of the PDTC component.*
(Right) *Strong and diffuse immunopositivity for TTF-1 is commonly seen in PDTC. This finding helps differentiate from other tumors as anaplastic thyroid carcinoma typically does not express immunoreactivity for thyroglobulin, pax-8, and TTF-1.*

p53 in PDTC

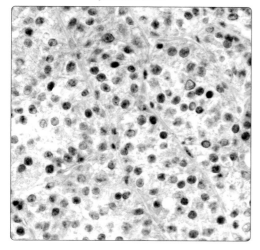

Proliferative Index by Ki-67

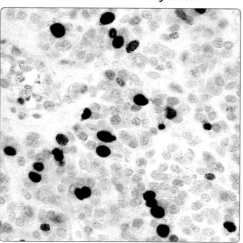

(Left) *Variable nuclear immunostain for p53 may be seen in PDTC, as shown in this insular growth patterned tumor. Gain-of-function mutations in p53 have been shown to occur preferentially in poorly differentiated and anaplastic thyroid carcinomas.*
(Right) *Mitotic activity is an important diagnostic criterion defined by the Turin consensus meeting. High proliferative index is characteristic of poorly differentiated carcinomas and can be assessed by Ki-67 immunostain, as shown.*

TERMINOLOGY

- Anaplastic thyroid carcinoma is highly aggressive thyroid malignancy composed of undifferentiated follicular thyroid cells

ETIOLOGY/PATHOGENESIS

- Most thyroid with anaplastic carcinoma have areas of differentiated thyroid carcinomas, suggesting high-grade evolution from these tumors

CLINICAL ISSUES

- Rapidly expanding neck mass
- No known genetic susceptibility findings specifically associated with development of nonsyndromic anaplastic thyroid carcinoma, but occurs in some inherited cancer syndromes

MICROSCOPIC

- Widely invasive, hypercellular neoplasm with extensive necrosis

- Morphological spectrum depends on admixture of 3 histological patterns
  - **Sarcomatoid form**: Features commonly seen in high-grade pleomorphic sarcoma
  - **Giant cell form**: Composed of highly pleomorphic malignant cells
  - **Epithelial form**: Manifests squamoid or squamous cohesive tumor nests

ANCILLARY TESTS

- Immunohistochemistry for p53 usually positive
- pax-8 positive in ~ 50% of ATC
- Ki-67 proliferative index > 80%
- Most consistent finding is association of ATC and *TP53* mutation, *BRAF*, β-catenin (*CTNNB1*), and *RAS* mutations
- Alterations in gene named "overexpressed in anaplastic thyroid carcinoma-1" (*PCLAF*)
- Copy-number gains in genes such as *EGFR*, *FLT1* (*VEGFR1*), *PDGFRB*, and *PIK3CA/B*

Gross Cut Surface

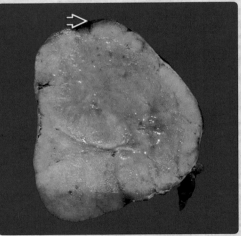

Extensive Areas of Necrosis

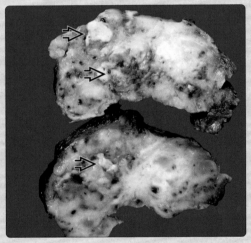

(Left) *Gross photograph shows an anaplastic thyroid carcinoma (ATC) with a fleshy cut surface as an incidental finding within a retrosternal thyroid goiter during cardiac surgery. A small rim of normal thyroid is seen ➡. In this case, there is no evidence of necrosis grossly.* (Right) *Gross cut surface of ATC shows a fleshy, variegated appearance with areas of degeneration, hemorrhage, and extensive areas of necrosis ➡. The tumor is usually nodular, bosselated, and highly infiltrative, extending into adjacent soft tissues.*

ATC With Residual PTC

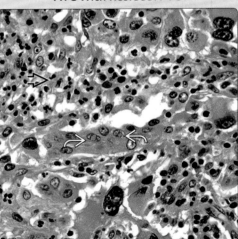

Immunopositivity for p53

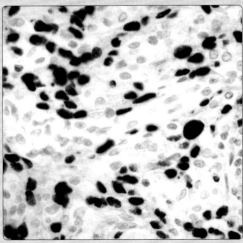

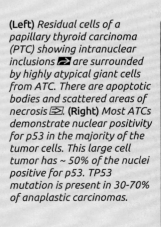

(Left) *Residual cells of a papillary thyroid carcinoma (PTC) showing intranuclear inclusions ➡ are surrounded by highly atypical giant cells from ATC. There are apoptotic bodies and scattered areas of necrosis ➡.* (Right) *Most ATCs demonstrate nuclear positivity for p53 in the majority of the tumor cells. This large cell tumor has ~ 50% of the nuclei positive for p53. TP53 mutation is present in 30-70% of anaplastic carcinomas.*

TERMINOLOGY

Abbreviations

- Anaplastic thyroid carcinoma (ATC)

Synonyms

- Undifferentiated thyroid carcinoma (UTC)
- Sarcomatoid carcinoma
- Metaplastic carcinoma
- Spindle cell carcinoma
- Giant cell carcinoma
- Dedifferentiated thyroid carcinoma
- Carcinosarcoma
- Pleomorphic carcinoma

Definitions

- ATC: Highly aggressive thyroid malignancy
  - Primarily composed of undifferentiated follicular thyroid cells that exhibit ultrastructural or immunohistochemical features of epithelial differentiation

ETIOLOGY/PATHOGENESIS

Environmental Exposure

- ~ 10% report radiation exposure
- Iodine deficiency for > 20 years in ~ 10%

Preexisting Poorly Differentiated or Well-Differentiated Thyroid Carcinoma

- Transformation or dedifferentiation of preexisting differentiated carcinoma
  - Papillary thyroid carcinoma can be identified in up to 80% of cases
  - Presence of differentiated carcinoma in up to 90% of anaplastic carcinomas
  - Presence of same mutation in differentiated component as in anaplastic carcinoma
    - *RAS* mutation present in ~ 60%
    - *BRAF* mutation V600E present in ~ 30%

Preexisting Benign Thyroid Disease

- Most patients with anaplastic carcinoma have longstanding history of nodular hyperplasia
- Background thyroid with multiple adenomatous nodules

CLINICAL ISSUES

Epidemiology

- Incidence
  - Accounts for < 5% of all malignant thyroid neoplasms, > 50% of deaths for thyroid cancer
    - Mortality rate > 90% and mean survival of 6 months
  - 1-2 cases per million annually
    - Incidence varies regionally
      - Higher in Europe than United States
      - Higher in endemic goiter due to iodine-deficient regions
- Age
  - Mean: Mid 60s
- Sex
  - F > M (2:1)

Presentation

- Rapidly expanding neck mass
- Usually patients present with long history of thyroid disease
- Usually present in patients with enlarged thyroid for years
- Single or multiple hard, fixed nodules
- Usually symptomatic
  - Hoarseness (80%), dysphagia (60%), vocal cord paralysis (50%), cervical pain (30%), and dyspnea (20%)
- Surrounding structures usually involved
  - Muscles, trachea, esophagus, laryngeal nerves, larynx
- Cervical lymphadenopathy present in many cases
- Metastases common at time of diagnosis: 30-40% of patients
  - Lung, bone, and brain
- Most tumors involve only 1 lobe
  - Tumors may be bilateral in 25%
  - Most tumors single; multifocal tumors accounts up to 40%
- Anaplastic thyroid carcinomas may occur in ectopic locations
  - Most common ectopic location retrosternal goiter

Treatment

- Options, risks, complications
  - Multimodality therapy required
  - Target therapy promising in some cases
- Surgical approaches
  - Surgery used to obtain diagnostic material and debulking for palliation of symptoms
- Adjuvant therapy
  - Poor response to chemotherapy
- Radiation
  - Used but with unpredictable response

Prognosis

- Overall poor
  - Mortality rate: > 90%
  - Mean survival: 1 year after diagnosis
  - Median 1-year survival: 10-20%
  - Overall 5-year survival: 0-14%
- Rapidly progressive local disease
- > 50% of patients have lymph node metastases at time of primary diagnosis
- Metastases to distant sites common: Lungs, bone, and brain
- Prognosis dependent on tumor confinement to capsule and percentage of anaplastic component in differentiated tumor
  - Worse prognosis in men and in patients > 60 years, with tumors > 5 cm, and with extensive local disease
- > 1/2 of deaths attributable to thyroid carcinomas result from ATC

Genetic Susceptibility

- No known genetic susceptibility findings specifically associated with development of nonsyndromic ATC
  - However, ATC occurs in inherited cancer syndromes
    - PTEN-hamartoma tumor syndrome/Cowden disease
    - Werner syndrome
    - Carney complex
    - Familial adenomatous polyposis

IMAGING

General Features

- Size
  - Tumors large, measuring up to 20 cm
- Infiltrative, heterogeneous mass with irregular borders, extensive necrosis, and calcifications
- CT shows extent of disease
- Calcification and necrosis may be identified

MACROSCOPIC

General Features

- Large, white-tan, fleshy tumors with variegated appearance with areas of necrosis and hemorrhage
- Replace most of normal thyroid parenchyma
- Infiltrative with irregular borders
- Invade into adjacent structures, including soft tissue, lymph nodes, larynx, pharynx, trachea, and esophagus

Size

- Mean: 6 cm (range: 1 to ~ 20 cm)

Sections to Be Submitted

- Sample entire tumor adequately to best classify these neoplasms and to identify preexisting and adjacent well-differentiated tumors

MICROSCOPIC

Histologic Features

- Widely invasive, hypercellular neoplasm with extensive necrosis
- Infiltrative pattern of growth
- Morphological spectrum depends on admixture of 3 histological patterns: Spindle cell sarcomatoid, giant cell, and epithelial components
  - **Sarcomatoid form**: Composed of malignant spindle cells with features commonly seen in high-grade pleomorphic sarcoma
  - **Giant cell form**: Composed of highly pleomorphic malignant cells, some of which contain multinucleated nuclei
  - **Epithelial form**: Manifests squamoid or squamous cohesive tumor nests with abundant eosinophilic cytoplasm; occasional keratinization may occur
- Diverse patterns depending on histological categories of epithelioid or sarcomatoid
  - Storiform, sheet-like, fascicular, angiomatoid, paucicellular
- Mixture of epithelioid cells, spindle cells, and pleomorphic giant cells
- Bizarre nuclei with prominent nucleoli
- Dense eosinophilic cytoplasm
- Increased mitotic activity
- Osteoclast-like giant cells common
- Extensive necrosis seen
- Inflammatory cells commonly present
  - Neutrophilic component may be present in some cases
- Colloid absent
- Desmoplastic stroma may be present

- Heterologous differentiation, as neoplastic bone and cartilage

Cytologic Features

- FNA can provide correct diagnosis in > 85% of cases
- Markedly pleomorphic nuclei with prominent nucleoli
- Multiple mitotic figures can be present
- Poorly differentiated cells: Can be spindled, polygonal, pleomorphic, epithelioid, and giant cell-like
- Background composed of necrotic cells and occasionally neutrophils

Lymphatic/Vascular Invasion

- Extensive lymphovascular invasion present
  - Numerous large vessels involved
  - Vessel walls invaded or destroyed by tumor

Predominant Pattern/Injury Type

- Anaplastic carcinomas grouped in 2 major categories: Sarcomatoid, giant cell, and epithelial
  - ATC with sarcomatoid appearance characterized by spindle cells and giant cells
    - Sarcomatoid appearance in tumors predominantly composed of spindle cells
      - □ Tumor cells can be arranged in fascicles in fascicular and storiform pattern of growth
      - □ Highly vascular tumors can show neoplastic cells in hemangiopericytoma-like arrangement
    - Giant cells shows marked pleomorphism and are interspersed among smaller cells
      - □ Osteoclast-like giant cells may be present
    - Heterologous elements may be present
      - □ Chondrosarcomatous and osteosarcomatous differentiation occur in > 5% ATC
      - □ Rhabdomyosarcoma differentiation can occur
  - ATC with epithelioid/squamoid appearance less heterogeneous than sarcomatoid tumors
    - Keratinization may occur in < 20% of these cases

UTC Variants

- Sarcomatoid/spindle cell variant
  - Atypical fascicles of spindle cells
- Giant cell (pleomorphic) variant
  - Sheets of highly pleomorphic cells
    - Some of which contain multiple nuclei
- Epithelial/squamoid variant
  - Nests or sheets of squamoid or squamous cohesive tumor nests with abundant eosinophilic cytoplasm
  - Hyalinization may be present
- Paucicellular variant
  - Hypocellular proliferation of mildly atypical tumor cells embedded in abundant dense, fibrous stroma
  - May be mistaken for Riedel thyroiditis/IgG4-related disease
- Angiomatoid variant
  - Anastomosing vascular spaces
- Rhabdoid variant
  - Composed of cells with eosinophilic cytoplasm and eccentric nucleus
- Lymphoepithelioma-like carcinoma
  - Resembles nasopharyngeal tumor, but EBER negative
- ATCs with heterologous differentiation

- o Presence of malignant cartilage or bone
- o Osteoclast-like Giant Cells
  - − Large numbers of osteoclast-like giant cells, positive for CD68

ANCILLARY TESTS

Cytology

- Highly cellular neoplasm with absent colloid
- Cells in clusters or sheets
- Marked cellular pleomorphism
- Ample eosinophilic cytoplasm
- Bizarre nuclei with prominent nucleoli
- Numerous mitotic figures
- Numerous apoptotic bodies
- Dirty background with necrotic debris and inflammatory cells

Electron Microscopy

- Undifferentiated cells with rare tight junctions, tonofilaments, and desmosomes
- Presence of complex cytoplasmic interdigitations
- Rare apical microvilli
- Incomplete basal lamina
- Some cells may show differentiation toward rhabdomyoblasts, lipoblasts, osteoblasts

Immunohistochemistry

- ATCs show variable immunophenotype; major role of IHC is to help distinguish ATC from other undifferentiated malignancies
- Keratin positive in ~ 80% of cases
  - o Keratin cocktails usually positive (CAM5.2 or AE1/AE3)
- Vimentin usually positive in majority of cases with spindle cell component
- EMA rarely positive, seen in up to 30-50% of cases
  - o EMA and CEA present in squamoid cells
  - o CEA rarely positive
- p53 usually diffusely positive in ATC
- p63 positive in up to 70% of cases, mostly in areas with squamoid differentiation
- Typically, ATC cells negative for TTF-1, thyroglobulin, and calcitonin
- pax-8 may be positive in ~ 50% of ATC
- Ki-67 proliferative index usually > 80%
- ATC has higher expression of cancer stem cell markers, such as aldehyde dehydrogenase 1(ALDH1) and CD133, than papillary thyroid carcinoma
  - o High expression of cancer stem cell markers related to adverse outcome

Flow Cytometry

- Tumors aneuploid

Genetic Testing

- Somatic gene mutations in components of principal oncogenic pathways occur with high frequency
- Conserved mutation pattern in well-differentiated and anaplastic components
  - o Undifferentiated component demonstrates increased mutation rates
  - o Confirm multistep dedifferentiation process

- Most consistent finding is association of ATC and *TP53* mutation
  - o 30-70% of ATC carry loss of function mutations in *TP53* gene
  - o *TP53* accumulated in nuclei
  - o p53 identified by immunohistochemistry in almost 100% of cases
  - o Identified by PCR in ~ 70-80% of cases
- *BRAF* and *RAS* mutations present in both differentiated and undifferentiated components
  - o *BRAF* present in ~ 20% of cases where papillary thyroid carcinoma was present
    - − In both tumor components, differentiated and undifferentiated
  - o RAS present
    - − *NRAS*, *KRAS*, or *HRAS* mutated in ~ 20% cases
    - − In both tumor components, differentiated and undifferentiated
- *RET/PTC* rearrangements rarely present in ATC
- β-catenin (*CTNNB1*) mutations also present in ATC
  - o Mutations of gene leading to constitutively active Wnt-signaling present in up to 60% of ATC
  - o Aberrant localization of β-catenin demonstrated in ~ 80% of cases
  - o β-catenin accumulated in nuclei due to altered degradation
- Alterations in gene named "overexpressed in anaplastic thyroid carcinoma-1" (*PCLAF*) associated with both de novo ATC and cases that arise in differentiated thyroid carcinoma
- Alterations in cell cycle control: Cyclin-D1, decreased expression of p27, and inactivation of p16 and *PTEN*
  - o Loss of function of *PTEN* gene present in 10-15% of ATC
- *FOXA1* DNA copy number gain within 14q21.1 locus in both ATC cell line and human ATC cases
- Complex and numerous chromosomal alterations, including numerical and structural aberrations
  - o Copy-number gains in genes such as *EGFR* (~ 45% cases), *FLT1* (VEGFR1) (45% of cases), *PDGFRB* (38% of cases), and *PIK3CA/B* (38% of cases)
  - o CGH demonstrates DNA imbalances at various chromosomal loci
  - o Median chromosomal gain: 10/case
- Allelic gains and losses at 1q, 1p, 5, 8, 9p, 11, 17p, 19p, 22q, 16p, and 18q

DIFFERENTIAL DIAGNOSIS

Primary Sarcoma

- Variety of primary thyroid sarcomas should be differentiated from UTC
  - o Synovial sarcoma, Ewing sarcoma, rhabdomyosarcoma, angiosarcoma, leiomyosarcoma, malignant peripheral nerve sheath tumor
  - o Differences in morphology, patterns of growth, cytologic appearance, molecular markers

Malignant Melanoma

- Positive immunohistochemistry for S100, Melan-A, Mart-1, HMB-45, and tyrosinase
- Similar genetic findings to UTC, as both have *BRAF* and *RAS* mutations

Riedel Thyroiditis

- Dense and hyalinized fibrous tissue (keloid-like), inflammatory cells, and vasculitis
- Rare or no atypical cells
- p53 negative
- Paucicellular variant of UTC may mimic Riedel thyroiditis

Poorly Differentiated Thyroid Carcinoma

- Variable histological appearance with 3 histological patterns
  o Solid, insular, or trabecular growth pattern
- Infiltrative growth pattern, necrosis and vascular invasion
- Monotonous population of neoplastic, nonpleomorphic cells
- Intermediate behavior between well-differentiated and undifferentiated thyroid carcinoma
- Ki-67 proliferative index around 10-30%
- TTF-1 and keratin positive

Spindle Cell Tumor With Thymus-Like Differentiation

- Usually in younger patients
- Spindle cell predominant pattern
  o Lacks pleomorphism, mitosis, and necrosis

Carcinoma With Thymus-Like Differentiation

- Nested and lobular pattern separated by fibrous stroma with inflammatory cells
- Squamoid cells lacking atypia; CD5 and 34βE12 positive

Squamous Cell Carcinoma

- Composed entirely of cells with squamous cell differentiation
- Primary head and neck squamous cell carcinoma and metastatic lung carcinoma consistently pax-8 negative

Medullary Thyroid Carcinoma

- Malignant tumor with C-cell differentiation
  o Positive for chromogranin, synaptophysin, and calcitonin

Mucoepidermoid Carcinoma

- Composed of combination of epidermoid and mucinous components
- Low-grade thyroid neoplasm

Sclerosing Mucoepidermoid Carcinoma With Eosinophilia

- Fibrohyaline stroma with striking infiltration by eosinophils
- Mucin secretion often present

DIAGNOSTIC CHECKLIST

Pathologic Interpretation Pearls

- Variety of patterns with areas of necrosis, increased mitotic activity, and positivity for p53

Staging

- All anaplastic thyroid carcinomas considered T4 tumors by definition
  o T4a: Intrathyroidal anaplastic carcinoma (surgically resectable)
  o T4b: Extrathyroidal anaplastic carcinoma (surgically unresectable)
- All anaplastic thyroid carcinomas considered stage IV
  o Stage IVA: T4a
  o Stage IVB: T4b
  o Stage IVC: Any T with metastases

SELECTED REFERENCES

1. Ahn S et al: Comprehensive screening for PD-L1 expression in thyroid cancer. Endocr Relat Cancer. 24(2):97-106, 2017
2. Bonhomme B et al: Molecular pathology of anaplastic thyroid carcinomas: a retrospective study of 144 cases. Thyroid. 27(5):682-692, 2017
3. Gibson WJ et al: Genomic heterogeneity and exceptional response to dual pathway inhibition in anaplastic thyroid cancer. Clin Cancer Res. 23(9):2367-2373, 2017
4. Gupta AJ et al: Primary sarcomas of thyroid gland-series of three cases with brief review of spindle cell lesions of thyroid. J Clin Diagn Res. 11(2):ER01-ER04, 2017
5. Molinaro E et al: Anaplastic thyroid carcinoma: from clinicopathology to genetics and advanced therapies. Nat Rev Endocrinol. ePub, 2017
6. Pezzi TA et al: Radiation therapy dose is associated with improved survival for unresected anaplastic thyroid carcinoma: outcomes from the National Cancer Data Base. Cancer. 123(9):1653-1661, 2017
7. Sandulache VC et al: Real-time genomic characterization utilizing circulating cell-free DNA in patients with anaplastic thyroid carcinoma. Thyroid. 27(1):81-87, 2017
8. Teng L et al: Hobnail variant of papillary thyroid carcinoma: molecular profiling and comparison to classical papillary thyroid carcinoma, poorly differentiated thyroid carcinoma and anaplastic thyroid carcinoma. Oncotarget. 8(13):22023-22033, 2017
9. Weinberger P et al: Cell cycle M-phase genes are highly upregulated in anaplastic thyroid carcinoma. Thyroid. 27(2):236-252, 2017
10. Zwaenepoel K et al: CD70 and PD-L1 in anaplastic thyroid cancer - promising targets for immunotherapy. Histopathology. ePub, 2017
11. Bible KC et al: Evolving molecularly targeted therapies for advanced-stage thyroid cancers. Nat Rev Clin Oncol. 13(7):403-16, 2016
12. Liu G et al: Elucidation of the molecular mechanisms of anaplastic thyroid carcinoma by integrated miRNA and mRNA analysis. Oncol Rep. 36(5):3005-3013, 2016
13. Penna GC et al: Molecular markers involved in tumorigenesis of thyroid carcinoma: focus on aggressive histotypes. Cytogenet Genome Res. 150(3-4):194-207, 2016
14. Xu B et al: Clinicopathologic features of fatal non-anaplastic follicular cell-derived thyroid carcinomas. Thyroid. 26(11):1588-1597, 2016
15. Kunstman JW et al: Characterization of the mutational landscape of anaplastic thyroid cancer via whole-exome sequencing. Hum Mol Genet. 24(8):2318-29, 2015
16. Smith N et al: Personalized therapy in patients with anaplastic thyroid cancer: targeting genetic and epigenetic alterations. J Clin Endocrinol Metab. 100(1):35-42, 2015
17. Amacher AM et al: Prevalence of a hobnail pattern in papillary, poorly differentiated, and anaplastic thyroid carcinoma: a possible manifestation of high-grade transformation. Am J Surg Pathol. ePub, 2014
18. Dibelius G et al: Noninvasive anaplastic thyroid carcinoma: report of a case and literature review. Thyroid. 24(8):1319-24, 2014
19. Charles RP et al: Activating BRAF and PIK3CA mutations cooperate to promote anaplastic thyroid carcinogenesis. Mol Cancer Res. 12(7):979-86, 2014
20. Ragazzi M et al: Update on anaplastic thyroid carcinoma: morphological, molecular, and genetic features of the most aggressive thyroid cancer. Int J Endocrinol. 2014:790834, 2014
21. Onoda N et al: Establishment, characterization and comparison of seven authentic anaplastic thyroid cancer cell lines retaining clinical features of the original tumors. World J Surg. 38(3):688-95, 2014
22. Pita JM et al: Cell cycle deregulation and TP53 and RAS mutations are major events in poorly differentiated and undifferentiated thyroid carcinomas. J Clin Endocrinol Metab. 99(3):E497-507, 2014
23. Yun JY et al: Expression of cancer stem cell markers is more frequent in anaplastic thyroid carcinoma compared to papillary thyroid carcinoma and is related to adverse clinical outcome. J Clin Pathol. 67(2):125-33, 2014
24. Wagle N et al: Response and acquired resistance to everolimus in anaplastic thyroid cancer. N Engl J Med. 371(15):1426-33, 2014
25. Deshpande HA et al: New targeted therapies and other advances in the management of anaplastic thyroid cancer. Curr Opin Oncol. 25(1):44-9, 2013
26. Walts AE et al: BRAF genetic heterogeneity in papillary thyroid carcinoma and its metastasis. Hum Pathol. 45(5):935-41, 2014
27. Granata R et al: Therapeutic strategies in the management of patients with metastatic anaplastic thyroid cancer: review of the current literature. Curr Opin Oncol. 25(3):224-8, 2013

28. Besic N et al: Sites of metastases of anaplastic thyroid carcinoma: autopsy findings in 45 cases from a single institution. Thyroid. 23(6):709-13, 2013

29. Buehler D et al: Expression of epithelial-mesenchymal transition regulators SNAI2 and TWIST1 in thyroid carcinomas. Mod Pathol. 26(1):54-61, 2013

30. Chernock RD et al: Napsin A expression in anaplastic, poorly differentiated, and micropapillary pattern thyroid carcinomas. Am J Surg Pathol. 37(8):1215-22, 2013

31. Guerra A et al: Genetic mutations in the treatment of anaplastic thyroid cancer: a systematic review. BMC Surg. 13 Suppl 2:S44, 2013

32. Chen JH et al: Clinicopathological and molecular characterization of nine cases of columnar cell variant of papillary thyroid carcinoma. Mod Pathol. 24(5):739-49, 2011

33. Kojic SL et al: Anaplastic thyroid cancer: a comprehensive review of novel therapy. Expert Rev Anticancer Ther. 11(3):387-402, 2011

34. Kao CS et al: NUT protein is not expressed in undifferentiated (anaplastic) thyroid carcinoma. Histopathology. 63(3):429-30, 2013

35. Rossi ED et al: Diagnostic and prognostic role of HBME-1, galectin-3, and β-catenin in poorly differentiated and anaplastic thyroid carcinomas. Appl Immunohistochem Mol Morphol. 21(3):237-41, 2013

36. Bellelli R et al: FOXM1 is a molecular determinant of the mitogenic and invasive phenotype of anaplastic thyroid carcinoma. Endocr Relat Cancer. 19(5):695-710, 2012

37. Smallridge RC et al: American Thyroid Association guidelines for management of patients with anaplastic thyroid cancer. Thyroid. 22(11):1104-39, 2012

38. Nosé V: Familial thyroid cancer: a review. Mod Pathol. 24 Suppl 2:S19-33, 2011

39. Nucera C et al: B-Raf(V600E) and thrombospondin-1 promote thyroid cancer progression. Proc Natl Acad Sci U S A. 107(23):10649-54, 2010

40. Roche B et al: Epidemiology, clinical presentation, treatment and prognosis of a regional series of 26 anaplastic thyroid carcinomas (ATC). Comparison with the literature. Ann Endocrinol (Paris). 71(1):38-45, 2010

41. Smallridge RC et al: Anaplastic thyroid carcinoma: pathogenesis and emerging therapies. Clin Oncol (R Coll Radiol). 22(6):486-97, 2010

42. Ito Y et al: Investigation of the validity of UICC stage grouping of anaplastic carcinoma of the thyroid. Asian J Surg. 32(1):47-50, 2009

43. Nucera C et al: A novel orthotopic mouse model of human anaplastic thyroid carcinoma. Thyroid. 19(10):1077-84, 2009

44. Nucera C et al: FOXA1 is a potential oncogene in anaplastic thyroid carcinoma. Clin Cancer Res. 15(11):3680-9, 2009

45. Smallridge RC et al: Anaplastic thyroid cancer: molecular pathogenesis and emerging therapies. Endocr Relat Cancer. 16(1):17-44, 2009

46. Olthof M et al: Anaplastic thyroid carcinoma with rhabdomyoblastic differentiation: a case report with a good clinical outcome. Endocr Pathol. 19(1):62-5, 2008

47. Tong GX et al: Fine-needle aspiration biopsy of primary osteosarcoma of the thyroid: report of a case and review of the literature. Diagn Cytopathol. 36(8):589-94, 2008

48. Won YS et al: A case of Riedel's thyroiditis associated with benign nodule: mimic of anaplastic transformation. Int J Surg. 6(6):e24-7, 2008

49. Zito G et al: In vitro identification and characterization of CD133(pos) cancer stem-like cells in anaplastic thyroid carcinoma cell lines. PLoS One. 3(10):e3544, 2008

50. Cerilli LA et al: Anaplastic carcinoma of the thyroid with chondroblastoma features mimicking papillary carcinoma: a case report. Acta Cytol. 51(5):825-8, 2007

51. Cornett WR et al: Anaplastic thyroid carcinoma: an overview. Curr Oncol Rep. 9(2):152-8, 2007

52. Lee JJ et al: Molecular cytogenetic profiles of novel and established human anaplastic thyroid carcinoma models. Thyroid. 17(4):289-301, 2007

53. Salvatore G et al: A cell proliferation and chromosomal instability signature in anaplastic thyroid carcinoma. Cancer Res. 67(21):10148-58, 2007

54. Takano T et al: BRAF V600E mutation in anaplastic thyroid carcinomas and their accompanying differentiated carcinomas. Br J Cancer. 96(10):1549-53, 2007

55. Wiseman SM et al: Anaplastic thyroid carcinoma: expression profile of targets for therapy offers new insights for disease treatment. Ann Surg Oncol. 14(2):719-29, 2007

56. Wiseman SM et al: Identification of molecular markers altered during transformation of differentiated into anaplastic thyroid carcinoma. Arch Surg. 142(8):717-27; discussion 727-9, 2007

57. Yassa L et al: Long-term assessment of a multidisciplinary approach to thyroid nodule diagnostic evaluation. Cancer. 111(6):508-16, 2007

58. Papi G et al: Primary spindle cell lesions of the thyroid gland; an overview. Am J Clin Pathol. 125 Suppl:S95-123, 2006

59. Reimann JD et al: Carcinoma showing thymus-like differentiation of the thyroid (CASTLE): a comparative study: evidence of thymic differentiation and solid cell nest origin. Am J Surg Pathol. 30(8):994-1001, 2006

60. Saltman B et al: Patterns of expression of cell cycle/apoptosis genes along the spectrum of thyroid carcinoma progression. Surgery. 140(6):899-905; discussion 905-6, 2006

61. Untch BR et al: Anaplastic thyroid carcinoma, thyroid lymphoma, and metastasis to thyroid. Surg Oncol Clin N Am. 15(3):661-79, x, 2006

62. Mizutani K et al: Overexpressed in anaplastic thyroid carcinoma-1 (OEATC-1) as a novel gene responsible for anaplastic thyroid carcinoma. Cancer. 103(9):1785-90, 2005

63. O'Neill JP et al: Anaplastic (undifferentiated) thyroid cancer: improved insight and therapeutic strategy into a highly aggressive disease. J Laryngol Otol. 119(8):585-91, 2005

64. Nikiforov YE: Genetic alterations involved in the transition from well-differentiated to poorly differentiated and anaplastic thyroid carcinomas. Endocr Pathol. 15(4):319-27, 2004

Immunohistochemistry

Antibody	Reactivity	Staining Pattern	Comment
pax-8	Positive	Nuclear	Retained in ~ 50% of ATC
TTF-1	Negative	Nuclear	Very rare cells may express weak reactivity
Thyroglobulin	Negative	Cytoplasmic	If positive, due to diffusion from entrapped nonneoplastic thyroid
AE1/AE3	Positive	Cytoplasmic	Positive in ~ 80% of cases
p53	Positive	Nuclear	70-100% positivity in anaplastic carcinoma
Ki-67	Positive	Nuclear	High; ~ 80% proliferative index
CEA-M	Positive	Cell membrane & cytoplasm	Rare; 10% predominantly in tumors with squamoid features
p63	Positive	Nuclear	
Desmin	Negative	Cytoplasmic	Useful for differentiating from rhabdomyosarcomas, as is myogenin
HMB-45	Negative	Cell membrane & cytoplasm	Along with S100 and Melan-A, assists in distinguishing from melanoma
CD31	Negative	Cell membrane	Differentiating between angiosarcomas, also factor VIII and CD34
CD34	Negative	Cell membrane	Use to exclude large cell lymphoma
BRAF	Positive	Cytoplasmic	~ 30% of ATC positive
ret	Negative		

Variants of Anaplastic Thyroid Carcinoma

Variants	Morphological Features
Sarcomatoid/spindle cell variant	Most common variant; has histological features of high-grade sarcoma
Giant cell variant/pleomorphic	2nd most common, composed of pleomorphic and bizarre cells with multinucleation
Epithelial/squamoid cell variant	Tumor shows sheets of cells with squamoid differentiation, desmoplastic stroma, and dyskeratosis
Osteoclast-like variant	Large numbers of multinucleated osteoclastic-like giant cells
Paucicellular variant	Tumor composed by extensive fibrous proliferation with scanty tumor cells with scattered inflammatory cells; difficult differential diagnosis with Riedel thyroiditis
Carcinosarcoma variant	Pleomorphic cells show variable differentiation with epithelioid areas intermixed with sarcomatous component, usually osteosarcoma, chondrosarcoma, rhabdomyosarcoma
Lymphoepithelioma-like variant	Resembles nasopharyngeal lymphoepithelioma but negative for EBER
Angiomatoid variant	Anastomosing vascular spaces with hemangiopericytoma-like pattern or staghorn pattern
Rhabdoid variant	Cells with eosinophilic hyaline-like cytoplasm and exocentric nucleus

Papillary Carcinoma and ATC

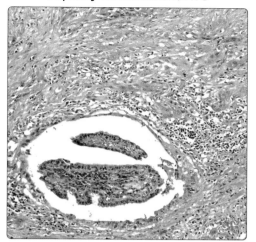

Spindle Cells Appearance in ATC

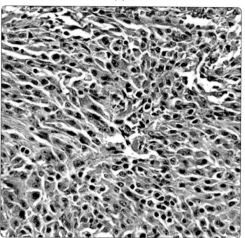

(Left) *ATC exhibits malignant cells adjacent to a papillary thyroid carcinoma, classical type. This undifferentiated tumor most likely arose from the differentiated component.* **(Right)** *Spindle cells are frequently seen in ATC. This figure shows fascicles of highly atypical spindle cells around small capillaries. There is pleomorphism, mitosis, apoptotic bodies, and focal necrosis.*

Paucicellular Variant of ATC

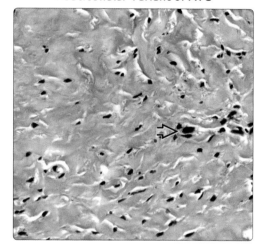

Combination of Patterns

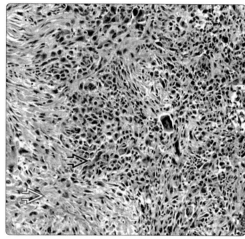

(Left) *Paucicellular variant of ATC shows scattered atypical spindle-shaped cells within abundant fibrous tissue with only occasional single highly atypical cells ➡️. Histologically, this variant mimics Riedel thyroiditis but is positive for p53.* **(Right)** *H&E of ATC shows a mixed cellularity pattern with less cellular ➡️ areas with fibrosis sharply demarcated from highly cellular areas ➡️ formed by pleomorphic cells with scattered giant cells.*

Abundant Fibrous Tissue

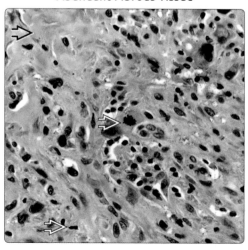

Mitotically Active Pleomorphic Tumor Cells

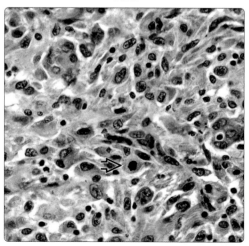

(Left) *This picture of an ATC shows extensive fibrosis and keloid-like hyalinization ➡️. There are scattered pleomorphic cells, giant cells, and mitotic figures ➡️.* **(Right)** *H&E shows ATC, pleomorphic variant with highly cellular areas formed by pleomorphic cells with scattered giant cells and numerous mitosis ➡️, with admixed inflammatory cells.*

Epithelioid Cells

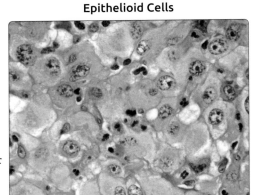

Spindle Cells

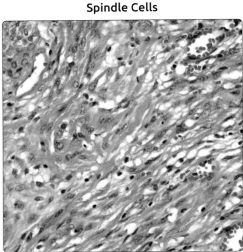

(Left) *The epithelial ATC form is composed of squamous cohesive epithelial cells with abundant eosinophilic cytoplasm. Occasional keratinization may be found. Necrosis and acute inflammatory cells are present.* (Right) *This ATC is composed of malignant spindle cells with features commonly seen in pleomorphic sarcoma. There is inflammatory infiltration within tumor cells, as well as ecstatic small vessels.*

Osteoid Formation in ATC

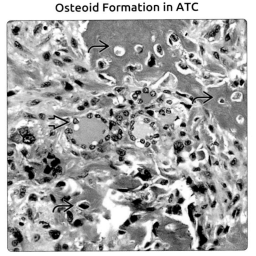

Osteoid and Atypical Cells

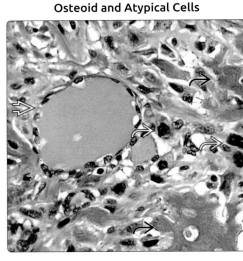

(Left) *In ATC, carcinosarcoma variant, the presence of malignant osteoid and osteoblasts can be identified around residual thyroid follicles ⊡. There is malignant osteoid with new bone formation ⊡ and prominent osteoblastic activity.* (Right) *ATC, carcinosarcoma variant shows an osteosarcoma component intermixed with residual normal thyroid follicles ⊡. There is new bone formation ⊡ and highly atypical cells ⊡.*

Heterologous Differentiation

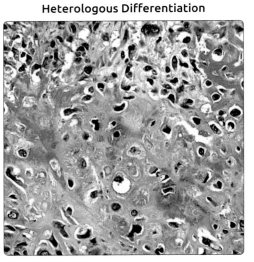

Rhabdomyoblastic Differentiation

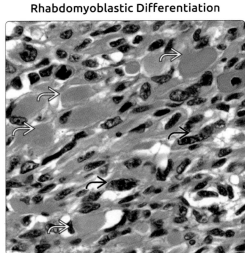

(Left) *Neoplastic bone & cartilage are 2° features of ATCs. Image illustrates an area of chondrosarcoma differentiation within ATC. The presence of osteosarcoma & chondrosarcoma are common components of ATCs.* (Right) *Within 2° features of ATCs are heterologous differentiation. Rhabdomyoblastic differentiation is focally seen in this ATC with rhabdomyoblasts containing ample granular eosinophilic cytoplasm ⊡ intermixed with other highly pleomorphic tumor cells ⊡.*

BRAF Immunoreactivity in ATC

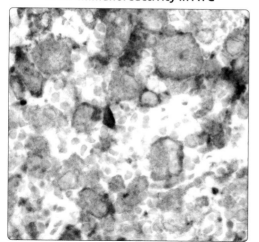

Immunoexpression of Keratin

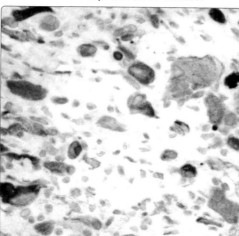

(Left) In ~ 20-30% of ATCs, there is an association with papillary thyroid carcinoma and with immunoexpression of BRAF by the tumor cells. Mutation of BRAF V600E is a recurring alteration present in ATC in ~ 20% of cases. (Right) Positive cytokeratin expression supports the epithelial nature of ATC. The expression may be focal and seen only in scattered tumor cells. Negative keratin staining does not rule out the diagnosis.

pax-8 Immunoreactivity

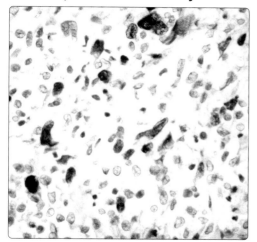

Loss of TTF-1 Stain by ATC Cells

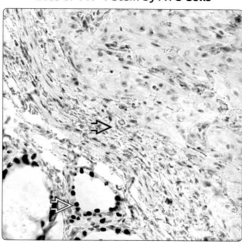

(Left) Common thyroid-lineage markers, as TTF1 and thyroglobulin, are usually absent or only focally present; however, pax-8 is retained in ~ 50% of ATCs. The stain may be in present in only some tumor cells, as illustrated in this figure. (Right) TTF-1 immunostain is usually negative in ATC neoplastic nuclei ⊳. It is positive in adjacent follicular cells ⊳. pax-8 is usually retained in ~ 50% of ATCs.

p53 Immunopositivity

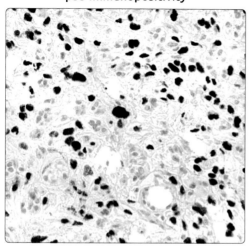

High Ki-67 Proliferative Index

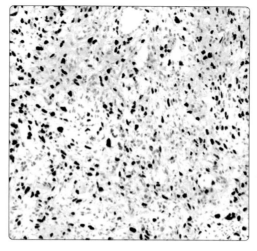

(Left) Most ATCs demonstrate nuclear positivity for p53. This immunostain is particularly useful when working with the paucicellular variant of anaplastic carcinoma. The most frequently mutated gene in ATCs is TP53, present in ~ 70% cases. (Right) Low-power view shows an ATC with a high proliferative index, highlighted by Ki-67 immunohistochemical stain. Most ATCs have a proliferative index > 70%.

ETIOLOGY/PATHOGENESIS

- Radiation exposure
- **Familial syndromes**
  - PTEN hamartoma tumor syndrome
  - Familial adenomatous polyposis (FAP) coli
  - Carney complex
  - Werner syndrome
  - Multiple endocrine neoplasia 2A
  - DICER1 syndrome
  - Familial papillary thyroid carcinoma (PTC) syndromes
- **Somatic mutations and rearrangements**
  - *BRAF* mutations
  - *RET* gene rearrangements
  - RAS mutations
  - *TERT* promoter
  - *ALK*

MICROSCOPIC

- In tumors without classical papillary architecture, diagnosis relies heavily on set of characteristic nuclear features, grouped in 3 categories
  - **Changes in size and shape**
    - Large ovoid nuclei
    - Nuclei are crowded and frequently overlap
    - Nuclear elongation
  - **Irregularities of membranes**
    - Marked remodeling of nuclear envelope
    - Abundant nuclear grooves, resulting from infolding of nuclear membrane
    - Highly irregular nuclear contours
    - Nuclear pseudoinclusions
  - **Chromatin characteristics**
    - Empty appearance of nucleoplasm
    - Powdery, optically clear nuclei; ground-glass (Orphan Annie) nuclei

Circumscribed Thyroid Carcinoma

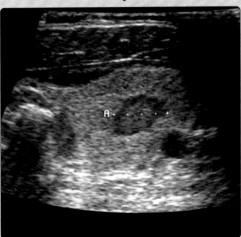

Gross Appearance of Papillary Carcinoma

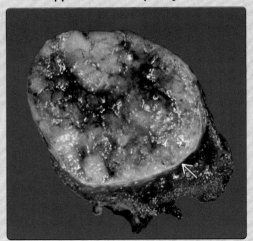

(Left) *Ultrasound shows the thyroid of a patient with a thyroid nodule on clinical exam. The nodule is hypoechoic and was histologically determined to be a follicular variant of papillary thyroid carcinoma (PTC).* **(Right)** *The cut surface of a PTC shows a granular appearance. The lesion is well circumscribed and has a thin capsule ➡ separating it from the adjacent normal parenchyma.*

Nuclear Features

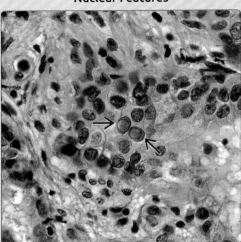

BRAF in Papillary Thyroid Carcinoma

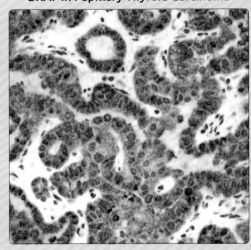

(Left) *Intranuclear inclusions ➡ are demonstrated in this photomicrograph. Note the crisp, punched-out border and eosinophilic color. Inclusions are typically round to oval in shape. They represent invaginations of the nuclear membrane.* **(Right)** *Immunostain for BRAF shows a cytoplasmatic positivity of neoplastic cells in some variants of PTC.*

TERMINOLOGY

Abbreviations

- Papillary thyroid carcinoma (PTC)

Synonyms

- Papillary carcinoma
- Thyroid papillary carcinoma
- Papillary thyroid adenocarcinoma

Definitions

- Malignant epithelial tumor showing evidence of follicular cell differentiation and set of distinctive nuclear features
- Papillae, invasions, or cytological features of PTC are required (WHO 2017)

ETIOLOGY/PATHOGENESIS

Environmental Exposure

- Radiation exposure
  - PTC is closely linked to ionizing radiation exposure
    - External sources (radioactive fallout)
    - Internal sources (radioactive iodine treatment)
  - Linear dose-response to radiation exposure is seen in all age groups
  - Only known predisposing factor in childhood development of PTC
- Iodine excess
  - Incidence of papillary carcinoma is higher in areas with high dietary iodine intake (Japan, Iceland)
  - In areas of endemic goiter, papillary carcinomas are more commonly seen after dietary iodine administration
    - These carcinomas are typically less aggressive and have better prognosis

Preexisting Benign Thyroid Disease

- Lymphocytic thyroiditis
  - Significant association between PTC and chronic lymphocytic thyroiditis
    - Hypothesized to be result of carcinoma, inducing autoimmune response or having pathogenetic mechanism
- Thyroid nodules
  - Risk of carcinoma increased 6x with multiple thyroid nodules
  - Single nodule is 38x more likely to be carcinoma than with multiple nodules

Familial Syndromes and Somatic Mutations and Rearrangements

- Familial syndromes
  - **PTEN hamartoma tumor syndrome**
    - Caused by germline mutation of *PTEN* tumor suppressor gene (10q23.3)
    - Encompasses both Cowden syndrome and Bannayan-Riley-Ruvalcaba syndrome (BRRS)
    - Patients affected by Cowden syndrome show multiple benign and malignant tumors in various tissues (breast, uterus, thyroid) and mucocutaneous hamartomas
    - Individuals with BRRS have macrocephaly, lipomatosis, hemangiomas, and penile macules

- Both syndromes are characterized by multiple thyroid nodules
- Grossly, these nodules diffusely involve gland (can show > 100 distinct nodules)
- Histologically, these nodules are follicular adenomas, follicular carcinomas, and, rarely, PTC
- C-cell hyperplasia is also associated with PTEN hamartoma tumor syndrome and is thought to be reactive rather than neoplastic in nature
  - **Familial adenomatous polyposis coli (FAP)**
    - Autosomal dominant syndrome caused by inherited germline mutations of *APC* gene (5q21)
    - Carriers develop hundreds of adenomatous colonic polyps during early childhood
    - Extracolonic manifestations include epidermal cysts, osteomas, desmoid tumors, hamartomas, hypertrophy of retinal pigmented epithelium, hepatoblastomas, and PTCs
    - FAP-associated PTC occurs in ~ 2% of patients
    - Risk of developing PTC is 160x greater in young women with FAP than in general population
    - FAP-associated carcinomas are typically bilateral and multifocal
    - Great majority (90%) of these tumors are cribriform morular variant of PTC
    - Characteristic nuclear features of PTC are rare to absent, and tumors show cribriform, morular, and solid areas
    - Prognosis is similar to that of conventional PTC
  - **Carney complex**
    - Autosomal dominant disease process
    - Characterized by skin and mucosal pigmentation, pigmented skin lesions, and various neoplasias (Sertoli-Leydig cell tumors, pituitary adenomas, pigmented nodular adrenal disease, and thyroid tumors)
    - Resected thyroids are multinodular and house multiple adenomatous nodules, follicular adenomas, follicular carcinoma, and PTC
  - **Familial PTC syndromes**
    - a.k.a. **familial nonmedullary thyroid carcinoma syndrome** (FNMTC)
    - Diagnosis is made when 3 or more family members have nonmedullary thyroid carcinomas in absence of other known tumor syndromes
    - Genetic inheritance is unknown
    - Typically multifocal and associated with benign nodules as well
    - PTC in FNMTC is usually bilateral, multicentric, and locally invasive with extrathyroid extension
    - Lymph node metastases and recurrence are common
    - Prognosis is worse than that of sporadic PTC
  - **Werner syndrome**
    - Autosomal recessive disorder
    - Affected individuals show premature aging, gray hair, skin atrophy, and bilateral cataracts
    - Patients have increased risk of various neoplasias, including benign thyroid lesions and PTC
  - **Multiple endocrine neoplasia 2A**
    - *RET* germline mutation
    - Microscopic PTC is seen with increased frequency

– Patients usually have multiple microscopic PTCs
- o **DICER1 syndrome**
  - – Features number of highly characteristic tumors and tumors-like conditions due to *DICER1* mutations
  - – Most important endocrine manifestations are multinodular hyperplasia and PTC
- **Somatic mutations and rearrangements**
  - o *BRAF* **mutations**
    - – Activating point mutations of *BRAF* gene
    - – Found in up to 90% of PTCs
    - – V600E point mutation accounts for 90% of *BRAF* mutations
    - – In radiation-induced PTC, *BRAF/AKAP9* intrachromosomal rearrangement also leads to constitutively active form of *BRAF*
    - – Confers worse prognosis
  - o *RET* gene **rearrangements**
    - – Most common chromosomal structural alteration in PTC
    - – 5-35% of sporadic adult cases, higher in children and adolescents (45-60%)
    - – Increased in population subject to radiation (50-80%)
    - – Several forms of *RET* gene rearrangements have been identified
  - o RAS **mutations**
    - – Activating point mutation of protooncogene
    - – Present in 0-35% of all PTCs but up to 40% of follicular variant of PTC
  - o *TERT* **promoter**
    - – Present in 5-25% of all PTCs
  - o *ALK*
    - – Present in 0-5% of all PTCs
  - o MicroRNA expression
    - – May serve as novel marker of PTC

CLINICAL ISSUES

Epidemiology
- Incidence
  - o Most common endocrine malignancy
  - o Most common type of thyroid cancer
  - o Incidence is increasing worldwide
    - – Incidence of thyroid cancer in USA in 2000 was 7.85 per 100,000, and in 2007, it was 11.99 per 100,000
    - – 80% of these cases are PTC
  - o Estimated number of cases of PTC in USA in 2010 was > 30,000
    - – 2014: > 62,280 new cases/year in USA
  - o Prevalence is 5-35%
- Age
  - o Most occur between 20-50 years; mean: 43 years
  - o Rare before 15 years
  - o Most common pediatric thyroid malignancy
    - – Commonly multifocal and biologically more aggressive in pediatric patients
- Sex
  - o Female:male = 4:1
    - – > 50 years of age, female preponderance is less pronounced
  - o Males typically have worse prognosis

- o In children, tumor distribution is almost equal
- Ethnicity
  - o Occurs more often in whites than blacks

Presentation
- Typically presents as palpable thyroid mass
- More distinctive nodule within goiter
- May present with enlarged cervical lymph nodes as well
- Can have compressive symptoms if mass is large or associated with goiter
  - o Dysphagia, odynophagia, cough, stridor, and shortness of breath
- Rarely interferes with thyroid function

Laboratory Tests
- Typically euthyroid
  - o Rarely can be hyper-/hypothyroid
- Serum thyroglobulin test can be used to monitor disease

Natural History
- Varies; some variants are more aggressive, while others are more indolent

Treatment
- Surgical approaches
  - o Surgical intervention is treatment of choice
    - – Extent of surgery is controversial
  - o Lymph node dissection
    - – Clinical or radiologic evidence of enlargement
- Radiation
  - o Radioactive iodine ablation is instituted after thyroidectomy
    - – Tumors must show radiolabel uptake in order to respond to radioablative therapies

Prognosis
- Prognosis is excellent
  - o 5-year survival: ~ 96%; 10-year survival: ~ 93%
- Prognosis correlates with risk group definition
  - o Risk groups defined by age, gender, tumor size, extrathyroid extension, metastasis, and completeness of resection
- Older patients typically have more advanced disease with larger tumor size and frequent extrathyroidal extension
- Vascular invasion and nuclear atypia are poor prognostic signs
- Certain variants carry worse prognosis (tall cell, diffuse sclerosing, hobnail, and columnar cell variants)
- Certain genetic mutations/rearrangements confer worse prognosis
  - o *BRAF* mutation is seen in more aggressive tumors

IMAGING

Radiographic Findings
- CT and MR are useful for imaging enlarged lymph nodes and extrathyroid extension
  - o CT preferred for imaging extent of suspected tracheal or mediastinal involvement
  - o Calcifications are highlighted on CT
    - – Psammoma bodies can be seen as calcifications on imaging

– Degenerative changes can also be associated with calcification seen on radiographic imaging
- Radioisotope uptake scans typically show "cold" nodule

Ultrasonographic Findings

- Useful for guiding FNA biopsies
- Useful for determining size and solid vs. cystic lesions
- Typically a hypo- or isoechoic nodule with ill-defined borders
- Central blood flow seen more commonly in PTC on color Doppler

MACROSCOPIC

General Features

- Can be solitary nodule; however, multifocality is common (up to 65%)
- Various gross appearances
  ○ Can be solid or cystic
  ○ Typically firm, pale tan to white nodules (hemorrhagic areas can also be present)
  ○ Appear granular or shaggy due to presence of papillae
- Usually infiltrative with poorly defined borders but can be circumscribed and rarely encapsulated (< 10%)
- Cut surface may be gritty due to presence of psammoma bodies
- Areas of fibrosis may be present
- Can show infiltration into perithyroidal skeletal muscle, adipose tissue, esophagus, trachea, or larynx
- Lymph node metastasis usually solid, whitish, firm lesions, but cystic metastases do occur

Size

- Varies widely, from microscopic up to 10 cm
- Mean: 1-3 cm

Sections to Be Submitted

- Record weight and dimensions
- Specimens should be inked and serially sectioned through entire gland
- Section of grossly apparent biopsy site should be taken if present
- Must include tumor and parenchyma interface
- Typically submit 1 section per cm of tumor
  ○ More sections can be submitted if grossly different areas are present
- If lesion is encapsulated, entire capsule should be submitted
- Areas of fibrosis must be sampled
- If any perithyroid soft tissue is attached, include sections showing relation to tumor to evaluate involvement
- Include en face isthmic resection margin if applicable
- Include sections of normal thyroid parenchyma from both lobes
- Submit lymph nodes &/or parathyroid glands, if present

MICROSCOPIC

Histologic Features

- Usually infiltrative but can be well circumscribed, encapsulated, or cystic

- Multiple different architectural patterns can be seen within same tumor (papillary, solid, trabecular, macro- and microfollicular, cystic)
  ○ Typically have branching papillae
    – Delicate arborizing fronds with thin fibrovascular cores
    – Monolayer of neoplastic cells surround papillae with haphazard nuclear arrangement
    – Stroma of papillae may be edematous, loose, myxoid, or hyalinized
  ○ Follicles are often present
    – Contain thick eosinophilic colloid within their lumina
    – Follicles may be enlarged, elongated, or irregularly shaped
- Characteristic nuclear features must be present in majority of tumor cells
  ○ In tumors without classic papillary architecture, diagnosis relies heavily on these characteristic nuclear features
  ○ Large ovoid nuclei with irregularly shaped nuclear membranes
    – Nuclei may be oval, elongated, crescent-shaped, asymmetric, angulated, or convoluted
  ○ Nuclei are crowded and frequently overlap
  ○ Powdery, ground-glass ("Orphan Annie") nuclei
    – Clear with accentuated nuclear borders
    – May be artifact of formalin fixation, as this feature is not seen with cytology preparations
  ○ Abundant nuclear grooves are present, resulting from infolding of nuclear membrane
    – Found in almost all cases
    – Discrete, longitudinal groove through long axis of nucleus, resembling coffee beans
  ○ Nuclear pseudoinclusions are usually present in few tumor cells
    – Pale-staining, well-demarcated vacuoles resulting from nuclear herniations of cytoplasm
    – May not be present in some variants
    – Less frequently seen nuclear features
- Neoplastic cells can be polygonal, cuboidal, flattened, columnar, or hobnailed
- Cytoplasm is typically lightly eosinophilic but can also be oxyphilic or clear
- Neoplastic cells are 2-3x larger than normal follicular cells
  ○ Nuclear:cytoplasmic ratio is increased
- Other morphologic features can be seen with specific variants
- Psammoma bodies are found in ~ 1/2 of all cases
  ○ Round, deep purple with concentric laminations
  ○ Seen within tumor, in association with tumor cells, or in lymphatic channels
  ○ May be only evidence of intrathyroid lymphatic spread or metastasis to lymph nodes
- Neoplastic nodules frequently associated with sclerotic or hyalinized stroma
- Encapsulated variants are surrounded by fibrous capsule, typically thin
- Colloid is intensely eosinophilic when compared to surrounding nonneoplastic gland
  ○ Colloid is thicker and may even be scalloped along edges
- Squamous metaplasia is common (~ 20% of cases)

- Usually associated with patchy, chronic inflammation and may be seen in background of lymphocytic thyroiditis
  - Lymphocytes, plasma cells, and histiocytes
- Multinucleated giant cells are almost pathognomonic for PTC
- Biopsy site changes are typically seen in association with papillary carcinoma
  - Includes hemorrhage, fibrosis, dystrophic calcification
- If tumor size is large, degenerative changes may also be present within tumor itself
  - Cystic changes, dystrophic calcification, hyalinization, fibrosis
  - Stellate fibrosis can be seen and may extend beyond tumor into adjacent gland

Lymphatic/Vascular Invasion

- Seen in large number of cases
- Lymphatic invasion is most commonly seen

Margins

- Important to sample to determine completeness of excision and presence of extrathyroid extension of tumor

Lymph Nodes

- Metastatic disease is common
- Metastatic deposits can be solid or cystic
- Psammoma bodies may be sole evidence of metastatic disease
- Benign follicular inclusions in lymph nodes do not exist and should be considered metastases

Variants

- Many histopathological variants of PTC exist, typically found in combination with each other
- Tumor should be dominated by certain features to be categorized as specific variant
- Papillae, invasion, or nuclear features of PTC are required
- **Classification of PTC** (based on WHO, 2017)
  - **Classic/conventional type**
  - **Papillary microcarcinoma**
  - **Follicular variant, encapsulated/well circumscribed, with invasion**
  - **Follicular variant, infiltrative**
  - **Macrofollicular variant**
  - **Diffuse sclerosing variant**
  - **Tall cell variant**
  - **Columnar cell variant**
  - **Cribriform-morular variant**
  - **Hobnail variant**
  - **Solid/trabecular variant**
  - **Oncocytic variant**
  - **Spindle cell variant**
  - **Clear cell variant**
  - **Warthin-like variant**
- **Microcarcinoma**
  - ≤ 1.0 cm in size
  - May show features of any variant, though usually follicular or papillary in architecture
  - Must be distinguished from intrathyroid spread
  - Treatment currently controversial
- **Diffuse sclerosing variant**

  - Diffuse involvement of 1 or both thyroid lobes, often with extrathyroid extension of tumor
  - Seen in younger patients
  - Most have *BRAF* mutation
  - Papillary and follicular architectures seen
  - Squamous metaplasia must be present and is often extensive
  - Lymphocytic infiltrate is seen
  - Psammoma bodies are abundant
  - Stromal fibrosis present
  - Regional and distant metastases are common
- **Follicular variant**
  - Common variants of PTC: Encapsulated/well-circumscribed and infiltrative
  - Composed of irregularly shaped follicles with few papillary structures
  - Eosinophilic colloid
  - Psammoma bodies rare
  - Intranuclear inclusions rare
  - May be completely encapsulated
  - HBME-1 and galectin-3 are useful for differentiating from follicular carcinoma
- **Macrofollicular variant**
  - Rarest variant of PTC
  - Composed largely of macrofollicles (> 250 micrometers)
  - Nuclear features show characteristic PTC morphology
  - Some nuclei are hyperchromatic
  - Peripheral vacuolization of colloid may be seen
  - Lymph node metastasis uncommon; however, metastases show macrofollicular architecture
- **Tall cell variant**
  - Aggressive variant
  - Less common
  - Cells have height 3x width
  - Papillary, follicular, and trabecular architecture
  - Nuclei show characteristic PTC features
  - Abundant nuclear pseudoinclusions and grooves
  - Nuclei are centrally located
  - Granular eosinophilic cytoplasm
  - Typically show extrathyroid extension and lymph node metastasis
  - *BRAF* mutation in up to 80% of cases
- **Columnar cell variant**
  - Rare, aggressive variant
  - Pseudostratified columnar cells with eosinophilic cytoplasm
  - Supra- and subnuclear cytoplasmic vacuoles present
  - Nuclei are hyperchromatic; characteristic papillary carcinoma nuclear features are rare
  - Papillary, follicular, trabecular, and solid architectures can be seen
  - Metastatic deposits often confused with metastasis from gastrointestinal, lung, or endometrial sites
  - Extrathyroid extension and metastasis more commonly seen
  - 2 subtypes are seen: Circumscribed lesions in young females; widely invasive lesions in older males
- **Cribriform morular variant**
  - Rare, 0.1-0.2% of all PTC cases
  - Typically seen in patients with Gardner syndrome or FAP

- More often seen in young women
- Typically multifocal when associated with syndromes, though solitary sporadic tumors do occur
- Cribriform features, focal papillary architecture, squamoid morules, solid and spindled areas present
- Most nuclei are hyperchromatic; however, some are clear and grooved
- β-catenin nuclear positivity
- **Hobnail variant**
  - Aggressive variant
  - Papillary pattern architecture with complex and micropapillary structures with fibrovascular cores
  - Cuboidal or oval epithelium lines papillae
  - Cells have increased nuclear:cytoplasmic ratio
  - Focal, characteristic, classic PTC nuclear features
  - Nuclei apically placed, producing bulge that leads to hobnail pattern appearance
  - Areas of cellular dyscohesiveness
  - Commonly associated with angiolymphatic invasion and lymph node metastasis
- **Solid/trabecular variant**
  - Solid sheets of tumor cells with characteristic papillary carcinoma features
  - More common in children
  - Should be distinguished from poorly differentiated/insular carcinoma
- **Oncocytic variant**
  - Characteristic mahogany brown color grossly, though some tumors may be grayish white
  - Papillary or follicular architecture
  - Cells are polygonal in shape
  - Nuclei are apically located
  - Have characteristic nuclear features
  - Abundant granular eosinophilic cytoplasm
- **Spindle cell variant**
  - Spindle cells may constitute < 5% to 85% of tumor
  - Spindle cells stain for TTF-1 and cytokeratin
  - Bland cytology and absence of mitosis or necrosis
- **Clear cell variant**
  - Uncommon
  - Usually papillary or follicular in architecture
  - Cells have abundant vacuolated, clear cytoplasm but may also be oncocytic
  - Nuclear features of conventional papillary carcinoma
- **Warthin-like variant**
  - Predominant lymphoid stroma
  - Eosinophilic elongated cells with abundant cytoplasm

ANCILLARY TESTS

Cytology

- FNA is typically initial diagnostic test for PTC
  - Sensitivity is ~ 83% and specificity 92%
- Typically performed with 27- to 25-gauge needle and guided by ultrasound
- Adequate samples must contain at least 6 groups of cells with 15-20 follicular cells per group
- Categorized using Bethesda system as benign, suspicious, indeterminate, or malignant
- Aspirates are obtained from FNA biopsies and are diagnostic test of choice

- Typically, aspirates are very cellular
  - Arranged in groups, sheets, and papillary tissue fragments
- Cells are enlarged and may be irregularly shaped
  - Usually cuboidal but can be polygonal, columnar, spindled, or squamoid
- Nuclei are enlarged and irregular in shape
  - Nuclear grooves are present
  - Chromatin is powdery
  - Small nucleoli may be present and are typically peripherally located
  - Nuclear pseudoinclusions are quite helpful when seen
- Colloid is thick and ropy, resembling chewing gum
- Psammoma bodies may also be present
- Multinucleated giant cells are another helpful finding

Frozen Sections

- Not as common since use of FNA
- Should only be performed when FNA is suspicious
- Touch preps performed at time of frozen section are useful adjunct

Immunohistochemistry

- Rarely of value
  - May help define malignancy in few cases
  - Can aid in defining thyroid origin
  - Positive stains
    - Thyroglobulin, TTF-1, pax-8, CK7, CK19, HBME-1, galectin-3, and CITED-1
    - Some variants are immunopositive for BRAF immunostain (v600e)

Genetic Testing

- Can be performed on paraffin blocks
- *BRAF*
  - Predominant serine-threonine kinase in thyroid follicular cells
  - T to A transversion at position 1799 leads to valine to glutamate substitution at residue 600 (V600E) in activating loop
    - Destabilizes inactive form of kinase
    - Some *BRAF* mutations alter kinase into catalytic form
  - Studies show *BRAF* mutation is present in 30-90% of PTC cases
  - Frequency varies among different variants of PTC
  - Uncommon in radiation-induced cases
  - *BRAF* mutations in PTC are associated with low expression of sodium iodide symporter genes, making these tumors refractory to radioactive iodine therapy
  - Associated with poor prognosis
    - Significant predictor of lymph node metastasis
    - Significant association with PTC-related mortality
- RAS
  - Protooncogenes belonging to family of G proteins
    - *HRAS*, *KRAS*, and *NRAS*
  - Plasma membrane GTPases
  - Mutations favor their GTP-bound, constitutively active form
  - Seen in 10-15% of PTC cases, predominantly in follicular variant (though more common in follicular adenomas/carcinomas)

- Most commonly *NRAS* and *HRAS*, though mutations of all RAS genes have been identified
  - o Some studies suggest that tumors harboring RAS mutations are clinically more aggressive
- *RET*
  - o Mutation leads to activation of *RET* protooncogene
  - o Intrachromosomal transversion or chromosomal translocation
  - o Fusion of tyrosine kinase region of *RET* with various activating sequences in thyroid follicular cells
    - e.g., *PTC1* inv(10)(q11.2q21)
  - o Fusion of activating gene alters RET protein leading to constitutive activation of tyrosine kinase-dependent portion
  - o At least 12 forms of *RET* gene rearrangements have been identified so far
    - *RET* and *PTC1* gene rearrangement is associated with classic type
    - *RET* and *PTC3* gene rearrangement is associated with solid variant
  - o Research suggests that *RET* gene rearrangements are early events in development of malignancy
    - High prevalence in occult or microcarcinomas
  - o Associated with exposure to ionizing radiation
  - o Present in less-aggressive forms of disease
- *TRK*
  - o Neurotropic receptor tyrosine kinase 1 (*NTRK1*) located on chromosome 1q22
  - o Chromosome rearrangement enables oncogenic activation
  - o Seen in ~ 3% of post-Chernobyl cases
- Multifocal PTC have been found to have differing cytogenetic profiles
  - o Independent clonal origin
  - o Develop through distinct mutational mechanisms
    - Multiple synchronous primary tumors

DIFFERENTIAL DIAGNOSIS

Papillary Hyperplasia

- Papillary fronds extending into follicles
- Epithelium overlying papillae do **not** have features of PTC
- Nuclei are hyperchromatic and basally oriented

Hashimoto Thyroiditis

- Nuclear clearing of follicular cells may be present
- Nuclei are enlarged compared to normal follicular cells
- Nuclei are typically uniform and round; do not vary in size and shape as seen in PTC
- Lack nuclear grooves and inclusions seen in PTC
- No mass lesion is seen
- Be cautious when diagnosing PTC in background of Hashimoto thyroiditis

Artifact/FNA Site Changes

- Areas of fibrosis, calcification, and hemorrhage seen following FNA biopsy
- Islands of follicular cells can be found within fibrotic areas
- Nuclei may be enlarged and pale staining
- Nuclei are round, not crowded, and lack nuclear grooves and inclusions or other features of PTC

Adenomatous Nodule

- Nodule composed of cells arranged in follicular pattern
- Cells are enlarged when compared to normal follicular cells
- Nuclei may be atypical but do not show characteristic PTC features
  - o Small number of cells may have nuclear clearing as fixation artifact but are few in number and usually centrally located

Follicular Thyroid Carcinoma

- Encapsulated lesions
- Neoplastic cells breach capsule
- Cells are arranged in follicular pattern
- Nuclei are round with granular chromatin
- Prominent nucleoli are seen
- Lack characteristic nuclear features of papillary carcinoma
  - o Though cells with nuclear clearing may be seen in less well-preserved areas of tumor

Medullary Carcinoma

- Sheets or islands of irregular cells separated by thin fibrovascular septa
  - o Other architectures may be seen (trabecular, papillary, cribriform, etc.)
- Cells are polygonal or spindly
- Nuclei are round to oval with fine chromatin
- Pleomorphism is not obvious
- Cytoplasm is granular, and mucin can be seen in ~ 1/2 of all tumor cells
- Amyloid stroma present in up to 80% of cases
- Calcitonin positive

Hyalinizing Trabecular Tumor

- Hyalinized amyloid stroma
- Polygonal cells arranged in trabeculae with intratrabecular and intertrabecular hyalinization
  - o Tumor cells are aligned perpendicularly in trabeculae
- Cell nuclei have longitudinal grooves and pseudoinclusions
- Perinuclear cytoplasmic bodies are present
  - o Pale yellow, spherical, and refractile
- Psammoma bodies may be present
- Nuclei are not optically clear like classic PTC nuclei

DIAGNOSTIC CHECKLIST

Clinically Relevant Pathologic Features

- Certain pathologic findings confer worse prognosis
  - o Extrathyroid extension, lymphovascular invasion, and lymph node metastasis are all independently associated with poorer clinical outcome
    - These findings must always be reported
- Some variants are more aggressive and are thus important with regard to prognosis
  - o Tall cell variant, hobnail variant, diffuse sclerosing variant, and columnar variant are typically more aggressive
  - o Extrathyroid extension, metastatic disease, and lymphovascular invasion are commonly seen in these variants
- Some variants/features are associated with genetic syndromes or tumor syndromes, and their presence should warrant further clinical work-up
  - o Columnar cell variant often clusters in families

- o Cribriform morular variant is seen in patients with FAP or Gardner syndrome
- o Multiple foci of papillary carcinoma should raise possibility of familial syndrome

Pathologic Interpretation Pearls

- When classic papillary architecture is not present, nuclear features become extremely important
- Characteristic PTC nuclear features must be present in majority of tumor cells
- Each variant has its own specific features required for diagnosis

STAGING

AJCC/TNM Staging (7th edition, 2010)

- Primary tumor
  - o TX: Primary tumor cannot be assessed
  - o T0: No evidence of primary tumor
  - o T1: Tumor < 2 cm, limited to thyroid
    - – T1a: Tumor ≤ 1 cm
    - – T1b: Tumor > 1 cm and < 2 cm
  - o T2: Tumor > 2 cm and < 4 cm, limited to thyroid
  - o T3: Tumor > 4 cm or any size tumor with extrathyroid extension
  - o T4: Advanced disease
    - – T4a: Moderately advanced disease: Tumor of any size with involvement of subcutaneous soft tissues, trachea, larynx, esophagus, or recurrent laryngeal nerve
    - – T4b: Very advanced disease: Tumor of any size involving prevertebral fascia, encasing carotid artery, or mediastinal vessels
- Lymph nodes
  - o NX: Regional lymph nodes cannot be assessed
  - o N0: No regional lymph node metastases
  - o N1a: Metastasis to level VI lymph nodes (pretracheal, paratracheal, and prelaryngeal/delphian nodes)
  - o N1b: Metastasis to unilateral, contralateral, or bilateral cervical (levels I, II, III, IV, V) or retropharyngeal or superior mediastinal (level VII) lymph nodes
- Distant metastasis
  - o M0: No distant metastasis
  - o M1: Distant metastasis

SELECTED REFERENCES

1. Choi EK et al: Clinicopathological characteristics including BRAF V600E mutation status and PET/CT findings in papillary thyroid carcinoma. Clin Endocrinol (Oxf). 87(1):73-79, 2017
2. Fakhruddin N et al: BRAF and NRAS mutations in papillary thyroid carcinoma and concordance in BRAF mutations between primary and corresponding lymph node metastases. Sci Rep. 7(1):4666, 2017
3. Geng J et al: Correlation between BRAF V600E mutation and clinicopathological features in pediatric papillary thyroid carcinoma. Sci China Life Sci. 60(7):729-738, 2017
4. Hardee S et al: Pathologic characteristics, natural history, and prognostic implications of BRAFV600E mutation in pediatric papillary thyroid carcinoma. Pediatr Dev Pathol. 20(3):206-212, 2017
5. Iyama K et al: Identification of three novel fusion oncogenes, SQSTM1/NTRK3, AFAP1L2/RET, and PPFIBP2/RET, in thyroid cancers of young patients in Fukushima. Thyroid. 27(6):811-818, 2017
6. Lloyd RV et al: WHO Classification oIf Tumours of Endocrine Organs. Lyon, France: IARC Press, 2017
7. Morandi L et al: Somatic mutation profiling of hobnail variant of papillary thyroid carcinoma. Endocr Relat Cancer. 24(2):107-117, 2017
8. Oishi N et al: Frequent BRAF V600E and absence of TERT promoter mutations characterize sporadic pediatric papillary thyroid carcinomas in Japan. Endocr Pathol. 28(2):103-111, 2017
9. Paja Fano M et al: Immunohistochemical detection of the BRAF V600E mutation in papillary thyroid carcinoma. Evaluation against real-time polymerase chain reaction. Endocrinol Diabetes Nutr. 64(2):75-81, 2017
10. Vuong HG et al: Prognostic implication of BRAF and TERT promoter mutation combination in papillary thyroid carcinoma - a meta-analysis. Clin Endocrinol (Oxf). ePub, 2017
11. Xu B et al: Primary thyroid carcinoma with low-risk histology and distant metastases: clinicopathologic and molecular characteristics. Thyroid. 27(5):632-640, 2017
12. Gertz RJ et al: Mutation in BRAF and other members of the MAPK pathway in papillary thyroid carcinoma in the pediatric population. Arch Pathol Lab Med. 140(2):134-9, 2016
13. Nikiforov YE et al: Nomenclature revision for encapsulated follicular variant of papillary thyroid carcinoma: a paradigm shift to reduce overtreatment of indolent tumors. JAMA Oncol. 2(8):1023-9, 2016
14. Prasad ML et al: NTRK fusion oncogenes in pediatric papillary thyroid carcinoma in northeast United States. Cancer. 122(7):1097-107, 2016
15. Torregrossa L et al: Papillary thyroid carcinoma with rare exon 15 BRAF mutation has indolent behavior: a single-institution experience. J Clin Endocrinol Metab. 101(11):4413-4420, 2016
16. Armstrong MJ et al: PAX8/PPARγ rearrangement in thyroid nodules predicts follicular-pattern carcinomas, in particular the encapsulated follicular variant of papillary carcinoma. Thyroid. 24(9):1369-74, 2014
17. Cancer Genome Atlas Research Network: Integrated genomic characterization of papillary thyroid carcinoma. Cell. 159(3):676-90, 2014
18. Giordano TJ et al: Molecular testing for oncogenic gene mutations in thyroid lesions: a case-control validation study in 413 postsurgical specimens. Hum Pathol. 45(7):1339-47, 2014
19. Hsiao SJ et al: Molecular approaches to thyroid cancer diagnosis. Endocr Relat Cancer. 21(5):T301-13, 2014
20. Jung CK et al: The increase in thyroid cancer incidence during the last four decades is accompanied by a high frequency of BRAF mutations and a sharp increase in RAS mutations. J Clin Endocrinol Metab. 99(2):E276-85, 2014
21. Radkay LA et al: Thyroid nodules with KRAS mutations are different from nodules with NRAS and HRAS mutations with regard to cytopathologic and histopathologic outcome characteristics. Cancer Cytopathol. ePub, 2014
22. Xing M et al: Association between BRAF V600E mutation and recurrence of papillary thyroid cancer. J Clin Oncol. 122(12):873-82, 2014
23. Nikiforov YE et al: New strategies in diagnosing cancer in thyroid nodules: impact of molecular markers. Clin Cancer Res. 19(9):2283-8, 2013
24. Xing M et al: Association between BRAF V600E mutation and mortality in patients with papillary thyroid cancer. JAMA. 309(14):1493-501, 2013
25. Asioli S et al: Papillary thyroid carcinoma with prominent hobnail features: a new aggressive variant of moderately differentiated papillary carcinoma. A clinicopathologic, immunohistochemical, and molecular study of eight cases. Am J Surg Pathol. 34(1):44-52, 2010
26. Nosé V: Familial follicular cell tumors: classification and morphological characteristics. Endocr Pathol. 21(4):219-26, 2010
27. Nosé V: Thyroid cancer of follicular cell origin in inherited tumor syndromes. Adv Anat Pathol. 17(6):428-36, 2010
28. Proietti A et al: BRAF status of follicular variant of papillary thyroid carcinoma and its relationship to its clinical and cytological features. Thyroid. 20(11):1263-70, 2010
29. Zhu X et al: Diagnostic significance of CK19, RET, galectin-3 and HBME-1 expression for papillary thyroid carcinoma. J Clin Pathol. 63(9):786-9, 2010
30. Ghossein R: Problems and controversies in the histopathology of thyroid carcinomas of follicular cell origin. Arch Pathol Lab Med. 133(5):683-91, 2009
31. Nikiforova MN et al: Molecular diagnostics and predictors in thyroid cancer. Thyroid. 19(12):1351-61, 2009
32. Dotto J et al: Familial thyroid carcinoma: a diagnostic algorithm. Adv Anat Pathol. 15(6):332-49, 2008
33. Fagin JA et al: Molecular pathology of thyroid cancer: diagnostic and clinical implications. Best Pract Res Clin Endocrinol Metab. 22(6):955-69, 2008
34. Williams ED et al: Morphologic characteristics of Chernobyl-related childhood papillary thyroid carcinomas are independent of radiation exposure but vary with iodine intake. Thyroid. 18(8):847-52, 2008
35. Schmidt J et al: BRAF in papillary thyroid carcinoma of ovary (struma ovarii). Am J Surg Pathol. 31(9):1337-43, 2007
36. Adeniran AJ et al: Correlation between genetic alterations and microscopic features, clinical manifestations, and prognostic characteristics of thyroid papillary carcinomas. Am J Surg Pathol. 30(2):216-22, 2006
37. DeLellis RA: Pathology and genetics of thyroid carcinoma. J Surg Oncol. 94(8):662-9, 2006
38. Lloyd RV et al: Observer variation in the diagnosis of follicular variant of papillary thyroid carcinoma. Am J Surg Pathol. 28(10):1336-40, 2004

Immunohistochemistry

Antibody	Reactivity	Staining Pattern	Comment
HBME-1	Positive	Cell membrane	More specific; also stains colloid
Galectin-3	Positive	Nuclear & cytoplasmic	Positive staining in nearly all papillary thyroid carcinomas
CK19	Positive	Cytoplasmic	Strong, can also be positive in reactive processes and chronic lymphocytic thyroiditis
MSG1	Positive	Nuclear & cytoplasmic	Equivalent to CITED-1; should be used with other immunohistochemical stains
FN1	Positive	Cell membrane	Luminal accentuation seen
TTF-1	Positive	Nuclear	Strong, diffuse nuclear staining
Thyroglobulin	Positive	Cytoplasmic	Artifact can be problem; staining may be lost in areas of squamous differentiation
pax-8	Positive	Nuclear	
Cyclin-D1	Positive	Nuclear	Positive metastatic disease and negative in nonmetastatic papillary carcinomas
CK7	Positive	Cytoplasmic	Stains almost all cells
AE1/AE3	Positive	Cytoplasmic	Stains almost all cells
Calcitonin	Negative		Useful for distinguishing from medullary thyroid carcinoma
CK20	Negative		
BRAF	Positive	Cytoplasmic	In majority of cases

Mutations in Papillary Thyroid Carcinoma

Mutation	Gene Rearrangement	Percentage of Cases	Comment
BRAF V600E point mutation	n/a	30-90%	Poorer prognosis, older age, locally more advanced disease, 15% are tall cell variant
RAS mutations	n/a	0-35%	More common in follicular variant; more common in women than men
RET gene rearrangements	10q11	5-35%	Radiation-associated carcinomas; more common in younger patients (40-60%)
NTRK1 fusion oncogene	1q21 rearrangement	10%	
TERT Promoter		5-25%	
ALK		0-5%	

Comparison of Selected Papillary Thyroid Carcinoma Variants

	Classic Variant	Follicular Variant	Tall Cell Variant	Diffuse Sclerosing Variant	Columnar Cell Variant
Age at presentation	Mean: 48 years	Mean: 48 years	Mean: 49 years	Mean: 29 years	Mean: 47 years
Size	Highly variable	Variable	Mean: 3.0 cm	Mean: 0.7 cm	Mean: 3.8 cm
Focality	Multifocality common	Unifocal	Unifocal	Multifocality common	Unifocal
Psammoma bodies	Variable	Absent	Absent	Abundant	Absent
Extrathyroid extension	Variable	Variable	Common	Common	Common
Lymph-vascular invasion	Variable	Variable	Widespread	Widespread	Widespread
Lymph node metastasis	Common	Not as common as other variants	Common	Common	Common
Distant metastasis	Rare	Occasional	Common	Common	Common
Recurrence	Rare	Rare	Common	Rare	Common
Prognosis	Good	Good	Poor	Good	Poor

US of Papillary Thyroid Carcinoma

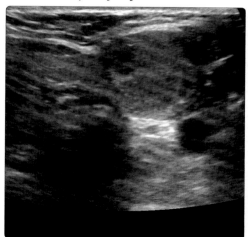

CT Scan of Papillary Thyroid Carcinoma

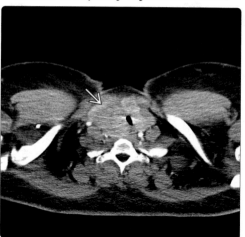

(Left) *Ultrasound shows a thyroid nodule on imaging test. The nodule is hypoechoic with ill-defined borders. Central blood flow is best seen on color Doppler and is a common finding in PTC.* **(Right)** *CT scan shows a patient with a large right-sided thyroid nodule ➡. This image demonstrates the nodule compressing the trachea. This patient had a 4-cm nodule that was found to be a follicular variant of PTC.*

Gross Cut Surface of Papillary Carcinoma

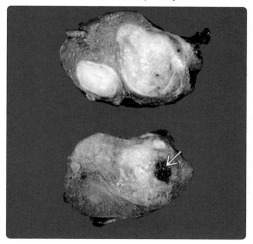

Cut Surface of Papillary Thyroid Carcinoma

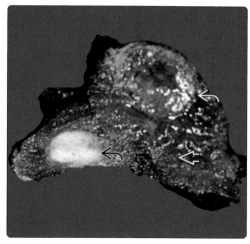

(Left) *Gross image of PTC shows multiple white-tan, pale, fleshy lesions. The bottom section shows a focus of hemorrhage ➡, most likely representing an FNA biopsy site or the degenerative changes commonly seen with larger lesions.* **(Right)** *Gross image shows 2 lesions with distinct gross morphology. Both lesions stand out from the background of unaffected thyroid parenchyma ➡. The nodular hyperplasia ➡ has a shiny beige appearance, while the papillary carcinoma has a white cut surface ➡.*

Cystic Papillary Thyroid Carcinoma

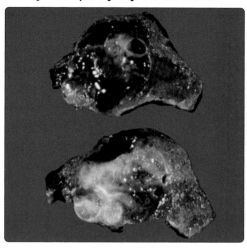

Cystic Papillary Thyroid Carcinoma

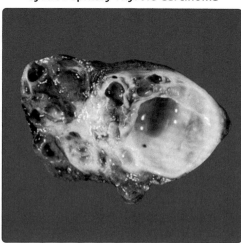

(Left) *Gross cut surface image of PTC illustrates that some lesions may be partially cystic in nature. Hemorrhage is readily identified within the cystic spaces.* **(Right)** *Gross photograph of PTC shows fibrosis and extensive cystic degeneration that may be seen in larger lesions.*

Papillary Thyroid Carcinoma Nuclei

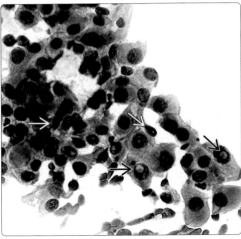

Cytology of Papillary Thyroid Carcinoma

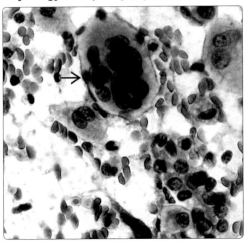

(Left) *Characteristic cytological features of PTC include enlarged tumor cells with abundant cytoplasm and nuclear inclusions ⊟. Nuclear grooves ➡ can also be seen within the nuclei of some cells.* (Right) *Cytologic preparation from PTC shows a multinucleated giant cell ⊟ and large, irregularly shaped cells with an increased nuclear:cytoplasmic ratio. The nuclei have irregular borders and conspicuous nucleoli.*

Cytology FNA Chart

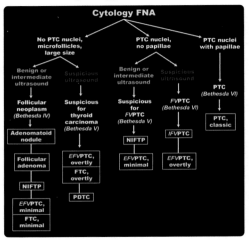

Papillary Thyroid Microcarcinoma

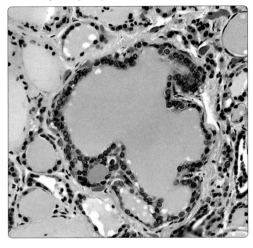

(Left) *This cytology fine needle aspiration flow chart, based on the nuclear features of PTC, helps in evaluation of the non-invasive follicular thyroid neoplasm with papillary-like nuclei (NIFTP) and other thyroid tumors.* (Right) *Papillary thyroid microcarcinoma photomicrograph demonstrates crowding and characteristic nuclear features of PTC. Nuclear clearing, nuclear overlapping, and occasional grooves are seen.*

Characteristic Nuclear Features

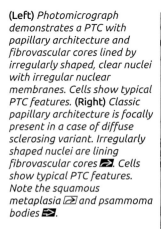

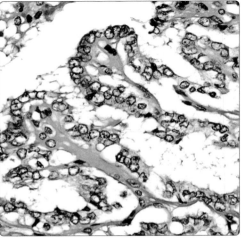

Squamous Metaplasia and Psammoma Bodies

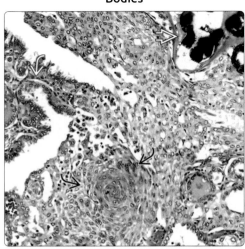

(Left) *Photomicrograph demonstrates a PTC with papillary architecture and fibrovascular cores lined by irregularly shaped, clear nuclei with irregular nuclear membranes. Cells show typical PTC features.* (Right) *Classic papillary architecture is focally present in a case of diffuse sclerosing variant. Irregularly shaped nuclei are lining fibrovascular cores ➡. Cells show typical PTC features. Note the squamous metaplasia ⊟ and psammoma bodies ➡.*

Papillary Thyroid Carcinoma Features

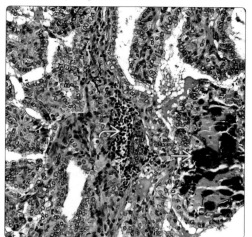

Psammoma Body and Fibrosis

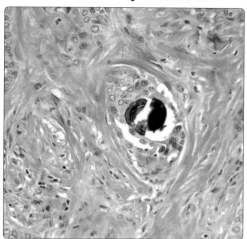

(Left) PTC (classic variant) demonstrates papillary architecture. Lymphoid infiltrate ➡ is often seen in association with tumor cells. Note the degenerating papillae on the right, which are forming calcified structures ➡. (Right) H&E of a PTC (diffuse sclerosing variant) demonstrates extensive fibrosis and a psammoma body with concentric laminations. Due to processing, psammoma bodies typically fragment and cause tissue artifacts.

Lymphoid-Rich Papillae

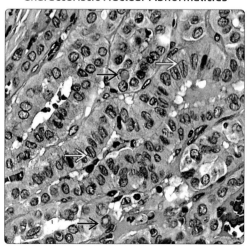

Nuclear Features of Papillary Thyroid Carcinoma

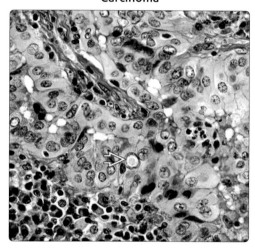

(Left) Warthin-like PTC has a papillary architecture. Eosinophilic cells surround papillae with lymphoid stroma, consisting primarily of plasma cells and lymphocytes. (Right) PTC (Warthin-like variant) is composed of large, irregularly shaped eosinophilic cells surrounding lymphoid stroma. Some cells show characteristic PTC nuclear features, while others are hyperchromatic. Numerous intranuclear inclusions are present ➡.

Characteristic Nuclear Abnormalities

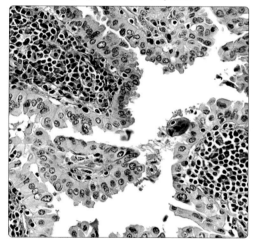

Marked Nuclear Enlargement

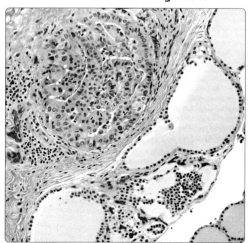

(Left) H&E of a tall cell variant shows tumor cells that are at least 3x as tall as they are wide. The cells have abundant eosinophilic cytoplasm, and the nuclei are centrally located. Nuclear grooves ➡ and pseudoinclusions ➡ are seen. Note the tram-tracking appearance that is characteristic of tall cell variant. (Right) A small focus of a tall cell variant is seen adjacent to normal thyroid parenchyma. The neoplastic cells are larger than the normal follicular cells.

(Left) *PTC (follicular variant) demonstrates a follicular architecture, increased nuclear:cytoplasmic ratio, and clear nuclei with irregular nuclear membranes. The follicles are small and have a thick eosinophilic colloid.* **(Right)** *H&E shows a PTC (follicular variant) in which nuclear membranous irregularity and enlarged clear nuclei of the neoplastic cells can be seen.*

Follicular-Patterned Tumor

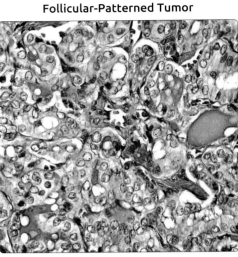

Papillary Thyroid Carcinoma Nuclei

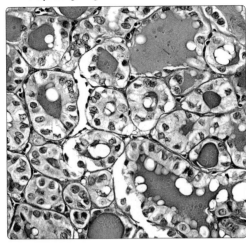

(Left) *PTC (follicular variant) is shown. The neoplastic cells are arranged in small follicles that contain deeply eosinophilic colloid. The nuclei are enlarged, optically clear, and have nuclear grooves.* **(Right)** *The tumor cells in the follicular variant of PTC are arranged in a follicular pattern. They demonstrate scalloping of colloid ➡, which is commonly seen in this variant. There is nuclear overlapping and marked nuclear clearing.*

Papillary Thyroid Carcinoma Nuclear Features

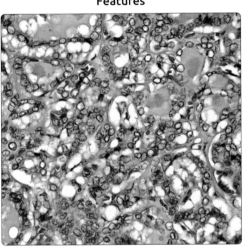
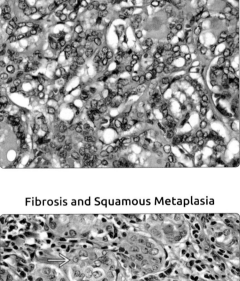

Nuclear Overlapping

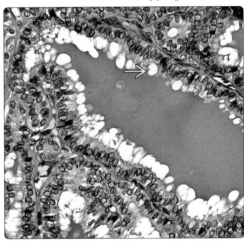

(Left) *Diffuse sclerosing variant of PTC demonstrates area of squamous metaplasia ➡ adjacent to tumor cells with characteristic papillary carcinoma features ➡. Lymphoid infiltrate is present in association with tumor cells.* **(Right)** *PTC (diffuse sclerosing variant) is characterized by thick fibrous bands associated with psammoma bodies ➡, lymphocytic infiltrate, variable architecture ➡, and squamous metaplasia.*

Fibrosis and Squamous Metaplasia

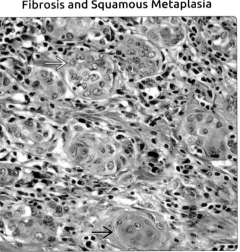

Papillary Thyroid Carcinoma

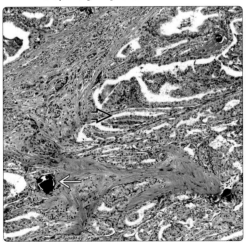

Cribriform Pattern and Lack of Colloid

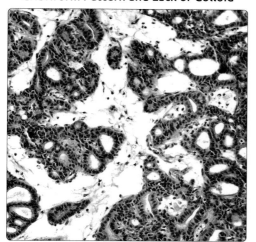

Cribriform Arrangement

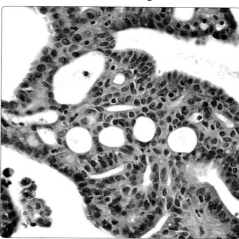

(Left) *H&E shows a cribriform morular variant of PTC with tumor cells arranged in a cribriform pattern, forming small, gland-like structures. These tumors are usually associated with a morular component.* **(Right)** *PTC (cribriform morular variant) demonstrates the characteristic punched-out cribriform pattern lacking colloid. The nuclei are enlarged and irregular but are not as clear as other subtypes of PTC.*

Oncocytic Papillary Thyroid Carcinoma

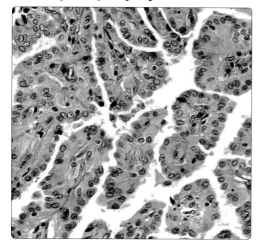

Oncocytic Papillary Carcinoma Cytoplasm

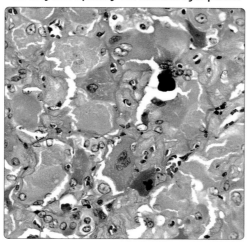

(Left) *Oncocytic variant of PTC contains tumor cells arranged in a papillary architecture with central vascular cores. The cytoplasm is ample, eosinophilic, and granular. The nuclei are pale staining compared to those of a normal follicle and are apically placed within the cells. Nuclear overlapping can also be noted.* **(Right)** *Oncocytic variant of PTC demonstrates abundant oncocytic granular cytoplasm and a pale-staining, optically clear nuclei.*

Overlapping Nuclei

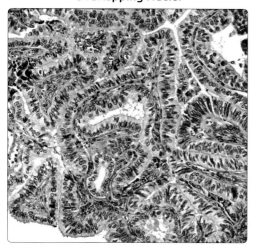

Extrathyroidal Extension

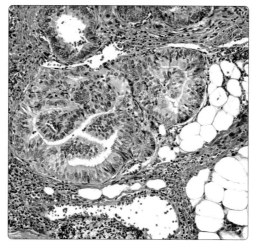

(Left) *PTC (columnar cell variant) demonstrates the neoplastic cells arranged in a pseudostratified pattern. The cells are enlarged and contain eosinophilic cytoplasm. The nuclei are basally located with supranuclear and subnuclear cytoplasmic vacuoles.* **(Right)** *Columnar cell variant (nonencapsulated) is an aggressive variant of PTC. Photomicrograph shows infiltration into the perithyroid adipose tissue.*

(Left) *H&E of a PTC metastatic to a lymph node demonstrates partial destruction of the lymph node architecture by tumor cells. This neoplasm has a diffuse and papillary architecture.* **(Right)** *Photomicrograph illustrates a tall cell variant of PTC metastatic to the lung. This example shows normal lung parenchyma ⇥ with the elongated tumor cells involving alveolar spaces. A psammoma body is present ⇥.*

Lymph Node Metastases

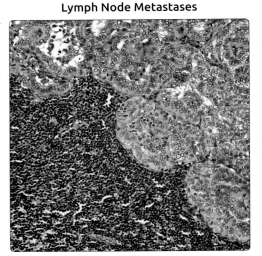

Lung Metastases

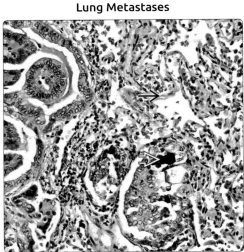

(Left) *Papillary carcinoma is shown invading the tracheal cartilage. These locally aggressive &/or very large lesions are often symptomatic. Patients typically present with dysphagia, dysphonia, and dyspnea as the lesions enlarge and encroach on surrounding structures.* **(Right)** *H&E shows PTC metastatic to a lymph node. The metastatic tumor demonstrates cystic change. Microscopically, this cystic structure is lined by cells with nuclear features characteristic of PTC.*

Tracheal Cartilage Invasion

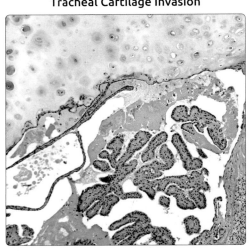

Cystic Papillary Thyroid Carcinoma

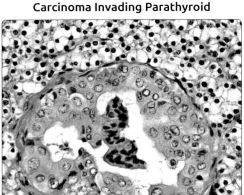

(Left) *H&E shows an invasive PTC infiltrating fibrous tissue and approaching skeletal muscle.* **(Right)** *Papillary carcinoma involving a parathyroid gland is shown. Normal parathyroid parenchyma is seen surrounding this tumor nodule. The neoplastic cells were histologically similar to the thyroid tumor.*

Extrathyroidal Extension

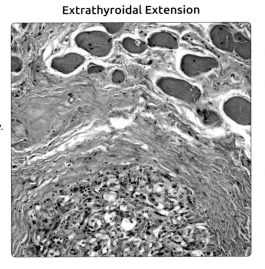

Carcinoma Invading Parathyroid

Papillary Thyroid Carcinoma

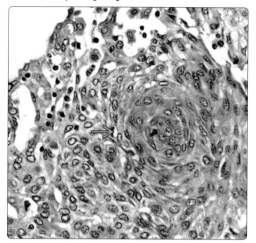

CK5/6 in Papillary Thyroid Carcinoma

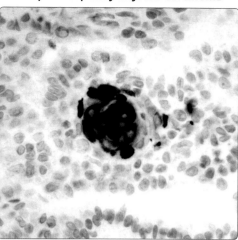

(Left) *This high-power H&E highlights an area of squamous metaplasia ⇥ in a diffuse sclerosing variant of a PTC This feature may often be extensive in this variant.* **(Right)** *Immunostain for CK5/6 highlights an area of squamous metaplasia in a diffuse sclerosing variant of a PTC.*

CK5 in Papillary Thyroid Carcinoma

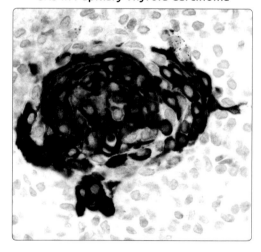

CD5 in Papillary Thyroid Carcinoma

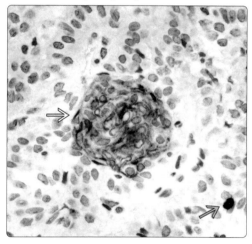

(Left) *Immunostain for CK5 highlights an area of squamous metaplasia within the tumor. Squamous metaplasia is 1 of the findings that may be present in the diffuse sclerosing variant of PTC.* **(Right)** *Immunohistochemical stain for CD5 shows an area of squamoid metaplasia ⇥ in a diffuse sclerosing variant of PTC. Note a lymphocyte ⇥ as internal control.*

Papillary Carcinoma in Parathyroid

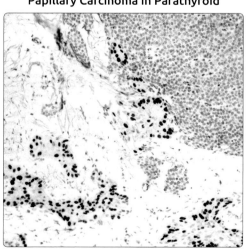

Invasion Into Parathyroid

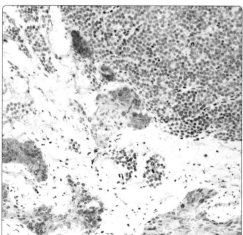

(Left) *Photomicrograph reveals a parathyroid gland with TTF-1-positive cells invading the parathyroid parenchyma, representing PTC.* **(Right)** *This PTC is invading into the adjacent parathyroid gland. The foci of tumor cells are highlighted by the immunopositivity for BRAF.*

HBME-1 Papillary Thyroid Carcinoma

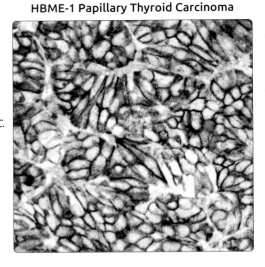

HBME-1

(Left) *HBME-1 immunostain demonstrates the characteristic membranous and luminal border staining pattern in PTC.* **(Right)** *Immunohistochemistry for HBME-1 shows characteristic membranous and luminal border staining pattern in PTC.*

Predominantly Luminal HBME-1

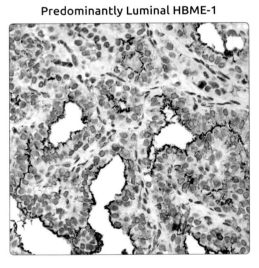

CITED-1 in Papillary Thyroid Carcinoma

(Left) *Photomicrography also shows the luminal pattern of an HBME-1 immunostain in a PTC. This pattern is usually seen in follicular variant of PTC.* **(Right)** *CITED-1 immunohistochemistry shows diffuse cytoplasmic staining in PTC. The stain intensity is characteristically variable between the tumor cells. This marker helps differentiate between the follicular variant of papillary thyroid carcinoma and follicular adenoma.*

CK19 in Papillary Thyroid Carcinoma

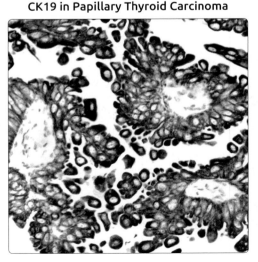

Galectin-3 in Papillary Thyroid Carcinoma

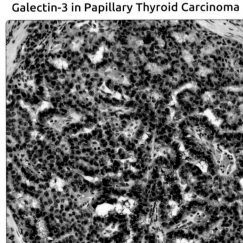

(Left) *Immunostain for CK19 shows a pattern of staining typical of PTC with strong fibrillary cytoplasmic staining of neoplastic cells.* **(Right)** *Follicular variant of PTC is usually characterized by an immunostain panel, including HBME-1, galectin-3, and CK19. This panel has 87% sensitivity and 89% specificity for PTC (follicular variant), while positive in only ~ 11% of follicular adenomas. Galectin-3 immunostaining is strong and cytoplasmic.*

BRAF in Papillary Thyroid Carcinoma

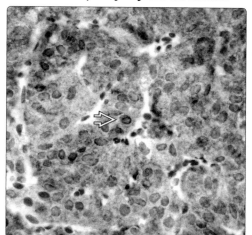

Granular Cytoplasmic positivity for BRAF

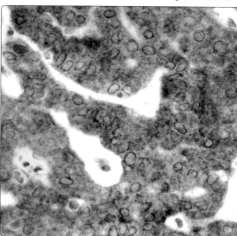

(Left) *This tall cell variant shows diffuse cytoplasmic immunoreactivity for BRAF. Note the intranuclear pseudoinclusion* ➡ *in 1 of the tumor cells. BRAF is usually positive in this variant.* **(Right)** *This PTC (tall cell variant) shows diffusely granular intracytoplasmic immunostaining for BRAF.*

BRAF Highlights Tumor

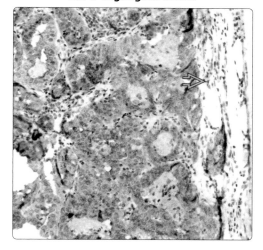

Specific Immunostain

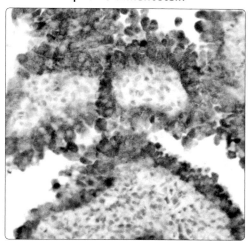

(Left) *BRAF immunohistochemistry shows diffuse cytoplasmic staining in PTC (mixed follicular variant and classic variant). Note that the normal follicles* ➡ *are negative for BRAF.* **(Right)** *BRAF immunostain shows a diffuse granular cytoplasmic positivity pattern in this PTC. The immunopositivity is granular in the cytoplasm. The lymphocytes are negative.*

BRAF Positivity in Tumor

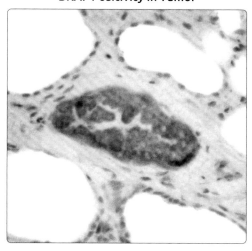

BRAF in Papillary Thyroid Microcarcinoma

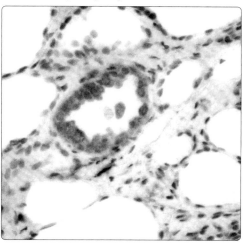

(Left) *Photomicrography shows a lymphovascular invasion of a PTC highlighted with a BRAF stain. The original tumor was a tall cell variant.* **(Right)** *This papillary thyroid microcarcinoma is very small and is highlighted with a BRAF immunostain.*

Papillary Thyroid Carcinoma, Classic Variant

TERMINOLOGY

- Malignant epithelial tumor showing evidence of follicular cell differentiation and characterized by distinctive nuclear features

CLINICAL ISSUES

- Most common in 3rd and 4th decades
- More common in women than in men (F:M = 4:1)
- Treatment involves partial or total thyroidectomy based on extent of disease
- Prognosis for this variant of papillary thyroid carcinoma (PTC) is usually excellent

MICROSCOPIC

- 2 cardinal morphological features of conventional/classic PTC: Papillae and characteristic nuclear changes
- Papillary architecture predominates; can contain foci of other patterns

- Characteristic cytological features are essential for diagnosis of PTC
- Nuclear changes can be grouped in 3 categories
  - **Changes in size and shape**: Nuclear enlargement, overlapping, elongation
  - **Irregularities of nuclear membrane**: Irregular nuclear membranes, longitudinal grooves, and intranuclear pseudoinclusions
  - **Chromatin characteristics:** Empty appearance of nucleoplasm, optically clear nuclei
- Psammoma bodies are often present
  - May be only evidence of angiolymphatic space invasion or lymph node metastases
- Background thyroid may be normal, multinodular, or show signs of lymphocytic thyroiditis

ANCILLARY TESTS

- HBME-1
- BRAF

Cut Surface of Encapsulated Papillary Thyroid Carcinoma

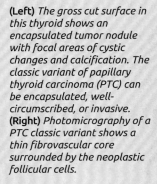

(Left) *The gross cut surface in this thyroid shows an encapsulated tumor nodule with focal areas of cystic changes and calcification. The classic variant of papillary thyroid carcinoma (PTC) can be encapsulated, well-circumscribed, or invasive.* (Right) *Photomicrography of a PTC classic variant shows a thin fibrovascular core surrounded by the neoplastic follicular cells.*

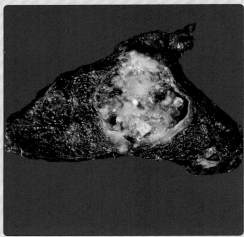

Papillae

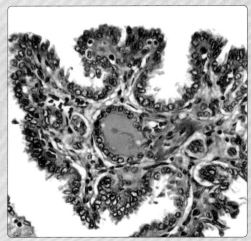

Intranuclear Pseudoinclusions

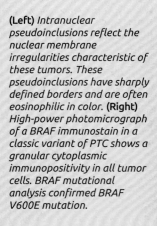

(Left) *Intranuclear pseudoinclusions reflect the nuclear membrane irregularities characteristic of these tumors. These pseudoinclusions have sharply defined borders and are often eosinophilic in color.* (Right) *High-power photomicrograph of a BRAF immunostain in a classic variant of PTC shows a granular cytoplasmic immunopositivity in all tumor cells. BRAF mutational analysis confirmed BRAF V600E mutation.*

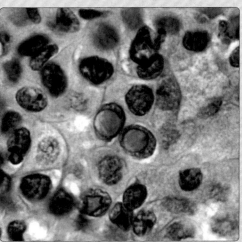

Granular Cytoplasmic BRAF Staining

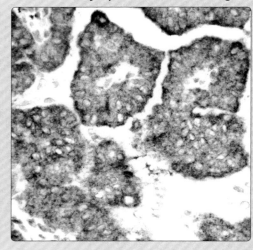

TERMINOLOGY

Abbreviations

- Papillary thyroid carcinoma (PTC)

Synonyms

- Classic PTC
- Conventional PTC
- PTC, classic, conventional, or usual variant

Definitions

- Malignant epithelial tumor showing evidence of follicular cell differentiation and characterized by distinctive nuclear features
- Papillae, invasion, or cytological features of PTC are required

ETIOLOGY/PATHOGENESIS

Multiple Causes

- Associated with radiation exposure, iodine deficiency, and lymphocytic thyroiditis

CLINICAL ISSUES

Epidemiology

- Incidence
  - Most common variant of PTC
  - There is increased in reported incidence of thyroid cancer since introduction of new imaging techniques
    - In USA, incidence rate tripled over last 30 years
- Age
  - Most common in 3rd and 4th decades
- Sex
  - More common in women than in men (F:M = 3-4:1)

Presentation

- Many cases are subclinical
- Patients may present with thyroid mass or unilateral neck mass
  - Tumors involving surrounding structures can be symptomatic (hoarseness, dysphagia, stridor, etc.)

Treatment

- Treatment involves partial or total thyroidectomy based on extent of disease
- Cervical lymph node dissection is indicated when there is radiologic evidence of metastatic involvement
- RAI therapy may also be treatment option

Prognosis

- Depends on age and stage; however, prognosis for this variant of PTC is usually excellent

MACROSCOPIC

General Features

- Tumors may be encapsulated, well circumscribed, or infiltrative
- Usually pale tan to white in color
- Usually solid and firm or friable and coarsely granular in appearance
- Cut surface may be gritty due to presence of psammoma bodies
- Cystic changes are seen in encapsulated tumors
- Calcifications may be apparent grossly

Size

- Variable
  - Range in size from few mm to several cm
  - Mean diameter: 2-3 cm

MICROSCOPIC

Histologic Features

- Tumors may be circumscribed, encapsulated, or infiltrative
- 2 cardinal morphological features of conventional/classic PTC are papillae and characteristic nuclear changes
  - This form of PTC shows great predominance of papillary structures throughout tumor
    - However, only few tumors are composed exclusively of papillae
- Papillae have central fibrovascular core covered by neoplastic follicular cells
- Papillary architecture predominates, though can contain foci of other patterns
  - Complex, branching forms
  - Fibrovascular cores
  - Edematous papillae
  - May be long, straight, or arborizing
  - Arranged in parallel, regimented fashion
  - Papillae can be short
  - Tightly packed
  - Thickness and composition of papillae is quite variable
- Nuclei of cells of PTC display characteristic set of nuclear changes
- Nuclear changes can be grouped in 3 categories
  - **Changes in size and shape**: Nuclear enlargement, overlapping, elongation
  - **Irregularities of nuclear membrane**: Irregular nuclear membranes, longitudinal grooves, and intranuclear pseudoinclusions
  - **Chromatin characteristics**: Empty appearance of nucleoplasm, optically clear nuclei
- Cytoplasm is slightly eosinophilic
- Stalk is made up of loose connective tissue and thin-walled vessels
- Psammoma bodies are often present in ~ 50% of cases
  - Have concentric laminations
  - Can create shattered appearance on H&E
  - May be only evidence of angiolymphatic space invasion or lymph node metastases
- Multinucleated giant cells may be present within tumor
- Mitosic figures are rare in conventional PTC
- Foci of squamous metaplasia is, 20-40% cases common
- Cystic changes are usually present
- Background thyroid may be normal, multinodular, or show signs of lymphocytic thyroiditis

Cytologic Features

- Characteristic cytologic features on H&E are essential for diagnosis of PTC
- Neoplastic cells are polygonal in shape
- Cytoplasm is eosinophilic or amphophilic
- Classic PTC nuclear features predominate on H&E

- o Tumor nuclei are enlarged, overlapping, and oval to irregular in shape
- o Chromatin is dusty, powdery, or ground-glass in appearance (clear Orphan Annie nuclei)
- o Nuclear grooves and pseudoinclusions are present
  - These reflect nuclear membrane irregularities
  - Nuclear pseudoinclusions have sharply defined border and are often eosinophilic in color

ANCILLARY TESTS

Cytology

- Fine-needle aspiration is useful in diagnosing PTC
  - o Aspirates are usually cellular
  - o Cells are arranged in papillary tissue fragments, 3-dimensional clusters, and monolayered sheets
  - o Neoplastic cells are cuboidal/polygonal in shape
  - o Nuclei are enlarged and irregular
  - o Chromatin is dusty or powdery with small nucleoli adjacent to nuclear membrane
  - o Nuclear grooves and pseudoinclusions are common
  - o Background colloid may be thick or ropy in appearance
  - o Psammoma bodies are occasionally seen in aspirates or touch imprints
  - o Multinucleated giant cells are helpful when identified

Frozen Sections

- Frozen section interpretation is difficult as freezing artifact can mimic PTC nuclear features

Immunohistochemistry

- IHC is not typically needed for diagnosis
- Positive immunohistochemical stains
  - o Thyroglobulin
  - o TTF-1
  - o pax-8
  - o HBME-1
  - o Galectin-3
  - o CITED1
  - o CK19
  - o Cytokeratins (CK7, CAM5.2, AE1/AE3)
  - o BRAF
- Negative for
  - o CK20
  - o Calcitonin
  - o Neuroendocrine markers

Genetic Testing

- Mutations in few tumor pathways are observed in this variant
  - o *BRAF*
    - Prevalence: 45-50%
  - o *RET/PTC* rearrangement: 5-25%
  - o RAS
  - o *NTRK1*
  - o Other: *ALK*
- Genetic alterations of PTC have been reported to change over past few decades
  - o Increasing trend of *BRAF* and decreasing trend of *RET/PTC* prevalence over time in classic PTCs

- o Accompanied by older age of PTC patients, increase in proportion of papillary thyroid microcarcinoma, and less aggressive behaviors of tumors

DIFFERENTIAL DIAGNOSIS

Papillary Hyperplasia

- Basally oriented round nuclei, lacking features of papillary carcinoma

Papillary Thyroid Carcinoma, Tall Cell Variant

- Tumor cells are eosinophilic; cell height at least 3x width

Papillary Thyroid Carcinoma, Columnar Cell Variant

- Tumor cells show stratified nuclei with supra- and subnuclear vacuoles

Papillary Thyroid Carcinoma, Oncocytic Variant

- Cells have granular eosinophilic cytoplasm

Papillary Thyroid Carcinoma, Hobnail Variant

- Large cells with eosinophilic cytoplasm and lack of cohesion

SELECTED REFERENCES

1. Alzahrani AS et al: Single point mutations in pediatric differentiated thyroid cancer. Thyroid. 27(2):189-196, 2017
2. Liu Z et al: A comparison of the clinicopathological features and prognoses of the classical and the tall cell variant of papillary thyroid cancer: a meta-analysis. Oncotarget. 8(4):6222-6232, 2017
3. Ohashi R et al: Clinicopathological significance of a solid component in papillary thyroid carcinoma. Histopathology. 70(5):775-781, 2017
4. Vuong HG et al: The changing characteristics and molecular profiles of papillary thyroid carcinoma over time: a systematic review. Oncotarget. 8(6):10637-10649, 2017
5. Xu B et al: Primary thyroid carcinoma with low-risk histology and distant metastases: clinicopathologic and molecular characteristics. Thyroid. 27(5):632-640, 2017
6. Martinuzzi C et al: A combination of immunohistochemistry and molecular approaches improves highly sensitive detection of BRAF mutations in papillary thyroid cancer. Endocrine. 53(3):672-80, 2016
7. Sung TY et al: Prognostic value of the number of retrieved lymph nodes in pathological Nx or N0 classical papillary thyroid carcinoma. World J Surg. 40(8):2043-50, 2016
8. Yazgan A et al: The correlation of sodium iodide symporter and BRAF(V600E) mutation in classical variant papillary thyroid carcinoma. Ann Diagn Pathol. 22:58-62, 2016
9. Yang J et al: Comparison of the clinicopathological behavior of the follicular variant of papillary thyroid carcinoma and classical papillary thyroid carcinoma: a systematic review and meta-analysis. Mol Clin Oncol. 3(4):753-764, 2015
10. Hsiao SJ et al: Molecular approaches to thyroid cancer diagnosis. Endocr Relat Cancer. 21(5):T301-13, 2014
11. Ohori NP et al: BRAF mutation detection in indeterminate thyroid cytology specimens: underlying cytologic, molecular, and pathologic characteristics of papillary thyroid carcinoma. Cancer Cytopathol. 121(4):197-205, 2013
12. Virk RK et al: BRAFV600E mutation in papillary thyroid microcarcinoma: a genotype-phenotype correlation. Mod Pathol. 26(1):62-70, 2013
13. Li C et al: BRAF V600E mutation and its association with clinicopathological features of papillary thyroid cancer: a meta-analysis. J Clin Endocrinol Metab. 97(12):4559-70, 2012
14. Khanafshar E et al: The spectrum of papillary thyroid carcinoma variants. Adv Anat Pathol. 18(1):90-7, 2011
15. Lin JD et al: Papillary thyroid carcinoma with different histological patterns. Chang Gung Med J. 34(1):23-34, 2011
16. LiVolsi VA: Papillary thyroid carcinoma: an update. Mod Pathol. 24 Suppl 2:S1-9, 2011
17. Ghossein R: Encapsulated malignant follicular cell-derived thyroid tumors. Endocr Pathol. 21(4):212-8, 2010
18. Nosé V: Thyroid cancer of follicular cell origin in inherited tumor syndromes. Adv Anat Pathol. 17(6):428-36, 2010
19. Sobrinho-Simões M et al: Hot topics in papillary thyroid carcinoma. Int J Surg Pathol. 18(3 Suppl):190S-193S, 2010
20. Tang KT et al: BRAF mutation in papillary thyroid carcinoma: pathogenic role and clinical implications. J Chin Med Assoc. 73(3):113-28, 2010

Most Relevant Genetic Alterations in Papillary Thyroid Carcinoma

PTC Variant	BRAF	RET/PTC	RAS	TERT Promoter	ALK
Conventional/classic type	45-80%	5-25%	0-15%	5-15%	Unknown
Follicular variant	5-25%	5-25%	15-35%	5-15%	Unknown
Tall cell variant	60-95%	35%	0%	5-30%	Unknown
All PTC histiotypes	30-90%	5-35%	0-35%	5-25%	0-5%

Papillary thyroid carcinoma = PTC.

Modified from Lloyd RV et al: WHO Classification of Tumours of Endocrine Organs. 4th ed. Paris: IARC Press, 2017.

Immunohistochemistry in Classic Type

Antibody	Reactivity	Staining Pattern	Comment
Thyroglobulin	Positive	Cytoplasmic	
pax-8	Positive	Nuclear	
TTF-1	Positive	Nuclear	
CK7	Positive	Cytoplasmic	
AE1/AE3	Positive	Cytoplasmic	
CK20	Negative		
BRAF	Positive	Cytoplasmic	
HBME-1	Positive	Cell membrane	Membranous HBME-1 staining is the most specific stain and typically seen in conventional PTC
Galectin-3	Positive	Nuclear & cytoplasmic	Present in most conventional PTC
CK19	Positive	Cytoplasmic	Least specific marker
Calcitonin	Negative		
Chromogranin-A	Negative		
Synaptophysin	Negative		
CD56	Negative		

Papillary thyroid carcinoma = PTC.

21. Lanzilotta SG et al: BRAF in papillary thyroid carcinoma. Cell Oncol. 29(4):269-77, 2007
22. Al-Brahim N et al: Papillary thyroid carcinoma: an overview. Arch Pathol Lab Med. 130(7):1057-62, 2006
23. Albores-Saavedra J et al: The many faces and mimics of papillary thyroid carcinoma. Endocr Pathol. 17(1):1-18, 2006
24. Baloch ZW et al: Cytologic and architectural mimics of papillary thyroid carcinoma. Diagnostic challenges in fine-needle aspiration and surgical pathology specimens. Am J Clin Pathol. 125 Suppl:S135-44, 2006

(Left) *Grossly, the classic variant of PTC can be encapsulates, well-circumscribed, or invasive with poorly defined margins. This gross cut surface shows an encapsulated with firm nodule with extensive central cystic changes.* **(Right)** *Grossly, these tumors are usually white to tan and firm. Note the difference in the gross appearance of the tumor ➡, the background thyroid, and an incidental hyperplastic nodule ➡.*

Encapsulate Cystic Neoplasm

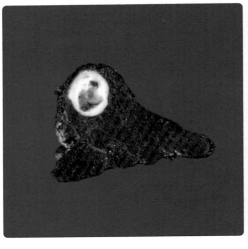

Gross Cut Surface of Papillary Thyroid Carcinoma

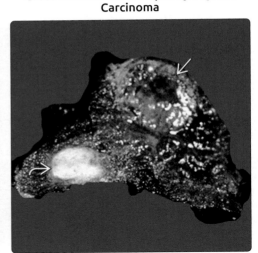

(Left) *Grossly, the classic/conventional PTC has distinct features: Encapsulated, well circumscribed, or invasive with poorly defined margins. The tumor in this figure is an encapsulated PTC with capsular invasion.* **(Right)** *Occasionally, these tumors will have a granular appearance grossly and may be quite friable. This results from the papillary architecture that is seen microscopically. A thin capsule demarcates the tumor from the normal thyroid parenchyma.*

Encapsulated Papillary Thyroid Carcinoma With Gross Invasion

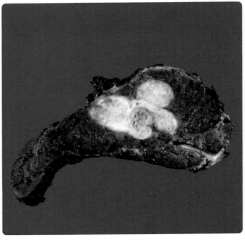

Cut Surface Appearance

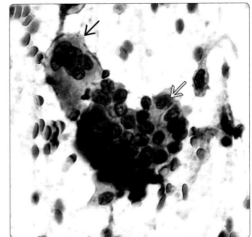

(Left) *This touch prep was taken at the time of intraoperative consultation. The tumor cells have abundant cytoplasm, and intranuclear pseudoinclusions are conspicuous.* **(Right)** *Fine-needle aspirate smears are usually cellular with clusters of cells &/or tissue fragments. The nuclear features of PTC (pale-staining irregular nuclei with nuclear grooves ➡) are nicely demonstrated in this aspirate. A multinucleated giant cell ➡ is also seen here.*

Cytology of Classic Variant

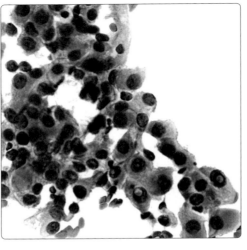

Cytological Features

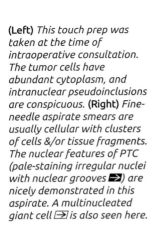

Papillary Thyroid Carcinoma, Classic Variant

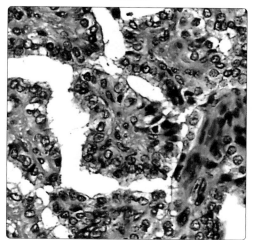

Histopathology Features of Classic Variant

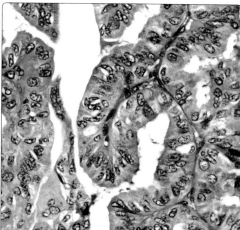

(Left) *This example shows papillary stalks that are thicker and more fibrous in appearance. The tumor cells show classic papillary thyroid carcinoma features.* **(Right)** *Photomicrography of a PTC, classic variant shows a thin fibrovascular core surrounded by the neoplastic follicular cells.*

Papillary Thyroid Carcinoma, Classic Variant

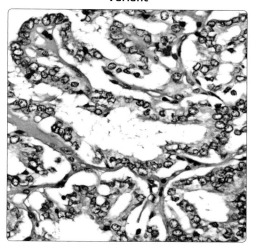

Morphology of Classic Variant

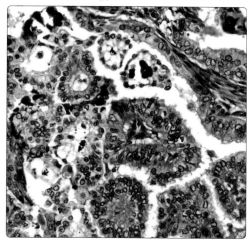

(Left) *This high-power view of a classic-type PTC reveals the typical papillary architectures and the characteristic nuclear features of PTC: Nuclear clearing, nuclear membrane irregularities, and nuclear grooves.* **(Right)** *This classic variant of a PTC shows classic nuclear features, calcification, and a papillary stalk with delicate fibrovascular core.*

Morphology of Classic Variant

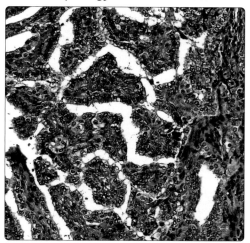

Nuclear Features

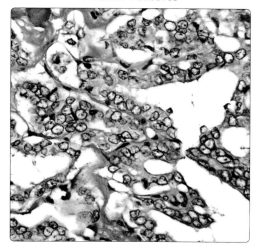

(Left) *PTC, classic variant, shows nuclei clearing, overlapping, and membrane irregularities. The papillary stalks have a delicate fibrovascular core.* **(Right)** *These papillae are composed of delicate fibrovascular cores surrounded by tumor cells that have distinct nuclear features. The nuclei are clear, overlapping, and have obvious membrane irregularities.*

(Left) *The papillary structures in classic PTC are typically described as having thin or delicate fibrovascular cores. In this example, the papillae are edematous and expanded, and lined by cells with characteristic PTC nuclei.* **(Right)** *These tumors are defined by their characteristic nuclear features. The nuclei are enlarged, overlapping, and have irregular contours. The tumor nuclei show the classic clear (ground-glass) chromatin pattern characteristic of this tumor.*

Nuclear Features of Classic Papillary Thyroid Carcinoma

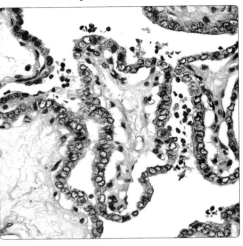

Characteristic Nuclear Features

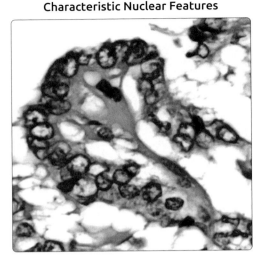

(Left) *Psammoma bodies are a common feature seen in PTC classic variant and are calcified remnants of degenerated papillae. This example shows multiple psammoma bodies. Nuclear grooves ➡ are apparent in these nuclei.* **(Right)** *This example of PTC classic variant shows multiple psammoma bodies, papillary stalks, and cells with marked nuclear membranous irregularity.*

Characteristic Nuclear Features and Psammoma Bodies

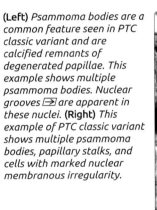
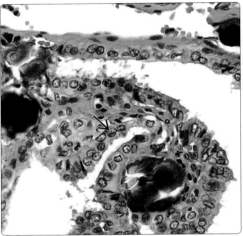

Papillary Thyroid Carcinoma, Classic Variant

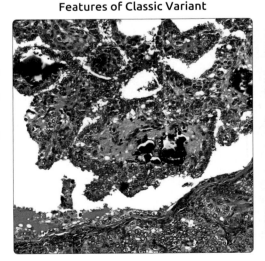

(Left) *Photomicrography shows a papillary structure commonly seen in classic variant, with delicate fibrovascular core, beside the psammoma bodies.* **(Right)** *Lymphovascular invasion and lymph node metastases are commonly seen in PTC. On occasion, a single psammoma body ➡ may be the only evidence of metastases or intrathyroid spread (as seen here). Resections and lymph nodes should be carefully examined for this finding.*

Features of Classic Variant

Intrathyroidal Spread

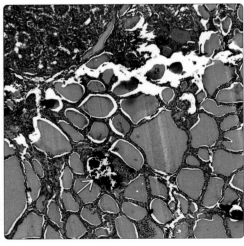

Classic Papillary Structures

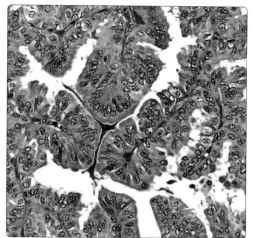

Extrathyroidal Extension

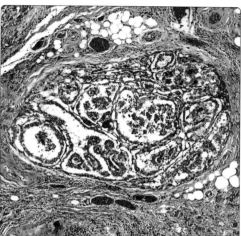

(Left) *Photomicrography of a PTC shows papillary structures commonly seen in classic variant with delicate fibrovascular core.* (Right) *Extension of tumor into perithyroid soft tissue is an indicator of poor prognosis. This tumor is invading the fibroadipose tissue surrounding the thyroid gland. The tumor deposit shows classic PTC architecture.*

Galectin-3 Expression

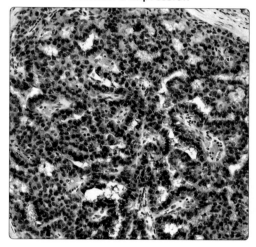

HBME-1 Characteristic Staining Pattern

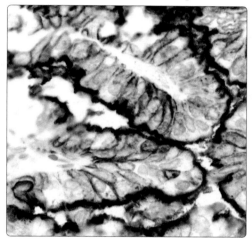

(Left) *Galectin-3 has a cytoplasmic staining pattern, as seen in this photograph. Galectin-3 is usually one of the immunohistochemical stains used as part of a panel.* (Right) *Immunohistochemical stains are generally not necessary when diagnosing this variant of PTC. However, PTC has a characteristic immunohistochemical profile in which it expresses HBME-1, galectin-3, CK19, TTF-1, and thyroglobulin. This image demonstrates the membranous staining pattern characteristic of HBME-1.*

BRAF Immunopositivity

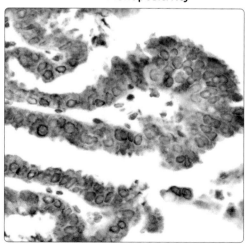

BRAF Cytoplasmic Immunopositivity

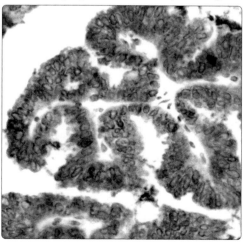

(Left) *BRAF immunostain shows a positive granular cytoplasmic stain in a classic variant of PTC. Note the negativity of the fibrovascular stalk.* (Right) *Photomicrograph of a BRAF immunostain in a classic variant of PTC shows a cytoplasmic immunopositivity. BRAF mutation analysis confirmed BRAF V600E mutation.*

KEY FACTS

TERMINOLOGY

- Variant of papillary thyroid carcinoma (PTC), encapsulated with invasion, composed entirely or almost entirely of variously sized follicles that have characteristic PTC nuclear features

ETIOLOGY/PATHOGENESIS

- Encapsulated follicular variant of PTC have molecular profile with high rate of RAS and absence of *BRAF* V600E mutations

CLINICAL ISSUES

- 2nd most common variant of PTC
- More common in women

MICROSCOPIC

- Tumors are well circumscribed or encapsulated with invasion
- Composed largely of irregularly shaped, small- to medium-sized follicles

- Characteristic PTC nuclear features are present
  - Clear, ground-glass chromatin, irregular membranes with nuclear grooves and with rare pseudoinclusions
  - These features may be present only focally, making this diagnosis difficult (so-called sprinkling sign)

ANCILLARY TESTS

- Positive: TTF-1, thyroglobulin, HBME-1, galectin-3, CK19
- BRAF negative

TOP DIFFERENTIAL DIAGNOSES

- Noninvasive follicular thyroid neoplasm with papillary-like nuclear features
  - Encapsulated or well-circumscribed, follicular-patterned neoplasm; no invasion
- Infiltrative follicular variant of PTC
  - Nuclei of cells lining follicles have features of conventional PTC
  - No capsule

Encapsulated Neoplasm

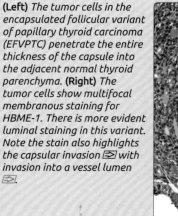

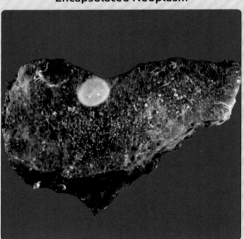

(Left) This gross cut surface of an encapsulated thyroid neoplasm shows a thick fibrous capsule surrounding the homogeneously tan tumor. There was no capsular invasion. As the tumor has nuclear features of papillary thyroid carcinoma, and is < 1 cm, the tumor is presently called microcarcinoma. (Right) The tumor capsule was penetrated and the tumor cells are seen within a vessel beyond the tumor capsule. Intravascular tumor cells are adherent to the vessel wall and covered by endothelial cells

Vascular Invasion

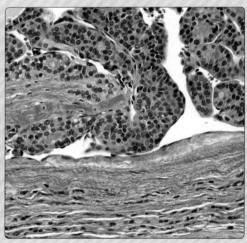

Capsular Invasion

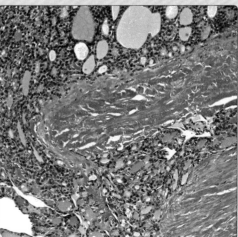

(Left) The tumor cells in the encapsulated follicular variant of papillary thyroid carcinoma (EFVPTC) penetrate the entire thickness of the capsule into the adjacent normal thyroid parenchyma. (Right) The tumor cells show multifocal membranous staining for HBME-1. There is more evident luminal staining in this variant. Note the stain also highlights the capsular invasion ⊡ with invasion into a vessel lumen ⊡.

HBME-1 Expression

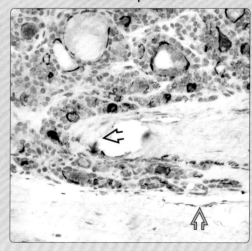

TERMINOLOGY

Abbreviations

- Papillary thyroid carcinoma, encapsulated follicular variant (EFVPTC)

Synonyms

- Encapsulated follicular variant of papillary thyroid carcinoma (EFVPTC) with invasion

Definitions

- Variant of papillary thyroid carcinoma, encapsulated, with invasion, composed entirely or almost entirely of variously sized follicles that have characteristic papillary thyroid carcinoma (PTC) nuclear features

ETIOLOGY/PATHOGENESIS

Environmental Exposure

- Associated with exposure to ionizing radiation

Genetics

- *RET* rearrangement
  - *RET* gene activation via rearrangement
  - Most common genetic abnormality in PTC
  - Associated with ionizing radiation
  - 9 different rearrangements have been identified
    - Most common is *RET/PTC1* (60-70%) followed by *RET/PTC3* (20-30%)
  - Found in 10-26% of follicular variant PTC (slightly lower than classic variant)
    - *RET/PTC1* most often associated
  - Research suggests prognosis is favorable with follicular variant when tumors harbor *RET/PTC* rearrangements
- RAS
  - Point mutation of activating protooncogene
  - Mutations are classified as *NRAS*, *KRAS*, and *HRAS*
  - Found in 10-20% of all PTC cases
    - Tumors with RAS mutations are almost always follicular variant
  - Prognosis usually better when this mutation present
    - Encapsulated tumors
    - Decreased incidence of lymph node metastases have been reported
  - Associated with less prominent characteristic PTC nuclei
  - Encapsulated follicular variant of PTC has molecular profile very close to follicular adenomas/carcinomas with high rate of RAS and absence of *BRAF* mutations
- *BRAF* V600E
  - Mutation in few cases reported
  - Not common
  - Usually present in infiltrative follicular variant of PTC and is associated with poor prognosis, as metastases, extrathyroid extension
  - With few reported cases of *BRAF* V601E mutation
- *NTRK1* and *NTRK3*
  - Rare type of tyrosine kinase receptor mutation
  - Seen in follicular variant as well as other variants of papillary carcinoma
  - Literature suggests worse prognosis in association with *NTRK1* mutation

- Cancer Genome Atlas study of PTC has shown at genomic level to consist of 2 highly distinct classes
  - Tumors with true papillary architecture were dominated by *BRAF* V600E mutations and *RET* kinase fusions and were designated as BRAF(V600E)-like
  - Tumors with follicular architecture were conversely dominated by RAS mutations and were designated as RAS-like
  - Given genotype:phenotype correlation, separation of BRAF(V600E)-like and RAS-like tumors has implications in classification, especially follicular variant of papillary carcinoma

CLINICAL ISSUES

Epidemiology

- Incidence
  - 2nd most common variant of PTC
  - Comprises ~ 30% of all PTC cases
- Age
  - Mean at presentation is 47.9 years
- Sex
  - More common in women

Presentation

- Typically present as palpable nodule on physical exam
- May present as painless, enlarging mass
  - May also present as unilateral neck swelling when due to lymph node metastasis
- May have compressive symptoms if involving surrounding structures
- May be found incidentally on imaging studies

Treatment

- Surgical treatment options vary depending on stage of disease
  - Lobectomy vs. total thyroidectomy
  - Neck dissection indicated when cervical lymph node metastases are present
- RAI therapy post surgery

Prognosis

- Encapsulated forms generally have better prognosis
  - Invasion of capsule, especially when multifocal, is associated with more aggressive behavior
- Nonencapsulated tumors usually behave more aggressively
  - Involve adjacent structures
  - Lymph node metastases more common
    - Present in 65% of cases vs. 5% of encapsulated tumors
- Certain molecular/genetic findings may portend worse prognosis (*BRAF*, *NTRK1*)

MACROSCOPIC

General Features

- Grossly may be encapsulated, well circumscribed, or infiltrative
- Typically white to tan in color
- Usually firm and solid in consistency
- Cystic cavities with hemorrhage and calcification may also be identified grossly

Size

- Can vary greatly

MICROSCOPIC

Histologic Features

- Tumors are well circumscribed or encapsulated with invasion
- Stromal sclerosis/fibrosis may be present
- Composed largely of irregularly shaped, small- to medium-sized follicles
  - Majority of tumor must be composed of follicles
- Hypereosinophilic colloid with scalloped edges
- Colloid may also be pale or watery in appearance
- Intrafollicular multinucleated giant cells are occasionally present
- Macrophages can be present within follicles
- Rare psammoma bodies
- Peritumoral lymphocytic infiltration may be present

Cytologic Features

- Neoplastic cells are cuboidal in shape
  - Larger when compared to cells comprising normal nonneoplastic follicles
- Individual cell contours may be irregular (cuboidal, polygonal)
- Cells may have eosinophilic, amphophilic, or clear cytoplasm
- Nuclei are enlarged
- Characteristic PTC nuclear features are present
  - These features may be present only focally, making this diagnosis difficult
  - Nuclei have clear, ground-glass chromatin
    - Optically clear, "Orphan Annie" nuclei
    - Nucleoli may be present focally
  - Nuclei have irregular membranes
    - Polygonal shape
    - Nuclear grooves
    - Intranuclear pseudoinclusions (less common than in classic variant PTC)
  - Occasionally characteristic PTC nuclear features are not present
    - Nuclei will have fine chromatin with prominent nucleoli
- Nuclei are back-to-back
  - Typically do not overlap or stratify (characteristic of classic variant)

ANCILLARY TESTS

Cytology

- Noncohesive cells are present
- Cells arranged in follicles
- Colloid is scant in background
- Nuclear features of PTC
  - Powdery chromatin
  - Irregular nuclear borders
  - Nuclear grooves
  - Rare nuclear inclusions

Frozen Sections

- Caution should be used as frozen section artifact can mimic nuclear features of PTC

Immunohistochemistry

- Positive
  - TTF-1 (nuclear), thyroglobulin (cytoplasmic), HBME-1 (luminal/membranous), galectin-3 (cytoplasmic), CK19 (cytoplasmic)
  - Immunohistochemistry can be quite useful when differentiating encapsulated tumors from follicular carcinomas/adenomas
- Negative
  - Calcitonin, chromogranin, synaptophysin, β-catenin, p53
  - BRAF

Cytogenetics

- Genetic analysis of tumors can be important for prognosis
- RAS protooncogene activating point mutations are frequently associated with follicular variant PTC
  - Reported in as many as 40% of cases
- RET rearrangement is found in ~ 10-26% of follicular variant of PTC
- BRAF K601N mutation may be found
  - BRAF V600E mutation is occasionally found
- Encapsulated follicular variant of PTC has molecular profile very close to follicular adenomas/carcinomas (high rate of RAS and absence of BRAF mutations)
  - Infiltrative follicular variant has opposite molecular profile closer to classic PTC than to follicular adenoma/carcinoma (BRAF > RAS mutations)
    - Molecular profile of encapsulated and infiltrative follicular variant parallels their biological behavior
- Testing for familial tumor syndromes may be necessary

DIFFERENTIAL DIAGNOSIS

Noninvasive Follicular Thyroid Neoplasm With Papillary-like Nuclear Features

- Encapsulated or well-circumscribed, follicular-patterned neoplasm
- Presence of PTC nuclear features
- No invasion present

Follicular Thyroid Carcinoma

- Encapsulated malignant neoplasm
- Capsular invasion must be present
- Architecture and cytologic features are different from those in surrounding tissue
  - May have follicular, trabecular, or solid growth patterns
- Nuclei are enlarged, hyperchromatic, and round
- Characteristic nuclear features of papillary carcinoma are absent
- Distinguished from follicular adenoma by presence of capsular invasion or metastases

Follicular Thyroid Adenoma

- Benign, encapsulated neoplasm
- Composed of many small follicles, trabeculae, or solid sheets of cells
- Nuclei are uniform, dark, and round
- Lack characteristic PTC nuclear features

Differential Diagnosis of Papillary Thyroid Carcinoma, Follicular Variant

Characteristic	Follicular Variant PTC	Follicular Thyroid Carcinoma	Follicular Thyroid Adenoma	Noninvasive Follicular Thyroid Neoplasm with Papillary-Like Nuclear Features (NIFTP)
Follicular architecture	Present	Always present	Always present	Present
Capsular invasion	May be present	Always present	Never present	Never present
Nuclear shape	Irregular, polygonal	Round	Round	Irregular, polygonal
Chromatin pattern	Ground-glass	Dense, hyperchromatic	Dense, hyperchromatic	Ground-glass
Nuclear grooves	Present	Absent	Absent	Present
Nuclear pseudoinclusions	Present	Absent	Absent	Present
Metastatic pattern	Lymphatics	Hematogenous	N/A	N/A
Background thyroid	Goiter, thyroiditis	Multinodular goiter	Normal	Normal
Immunohistochemistry	HBME-1, galectin-3(+)	HBME-1 and galectin-3(+/-); β-catenin(+)	HBME-1, galectin-3(+/-)	HBME-1, galectin-3 (+)
Molecular findings	RAS, RET/PTC may have BRAD 601	RAS, PPARγ, PTEN, CTNNB1, TP53	RAS, PPARγ	RAS

Infiltrative Follicular Variant of Papillary Thyroid Carcinoma

- Shares many features with classic/conventional PTC
- Nuclei of cells lining follicles have features of conventional PTC
- Has no capsule

DIAGNOSTIC CHECKLIST

Pathologic Interpretation Pearls

- Encapsulated, with capsular &/or vascular invasion
- Has exclusively or almost exclusively follicular growth pattern
- Nuclear features of PTC

SELECTED REFERENCES

1. Basolo F et al: The molecular landscape of noninvasive follicular thyroid neoplasm with papillary-like nuclear features (NIFTP): a literature review. Adv Anat Pathol. 24(5):252-258, 2017
2. Giannini R et al: Identification of two distinct molecular subtypes by digital RNA counting of "non-invasive follicular tumour with papillary-like nuclear features (NIFTP)". Thyroid. ePub, 2017
3. Haugen BR Md et al: The ATA Guidelines on Management of Thyroid Nodules and Differentiated Thyroid Cancer Task Force review and recommendation on the proposed renaming of FVPTC without invasion to NIFTP. Thyroid. 27(4):481-483, 2017
4. Scharpf J et al: The follicular variant of papillary thyroid cancer and noninvasive follicular thyroid neoplasm with papillary-like nuclear features (NIFTP). Curr Opin Oncol. 29(1):20-24, 2017
5. Sullivan MC et al: Prevalence of contralateral tumors in patients with follicular variant of papillary thyroid cancer. J Am Coll Surg. 224(6):1021-1027, 2017
6. Xu B et al: Primary thyroid carcinoma with low-risk histology and distant metastases: clinicopathologic and molecular characteristics. Thyroid. 27(5):632-640, 2017
7. Giordano TJ: Follicular cell thyroid neoplasia: insights from genomics and The Cancer Genome Atlas research network. Curr Opin Oncol. 28(1):1-4, 2016
8. Gucer H et al: The value of HBME-1 and Claudin-1 expression profile in the distinction of BRAF-like and RAS-like phenotypes in papillary thyroid carcinoma. Endocr Pathol. 27(3):224-32, 2016
9. Hodak S et al: Changing the cancer diagnosis: the case of follicular variant of papillary thyroid cancer-primum non nocere and NIFTP. Thyroid. 26(7):869-71, 2016
10. Jeon MJ et al: Impact of reclassification on thyroid nodules with architectural atypia: from non-invasive encapsulated follicular variant papillary thyroid carcinomas to non-invasive follicular thyroid neoplasm with papillary-like nuclear features. PLoS One. 11(12):e0167756, 2016
11. Krane JF et al: Coming to terms with NIFTP: a provisional approach for cytologists. Cancer Cytopathol. 124(11):767-772, 2016
12. Nikiforov YE et al: Nomenclature revision for encapsulated follicular variant of papillary thyroid carcinoma: a paradigm shift to reduce overtreatment of indolent tumors. JAMA Oncol. 2(8):1023-9, 2016
13. Strickland KC et al: Preoperative cytologic diagnosis of noninvasive follicular thyroid neoplasm with papillary-like nuclear features: a prospective analysis. Thyroid. 26(10):1466-1471, 2016
14. Schulten HJ et al: Comparison of microarray expression profiles between follicular variant of papillary thyroid carcinomas and follicular adenomas of the thyroid. BMC Genomics. 16 Suppl 1:S7, 2015
15. Dettmer M et al: Comprehensive MicroRNA expression profiling identifies novel markers in follicular variant of papillary thyroid carcinoma. Thyroid. 23(11):1383-9, 2013
16. Lee SR et al: Molecular genotyping of follicular variant of papillary thyroid carcinoma correlates with diagnostic category of fine-needle aspiration cytology: values of RAS mutation testing. Thyroid. 23(11):1416-22, 2013
17. Park JY et al: BRAF and RAS mutations in follicular variants of papillary thyroid carcinoma. Endocr Pathol. 24(2):69-76, 2013
18. Rivera M et al: Molecular genotyping of papillary thyroid carcinoma follicular variant according to its histological subtypes (encapsulated vs infiltrative) reveals distinct BRAF and RAS mutation patterns. Mod Pathol. 23(9):1191-200, 2010
19. Ghossein R: Encapsulated malignant follicular cell-derived thyroid tumors. Endocr Pathol. 21(4):212-8, 2010
20. Faquin WC: Diagnosis and reporting of follicular-patterned thyroid lesions by fine needle aspiration. Head Neck Pathol. 3(1):82-5, 2009
21. Ghossein R: Problems and controversies in the histopathology of thyroid carcinomas of follicular cell origin. Arch Pathol Lab Med. 133(5):683-91, 2009
22. Salajegheh A et al: Follicular variant of papillary thyroid carcinoma: a diagnostic challenge for clinicians and pathologists. Postgrad Med J. 84(988):78-82, 2008
23. Albores-Saavedra J et al: The many faces and mimics of papillary thyroid carcinoma. Endocr Pathol. 17(1):1-18, 2006
24. Suster S: Thyroid tumors with a follicular growth pattern: problems in differential diagnosis. Arch Pathol Lab Med. 130(7):984-8, 2006
25. Giordano TJ et al: Molecular classification of papillary thyroid carcinoma: distinct BRAF, RAS, and RET/PTC mutation-specific gene expression profiles discovered by DNA microarray analysis. Oncogene. 24(44):6646-56, 2005
26. Baloch ZW et al: Follicular-patterned lesions of the thyroid: the bane of the pathologist. Am J Clin Pathol. 117(1):143-50, 2002

(Left) *This photograph demonstrates gross features commonly seen in the EFVPTC, with solid, white-tan nodules. A thin capsule ➡ can be identified, but invasion into the adjacent thyroid can be appreciated.* **(Right)** *This EFVPTC shows a complete capsule invasion, and the tumor cells are seen within a vessel lumen ➡. Intravascular tumor cells are adherent to the vessel wall and covered by endothelial cells ➡.*

Encapsulated Tumor With Invasion

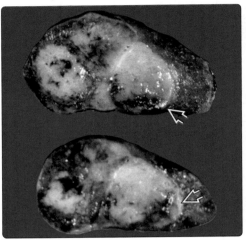

Vascular Invasion With Tumor Adherent to Wall

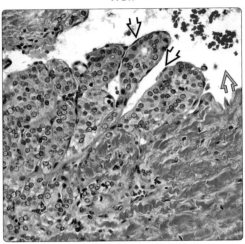

(Left) *This photomicrograph shows an EFVPTC with both capsular and vascular invasion. This lower power view from the following figure shows encapsulated tumor penetrating through the capsule ➡ into an extracapsular vessel ➡.* **(Right)** *This high-power figure illustrates the encapsulated tumor penetrating through the capsule ➡ into an extracapsular vessel ➡. Intravascular tumor cells are adherent to the vessel wall and are covered by endothelial cells.*

Capsular and Lymphovascular Invasion

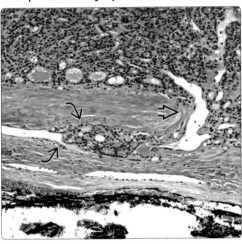

Capsular and Lymphovascular Invasion

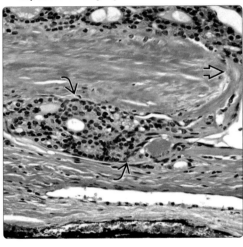

(Left) *There is capsular invasion ➡ with tumor cells going through the thick capsule. The tumor has a follicular architecture and is composed of cells with nuclear features of papillary thyroid carcinoma (PTC). The follicles are filled with dark staining colloid.* **(Right)** *This encapsulated follicular-patterned neoplasm is surrounded by a thick fibrous capsule, which shows focal calcification ➡. There is complete capsular invasion ➡ with tumor cells going through the thick capsule.*

Capsular Invasion

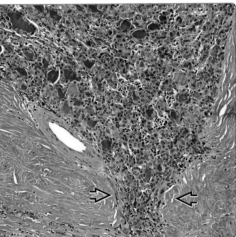

Capsular Invasion

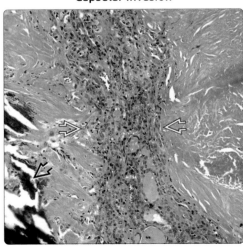

Typical Nuclear Features of PTC

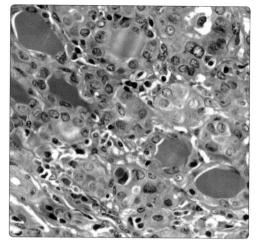

Characteristic Nuclear Features

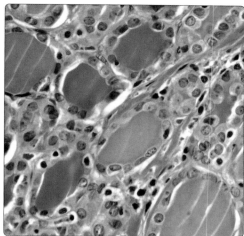

(Left) *EFVPTC usually has the characteristic nuclear features of PTC, as nuclear overlapping, nuclear enlargement, nuclear clearing, and nuclear membrane irregularities.* **(Right)** *The nuclei of the cells of PTC display a characteristic set of abnormalities, grouped as changes in size and shape, irregularities of the nuclear membranes, and characteristic chromatin. There is nuclear enlargement and overlapping, nuclear grooves and pseudoinclusions, as well as empty appearance of the nuclei.*

Nuclear Features and Dark Colloid

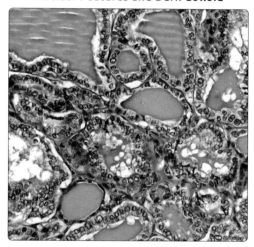

Dark Colloid With Scalloping

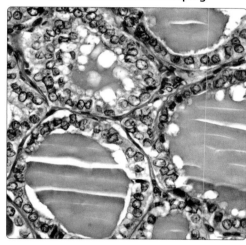

(Left) *H&E shows characteristic features of the follicular variant of PTC. The tumor cells are arranged in follicles of varying sizes and shapes, with classic PTC nuclear features.* **(Right)** *This high-power image highlights nuclear and morphological features seen in this variant of PTC. The nuclei are enlarged and have ground-glass chromatin with nuclear grooves and irregular nuclear contours. The colloid is deeply eosinophilic. Scalloping of colloid is also present.*

Giant Cell

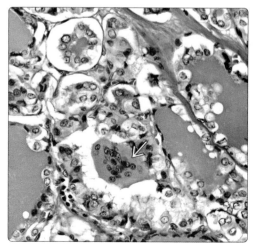

Nuclei of PTC

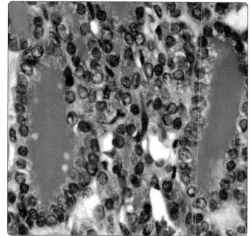

(Left) *H&E demonstrates a multinucleated giant cell* ➡ *present within a follicle in papillary carcinoma, follicular variant. This finding on FNA is almost pathognomonic for PTC.* **(Right)** *The nuclei of the cells of PTC display a set of abnormalities grouped in 3 categories: (1) changes in size and shape (nuclear enlargement and overlapping); (2) irregularities of the membrane (irregular nuclear contours and pseudoinclusions); and (3) chromatin changes (empty appearance of the nucleoplasm).*

Papillary Nuclear Features

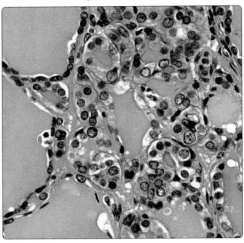

Sprinkling Sign

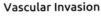

(Left) *Follicular variant of PTC is composed of irregular follicles, which contain hypereosinophilic colloid. The nuclei have characteristic features of papillary carcinoma.* **(Right)** *High-power image shows the enlarged neoplastic cells present in this variant of PTC. The neoplastic thyroid follicles have classic cytomorphological features: Enlarged nuclei with irregular nuclear membranes, nuclear grooves, and pale-staining ground-glass chromatin.*

Vascular Invasion

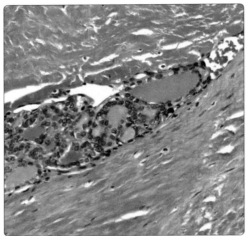

Invasion Into Adjacent Tissues

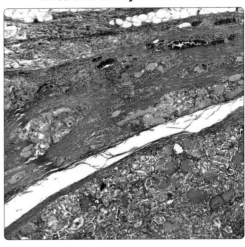

(Left) *Intravascular tumor cells are (1) adherent to the vessel wall, (2) covered by endothelial cells, and (3) present in a vessel beyond the tumor capsule. These 3 criteria for true vascular invasion should be present.* **(Right)** *The encapsulated variant of PTC may show the invasion of the tumor capsule in multiple places and may be associated with extrathyroidal extension.*

EFVPTC Adjacent to Parathyroid

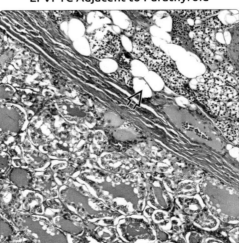

Tumor Extending Outside Tumor Capsule

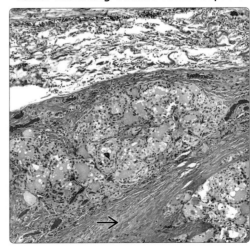

(Left) *This EFVPTC is approaching the adjacent parathyroid gland ⊟. Clear nuclear features of papillary carcinoma are seen in this large tumor nodule.* **(Right)** *Low-power image shows a follicular variant of PTC with tumor cells that have traversed a thick fibrous capsule ⊟, having tumor present on both sides. This tumor also extends to the perithyroidal soft tissues. Both of these features are associated with less favorable prognosis.*

Capsular and Vascular Invasion

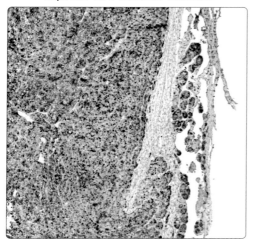

EFVPTV With Vascular Invasion

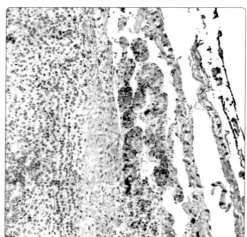

(Left) *This image shows cyclin-D1 immunohistochemistry staining seen in encapsulated follicular variant of PTC with both capsular and vascular invasion. Positive staining is useful when used in conjunction with other immunohistochemical stains.* (Right) *CK19 has a cytoplasmic staining pattern in these tumors. Immunohistochemistry is not usually required for diagnosis, but when used it should incorporate a panel of antibodies that typically consists of HBME-1, galectin-3, CK19, CITED-1, and cyclin-D1.*

HBME-1 in Follicular Variant of PTC

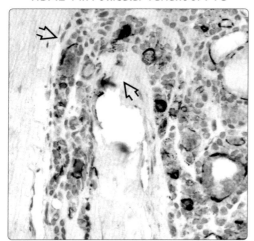

Patchy HBME1 Membranous Staining

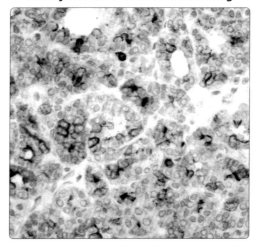

(Left) *HBME-1 stain highlights the capsular invasion ⊡ on the EFVPTC. The staining is present on the membranes of the neoplastic cells and seen here predominantly within the luminal border of the follicles.* (Right) *Immunohistochemistry shows a characteristic patchy membranous pattern seen in the follicular variant of PTC. The stain is present multifocally on the membranes of the neoplastic cells, in a patchy way, and not in a diffuse pattern, as seen in the classic and tall cell variants.*

Membranous And Luminal HBME-1 Stain

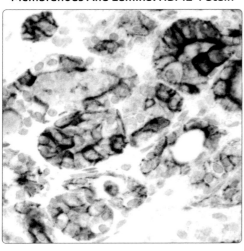

Galectin-3 in EFVPTV

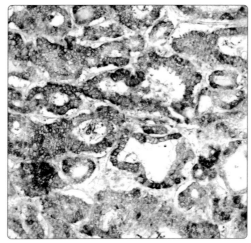

(Left) *Immunohistochemistry shows the diagnostic luminal border and membranous staining of HBME-1. Not all tumor cells are positive. This is the classic staining pattern seen in the follicular variant of PTC.* (Right) *Galectin-3 is usually positive in the cytoplasm of PTC tumor cells. Follicular variant of PTC usually shows only focal and weak staining. A panel with positivity for HBME-1, CITED-1, CK19, and galectin-3 is sensitive and specific for papillary carcinoma.*

Papillary Thyroid Carcinoma, Follicular Variant, Infiltrative

TERMINOLOGY

- Variant of papillary thyroid carcinoma, infiltrative and unencapsulated, composed mostly of variously sized follicles that have nuclei with features of conventional papillary thyroid carcinoma

CLINICAL ISSUES

- *BRAF* mutation present in ~ 25%

MICROSCOPIC

- Tumors may be microcarcinoma, widely invasive, and infiltrative
- Composed largely of irregularly shaped small- to medium-sized follicles
- Characteristic conventional papillary thyroid carcinoma nuclear features
  - Clear, ground-glass chromatin, irregular membranes with nuclear grooves and pseudoinclusions
- These features may be present only focally: Sprinkling sign

ANCILLARY TESTS

- Immunohistochemistry
  - Positive: TTF-1, pax-8, thyroglobulin, HBME-1, galectin-3, CK19, CITED1
- BRAF immunohistochemistry is positive in ~ 25%
  - *BRAF* V600E mutation is associated with infiltrative FVPTC and aggressive histopathological tumor features

DIAGNOSTIC CHECKLIST

- FVPTC is heterogeneous disease composed of 2 distinct groups
  - Infiltrative/diffuse nonencapsulated variant, which resembles classic papillary carcinoma
  - Encapsulated variant, which behaves more like follicular thyroid carcinoma
  - Variants identified by *BRAF* V600E mutation
    - *BRAF* V600E mutation is associated with unencapsulated FVPTC

Gross Cut Surface

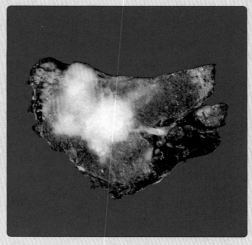

Histologic Features

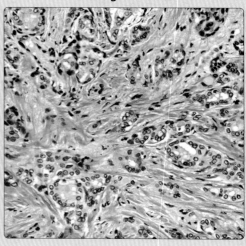

(Left) The gross thyroid cut surface highlights characteristic gross aspect usually identified in the infiltrative follicular variant of papillary thyroid carcinoma (FVPTC). No capsule is identified and the tumor has infiltrative borders. *(Right)* This image highlights characteristic infiltrative growth pattern and the characteristic nuclear features present in the infiltrative FVPTC. Dense collagen fibers can be seen intervening between neoplastic follicles.

Perineural Invasion

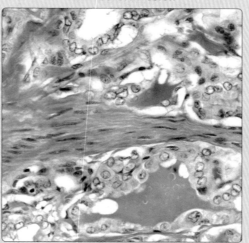

S100 in Perineural Invasion

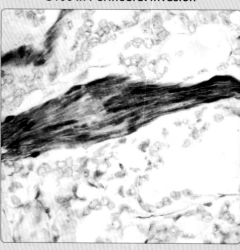

(Left) This image demonstrates characteristic papillary thyroid carcinoma (PTC) nuclear features present in the infiltrative FVPTC, showing tongues of tumor infiltrating the perineural spaces. *(Right)* Infiltrative follicular variant of PTC shows a tumor growing in a follicular pattern with marked fibrosis and with a perineural infiltration. The perineural invasion is highlighted by the S100 immunohistochemical stain.

TERMINOLOGY

Synonyms

- Infiltrative follicular variant of papillary thyroid carcinoma (FVPTC)

Definitions

- Variant of papillary thyroid carcinoma (PTC), infiltrative and unencapsulated, composed mostly of variously sized follicles that have nuclei with features of conventional PTC

ETIOLOGY/PATHOGENESIS

Environmental Exposure

- Associated with exposure to ionizing radiation

Genetics

- Infiltrative follicular variant has molecular profile closer to classic PTC than to follicular adenoma/carcinoma: *BRAF* V600E > *RAS* mutations
  - Encapsulated follicular variant of PTCs have molecular profile very close to follicular adenomas/carcinomas: High rate of RAS and absence of *BRAF* mutations
  - Molecular profile of encapsulated and infiltrative follicular variant parallels their biological behavior (i.e., metastatic nodal and invasive patterns)
- *BRAF*
  - *BRAF* V600E mutation was found in ~ 25% of infiltrative tumor and not in encapsulated carcinomas
  - Associated with poor prognosis (metastases, extrathyroid extension)
- RAS
  - RAS mutations were observed in ~ 35% of encapsulated tumors and in only ~ 10% of infiltrative tumors
  - Associated with less prominent characteristic PTC nuclei
- *RET* rearrangement
  - Research suggests prognosis is favorable with follicular variant when tumors harbor *RET* rearrangements

CLINICAL ISSUES

Epidemiology

- Age
  - Mean at presentation: ~ 50 years

Presentation

- Typically present as palpable nodule on physical exam
- May present as painless, enlarging mass
  - May also present as unilateral neck swelling when due to lymph node metastasis
- May have compressive symptoms if involving surrounding structures
- May be found incidentally on imaging studies
- Infiltrative carcinomas had much higher frequency of extrathyroidal extension, positive margins, and nodal metastases than encapsulated tumors

Treatment

- Surgical treatment options vary depending on stage of disease
  - Lobectomy vs. total thyroidectomy
  - Neck dissection indicated when cervical lymph node metastases are present
- RAI therapy post surgery

Prognosis

- Infiltrative, nonencapsulated tumors usually behave more aggressively
  - Involve adjacent structures
  - Lymph node metastases more common
    - Present in 65% of cases vs. 5% of encapsulated tumors
  - Perineural invasion is present
  - In comparison, encapsulated forms generally have better prognosis
    - Invasion of capsule, especially when multifocal, is associated with more aggressive behavior
- Certain molecular genetic findings may portend worse prognosis (*BRAF*)

MACROSCOPIC

General Features

- Grossly are infiltrative
- Typically white to tan in color
- Usually firm and solid in consistency
- Cystic cavities with hemorrhage and calcification may also be identified grossly

Size

- Can vary greatly

MICROSCOPIC

Histologic Features

- Tumors are widely invasive, infiltrating
- Stromal sclerosis/fibrosis may be present
- Tongues of tumor-infiltrating nonneoplastic thyroid without interposition of capsule
- Tumor growing in follicular pattern with marked fibrosis and infiltrating advancing front
  - Exclusively or almost exclusively follicular growth pattern
  - Composed largely of irregularly shaped small- to medium-sized follicles
    - Majority of tumor must be composed of follicles
- Hypereosinophilic colloid with scalloped edges
  - Colloid may also be pale or watery in appearance
- Rare psammoma bodies
- Infiltration into perithyroidal soft tissue
- Perineural invasion usually identified

Cytologic Features

- Neoplastic cells are cuboidal in shape
  - Larger when compared to cells comprising normal nonneoplastic follicles
- Individual cell contours may be irregular (cuboidal, polygonal)
- Cells may have eosinophilic, amphophilic, or clear cytoplasm
- Nuclear features of conventional PTC: Overlapping nuclei with irregular nuclear membranes, clearing with ground-glass chromatin and grooves
  - Characteristic PTC nuclear features are present, but these features may be only focal (sprinkling sign)

ANCILLARY TESTS

Cytology

- Cells arranged in follicles
- Colloid is scant in background
- Nuclear features of PTC
  - Powdery chromatin
  - Irregular nuclear borders
  - Nuclear grooves
  - Rare nuclear inclusions

Frozen Sections

- Caution should be used as frozen section artifact can mimic nuclear features of PTC

Immunohistochemistry

- Positive
  - TTF-1, pax-8, thyroglobulin, HBME-1, galectin-3, CK19, MSG1
  - BRAF in ~ 25%
- Negative
  - Calcitonin, chromogranin, synaptophysin, β-catenin

Genetic Testing

- Genetic analysis of tumors can be important for prognosis
  - *BRAF* V600E mutation is present in ~ 25%
  - RAS protooncogene activating point mutations is present in ~ 10% of infiltrative FVPTC
  - *RET* rearrangement is not common in infiltrative FVPTC

DIFFERENTIAL DIAGNOSIS

Follicular Thyroid Carcinoma

- Encapsulated malignant neoplasm with capsular invasion
- Characteristic nuclear features of PTC are absent

Follicular Thyroid Adenoma

- Benign, encapsulated neoplasm
- Lack characteristic PTC nuclear features

Encapsulated FVPTC With Invasion

- Encapsulated PTC with invasion

Noninvasive Follicular Thyroid Neoplasm With Papillary-Like Nuclear Features

- Encapsulated follicular patterned neoplasm with no invasion

DIAGNOSTIC CHECKLIST

FVPTC Has 2 Subvariants: Infiltrative and Encapsulated With Invasion

- FVPTC is heterogeneous disease composed of 2 distinct groups
  - Infiltrative nonencapsulated variant, which resembles classic papillary carcinoma in its nuclear features, metastatic lymph node pattern, and invasive growth
  - Encapsulated form, which behaves more like follicular thyroid carcinoma
- *BRAF* V600E mutation is associated with infiltrative type and aggressive histopathologic tumor features
  - *BRAF* K601E is strongly associated with follicular-patterned cancer, particularly with encapsulated FVPTC

- Correct classification has correlation with prognosis

SELECTED REFERENCES

1. Xu B et al: Evolution of the histologic classification of thyroid neoplasms and its impact on clinical management. Eur J Surg Oncol. ePub, 2017
2. Xu B et al: Primary thyroid carcinoma with low-risk histology and distant metastases: clinicopathologic and molecular characteristics. Thyroid. 27(5):632-640, 2017
3. Nikiforov YE et al: Nomenclature revision for encapsulated follicular variant of papillary thyroid carcinoma: a paradigm shift to reduce overtreatment of indolent tumors. JAMA Oncol. 2(8):1023-9, 2016
4. Shi X et al: Differential clinicopathological risk and prognosis of major papillary thyroid cancer variants. J Clin Endocrinol Metab. 101(1):264-74, 2016
5. Abd-El Raouf SM et al: Immunohistochemical expression of HBME-1 and galectin-3 in the differential diagnosis of follicular-derived thyroid nodules. Pathol Res Pract. 210(12):971-8, 2014
6. Armstrong MJ et al: PAX8/PPARγ rearrangement in thyroid nodules predicts follicular-pattern carcinomas, in particular the encapsulated follicular variant of papillary carcinoma. Thyroid. 24(9):1369-74, 2014
7. Asa SL et al: Implications of the TCGA genomic characterization of papillary thyroid carcinoma for thyroid pathology: does follicular variant papillary thyroid carcinoma exist? Thyroid. 25(1):1-2, 2014
8. Chai YJ et al: BRAF mutation in follicular variant of papillary thyroid carcinoma is associated with unfavourable clinicopathological characteristics and malignant features on ultrasonography. Clin Endocrinol (Oxf). 81(3):432-9, 2014
9. Jung CK et al: The increase in thyroid cancer incidence during the last four decades is accompanied by a high frequency of BRAF mutations and a sharp increase in RAS mutations. J Clin Endocrinol Metab. 99(2):E276-85, 2014
10. McFadden DG et al: Identification of oncogenic mutations and gene fusions in the follicular variant of papillary thyroid carcinoma. J Clin Endocrinol Metab. 99(11):E2457-62, 2014
11. Pusztaszeri M: Follicular variant of papillary thyroid carcinoma: distinct biologic behavior based on ultrasonographic features. Thyroid. 24(6):1067-8, 2014
12. Dettmer M et al: Comprehensive MicroRNA expression profiling identifies novel markers in follicular variant of papillary thyroid carcinoma. Thyroid. 23(11):1383-9, 2013
13. Lee SR et al: Molecular genotyping of follicular variant of papillary thyroid carcinoma correlates with diagnostic category of fine-needle aspiration cytology: values of RAS mutation testing. Thyroid. 23(11):1416-22, 2013
14. Park JY et al: BRAF and RAS mutations in follicular variants of papillary thyroid carcinoma. Endocr Pathol. 24(2):69-76, 2013
15. Vanzati A et al: The "sprinkling" sign in the follicular variant of papillary thyroid carcinoma: a clue to the recognition of this entity. Arch Pathol Lab Med. 137(12):1707-9, 2013
16. Ghossein R: Encapsulated malignant follicular cell-derived thyroid tumors. Endocr Pathol. 21(4):212-8, 2010
17. Rivera M et al: Molecular genotyping of papillary thyroid carcinoma follicular variant according to its histological subtypes (encapsulated vs infiltrative) reveals distinct BRAF and RAS mutation patterns. Mod Pathol. 23(9):1191-200, 2010
18. Ghossein R: Problems and controversies in the histopathology of thyroid carcinomas of follicular cell origin. Arch Pathol Lab Med. 133(5):683-91, 2009
19. Salajegheh A et al: Follicular variant of papillary thyroid carcinoma: a diagnostic challenge for clinicians and pathologists. Postgrad Med J. 84(988):78-82, 2008
20. Wreesmann VB et al: Follicular variant of papillary thyroid carcinoma: genome-wide appraisal of a controversial entity. Genes Chromosomes Cancer. 40(4):355-64, 2004

Histologic Features

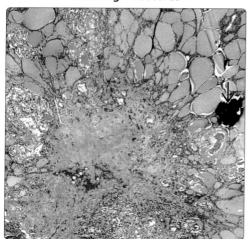

BRAF in Infiltrative FVPTC

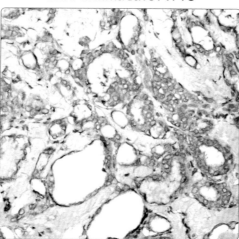

(Left) Low-power view demonstrates the infiltrative FVPTC. Note the thick stellate intratumoral fibrosis extending into the adjacent thyroid. The neoplastic follicles are also infiltrating the adjacent normal thyroid. A psammoma body ⇨ can be seen at the periphery. (Right) The infiltrative FVPTC shows BRAF mutation in ~ 25%, while the encapsulated variant is negative for the mutation. Immunohistochemistry for BRAF shows positive staining in the tumor cells.

Nuclear Features in Infiltrative FVPTC

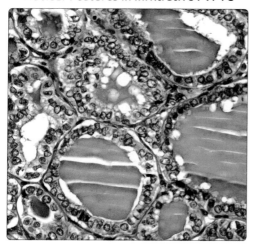

Histologic Features

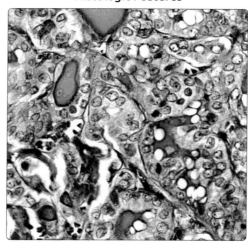

(Left) This high-power image highlights nuclear and morphologic features seen in this variant of PTC. The nuclei are enlarged and have ground-glass chromatin with nuclear grooves and irregular nuclear contours. The colloid is deeply eosinophilic. Scalloping of colloid is also present. (Right) FVPTC of the infiltrative subtype is composed of irregular follicles lined by cells with nuclei that have the characteristic features of the conventional PTC.

BRAF Staining

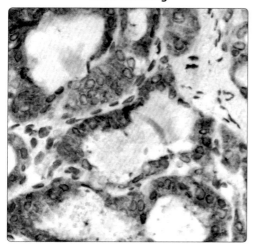

HMBE-1 Staining

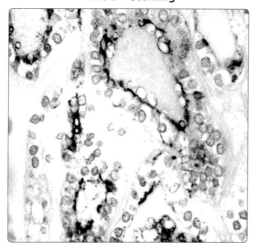

(Left) Immunohistochemistry for BRAF shows positive staining in the tumor cells. Note the negative stain in the endothelial cells and lymphocytes. About 25% of the tumors of this variant are BRAF mutant. (Right) Immunohistochemistry shows the diagnostic luminal border staining of HBME-1. This is the classic staining pattern seen in the FVPTC. The stain is present on the membranes of the neoplastic cells but is most prominently seen within the lumina of the follicles.

Papillary Thyroid Carcinoma, Macrofollicular Variant

TERMINOLOGY

- Variant of papillary thyroid carcinoma composed exclusively or predominantly (> 50%) of macrofollicles > 200 μm in > 50% of cross-sectional area

CLINICAL ISSUES

- More common in 3rd and 4th decades of life
- More commonly seen in female patients
- ~ 1% of papillary carcinoma cases

MICROSCOPIC

- Follicular architecture
- Composed predominantly of macrofollicles (> 200 μm)
- Eosinophilic colloid compared to normal thyroid
- Prominent peripheral scalloping of colloid
- Minute neoplastic follicles are scattered in background of cystically dilated follicles
- Nuclear features of PTC are focal
  - Nuclei are optically clear ("ground glass"), mostly within sprinkling areas
  - Abundant nuclear grooves are present
  - Nuclear membrane's irregularities
- Metastatic tumor deposits usually have macrofollicles

ANCILLARY TESTS

- HBME-1: focal; mostly identified in cells of sprinkling sign areas

TOP DIFFERENTIAL DIAGNOSES

- Its characteristic histologic pattern can be mistaken by adenoma or hyperplastic nodule

DIAGNOSTIC CHECKLIST

- > 50% of cross-sectional area must be composed of macrofollicles (> 200 μm)
- Characteristic nuclear features of PTC may only be focal
- Sprinkling sign: Presence of multiple scattered dark small spots in what appears to be benign follicular nodule

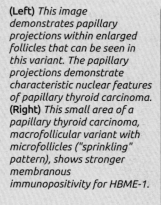

(Left) This gross picture of a macrofollicular variant of papillary thyroid carcinoma shows a thin fibrous capsule. These tumors are usually > 2 cm and may grossly mimic a hyperplastic nodule. (Right) The previous image shows large macrofollicles characteristic of papillary thyroid carcinoma macrofollicular variant. Macrofollicles represent at least 50% of the cross-sectional area in this image.

Gross Appearance

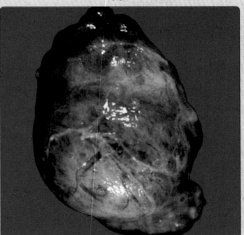

Low-Power View of Tumor

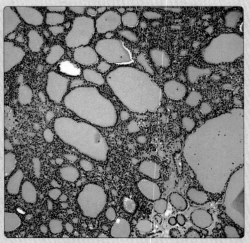

(Left) This image demonstrates papillary projections within enlarged follicles that can be seen in this variant. The papillary projections demonstrate characteristic nuclear features of papillary thyroid carcinoma. (Right) This small area of a papillary thyroid carcinoma, macrofollicular variant with microfollicles ("sprinkling" pattern), shows stronger membranous immunopositivity for HBME-1.

Focal Hyperplastic Areas

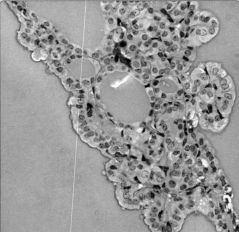

HBME-1 Stain

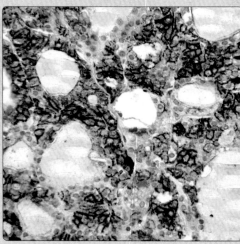

TERMINOLOGY

Abbreviations

- Papillary thyroid carcinoma, macrofollicular variant (PTC-MFV)

Synonyms

- Macrofollicular variant of papillary carcinoma (MFPC)
- Macrofollicular encapsulated variant of papillary carcinoma (MEPC)

Definitions

- Variant of papillary thyroid carcinoma composed either exclusively or predominantly (> 50% of cross-sectional area) of macrofollicles > 200 μm

CLINICAL ISSUES

Epidemiology

- Incidence
  - Rare
  - < 0.5% of all papillary carcinoma cases
- Age
  - More common in 3rd and 4th decades of life
  - Age at presentation varies from teens to 7th decade
- Sex
  - More commonly seen in female patients

Presentation

- Most commonly presents as painless neck mass
- Obstructive symptoms can be present with larger tumor size
  - Hoarseness, dysphagia, shortness of breath
- Cold on uptake scans
- Enlarged cervical lymph nodes may be present due to presence of metastases

Treatment

- Surgical approaches
  - Partial or total thyroidectomy
  - Lymph node dissection if indicated

Prognosis

- Indolent disease
- Good prognosis
  - Except with presence of insular component
  - Extrathyroid extension and lymphovascular invasion confer worse prognosis
- Moderate metastatic risk
  - Lymph node metastases seen in ~ 20% of cases
  - Few cases with lung and bony metastases have been reported
  - Metastases are more likely to occur in patients who have extrathyroid extension and vascular invasion

IMAGING

Ultrasonographic Findings

- Can appear benign or malignant
  - Well defined, smooth borders, homogeneous echogenicity
  - Irregular borders with heterogeneous echogenicity

MACROSCOPIC

General Features

- Well circumscribed, encapsulated, or infiltrative
- Capsule can be partial or complete
  - Variable capsule thickness
- Mostly solid in consistency
  - Cysts may be present
- Abundant colloid appearance
  - Macrofollicles may be seen grossly
- Light to dark brown cut surface
- Occasional foci of hemorrhage are present

Size

- Generally > 2.0 cm in size
  - Tumors can become quite large, up to 11 cm
  - Average size is 4.8 cm

MICROSCOPIC

Histologic Features

- Follicular architecture, with follicles of varying sizes
  - Composed predominantly of macrofollicles (> 200 micrometers)
- Follicles vary in shape
  - Neoplastic follicles are cystically dilated
    - They simulate nodular hyperplasia
- Encapsulated or well circumscribed
  - Capsule thickness varies greatly
  - Capsular invasion is fairly common
- Neoplastic cells may be flat to cuboidal in shape
- Few papillary projections may be seen within macrofollicles
- Dense eosinophilic colloid distends macrofollicles
- Prominent peripheral scalloping of colloid
- Minute neoplastic follicles are scattered in background of normal-appearing follicles
  - Sprinkling sign is noted on low-power examination
    - Presence of multiple scattered dark small spots in what appears otherwise to be unremarkable benign follicular nodule
- Macrophages are usually present within neoplastic follicles
- Psammoma bodies are rare
- Randomly distributed foci of conventional and follicular variants of papillary carcinoma may be present
- Lack of desmoplastic stromal response
- Intrathyroid spread may be present
  - Multicentric follicles lacking desmoplastic response in contralateral lobe

Cytologic Features

- 3 types of nuclear features are present
  - Large cuboidal cells with ground-glass nuclei (characteristic PTC nuclear features)
    - Back to back, overlapping nuclei
    - Few nuclear pseudoinclusions
    - Irregular contour of nuclear membranes, with abundant nuclear grooves
    - Elevated N:C ratio
  - Cuboidal cells with large, but less pale, nuclei
    - Finely granular to stippled chromatin pattern
    - Peripheral nucleoli present

- o Low cuboidal cells with hyperchromatic nuclei
- PTC nuclear features may be focal
- Each macrofollicle usually composed of 1 type of nucleus
  - o However, 2 or all 3 types of nuclear features may be present within same follicle

Lymph Nodes

- Metastatic tumor deposits usually have macrofollicles
- Desmoplastic stromal response absent
- Nuclear features are similar to primary tumor

ANCILLARY TESTS

Cytology

- Diagnosis of PTC-MFV via cytology specimens is difficult
  - o FNA has low sensitivity for PTC-MFV
- Specimens usually moderate to high cellularity
- Follicles of different sizes present
- Nuclei may have features of papillary thyroid carcinoma
  - o Nuclear grooves
  - o Nuclear pseudoinclusions can be seen
  - o Overlapping nuclei
  - o Small peripheral nucleoli common
- Ground-glass chromatin
- Papillary architecture is absent
- Macrophages generally present
- Colloid can be thick or watery

Frozen Sections

- Should not be performed as diagnosis is often inaccurate
  - o Misdiagnosed as benign follicular lesions

Immunohistochemistry

- Positive
  - o HBME-1: Membranous/luminal and focal; mostly identified in areas of sprinkling sign follicles
  - o pax-8
  - o TTF-1
  - o Thyroglobulin
  - o AE1/AE3
  - o Galectin-3
  - o CK19
  - o ret
- Negative
  - o BRAF

Genetic Testing

- *BRAF*
  - o Has been reported as negative
    - – *BRAF* and RAS mutations has not been found in PTC-MFV

DIFFERENTIAL DIAGNOSIS

Benign Thyroid Nodules

- Characteristic histologic pattern could be mistaken for that of adenoma or hyperplastic nodule

Multinodular Hyperplasia

- Follicles of varying sizes
  - o Numerous large follicles
- Diffuse architecture

- Multinodular with fibrous bands separating nodules
- Lacks capsule
- Watery colloid
- Peripheral scalloping of colloid
- Low cuboidal to flat nuclei of variable size
- Nuclei are hyperchromatic and lack characteristic nuclear features of papillary carcinoma

Follicular Adenoma

- Encapsulated nodules
- Can be composed of large follicles
- Lined by flat/cuboidal epithelial cells
- Hyperchromatic nuclei
- Lack characteristic papillary carcinoma nuclear features
- Nuclei do not overlap as they do in papillary carcinoma
- No foci of classic or follicular papillary carcinoma

DIAGNOSTIC CHECKLIST

Pathologic Interpretation Pearls

- > 50% of cross-sectional area must be composed of macrofollicles (> 200 μm)
  - o Macrofollicles may be present in classic and follicular variants of papillary thyroid carcinoma
- Characteristic nuclear features of PTC may only be focal
- Sprinkling sign: Presence of multiple scattered dark small spots in what appears otherwise benign follicular nodule

SELECTED REFERENCES

1. Asa SL et al: The epigenetic landscape of differentiated thyroid cancer. Mol Cell Endocrinol. ePub, 2017
2. Cracolici V et al: Synchronous and metastatic papillary and follicular thyroid carcinomas with unique molecular signatures. Endocr Pathol. ePub, 2017
3. Rossi ED et al: The cytological diagnosis of a 'benign thyroid lesion': is it a real safe diagnosis for the patient? Cytopathology. 27(3):168-75, 2016
4. Armstrong MJ et al: PAX8/PPARγ rearrangement in thyroid nodules predicts follicular-pattern carcinomas, in particular the encapsulated follicular variant of papillary carcinoma. Thyroid. 24(9):1369-74, 2014
5. Chai YJ et al: BRAF mutation in follicular variant of papillary thyroid carcinoma is associated with unfavourable clinicopathological characteristics and malignant features on ultrasonography. Clin Endocrinol (Oxf). 81(3):432-9, 2014
6. Erol V et al: Papillary thyroid cancer, macrofollicular variant: the follow-up and analysis of prognosis of 5 patients. J Thyroid Res. 2014:818134, 2014
7. Jung CK et al: The increase in thyroid cancer incidence during the last four decades is accompanied by a high frequency of BRAF mutations and a sharp increase in RAS mutations. J Clin Endocrinol Metab. 99(2):E276-85, 2014
8. Marques P et al: Remarkable response to radioiodine therapy in a case of metastatic macrofollicular variant of papillary thyroid carcinoma. Clin Nucl Med. 39(2):219-21, 2014
9. Pusztaszeri M: Follicular variant of papillary thyroid carcinoma: distinct biologic behavior based on ultrasonographic features. Thyroid. 24(6):1067-8, 2014
10. Yeo MK et al: Macrofollicular variant of papillary thyroid carcinoma with extensive lymph node metastases. Endocr Pathol. 25(3):265-72, 2014
11. Policarpio-Nicolas ML et al: Macrofollicular variant of papillary carcinoma, a potential diagnostic pitfall: a report of two cases including a review of literature. Cytojournal. 10:16, 2013
12. Pusztaszeri M et al: A noninvasive encapsulated macrofollicular variant of papillary thyroid carcinoma presenting with gross lymph node metastasis: a case report and literature review. Thyroid. 23(9):1178-9, 2013
13. Vanzati A et al: The "sprinkling" sign in the follicular variant of papillary thyroid carcinoma: a clue to the recognition of this entity. Arch Pathol Lab Med. 137(12):1707-9, 2013
14. Vanzati A et al: The "sprinkling" sign in the follicular variant of papillary thyroid carcinoma: a clue to the recognition of this entity. Arch Pathol Lab Med. 137(12):1707-9, 2013
15. Emad R et al: Three cases of macrofollicular variant of papillary thyroid carcinoma. Ann Saudi Med. 31(6):644-7, 2011
16. Laury AR et al: Thyroid pathology in PTEN-hamartoma tumor syndrome: characteristic findings of a distinct entity. Thyroid. 21(2):135-44, 2011

Differential Diagnosis

Characteristic	Macrofollicular Variant of Papillary Thyroid Carcinoma	Follicular Adenoma	Multinodular Hyperplasia
Capsule	Partial or complete	Complete	Absent
Capsular invasion	Occasional	Absent	N/A
Chromatin	Ground glass, clear	Hyperchromatic	Hyperchromatic
Nuclear shape	Cuboidal	Flat	Flat
Nuclear grooves	Present	Absent	Absent
Nuclear pseudoinclusions	Present	Absent	Absent
Psammoma bodies	Rare	Absent	Absent
Colloid	Dense, eosinophilic		Watery
Papillary projections	Uncommon	Absent	Common
Immunohistochemistry			
Thyroglobulin	Positive	Positive	Positive
TTF-1	Positive	Positive	Positive
pax-8	Positive	Positive	Positive
HBME-1*	Positive	Negative	Negative
Galectin-3+	Positive	Negative	Negative
CITED1	Positive	Negative	Negative

Membranous HBME-1 staining is most specific; it is typically present in the conventional PTC, as well as the diffuse sclerosing and tall cell variants, and with lower frequency in follicular variant. HBME-1 staining is mostly present in follicular cells within areas of the "sprinkling sign." Galectin-3(+) should be both nuclear and cytoplasmic.

17. Maruta J et al: Improving the diagnostic accuracy of thyroid follicular neoplasms: cytological features in fine-needle aspiration cytology. Diagn Cytopathol. 39(1):28-34, 2011

18. Nosé V: Familial thyroid cancer: a review. Mod Pathol. 24 Suppl 2:S19-33, 2011

19. Cardenas MG et al: Two patients with highly aggressive macrofollicular variant of papillary thyroid carcinoma. Thyroid. 19(4):413-6, 2009

20. Fukushima M et al: Macrofollicular variant of papillary thyroid carcinoma: its clinicopathological features and long-term prognosis. Endocr J. 56(3):503-8, 2009

21. Chung D et al: Macrofollicular variant of papillary carcinoma: a potential thyroid FNA pitfall. Diagn Cytopathol. 35(9):560-4, 2007

22. Albores-Saavedra J et al: The many faces and mimics of papillary thyroid carcinoma. Endocr Pathol. 17(1):1-18, 2006

23. Rossi ED et al: Simultaneous immunohistochemical expression of HBME-1 and galectin-3 differentiates papillary carcinomas from hyperfunctioning lesions of the thyroid. Histopathology. 48(7):795-800, 2006

24. Lugli A et al: Macrofollicular variant of papillary carcinoma of the thyroid: a histologic, cytologic, and immunohistochemical study of 3 cases and review of the literature. Arch Pathol Lab Med. 128(1):54-8, 2004

25. Fadda G et al: Macrofollicular encapsulated variant of papillary thyroid carcinoma as a potential pitfall in histologic and cytologic diagnosis. A report of three cases. Acta Cytol. 46(3):555-9, 2002

26. Hernández-Ortiz MJ et al: Fine needle aspiration cytology of macrofollicular variant of thyroid papillary carcinoma in a male. Acta Cytol. 45(3):483-6, 2001

27. Goodell WM et al: Fine-needle aspiration diagnosis of the follicular variant of papillary carcinoma. Cancer. 84(6):349-54, 1998

28. Hirokawa M et al: Macrofollicular variant of papillary thyroid carcinoma. Report of a case with fine needle aspiration biopsy findings. Acta Cytol. 42(6):1441-3, 1998

29. Mesonero CE et al: Fine-needle aspiration of the macrofollicular and microfollicular subtypes of the follicular variant of papillary carcinoma of the thyroid. Cancer. 84(4):235-44, 1998

30. Nakamura T et al: Macrofollicular variant of papillary thyroid carcinoma. Pathol Int. 48(6):467-70, 1998

31. Woyke S et al: Macrofollicular variant of papillary thyroid carcinoma diagnosed by fine needle aspiration biopsy: a case report. Acta Cytol. 42(5):1184-8, 1998

32. Gamboa-Dominguez A et al: Macrofollicular variant of papillary thyroid carcinoma: a case and control analysis. Endocr Pathol. 7(4):303-308, 1996

33. Albores-Saavedra J et al: The macrofollicular variant of papillary thyroid carcinoma: a study of 17 cases. Hum Pathol. 22(12):1195-205, 1991

Papillary Thyroid Carcinoma, Macrofollicular Variant

Gross Cut Surface

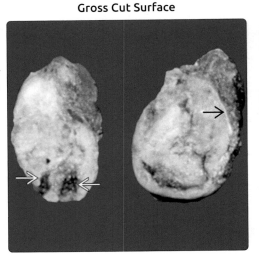

(Left) *This gross image demonstrates characteristic gross cut surface features of this variant. The tumor is solid, light tan to brown, with foci of hemorrhage ➡. A thin capsule ⇥ is present focally.* **(Right)** *This higher power image highlights characteristic nuclear features of papillary carcinoma. Some nuclei are enlarged and are optically clear; nuclear membranes are irregularly shaped, and nuclear grooves are present.*

Focal Nuclear Features

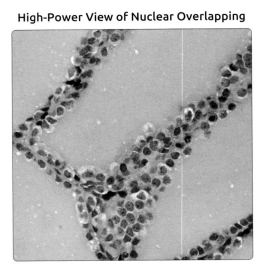

Macrofollicles With Scalloping of Colloid

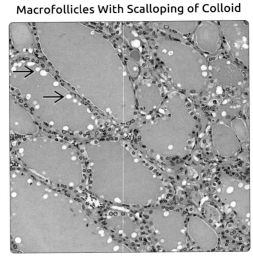

(Left) *This image shows scalloping of colloid ⇥ that is common in this variant. The cells lining the neoplastic follicles are cuboidal and occasionally flat in shape. Some ground-glass nuclei are visible in this image.* **(Right)** *The nuclei are enlarged and the nuclear:cytoplasmic ratio is increased. Note that the cells do not demonstrate grooves or optical clearing. The nuclear membranes are irregularly shaped and there is nuclear overlapping.*

High-Power View of Nuclear Overlapping

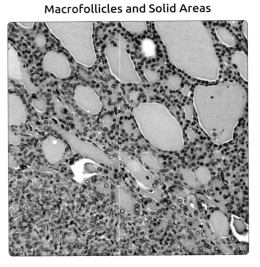

Macrofollicles and Solid Areas

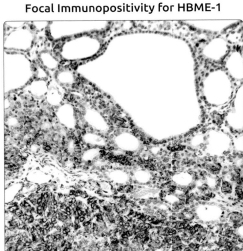

(Left) *The upper half of this section demonstrates macrofollicles adjacent to smaller follicles in the lower half that are considered as the sprinkling sign. Macrofollicles should be present in at least 50% of the cross-sectional area of the sampled tumor.* **(Right)** *HBME-1 immunohistochemical stain shows membranous staining of neoplastic cells. Luminal staining can also be seen (membrane staining more prominent in luminal borders of neoplastic follicles).*

Focal Immunopositivity for HBME-1

Macrofollicles

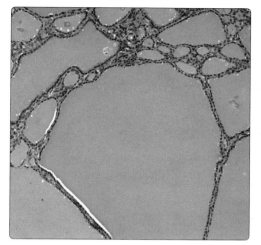

Sprinkling Sign

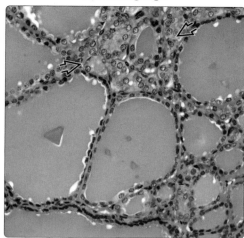

(Left) *Low-power view of this encapsulated nodule shows large macrofollicles characteristic of the macrofollicular variant of papillary thyroid carcinoma. For this diagnosis, macrofollicles should be present in at least 50% of the tumor.* **(Right)** *In focal areas of the macrofollicular-predominant tumor, there are foci of small follicles composed by cells with characteristic nuclear features of papillary thyroid carcinoma (so-called sprinkling sign) ⇗. These foci are known to support the diagnosis of PTC.*

Minute Neoplastic Follicle

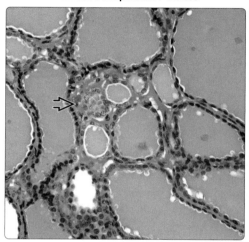

High-Power View of Area of Sprinkling Sign

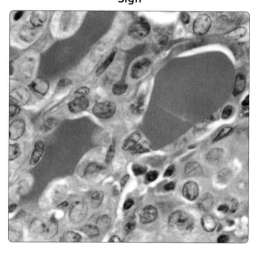

(Left) *The neoplastic follicles are mildly cystically dilated, mimicking nodular hyperplasia. Minute neoplastic follicles are scattered in a background of normal-looking thyroid follicles (so-called sprinkling sign) ⇗.* **(Right)** *Minute foci of small follicles surrounded by cystically dilated follicles are present in the macrofollicular variant of PTC. These foci show better conventional PTC nuclear features.*

BRAF Negative

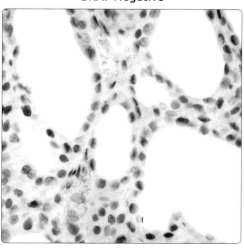

Focal HBME1 Stain

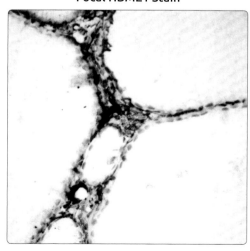

(Left) *In the macrofollicular variant of papillary thyroid carcinoma, there is no immunoexpression of BRAF in the tumor, including in areas of more PTC nuclear features.* **(Right)** *HBME-1 immunohistochemical stain reveals only focal membranous staining of neoplastic cells. The stain is more prominent within areas of microfollicles and with more prominent nuclear features of PTC.*

Papillary Thyroid Carcinoma, Diffuse Sclerosing Variant

TERMINOLOGY

- Aggressive variant of papillary carcinoma characterized by prominent stromal fibrosis, dense lymphocytic infiltrates, numerous psammoma bodies, and squamous metaplasia

CLINICAL ISSUES

- Rare; comprises ~ 2% of all papillary thyroid carcinoma cases
- Accounts for ~ 30% of papillary carcinoma cases in patients younger than 20
- Usually present with rapid and diffuse thyroid enlargement (most commonly in women)
- Although these tumors are biologically aggressive, prognosis remains favorable

MACROSCOPIC

- Tumors are quite large, diffusely involving thyroid gland

MICROSCOPIC

- Dense bands of fibrosis/sclerosis that separate thyroid into nodules
- Solid, papillary, or follicular arrangement of neoplastic thyroid cells with characteristic papillary carcinoma nuclear features
- Innumerable psammoma bodies (present in both lobes of thyroid)
- Extensive lymphoplasmacytic infiltrate
- Foci of squamous metaplasia
- Infiltration into perithyroid soft tissues is common
- Vascular invasion is hallmark feature of this variant

TOP DIFFERENTIAL DIAGNOSES

- Lymphocytic thyroiditis
- Classic variant of papillary thyroid carcinoma
- Primary squamous cell carcinoma of thyroid
- Metastases

Characteristic Histological Features

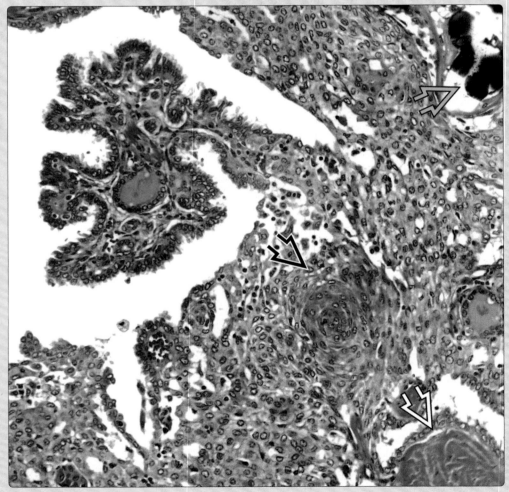

This image shows a focus of squamous metaplasia ⊳. Squamous metaplasia is one of the criteria present in the diffuse sclerosing variant. Additionally, psammoma bodies ⊳, classic papillary fronds, follicles, sclerosis ⊳, and a lymphocytic infiltrate are present.

TERMINOLOGY

Abbreviations

- Diffuse sclerosing variant of papillary thyroid carcinoma (DSVPTC)

Synonyms

- Diffuse sclerosing variant (DSV)
- Diffuse sclerosing papillary carcinoma
- Diffuse sclerosing papillary thyroid carcinoma

Definitions

- Aggressive variant of papillary carcinoma characterized by prominent stromal fibrosis, dense lymphocytic infiltrates, numerous psammoma bodies, and squamous metaplasia

ETIOLOGY/PATHOGENESIS

Association With Ionizing Radiation

- Found in few patients after Chernobyl accident

Genetics

- *RET/PTCH1* gene rearrangements seen in 30% of cases
- *BRAF* mutation

Associated Conditions

- Often associated with lymphocytic thyroiditis or autoimmune thyroiditis

CLINICAL ISSUES

Epidemiology

- Incidence
  - Rare; comprises ~ 2% of all papillary thyroid carcinoma cases
- Age
  - Occurs in younger patients
    - Accounts for ~ 30% of papillary carcinoma cases in patients younger than 20
  - Commonly seen in adolescents
  - Age at presentation is younger in women than men
    - Women: Average age 25
    - Men: Average age 38
- Sex
  - More common in women than in men

Presentation

- Usually present with rapid and diffuse thyroid enlargement (most commonly in women)
  - Often patients complain of compressive symptoms associated with tumor infiltration of surrounding structures
    - Hoarseness, dysphagia, dyspnea, difficulty breathing or swallowing
  - May present with neck enlargement due to cervical lymph node metastases
- Patients may also be asymptomatic
  - Often found on school-required routine physical exam
- Patients are most often euthyroid
  - May be hypothyroid as this variant is occasionally seen in association with lymphocytic thyroiditis
- Clinically may be mistaken for autoimmune thyroiditis

- Antimitochondrial and antithyroid antibodies may be present

Treatment

- Early total thyroidectomy with lymph node dissection
- Radioactive iodine ablation post operation
- External radiotherapy may be indicated if tumor extends beyond thyroid

Prognosis

- Compared with conventional PTC, DSVPTC is associated with higher incidence of
  - Extrathyroidal extension
  - Cervical lymph nodes metastases
  - Distant metastases, primarily to lungs (~ 10-15%)
- Recurrence rate is higher than classic variant
- Mortality rate is comparable with classic variant
- DSVPTC is also associated with shorter disease-free survival
- Although these tumors are biologically aggressive, prognosis remains favorable, with 93% 10-year disease-specific survival rate

IMAGING

Radiographic Findings

- Punctate calcification are seen on x-ray due to numerous calcifications

Ultrasonographic Findings

- Ultrasound can demonstrate solid mass with ill-defined borders
  - Masses may also be partially or entirely cystic
- Occasionally, no mass is identified on ultrasound due to diffuse involvement of entire gland (heterogeneous appearance of thyroid gland)
- Characteristic snowstorm appearance is common due to innumerable calcifications seen within tumor
- Lymph node metastases may be identified via ultrasound

CT Findings

- CT scan is useful for demonstrating involvement of surrounding structures and lymph node metastases
- Snowstorm appearance due to abundant microcalcifications is commonly demonstrated on CT scan

Radioactive Iodine Uptake

- Usually "cold" nodule on RAI uptake scans, though scan may be normal

MACROSCOPIC

General Features

- Tumors are quite large
  - Average tumor size is 5.8 cm
- Diffusely involves gland
  - Commonly involves both lobes of thyroid
- No obvious circumscription or encapsulation
- Tumors are lobulated, nodular, and often multifocal
- Masses are firm to hard in consistency
- Pale gray to white in color, occasionally showing mottled appearance
- Fish flesh appearance may be present, reflecting lymphocytic thyroiditis

- Cut surface is gritty due to numerous psammoma bodies
- Extension into perithyroidal soft tissues may be evident grossly
- Cystic degeneration is usually present
- Involved lymph nodes are grossly replaced by tumor and often show cystic changes

Size

- Tumors are quite large
  o Average tumor size is 5.8 cm (range of 3-8 cm)
    – Smaller and larger lesions can be seen
- For this variant, size is less significant prognostic feature

MICROSCOPIC

Histologic Features

- There is diffuse involvement of lobe or entire thyroid gland
- Ill-defined nodule replacing most of parenchyma
- Infiltration into perithyroid soft tissues is common
- Vascular invasion is hallmark feature of this variant
- Usually has
  o Dense bands of fibrosis/sclerosis that separate thyroid into nodules
  o **Solid, papillary, or follicular** arrangement of neoplastic thyroid cells with characteristic papillary carcinoma morphologic features
    – Areas of **tall cell variant** are usually present
  o Innumerable psammoma bodies
    – Presence of calcifications often leads to shattered appearance of histologic sections
    – Psammoma bodies are present in both lobes of gland and are quite often only evidence of lymphovascular invasion
  o Foci of squamous metaplasia
    – Squamous metaplasia can transform into squamous cell carcinoma
  o Extensive lymphoplasmacytic infiltrate
    – Often has appearance of lymphocytic thyroiditis (lymphoid follicles with germinal center formation)
- Papillary structures are often found within dilated lymphatics
  o Psammoma bodies may be present within lymphatics without adherent tumor cells
- Uninvolved thyroid parenchyma may be atrophic

Cytologic Features

- Tumor cells show characteristic papillary thyroid carcinoma cytomorphologic features
  o Enlarged cells with irregular contours
  o Nuclei are enlarged and optically clear
    – Nuclear membranes are irregular
  o Nuclear grooves and pseudoinclusions are common

Lymph Nodes

- Lymph node metastases are found in at least 80% of cases
  o Unilateral or bilateral
- Metastases may resemble any of various histologic components found in this tumor
  o Overt papillary thyroid carcinoma
  o Squamous metaplasia
  o Psammoma bodies

ANCILLARY TESTS

Cytology

- Papillary structures and sheets of cells may be present
- Neoplastic cells demonstrate papillary carcinoma nuclear features
  o Enlarged pale nuclei, irregular nuclear membranes, nuclear grooves and inclusions
- Psammoma bodies are abundant
  o May be seen individually or within tissue fragments/sheets of cells
- Metaplastic squamous epithelium may be present in aspirates
- Variable amount of lymphocytes in background
  o Lymphocytes may be admixed within clusters of tumor cells
- Overwhelming presence of these characteristics may allow diagnosis of DSV on FNA cytology
- Multinucleated giant cells may be seen
- Colloid is usually scant
- Sampling error is pitfall of cytology

Immunohistochemistry

- Diagnosis is made based in morphologic characteristics, though IHC is occasionally used
- Positive immunostains
  o In both PTC follicular cells lining follicles and papillae and in areas of squamous metaplasia
    – Keratin
    – CK19
    – Thyroglobulin
    – TTF-1
    – pax-8
  o In areas of squamous metaplasia
    – p63
    – CK5/6
    – May be CD5(+)
  o EMA, galectin-3, CITED-1, and HBME-1 may be positive
  o S100 positivity purported to be associated with better prognosis
  o BRAF immunopositivity

Genetic Testing

- Show *RET/PTCH1* rearrangements in ~ 30% of cases
- *BRAF* is found in this variant in older patients

DIFFERENTIAL DIAGNOSIS

Lymphocytic Thyroiditis

- Diffuse involvement of gland; lymphoid follicles contain germinal centers
- Lacks squamous metaplasia and psammoma bodies
- No oncocytic cell changes are seen in DSV

Classic Variant of Papillary Thyroid Carcinoma

- Lacks squamous metaplasia
- Extensive lymphovascular invasion is not usually seen in classic variant
- May be associated with fibrosis, though not as diffuse as with DSV

Primary Squamous Cell Carcinoma of Thyroid

- Does not have papillary thyroid carcinoma nuclear features
- Does not show extensive lymphovascular involvement
- Psammoma bodies are absent

Lymphoma

- Lacks papillary thyroid carcinoma foci
- Squamous metaplasia absent
- Psammoma bodies are not present in lymphoma
- Not associated with dense fibrosis

Metastases

- If few foci of tumor are present, metastases may be considered in differential
- Immunohistochemistry may be helpful in differentiating metastatic tumors (thyroglobulin is negative in pulmonary adenocarcinoma)
- Generally not associated with fibrosis
- Squamous metaplasia is absent

Mucoepidermoid Carcinoma of Thyroid Gland

- Psammoma bodies are absent
- Extensive lymphovascular invasion is absent
- Lymph node metastases are absent

DIAGNOSTIC CHECKLIST

Pathologic Interpretation Pearls

- Dense bands of fibrosis/sclerosis that separate thyroid into nodules
- Solid, papillary, or follicular arrangement of neoplastic thyroid cells with characteristic papillary carcinoma morphologic features
  - Areas of tall cell variant are usually present
  - Squamoid morules are present
- Innumerable psammoma bodies
- Foci of squamous metaplasia
- Variable amount of lymphocytic infiltrate

SELECTED REFERENCES

1. Lloyd RV et al: WHO Classification of Tumours of Endocrine Organs. Lyon, France: IARC Press, 2017
2. Russo M et al: Tall cell and diffuse sclerosing variants of papillary thyroid cancer: outcome and predicting value of risk stratification methods. J Endocrinol Invest. ePub, 2017
3. Vuong HG et al: Prognostic significance of diffuse sclerosing variant papillary thyroid carcinoma: a systematic review and meta-analysis. Eur J Endocrinol. 176(4):431-439, 2017
4. Chereau N et al: Diffuse sclerosing variant of papillary thyroid carcinoma is associated with aggressive histopathological features and a poor outcome: results of a large multicentric study. J Clin Endocrinol Metab. 101(12):4603-4610, 2016
5. Joung JY et al: Diffuse sclerosing variant of papillary thyroid carcinoma: major genetic alterations and prognostic implications. Histopathology. 69(1):45-53, 2016
6. Low S et al: High endothelial venule-like vessels and lymphocyte recruitment in diffuse sclerosing variant of papillary thyroid carcinoma. Pathology. 48(7):666-674, 2016
7. Akaishi J et al: Clinicopathologic features and outcomes in patients with diffuse sclerosing variant of papillary thyroid carcinoma. World J Surg. 39(7):1728-35, 2015
8. Pillai S et al: Diffuse sclerosing variant of papillary thyroid carcinoma–an update of its clinicopathological features and molecular biology. Crit Rev Oncol Hematol. 94(1):64-73, 2015
9. Takagi N et al: Diffuse sclerosing variant of papillary thyroid carcinoma: a study of fine needle aspiration cytology in 20 patients. Cytopathology. 25(3):199-204, 2014
10. Lim JY et al: Clinicopathologic implications of the BRAF(V600E) mutation in papillary thyroid cancer: a subgroup analysis of 3130 cases in a single center. Thyroid. 23(11):1423-30, 2013
11. Lin JD et al: Papillary thyroid carcinoma with different histological patterns. Chang Gung Med J. 34(1):23-34, 2011
12. Lloyd RV et al: Papillary thyroid carcinoma variants. Head Neck Pathol. 5(1):51-6, 2011
13. Regalbuto C et al: A diffuse sclerosing variant of papillary thyroid carcinoma: clinical and pathologic features and outcomes of 34 consecutive cases. Thyroid. 21(4):383-9, 2011
14. Silver CE et al: Aggressive variants of papillary thyroid carcinoma. Head Neck. 33(7):1052-9, 2011
15. Asioli S et al: Papillary thyroid carcinoma with prominent hobnail features: a new aggressive variant of moderately differentiated papillary carcinoma. A clinicopathologic, immunohistochemical, and molecular study of eight cases. Am J Surg Pathol. 34(1):44-52, 2010
16. Kim HS et al: Papillary thyroid carcinoma of a diffuse sclerosing variant: ultrasonographic monitoring from a normal thyroid gland to mass formation. Korean J Radiol. 11(5):579-82, 2010
17. Koo JS et al: Immunohistochemical characteristics of diffuse sclerosing variant of papillary carcinoma: comparison with conventional papillary carcinoma. APMIS. 118(10):744-52, 2010
18. Regalbuto C et al: An unusual presentation of diffuse sclerosing variant of papillary thyroid carcinoma. J Endocrinol Invest. 33(6):434-5, 2010
19. Bongiovanni M et al: Fine-needle aspiration of the diffuse sclerosing variant of papillary thyroid carcinoma masked by florid lymphocytic thyroiditis; a potential pitfall: a case report and review of the literature. Diagn Cytopathol. 37(9):671-5, 2009
20. Fukushima M et al: Clinicopathologic characteristics and prognosis of diffuse sclerosing variant of papillary thyroid carcinoma in Japan: an 18-year experience at a single institution. World J Surg. 33(5):958-62, 2009
21. Koo JS et al: Diffuse sclerosing variant is a major subtype of papillary thyroid carcinoma in the young. Thyroid. 19(11):1225-31, 2009
22. Gilbert MP et al: Visual vignette. Diffuse sclerosing variant of papillary thyroid carcinoma. Endocr Pract. 14(7):950, 2008
23. Lin X et al: Molecular analysis of multifocal papillary thyroid carcinoma. J Mol Endocrinol. 41(4):195-203, 2008
24. Lee JY et al: Diffuse sclerosing variant of papillary carcinoma of the thyroid: imaging and cytologic findings. Thyroid. 17(6):567-73, 2007
25. Sheu SY et al: Diffuse sclerosing variant of papillary thyroid carcinoma: lack of BRAF mutation but occurrence of RET/PTC rearrangements. Mod Pathol. 20(7):779-87, 2007
26. Simpson KW et al: Unusual findings in papillary thyroid microcarcinoma suggesting partial regression: a study of two cases. Ann Diagn Pathol. 11(2):97-102, 2007
27. Falvo L et al: Prognostic importance of sclerosing variant in papillary thyroid carcinoma. Am Surg. 72(5):438-44, 2006
28. Lam AK et al: Diffuse sclerosing variant of papillary carcinoma of the thyroid: a 35-year comparative study at a single institution. Ann Surg Oncol. 13(2):176-81, 2006
29. Thompson LD et al: Diffuse sclerosing variant of papillary thyroid carcinoma: a clinicopathologic and immunophenotypic analysis of 22 cases. Endocr Pathol. 16(4):331-48, 2005
30. Hirokawa M et al: Morules in cribriform-morular variant of papillary thyroid carcinoma: Immunohistochemical characteristics and distinction from squamous metaplasia. APMIS. 112(4-5):275-82, 2004
31. Chow SM et al: Diffuse sclerosing variant of papillary thyroid carcinoma–clinical features and outcome. Eur J Surg Oncol. 29(5):446-9, 2003
32. Triggiani V et al: Papillary thyroid carcinoma, diffuse sclerosing variant, with abundant psammoma bodies. Acta Cytol. 47(6):1141-3, 2003
33. Caplan RH et al: Diffuse sclerosing variant of papillary thyroid carcinoma: case report and review of the literature. Endocr Pract. 3(5):287-92, 1997
34. Schröder S: Diffuse sclerosing variant of papillary thyroid carcinoma. Am J Surg Pathol. 15(5):492-3, 1991
35. Schröder S et al: Diffuse sclerosing variant of papillary thyroid carcinoma. S-100 protein immunocytochemistry and prognosis. Virchows Arch A Pathol Anat Histopathol. 416(4):367-71, 1990
36. Carcangiu ML et al: Diffuse sclerosing variant of papillary thyroid carcinoma. Clinicopathologic study of 15 cases. Am J Surg Pathol. 13(12):1041-9, 1989
37. Soares J et al: Diffuse sclerosing variant of papillary thyroid carcinoma. A clinicopathologic study of 10 cases. Pathol Res Pract. 185(2):200-6, 1989

Gross Cut Surface of DSVPTC

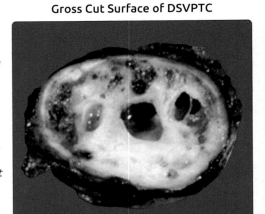

Gross Features of DSVPTC

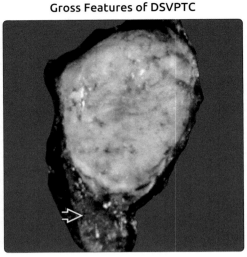

(Left) This gross image demonstrates diffuse involvement of the thyroid lobe, which is a typical finding seen in the diffuse sclerosing variant of papillary thyroid carcinoma (DSVPTC). There are cystic spaces, extensive fibrosis, and focal areas of hemorrhage. (Right) Grossly these tumors typically involve &/or replace the majority of the thyroid gland. An adjacent rim of normal thyroid parenchyma is present ➡ in this example.

Fibrosis and Psammoma Body

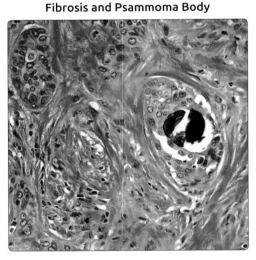

Nuclear Features

(Left) Photomicrography of a DSVPTC demonstrates the extensive fibrosis seen in this variant. A psammoma body with concentric laminations. Due to processing, they typically fragment and cause artifacts and irregularities. (Right) This area of a DSVPTC shows cells with typical papillary thyroid carcinoma nuclear features ➡. A focus of squamous metaplasia ➡ is present.

Characteristics of DSVPTC

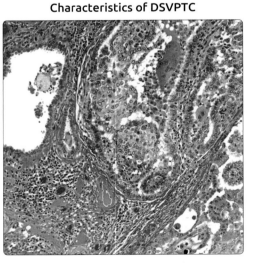

CK5/6 in Squamous Metaplasia

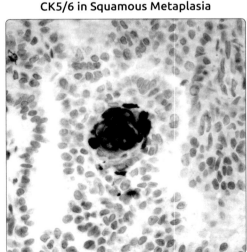

(Left) The histopathological features of the DSVPTC, as both papillary and follicular architectures, foci of squamous metaplasia, lymphocytic infiltrate is seen, presence of psammoma bodies, and stromal fibrosis are present in this picture. (Right) Immunostain for CK5/6 highlights an area of squamous metaplasia within the tumor. Squamous metaplasia is one of the findings that may be present in the DSVPTC.

Histologic Features

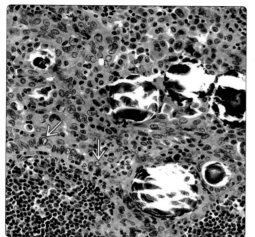

Extrathyroidal Extension

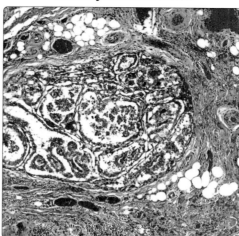

(Left) *Multiple psammoma bodies showing concentric laminations are seen here. A dense lymphocytic infiltrate is present in the lower corners. The classic piled-up "Orphan Annie" nuclei ➡ of PTC are also shown in this image.* (Right) *DSVPTC is characterized by locally aggressive behavior. Very often, these tumors can be found infiltrating the perithyroid soft tissues, a feature that is shown in this image. This particular focus of tumor had a papillary architecture.*

BRAF in Tumor Cells Invading Parathyroid

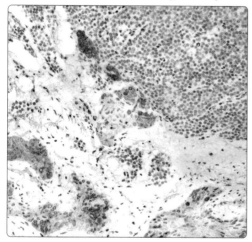

TTF1 in Tumor Cells Invading Parathyroid

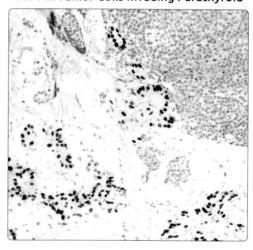

(Left) *Group of tumor cells from a DSVPTC are invading into the adjacent parathyroid gland. The foci of tumor cells are highlighted by the immunopositivity for BRAF.* (Right) *This photomicrograph reveals a parathyroid gland with TTF1(+) cells invading the parathyroid parenchyma. The primary tumor is a DSVPTC.*

Granular BRAF Positivity

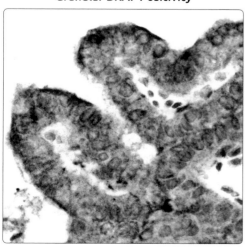

Cytoplasmic BRAF Immunoreactivity

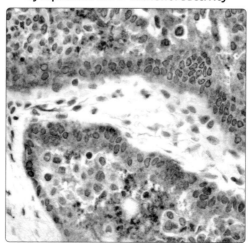

(Left) *BRAF immunohistochemistry shows diffuse cytoplasmic staining in DSVPTC.* (Right) *BRAF immunostain shows a diffuse granular cytoplasmic positivity pattern in this papillary thyroid carcinoma. The immunopositivity is granular in the cytoplasm. The lymphocytes and stromal cells are negative.*

Papillary Thyroid Carcinoma, Oncocytic Variant

TERMINOLOGY

- Papillary thyroid carcinoma (PTC): Malignant follicular neoplasm characterized by cells with oncocytic cytoplasm and PTC nuclear features

CLINICAL ISSUES

- In pure form, this variant is rare
- Tumors less responsive to radioactive iodine therapy

MICROSCOPIC

- Generally well circumscribed
- Architecture primarily papillary or follicular
  - Both forms can be present in varying amounts
- Tumor often associated with lymphocytic thyroiditis
- Cells enlarged and polygonal
- Abundant granular eosinophilic cytoplasm
- Characteristic PTC nuclear features present
  - May be quite subtle
  - Nuclear clearing, irregular nuclear contours with nuclear grooves and pseudoinclusions

ANCILLARY TESTS

- Immunohistochemistry for HBME1 may be useful for diagnosing an oncocytic tumor as oncocytic variant of PTC
- Mutations in complex 1 subunit encoded by *NDUFA13* (a.k.a. GRIM-19) nuclear gene specific for oncocytic tumors
  - Found in ~ 10% of oncocytic variant of PTC
- *BRAF* V600E mutation
- *TERT* promoter mutation
- *RET* gene rearrangements

TOP DIFFERENTIAL DIAGNOSES

- PTC, tall cell variant
- PTC, Warthin-like variant
- Follicular carcinoma, oncocytic
- Follicular adenoma, oncocytic

Encapsulated Oncocytic Variant of PTC

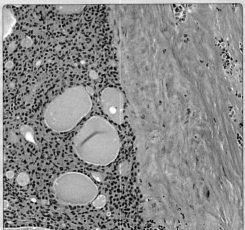

PTC Nuclear Features

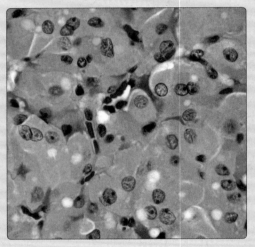

(Left) This example shows an encapsulated oncocytic variant of papillary thyroid carcinoma (PTC) composed of markedly eosinophilic tumor cells. The fibrous capsule shows focal hyalinization and separates the tumor from adjacent parenchyma. (Right) This variant of PTC is characterized by large eosinophilic cells that have characteristic papillary carcinoma nuclear features including clearing, nuclear membrane irregularities, and intranuclear grooves. Note the small, pink nucleoli seen in some of the nuclei.

Hemosiderin Deposition

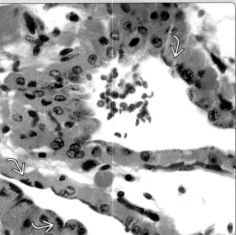

Membranous HBME1 Pattern

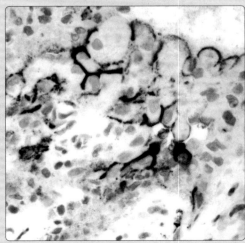

(Left) Papillary carcinoma nuclear features are seen in this figure, including clearing, nuclear membrane irregularities, and nuclear overlapping. Also identified is the brown hemosiderin ⟹ deposition within the follicular cells. (Right) Immunohistochemistry for HBME1 shows membranous staining on papillary thyroid carcinomas. This marker is useful for diagnosing an oncocytic tumor as oncocytic variant of PTC, distinguishing it from other oncocytic neoplasms.

Papillary Thyroid Carcinoma, Oncocytic Variant

TERMINOLOGY

Synonyms

- Papillary thyroid carcinoma (PTC), Hürthle variant

Definitions

- Malignant follicular neoplasm characterized by cells with eosinophilic granular cytoplasm and papillary thyroid carcinoma nuclear features

CLINICAL ISSUES

Epidemiology

- Incidence
  - In pure form, this variant is extremely rare (WHO 2017)
    - Oncocytic change found in 45.8% (65/142) of PTC patients
      - Proportion of patients with oncocytic change higher in obese patients than in lean patients and shows significant correlation with BMI
    - May account for < 10% of all PTC diagnoses
- Age
  - Average at presentation: Usually 5th decade
- Sex
  - More common in women

Presentation

- Often with neck mass
  - May have compressive/obstructive symptoms if large

Treatment

- Treatment involves surgical resection
- Lymph node dissection performed when indicated
- These tumors show decreased uptake of radioactive iodine, thus they are less responsive to radioactive iodine therapy

Prognosis

- Controversial
  - Some authors suggest prognosis similar to conventional PTC, while others feel these tumors more aggressive
  - Presence of *BRAF* mutation, extrathyroid extension, and vascular invasion associated with worse prognosis
  - Thyroid carcinomas that harbor *TERT* (C228T) mutation associated with recurrence
  - Coexistence of *TERT* (C228T) and *BRAF* V600E mutations found in ~ 13% of PTCs
    - Significantly associated with older age and advanced stage compared with group negative for either mutation
  - PTC patients with oncocytic changes show higher recurrence rate than PTC patients without oncocytic change
    - Presence of oncocytic change poor prognostic factor in PTC patients
      - Even if oncocytic change involves < 75% of tumor

MACROSCOPIC

General Features

- Well circumscribed and may be encapsulated
  - Characteristic brown color grossly (reflecting oncocytic appearance microscopically)

Size

- Average: 2.5 cm

MICROSCOPIC

Histologic Features

- May be encapsulated and are well circumscribed
- Architecture primarily papillary or follicular (both forms can be present in varying amounts)
  - Papillae have true fibrovascular cores
  - Follicles may be micro- or macrofollicular
- Architecture may be solid or trabecular
- Tumors markedly eosinophilic
- Colloid present in variable amounts
- Psammoma bodies absent
- Tumor often associated with lymphocytic thyroiditis
- Extrathyroid extension not often seen
- Angiolymphatic invasion rare
- Areas of hemorrhage usually present
- Hemosiderin deposition seen within stroma and within tumor cells lining papillae
  - Mostly seen in cytoplasmic borders

Cytologic Features

- Cells enlarged and polygonal
- Abundant granular eosinophilic cytoplasm
- Nuclei enlarged and pleomorphic
- Characteristic PTC nuclear features present
  - May be quite subtle
    - Irregular nuclear contours with nuclear grooves and pseudoinclusions (rare)
    - Chromatin pale staining, though often more basophilic than in conventional PTC
    - Nucleoli almost always present and are peripherally located
- Cells without PTC nuclear features have large, pleomorphic, and hyperchromatic nuclei with prominent nucleoli

Other

- Oncocytic changes in follicular cells occur in inflammatory, hyperplastic, and neoplastic settings, including both benign and malignant tumors
- Oncocytic variant of papillary thyroid carcinoma may show papillae, follicles, have solid arrangement
  - Composed by cells with large oncocytic granular cytoplasm featuring clear PTC nuclear features
- Morphologically similar but biologically distinct lesion is encapsulated papillary oncocytic neoplasia

ANCILLARY TESTS

Cytology

- Aspirates very cellular
- Sheets of cells, papillary fragments and clusters, or single cells present
- Papillary fragments have fibrovascular cores
- Cells enlarged and polygonal in shape
- Cytoplasm granular and eosinophilic
- Nuclei enlarged and pleomorphic
- Cells may have pale-staining chromatin with prominent nucleoli
- Rare nuclear grooves and pseudoinclusions present

- Colloid also present in varying amounts
- Lymphocytes may be present when associated with lymphocytic thyroiditis

Immunohistochemistry

- Panel of immunohistochemical stains may be useful in diagnosing oncocytic variant of PTC
  - Positive
    - HBME-1
    - Galectin-3
    - CK19
    - CITED-1
    - TTF-1
    - Thyroglobulin
    - BRAF
      - Other antibodies directed to proteins generated by mutated genes may represent cost-effective method for diagnosing and managing patients with thyroid tumor

Genetic Testing

- Oncocytic cell tumors have higher frequency of mitochondrial DNA mutations than nononcocytic tumors
- *BRAF* V600E mutation found in up to 55% of these tumors
- Mutations in complex 1 subunit encoded by *NDUFA13* (a.k.a. *GRIM-19*) nuclear gene specific for oncocytic tumors
  - Found in ~ 10% of oncocytic variant of PTC
- *TERT* promoter mutation
- *RET* gene rearrangements also found in some tumors

DIFFERENTIAL DIAGNOSIS

Papillary Thyroid Carcinoma, Tall Cell Variant

- Cell height is 3x width
- PTC nuclear features predominate, and pseudoinclusions abundant

Papillary Thyroid Carcinoma, Warthin-Like Variant

- Papillae have stroma filled with lymphocytes and plasma cells

Follicular Carcinoma, Oncocytic

- Encapsulated tumors showing capsular &/or vascular invasion
- Lack PTC nuclear features and papillary architecture

Follicular Adenoma, Oncocytic

- Encapsulated neoplasm
- Lacks PTC nuclear features and papillary architecture
- Immunohistochemistry may be useful for differentiating from oncocytic variant of PTC

SELECTED REFERENCES

1. Evranos B et al: Bethesda classification is a valuable guide for fine needle aspiration reports and highly predictive especially for diagnosing aggressive variants of papillary thyroid carcinoma. Cytopathology. 28(4):259-267, 2017
2. Glomski K et al: Metastatic follicular thyroid carcinoma and the primary thyroid gross examination: institutional review of cases from 1990 to 2015. Endocr Pathol. 28(2):177-185, 2017
3. Hirokawa M et al: Chromophobe renal cell carcinoma-like thyroid carcinoma: a novel clinicopathologic entity possibly associated with tuberous sclerosis complex. Endocr J. ePub, 2017
4. Seethala RR et al: Clinical and morphologic features of ETV6-NTRK3 translocated papillary thyroid carcinoma in an adult population without radiation exposure. Am J Surg Pathol. ePub, 2017
5. Hong JH et al: Implications of oncocytic change in papillary thyroid cancer. Clin Endocrinol (Oxf). 85(5):797-804, 2016
6. Lee SE et al: Prognostic significance of TERT promoter mutations in papillary thyroid carcinomas in a BRAF(V600E) mutation-prevalent population. Thyroid. 26(7):901-10, 2016
7. Peckova K et al: Selected case from the Arkadi M. Rywlin International Pathology Slide Seminar: Benign Warthin Tumor of the Thyroid. Adv Anat Pathol. 23(5):339-42, 2016
8. Wei S et al: STK11 Mutation identified in thyroid carcinoma. Endocr Pathol. 27(1):65-9, 2016
9. Yazici P et al: Malignancy risk of oncocytic changes in thyroid nodules: who should we offer surgery to? Acta Chir Belg. 116(1):30-5, 2016
10. Deshmukh SD et al: Oncocytic adenoma of thyroid with papillary architecture: a diagnostic dilemma. South Asian J Cancer. 4(1):50-1, 2015
11. Fadda G et al: Immunohistochemical diagnosis of thyroid tumors. Surg Pathol Clin. 7(4):491-500, 2014
12. Givens DJ et al: BRAF V600E does not predict aggressive features of pediatric papillary thyroid carcinoma. Laryngoscope. 124(9):E389-93, 2014
13. Hsiao SJ et al: Molecular approaches to thyroid cancer diagnosis. Endocr Relat Cancer. 21(5):T301-13, 2014
14. Radkay LA et al: Thyroid nodules with KRAS mutations are different from nodules with NRAS and HRAS mutations with regard to cytopathologic and histopathologic outcome characteristics. Cancer Cytopathol. ePub, 2014
15. Lee KH et al: Predictive factors of malignancy in patients with cytologically suspicious for Hurthle cell neoplasm of thyroid nodules. Int J Surg. 11(9):898-902, 2013
16. Rossi ED et al: The cytologic category of oncocytic (Hurthle) cell neoplasm mostly includes low-risk lesions at histology: an institutional experience. Eur J Endocrinol. 169(5):649-55, 2013
17. Xing M et al: Association between BRAF V600E mutation and mortality in patients with papillary thyroid cancer. JAMA. 309(14):1493-501, 2013
18. Bellevicine C et al: Multicentric encapsulated papillary oncocytic neoplasm of the thyroid: a case diagnosed by a combined cytological, histological, immunohistochemical, and molecular approach. Diagn Cytopathol. 40(5):450-4, 2012
19. Bellevicine C et al: Multicentric encapsulated papillary oncocytic neoplasm of the thyroid: A case diagnosed by a combined cytological, histological, immunohistochemical, and molecular approach. Diagn Cytopathol. 40(5):450-4, 2012
20. Lloyd RV et al: Papillary thyroid carcinoma variants. Head Neck Pathol. 5(1):51-6, 2011
21. Woodford RL et al: Encapsulated papillary oncocytic neoplasms of the thyroid: morphologic, immunohistochemical, and molecular analysis of 18 cases. Am J Surg Pathol. 34(11):1582-90, 2010
22. Gross M et al: Clinicopathologic features and outcome of the oncocytic variant of papillary thyroid carcinoma. Ann Otol Rhinol Laryngol. 118(5):374-81, 2009
23. Lee J et al: Oncocytic variant of papillary thyroid carcinoma associated with Hashimoto's thyroiditis: a case report and review of the literature. Diagn Cytopathol. 37(8):600-6, 2009
24. Ito Y et al: Prevalence and biological behaviour of variants of papillary thyroid carcinoma: experience at a single institute. Pathology. 40(6):617-22, 2008
25. Montone KT et al: The thyroid Hürthle (oncocytic) cell and its associated pathologic conditions: a surgical pathology and cytopathology review. Arch Pathol Lab Med. 132(8):1241-50, 2008
26. Sobrinho-Simões M et al: Hürthle (oncocytic) cell tumors of thyroid: etiopathogenesis, diagnosis and clinical significance. Int J Surg Pathol. 13(1):29-35, 2005
27. Trovisco V et al: Type and prevalence of BRAF mutations are closely associated with papillary thyroid carcinoma histotype and patients' age but not with tumour aggressiveness. Virchows Arch. 446(6):589-95, 2005

Edematous Papillae and Hemosiderin

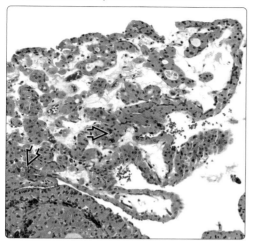

Intranuclear Grooves

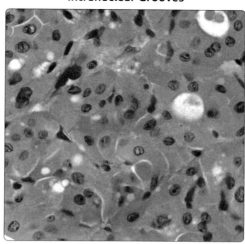

(Left) *The oncocytic variant of PTC is usually well circumscribed or encapsulated. The architectural pattern is a mixture of follicles and papillary structures. Almost no colloid is seen here. Hemosiderin deposition ⊠ is a frequent finding.* (Right) *Some of the oncocytic variants of papillary thyroid carcinoma are unencapsulated and have a predominant diffuse pattern. This photomicrograph shows large cells with abundant oncocytic cytoplasm and PTC nuclear changes including numerous intranuclear grooves.*

Nuclear Grooves

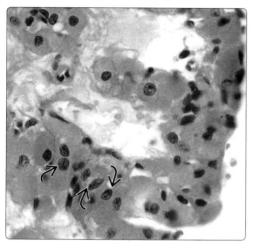

Follicular Cell Characteristics

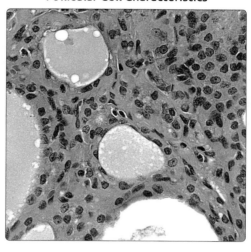

(Left) *The papillary carcinoma nuclear features are seen in this edematous papilla, including overlapping, nuclear membrane irregularities, and numerous intranuclear grooves ⊠.* (Right) *PTC, oncocytic variant is characterized by large, eosinophilic cells with granular cytoplasm. The tumor cells have characteristic PTC nuclear features.*

Large Oncocytic Tumor Cells

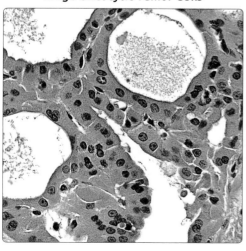

Membranous HBME1 Staining

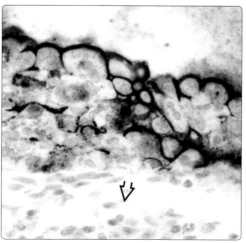

(Left) *PTC nuclear features may be quite subtle in the oncocytic variant. This example shows large, irregular nuclei that are pale staining when compared to normal follicular cells. Nucleoli are a characteristic finding of this variant.* (Right) *Oncocytic PTC shows a characteristic membranous staining for HBME-1 on the oncocytic tumor cells lining a papillae. Note that the cells in the stroma ⊠ are negative for this marker.*

Papillary Thyroid Carcinoma, Tall Cell Variant

TERMINOLOGY

- Aggressive variant of papillary thyroid carcinoma (PTC) predominantly composed of elongated neoplastic follicular cells with abundant eosinophilic cytoplasm, scant colloid, and characteristic papillary nuclear features
- Extrathyroidal extension and metastatic disease are more frequently observed in this variant than in classic PTC

MACROSCOPIC

- Tumors are large, usually > 4 cm
- Infiltrative growth pattern

MICROSCOPIC

- Tumor composed of cells with height 2-3x their width, show abundant eosinophilic (oncocytic-like) cytoplasm, and characteristic nuclear features (WHO 2017)
- Tall cells must account for > 30% of all tumor cells for diagnosis of tall cell variant (WHO 2017)
- Papillary, trabecular, and cord-like patterns most common
  - Cord-like pattern is known as "tram-tracking"
- Numerous nuclear pseudoinclusions are easily found
  - Pseudoinclusions are more common in this variant than any other, including classic variant PTC

ANCILLARY TESTS

- Increased incidence of *BRAF* V600E mutation compared to classic variant and other variants
  - *BRAF* V600E is most common mutation present in tall cell variant PTC
    - Present in 60-95% of cases
- ~ 5-30% of cases have *TERT* promoter mutation
  - *TERT* mutation predicts highly significant tumor relapse
- *RET* gene rearrangement is seen in ~ 35% cases
- *RAS* is not identified in tall cell variant cases
- Immunohistochemistry
  - HBME1
  - BRAF
  - High Ki-67 proliferative index

Intranuclear Inclusions and Mitosis

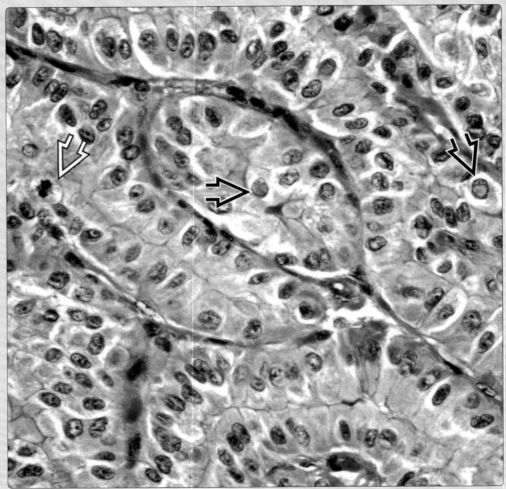

In this picture, the tumor has at least 50% of tumor cells have height 3x their width. Tumor cells have abundant eosinophilic cytoplasm. The nuclei are similar to conventional papillary thyroid carcinoma (PTC) and nuclear pseudoinclusions ⊃ are usually easily identified. One mitosis is present ⇒.

TERMINOLOGY

Abbreviations

- Papillary thyroid carcinoma, tall cell variant (PTCTCV) or (TCVPTC)

Synonyms

- Tall cell papillary carcinoma

Definitions

- Aggressive variant of papillary thyroid carcinoma (PTC) predominantly composed of cells with height 2-3x their width, show abundant eosinophilic (oncocytic-like) cytoplasm, and characteristic nuclear features (WHO 2017)
  - Tall cells must account for > 30% of tumor cells for diagnosis of tall cell variant (WHO 2017)
  - Nuclear pseudoinclusions are usually easily found

ETIOLOGY/PATHOGENESIS

Genetic

- Increased incidence of *BRAF* mutation compared to classic variant
  - Present in 60-95% of cases
- *RET/NCOA4* gene rearrangement is seen in tall cell variant cases associated with radiation exposure (~ 35% cases)
- *TERT* promoter present in 5-30% cases
- *RAS* is not identified in tall cell variant cases

CLINICAL ISSUES

Epidemiology

- Incidence
  - Most common **aggressive** variant of PTC
    - Represents 4-19% of papillary thyroid carcinomas
  - Widely known to be underdiagnosed
    - Multiple authors report that majority of tall cell variant cases are missed by pathologists
- Age
  - Presents later in life
    - Average age at presentation is 55 years vs. 46 years for classic variant PTC
- Sex
  - More common in males

Presentation

- Generally present as neck masses
- Patients commonly present with symptoms related to involvement of surrounding structures
  - Stridor, dysphagia, odynophagia, hoarseness

Treatment

- Thyroidectomy is surgical treatment of choice
- Lymph node dissection if clinically indicated (lymph node involvement)
- External radiotherapy for residual disease after thyroidectomy
- Systemic radioactive iodine therapy for metastatic disease
  - 20% of cases are refractory to radioactive iodine ablation

Prognosis

- Tall cell variant of papillary thyroid carcinoma is more aggressive than classic PTC

- However, percentage of tall cells needed to diagnose TCVPTC remains controversial
- Typically prognosis is poor
- Lymph node metastasis rate is higher than classic variant PTC
- Extrathyroid extension is common and associated with poorer prognosis
- Tall cell histology alone is recognized as significant prognostic factor for disease-specific death
  - Even gland-defined tumors without extrathyroid extension behave aggressively
- Increased risk of recurrence

IMAGING

CT Findings

- Imaging is helpful in demonstrating involvement of surrounding structures
- Involvement of lymph nodes may also be seen on imaging

MACROSCOPIC

General Features

- Tumors are large, usually > 4 cm
- Infiltrative growth pattern
  - Extension beyond thyroid is common
- Usually solid firm lesions
- Areas of frank necrosis may be visible grossly
- Pale tan to white in color
- Foci of hemorrhage are common

Size

- Typically 4 cm or greater

MICROSCOPIC

Histologic Features

- Tumor composed of cells that are 2-3x as tall as they are wide, and show abundant eosinophilic cytoplasm
- Tall cells must account for > 30% of all tumor cells for diagnosis of tall cell variant (WHO 2017)
- Papillary, trabecular, and cord-like patterns most common
  - Papillary structures are elongated
  - Cord-like pattern is known as "tram-tracking"
- Typical nuclear features of PTC are present
- Numerous nuclear pseudoinclusions are easily found
  - Pseudoinclusions are more common in this variant than any other, including classic variant PTC
- Follicular structures are rare
- May be associated with fibrosis
- Extrathyroid extension is common (more frequently than conventional/classic variant PTC)
- Psammoma bodies are less common
- Necrosis is commonly seen
- Scant or absent colloid

Cytologic Features

- At least 30% of tumor cells have height 2-3x their width
- Tumor cells have abundant eosinophilic cytoplasm
  - Cytoplasm is not granular and thus are not true Hürthle cells
- Nuclei tend to be basally oriented

- Nuclei are similar to conventional PTC
  - Nuclei have ground-glass chromatin, though some may be hyperchromatic
  - Nuclei are enlarged
  - Membrane contours are irregular
  - Nuclear pseudoinclusions are abundant
    - Pseudoinclusions are more common in this variant than any other, including classic variant PTC
  - Nuclear grooves are abundant
- Nuclei do not overlap due to abundant cytoplasm
- Mitotic figures are common

ANCILLARY TESTS

Cytology

- Fine-needle aspiration is useful for diagnosis
- Cells are arranged in monolayer sheets
  - Usually small and flat
- Occasionally papillary structures are present
- Cells are larger than in classic variant
- Cells are elongated, polygonal, and columnar in shape
- Abundant eosinophilic cytoplasm
- Prominent cytoplasmic borders
- Nuclei usually centrally located
- Nuclei may be more granular than classic papillary carcinoma
- Nuclear grooves are prominent
- Pseudoinclusions are strikingly common
  - Multiple pseudoinclusions may be present within single nucleus (soap bubble)
- Psammoma bodies are rare
- Multinucleated cells may be present within aspirate
- Variable amount of colloid in background

Immunohistochemistry

- Staining pattern is similar to that of conventional PTC
- Positive
  - Thyroglobulin (cytoplasmic)
  - TTF-1 (nuclear)
  - pax-8
  - HBME-1 (membranous/luminal)
  - Galectin-3 (cytoplasmic)
  - p53 may be positive
  - Ki-67 proliferative index usually higher than other PTC variants
- Negative
  - Calcitonin
  - CDX-2
- BRAF is positive in vast majority of tall cell variant

Genetic Testing

- Presence of tall cells is associated with *BRAF* V600E and telomerase reverse transcriptase (*TERT*) promoter mutations
  - *BRAF* V600E is most common mutation present in tall cell variant PTC
    - *BRAF* mutation is found in 60-95% of cases
      - Presence of this mutation is associated with poor prognosis (vascular invasion, metastases, extrathyroidal extension)
  - ~ 5-30% of cases have *TERT* promoter mutation

- *TERT* mutation predicts highly significant tumor relapse
  - *RET* seen in ~ 35% cases

DIFFERENTIAL DIAGNOSIS

Conventional Variant of Papillary Thyroid Carcinoma

- Nuclei are round to oval in shape
- Nuclei overlap and have pale, optically clear nuclei with ground-glass chromatin
- Nuclear membranes are irregular, with abundant grooves and pseudoinclusions
- Cells are usually cuboidal in shape

Follicular Oncocytic Carcinoma

- Encapsulated follicular cell tumors
- Follicular architecture
- Granular eosinophilic cytoplasm
- Lack characteristic PTC nuclear features

Oncocytic Papillary Thyroid Carcinoma

- Papillary architecture with fibrovascular cores
- Tumor cells have granular eosinophilic cytoplasm
- Cells are polygonal in shape
- Exhibit classic papillary carcinoma nuclear features
- Usually well defined or encapsulated

Warthin-Like Papillary Thyroid Carcinoma

- Usually papillary in architecture
- Eosinophilic cells line papillae composed of lymphoid stroma
- Nuclear grooves and inclusions are less common in this variant

Columnar Cell Variant of Papillary Thyroid Carcinoma

- Nuclei are elongated and hyperchromatic
- Nuclei are centrally located and pseudostratified
- Subnuclear and supranuclear vacuoles are present
- Absence of nuclear pseudoinclusions

DIAGNOSTIC CHECKLIST

Clinically Relevant Pathologic Features

- Extrathyroid extension and lymphovascular invasion are common
- In metastasis or recurrence, tall cell feature may be more prominent
- Even small foci (< 30%) should be mentioned, as prognosis is worse in this population

Pathologic Interpretation Pearls

- Tumor composed of cells that are 2-3x as tall as they are wide and show abundant eosinophilic cytoplasm
- Morphologic tall cell features must be present in at least 30% of tumor cells for diagnosis

SELECTED REFERENCES

1. Ito Y et al: Prognostic significance of the proportion of tall cell components in papillary thyroid carcinoma. World J Surg. 41(3):742-747, 2017
2. Liu Z et al: A comparison of the clinicopathological features and prognoses of the classical and the tall cell variant of papillary thyroid cancer: a meta-analysis. Oncotarget. 8(4):6222-6232, 2017
3. Lloyd RV et al: WHO Classification of Tumours of Endocrine Organs. Lyon, France: IARC Press, 2017

Differential Diagnosis of Tall Cell Variant

Feature	Tall Cell Variant	Classic Variant	Columnar Cell Variant	Warthin-Like Variant	Oncocytic Variant
Architecture	Papillary, follicular, tram-tracking	Papillary	Papillary	Papillary	Papillary
Cell shape	Elongated, height 3x width	Polygonal, cuboidal	Columnar	Polygonal, columnar	Polygonal, columnar
Cytoplasm	Eosinophilic	Amphophilic	Eosinophilic	Eosinophilic	Eosinophilic, granular
Nucleus shape	Oval, basally located	Irregular, angulated	Elongated, centrally located	Polygonal	Round to polygonal
Chromatin pattern	Powdery, ground-glass	Powdery, ground-glass	Hyperchromatic, focally powdery	Powdery, ground-glass	Powdery, ground-glass
Nuclear grooves	Abundant	Abundant	Occasional	Common	Common
Nuclear pseudoinclusions	Abundant	Common	Rare	Common	Common
Psammoma bodies	Occasional	Common	Rare	Rare to absent	Rare to absent
Miscellaneous			Supra- and subnuclear vacuoles	Lymphoid stroma	
Cytogenetics	*BRAF* (60-95%), *RET* (35%), *RAS* (0%)	*BRAF* (45-80%), *RET* (5-25%), *RAS* (0-15%)	*BRAF*	*BRAF*	

4. Patten DK et al: Anaplastic spindle cell squamous carcinoma arising from tall cell variant papillary carcinoma of the thyroid gland: a case report and review of the literature. Case Rep Endocrinol. 2017:4581626, 2017

5. Russo M et al: Tall cell and diffuse sclerosing variants of papillary thyroid cancer: outcome and predicting value of risk stratification methods. J Endocrinol Invest. ePub, 2017

6. Villar-Taibo R et al: Aggressiveness of the tall cell variant of papillary thyroid carcinoma is independent of the tumor size and patient age. Oncol Lett. 13(5):3501-3507, 2017

7. Fridman M et al: Characteristics of young adults of Belarus with post-Chernobyl papillary thyroid carcinoma: a long-term follow-up of patients with early exposure to radiation at the 30th anniversary of the accident. Clin Endocrinol (Oxf). 85(6):971-978, 2016

8. Wang X et al: Tall cell variant of papillary thyroid carcinoma: current evidence on clinicopathologic features and molecular biology. Oncotarget. 7(26):40792-40799, 2016

9. Dettmer MS et al: Tall cell papillary thyroid carcinoma: new diagnostic criteria and mutations in BRAF and TERT. Endocr Relat Cancer. 22(3):419-29, 2015

10. Okuyucu K et al: Clinicopathologic features and prognostic factors of tall cell variant of papillary thyroid carcinoma: comparison with classic variant of papillary thyroid carcinoma. Nucl Med Commun. 36(10):1021-5, 2015

11. Boutzios G et al: Higher incidence of tall cell variant of papillary thyroid carcinoma in Graves' Disease. Thyroid. 24(2):347-54, 2014

12. Collini P et al: Tall cell variant of papillary thyroid carcinoma in children: report of three cases with long-term follow-up from a single institution. Int J Surg Pathol. 22(6):499-504, 2014

13. Ganly I et al: Prognostic implications of papillary thyroid carcinoma with tall-cell features. Thyroid. 24(4):662-70, 2014

14. Lee SH et al: Liquid-based cytology improves preoperative diagnostic accuracy of the tall cell variant of papillary thyroid carcinoma. Diagn Cytopathol. 42(1):11-7, 2014

15. Oh WJ et al: Classic papillary thyroid carcinoma with tall cell features and tall cell variant have similar clinicopathologic features. Korean J Pathol. 48(3):201-8, 2014

16. Beninato T et al: Ten percent tall cells confer the aggressive features of the tall cell variant of papillary thyroid carcinoma. Surgery. 154(6):1331-6; discussion 1336, 2013

17. Bernstein J et al: Tall cell variant of papillary thyroid microcarcinoma: clinicopathologic features with BRAF(V600E) mutational analysis. Thyroid. 23(12):1525-31, 2013

18. Guan H et al: Can the tall cell variant of papillary thyroid carcinoma be distinguished from the conventional type in fine needle aspirates? A cytomorphologic study with assessment of diagnostic accuracy. Acta Cytol. 57(5):534-42, 2013

19. Min HS et al: Correlation of immunohistochemical markers and BRAF mutation status with histological variants of papillary thyroid carcinoma in the Korean population. J Korean Med Sci. 28(4):534-41, 2013

20. Virk RK et al: BRAFV600E mutation in papillary thyroid microcarcinoma: a genotype-phenotype correlation. Mod Pathol. 26(1):62-70, 2013

21. Nosé V: Familial thyroid cancer: a review. Mod Pathol. 24 Suppl 2:S19-33, 2011

22. LiVolsi VA: Papillary carcinoma tall cell variant (TCV): a review. Endocr Pathol. 21(1):12-5, 2010

23. Morris LG et al: Tall-cell variant of papillary thyroid carcinoma: a matched-pair analysis of survival. Thyroid. 20(2):153-8, 2010

24. Urano M et al: Tall cell variant of papillary thyroid carcinoma: its characteristic features demonstrated by fine-needle aspiration cytology and immunohistochemical study. Diagn Cytopathol. 37(10):732-7, 2009

25. Frasca F et al: BRAF(V600E) mutation and the biology of papillary thyroid cancer. Endocr Relat Cancer. 15(1):191-205, 2008

26. Ito Y et al: Prevalence and biological behaviour of variants of papillary thyroid carcinoma: experience at a single institute. Pathology. 40(6):617-22, 2008

27. Ito Y et al: Prevalence and prognostic significance of poor differentiation and tall cell variant in papillary carcinoma in Japan. World J Surg. 32(7):1535-43; discussion 1544-5, 2008

28. Leung AK et al: Clinical features and outcome of the tall cell variant of papillary thyroid carcinoma. Laryngoscope. 118(1):32-8, 2008

29. Ghossein RA et al: Tall cell variant of papillary thyroid carcinoma without extrathyroid extension: biologic behavior and clinical implications. Thyroid. 17(7):655-61, 2007

(Left) *This gross image shows a large tumor occupying almost the entire thyroid lobe. Tall cell variant tumors are usually large with an infiltrative growth pattern and extrathyroidal extension.*
(Right) *This variant of PTC is characterized by cells with ample eosinophilic cytoplasm with well-defined, cytoplasmic borders. The cells nuclei show a powdery, almost ground-glass chromatin. Colloid is often scant or absent in this variant.*

Gross Cut Surface

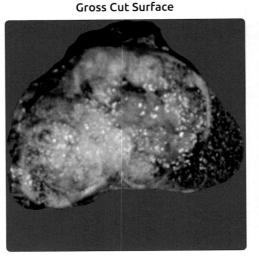

Ample Eosinophilic Cytoplasm

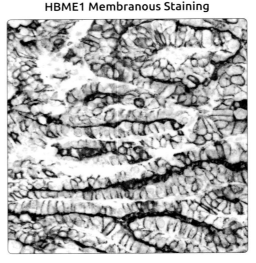

(Left) *This high-power view of the tall cell variant of PTC shows the characteristic trabecular ("tram-tracking") arrangement, often present in this variant of papillary carcinoma. The cells are at least 3x as tall as they are wide and have abundant eosinophilic cytoplasm. Intranuclear pseudoinclusions ⊠ are easily identified in this subtype.* **(Right)** *BRAF immunostain shows a diffuse granular cytoplasmic positivity in this TCVPTC. The immunopositivity is granular in the cytoplasm.*

Intranuclear Pseudoinclusions

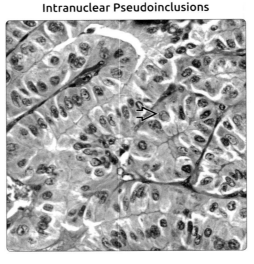

Granular Cytoplasmic BRAF Stain

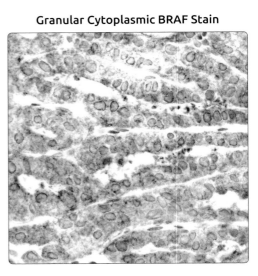

(Left) *HBME-1 demonstrates a membranous staining pattern in PTC. It also has a luminal staining pattern in PTC with follicular architecture. This image demonstrates the membranous staining pattern seen in the tall cell variant tumor cells.* **(Right)** *Immunohistochemistry shows diffuse cytoplasmic staining in this focus of the tall cell variant of PTC within lymphovascular spaces. The adjacent thyroid is negative.*

HBME1 Membranous Staining

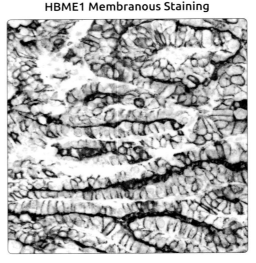

BRAF in Tumor Within Lymphatics

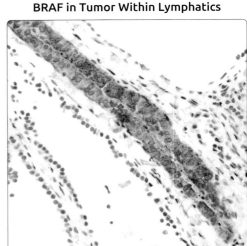

Trabecular and Follicular Architecture

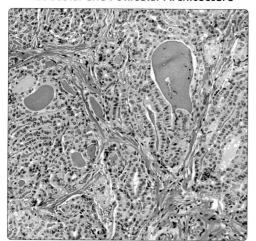

Cellular Characteristics

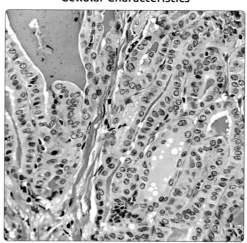

(Left) *This medium-power image demonstrates the follicular and cord-like patterns (also known as "tram-tracking") commonly seen in tall cell variant PTC. The cells also appear elongated. Hypereosinophilic colloid can be seen within the follicles.* **(Right)** *At higher power, characteristic PTC nuclear features become more evident. The cells are elongated and contain oncocytic cytoplasm. The nuclei are oval to polygonal in shape and with prominent nuclear grooves.*

Mitoses

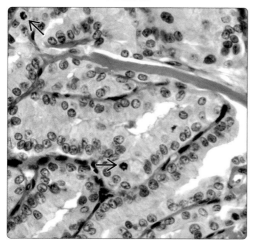

Numerous Pseudoinclusions

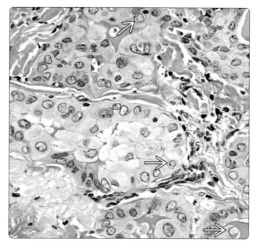

(Left) *Mitotic activity is common in this aggressive variant. This image demonstrates multiple mitotic figures* ➡ *and basal location of nuclei. The tumor cells are quite elongated with distinct cytoplasmic borders. The chromatin is pale staining and nuclear grooves are identified.* **(Right)** *Nuclear pseudoinclusions* ➡ *are quite common in this variant of PTC. Three can be clearly seen in this image. Irregular nuclear membranes and ground-glass chromatin are also evident.*

Small Focus of Carcinoma

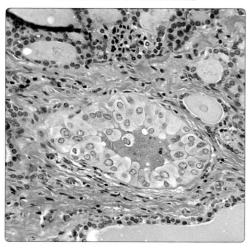

Sclerosis

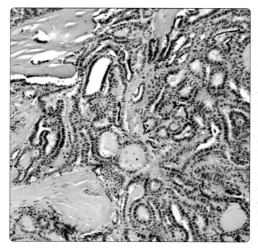

(Left) *This image demonstrates a micropapillary carcinoma (< 1 cm) with tall cell features. Tall cell variant microcarcinomas are rare, and a lymphovascular invasion from a larger tumor should be ruled out. Many of these carcinomas are located toward the periphery of the gland and may show extrathyroid extension.* **(Right)** *Tall cell variant PTC may be associated with fibrosis and sclerosis as seen in this photograph. The sclerotic bands can be seen between tumor follicles.*

Lymph Node Metastasis

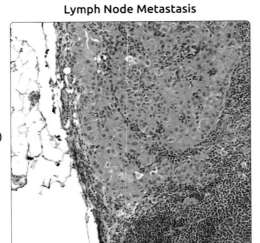

Lung Metastases

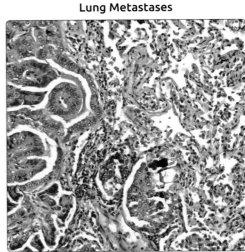

(Left) *Patients that develop papillary carcinoma are often found to have lymph node metastases at the time of diagnosis. These metastatic tumor deposits show characteristic tall cell variant features (elongated "tall" cells, eosinophilic cytoplasm, and nuclear inclusions).* (Right) *Tall cell variant commonly metastasizes to distant locations. This image was taken from a lung nodule in a patient with a history of PTC. Tumor cells with tall cell features are seen infiltrating lung tissue.*

Tumor Infiltrating Parathyroid

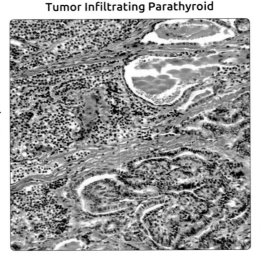

PTC Within Parathyroid

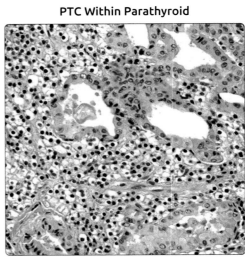

(Left) *This variant is known to be locally aggressive and frequently invades adjacent structures. This image demonstrates a tall cell variant PTC tumor infiltrating into the adjacent parathyroid gland (located top left corner).* (Right) *Higher power image shows multiple tumor follicles with tall cell variant features invading the parathyroid gland. Specimens should be carefully examined for both the presence of parathyroid glands and their involvement by tumor.*

Invasion Into Tracheal Cartilage

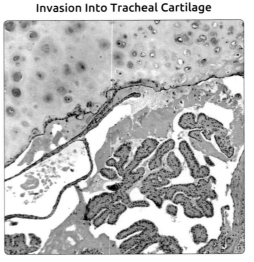

PTC Involving Pyriform Sinus

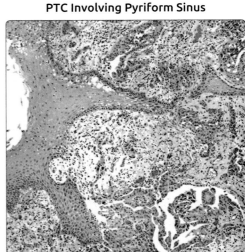

(Left) *This locally aggressive tumor was found to be invading into the trachea. A ring of cartilage is shown being eroded by tumor cells. Clinically, this patient presented with compressive symptoms and a large immobile neck mass.* (Right) *This image shows tumor cells invading into the pyriform sinus. This patient presented with dysphagia and hoarseness. On endoscopic exam, the vocal cord was fixed/immobile and was histologically shown to be involved by tumor.*

Trabecular Arrangement

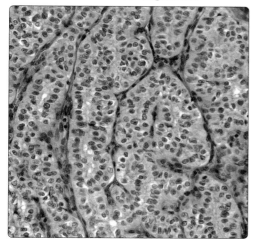

Galectin-3 Immunopositivity

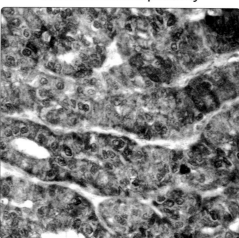

(Left) *H&E shows the tram-tracking pattern commonly seen in this variant of papillary carcinoma. The cells are at least 3x as tall as they are wide and have abundant eosinophilic cytoplasm.* (Right) *This image demonstrates the strong cytoplasmic staining pattern of galectin-3, highlighting the tall cell morphology seen here. Galectin-3 should be used in conjunction with other immunohistochemical stains for diagnosing PTC.*

Membranous HBME-1 Staining

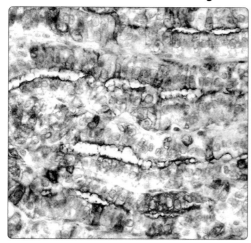

Patchy Thyroglobulin

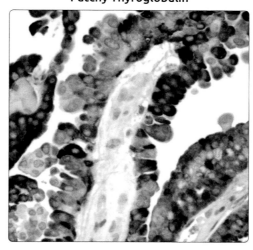

(Left) *HBME-1 demonstrates a membranous staining pattern in PTC and in tall cell variant tumor cells. It also has a luminal staining pattern in PTC with follicular architecture.* (Right) *Thyroglobulin is useful for confirming neoplasms of thyroid origin. Thyroglobulin has a cytoplasmic staining pattern, which is demonstrated in this image.*

TTF-1

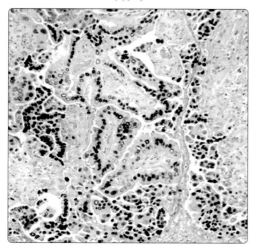

Cytologic Features

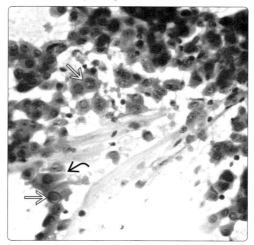

(Left) *TTF-1 has a nuclear staining pattern. Use of this immunostain should be used in conjunction with other immunostains (i.e., thyroglobulin and pax-8) to definitively confirm tumors of thyroid origin.* (Right) *This touch prep is from a tumor with tall cell variant histology. There are many cells arranged in a vague papillary architecture. The cells have abundant eosinophilic cytoplasm. Some of the cells at the periphery are elongated ➔. Nuclear pseudoinclusions ➡ are present.*

Papillary Thyroid Carcinoma, Columnar Cell Variant

TERMINOLOGY

- Rare variant of papillary thyroid carcinoma (PTC) composed of columnar shaped cells with pseudostratified hyperchromatic nuclei
- Can be further classified as indolent or aggressive

CLINICAL ISSUES

- Neoplasms that behave indolently or aggressively characterized by recognition of clinicopathological characteristics and molecular features

MICROSCOPIC

- Varied architectural arrangements often identified
- Nuclei usually lack conventional characteristics of conventional PTC nuclei
  - Nuclei show characteristic stratification
  - Hyperchromatic, elongated nuclei
  - Presence of supranuclear and subnuclear cytoplasmic vacuoles

- Lymphovascular invasion common
- Extrathyroid extension commonly seen in unencapsulated forms

ANCILLARY TESTS

- Immunohistochemistry
  - Positive: TTF-1, pax-8, cyclin-D1, ER, PR
    - BRAF positive in ~ 1/2 of cases
    - CDX-2 (very rare cases)
- Genetic:
  - *BRAF* V600E mutation may be present
    - Typically found in invasive aggressive tumors

TOP DIFFERENTIAL DIAGNOSES

- Tall cell variant, PTC classic variant, metastases from colon or endometrium

---

Well-Circumscribed Tumor

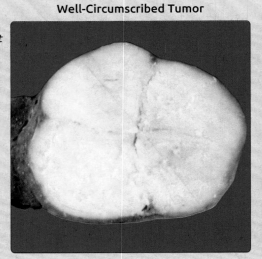

Pseudostratified Cellular Arrangement

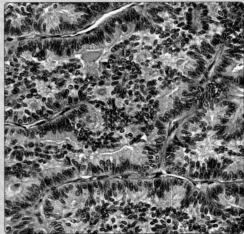

(Left) *The tumor is white and solid in consistency and almost entirely replaces the thyroid lobe. Adjacent normal thyroid parenchyma is visible on the left. This example shows a fairly well-circumscribed nodule.* (Right) *H&E demonstrates characteristic columnar-shaped cells with stratified, hyperchromatic nuclei and clear to lightly eosinophilic cytoplasm. The nuclei are central to basally located.*

Cytoplasmic Vacuolization

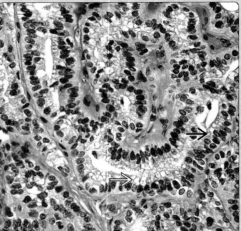

HBME-1 Luminal Expression

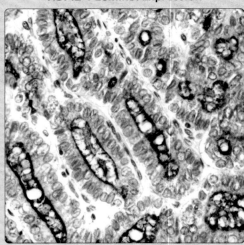

(Left) *High-power view shows clear supranuclear vacuoles ➡ that can be seen in columnar variant papillary thyroid carcinoma (PTC). Also note the stratification ➡ of the nuclei. The cells in this example have lightly eosinophilic to clear cytoplasm with basally oriented nuclei.* (Right) *HBME-1 stains luminal borders in variants of papillary carcinoma with follicular structures. This example shows columnar cell variant with follicular architecture.*

TERMINOLOGY

Abbreviations

- Papillary thyroid carcinoma, columnar cell variant (PTCCCV)

Synonyms

- Columnar cell variant papillary thyroid carcinoma (CCVPTC)

Definitions

- Rare, aggressive variant of papillary thyroid carcinoma (PTC) composed of columnar-shaped cells with pseudostratified hyperchromatic nuclei
- Cells lack conventional nuclear features of PTC
- Can be further classified as indolent or aggressive

CLINICAL ISSUES

Epidemiology

- Incidence
  - Rare, accounting for 0.15-0.20% of all PTC cases
- Age
  - More common in 4th and 5th decades
    - Average: 49 years; range: 17-76
- Sex
  - 2x as common in women

Presentation

- Can be asymptomatic
- May present with neck pain
- Gradually enlarging neck mass
- May be fixed if involvement of surrounding structures present
- Involvement of adjacent structures presents via hoarseness, stridor, dysphagia, dysphonia, or dyspnea
- Involvement of cervical nodes commonly seen
- Distant metastases to brain, lung, and bone are frequent

Treatment

- Total thyroidectomy
- En bloc resection if surrounding structures involved
- Neck dissection indicated with presence of lymphadenopathy
- Radioiodine treatment may be given
- External beam radiation therapy for residual invasive disease or poor response to radioiodine therapy

Prognosis

- These neoplasms may behave indolently or aggressively based on pathological features, clinical data, and molecular findings
- Indolent tumors typically small, circumscribed or encapsulated, and occur more frequently in younger female patients
  - Encapsulated form shows better prognosis
    - Literature reports patients to be disease free at average of 5 years after initial surgery
- Aggressive tumors large, locally aggressive, associated with regional and distant metastasis, and occur in older male patients
  - Worse prognosis in nonencapsulated disease
    - Up to 67% of cases had extrathyroid extension at time of surgery
    - Distant metastases found in up to 87% of cases
  - Studies report mortality rate as high as 60-70% (40-month follow-up)
  - Locoregional recurrence in up to 1/3 of cases

MACROSCOPIC

General Features

- Typically unifocal
- Grayish tan to white lesions
- Usually solid
- Firm in consistency
- Tumors may be encapsulated (usually in younger patients)
- Tumors may be widely invasive (usually in older patients)
  - Extrathyroid extension may be identified grossly
  - Irregular in contour
- Foci of hemorrhage are also commonly seen

Size

- Encapsulated tumors usually smaller
- Large tumors (average: 3.8 cm)
  - Range: 1.5-10.0 cm

MICROSCOPIC

Histologic Features

- May be either encapsulated or unencapsulated, widely invasive
- Hypercellular neoplasm showing thin papillae or glandular-like spaces lined by pseudostratified epithelium
- Varied architectural arrangements often identified
  - Trabecular
  - Papillary with fibrovascular cores
  - Follicular or microfollicular, tubular
  - Cord-like
  - Solid
  - Cribriform
- Subnuclear vacuolization or clear cytoplasm reminiscent of endometrioid or intestinal carcinoma
- Extrathyroid extension commonly seen in unencapsulated forms
- Lymphovascular invasion common
- Necrosis may be present
- Colloid may be present within follicles
- Multinucleated giant cells occasionally present
- Desmoplasia and fibrosis in relation to tumor
- Psammoma bodies absent (except where associated with classic variant PTC)
- Association with squamous morules has been reported

Cytologic Features

- Characteristic columnar cells must be present in at least 30% of sampled tumor
- Cells elongated; height at least 2x width
  - Cells more elongated than tall cell variant
- Cytoplasm amphophilic to clear in color
  - Supranuclear and subnuclear cytoplasmic vacuoles typically present
  - Cytoplasmic glycogen may be apparent
- Lack characteristic conventional PTC nuclei
  - Nuclei show characteristic stratification
  - Nuclei usually slim and elongated

- o Hyperchromatic to stippled, vesicular nuclei
- o Nuclei typically centrally located
- o Rarely will have large, ground-glass nuclei with nuclear grooves and pseudoinclusions
- Increased mitotic activity common

Lymph Nodes

- Metastases to cervical lymph nodes common
- Metastases to mediastinal nodes have also been documented
- Metastatic deposits show characteristic columnar cell morphology
  - o Lymph node metastases may be confused with metastatic adenocarcinoma from other sites
    - – Immunohistochemistry helpful

ANCILLARY TESTS

Cytology

- Diagnosis by fine-needle aspiration not sensitive
- Smears moderately cellular
- Colloid usually absent
- Papillary fragments with fibrovascular cores may be present
- Homogeneous columnar cells arranged in monolayers
- Nuclei oval and elongated
- Stratification of nuclei may be present in tissue fragments
- Cytoplasmic vacuoles can be seen
- Cells lack grooves and intranuclear inclusions

Immunohistochemistry

- Positive
  - o TTF-1, pax-8, cyclin-D1, ER, PR
  - o May be positive for CDX-2 in rare cases
    - – CDX-2 does not play role in intestinal phenotype of these tumors
  - o BRAF positive in most cases, predominantly in invasive tumors in older patients
- Negative
  - o CEA, p53, calcitonin
  - o β-catenin (membranous)

Genetic Testing

- *BRAF* V600E mutation may be present
  - o Typically found in tumors of older male patients
  - o Associated with distant metastases and aggressive behavior

DIFFERENTIAL DIAGNOSIS

Tall Cell Variant

- Cells tall (height 3x width)
- Nuclear grooves abundant
- Numerous nuclear pseudoinclusions seen
- Nuclei basally located
- No pseudostratification of nuclei
- Cytoplasm eosinophilic

Papillary Thyroid Carcinoma, Classic Variant

- Conventional papillary carcinoma nuclei
- Papillary architecture predominates
- Cyclin-D1 negative

Metastases

- Must rule out metastases from other sites of origin that may have similar morphology
  - o Endometrial
  - o Colorectal
  - o Immunohistochemistry for TTF-1 and pax-8 may be useful

DIAGNOSTIC CHECKLIST

Clinically Relevant Pathologic Features

- Gross appearance
  - o Well-circumscribed and partially encapsulated (clinically indolent)
  - o Diffusely infiltrative (clinically aggressive)

Pathologic Interpretation Pearls

- Follicular cells with pseudostratified, hyperchromatic nuclei and supranuclear and subnuclear vacuoles

SELECTED REFERENCES

1. Bongiovanni M et al: Columnar cell variant of papillary thyroid carcinoma: Cytomorphological characteristics of 11 cases with histological correlation and literature review. Cancer. 125(6):389-397, 2017
2. Rottuntikarn W et al: Cytomorphology and immunocytochemistry of columnar cell variant of papillary thyroid carcinoma. Cytopathology. ePub, 2017
3. Afrogheh AH et al: Molecular characterization of an endometrial endometrioid adenocarcinoma metastatic to a thyroid Hürthle cell adenoma showing cancerization of follicles. Endocr Pathol. 27(3):213-9, 2016
4. Verma R et al: Columnar cell variant of papillary thyroid carcinoma: A diagnostic dilemma in fine-needle aspiration cytology. Diagn Cytopathol. 44(10):816-9, 2016
5. Bongiovanni M et al: CDX2 expression in columnar variant of papillary thyroid carcinoma. Thyroid. 23(11):1498-9, 2013
6. Sujoy V et al: Columnar cell variant of papillary thyroid carcinoma: a study of 10 cases with emphasis on CDX2 expression. Thyroid. 23(6):714-9, 2013
7. Enriquez ML et al: CDX2 expression in columnar cell variant of papillary thyroid carcinoma. Am J Clin Pathol. 137(5):722-6, 2012
8. Chen JH et al: Clinicopathological and molecular characterization of nine cases of columnar cell variant of papillary thyroid carcinoma. Mod Pathol. 24(5):739-49, 2011
9. Lloyd RV, Buehler D, Khanafshar E. Papillary thyroid carcinoma variants. Head Neck Pathol. 2011 Mar;5(1):51-6. Epub 2011 Jan 8. Review. PubMed PMID: 21221869; PubMed Central PMCID: PMC3037461.
10. Silver CE et al: Aggressive variants of papillary thyroid carcinoma. Head Neck. 33(7):1052-9, 2011
11. Albores-Saavedra J et al: The many faces and mimics of papillary thyroid carcinoma. Endocr Pathol. 17(1):1-18, 2006
12. Barton CP 3rd et al: Columnar cell variant of papillary thyroid carcinoma. Ear Nose Throat J. 85(10):640, 643, 2006
13. Wenig BM et al: Thyroid papillary carcinoma of columnar cell type: a clinicopathologic study of 16 cases. Cancer. 82(4):740-53, 1998
14. Fukunaga M et al: Columnar cell carcinoma of the thyroid. Pathol Int. 47(7):489-92, 1997
15. Evans HL: Encapsulated columnar-cell neoplasms of the thyroid. A report of four cases suggesting a favorable prognosis. Am J Surg Pathol. 20(10):1205-11, 1996
16. Ferreiro JA et al: Columnar cell carcinoma of the thyroid: report of three additional cases. Hum Pathol. 27(11):1156-60, 1996
17. Gaertner EM et al: The columnar cell variant of thyroid papillary carcinoma. Case report and discussion of an unusually aggressive thyroid papillary carcinoma. Am J Surg Pathol. 19(8):940-7, 1995
18. Mizukami Y et al: Columnar cell carcinoma of the thyroid gland: a case report and review of the literature. Hum Pathol. 25(10):1098-101, 1994

Gross Features

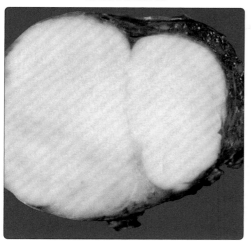

Papillae and Pseudostratification

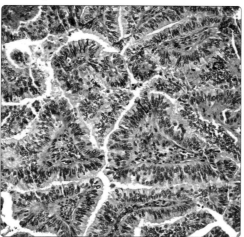

(Left) *Gross cut surface shows a large, bosselated tumor with a white and solid well-circumscribed surface that almost entirely replaces the thyroid lobe.* (Right) *H&E highlights the classic nuclear stratification seen in this variant. The nuclei are elongated in this example, and the cells have eosinophilic cytoplasm. Note the papillary architecture with fibrovascular cores.*

Pseudostratified Epithelium

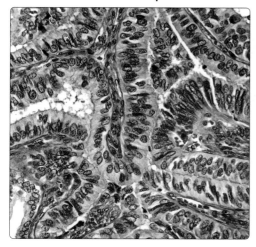

Extrathyroidal Extension

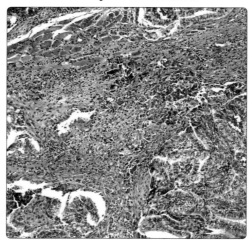

(Left) *The neoplastic follicular cells have basally pseudostratified and hyperchromatic nuclei with a pale eosinophilic cytoplasm and are arranged in a trabecular pattern. There is only focal nuclear clearing.* (Right) *H&E demonstrates involvement of perithyroid soft tissues. Here, tumor can be seen infiltrating skeletal muscle. The tumor cells show characteristic features of the columnar cell variant of PTC.*

Invasion into Fibroadipose Tissue

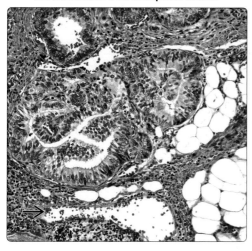

TTF-1 Staining

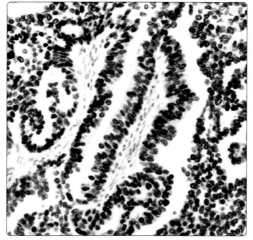

(Left) *These tumors are more aggressive when nonencapsulated. Tumor cells can be seen directly adjacent to adipose tissue. The tumor cells are approaching (but not involving) a vessel ➡.* (Right) *This variant characteristically stains positively for TTF-1, demonstrating strong nuclear staining. The staining pattern also highlights the stratified pattern of the nuclei. TTF-1 is useful for differentiating primary thyroid carcinoma from metastases from other sites.*

ETIOLOGY/PATHOGENESIS

- Clear cell variant is related to oncocytic variant, and tumors with clear cells usually have oncocytic cells as well
- Clear cell appearance believed to be due to mitochondrial expansion or accumulation of glycogen or mucin
  - Clear change has been attributed to dilated mitochondria

CLINICAL ISSUES

- Frequency is reported to be 1.7% of all papillary thyroid carcinoma (PTC) cases
- Appears to be same as in conventional PTC
- Extrathyroid extension, angiolymphatic invasion, and lymph node metastases are associated with poorer prognosis

MACROSCOPIC

- Solid in consistency; pale to white
- May be well circumscribed or infiltrating upon gross inspection

MICROSCOPIC

- Cells show cytoplasmic clearing
  - Range from water clear to granular in appearance
  - Usually associated with oncocytic cells
- Nuclear features of PTC are present
- Papillary, solid, or follicular architecture
- Varying amounts of colloid may be present
- May be associated with background lymphocytic thyroiditis

ANCILLARY TESTS

- TTF-1 and thyroglobulin (+)
- Alcian blue, PAS, and mucicarmine (+)

TOP DIFFERENTIAL DIAGNOSES

- Clear cell medullary thyroid carcinoma
- Follicular carcinoma
- Undifferentiated thyroid carcinoma
- Metastatic renal cell carcinoma

Clear Cell Follicular Variant

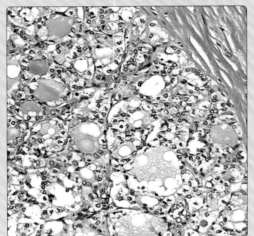

Cellular Characteristics

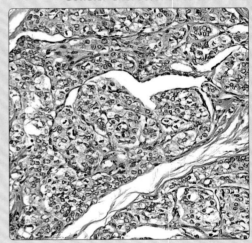

(Left) Papillary thyroid carcinoma (PTC), clear cell variant, is characterized by tumor cells with clear cytoplasm. This clear cell tumor has a predominant follicular architecture and is encapsulated. (Right) Clear cell-variant PTC may have a solid architecture. The nuclei are pale staining with irregular contours. The cytoplasm of the tumor cells ranges from water clear to granular in appearance.

Clear Cells Intermixed With Nonclear Cells

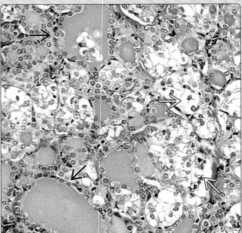

HBME-1 Immunopositivity in Clear Cells

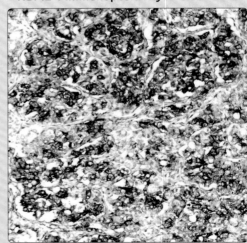

(Left) H&E demonstrates the cytologic and cytoplasmic characteristics in different areas of this PTC with follicular ➡ and clear cell ➡ components. The clear cells have abundant clear cytoplasm, while the nonclear cells show an oncocytic staining pattern. (Right) Clear cells may be present in thyroid carcinomas, including medullary carcinoma, papillary carcinoma, and follicular carcinoma. HBME-1 membranous staining is characteristic of PTC.

TERMINOLOGY

Definitions

- Malignant neoplasm composed predominantly of tumor cells with clear cytoplasm and papillary thyroid carcinoma (PTC) nuclear features

ETIOLOGY/PATHOGENESIS

Pathogenesis

- Clear cell appearance believed to be due to mitochondrial expansion or accumulation of glycogen or mucin
  - Electron microscopy reveals dilated empty mitochondria
- Also believed to be related to TSH overstimulation

CLINICAL ISSUES

Epidemiology

- Incidence
  - Rare variant of PTC: ~ 1.5% of all PTC

Presentation

- Present as neck mass
  - If tumors are large, patients may present with obstructive symptoms
- Patient may be asymptomatic with nodule found on physical exam

Treatment

- Includes surgical resection
- Lymph node dissection if indicated
- Radioactive iodine therapy may be used as adjunct to surgical therapy

Prognosis

- Appears to be same as in conventional PTC
- Extrathyroid extension, angiolymphatic invasion, and lymph node metastases are associated with poorer prognosis

MACROSCOPIC

General Features

- Solid in consistency; pale to white
- May be well circumscribed or infiltrating upon gross inspection

MICROSCOPIC

Histologic Features

- Often found in conjunction with other variants of PTC
- Tumors may be well circumscribed or infiltrative
- May be encapsulated
- Papillary, solid, or follicular architecture
  - Papillary architecture is less common than follicular and solid
  - Microfollicular pattern may also be seen
- Fibrous septa present between follicles or nests of cells
- Varying amounts of colloid may be present
- Psammoma bodies may be present
- Necrosis is absent
- May be associated with background lymphocytic thyroiditis

Cytologic Features

- Cells are cuboidal to columnar in shape
  - Cuboidal in solid and follicular areas
  - Cuboidal to low columnar in papillary areas
- Cells show cytoplasmic clearing
  - Range from water clear to granular in appearance
  - In columnar cells, only apical clearing of cytoplasm may be evident, which contrasts with oncocytic basal cytoplasm
- Prominent cell membranes
- Nuclear features of PTC are present
  - May only be present focally
  - Clear, pale-staining chromatin
  - Irregular nuclear membranes with nuclear grooves
  - Otherwise, nuclei are round with prominent nucleoli
- Nuclei are centrally located
  - May be basally or centrally located in papillary structures

ANCILLARY TESTS

Histochemistry

- Alcian blue, PAS, and mucicarmine (+)

Immunohistochemistry

- Positive for
  - TTF-1 (nuclear)
  - Thyroglobulin (cytoplasmic and in colloid)

DIFFERENTIAL DIAGNOSIS

Follicular Carcinoma

- Encapsulated tumors with capsular ± vascular invasion
- Lacks PTC nuclear features

Undifferentiated Thyroid Carcinoma

- Lacks PTC nuclear features

Metastatic Carcinoma

- Lacks PTC nuclear features
- Immunohistochemistry is useful
  - TTF-1 and thyroglobulin are useful for differentiating primary and metastatic disease
- Metastatic renal cell carcinoma is positive for CD10 and renal cell antigen

SELECTED REFERENCES

1. Cipriani NA et al: Clear cell change in thyroid carcinoma: a clinicopathologic and molecular study with identification of variable genetic anomalies. Thyroid. 27(6):819-824, 2017
2. Tong GX et al: Mutations of TSHR and TP53 genes in an aggressive clear cell follicular carcinoma of the thyroid. Endocr Pathol. 26(4):315-9, 2015
3. Yazici B et al: A clear cell variant of papillary thyroid microcarcinoma with lung, bone, and soft tissue metastases. Clin Nucl Med. 40(11):885-7, 2015
4. Sayar I et al: Clear cell variant of follicular thyroid carcinoma with normal thyroid-stimulating hormone value: a case report. J Med Case Rep. 8:160, 2014
5. Albores-Saavedra J et al: The many faces and mimics of papillary thyroid carcinoma. Endocr Pathol. 17(1):1-18, 2006
6. Asanuma K et al: Pure clear cell papillary thyroid carcinoma with chronic thyroiditis: report of a case. Surg Today. 28(4):464-6, 1998
7. Carcangiu ML et al: Clear cell change in primary thyroid tumors. a study of 38 cases. Am J Surg Pathol. 9(10):705-22, 1985
8. Dickersin GR et al: Papillary carcinoma of the thyroid, oxyphil cell type, "clear cell" variant: a light- and electron-microscopic study. Am J Surg Pathol. 4(5):501-9, 1980

TERMINOLOGY

- Term solid variant should be used when all or nearly all of tumor not belonging to any of other variants has solid, trabecular, or nested/insular appearance

ETIOLOGY/PATHOGENESIS

- Strongly associated with exposure to ionizing radiation, though sporadic cases occur

CLINICAL ISSUES

- Rare, accounting for 1-3% of all adult PTC cases
- Comprise ~ 1/2 of cases of post-Chernobyl radiation exposure, mostly in children
- These tumors appear to be more frequently associated with lung metastases and may confer slightly higher mortality rate in adults
- This variant has high propensity for extrathyroidal extension and cervical lymph node metastases

MACROSCOPIC

- Tumors are usually solitary, well circumscribed, but unencapsulated

MICROSCOPIC

- Tumor shows predominantly solid architecture
- Tumor cells are arranged in solid sheets, nests, or cord-like trabeculae
- Cells have classic papillary thyroid carcinoma nuclear features
- Psammoma bodies are seen in < 50% of cases
- Fibrosis is common in varying amounts

ANCILLARY TESTS

- This variant is frequently associated with *RET/NCOA4* fusions in radiation-associated and pediatric cases
- Rearrangement of the *RET* gene is not associated in tumors in adult population
- Tumor cells are positive for TTF-1, pax-8, and thyroglobulin

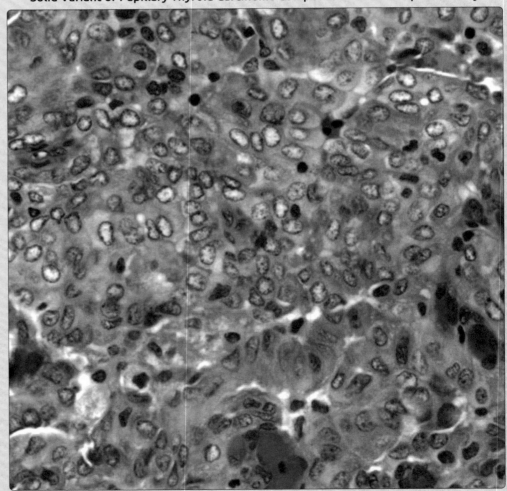

Solid Variant of Papillary Thyroid Carcinoma Composed of Solid Component Only

Solid variant papillary thyroid cancer (SVPTC) is a rare type of thyroid malignancy that is composed of (or predominately of) a solid component. This papillary thyroid carcinoma (PTC) should be differentiated from the poorly differentiated carcinoma that has the same growth pattern but is characterized by cells that lack the nuclear features of PTC, necrosis and high mitotic activity.

TERMINOLOGY

Abbreviations

- Solid variant papillary thyroid cancer (SVPTC)

Synonyms

- Solid variant of papillary thyroid carcinoma (PTC)
- Solid/trabecular variant of PTC
- Trabecular variant of PTC

Definitions

- Malignant neoplasm composed predominantly of solid sheets, nests, or cords of cells that have PTC nuclear features
- Term solid variant should be used when all or nearly all of tumor not belonging to any of other variants has solid, trabecular, or nested/insular appearance

ETIOLOGY/PATHOGENESIS

Environmental Exposure

- Strongly associated with exposure to ionizing radiation, though sporadic cases occur

CLINICAL ISSUES

Epidemiology

- Incidence
  - Rare, accounting for 1-3% of all PTC cases of adult PTCs
  - Comprise ~ 37% of cases of post-Chernobyl radiation exposure (mostly in children)
  - In children, 4% of all PTC cases are this subtype
- Age
  - In adults, these tumors occur in later half of 5th decade
  - In children, most affected are < 5 years old
- Sex
  - In sporadic cases, F:M = 9:1
  - No gender predilection for tumors related to radiation exposure
- Ethnicity
  - More common in Japan (reported up to 16% of cases)

Presentation

- Usually present as solitary thyroid nodule
- Neck swelling may be present with lymph node metastases

Treatment

- Total or near total thyroidectomy with en bloc resection of gross disease
- Modified radical neck dissection when cervical lymph node metastases are present
- Radioactive iodine ablation may be considered following surgery

Prognosis

- This variant has high propensity for extrathyroidal extension and cervical lymph node metastases
- Some studies report prognosis similar to that of classic PTC while other authors report more aggressive disease
- These tumors appear to be more frequently associated with lung metastases and may confer slightly higher mortality rate in adults

- Various features associated with poor prognosis are common
  - Extrathyroid extension is seen in up to 84% of cases
  - As many as 83% of cases have lymph node metastases
  - Distant metastases reported in 17-21% of cases
- Recurrence rate reported to be as high as 33%

MACROSCOPIC

General Features

- Tumors are usually solitary, well circumscribed, but unencapsulated
- White and firm and may be associated with fibrosis grossly

Size

- Usually < 2 cm

MICROSCOPIC

Histologic Features

- Tumor shows predominantly solid architecture
  - Tumor cells are arranged in solid sheets, nests, or cord-like trabeculae
  - Variable amount of intermixed follicles
- Nuclear features of PTC are present
  - Intranuclear pseudoinclusion is rarely present
- Psammoma bodies are seen in < 50% of cases
- Fibrosis is common in varying amounts
  - Ranges from delicate bands between nests of cells to broad bands of fibrosis
- Lack fibrous capsule
- Necrosis is uncommon

Cytologic Features

- Cells have classic PTC nuclear features
  - Ground-glass chromatin pattern
  - Irregular nuclear membranes
    - Contain nuclear grooves and pseudoinclusions
  - Nuclear crowding and overlap are common
- Mitoses are rare

ANCILLARY TESTS

Cytology

- Sheets or groups of cells are arranged in loosely cohesive clusters
- May show thick, tightly cohesive anastomotic cords
- Single cells are also common
- Cells are polygonal in shape
- Cytoplasm is eosinophilic and granular
- Cells have characteristic PTC nuclear findings

Immunohistochemistry

- Tumor cells are positive for TTF-1, pax-8, and thyroglobulin

Genetic Testing

- This variant is frequently associated with rearrangement of the *RET* gene in radiation-associated and pediatric cases
  - Most commonly associated with *RET/NCOA4* mutation
    - Paracentric chromosomal inversion involving *RET* protooncogene
    - Fusion of 3' portion of *RET* to 5' region of unrelated genes

– Leads to activation of *RET* tyrosine kinase and MAPK signaling pathways and subsequent tumorigenesis of follicular-derived cells
- *RET* gene fusion is not associated in tumors in adult population

DIFFERENTIAL DIAGNOSIS

Poorly Differentiated Thyroid Carcinoma

- Lacks classic PTC nuclear features
- Associated with necrosis
- Usually associated with high mitotic activity
- Usually cyclin-D1 and p53 (+)

DIAGNOSTIC CHECKLIST

Pathologic Interpretation Pearls

- SVPTC is rare type of thyroid malignancy that is composed by (or predominately by) solid component
- Term "solid variant" should be used when all or nearly all of tumor not belonging to any of other variants has solid, trabecular, or nested appearance
- This PTC should be differentiated from poorly differentiated carcinoma
  o Has same growth pattern
  o Characterized by cells that lack nuclear features of conventional PTC
  o Lack necrosis
  o Lack high mitotic activity

SELECTED REFERENCES

1. Li W et al: A rare case report of very low thyroglobulin and a negative whole-body scan in a patient with a solid variant of papillary thyroid carcinoma with distant metastases. Medicine (Baltimore). 96(7):e6086, 2017
2. Lloyd RV et al: WHO Classification of Tumours of Endocrine Organs. Lyon, France: IARC Press, 2017
3. Ohashi R et al: Clinicopathological significance of a solid component in papillary thyroid carcinoma. Histopathology. 70(5):775-781, 2017
4. Ohashi R et al: Expression of MRP1 and ABCG2 is associated with adverse clinical outcomes of the papillary thyroid carcinoma with a solid component. Hum Pathol. ePub, 2017
5. Ohashi R et al: Fine needle aspiration cytology of the papillary thyroid carcinoma with a solid component: a cytological and clinical correlation. Diagn Cytopathol. 45(5):391-398, 2017
6. Paulson VA et al: NIFTP accounts for over half of "carcinomas" harboring RAS mutations. Thyroid. 7(4):506-511, 2017
7. Collini P et al: Histopathology, immunohistochemistry and molecular biology of follicular epithelium-derived pediatric thyroid carcinomas. Curr Pediatr Rev. 12(4):272-279, 2016
8. Higuchi M et al: Cytological features of solid variants of papillary thyroid carcinoma: a fine needle aspiration cytology study of 18 cases. Cytopathology. 28(4):268-272, 2016
9. Onder S et al: Classic architecture with multicentricity and local recurrence, and absence of TERT promoter mutations are correlates of BRAF (V600E) harboring pediatric papillary thyroid carcinomas. Endocr Pathol. 27(2):153-61, 2016
10. Prasad ML et al: NTRK fusion oncogenes in pediatric papillary thyroid carcinoma in northeast United States. Cancer. 122(7):1097-107, 2016
11. Ritterhouse LL et al: ROS1 rearrangement in thyroid cancer. Thyroid. 26(6):794-7, 2016
12. Giorgadze TA et al: Fine-needle aspiration cytology of the solid variant of papillary thyroid carcinoma: a study of 13 cases with clinical, histologic, and ultrasound correlations. Cancer Cytopathol. 123(2):71-81, 2015
13. Abdul Rahman WF et al: Solid variant of papillary thyroid carcinoma in a 14-year-old girl. BMJ Case Rep. 2013, 2013
14. Kakudo K et al: Classification of thyroid follicular cell tumors: with special reference to borderline lesions [Review]. Endocr J. 59(1):1-12, 2011
15. Damle N et al: Solid variant of papillary carcinoma thyroid in a child with no history of radiation exposure. Indian J Nucl Med. 26(4):196-8, 2011
16. LiVolsi VA et al: The Chernobyl thyroid cancer experience: pathology. Clin Oncol (R Coll Radiol). 23(4):261-7, 2011
17. Lloyd RV et al: Papillary thyroid carcinoma variants. Head Neck Pathol. 5(1):51-6, 2011
18. Silver CE et al: Aggressive variants of papillary thyroid carcinoma. Head Neck. 33(7):1052-9, 2011
19. Chiosea S et al: A novel complex BRAF mutation detected in a solid variant of papillary thyroid carcinoma. Endocr Pathol. 20(2):122-6, 2009
20. Troncone G et al: Cytological and molecular diagnosis of solid variant of papillary thyroid carcinoma: a case report. Cytojournal. 5:2, 2008
21. Volante M et al: A practical diagnostic approach to solid/trabecular nodules in the thyroid. Endocr Pathol. 19(2):75-81, 2008
22. Volante M et al: Poorly differentiated thyroid carcinoma: the Turin proposal for the use of uniform diagnostic criteria and an algorithmic diagnostic approach. Am J Surg Pathol. 31(8):1256-64, 2007
23. Albores-Saavedra J et al: The many faces and mimics of papillary thyroid carcinoma. Endocr Pathol. 17(1):1-18, 2006
24. Collini P et al: Papillary carcinoma of the thyroid gland of childhood and adolescence: Morphologic subtypes, biologic behavior and prognosis: a clinicopathologic study of 42 sporadic cases treated at a single institution during a 30-year period. Am J Surg Pathol. 30(11):1420-6, 2006
25. Nguyen GK et al: Solid/trabecular variant papillary carcinoma of the thyroid: report of three cases with fine-needle aspiration. Diagn Cytopathol. 34(10):712-4, 2006
26. Trovisco V et al: A new BRAF gene mutation detected in a case of a solid variant of papillary thyroid carcinoma. Hum Pathol. 36(6):694-7, 2005
27. Massi D et al: Ultrastructural features of solid/trabecular areas in differentiated thyroid carcinoma. Ultrastruct Pathol. 25(1):13-20, 2001
28. Nair M et al: Papillary carcinoma of the thyroid and its variants: a cytohistological correlation. Diagn Cytopathol. 24(3):167-73, 2001
29. Nikiforov YE et al: Solid variant of papillary thyroid carcinoma: incidence, clinical-pathologic characteristics, molecular analysis, and biologic behavior. Am J Surg Pathol. 25(12):1478-84, 2001
30. Nikiforov YE et al: Distinct pattern of ret oncogene rearrangements in morphological variants of radiation-induced and sporadic thyroid papillary carcinomas in children. Cancer Res. 57(9):1690-4, 1997
31. Mizukami Y et al: Papillary thyroid carcinoma in Kanazawa, Japan: prognostic significance of histological subtypes. Histopathology. 20(3):243-50, 1992

Well-Circumscribed Tumor

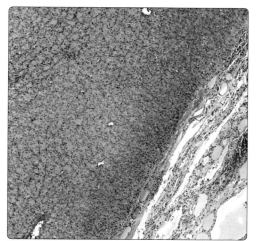

Solid and Trabecular Pattern

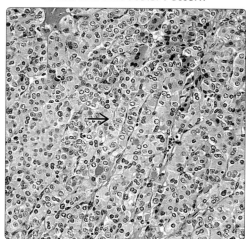

(Left) The solid variant of PTC is often characterized by solid sheets of tumor cells. There is little to no colloid present, in contrast to the adjacent normal thyroid. (Right) Architecturally, these tumors are composed of solid sheets, nests, or cord-like trabeculae ➡. Tram-track-like trabeculae are seen in the center of this image. The classic nuclear features of PTC, nuclear clearing, and nuclear grooves are present.

Fibrous Stroma

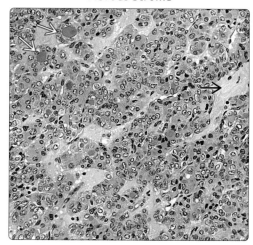

SVPTC Nuclear Features

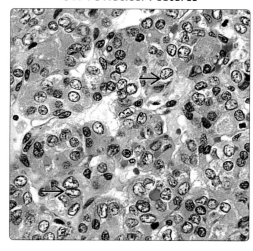

(Left) This example shows nests of tumor cells that lack colloid, though a few residual follicles ➡ are present. The solid nests are surrounded by delicate fibrohyaline stroma and are also associated with varying amounts of fibrosis ➡. (Right) At higher magnification note the classic nuclear features of PTC: Nuclear clearing, intranuclear grooves, and abundant pale eosinophilic cytoplasm with indistinct borders. The nuclei are enlarged, crowded, and irregular in shape with pale chromatin and nuclear grooves ➡.

Solid Arrangement With Psammoma Body

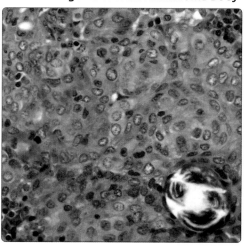

Cell Characteristics

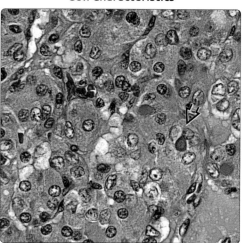

(Left) Solid variant of PTC showing the solid nests composed by cells with classic PTC nuclear features. No papillary growth is present, and a psammoma body is seen. These are usually present in < 50% of cases. (Right) The high-power view of this tumor shows the characteristic findings of the solid variant. There is a predominantly solid architecture, and the tumor cells are arranged in solid sheets, nests, or cord-like trabeculae. There is an intermixed small follicle ➡, and the nuclear features of PTC are present.

Papillary Thyroid Carcinoma, Cribriform-Morular Variant

TERMINOLOGY

- Rare variant of thyroid carcinoma characterized by cribriform architecture with squamous morules and lacking colloid and characteristic nuclear features of papillary thyroid carcinoma (PTC)
- It can occur in sporadic form or as part of familial adenomatous polyposis (FAP) syndrome

ETIOLOGY/PATHOGENESIS

- Associated with FAP
  o Found in ~ 12% of FAP patients
- Sporadic

CLINICAL ISSUES

- When associated with FAP, these tumors are usually bilateral, present at younger age, and are 10x more common in female patients

MICROSCOPIC

- Tumors are either single (sporadic cases) or, multifocal and bilateral (FAP-associated tumors)
- Combination of cribriform, morular, solid, follicular, papillary, spindled, or trabecular patterns of growth
- Squamous morules with peculiar nuclear clearing

ANCILLARY TESTS

- Aberrant nuclear and cytoplasmic expression of β-catenin in cribriform and morular areas
- Squamoid morules are positive for CK5/6 and for CD5

TOP DIFFERENTIAL DIAGNOSES

- Tall cell variant of PTC
- Columnar cell variant of PTC
- Hyalinizing trabecular tumor

DIAGNOSTIC CHECKLIST

- Any patient with diagnosis of cribriform-morular variant should be screened for FAP

Multiple Small Thyroid Tumors in Familial Adenomatous Polyposis

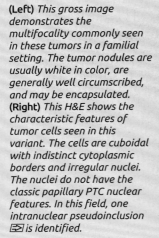

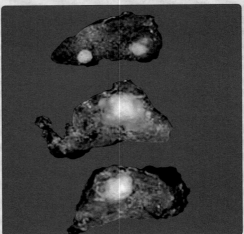

Characteristic Cytological Features

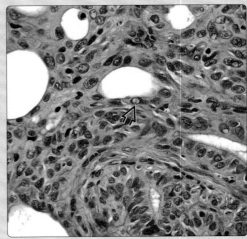

(Left) This gross image demonstrates the multifocality commonly seen in these tumors in a familial setting. The tumor nodules are usually white in color, are generally well circumscribed, and may be encapsulated. (Right) This H&E shows the characteristic features of tumor cells seen in this variant. The cells are cuboidal with indistinct cytoplasmic borders and irregular nuclei. The nuclei do not have the classic papillary PTC nuclear features. In this field, one intranuclear pseudoinclusion ⊵ is identified.

Strong Nuclear and Cytoplasmic Stain

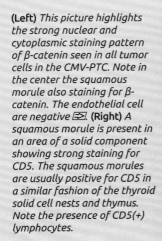

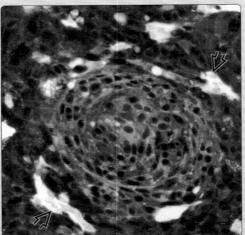

CD5 in Squamous Morule

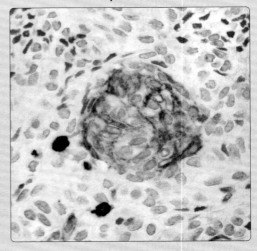

(Left) This picture highlights the strong nuclear and cytoplasmic staining pattern of β-catenin seen in all tumor cells in the CMV-PTC. Note in the center the squamous morule also staining for β-catenin. The endothelial cell are negative ⊵. (Right) A squamous morule is present in an area of a solid component showing strong staining for CD5. The squamous morules are usually positive for CD5 in a similar fashion of the thyroid solid cell nests and thymus. Note the presence of CD5(+) lymphocytes.

TERMINOLOGY

Abbreviations

- Papillary thyroid carcinoma, cribriform-morular variant (PTC-CMV) or (CMV PTC)

Synonyms

- Cribriform morular carcinoma

Definitions

- Rare variant of thyroid carcinoma characterized by cribriform architecture with squamous morules lacking colloid and characteristic nuclear features of papillary thyroid carcinoma (PTC)
- Considered to constitute distinct category of thyroid carcinoma
- It can occur in sporadic form or as part of familial adenomatous polyposis (FAP) syndrome

ETIOLOGY/PATHOGENESIS

Familial

- Associated with FAP
  - Found in ~ 12% of FAP patients
- Accounts for 90% of cases of patients who have FAP and synchronous papillary thyroid carcinoma
- Associated with germline mutations in *APC* gene
- 1/6 of patients with CMV-PTC may have occult FAP
- Younger patients
- More likely to have multicentric tumors than those with sporadic CMV-PTC
- RAS mutation may be detected

Sporadic

- Occur at later age than in familial counterpart
- Not all cases of PTC-CMV are associated with FAP; some are considered sporadic
- Rare cases are associated with somatic mutations in *APC* gene
- Tumors are single and larger than familial tumors

APC Gene Mutation

- *APC* gene is located on chromosome 5q21-q22
- Mutations of *APC* are common in adenomatous familial polyposis and are found in tumors showing PTC-CMV phenotype
  - More commonly, *APC* germline mutations are identified; rarely, somatic mutations can be present as well
- *APC* gene is normally active and causes degradation of β-catenin preventing its accumulation in cells, thus inhibiting Wnt signaling
  - β-catenin is normally present in low levels within cytoplasm and is mainly expressed in cell membranes
  - Activation of Wnt signaling leads to accumulation of β-catenin in nucleus
    - β-catenin accumulation can be visualized via immunohistochemistry
- *APC* plays significant role in Wnt pathway, which is responsible for embryonic development of tissues and causes tumorigenesis when aberrantly activated
  - Inappropriate activation of Wnt pathway through loss of *APC* function contributes to cancer progression, as in FAP
  - Wnt signaling is transmitted to nuclei by cytoplasmic β-catenin
    - β-catenin is protein encoded by *CTNNB1* gene

CLINICAL ISSUES

Epidemiology

- Incidence
  - Very rare, accounting for 0.1-0.2% of papillary thyroid carcinoma cases
- Age
  - Familial tumors occurs in young female patients, while sporadic tumors occur in older patients
  - Usually present in patients younger than 30 years
- Sex
  - Occurs almost exclusively in females when associated with FAP

Presentation

- When associated with FAP, these tumors are usually bilateral, present at younger age, and are 10x more common in female patients
- Usually present as painless thyroid nodule
- May be found incidentally on routine physical exam

Treatment

- Surgical approaches
  - Total thyroidectomy is usually performed due to high incidence of bilaterality
- Radiation
  - Locoregional radiation therapy may be indicated in some cases
- Further testing
  - Patients found to have PTC-CMV should have colon screening
  - Clinicians may also recommend both colorectal screening and genetic counseling for family members if indicated

Prognosis

- Overall prognosis is similar to that of classic variant of PTC
- Low risk for metastases
- < 10% of cases show aggressive behavior

IMAGING

Ultrasonographic Findings

- May reveal single or multiple thyroid nodules that are usually well circumscribed or encapsulated

MACROSCOPIC

General Features

- Tumors are usually multifocal and vary in size
  - Most patients have multiple and bilateral tumor nodules
- Tumor foci are well circumscribed
- Pale brown to tan in color
- May be solid or cystic
  - Cysts are thin walled and filled with hemorrhagic fluid
- Necrosis and calcifications are absent
- Some nodules are white, firm, and fibrotic

Size

- Tumor foci vary greatly in size
  - Foci can range from microcarcinomas (< 1.0 cm) to 3.0 cm

MICROSCOPIC

Histologic Features

- Tumors are either single (sporadic) or multifocal and bilateral (familial)
- When encapsulated, tumors may invade through capsule
  - Angioinvasion may be present within capsule
- Typical cribriform morular carcinoma are easily recognized in low-power microscopy
- Combination of cribriform, morular, solid, follicular, papillary, spindled, or trabecular patterns of growth
  - These various growth patterns merge intricately together
- Cribriform architecture formed by anastomosing bars or arches 1-2 cell layers thick
  - Lack fibrovascular stroma
- Follicular structures are devoid of colloid, though few may have histiocytes within their lumina
  - Angulated and elongated
- Squamous morules with intranuclear inclusions (a.k.a. peculiar nuclear inclusions)
  - Not early form of squamous metaplasia (immunohistochemical profile is different)
- Very little colloid is found within tumor deposits
- Sclerotic/fibrotic bands may give tumor nodular appearance
- Hyalinized material is frequently found in these tumors
- Psammoma bodies are absent though calcifications are rare
- Necrosis is absent
- Background thyroid may be normal, multinodular, or show lymphocytic thyroiditis

Cytologic Features

- Tumor cells lining papillary or tubular structures are cuboidal or elongated in shape
  - Contain abundant cytoplasm
  - Show nuclear pseudostratification
  - Nuclei are hyperchromatic in these areas
    - Have small nucleoli
- Cells are amphophilic to eosinophilic in color
- Few cells may have spindled shape
  - Typically in solid areas and are arranged in whorling pattern, forming morules
- Cells have eosinophilic cytoplasm
- Morular cells show peculiar nuclear clearing
  - Majority of nucleus is occupied by clear area with condensed chromatin at periphery
- Nuclei may have grooves
- Lack of colloid

ANCILLARY TESTS

Cytology

- FNA specimens are generally quite cellular
- Large 3-dimensional clusters and monolayered sheets are abundant

- Branching tissue fragments with fibrovascular cores may be appreciated
- Cribriform architecture can be appreciated
  - Round to oval slit-like spaces formed by spindle to ovoid cells within tissue fragments
- Squamoid morules may be identified on cytology
  - Cell clusters with eddy formation
  - Composed of spindled and oval tumor cells
- Tumor cells are mostly round to ovoid, though few columnar or spindle-shaped cells may be present
- Cytoplasm tends to be eosinophilic
- Nuclei tend to be eccentrically placed
- Some cells have elongated cytoplasmic tails
- Nuclei are round to oval in shape
  - Though spindle-shaped cells have spindle-shaped nuclei
- Nuclei have grooves and indentations
- Peculiar nuclear clearings may be seen
  - Pale-staining area occupying most of nuclei accompanied by dense chromatin at periphery
- Absence of nuclear inclusions
- Generally lack ground-glass chromatin pattern
- Background is typically clean
  - May contain few macrophages (± hemosiderin)
  - Colloid, psammoma bodies, and multinucleated giant cells are absent
- β-catenin stain may help

Immunohistochemistry

- Aberrant nuclear and cytoplasmic expression of β-catenin in cribriform and morular areas
  - Nontumor follicular cells show membranous staining
  - Can be positive on cytology aspirate specimens
- Other positive stains
  - Squamoid morules are positive for CK5/6 and for CD5
  - TTF-1, pax-8, ER, PR, Bcl-2 (nuclear), E-cadherin, galectin-3, p53, cyclin-D1, CK7, CK19, Ki-67
- Negative immunostains
  - Usually negative: HBME-1, thyroglobulin

Genetic Testing

- Germline mutation in *APC* gene in familial forms associated with FAP
- Somatic mutation in *APC* gene in sporadic cases
- *CTNNB1* and *PI3KCA* mutations have been reported
- *RET* rearrangement is negative (occurs in sporadic tumors occurring in FAP patients)
- RAS mutation is usually negative with very rare reported positive cases
- *BRAF* V600E mutation is negative

DIFFERENTIAL DIAGNOSIS

Tall Cell Variant of Papillary Thyroid Carcinoma

- Neoplastic cells have height that is 3x width
- Eosinophilic cytoplasm
- Nuclei have characteristic PTC features
- Abundant nuclear inclusions
- Lacks squamous morules and cribriform pattern seen in PTC-CMV

Columnar Cell Variant of Papillary Thyroid Carcinoma

- Neoplastic cells have columnar shape

- Nuclei are centrally located
- Lacks squamous morules and cribriform architecture

Hyalinizing Trabecular Tumor

- Lacks squamous morules
- Hyalinized stroma is present

DIAGNOSTIC CHECKLIST

Clinically Relevant Pathologic Features

- Any patient with diagnosis of cribriform-morular variant should be screened for FAP
  - Diagnosis of PTC-CMV may predate diagnosis of FAP by as many as 12 years

SELECTED REFERENCES

1. Lam AK et al: Cribriform-morular variant of papillary thyroid carcinoma: a distinctive type of thyroid cancer. Endocr Relat Cancer. 24(4):R109-R121, 2017
2. Priyani AA et al: Cribriform morular variant of papillary thyroid carcinoma: cytomorphology, differential diagnosis and diagnostic implications in patients with adenomatous polyposis coli. J Cytol. 33(4):235-238, 2016
3. Kwon MJ et al: Cribriform-morular variant of papillary thyroid carcinoma: a study of 3 cases featuring the PIK3CA mutation. Hum Pathol. 46(8):1180-8, 2015
4. Perea Del Pozo E et al: Cribiform variant of papillary thyroid cancer and familial adenomatous polyposis. Int J Surg Case Rep. 16:192-4, 2015
5. Pradhan D et al: Cribriform-morular variant of papillary thyroid carcinoma. Pathol Res Pract. 211(10):712-6, 2015
6. Giannelli SM et al: Familial adenomatous polyposis-associated, cribriform morular variant of papillary thyroid carcinoma harboring a K-RAS mutation: case presentation and review of molecular mechanisms. Thyroid. 24(7):1184-9, 2014
7. Levy RA et al: Cribriform-morular variant of papillary thyroid carcinoma: an indication to screen for occult FAP. Fam Cancer. 13(4):547-51, 2014
8. Boonyaarunnate T et al: Cribriform morular variant of papillary thyroid carcinoma: clinical and cytomorphological features on fine-needle aspiration. Acta Cytol. 57(2):127-33, 2013
9. Nakazawa T et al: Cribriform-morular variant of papillary thyroid carcinoma displaying poorly differentiated features. Int J Surg Pathol. 21(4):379-89, 2013
10. Cetta F et al: Familial adenomatous polyposis-associated papillary thyroid carcinoma shows an indolent course and usually, but not always, belongs to the cribriform-morular variant of papillary thyroid carcinoma. Acta Cytol. 56(1):107-8, 2012
11. Rossi ED et al: Cribriform-morular variant of papillary thyroid carcinoma in an 8-year-old girl: a case report with immunohistochemical and molecular testing. Int J Surg Pathol. 20(6):629-32, 2012
12. Ito Y et al: Our experience of treatment of cribriform morular variant of papillary thyroid carcinoma; difference in clinicopathological features of FAP-associated and sporadic patients. Endocr J. 58(8):685-9, 2011
13. Laury AR et al: Thyroid pathology in PTEN-hamartoma tumor syndrome: characteristic findings of a distinct entity. Thyroid. 21(2):135-44, 2011
14. Nosé V: Familial thyroid cancer: a review. Mod Pathol. 24 Suppl 2:S19-33, 2011
15. Smith JR et al: Thyroid nodules and cancer in children with PTEN hamartoma tumor syndrome. J Clin Endocrinol Metab. 96(1):34-7, 2011
16. Zhang Y et al: Endocrine tumors as part of inherited tumor syndromes. Adv Anat Pathol. 18(3):206-18, 2011
17. Hirokawa M et al: Cribriform-morular variant of papillary thyroid carcinoma–cytological and immunocytochemical findings of 18 cases. Diagn Cytopathol. 38(12):890-6, 2010
18. Nosé V: Thyroid cancer of follicular cell origin in inherited tumor syndromes. Adv Anat Pathol. 17(6):428-36, 2010
19. Cameselle-Teijeiro J et al: Cribriform-morular variant of papillary thyroid carcinoma: molecular characterization of a case with neuroendocrine differentiation and aggressive behavior. Am J Clin Pathol. 131(1):134-42, 2009
20. Dong Y et al: Cribriform-morular variant of papillary thyroid carcinoma: report of three cases and review of the literature. Pathology. 41(5):509-12, 2009
21. Donnellan KA et al: Papillary thyroid carcinoma and familial adenomatous polyposis of the colon. Am J Otolaryngol. 30(1):58-60, 2009
22. Jung CK et al: The cytological, clinical, and pathological features of the cribriform-morular variant of papillary thyroid carcinoma and mutation analysis of CTNNB1 and BRAF genes. Thyroid. 19(8):905-13, 2009
23. Rivera M et al: Encapsulated papillary thyroid carcinoma: a clinico-pathologic study of 106 cases with emphasis on its morphologic subtypes (histologic growth pattern). Thyroid. 19(2):119-27, 2009
24. Schuetze D et al: The T1799A BRAF mutation is absent in cribriform-morular variant of papillary carcinoma. Arch Pathol Lab Med. 133(5):803-5, 2009
25. Costa AM et al: BRAF mutation associated with other genetic events identifies a subset of aggressive papillary thyroid carcinoma. Clin Endocrinol (Oxf). 68(4):618-34, 2008
26. Dotto J et al: Familial thyroid carcinoma: a diagnostic algorithm. Adv Anat Pathol. 15(6):332-49, 2008
27. Groen EJ et al: Extra-intestinal manifestations of familial adenomatous polyposis. Ann Surg Oncol. 15(9):2439-50, 2008
28. Nosé V: Familial non-medullary thyroid carcinoma: an update. Endocr Pathol. 19(4):226-40, 2008
29. Herraiz M et al: Prevalence of thyroid cancer in familial adenomatous polyposis syndrome and the role of screening ultrasound examinations. Clin Gastroenterol Hepatol. 5(3):367-73, 2007
30. Subramaniam MM et al: Clonal characterization of sporadic cribriform-morular variant of papillary thyroid carcinoma by laser microdissection-based APC mutation analysis. Am J Clin Pathol. 128(6):994-1001, 2007
31. Dalal KM et al: Clinical curiosity: cribriform-morular variant of papillary thyroid carcinoma. Head Neck. 28(5):471-6, 2006
32. Uchino S et al: Mutational analysis of the APC gene in cribriform-morula variant of papillary thyroid carcinoma. World J Surg. 30(5):775-9, 2006
33. Chuah KL et al: Cytologic features of cribriform-morular variant of papillary carcinoma of the thyroid: a case report. Acta Cytol. 49(1):75-80, 2005
34. Chikkamuniyappa S et al: Cribriform-morular variant of papillary carcinoma: association with familial adenomatous polyposis - report of three cases and review of literature. Int J Med Sci. 1(1):43-49, 2004
35. Hirokawa M et al: Morules in cribriform-morular variant of papillary thyroid carcinoma: Immunohistochemical characteristics and distinction from squamous metaplasia. APMIS. 112(4-5):275-82, 2004
36. Kameyama K et al: Cribriform-morular variant of papillary thyroid carcinoma: ultrastructural study and somatic/germline mutation analysis of the APC gene. Ultrastruct Pathol. 28(2):97-102, 2004
37. Tomoda C et al: Cribriform-morular variant of papillary thyroid carcinoma: clue to early detection of familial adenomatous polyposis-associated colon cancer. World J Surg. 28(9):886-9, 2004
38. Ng SB et al: Cribriform-morular variant of papillary carcinoma: the sporadic counterpart of familial adenomatous polyposis-associated thyroid carcinoma. A case report with clinical and molecular genetic correlation. Pathology. 35(1):42-6, 2003
39. Xu B et al: Cribriform-morular variant of papillary thyroid carcinoma: a pathological and molecular genetic study with evidence of frequent somatic mutations in exon 3 of the beta-catenin gene. J Pathol. 199(1):58-67, 2003
40. Cameselle-Teijeiro J et al: Somatic but not germline mutation of the APC gene in a case of cribriform-morular variant of papillary thyroid carcinoma. Am J Clin Pathol. 115(4):486-93, 2001
41. Francesco C et al: Correspondence re: Cameselle-Teijeiro J, Chan JKC: Cribriform-morular variant of papillary carcinoma: a distinctive variant representing the sporadic counterpart of familial adenomatous polyposis-associated thyroid carcinoma? Mod Pathol. 13(3):363-5, 2000
42. Cameselle-Teijeiro J et al: Cribriform-morular variant of papillary carcinoma: a distinctive variant representing the sporadic counterpart of familial adenomatous polyposis-associated thyroid carcinoma? Mod Pathol. 12(4):400-11, 1999
43. Hizawa K et al: Association between thyroid cancer of cribriform variant and familial adenomatous polyposis. J Clin Pathol. 49(7):611-3, 1996
44. Harach HR et al: Familial adenomatous polyposis associated thyroid carcinoma: a distinct type of follicular cell neoplasm. Histopathology. 25(6):549-61, 1994

Polyps in Familial Adenomatous Polyposis

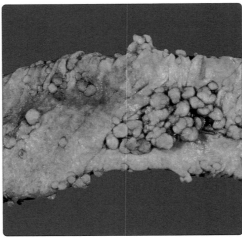

Retina

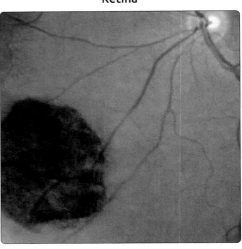

(Left) *This colon was resected from a patient with familial adenomatous polyposis. Note the numerous polyps present on the mucosal surface. These patients have an increased risk of developing PTC-CMV.* (Right) *This clinical photograph shows congenital hypertrophy of the pigmented retinal epithelium. This condition is benign and is often found in up to 2/3 of patients who have familial adenomatous polyposis (FAP). When associated with FAP, these lesions may be multiple and bilateral.*

Encapsulated Tumor

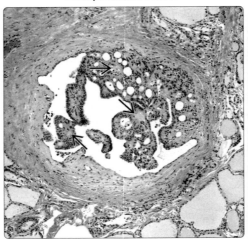

Thick Fibrous Capsule

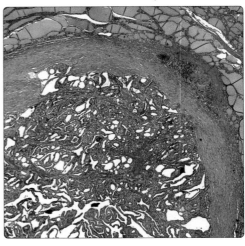

(Left) *Encapsulation is common among this subtype of tumor. This particular example shows a thick fibrous band encapsulating the tumor. Note the papillary and cribriform architecture. Also shown are eosinophilic foci of sclerosis/hyalinization ➡ within the stroma. This focus of tumor was less than 1 cm, classifying it as a microcarcinoma.* (Right) *These tumors are usually encapsulated. This H&E section demonstrates a very thick capsule, which is often seen in these tumors. Note the adjacent normal thyroid.*

Cribriform Growth Pattern

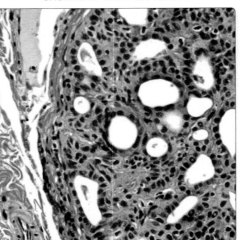

Peculiar Nuclear Clearing

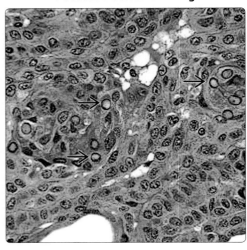

(Left) *This H&E shows the cytologic features of tumor cells typically seen in this variant. The cells are cuboidal with basophilic cytoplasm and hyperchromatic nuclei. Note the absence of classic PTC nuclei and the absence of a capsule.* (Right) *This H&E demonstrates the characteristic peculiar nuclear clearing (PNC) ➡ seen within some of the nuclei in these tumors. These PNCs are found within squamous morules and are usually not as abundant as is seen in this example.*

Large Unifocal Tumor in Sporadic Setting

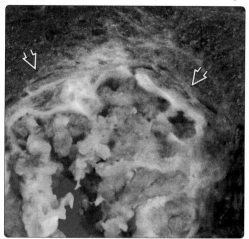

Multifocal Tumors in Familial Setting

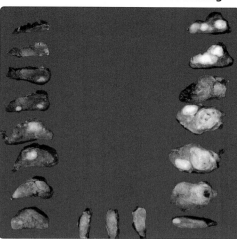

(Left) *This gross cut surface picture shows a large, well-circumscribed, and partially encapsulated thyroid tumor* ➡ *with a pale and friable appearance. This PTC-CMV was identified on a patient with no history and no findings of FAP.* (Right) *This gross image demonstrates multiple tumor nodules seen in the cribriform variant of PTC present in a familial setting. Sporadic tumors are usually solitary and larger than the tumors occurring in FAP patients.*

Solid Growth Pattern

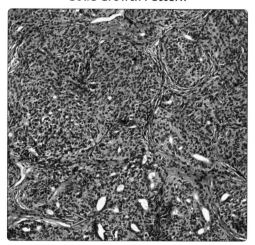

Small Cribriform and Solid Tumor

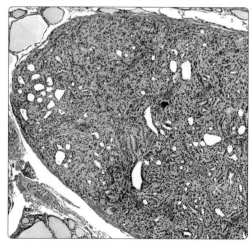

(Left) *This H&E demonstrates the solid pattern seen in PTC-CMV. An area with the more common cribriform pattern* ➡ *is seen in the lower right-hand corner of the image.* (Right) *This photomicrograph illustrates an example of PTC-CMV, well circumscribed, without a fibrous capsule. It also highlights the solid areas often seen in these types of tumors. This tumor shows areas of both cribriform pattern and solid pattern, however this tumor has a predominantly solid architecture.*

Lymphovascular Invasion

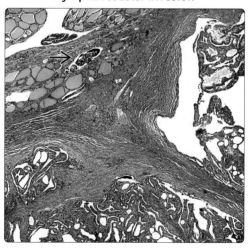

Metastatic Tumor to Lymph Node

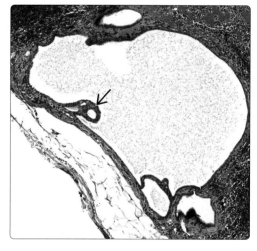

(Left) *Low-power H&E demonstrates a focus of lymphovascular invasion* ➡, *an unusual finding in cribriform-morular variant of PTC. This tumor also had bands of fibrosis. Note the cribriform and papillary-type architectures seen in this example.* (Right) *This H&E shows a metastatic tumor focus in a lymph node, an unusual finding in cribriform-morular variant of PTC. The tumor deposit is largely cystic, though a small papillary structure with cribriform-appearing areas* ➡ *is present.*

Aberrant β-Catenin Expression

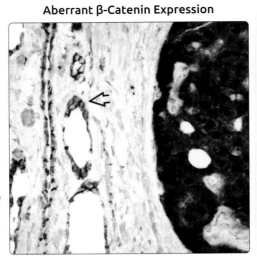

Aberrant Nuclear β-Catenin

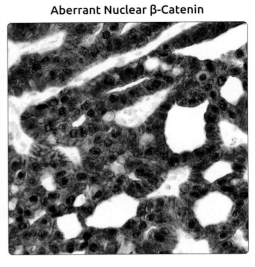

(Left) This image demonstrates the strong nuclear and cytoplasmic staining pattern of β-catenin seen in CMV-PTC. Note how this differs from the membranous staining pattern seen in the adjacent normal thyroid parenchyma (left) ⇨. (Right) This higher power image demonstrates the staining pattern of β-catenin that is characteristic in this variant of PTC. Note the diffuse cytoplasmic and strong nuclear staining, resulting from aberrant accumulation within the nucleus.

Estrogen Receptor in CMVPTC

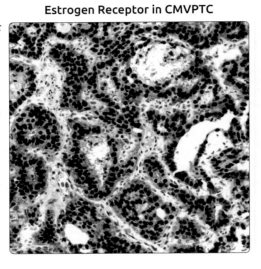

Progesterone Receptor

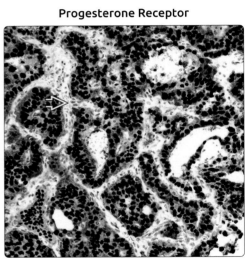

(Left) One of the characteristic findings in the cribriform-morular variant of PTC is that the neoplastic cells stain for estrogen receptor (ER). Most of the cribriform-morular variants show moderate to strong nuclear positivity in the many different areas of the tumor. (Right) Another characteristic of the cribriform-morular variant is strong nuclear positivity for progesterone receptor (PR) by immunohistochemistry. The lymphocytes ⇨ in the intervening stroma are negative.

Cyclin-D1 Staining

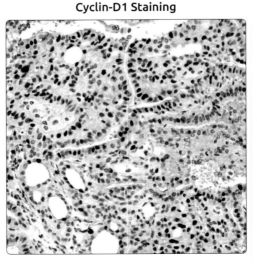

p53 Expression

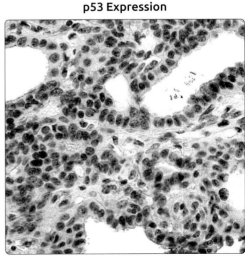

(Left) Cyclin-D1 is a useful immunohistochemical stain used to better characterize cribriform-morular variant of PTC. This variant has a moderate to strong nuclear staining pattern. (Right) The immunoexpression of p53 in PTCs is rarely present. The cribriform-morular variant of PTC usually presents with a low and multifocal immunoexpression of this antigen, as highlighted in this image.

Epithelial Morule With PNC

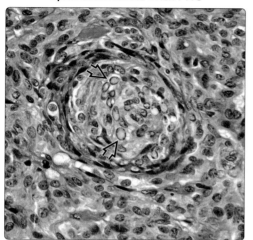

Squamous Morule

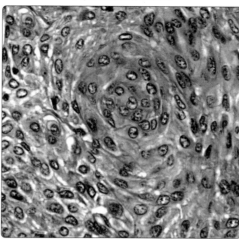

(Left) This H&E demonstrates nuclei of the atypical cells presenting in the whorl formations, forming a squamous morule present with the characteristic peculiar nuclear clearing (PNC) ➡, a characteristic finding seen in these PTC-CMV tumor cells. The squamous morule is within a background of solid growth pattern. (Right) A squamous morule is present in an area of a solid component showing the characteristic peculiar nuclear clearing. The squamous morules may be very frequently present in PTC-CMV.

β-Catenin Staining in CMV PTC

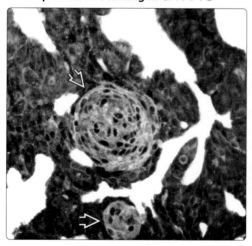

β-Catenin in Squamous Morules

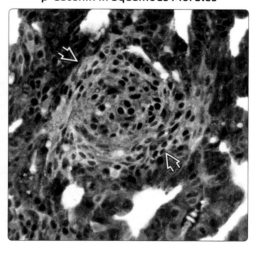

(Left) In this high-power picture of the PTC-CMV, 2 squamoid morules ➡ are present and showing the characteristic nuclear and cytoplasmic staining for β-catenin. The cytoplasm of the squamous morules stains less intensely than the cytoplasm within the cribriform areas. (Right) A squamous morule is present in an area of a cribriform component showing the characteristic nuclear and cytoplasmic staining for β-catenin. The squamous morule ➡ is distinct from the cribriform component.

CK5/6 in Squamous Morule

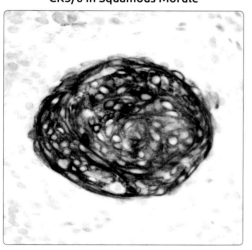

Squamous Morule Highlighted By CD5

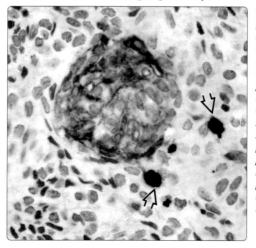

(Left) In this high-power picture of the PTC-CMV, the squamoid morules show the characteristic keratin pattern of the stain. The cribriform and solid areas are negative for CK5/6. (Right) A squamous morule is present in an area of a solid component showing strong staining for CD5. The squamous morules are usually positive for CD5 in a similar fashion of the thyroid solid cell nests and thymus. Note the presence of CD5(+) lymphocytes ➡ adjacent to the morule.

Papillary Thyroid Carcinoma, Hobnail Variant

CLINICAL ISSUES

- Mean age at presentation: 57.6 years
- Rare, likely accounting for < 1% of all PTC cases
- These tumors are aggressive with relatively poor prognosis

MACROSCOPIC

- Most often described as multifocal and present within both thyroid lobes
- Range in size from 1-4 cm (average is 2.5 cm)

MICROSCOPIC

- Defined by > 30% of cells with hobnail features
- Main architectural growth pattern for HVPTC is micropapillary
  - Small components of follicular pattern or clustered pattern may be present
- Other common characteristics include
  - Loss or inversion of cellular polarity
- Cells have dense eosinophilic cytoplasm and well-defined cell membranes
- Increased nuclear:cytoplasmic ratios
- Pleomorphic nuclei mostly located in apex of cytoplasm that gives characteristic hobnail appearance
- Nuclear atypia is moderate to severe
- Nuclear features of conventional PTC are present, though may be only focal
- Loss of cellular cohesion

ANCILLARY TESTS

- *BRAF* V600E mutation was most common mutation, present in ~ 95% HVPTC cases
- *TP53* mutations are commonly seen
- *TERT* promoter mutation in ~ 50% tumors
- Mutations in *PIK3CA* in ~ 30%, *CTNNB1* in ~ 20%, and *EGFR* in ~ 10% tumors
- No RAS mutation

Papillary and Micropapillary Structures With Loss of Cellular Polarity

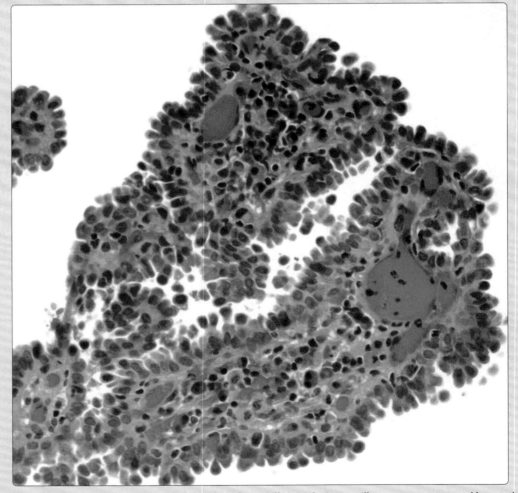

The hobnail variant of papillary thyroid carcinoma exhibits complex papillary and micropapillary structures covered by neoplastic follicular cells containing eosinophilic cytoplasm and apically located nuclei.

TERMINOLOGY

Abbreviations

- Papillary thyroid carcinoma, hobnail variant (PTC-HV) or (HVPTC)

Synonyms

- Papillary thyroid carcinoma with prominent hobnail features
- Hobnail variant of papillary thyroid carcinoma
- Papillary thyroid carcinoma with hobnail/micropapillary features

Definitions

- Variant of papillary thyroid carcinoma characterized by loss of cellular polarity/cohesiveness with hobnail features in > 30% of neoplastic cells (who 2017)

ETIOLOGY/PATHOGENESIS

Environmental Exposure

- Currently no known associations with environmental exposure

Genetic Alterations

- *BRAF* mutation present in ~ 95%
- *TP53* mutation
- *TERT* promoter mutation in ~ 50%

CLINICAL ISSUES

Epidemiology

- Incidence
  - Rare, likely accounting for < 1% of all PTC cases
- Age
  - Mean age at presentation: 57.6 years
    - Age at initial diagnosis ranges from 28-78 years
- Sex
  - More common in females than males (~ 3:1)

Presentation

- Patients most commonly present with neck mass
  - May cause compressive symptoms
    - Dysphagia, dyspnea, stridor, hoarseness
- Also commonly presents with cervical lymphadenopathy

Treatment

- Thyroidectomy (with cervical lymph node dissection where indicated)
- Surgery may be followed by RAI therapy

Prognosis

- Tumors are aggressive with relatively poor prognosis
  - Most are aggressive with distant metastases, lymph node metastases, &/or local recurrence
  - Lung, brain, and bone are most common sites of distant metastases
- Significantly increased mortality risk in patients harboring *BRAF* mutation and *BRAF* mutation associated with *TP53* &/or *PIK3CA* mutation

IMAGING

General Features

- Ultrasound may be used for needle-guided biopsy and identification of mass
- CT scan is useful for evaluating extent of disease (extrathyroid extension/lymph node metastases)

MACROSCOPIC

General Features

- Most often described as multifocal and present within both thyroid lobes
  - Can also be unifocal and encapsulated
- Infiltrative appearance may be evident on gross inspection
- May show signs of hemorrhagic degeneration

Size

- Range in size from 1-4 cm
  - Average size is 2.5 cm

MICROSCOPIC

Histologic Features

- Defined by > 30% of cells with hobnail features
- Tumors have invasive growth pattern and show 3 main architectural patterns
  - Papillary and micropapillary pattern
    - Variably sized papillae have prominent vascular cores and are lined by layer of epithelium 1-4 cells thick
    - Papillary structures are lined by cuboidal to oval cells with increased nuclear to cytoplasmic ratio
  - Follicular pattern
    - Variably sized follicles with little to no colloid
    - Follicles may be micro- or macrofollicular in appearance
    - Lined by same hobnail cells as seen in other patterns
  - Clustered pattern
    - Many clusters of malignant cells with hobnail appearance
    - Form papillary structures without fibrovascular cores
- Pleomorphic nuclei mostly located in apex of cytoplasm that gives characteristic hobnail appearance
- All cases show loosely and individually arranged neoplastic cells
  - Loss of cellular cohesion
- Invasive front of tumor shows nuclear atypia
- Psammoma bodies are rare
- Lymphovascular invasion is identified in almost all cases
- Colloid is limited to absent
- Necrosis may be present
- May be associated with other variants of PTC

Cytologic Features

- Neoplastic cells have same cytologic features on H&E regardless of architectural pattern
- Cells have dense eosinophilic cytoplasm and well-defined cell membranes
- Loss of cellular cohesion
- Nuclear atypia is moderate to severe
- Nuclei are located in apical or mid portions of cytoplasm of neoplastic cells

- o Gives rise to hobnailed or matchstick appearance
- Nuclear features of PTC are present, though may be only focal
  - o Nuclear enlargement, overlap and stratification are common
  - o Nuclei may have irregular contours
    - – Membrane irregularity reflected by grooves and pseudoinclusions
  - o Ground-glass chromatin pattern
- Mitosis are present (with rare atypical mitotic figures)

Lymph Nodes

- Metastases to lymph nodes and distant organs show hobnail pattern

ANCILLARY TESTS

Cytology

- Not described fully in literature

Immunohistochemistry

- Positive immunostains
  - o Thyroglobulin (cytoplasmic focal)
  - o TTF-1
  - o pax-8
  - o CK19
  - o CK7
  - o EMA
  - o HBME-1
  - o p53
  - o Ki-67 (approximate proliferative index 10%)

Genetic Testing

- BRAF V600E mutation was most common mutation, which is present in ~ 95% HVPTC cases
  - o Kinase encoding gene from RAF/RAS/MAPK pathway
  - o Associated with vascular invasion, lymph node metastases, and less commonly, extrathyroid extension
- TP53 mutations are commonly seen
- BRAF and TP53 mutations are by far most common genetic alterations in primary HPTC
- TERT promoter mutation in ~ 50%
- Mutations in PIK3CA (~ 30%), CTNNB1 (~ 20%), EGFR (~ 10%), AKT1 (~ 5%) and NOTCH1 (~ 5%) have been found
- No RAS mutation: Negativity for NRAS, HRAS, and KRAS mutations
- Negativity for RET/PTCH1, RET/NCOA4 rearrangements and PAX8/PPARG rearrangements
  - o RET rearrangements have been described in one report

DIFFERENTIAL DIAGNOSIS

Papillary Thyroid Carcinoma, Classic Variant

- Predominant papillary architecture
- Almost all tumor cells demonstrate conventional PTC nuclear features
- Lack apical tufting (hobnailing) seen in Hobnail variant
  - o Nuclei are generally not apically located

Papillary Thyroid Carcinoma, Tall Cell Variant

- Tumor cells are eosinophilic with height at least 3x width
  - o Lack dyscohesive and hobnail appearance
- Neoplastic nuclei show PTC nuclear features

- Abundant nuclear pseudoinclusions and grooves

Papillary Thyroid Carcinoma, Oncocytic Variant

- Cells have granular eosinophilic cytoplasm
- PTC nuclear features are present, though may be subtle
- Tumor cells have prominent nucleoli, characteristic finding
- May show focal hobnail pattern
- Lack aggressive histologic features (loss of cohesiveness, extrathyroid extension, angiolymphatic invasion)

Papillary Thyroid Carcinoma, Columnar Cell Variant

- Characterized by pseudostratified columnar cells
- Supra and subnuclear vacuoles
- Nuclei are predominantly hyperchromatic with focal conventional PTC nuclear features

Metastases

- Will have immunophenotype of primary malignancy
- Panel of immunostains including thyroid markers should be used when considering nonthyroid primaries

DIAGNOSTIC CHECKLIST

Clinically Relevant Pathologic Features

- Loss of polarity and presence of dyscohesive cells are suggested to be associated with worse prognosis
- Extrathyroid extension and angiolymphatic invasion are associated with poor prognosis
- Presence of BRAF mutation confers worse prognosis
  - o Significantly increased mortality risk in patients harboring BRAF mutation and BRAF mutation associated with TP53 &/or PIK3CA mutation

Pathologic Interpretation Pearls

- Predominant growth pattern for HVPTC is micropapillary
  - o Papillary, follicular, and dyscohesive pattern
- Large eosinophilic cytoplasm
- Nuclei are located in apical or mid portions of cytoplasm, giving hobnail appearance
  - o Loss of polarity
  - o Clusters of dyscohesive cells present
- Nuclear features of conventional PTC are present, though may be only focal
- Pleomorphic nuclei
- Almost always associated with extrathyroid extension and vascular invasion

SELECTED REFERENCES

1. Cameselle-Teijeiro JM et al: Hobnail variant of papillary thyroid carcinoma: clinicopathologic and molecular evidence of progression to undifferentiated carcinoma in 2 cases. Am J Surg Pathol. 41(6):854-860, 2017
2. Morandi L et al: Somatic mutation profiling of hobnail variant of papillary thyroid carcinoma. Endocr Relat Cancer. 24(2):107-117, 2017
3. Teng L et al: Hobnail variant of papillary thyroid carcinoma: molecular profiling and comparison to classical papillary thyroid carcinoma, poorly differentiated thyroid carcinoma and anaplastic thyroid carcinoma. Oncotarget. 8(13):22023-22033, 2017
4. Ieni A et al: The micropapillary/hobnail variant of papillary thyroid carcinoma: a review of series described in the literature compared to a series from one southern Italy pathology institution. Rev Endocr Metab Disord. 17(4):521-527, 2016
5. Lee YS et al: Cytologic, clinicopathologic, and molecular features of papillary thyroid carcinoma with prominent hobnail features: 10 case reports and systematic literature review. Int J Clin Exp Pathol. 8(7):7988-97, 2015
6. Schwock J et al: Hobnail-variant of papillary thyroid carcinoma in liquid-based cytology. Diagn Cytopathol. 43(12):990-2, 2015

Differential Diagnosis of Hobnail Variant

Feature	Hobnail Variant	Classic Variant	Tall Cell Variant	Columnar Cell Variant	Oncocytic Variant
Age	Mean 57.6 years	Mean 48 years	Mean 49 years	Mean 47 years	Mean 57 years
Size	2.5 cm average	Variable	2.8 cm average	3.8 cm average	2.5 cm average
Multifocal	Rarely	Common	Rarely	Rarely	Rarely
Extrathyroid extension	Common	Variable	Common	Common	Occasional
Lymphovascular invasion	Extensive	Minimal	Extensive	Extensive	Minimal
Necrosis	Common	Minimal	Common	Occasional	Minimal
Mitotic activity	Common	Rare	Common	Common	Rare
Cell shape	Stratified, hobnail	Cuboidal or polygonal	Height 3x width	Columnar	Polygonal
Nuclear features	Focal PTC	PTC	PTC	Focal PTC	PTC
Cytoplasm	Eosinophilic	Amphophilic	Eosinophilic, granular	Eosinophilic	Eosinophilic, granular
Other diagnostic features	Dyscohesive cells, loss of polarity		Abundant nuclear pseudoinclusions	Supra & subnuclear vacuoles	Prominent nucleoli
Recurrence	Common	Rare	Common	Common	Rare
Prognosis	Poor	Good	Poor	Poor	Good
Cytogenetics	*BRAF*	*BRAF, RAS,* and *RET* rearrangement	*BRAF* and *RET* rearrangement	*BRAF*	*BRAF* and *RET* rearrangement

PTC = papillary thyroid carcinoma.

7. Asioli S et al: Cytomorphologic and molecular features of hobnail variant of papillary thyroid carcinoma: case series and literature review. Diagn Cytopathol. 42(1):78-84, 2014

8. Lubitz CC et al: Hobnail variant of papillary thyroid carcinoma: an institutional case series and molecular profile. Thyroid. 24(6):958-65, 2014

9. Asioli S et al: Papillary thyroid carcinoma with hobnail features: histopathologic criteria to predict aggressive behavior. Hum Pathol. 44(3):320-8, 2013

10. Yang GC et al: Cytological features of clear cell thyroid tumors, including a papillary thyroid carcinoma with prominent hobnail features. Diagn Cytopathol. 41(9):757-61, 2013

11. Bellevicine C et al: Cytological and molecular features of papillary thyroid carcinoma with prominent hobnail features: a case report. Acta Cytol. 56(5):560-4, 2012

12. Kakudo K et al: Classification of thyroid follicular cell tumors: with special reference to borderline lesions [Review]. Endocr J. Epub, 2011

13. Lino-Silva LS et al: Thyroid gland papillary carcinomas with "micropapillary pattern," a recently recognized poor prognostic finding: clinicopathologic and survival analysis of 7 cases. Hum Pathol. 43(10):1596-600, 2012

14. Liu Z et al: Loss of cellular polarity/cohesiveness in the invasive front of papillary thyroid carcinoma, a novel predictor for lymph node metastasis; possible morphological indicator of epithelial mesenchymal transition. J Clin Pathol. 64(4):325-9, 2011

15. Lloyd RV et al: Papillary thyroid carcinoma variants. Head Neck Pathol. 5(1):51-6, 2011

16. Albores-Saavedra J: Papillary thyroid carcinoma with prominent hobnail features: a new aggressive variant of moderately differentiated papillary carcinoma. A clinicopathologic, immunohistochemical, and molecular study of 8 cases. Am J Surg Pathol. 34(6):913; author reply 914, 2010

17. Asioli S et al: Papillary thyroid carcinoma with prominent hobnail features: a new aggressive variant of moderately differentiated papillary carcinoma. A clinicopathologic, immunohistochemical, and molecular study of eight cases. Am J Surg Pathol. 34(1):44-52, 2010

18. Bai Y et al: Loss of cellular polarity/cohesiveness in the invasive front of papillary thyroid carcinoma and periostin expression. Cancer Lett. 281(2):188-95, 2009

19. Motosugi U et al: Thyroid papillary carcinoma with micropapillary and hobnail growth pattern: a histological variant with intermediate malignancy? Thyroid. 19(5):535-7, 2009

20. Bai Y et al: Subclassification of non-solid-type papillary thyroid carcinoma identification of high-risk group in common type. Cancer Sci. 2008 Oct;99(10):1908-15. Erratum in: Cancer Sci. 99(12):2548, 2008

21. Kakudo K et al: Papillary carcinoma of the thyroid in Japan: subclassification of common type and identification of low risk group. J Clin Pathol. 57(10):1041-6, 2004

22. Hirokawa M et al: Dilated rough endoplasmic reticulum corresponding to septate cytoplasmic vacuoles in papillary thyroid carcinoma. Diagn Cytopathol. 23(5):351-3, 2000

(Left) *Micropapillary structures lined by cuboidal cells with apically placed nuclei (hobnail appearance) and loss of cellular cohesion are shown. The papillary architecture with focal micropapillary areas are best seen at low magnification.* **(Right)** *The papillary architecture and characteristic nuclear features of papillary carcinoma, pseudoinclusions and nuclear grooves, are shown. The hobnail pattern in this example is less pronounced.*

Micropapillae and Papillae

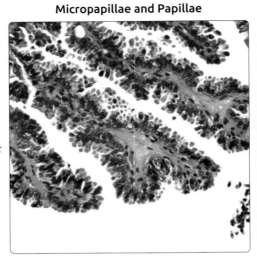

Hobnail and Micropapillary Pattern

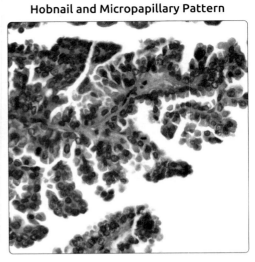

(Left) *H&E shows tumor cells with nuclei exhibiting classic papillary thyroid carcinoma nuclear features. An intranuclear inclusion ➡ is present.* **(Right)** *This variant of papillary thyroid carcinoma is characterized by 3 main architectural patterns: Papillary, follicular, and clustered. This image shows both the papillary and clustered ➡ patterns. Both subtypes are characterized by a papillary appearance. The papillary pattern has a true fibrovascular core, while the clustered type does not.*

Intranuclear Inclusion

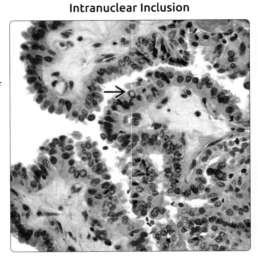

Hobnailing

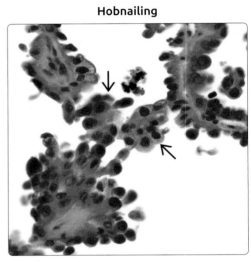

(Left) *Hobnail variant papillary thyroid carcinoma (HVPTC) shows the micropapillary architecture with a ventral core, lined by cells with eosinophilic cytoplasm with loss of cellular polarity with apocrine snouting of cells.* **(Right)** *Hobnail cells are characterized as cells with apically placed nuclei. They show a loss of polarity and have a matchstick appearance. These tumors have pleomorphic nuclei with focal papillary thyroid carcinoma features.*

Ample Eosinophilic Cytoplasm

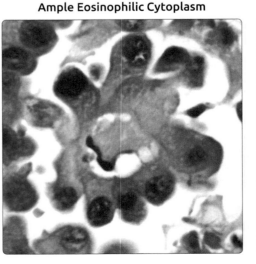

Loss of Polarity

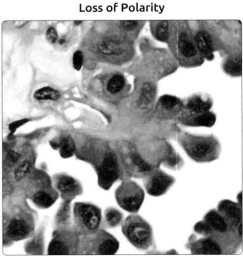

Nuclear Features in HVPTC

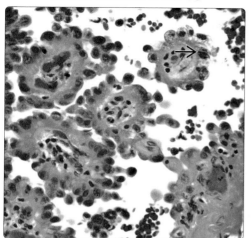

Classic Micropapillary Pattern

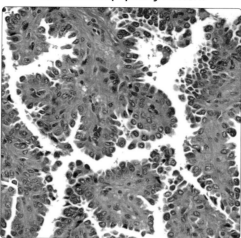

(Left) *The characteristic papillary thyroid carcinoma features may be present only focally in this variant. The nuclei in this example are enlarged and irregular in contour. Nuclear grooves ➡ can be seen in a few of the cells. The characteristic hobnail pattern is striking.* (Right) *Micropapillary structures lined by cuboidal cells with apically placed nuclei (hobnail appearance) and loss of cellular cohesion are shown.*

Cystic Changes With Flattened Cells

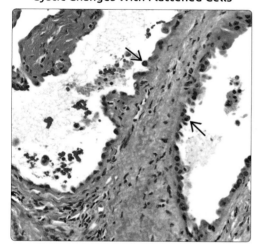

Clustered Pattern of Growth

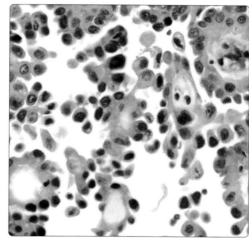

(Left) *Large cystic structures should be carefully examined, with particular attention to the lining epithelial cells. These cystic structures are lined by cells that have a hobnail appearance ➡. They show loss of polarity with apically placed nuclei.* (Right) *HVPTC shows the micropapillary architecture and loss of cellular polarity with apocrine snouting of cells.*

BRAF Positivity

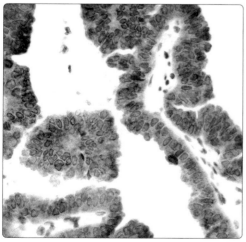

BRAF Granular Immunopositivity

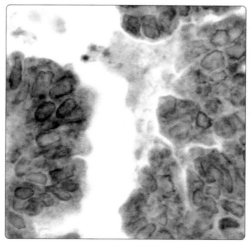

(Left) *The tumor cells in the HVPTC show diffuse granular immunopositivity for BRAF. The stroma and the cells within the papillary stalks are negative for BRAF.* (Right) *BRAF mutation is present in the majority of HVPTC. This high-power view highlights the granular cytoplasmic immunopositivity for BRAF.*

Papillary Thyroid Carcinoma, Warthin-Like Variant

TERMINOLOGY

- Malignant neoplasm composed predominantly of papillae filled with prominent lymphoplasmacytic component and lined by oncocytic cells with papillary thyroid carcinoma (PTC) nuclear features
  - Histological similarity to Warthin tumor of salivary glands

CLINICAL ISSUES

- Rare tumors, more common in women
- Average age at presentation is 48 years
- Frequently associated with Hashimoto thyroiditis
- Prognosis is very good
- These tumors behave similarly to usual papillary carcinoma

MICROSCOPIC

- Overall, tumors are well circumscribed
- Prominent papillary architecture
- Large, eosinophilic cells line papillae
- Papillary stalks are filled with inflammatory cells
- Inflammatory component predominantly lymphocytes with rare plasma cells
- Characteristic PTC nuclear features are present at least focally
- Nuclei without characteristic PTC features are large and pleomorphic
- Background thyroid with Hashimoto thyroiditis

TOP DIFFERENTIAL DIAGNOSES

- Tall cell variant PTC
  - Lacks lymphoplasmacytic infiltrate seen in WLPTC
- Lymphocytic thyroiditis
  - Lacks papillary architecture
  - Nuclear features of PTC are absent
- Oncocytic variant PTC
  - Not associated with prominent lymphoplasmacytic component
- Hobnail variant
  - Lacks lymphoplasmacytic infiltrate seen in WLPTC

Large Eosinophilic Cells Lining Papillae

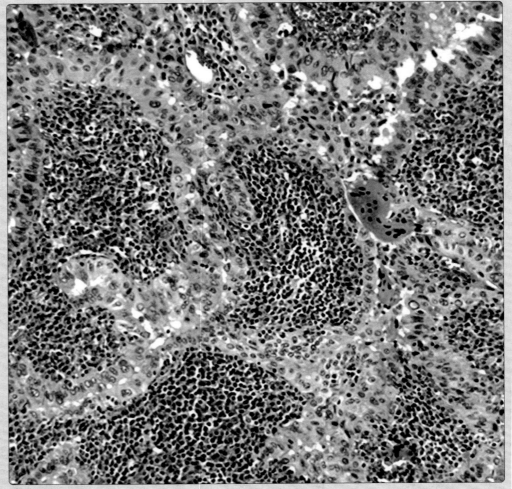

Photomicrograph of Warthin-like variant of papillary thyroid carcinoma (PTC) shows a lymphoplasmacytic infiltrate replacing the cores of papillae. The follicular tumor cells lining the papillae are eosinophilic and large, and the nuclei have the characteristic papillary carcinoma nuclei.

TERMINOLOGY

Abbreviations

- Warthin-like papillary thyroid carcinoma (WLPTC)

Synonyms

- Papillary Hürthle cell carcinoma with lymphoid stroma

Definitions

- Malignant neoplasm composed predominantly of papillae filled with prominent lymphoplasmacytic component and lined by oncocytic cells with papillary thyroid carcinoma (PTC) nuclear features
  - Histological similarity to Warthin tumor of salivary glands

CLINICAL ISSUES

Epidemiology

- Incidence
  - Rare
    - ~ 80 cases reported in literature
- Age
  - Average at presentation is 48 years
    - Range: 19-85 years
- Sex
  - More common in women than men
    - M:F = 1:8

Presentation

- Usually presents as palpable thyroid nodule
- Frequently associated with Hashimoto thyroiditis

Treatment

- Treatment usually involves thyroidectomy
- Lymph node dissection indicated when evidence of lymph node involvement on imaging

Prognosis

- Prognosis is very good (similar to that of classic PTC)

MACROSCOPIC

General Features

- Usually solitary nodules
- Well circumscribed
- May be encapsulated, though usually not
- Variety of gross appearances are possible
  - Solid, granular, papillary, cystic
  - Red-brown to tan or white in color

Size

- Tumors are generally small, averaging 2.3 cm in diameter
  - Range: 0.3-6.6 cm

MICROSCOPIC

Histologic Features

- Overall, tumors are well circumscribed
- May be encapsulated
- Prominent papillary architecture
  - Papillary stalks are filled with inflammatory cells
    - Inflammatory component is predominantly lymphocytes with rare plasma cells

- Lymphovascular invasion is almost always absent
- Large, eosinophilic cells line papillae
  - Cells are polygonal in shape and have distinct cytoplasmic borders
  - Abundant eosinophilic cytoplasm
- Characteristic PTC nuclear features are present at least focally
  - Nuclei are crowded, overlapping, show molding, and may demonstrate optical clearing
  - Nuclei are irregular, and grooves and pseudoinclusions may be seen
- Nuclei without characteristic PTC features are large, pleomorphic, and have prominent nucleoli
- Nuclei are usually arranged haphazardly within neoplastic cells
- Background thyroid with Hashimoto thyroiditis
  - WLPTCs are more commonly associated with Hashimoto thyroiditis than classic PTCs (93% vs. 36%, respectively) in one report

ANCILLARY TESTS

Cytology

- FNA specimens are usually cellular
- Composed of follicular cells in sheets, papillary fragments, and scattered single cells
- Numerous small lymphocytes and mature plasma cells in background
- Lymphocytes and plasma cells are also intimately associated with papillary fragments, filling stalks
- Cells have abundant granular eosinophilic cytoplasm with distinct cell borders
- Nuclei are enlarged, irregular in contour, and are eccentrically located
- Occasional nuclei show clearing, grooves, and pseudoinclusions
- Occasional prominent nucleoli

Immunohistochemistry

- Positive stains
  - Cytokeratin, thyroglobulin, HBME-1, galectin-3, Ki-67 (low), S100 (in Langerhans cells)
  - These tumors have similar staining pattern to classic variant PTC

Genetic Testing

- *BRAF* V600E present
  - May be seen in large majority of these tumors (up to 70% as reported in 1 study)
  - WLPTCs showed significantly lower rate of BRAF mutation when compared to classic PTCs (65% vs. 84%, respectively) in one report
- *RET/PTC* gene rearrangements also identified

DIFFERENTIAL DIAGNOSIS

Main DDx

- Warthin-like tumors can be mistaken for benign lymphoepithelial lesions of thyroid, oncocytic (Hürthle cell) carcinoma, and tall cell variant of papillary carcinoma in both FNA and histology specimens

Tall Cell Variant Papillary Thyroid Carcinoma

- Neoplastic cells have nuclei with height at least 3x width
- Lacks lymphoplasmacytic infiltrate seen in WLPTC

Lymphocytic Thyroiditis

- Lacks papillary architecture seen in Warthin-like variant
- Nuclear features of PTC are absent

Oncocytic Variant Papillary Thyroid Carcinoma

- Not associated with prominent lymphoplasmacytic component

Hobnail Variant

- Lacks lymphoplasmacytic infiltrate seen in WLPTC

DIAGNOSTIC CHECKLIST

Pathologic Interpretation Pearls

- Morphologically, it resembles Warthin tumors of salivary glands
- Hallmark histological feature of this variant is papillary folding lined by oncocytic neoplastic cells with clear nuclei and nuclear features of PTC, accompanied by prominent lymphocytic infiltrate in papillary stalks
- Numerous papillae lined by large cells with ample eosinophilic cytoplasm
- Tumor cells with distinct cell membranes
- Nuclear features of PTC
- T and B lymphocytes infiltrating stalks of papillae

Association with Hashimoto Thyroiditis

- Background thyroid with Hashimoto thyroiditis
- Patients with WLPTC have similar demographic, clinical, pathological, and molecular characteristics to those with classic PTC coexisting with Hashimoto thyroiditis

SELECTED REFERENCES

1. Vallonthaiel AG et al: Cytological features of warthin-like papillary thyroid carcinoma: a case report with review of previous cytology cases. Diagn Cytopathol. ePub, 2017
2. Dencic TM et al: Strong expression of HBME-1 associates with high-risk clinicopathological factors of papillary thyroid carcinoma. Pathol Oncol Res. 21(3):735-42, 2015
3. González-Colunga KJ et al: Warthin-like papillary thyroid carcinoma associated with lymphadenopathy and Hashimoto's thyroiditis. Case Rep Endocrinol. 2015:251898, 2015
4. Han F et al: Occult oncocytic papillary thyroid carcinoma with lymphoid stroma (Warthin-like tumor): report of a case with concomitant mutations of BRAF V600E and V600K. Int J Clin Exp Pathol. 8(5):5896-901, 2015
5. Yeo MK et al: The Warthin-like variant of papillary thyroid carcinoma: a comparison with classic type in the patients with coexisting Hashimoto's thyroiditis. Int J Endocrinol. 2015:456027, 2015
6. Jun HH et al: Warthin-like variant of papillary thyroid carcinoma: single institution experience. ANZ J Surg. ePub, 2014
7. Erşen A et al: Warthin-like papillary carcinoma of the thyroid: a case series and review of the literature. Turk Patoloji Derg. 29(2):150-5, 2013
8. Paker I et al: Oncocytic variant of papillary thyroid carcinoma with lymphocytic stroma (Warthin-like variant): report of a case with fine needle variant cytology and review of the literature. Cytopathology. 23(6):408-10, 2012
9. Paliogiannis P et al: Warthin-like papillary carcinoma of the thyroid gland: case report and review of the literature. Case Rep Oncol Med. 2012:689291, 2012
10. LiVolsi VA et al: The Chernobyl thyroid cancer experience: pathology. Clin Oncol (R Coll Radiol). 23(4):261-7, 2011
11. Panayiotides IG et al: Simultaneous occurrence of Warthin-like papillary carcinoma and lymphoma of the mucosa associated lymphoid tissue in Hashimoto thyroiditis. J Clin Pathol. 63(7):662-3, 2010
12. Abrosimov A et al: Different structural components of conventional papillary thyroid carcinoma display mostly identical BRAF status. Int J Cancer. 120(1):196-200, 2007
13. Abrosimov A et al: The cytoplasmic expression of MUC1 in papillary thyroid carcinoma of different histological variants and its correlation with cyclin D1 overexpression. Endocr Pathol. 18(2):68-75, 2007
14. Kim HH et al: Warthin-like tumor of the thyroid gland: an uncommon variant of papillary thyroid cancer. Ear Nose Throat J. 85(1):56-9, 2006
15. Ciampi R et al: Alterations of the BRAF gene in thyroid tumors. Endocr Pathol. 16(3):163-72, 2005
16. Trovisco V et al: Type and prevalence of BRAF mutations are closely associated with papillary thyroid carcinoma histotype and patients' age but not with tumour aggressiveness. Virchows Arch. 446(6):589-95, 2005
17. Mai KT et al: Pathologic study and clinical significance of Hürthle cell papillary thyroid carcinoma. Appl Immunohistochem Mol Morphol. 12(4):329-37, 2004
18. Trovisco V et al: BRAF mutations are associated with some histological types of papillary thyroid carcinoma. J Pathol. 202(2):247-51, 2004
19. Anwar F: The phenotype of Hurthle and Warthin-like papillary thyroid carcinomas is distinct from classic papillary carcinoma as to the expression of retinoblastoma protein and E2F-1 transcription factor. Appl Immunohistochem Mol Morphol. 11(1):20-7, 2003
20. Ludvíková M et al: Oncocytic papillary carcinoma with lymphoid stroma (Warthin-like tumour) of the thyroid: a distinct entity with favourable prognosis. Histopathology. 39(1):17-24, 2001
21. Urano M et al: Warthin-like tumor variant of papillary thyroid carcinoma: case report and literature review. Pathol Int. 51(9):707-12, 2001
22. D'Antonio A et al: Warthin-like tumour of the thyroid gland: RET/PTC expression indicates it is a variant of papillary carcinoma. Histopathology. 36(6):493-8, 2000
23. Baloch ZW et al: Fine-needle aspiration cytology of papillary Hurthle cell carcinoma with lymphocytic stroma "Warthin-like tumor" of the thyroid. Endocr Pathol. 9(1):317-323, 1998
24. Vasei M et al: Papillary Hürthle cell carcinoma (Warthin-like tumor) of the thyroid. Report of a case with fine needle aspiration findings. Acta Cytol. 42(6):1437-40, 1998
25. Vera-Sempere FJ et al: Warthin-like tumor of the thyroid: a papillary carcinoma with mitochondrion-rich cells and abundant lymphoid stroma. A case report. Pathol Res Pract. 194(5):341-7, 1998
26. Apel RL et al: Papillary Hürthle cell carcinoma with lymphocytic stroma. "Warthin-like tumor" of the thyroid. Am J Surg Pathol. 19(7):810-4, 1995

Gross Cut Surface

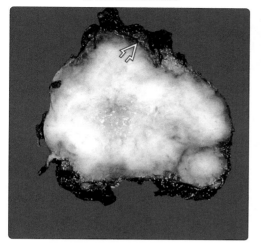

Low-Power View of WLPTC

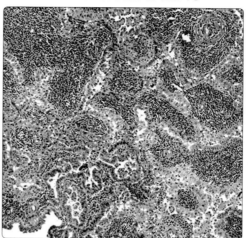

(Left) *Gross cut surface of Warthin-like variant of PTC is white-tan, firm, and typically small and well circumscribed. The residual uninvolved thyroid is compressed at the edge ➡.* (Right) *The distinguishing histological feature of this variant is papillary foldings lined by oncocytic neoplastic cells with clear nuclei, accompanied by prominent lymphoplasmacytic infiltrate in the papillary stalks.*

Characteristic Histological Features

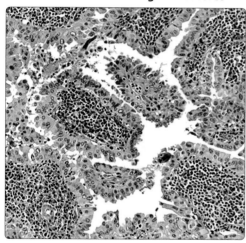

Nuclear Features of WLPTC

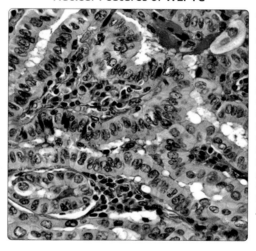

(Left) *Photomicrograph shows neoplastic oncocytic cells with clear nuclei and a few nuclear grooves lining the lymphoplasmacytic-rich papillary folds. A small proportion of these tumors may focally show features of hobnail variant of PTC.* (Right) *Highlighted here are the classic PTC nuclear features seen in this variant, including nuclear clearing, pseudoinclusions, grooves, molding, and overlap, and with a lymphoplasmacytic-rich fibrovascular stroma.*

High-Power View of Oncocytic Cells

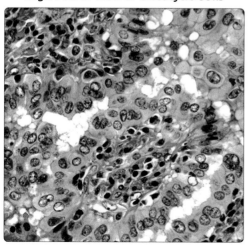

Nuclear Features of PTC

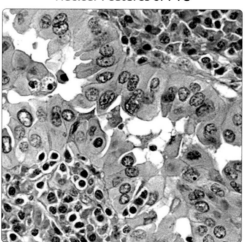

(Left) *WLPTC is a malignant neoplasm, with oncocytic cells that have PTC-like nuclear features that line papillae, which are filled with numerous inflammatory cells (lymphocytes and plasma cells).* (Right) *The histologic appearance of Warthin-like tumor variant is somewhat similar to tall cell variant of papillary carcinoma, including tall cell features and distinct cytoplasmic membranes. Some tumors may have hobnail-like features.*

Gross Cut Surface

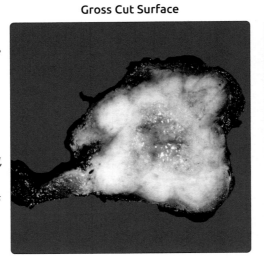

Cells With Oncocytic Cytoplasm

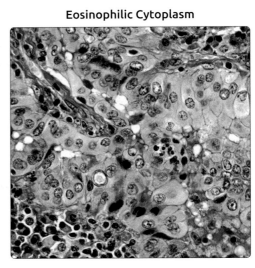

(Left) *This tumor grossly involves the majority of the thyroid lobe. These tumors are typically small, white-tan to red, and well circumscribed, traits that are not demonstrated in this image.* **(Right)** *The nuclei tend to overlap and are arranged haphazardly within the oncocytic cytoplasm. Some of the nuclei are basally oriented, while others are apically oriented. A degenerating multinucleated giant cell ➯ is seen.*

Intranuclear Inclusions

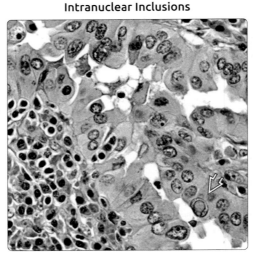

Eosinophilic Cytoplasm

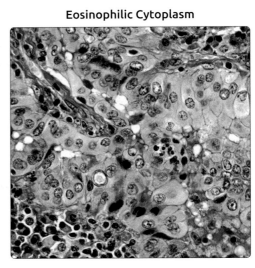

(Left) *Tumor cells have granular oncocytic cytoplasm and nuclear features of papillary carcinoma including optically clear nuclei, nuclear grooves, and intranuclear pseudoinclusions ➡. A dense lymphoplasmacytic infiltration is seen in the stalk.* **(Right)** *The Warthin-like variant of papillary carcinoma is associated with chronic lymphocytic (Hashimoto) thyroiditis. The tumor shows well-developed papillae lined by eosinophilic cells with well-defined cytoplasmic membranes.*

WLPTC Cytological Features

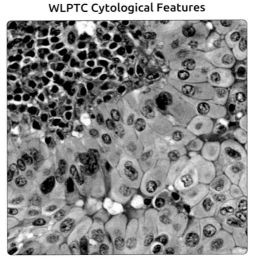

BRAF Positivity

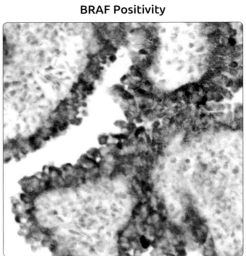

(Left) *Highlighted on this high-power view are the tumor cells with ample oncocytic cytoplasm and well-defined cytoplasmic membrane. Also present are the classic PTC nuclear features seen in this variant, with nuclear clearing, grooves, molding, and overlapping.* **(Right)** *A small proportion of the Warthin-like variant may have BRAF V600E mutation and demonstrates immunopositivity for BRAF. Note the lymphoplasmacytic infiltrate is negative.*

Granular Immunopositivity for BRAF

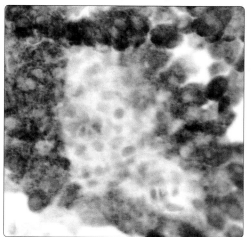

Cyclin-D1 Stain

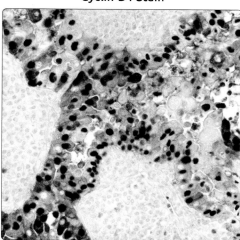

(Left) *Warthin-like variant may have BRAF V600E mutation. Immunohistochemistry for BRAF shows agranular intense cytoplasmic positivity.* (Right) *The immunohistological features of this variant are papillary foldings lined by oncocytic neoplastic cells with clear nuclei and nuclear pseudoinclusions, usually with nuclear positivity for cyclin-D1.*

EMA Stain

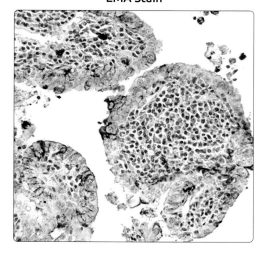

HBME-1 Stain

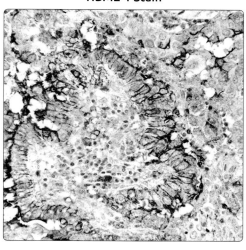

(Left) *WLPTC stained for epithelial membrane antigen shows a patchy membranous staining of the tumor cells.* (Right) *Photomicrograph of WLPTC shows the membranous staining of the tumor cells for HBME-1. There is a focal luminal pattern of staining.*

HBME-1 Membranous Immunopositivity

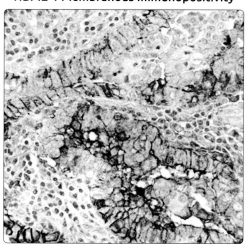

Patchy Galectin-3 Stain

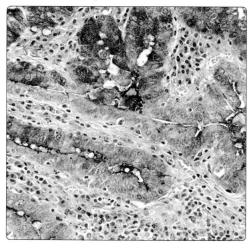

(Left) *High-power view of WLPTC shows patchy membranous staining of the tumor cells for HBME-1, and lymphoplasmacytic infiltrate replacing the cores of papillae is negative.* (Right) *High-power view of WLPTC shows cytoplasmic staining of the tumor cells for galectin-3. Note that the lymphoplasmacytic infiltrate is negative.*

Struma Ovarii, Struma Carcinoid, and Malignant Struma Ovarii

TERMINOLOGY

- Struma ovarii: Ovarian teratomas in which thyroid tissue is predominant (at least 50%) or sole tissue component
- Struma carcinoid: Ovarian tumor includes presence of thyroid tissue admixed with carcinoid tumor
- Malignant struma ovarii (MSO): Malignant ovarian teratomas in which malignant thyroid tumor [usually papillary thyroid carcinoma (PTC)] is intermixed or originating from thyroid tissue of struma ovarii
- Strumosis: Thyroid tissue from struma ovarii that spreads to peritoneum forming peritoneal implants

CLINICAL ISSUES

- Presentation is similar to ovarian teratoma
- Enlarging abdominal mass

MICROSCOPIC

- **Struma ovarii**: Normal-appearing thyroid follicular tissue

- **Struma carcinoid**: Characterized by presence of normal thyroid tissue admixed with carcinoid tumor
  - Diagnosis made as long as both components are present, not on whether one or other predominates
- **MSO**: Most MSO are histologically classified as PTCs
- Immunohistochemistry shows immunoexpression of HBME-1, cytokeratin-19, galectin-3, and CITED-1
- *BRAF* mutations present in 67% of MSO and absent in benign struma ovarii

ANCILLARY TESTS

- Immunohistochemistry: TTF-1, pax-8, thyroglobulin
  - Neuroendocrine markers also present in struma carcinoid
  - If MSO: HBME-1, galectin-3, CITED-1, BRAF
- *BRAF*: Includes V600E, K601E, and novel deletion/substitution TV599-600M

Struma Ovarii

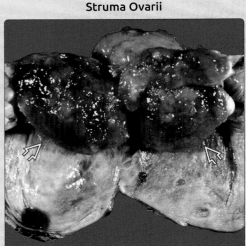

Papillary Thyroid Carcinoma

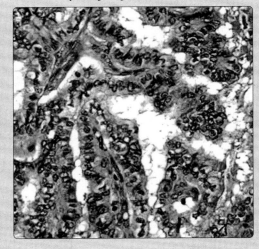

(Left) *Gross image shows a struma ovarii where the tumor nodule ➡ resembles normal thyroid as an homogeneous red-brown nodule within a cystic ovarian teratoma.* (Right) *Malignant struma ovarii (MSO) shows papillary thyroid carcinoma (PTC), classical variant, with papillae formation and characteristic nuclear features of PTC.*

HBME-1 Immunoexpression in Malignant Struma Ovarii

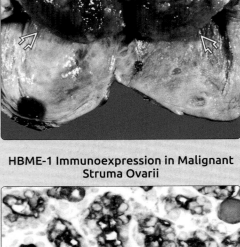

BRAF in Malignant Struma Ovarii

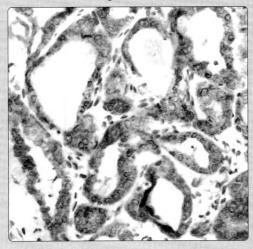

(Left) *This ovarian follicular variant of PTC shows membranous and luminal immunopositivity for HBME-1. MSO can be characterized by immunohistochemistry using a panel of antibodies including HBME-1.* (Right) *Immunohistochemistry using anti-BRAF V600E antibody (clone VE1) for specific detection of the BRAF V600E mutant protein is usually present in these tumors as a uniform cytoplasmic staining, in some MSO.*

Struma Ovarii, Struma Carcinoid, and Malignant Struma Ovarii

TERMINOLOGY

Definitions
- **Ovarian thyroid tissue**
  - Presence of thyroid parenchyma in setting of ovarian teratoma
  - Thyroid tissue represents only minor component of ovarian teratoma
- **Struma ovarii (SO)**
  - Ovarian teratomas in which thyroid tissue is predominant (at least 50%) or sole tissue component
- **Strumosis**
  - Thyroid tissue from SO that spread to peritoneum forming peritoneal implants
- **Struma carcinoid**
  - Ovarian tumor includes presence of thyroid tissue admixed with carcinoid tumor
    - In this setting, other teratomatous elements usually absent
- **Malignant struma ovarii (MSO)**
  - Malignant ovarian teratomas in which malignant thyroid tumor [usually papillary thyroid carcinoma (PTC)] is intermixed or originating from thyroid tissue in SO
  - MSO are rare tumors that arise from ectopic thyroid tissue in ovary (benign SO)

ETIOLOGY/PATHOGENESIS

Idiopathic
- No known associated causes or risk factors

CLINICAL ISSUES

Epidemiology
- Incidence
  - 5-15% of mature ovarian teratomas contain thyroid tissue
    - Identification may be function of adequate sampling
- Age
  - **SO**
    - May occur over wide range, between 2nd-9th decades
    - Occurs mostly > 40 yr
  - **Struma carcinoid**
    - Majority are postmenopausal
    - Occur over wide age range, from 3rd-8th decades
  - **MSO**
    - Usually occurs mostly > 40 yr
- Sex
  - Exclusively in women

Site
- Exclusively limited to ovary
  - Bilaterality may occur in up to 5% of cases

Presentation
- **SO**
  - Presentation is similar to ovarian teratoma
    - Enlarging abdominal mass
    - Incidental finding on routine gynecologic (or urologic) evaluation
  - Other (uncommon) clinical presentations may include
    - Symptoms related to function of thyroid component (hyperthyroidism); occur in < 10%
    - Ascites that, in presence of ovarian mass, may be suspicious for ovarian carcinoma
    - Ascites and hydrothorax (pseudo-Meigs syndrome) may occur
- **Struma carcinoid**
  - Presentation similar to ovarian teratoma
    - Abdominal mass
    - Acute abdominal pain
    - Incidental finding on routine gynecologic or urologic evaluation
    - Rarely, may initially be detected as ovarian mass complicating pregnancy
  - Other uncommon presentations may include
    - Constipation (peptide YY found in association with constipation)
    - Pain on defecation
    - Virilization, hirsutism
    - Symptoms related to hyperthyroidism rarely occur
  - Carcinoid syndrome
    - Occurs in 25-33% of cases
    - May include facial flushing, diarrhea, bronchospasm, hypertension
    - Rare occurrence of carcinoid heart disease reported; may include edema
- **MSO**
  - Rare tumor
    - Real incidence is unknown
  - Identification of malignancy in SO is related to tissue sampling
  - BRAF mutations present in 67% of MSO
    - BRAF mutations include V600E, K601E, and novel deletion/substitution TV599-600M
    - Oncogenic activation of BRAF (35-69%), RAS (10%), or RET (5-30%) is common in PTC

Laboratory Tests
- SO
  - Functional abnormalities may occur, including
    - Hyperthyroidism (rarely, SO may coexist with Graves disease)
    - Increased serum thyroglobulin may be present in metastatic thyroid carcinoma arising in SO
    - Increased serum CA-125 levels in pseudo-Meigs syndrome (ascites and hydrothorax)

Treatment
- **SO**
  - Surgical excision is treatment of choice
    - Unilateral salpingo-oophorectomy or total abdominal hysterectomy and salpingo-oophorectomy (uni- or bilateral)
  - In presence of normally situated (cervical) thyroid gland without abnormalities, surgical intervention not indicated
- **Struma carcinoid**
  - Unilateral salpingo-oophorectomy in younger patients
  - Bilateral oophorectomy and hysterectomy in older patients
- **MSO**

Thyroid

233

- o Surgical excision
  - – Unilateral salpingo-oophorectomy or total abdominal hysterectomy and salpingo-oophorectomy (uni- or bilateral)
- o Excision of metastases
- o Treatment for metastatic thyroid (papillary) carcinoma in SO may include
  - – Surgical removal ± supplemental radioactive iodine therapy
  - – Use of radioactive iodine therapy, which would necessitate ablation of cervical thyroid gland

Prognosis

- **SO**
  - o Surgical removal is curative
  - o Rare instances of non-Hodgkin malignant lymphomas reported in SO
- **Benign peritoneal strumosis or stromatosis**
  - o Mature thyroid follicular epithelium that spread within peritoneum
    - – These foci should be considered to represent spread from SO
- **Struma carcinoid**
  - o Prognosis considered excellent following surgical removal, even in presence of metastatic tumor
    - – Both struma and carcinoid components capable of giving rise to metastases
- **MSO**
  - o Prognosis considered excellent
  - o Recurrence or metastases may occur many years after original diagnosis
  - o Metastatic disease from papillary carcinoma may occur
    - – Found in contralateral ovary, peritoneum, regional lymph nodes, liver, and brain
  - o Prognosis associated with malignant thyroid tumors in SO considered good with overall survival rates of
    - – 89% at 10 yr
    - – 84% at 25 yr
    - – Although unusual, fatalities secondary to widespread metastatic disease have occurred
- Pathologic factors predictive of poorer prognosis include
  - o Large size (≥ 10 cm)
  - o Struma component > 80%
  - o Extensive papillary carcinoma, especially with solid areas
  - o Necrosis, ≥ 5 mitoses per 10 HPF

IMAGING

MR Findings

- Presence of multilocular cystic mass with variable signal intensity within loculi
- Loculi or small cysts within septations may show
  - o Low signal intensity on T1-weighted images
  - o Very low signal intensity on T2-weighted images
- Gd-DTPA-enhanced T1-weighted images may show
  - o Presence of thick septations
  - o Locally thickened wall with marked enhancement (corresponding microscopically to thyroid tissue)

MACROSCOPIC

General Features

- On gross examination, cystic strumas can be mistaken for mucinous or serous cystic tumors of other primary sites, depending on presence of mucoid or watery fluid
- **SO**
  - o Resembles normal thyroid
    - – Homogeneous red-brown nodule within teratoma
  - o May resemble nodular goiter, appearing as multiple glistening brown nodules
  - o Just as SO can mimic variety of other ovarian tumors, converse is also true
- **MSO**
  - o Usually as part of SO, identified as tan-white area within brown thyroid tissue

MICROSCOPIC

Histologic Features

- **SO**
  - o Normal-appearing thyroid follicular tissue (most common finding)
  - o Multinodular goiter with colloid-filled, variably sized follicles lined by flattened follicular epithelial cells
  - o Secondary degenerative changes (e.g., fibrosis, cyst formation, hemorrhage) may be present
  - o Changes of lymphocytic thyroiditis may be present
  - o Other less common findings
    - – Papillary hyperplasia of follicular epithelium, clear cells, signet ring cells
    - – Proliferative SO
      - □ Refers to discrete mass composed of densely cellular thyroid follicles (without evidence of malignancy)
- **Struma carcinoid**
  - o Characterized by presence of normal thyroid tissue admixed with carcinoid tumor
  - o Diagnosis made as long as both components are present, not on whether one or other predominates
  - o Carcinoid component shows
    - – Trabecular, organoid, and solid growth patterns
    - – Cells with small round to oval nuclei, dispersed (salt and pepper) nuclear chromatin
    - – Rarely, stromal amyloid deposition is present
    - – Rarely, carcinoid component may be mucinous type (mucus-secreting cells)
    - – Birefringent calcium oxalate monohydrate crystals may be identified in colloid material
  - o Just as SO can mimic variety of other ovarian tumors, reverse is also true
- **MSO**
  - o Rarely, thyroid neoplasms arise in setting of SO
  - o Most MSO are histologically classified as PTCs
    - – PTC can be of classical, follicular, or solid variants
  - o If thyroid neoplasms arise in setting of SO
    - – Diagnosis based on cytomorphologic (i.e., nuclear) features
    - – Invasive growth (vascular or stromal) not required for diagnosis of papillary carcinoma

- o Follicular carcinoma within SO is very difficult or impossible to diagnose
  - – Diagnosis based on presence of capsular or vascular invasion
- o Rare cases of anaplastic carcinoma are reported
- Concurrent neoplasms
  - o Concurrent described primary ovarian lesions included: Serous cystadenoma, mucinous cystadenoma, Brenner tumor, thecoma, ovarian fibroma, and focal hilus cell hyperplasia

ANCILLARY TESTS

Immunohistochemistry

- Struma carcinoid
  - o Thyroglobulin reactivity positive in follicular component
  - o TTF-1
    - – Expressed in follicular epithelial cells
    - – Thyroglobulin and TTF-1 negative in carcinoid component
  - o pax-8
  - o Chromogranin, synaptophysin, CD56, NSE, and serotonin positive
    - – Calcitonin only rarely found
  - o Neurohormonal peptides can be present
    - – Pancreatic polypeptide, vasoactive intestinal polypeptide, insulin, glucagon, substance-P, and somatostatin
- MSO
  - o PTC shows immunoexpression of HBME-1, CK19, galectin-3, CITED-1, and may express V600E BRAF

Genetic Testing

- *BRAF* mutation
  - o Positive in PTC arising in SO
  - o Present in 67% of MSO and absent in all benign SO
  - o Includes V600E, K601E, and novel deletion/substitution TV599-600M
- Development of MSO with PTC features is associated with unusual *BRAF* mutations
  - o *BRAF* mutation commonly observed in PTC, suggesting common pathogenesis for all PTCs regardless of location

DIFFERENTIAL DIAGNOSIS

Metastatic Thyroid Carcinoma to Ovary

- Extraordinarily rare occurrence
- In presence of malignant thyroid neoplasm in SO, detailed evaluation of thyroid gland proper indicated

Metastatic Neuroendocrine Carcinoma (Carcinoid) to Ovary

- Common feature from gastrointestinal neuroendocrine carcinoma (appendix, small intestine)
- Clues in support of metastasis include bilaterality, multinodularity, presence of peritoneal metastases

Clear Cell Carcinoma, Endometrioid Carcinoma, Sertoli-Leydig Cell Tumors, and Pregnancy Luteoma

- May contain cystic glands or follicle-like spaces filled with secretions resembling thyroid colloid, but identifying other features of such tumors permit their identification

Well-Differentiated Sertoli Cell Tumor

- In these cases, the following may be helpful in confirming follicular-derived tumor
  - o Association with dermoid cyst or teratomatous elements of another type
  - o Demonstration of foci of typical thyroid follicles
  - o Presence of eosinophilic secretions
  - o Immunoreactivity for thyroglobulin

Mucinous or Serous Cystic Tumors

- On gross examination, cystic strumas can be mistaken for mucinous or serous cystic tumors of other primary sites
- Green to brown color of fluid
- On microscopic examination, diagnosis is confirmed by presence or absence of thyroid follicles in wall

DIAGNOSTIC CHECKLIST

Clinically Relevant Pathologic Features

- Functional abnormalities may occur, including increased serum thyroglobulin in metastatic thyroid carcinoma arising in SO

SELECTED REFERENCES

1. Fukunaga M et al: Malignant struma ovarii with a predominant component of anaplastic carcinoma. Int J Gynecol Pathol. 35(4):357-61, 2016
2. Goffredo P et al: Malignant struma ovarii: a population-level analysis of a large series of 68 patients. Thyroid. 25(2):211-5, 2015
3. Tan A et al: Novel BRAF and KRAS mutations in papillary thyroid carcinoma arising in struma ovarii. Endocr Pathol. 26(4):296-301, 2015
4. Wei S et al: Pathology of struma ovarii: a report of 96 cases. Endocr Pathol. 26(4):342-8, 2015
5. Karagkounis G et al: Tall-cell variant papillary thyroid carcinoma arising from struma ovarll. Endocr Pract. 20(2):e24-7, 2014
6. Matsunami K et al: Peptide YY producing strumal carcinoid tumor of the ovary. Eur J Gynaecol Oncol. 32(2):201-2, 2011
7. Miñambres I et al: Unusual characteristics and fatal outcome of a malignant struma ovarii. Case report and literature review. Endocrinol Nutr. 58(7):377-9, 2011
8. Marcy PY et al: Lethal, malignant, metastatic struma ovarii. Thyroid. 20(9):1037-40, 2010
9. Michels A et al: Malignant struma ovarii. J Clin Endocrinol Metab. 95(4):1505, 2010
10. Shaco-Levy R et al: Natural history of biologically malignant struma ovarii: analysis of 27 cases with extraovarian spread. Int J Gynecol Pathol. 29(3):212-27, 2010
11. Roth LM et al: Highly differentiated follicular carcinoma arising from struma ovarii: a report of 3 cases, a review of the literature, and a reassessment of so-called peritoneal strumosis. Int J Gynecol Pathol. 27(2):213-22, 2008
12. Roth LM et al: Typical thyroid-type carcinoma arising in struma ovarii: a report of 4 cases and review of the literature. Int J Gynecol Pathol. 27(4):496-506, 2008
13. Ciampi R et al: RET/PTC rearrangements and BRAF mutations in thyroid tumorigenesis. Endocrinology. 148(3):936-41, 2007
14. Schmidt J et al: BRAF in papillary thyroid carcinoma of ovary (struma ovarii). Am J Surg Pathol. 31(9):1337-43, 2007
15. Xing M: BRAF mutation in papillary thyroid cancer: pathogenic role, molecular bases, and clinical implications. Endocr Rev. 28(7):742-62, 2007

Ovarian Cystic Mass

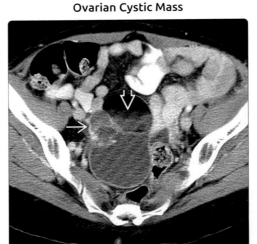

Multiloculated Ovarian Mass

(Left) *Axial CECT shows a complex cystic mass containing fat-fluid level ➡ and an avidly enhancing nodular soft tissue component ➡.* **(Right)** *Sagittal T2WI MR in the same patient confirms the presence of a large, multiloculated cystic mass ➡ within the pelvis. Pathology confirmed mature teratoma containing mainly thyroid tissue.*

Struma Ovarii

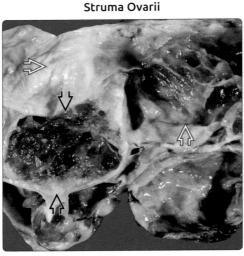

Malignant Struma Ovarii

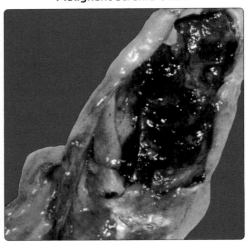
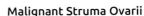
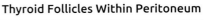

(Left) *This struma ovarii arising in a cystic teratoma ➡ has features resembling a nodular goiter. The cut surface of this area ➡ shows multiple glistening brown nodular areas with cystic changes.* **(Right)** *This struma ovarii, which had a microscopic focus of papillary thyroid carcinoma, grossly resembles normal thyroid tissue. The mass forms a homogeneous red-brown nodule within a teratoma.*

Papillary Tyroid Carcinoma Arising in Struma Ovarii

Thyroid Follicles Within Peritoneum

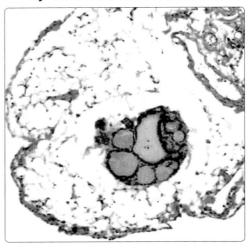

(Left) *Struma ovarii is shown with normal-appearing thyroid follicular tissue ➡ and a focus of PTC ➡. The tumor has a follicular architecture, increased nuclear:cytoplasmic ratio, and characteristic nuclear features of PTC.* **(Right)** *Strumosis is a term used for the presence of benign thyroid follicular epithelium within the peritoneum, usually as spread from struma ovarii. Metastatic thyroid carcinoma should be considered in the differential diagnosis.*

Malignant Struma Ovarii

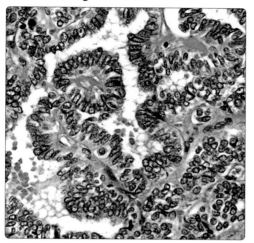

Papillary Tyroid Carcinoma, Classic

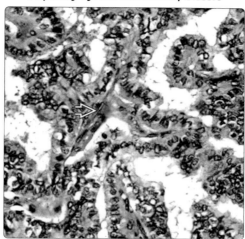

(Left) *This photomicrograph of an MSO demonstrates a PTC with papillary architecture and fibrovascular cores lined by irregularly shaped, clear nuclei with irregular nuclear membranes.* (Right) *This MSO demonstrates a PTC with papillary architecture and a thin fibrovascular core ➡ lined by irregularly shaped, clear nuclei with features of PTC.*

Characteristic Architecture

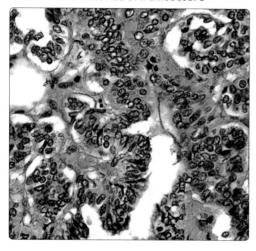

Malignant Struma Ovarii With Follicles

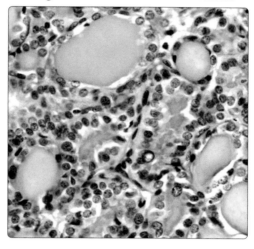

(Left) *The tumor cells in this example of a recurrent MSO with PTC are arranged in a follicular and tubercular pattern. Enlarged, irregularly shaped nuclei demonstrate the nuclear clearing and grooves characteristic of PTC.* (Right) *PTC, follicular variant, demonstrates a follicular architecture, increased nuclear:cytoplasmic ratio, and clear nuclei with irregular nuclear membranes. The follicles are small and have a thick eosinophilic colloid.*

Papillary Thyroid Carcinoma, Follicular Variant

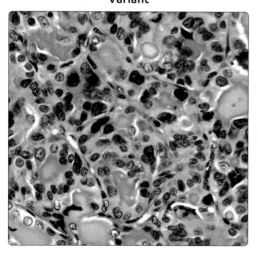

Papillary Thyroid Carcinoma, Follicular Variant

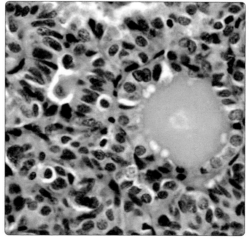

(Left) *The tumor cells in this MSO with a PTC are arranged in a follicular pattern. The follicles demonstrate dark colloid, which is commonly seen in this variant. There is nuclear overlapping and marked nuclear pleomorphism in this area.* (Right) *MSO with a PTC, follicular variant, demonstrates a follicular architecture, increased nuclear:cytoplasmic ratio, and clear nuclei with irregular nuclear membranes.*

Recurrent Malignant Struma Ovarii

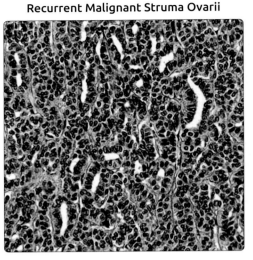

Galectin-3 Immunopositivity

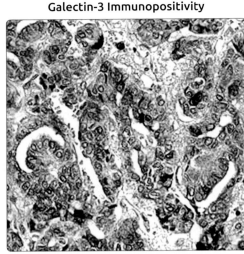

(Left) *The tumor cells of this recurrent MSO with PTC are arranged in an irregular trabecular pattern. The primary tumor of this patient had a follicular variant pattern.* (Right) *The PTC with trabecular and follicular pattern of this recurrent malignant struma ovarii is characterized by immunopositivity for HBME-1, galectin-3 (shown here), and CK19.*

Struma Carcinoid

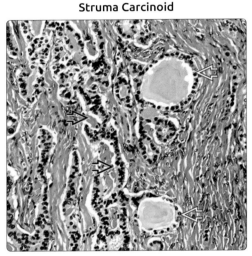

TTF-1 Nuclear Staining

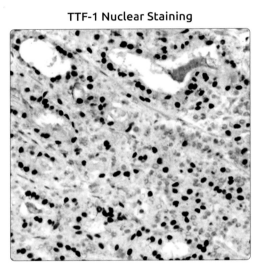

(Left) *Microscopic appearance of an ovarian struma carcinoid shows intimate admixture of thyroid follicles and carcinoid trabeculae. Some tumors may show a trabecular or mucinous appearance.* (Right) *Immunohistochemistry for TTF-1 of an ovarian struma carcinoid identifies the follicular cells and highlights the intimate admixture of thyroid follicles and carcinoid component.*

Struma Carcinoid

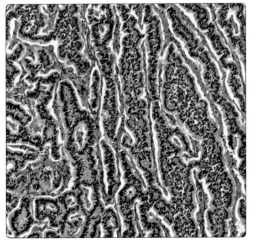

TTF-1 and Chromogranin Staining

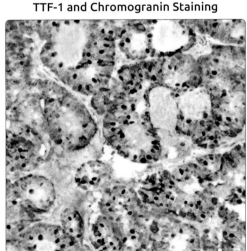

(Left) *One area of a struma carcinoid of the ovary is shown with a predominant neuroendocrine component. The tumor has a trabecular appearance, somewhat similar to carcinoid in the lung or rectum.* (Right) *Double immunohistochemistry stain for TTF-1 and chromogranin of a struma carcinoid highlights the 2 cellular components present in these tumors. There is an intimate admixture of follicular cells and neuroendocrine cells.*

Papillary Thyroid Carcinoma, Follicular Variant

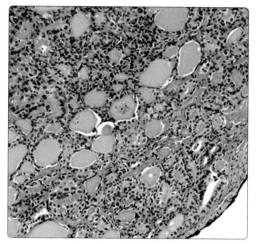

Galectin-3 Immunopositivity

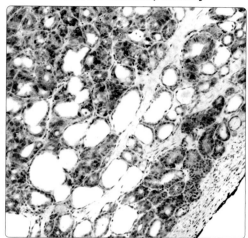

(Left) *MSO shows PTC arising within an ovarian teratoma. The neoplastic deposits show follicular architecture with nuclear features of PTC, i.e., nuclear clearing, overlap, and grooves.* (Right) *Immunohistochemistry shows diffuse cytoplasmic staining for galectin-3 in MSO cells. The stain intensity is characteristically variable between the tumor cells. These tumors can also be characterized using HBME-1, CITED-1, and CK19.*

HBME-1 Immunopositivity

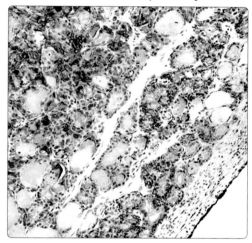

Negative Calcitonin Stain

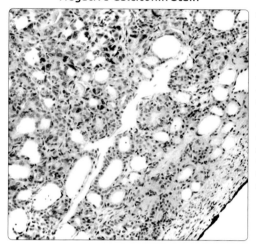

(Left) *HBME-1 immunostain in an MSO demonstrates the characteristic membranous staining pattern in the tumor cells. This pattern gives rise to the luminal border staining seen in the follicular variant of PTC.* (Right) *Calcitonin immunostain is negative in the benign and malignant struma ovarii. It can rarely be identified in struma carcinoid, which can be weakly positive in rare tumor cells showing ectopic hormone production.*

Cellular Characteristics

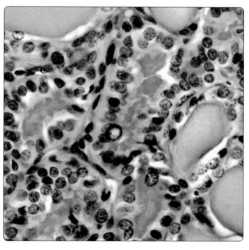

CITED-1 Immunopositivity

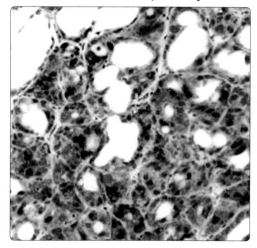

(Left) *High-power view of a PTC arising in a struma ovarii with a follicular architecture shows that the follicles are small and have a thick, eosinophilic colloid. The nuclei have the characteristic features of PTC.* (Right) *MSO can be characterized by immunohistochemistry using a panel of antibodies including HBME-1, galectin-3, CITED-1 (MSG1), and CK19. This panel has up to 90% sensitivity and specificity.*

KEY FACTS

TERMINOLOGY

- Malignant tumor of thyroid gland composed of cells with evidence of C-cell differentiation

CLINICAL ISSUES

- Germline mutations of *RET* protooncogene cause hereditary forms
- Somatic *RET* mutations can be present in sporadic forms of disease

MICROSCOPIC

- Finding neoplastic/primary C-cell hyperplasia (CCH) may serve as morphological marker for multiple endocrine neoplasia type 2 (MEN2)-associated medullary thyroid carcinoma (MTC)
- Neoplastic/primary CCH is precursor lesion in hereditary MTC
  - a.k.a. C-cell carcinoma in situ or medullary carcinoma in situ or thyroid intraepithelial neoplasia of C cells

- Distinguishing CCH from MMC may be difficult
  - Extension of C cells through basement membranes of expanded C-cell-filled follicles into surrounding interstitium
  - Loss of organoid arrangement of C-cell-filled follicles
  - Appearance of desmoplastic stromal reaction surrounding groups of infiltrating tumor cells
- Histologic appearance of MTC is quite variable
- Most common morphology is solid tumor (known as solid carcinoma)
  - MTC may also present as sheets, nests, trabeculae, or insular patterns
  - Rare variants: Pseudopapillary, tubular/glandular, follicular, spindle cell, clear cell, oncocytic, small cell, giant cell, melanotic, amphicrine, paraganglioma-like, oat cell carcinoma, angiosarcoma-like, and squamous cell variant
  - Staining for calcitonin is helpful in making distinction between MTC and other diverse tumors it may mimic

Cut Surface of Both Thyroid Lobes

(Left) The right ⇨ and left ⇨ thyroid lobes have firm, well-circumscribed, white-gray-yellow tumors. The 2 serial sections of the right lobe show a larger tumor than the sections on the left lobe in this patient with multiple endocrine neoplasia type 2 (MEN2) syndrome. (Right) Photomicrograph shows a thyroid from a patient with MEN2. The C-cell hyperplasia is easily identified by H&E ⇨. In inherited syndromes, the primary/neoplastic C-cell hyperplasia usually precedes neoplasia.

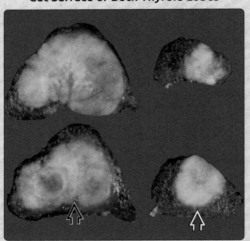

C-Cell Hyperplasia in MEN2

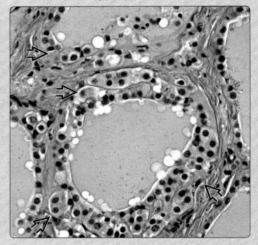

C Cells Associated With Solid Cell Nests

(Left) C cells are usually associated with solid cell nests. In this photomicrograph, the prominent C-cell population ⇨ on the lower left corner is adjacent to a solid cell nest ⇨. (Right) A medullary thyroid microcarcinoma is defined as a tumor measuring < 1.0 cm. Invasion of the adjacent tissue should be present, and desmoplasia may be present.

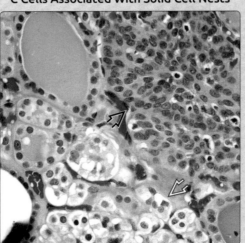

Medullary Thyroid Microcarcinoma

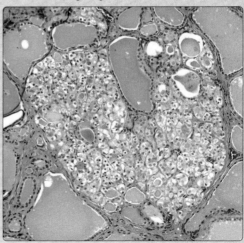

TERMINOLOGY

Abbreviations

- Medullary thyroid carcinoma (MTC)

Synonyms

- Solid carcinoma with amyloid stroma
- C-cell carcinoma
- Parafollicular cell carcinoma

Definitions

- Malignant tumor of thyroid gland composed of cells with evidence of C-cell differentiation
- MTCs measuring < 1 cm in diameter are called medullary thyroid microcarcinomas (MMC)

ETIOLOGY/PATHOGENESIS

Genetic Predisposition

- Hereditary forms of MTC are transmitted as autosomal dominant traits, usually with high penetrance
- Multiple endocrine neoplasia type 2 (MEN2) syndrome and familial MTC (FMTC)-only syndrome are caused by mutations in *RET* gene
  - Commonly activating point mutations
  - Exon 10 codons 609, 611, 618, 620, and exon 11 codon 634 responsible for majority of MEN2A and FMTC
    - MEN2A: Majority involve exon 11 codon 634
  - MEN2B: Majority associated with exon 16 codon 918 mutation
  - Fusion genes with tyrosine kinase domain of *RET* also occur
    - *RET* chromosomal rearrangements also associated with papillary carcinoma (*RET*/PTC)
  - Somatic *RET* mutations also present in up to ~ 50% of sporadic MTCs
- MTC is seen in setting of MEN2 syndromes
  - **MEN2A**
    - MTC, parathyroid hyperplasia, pheochromocytoma, and pancreatic endocrine tumors
    - ~ 100% of individuals with MEN2A develop MTC
  - **MEN2B**
    - MTC, pheochromocytoma, mucosal and soft tissue tumors (notably neuromas), marfanoid body habitus
    - Characterized by early development of aggressive form of MTC in ~ 100% of affected individuals
  - **FMTC-only syndrome**
    - MTC not associated with other tumors
    - Comprises ~ 10-20% of MEN2 cases

Precursor Lesions

- **Neoplastic or primary C-cell hyperplasia (CCH)**
  - Precursor lesion in hereditary MTC
  - Recognized on basis of expansile intrafollicular C-cell proliferation with varying degree of dysplasia
    - C-cell clusters surrounding or invading follicles
  - a.k.a. C-cell carcinoma in situ or medullary carcinoma in situ or thyroid intraepithelial neoplasia of C cells
  - These lesions harbor germline *RET* mutations
  - Postulated that CCH progresses to MMC and eventually to MTC
  - Found in vicinity of medullary carcinomas

- Distinguishing CCH from MMC may be difficult
  - Extension of C cells through basement membranes of expanded C-cell-filled follicles into surrounding interstitium
  - Loss of the organoid arrangement of C-cell-filled follicles
  - Appearance of desmoplastic stromal reaction surrounding groups of infiltrating tumor cells
- **Reactive or physiological CCH**
  - Increase in number of C cells secondary to associated
    - Thyroid disorder (nodules, papillary or follicular carcinoma, inflammatory or autoimmune, and PTEN hamartoma tumor syndrome)
    - Hypergastrinemia
    - Hyperparathyroidism
    - Hypercalcemic states
  - Clusters should have > 50 C cells per low-power (100x) magnification
  - Lacks pleomorphism, amyloid, fibrosis, or invasion of follicles
  - Difficult to visualize on H&E alone; requires calcitonin staining to identify C cells
  - Role of CCH in sporadic MTC remains unknown

Sporadic Medullary Thyroid Carcinoma

- Unknown etiology

CLINICAL ISSUES

Epidemiology

- Incidence
  - 2-3% of all thyroid malignancies
    - 70% are sporadic
    - 30% are hereditary
  - Variable incidence due to calcitonin-screening protocols and *RET* genetic testing and relative increased incidence of papillary thyroid carcinoma
    - Increase in prophylactic thyroidectomies
    - Mostly MMC identified in familial cases
- Age
  - In sporadic cases: 50-60 years
  - Familial cases can present from early childhood
    - MTC in MEN2B: ~ 5 years
    - MTC in MEN2A: 25-30 years
    - MTC in FMTC: ~ 50 years
- Sex
  - 1:1 in familial cases

Presentation

- Often presents as painless, "cold" nodule
- Up to 70% have nodal metastases
- Up to 10% may present with distant metastases
- Symptoms of carcinoid and Cushing syndromes may be present (production of ACTH or CRH)
- Large tumors may lead to dysphagia and upper airway obstruction
- Nonthyroid findings: Mucosal neuromas; parathyroid, adrenal, pituitary, and pancreatic tumors
- MTC tends to metastasize early: Liver, lungs, bone, soft tissue outside neck, brain, and bone marrow

Laboratory Tests

- Screening and monitoring tests are performed in patients at risk
  - History or presence of MEN
  - Family history of MEN2 or FMTC
  - Genetic counseling is recommended to assess patient-specific risk
  - Annual serum calcitonin screening should begin in children with MEN2B at 6 months, MEN2A at 3-5 years of age
- Increased serum calcitonin and CEA levels
  - Correlate with tumor burden
- Abnormal pentagastrin-stimulated calcitonin response
- *RET* molecular genetic testing indicated in all individuals with
  - Diagnosis of MTC
  - Clinical diagnosis of MEN2
  - Primary CCH
- *RET* gene mutation analysis
  - Most commonly exons 10, 11, 13, 14, and 16 in hereditary forms
  - Mutations in codons 768, 790, 791, and 804 may predispose to milder form of MTC with low penetrance, late onset, and without family history
  - Most common somatic mutation in sporadic MTC is M918T
- MEN2A: ~ 100% of families have *RET* mutation in exon 10 or 11
- FMTC: Families have almost 100% *RET* mutation
- MEN2B: Individuals with features of this syndrome should have mutation analysis or sequencing of exons 15 or 16 to detect p.M918T and p.A883F mutations
- Rarely, germline *RET* mutation may not be detected in family with clinical diagnosis of MEN2A, MEN2B, or FMTC

Treatment

- Surgical approaches
  - Total thyroidectomy offers best chance of cure
  - Associated neck dissections considered for tumors > 1 cm
  - American Thyroid Association Guidelines Task Force has classified mutations based on risk for aggressive MTC
    - May be used in predicting phenotype and recommendations for age at which to perform prophylactic thyroidectomy and to begin biochemical screening for associated diseases
  - Prophylactic thyroidectomy
    - Primary preventive measure for individuals with identified germline *RET* mutation
  - Prophylactic thyroidectomy recommendations for specific *RET* germline mutations
    - Codons 883, 918, or 922: Thyroidectomy by 1 year of age
    - Codons 609, 611, 618, 620, 630, or 634: Thyroidectomy before 5 years of age
    - Codons 786, 790, 791, 804, or 891: Consider surgery before age of 5; may delay surgery up to 10 years
    - Other mutations: Thyroidectomy once stimulated calcitonin screening turns abnormal

- Thyroidectomy for CCH, before progression to micromedullary carcinoma, may allow surgery to be limited to thyroidectomy alone, sparing of lymph nodes
- Adjuvant therapy
  - Targeted tyrosine kinase, hormone therapy, chemotherapy, and anti-CEA treatments can be considered
- Radiation
  - For residual disease and palliation

Prognosis

- Considerable variation
- Overall 5- and 10-year survivals of 60-80% and 40-70%, respectively
- 10-year survival by tumor stage
  - Stage I: Near 100%; stage II: 98%; stage III: 81%; stage IV: 28%
- Better prognostic factors are tumor stage, young age, women, and familial forms
- Poor prognostic factors are necrosis, squamous metaplasia, < 50% calcitonin immunoreaction, and CEA reactivity in absence of calcitonin

IMAGING

Scintigraphic Scan

- "Cold" nodule on iodine scan

MACROSCOPIC

General Features

- Typically at junction of upper and middle 1/3 of lobe
- Sporadic tumors tend to present as solitary mass
- Hereditary tumors seen in MEN are usually multicentric and bilateral
- Usually not encapsulated but well circumscribed
- Firm, grayish-tan to yellow-white, gritty cut surface

Size

- Ranges from grossly undetectable to large, replacing entire lobe
- Small tumors often seen in prophylactic thyroidectomy specimens from MEN2 patients

Sections to Be Submitted

- In high-risk patients (MEN2 and FMTC) who undergo prophylactic thyroidectomy, entire gland should be submitted to identify MMC and CCH
  - Specimen should be serially sectioned and submitted as whole from superior to inferior
  - C cells are normally situated in upper and middle portions of lobes; submit apparently normal thyroid for histological examination
    - Search for CCH

MICROSCOPIC

Histologic Features

- Tumors from patients with heritable forms and virtually indistinguishable from those occurring sporadically
  - Except for their bilaterality, multicentricity, and association with primary CCH

- MTC is diagnosed histologically when nests of C cells appear to extend beyond basement membrane and infiltrate and destroy thyroid follicles
  - Primary CCH can often be recognized by presence of expansile intrafollicular C-cell proliferation with varying degrees of dysplasia
    - Finding primary CCH may serve as morphological marker for MEN2-associated MTC
    - In MEN2, age of transformation from CCH to MTC varies with different germline *RET* mutation
- Most common prototypical morphology has solid, trabecular, or insular growth pattern
- Cells can be round, polygonal, plasmacytoid, or spindle-shaped, separated by thin fibrovascular cores
- Cytoplasm can be clear, amphophilic, or eosinophilic
- Nuclei are round to oval with small nucleoli
- Chromatin is fine granular and dispersed or coarsely clumped
- Vacuoles with mucin have been frequently described
- Psammoma-like concretions are occasionally seen
- Up to 90% show calcitonin-positive amyloid in stroma
- Histological appearance is quite variable and can mimic entire spectrum of thyroid malignancies
  - May mimic other thyroid carcinomas (follicular, papillary, poorly differentiated, anaplastic)

Histologic Variants

- Rare variants: Papillary, pseudopapillary, tubular/glandular, follicular, spindle cell, clear cell, oncocytic, small cell, giant cell, melanotic, amphicrine, paraganglioma-like, oat cell carcinoma, angiosarcoma-like, and squamous cell variant
- Variant patterns of MTC may resemble wide range of thyroid and extrathyroid tumors
  - Staining for calcitonin is helpful in making distinction between MTC and other diverse tumors it may mimic

ANCILLARY TESTS

Cytology

- Aspirates are hypercellular with loosely cohesive to noncohesive cells
- Spindle, polygonal, or bipolar cells, often with eccentric nuclei
- Hyperchromatic nuclei with granular chromatin and moderate pleomorphism
- Amyloid may be seen in 50-70% of tumors
- Multinucleated giant tumor cells are common
  - Despite well-known cytological features, only ~ 45% of cases are diagnosed in clinical practice
    - Highlighting difficulty in making this diagnosis

Histochemistry

- Congo red
  - Reactivity: Positive
  - Staining pattern: Amyloid shows light green birefringence with polarization

Immunohistochemistry

- Hallmark of MTC is positivity for calcitonin and calcitonin gene-related peptide
  - Cases with lack of calcitonin expression, may have immunoreactivity for calcitonin-gene-related peptide

- Tumor cells are also positive for neuroendocrine markers (chromogranin, synaptophysin) and CEA
- TTF-1 and pax-8 are positive but weak
- Progesterone receptor and S100 (in sustentacular cells) can be positive
- Other peptide products may be present: ACTH, somatostatin, gastrin-releasing peptide, neurotensin

Genetic Testing

- *RET* gene sequencing is important to determine prognosis and timing of prophylactic thyroidectomy
  - Exons 10, 11, 13, 14, 15, and 16 cover 95% of cases
  - M918T *RET* mutation in exon 16 is present in 98% of patients with MEN2B
  - MEN2A: 85% carry codon 634 mutation (associated with pheochromocytoma and hyperparathyroidism)
- Identify rearrangements involving *RET* gene
- Somatic *RET* mutations (M918T) have been reported in 40-60% of sporadic tumors
- Presence of *HRAS* and *KRAS* mutation in 56% and 12% of *RET*-negative sporadic MTCs, respectively
  - Mutual exclusivity suggests that RAS activation may constitute alternative molecular pathway for development of MTC
- *MYH13-RET* fusion found in sporadic MTC
- *GFPT1-ALK* fusion also found in sporadic MTC
- Programmed cell death 4 (*PDCD4*) is tumor-suppressor gene involved in tumorigenesis

Electron Microscopy

- Presence of neurosecretory granules confirms neuroendocrine origin of tumor
  - 2 types: 280 nm and 130 nm electron dense, membrane bound
- Amyloid material is detected as fine fibrillary material within parenchymal space

DIFFERENTIAL DIAGNOSIS

Intrathyroid Tumor

- **Metastatic neuroendocrine tumors**
  - Can be positive for calcitonin and CEA in rare cases
  - Clinical and radiologic correlation may help in differential
- **Paraganglioma**
  - Negative for calcitonin; zellballen with S100-positive sustentacular cells
- **Follicular carcinoma**
  - Thyroglobulin is positive
  - Nuclear features: Neuroendocrine chromatin in MTC compared with dark dense nuclei in follicular carcinoma
- **Undifferentiated carcinoma**
  - Hemorrhage, necrosis, and high mitotic activity seen in undifferentiated carcinoma
  - Negative for calcitonin
- **Papillary thyroid carcinoma (PTC)**
  - Intranuclear inclusions can be seen in both MTC and PTC
  - Nuclear features usually unique to PTC
  - PTC is calcitonin negative and thyroglobulin positive
- **Hyalinizing trabecular tumor**
  - Thyroglobulin positive, calcitonin negative
  - Hyaline material is not amyloid when stained by Congo red under polarized light

- **Intrathyroid parathyroid tumors**
  - Clear cytoplasm, defined cell border
  - PTH positive; calcitonin and thyroglobulin negative

Tumor in Lymph Nodes

- MTC metastatic to lymph nodes may be misdiagnosed as melanoma or metastatic neuroendocrine tumors
- Calcitonin and CEA immunostains should be performed in any suspicious case

Benign Conditions

- **Amyloid goiter**
  - May infiltrate fat, and Congo red is positive
  - Involves thyroid gland diffusely
  - Calcitonin stain is negative

Sporadic vs. Familial Medullary Thyroid Carcinoma

- There is only 1 genetic differential diagnosis for MTC: MEN2
- Important for medical management of individual and his/her family to distinguish MTC + MEN2 from truly sporadic MTC
- Germline mutations in *RET* gene in individuals with apparent sporadic MTC: 6.0-9.5%
- Sporadic tumors are usually
  - Solitary mass
  - Unilateral
  - Not associated with CCH
  - Histological findings: Same as familial

DIAGNOSTIC CHECKLIST

Pathologic Interpretation Pearls

- Finding CCH may serve as morphological marker for MEN2-associated MTC
- Desmoplasia and breakage of follicular basement membrane help differentiate CCH from MMC

SELECTED REFERENCES

1. Lloyd RV et al: WHO Classification of Tumours of Endocrine Organs. Lyon, France: IARC Press, 2017
2. Mathiesen JS et al: Distribution of RET mutations in multiple endocrine neoplasia 2 in Denmark 1994-2014: a nationwide study. Thyroid. 27(2):215-223, 2017
3. Mohammadi M et al: A brief review on the molecular basis of medullary tyroid carcinoma. Cell J. 18(4):485-492, 2017
4. Essig GF Jr et al: Multifocality in sporadic medullary thyroid carcinoma: an international multicenter study. Thyroid. 26(11):1563-1572, 2016
5. Kameda Y: Cellular and molecular events on the development of mammalian thyroid C cells. Dev Dyn. 245(3):323-41, 2016
6. Kasajima A et al: A calcitonin non-producing neuroendocrine tumor of the thyroid gland. Endocr Pathol. 27(4):325-331, 2016
7. Myoteri D et al: Mixed medullary and papillary thyroid carcinoma: a stepwise diagnosis. J BUON. 21(6):1561-1562, 2016
8. Parmer M et al: Calcitonin-negative neuroendocrine tumor of the thyroid: follicular or parafollicular cell of origin? Int J Surg Pathol. 25(2):191-194, 2016
9. Spinelli C et al: Surgical management of medullary thyroid carcinoma in pediatric age. Curr Pediatr Rev. 12(4):280-285, 2016
10. Kim GY et al: A calcitonin-negative neuroendocrine tumor derived from follicular lesions of the thyroid. Endocrinol Metab (Seoul). 30(2):221-5, 2015
11. Mathiesen JS et al: Aggressive medullary thyroid carcinoma in a ten-year-old patient with multiple endocrine neoplasia 2B due to the A883F mutation. Thyroid. 25(1):139-40, 2015
12. Pennelli G et al: The PDCD4/miR-21 pathway in medullary thyroid carcinoma. Hum Pathol. 46(1):50-7, 2015
13. Barbieri RB et al: Polymorphisms of cell cycle control genes influence the development of sporadic medullary thyroid carcinoma. Eur J Endocrinol. 171(6):761-7, 2014
14. Grubbs EG et al: RET fusion as a novel driver of medullary thyroid carcinoma. J Clin Endocrinol Metab. jc20144153, 2014
15. Jaskula-Sztul R et al: Tumor-suppressor role of Notch3 in medullary thyroid carcinoma revealed by genetic and pharmacological induction. Mol Cancer Ther. 14(2):499-512, 2014
16. Lyra J et al: mTOR activation in medullary thyroid carcinoma with RAS mutation. Eur J Endocrinol. 171(5):633-40, 2014
17. Perri F et al: Targeted therapy: a new hope for thyroid carcinomas. Crit Rev Oncol Hematol. 94(1):55-63, 2014
18. Romei C et al: 20 Years of lesson learning: how does the ret genetic screening test impact the clinical management of medullary thyroid cancer? Clin Endocrinol (Oxf). 82(6):892-9, 2014
19. Toledo RA et al: Comprehensive assessment of the disputed RET Y791F shows no association with MTC susceptibility. Endocr Relat Cancer. 22(1):65-76, 2014
20. Valdés N et al: RET Cys634Arg mutation confers a more aggressive multiple endocrine neoplasia type 2A phenotype than Cys634Tyr mutation. Eur J Endocrinol. 172(3):301-7, 2014
21. Viola D et al: Medullary thyroid carcinoma in children. Endocr Dev. 26:202-13, 2014
22. Yamazaki M et al: A newly identified missense mutation in RET codon 666 is associated with the development of medullary thyroid carcinoma Rapid Communication. Endocr J. 61(11):1141-4, 2014
23. Maliszewska A et al: Differential gene expression of medullary thyroid carcinoma reveals specific markers associated with genetic conditions. Am J Pathol. 182(2):350-62, 2013
24. Agarwal S et al: MEN 2A family–prophylactic thyroidectomy for asymptomatic siblings with positive 634 codon mutation. J Assoc Physicians India. 60:127-9, 2012
25. Martucciello G et al: Multiple endocrine neoplasias type 2B and RET proto-oncogene. Ital J Pediatr. 38:9, 2012
26. Shankar RK et al: Medullary thyroid cancer in a 9-week-old infant with familial MEN 2B: Implications for timing of prophylactic thyroidectomy. Int J Pediatr Endocrinol. 2012(1):25, 2012
27. Chernyavsky VS et al: Calcitonin-negative neuroendocrine tumor of the thyroid: a distinct clinical entity. Thyroid. 21(2):193-6, 2011
28. Marsh DJ et al: Multiple endocrine neoplasia: types 1 and 2. Adv Otorhinolaryngol. 70:84-90, 2011
29. Nosé V: Familial thyroid cancer: a review. Mod Pathol. 24 Suppl 2:S19-33, 2011
30. Waguespack SG et al: Management of medullary thyroid carcinoma and MEN2 syndromes in childhood. Nat Rev Endocrinol. 7(10):596-607, 2011
31. Eng C: Mendelian genetics of rare–and not so rare–cancers. Ann N Y Acad Sci. 1214:70-82, 2010
32. Pacini F et al: Medullary thyroid carcinoma. Clin Oncol (R Coll Radiol). 22(6):475-85, 2010
33. Phay JE et al: Targeting RET receptor tyrosine kinase activation in cancer. Clin Cancer Res. 16(24):5936-41, 2010
34. Richards ML: Familial syndromes associated with thyroid cancer in the era of personalized medicine. Thyroid. 20(7):707-13, 2010
35. Sadow PM et al: Mixed medullary-follicular-derived carcinomas of the thyroid gland. Adv Anat Pathol. 17(4):282-5, 2010
36. Torino F et al: Medullary thyroid cancer: a promising model for targeted therapy. Curr Mol Med. 10(7):608-25, 2010
37. American Thyroid Association Guidelines Task Force et al: Medullary thyroid cancer: management guidelines of the American Thyroid Association. Thyroid. 19(6):565-612, 2009
38. Cakir M et al: Medullary thyroid cancer: molecular biology and novel molecular therapies. Neuroendocrinology. 90(4):323-48, 2009
39. Cerrato A et al: Molecular genetics of medullary thyroid carcinoma: the quest for novel therapeutic targets. J Mol Endocrinol. 43(4):143-55, 2009
40. Wells SA Jr et al: Targeting the RET pathway in thyroid cancer. Clin Cancer Res. 15(23):7119-23, 2009
41. Etit D et al: Histopathologic and clinical features of medullary microcarcinoma and C-cell hyperplasia in prophylactic thyroidectomies for medullary carcinoma: a study of 42 cases. Arch Pathol Lab Med. 132(11):1767-73, 2008
42. Tischler AS et al: Prophylactic thyroidectomy in multiple endocrine neoplasia type 2A. N Engl J Med. 353(26):2817-8; author reply 2817-8, 2005
43. Baloch ZW et al: Neuroendocrine tumors of the thyroid gland. Am J Clin Pathol. 115 Suppl:S56-67, 2001
44. Moline J, Eng C. Multiple endocrine neoplasia type 2. 1993-, 1999
45. DeLellis RA: Multiple endocrine neoplasia syndromes revisited. Clinical, morphologic, and molecular features. Lab Invest. 72(5):494-505, 1995

Differential Diagnosis of Medullary Thyroid Carcinoma by Immunohistochemistry

Antibody	MTC	PTC	PDC	ATC	PA/C	Para	Met C
Cytokeratin	+	+	+	+/-	+	-	+
Thyroglobulin	-	+	+	-	-	-	-
TTF-1	+	+	+	-	-	-	-/+
Pax-8	+	+	+	+/-	-	-	-/+
Chromogranin	+	-	-	-	+	+	+/-
Synaptophysin	+	-	-	-	+/-	+	+/-
Calcitonin	+	-	-	-	-	-	-
PTH	-	-	-	-	+	-	-
S100	-	-	-	-	-	+	-

MTC = medullary thyroid carcinoma; PTC = papillary thyroid carcinoma; PDC = poorly differentiated carcinoma; ATC = anaplastic thyroid carcinoma; PA/C = parathyroid adenoma/carcinoma; para = paraganglioma; met C = metastatic carcinoma.

Pathological Features Distinguishing Familial From Sporadic Medullary Thyroid Carcinoma

Characteristics	Familial Medullary Thyroid Carcinoma	Sporadic Medullary Thyroid Carcinoma
Gross features	Multicentric and bilateral	Solitary mass; unilateral
Tumor characteristics	Small tumors in prophylactic thyroidectomy specimens	Usually large tumors
Microscopic features	Associated with neoplastic C-cell hyperplasia	Association with C-cell hyperplasia unknown
RET mutation	Present in majority of hereditary forms	May be present in sporadic cases

Differential Diagnosis of Medullary Thyroid Microcarcinoma

Characteristics	Familial	Sporadic
Multifocality	Frequent (~ 90%)	Rare (~ 10%)
Bilaterality	Common (~ 70%)	Rare (~ 10%)
Physiologic C-cell hyperplasia	Rare (~ 10%)	Common (~ 55%)
Neoplastic C-cell hyperplasia	Frequent (~ 90%)	Rare (~ 15%)

PET of Metastatic Carcinoma

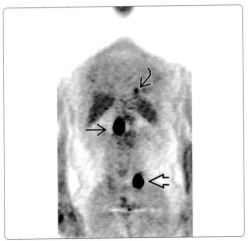

FDG PET/CT of Thyroid Tumor

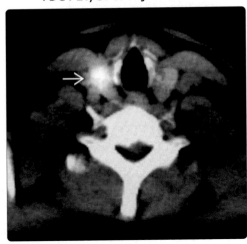

(Left) Coronal FDG PET shows hypermetabolic foci in an upper lumbar vertebra ⊡, left sacroiliac region ⊡, and left lung ⊡ in a patient with metastatic medullary thyroid cancer. Up to 20% of patients may have distant metastases at the time of presentation. (Right) FDG PET/CT shows a focal hypermetabolic mass ➡ in the right thyroid lobe in a patient with medullary thyroid cancer.

Nodular C-Cell Hyperplasia

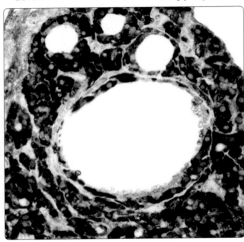

Calcitonin in Nodular C-Cell Hyperplasia

(Left) Unlike sporadic medullary thyroid carcinoma, MEN2 is frequently accompanied by neoplastic/primary C-cell hyperplasia. C cells are usually identified by calcitonin staining; however, in many cases of MEN2, C cells are easily identified by H&E. (Right) In MEN2 patients, foci of C-cell hyperplasia are typically present in the vicinity of the tumor as well as in the contralateral lobe. This photomicrograph shows calcitonin stain highlighting C-cell hyperplasia adjacent to a medullary thyroid carcinoma.

Cytological Features

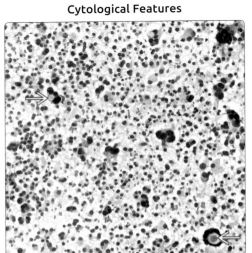

Calcitonin Immunostain in Cytology

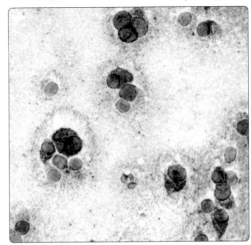

(Left) FNA of a medullary thyroid carcinoma shows a characteristic cellular specimen with clusters of loosely cohesive, round to oval cells of variable sizes. Amyloid spheres ➡ can be seen in the background or associated with clusters of malignant cells. Colloid is absent. (Right) Thyroid FNA specimen immunocytological stain for calcitonin shows coarse granular cytoplasmic staining. Here, medullary thyroid carcinoma cells demonstrate the characteristic coarse neuroendocrine-type nuclear chromatin.

Prophylactic Thyroidectomy Specimen

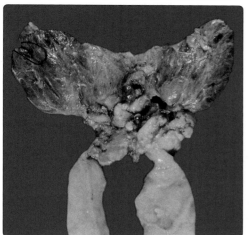

Medullary Thyroid Microcarcinoma

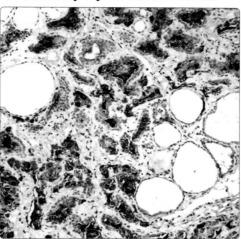

(Left) *Total prophylactic thyroidectomy with a portion of thymus from a patient with MEN2B and with mutation of the RET gene shows a grossly normal thyroid. However, on histological examination, C-cell hyperplasia and bilateral small medullary thyroid carcinomas were present.* **(Right)** *Calcitonin-stained thyroid section from a prophylactic thyroidectomy from a patient with RET mutation and family history of MEN2B shows C-cell hyperplasia and medullary thyroid microcarcinoma.*

C-Cell Hyperplasia in MEN2

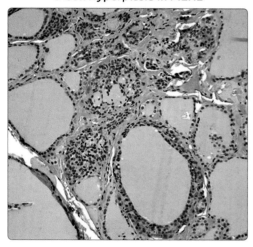

C-Cell Hyperplasia in MEN2

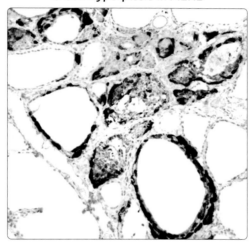

(Left) *Histological routine section reveals C-cell hyperplasia in a thyroid lobe of a patient with medullary thyroid carcinoma in the other lobe. Both were associated with MEN2 and RET mutation. Primary C-cell hyperplasia can be easily identified on H&E section on heritable cases.* **(Right)** *Primary/neoplastic C-cell hyperplasia highlighted by calcitonin staining shows the thyroid follicular cells replaced by an increased number of C cells.*

Plasmacytoid and Epithelioid Cells

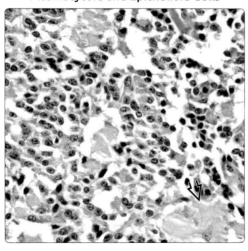

Spindle Cell Variant

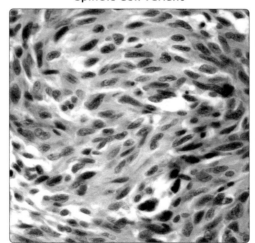

(Left) *This tumor is composed of epithelioid cells in a diffuse pattern. The cells are round to oval with large cytoplasm and nuclei with fine, granular, and dispersed chromatin. Amyloid is focally present ⇒. **(Right)** The histological appearance of medullary thyroid carcinomas is quite variable. This stain shows a spindle cell variant with characteristic neuroendocrine nuclear features.*

Gross Cut Surface of Sporadic MTC

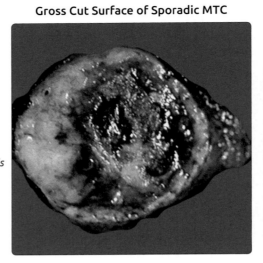

Extrathyroidal Extension

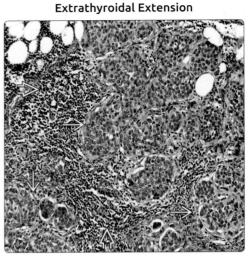

(Left) *Gross cut surface of a thyroid lobe shows a well-circumscribed, white-gray-yellow thyroid tumor. Medullary thyroid carcinomas are usually firm and gritty. Areas of hemorrhage are present.* (Right) *Medullary thyroid carcinoma extending into extrathyroidal fibroadipose tissue shows multiple nests ➡ of small cells with scant cytoplasm and regular, round nuclei, associated with marked inflammatory infiltrate ➡.*

Metastatic MTC to Ovary

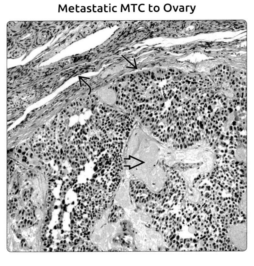

Metastases Highlighted by Calcitonin

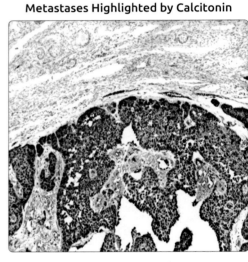

(Left) *This micrograph depicts an unusually aggressive case of medullary thyroid carcinoma metastatic to the ovary. A well-defined nodule of tumor cells ➡ with interspersed areas of amyloid deposition ➡ can be seen. Compressed normal ovarian parenchyma ➡ is present surrounding the tumor.* (Right) *Section of an ovary stained for calcitonin highlights the neoplasm (positive staining) and confirms medullary thyroid carcinoma as the origin of this metastatic lesion.*

Dual Stain for TTF-1 and Chromogranin

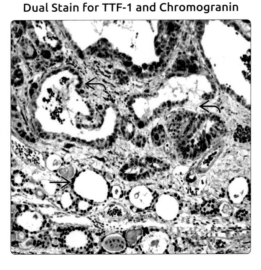

Variable Calcitonin Staining by Tumor Cells

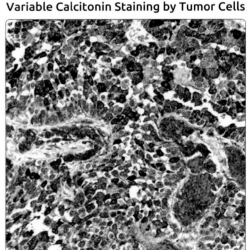

(Left) *Dual immunohistochemistry with chromogranin (red) and TTF-1 (brown) marks neuroendocrine-derived cells of medullary thyroid carcinoma ➡ from normal adjacent TTF-1(+) follicular cells ➡; medullary thyroid carcinoma cells are TTF-1 and chromogranin (+). Immunophenotypical distinction is key in follicular-patterned medullary thyroid carcinoma morphology.* (Right) *Variable cytoplasmic calcitonin immunostaining is typical of medullary thyroid carcinoma cells.*

Bilateral Tumors in Heritable Syndromes

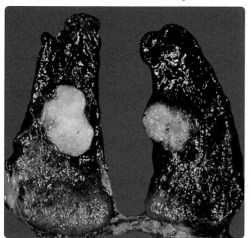

Synaptophysin Immunopositivity

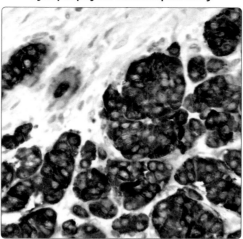

(Left) *Bilateral medullary thyroid carcinoma from a patient with MEN2A shows the characteristic well-circumscribed cut surface. MEN-associated tumors are usually bilateral and multifocal.* (Right) *Immunostaining for synaptophysin, as shown here, frequently gives strong diffuse cytoplasmic reactivity. This marker and other markers of neuroendocrine lineage can be helpful in establishing the diagnosis.*

Chromogranin Staining by Tumor Cells

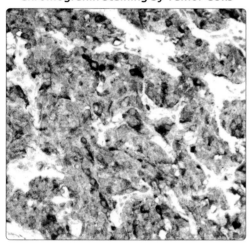

Calcitonin Immunostaining

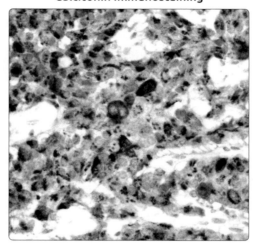

(Left) *Although calcitonin is the specific stain for medullary thyroid carcinoma, chromogranin immunostain, as a neuroendocrine marker, shows usually variable immunopositivity in the tumor cells.* (Right) *Variable cytoplasmic immunopositivity for calcitonin is present in the tumor cells of medullary thyroid carcinoma. This stain helps differentiate medullary thyroid carcinoma from many mimics.*

Congo Red Stain Showing Congophilia

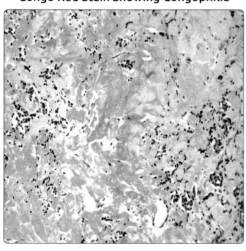

Polarized Congo Red Stain

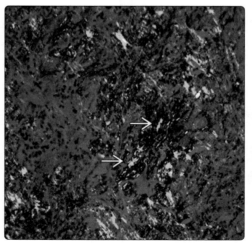

(Left) *Photomicrograph of a Congo red-stained tumor shows extensive deposition of dense amorphous material suggestive of amyloid. Although not essential for the diagnosis of medullary thyroid carcinoma, variable amounts of amyloid are commonly seen in these tumors.* (Right) *Congo red-stained medullary thyroid carcinoma under polarized light reveals the characteristic apple-green birefringence ➡, confirming amyloid deposition.*

Mixed Medullary and Follicular Cell Carcinoma

TERMINOLOGY

- Mixed medullary and follicular carcinoma (MMFCC): Primary malignant epithelial neoplasm of thyroid showing morphological and immunophenotypical evidence of coexistence of follicular and parafollicular cell-derived tumor populations within same lesion (WHO 2017)
  - Immunopositivity for calcitonin in C-cell component and thyroglobulin in follicular cell-derived carcinoma

CLINICAL ISSUES

- Extremely rare (< 0.15% of thyroid tumors; < 60 cases reported)

MICROSCOPIC

- Extremely heterogeneous group of tumors
  - Follicular-derived component can have follicular, tubular, solid, or papillary growth patterns
- Strict criteria ought to be applied for defining mixed tumors
- **Concurrent or synchronous**
  - Anatomically distinct papillary thyroid carcinoma (PTC) and medullary thyroid carcinoma (MTC)
- **Collision tumors**
  - MTC and PTC that merge with one another
- **True mixed MTC/follicular-derived carcinoma**
  - MTC and follicular cell-derived carcinoma that are intimately intermixed
- Mixed components may also be present in metastatic foci

ANCILLARY TESTS

- Amount of each component highly variable
- Immunohistochemistry better identifies both components
  - Follicular cell tumor: TTF-1 and thyroglobulin
  - MTC: TTF-1, calcitonin, chromogranin, and CEA
- No genetic data available on follicular counterpart
- Somatic *RET* mutations have been detected, mostly affecting codon 918

Coexistent Tumor Cell Populations

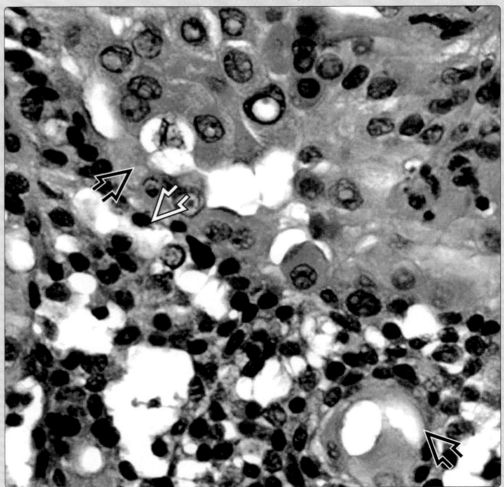

Mixed medullary and follicular carcinoma (MMFCC) shows morphological evidence of an intimate admixture of tumor composed of 2 components: C cells ➡ and follicular cells ➡.

TERMINOLOGY

Abbreviations

- Mixed medullary and follicular cell carcinoma (MMFCC)

Synonyms

- Combined papillary thyroid carcinoma (PTC) and medullary thyroid carcinoma (MTC)
- Composite/biphasic/stem cell thyroid carcinoma
- Mixed follicular and C-cell carcinoma
- Concurrent medullary-follicular thyroid carcinoma

Definitions

- MMFCC: Primary malignant epithelial neoplasm of thyroid showing morphological and immunophenotypical evidence of coexistence of follicular and parafollicular cell-derived tumor populations within same lesion (WHO 2017)
  - Tumors showing morphological features of both medullary carcinoma [calcitonin(+)] and follicular cell-derived carcinoma [thyroglobulin(+)]
- **Classification of concurrent medullary and follicular-derived carcinoma**
  - **Concurrent or synchronous**
    - Anatomically distinct PTC and MTC
  - **Collision tumors**
    - MTC and PTC that merge with one another
  - **True mixed MTC/follicular-derived carcinoma**
    - MTC and follicular cell-derived carcinoma that are intimately intermixed

ETIOLOGY/PATHOGENESIS

Developmental Anomaly

- Embryologically, thyroid gland forms through fusion of median thyroid anlage and ultimobranchial body (or lateral anlage)
  - Thyroid follicular epithelial cells most likely derived only from median thyroid anlage
  - Parafollicular cells of thyroid (C cells) embryologically derived from ultimobranchial body
- Anatomically, largest concentration of C cells seen in upper-outer superior 2/3 of thyroid lobes

Association of Neoplasms

- Concurrent finding of papillary carcinoma and medullary carcinoma in same thyroid gland not uncommon
- High rate of incidental PTC; finding of PTC in background thyroid of patients with resection for MTC is expected
  - Occult papillary carcinoma found in ~ 15% of cases of overt MTC and < 20% of cases with MTC or C-cell hyperplasia
- Rare tumors exist in thyroid that have both C-cell-derived components and follicular epithelial cell-derived components
  - These tumors are clearly separate primary lesions unrelated pathogenetically
- Other tumors seem to have mixtures of the 2 components, either only at interface zone (so-called collision tumors) or throughout lesion (true mixed tumors)

CLINICAL ISSUES

Epidemiology

- Incidence
  - Extremely rare (< 0.15% of thyroid tumors; < 60 cases reported)
- Age
  - Mean: 36 years
- Sex
  - M:F = 1.3:1

Presentation

- Thyroid mass
  - Usual presentation is "cold" nodule on scintigraph scan and solid on ultrasonography

Prognosis

- Few mixed medullary-follicular lesions have been described in the literature; prognosis and treatment options are not well understood
- Behavior seems similar to other conventional, pure medullary carcinoma, with high metastatic and recurrence rates
  - Relatively long-term poor prognosis as compared with well-differentiated follicular-derived carcinomas

MACROSCOPIC

General Features

- Overlap those of conventional medullary carcinoma and papillary carcinoma
- Solid, whitish, and firm unencapsulated mass

Size

- Mean diameter: 3.7 cm

MICROSCOPIC

Histologic Features

- Extremely heterogeneous group of tumors
- **Concurrent or synchronous MTC and PTC**
  - High rate of incidental PTC; finding of PTC in background thyroid of patients with resection for MTC is expected
  - Presence of PTC in gland removed for MTC
  - Distinct tumors
  - Medullary carcinomas may show mixture of C-cell-derived components and follicular-derived components
    - Whether these represent truly admixed tumors or are tumors mixed by chance (collision tumors) may not be determined from histology
- **Collision tumors and true mixed MTC/follicular-derived carcinoma**
  - Histologically, true mixed medullary-follicular tumors should have morphologic evidence of intimate admixture of 2 components
    - Medullary and follicular cells, along with immunohistochemical evidence of 2 different cell types by calcitonin and thyroglobulin stains
    - Amount of each component is highly variable
    - Follicular-derived component can have follicular, tubular, or solid growth, or it can show papillary growth with papillary carcinoma nuclear features

- Medullary carcinoma is composed of cell population with neuroendocrine differentiation
- Tumor cell morphology is highly variable, with different patterns including spindled, epithelioid, or plasmacytoid
- Amyloid will be detectable in ~ 80% of cases either on H&E stain or using Congo red stain
- Mixed components also seen in metastatic foci
  - Strict criteria ought to be applied for defining mixed tumors, with inclusion of only those tumors with immunohistochemical or molecular evidence of divergent differentiation
  - Mixed components may also be present in metastatic foci

ANCILLARY TESTS

Immunohistochemistry

- Amount of each component is highly variable from tumor to tumor; immunohistochemistry better identifies both components
- Follicular-derived component positive for TTF-1 and thyroglobulin
  - Thyroglobulin can be leaky; reliance on thyroglobulin positivity alone, particularly at edges of lesions, should be avoided
- C-cell-derived component is positive for TTF-1, chromogranin, calcitonin, and CEA
  - Expression of CEA by all MTCs is useful diagnostic immunohistochemical feature, using polyclonal CEA antibody
- Strict criteria should be applied for defining mixed tumors
  - Inclusion of only those tumors with immunohistochemical or molecular evidence of divergent differentiation
    - Away from edges of tumor or in metastatic foci

Genetic Testing

- No genetic data available on follicular counterpart
- Somatic *RET* mutations have been detected in some cases exclusively in MTC component, mostly affecting codon 918
- Clonality analysis showed that the 2 tumor components are unrelated
- **Mixed medullary-follicular tumors** studied at molecular level
  - Analysis of clonality by loss of heterozygosity and X-inactivation studies and *RET* mutational analysis
  - Suggested that follicular-derived component was clonally different from medullary carcinoma component
  - These interesting molecular results argue against either stem cell or divergent differentiation theories
- **Collision tumors** have been occasionally studied at molecular level
  - Spatially distinct MTC and PTC within same thyroid, medullary carcinoma component had *RET* mutations, and papillary carcinoma component had *BRAF* mutation
    - Supports histologic impression that these were separate, nonrelated tumors
  - *RET/PTC* translocations have not been well studied in setting of synchronous tumors

DIFFERENTIAL DIAGNOSIS

Pure Medullary Thyroid Carcinoma or Follicular Cell-Derived Carcinoma

- Immunohistochemistry will help differentiate
  - Chromogranin and calcitonin only for MTC

DIAGNOSTIC CHECKLIST

Pathologic Interpretation Pearls

- Concurrent finding of papillary carcinoma and medullary carcinoma in same thyroid gland may be seen
  - So-called collision tumors
    - Some tumors may have separate C-cell-derived components and follicular epithelial cell-derived components, only intermingle at interface zone
  - True mixed tumors
    - Other tumors seem to have mixtures of the 2 components throughout
- Histologically, true mixed medullary-follicular tumors should have morphologic evidence of intimate admixture of both cellular components
  - Medullary and follicular cell components
  - These tumors show immunohistochemical evidence of the 2 corresponding cell types of differentiation
    - Calcitonin stains C-cell-derived component and thyroglobulin stains follicular cell-derived component

SELECTED REFERENCES

1. Lloyd RV et al: WHO Classification of Tumours of Endocrine Organs. Lyon, France: IARC Press, 2017
2. Pereira F et al: Lymph node metastases in papillary and medullary thyroid carcinoma are independent of intratumoral lymphatic vessel density. Eur Thyroid J. 6(2):57-64, 2017
3. Nilsson M et al: On the origin of cells and derivation of thyroid cancer: C cell story revisited. Eur Thyroid J. 5(2):79-93, 2016
4. Erhamamci S et al: Simultaneous occurrence of medullary and differentiated thyroid carcinomas. Report of 4 cases and brief review of the literature. Hell J Nucl Med. 17(2):148-52, 2014
5. Tohidi M et al: Mixed medullary-follicular carcinoma of the thyroid. Case Rep Endocrinol. 2013:571692, 2013
6. Hanna AN et al: Mixed medullary-follicular carcinoma of the thyroid: diagnostic dilemmas in fine-needle aspiration cytology. Diagn Cytopathol. 39(11):862-5, 2011
7. Ueki I et al: A case of mixed medullary and follicular cell carcinoma of the thyroid. Intern Med. 50(12):1313-6, 2011
8. Sadow PM et al: Mixed medullary-follicular-derived carcinomas of the thyroid gland. Adv Anat Pathol. 17(4):282-5, 2010
9. Nangue C et al: Mixed medullary-papillary carcinoma of the thyroid: report of a case and review of the literature. Head Neck. 31(7):968-74, 2009
10. Papotti M et al: Thyroid carcinomas with mixed follicular and C-cell differentiation patterns. Semin Diagn Pathol. 17(2):109-19, 2000
11. Vitri P et al: Mixed follicular and parafollicular thyroid carcinoma. J Exp Clin Cancer Res. 18(4):567-9, 1999
12. Volante M et al: Mixed medullary-follicular thyroid carcinoma. Molecular evidence for a dual origin of tumor components. Am J Pathol. 155(5):1499-509, 1999
13. Wu CJ et al: Mixed medullary-follicular carcinoma and papillary carcinoma of the same thyroid. Intern Med. 37(11):955-7, 1998
14. Mizukami Y et al: Mixed medullary-follicular carcinoma of the thyroid gland: a clinicopathologic variant of medullary thyroid carcinoma. Mod Pathol. 9(6):631-5, 1996
15. Albores-Saavedra J et al: Mixed medullary-papillary carcinoma of the thyroid: a previously unrecognized variant of thyroid carcinoma. Hum Pathol. 21(11):1151-5, 1990

Lymph Node Metastases With Both Tumors

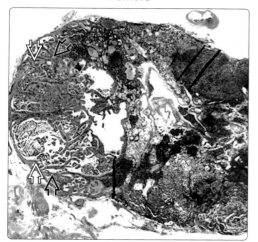

Classic PTC and Small Cell MTC

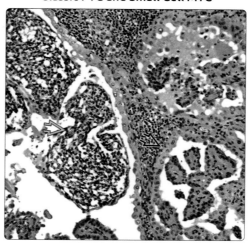

(Left) Lymph node shows that metastatic foci are formed by mixed components of medullary thyroid carcinoma (MTC) ➡ and follicular-derived carcinoma ➡. (Right) This lymph node with metastatic mixed medullary ➡ and papillary thyroid carcinoma (PTC) ➡ shows equal amounts of each component. The amount of each component is highly variable within these tumors.

PTC Nuclear Features

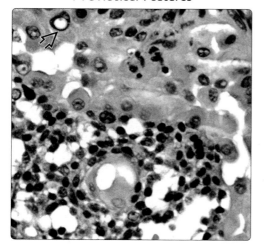

Predominantly Small Cell MTC

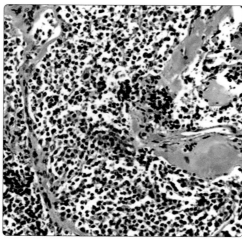

(Left) The follicular-derived component in MMFCC includes conventional or follicular variant of PTC or follicular carcinoma. Note PTC nuclear features ➡. (Right) This MMFCC is almost exclusively formed by tumor of C-cell origin. These mixed neoplasms are known to have different amounts of each tumor component.

Calcitonin(+) Tumor Cells

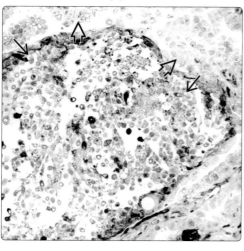

TTF-1 Positivity in Both Components

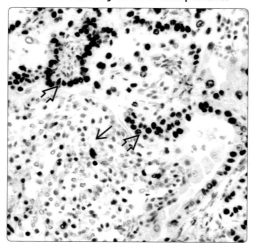

(Left) Calcitonin immunostaining of MMFCC highlights the tumor component formed by C cells ➡. The stain is negative in the follicular cell-derived carcinoma ➡. (Right) TTF-1 immunopositivity in MMFCC is variable in both intermixed tumor components; weaker staining is seen in the C-cell component ➡ and strong reactivity is present in the follicular cells ➡.

Spindle Epithelial Tumor With Thymus-Like Differentiation

TERMINOLOGY

- Spindle epithelial tumor with thymus-like differentiation
- Neoplasm with biphasic growth pattern, showing spindle-shaped epithelial cells that blend with scattered glandular structures

ETIOLOGY/PATHOGENESIS

- Considered to be derived from
  - Intrathyroidal ectopic thymic tissue
  - Remnants of branchial pouches that retained ability to differentiate into thymic-like tumor

CLINICAL ISSUES

- Characteristically present in young patients
- Presents usually with painless neck mass
- Tumor has indolent course; typically associated with delayed blood-borne metastases

MACROSCOPIC

- Grossly encapsulated, partially circumscribed, or infiltrative

- Cut surface shows lobulated grayish-white to tan firm mass with small cysts

MICROSCOPIC

- Most tumors are biphasic, spindled, and glandular
- Spindle cells with elongated nuclei with fine chromatin and inconspicuous nucleoli
- Glandular component is usually has tubules, papillae, cords, epithelium-lined cysts, and small pale-staining cellular islands
- Both spindle and glandular cells express cytokeratin

TOP DIFFERENTIAL DIAGNOSES

- Synovial sarcoma
  - Higher nuclear grade, presence of *SS18* gene translocation
- Solitary fibrous tumor
- Anaplastic thyroid carcinoma
- Ectopic thymoma

Fibrous Capsule

Spindle Cell Component

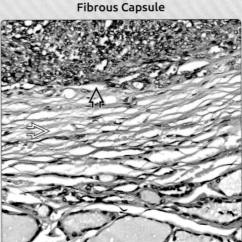
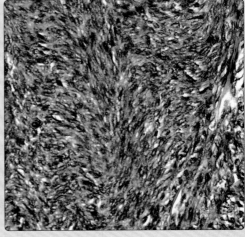

(Left) *Photomicrograph of a spindle cell tumor with thymus-like differentiation (SETTLE) shows a spindle cell neoplasm ⇗ separated from the thyroid by a well-developed acellular fibrous capsule ⇘.* (Right) *A spindle cell area of a biphasic SETTLE shows a cellular neoplasm composed of intersecting fascicles of spindle cells, which have elongated nuclei with fine chromatin. Pleomorphism is absent.*

Biphasic Epithelial Component

Cytokeratin Immunoreactivity

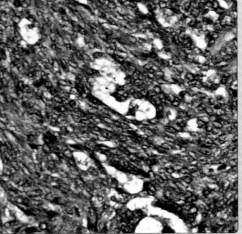
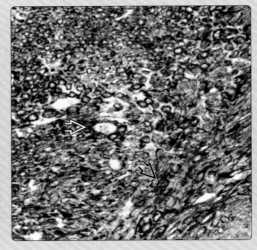

(Left) *SETTLE are usually biphasic. There are intersecting bundles of spindle-shaped cells blending with glandular and tubulopapillary structures. These glandular structures form cystic spaces that may contain mucin within the lumen.* (Right) *The diffuse and intense positivity for high molecular weight cytokeratin in both the spindle cell component ⇘ and the syncytial, epithelioid, and glandular components ⇘ is highlighted in this photomicrograph.*

TERMINOLOGY

Abbreviations

- Spindle epithelial tumor with thymus-like differentiation (SETTLE)

Synonyms

- Spindle cell tumor with thymus-like differentiation
- Spindle epithelial tumor with thymus-like elements

Definitions

- SETTLE is rare malignant tumor of thyroid characterized by lobulated architecture and biphasic cellular composition featuring spindled epithelial cells that merge into glandular structures

ETIOLOGY/PATHOGENESIS

Developmental Anomaly

- Considered to be derived from
  - Intrathyroidal ectopic thymic tissue
  - Remnants of branchial pouches that retained ability to differentiate into thymic-like tumor

CLINICAL ISSUES

Epidemiology

- Incidence
  - Very rare
- Age
  - Characteristically affects children and young adults, with mean age of 19 years
- Sex
  - Males are affected 1.5x more often than females

Presentation

- Presents usually with painless neck mass
- Less frequently, patients may present with
  - Rapidly enlarging painful mass
  - Localized tenderness mimicking thyroiditis
  - Signs of tracheal compression
- Symptoms may be present for weeks to years
- No associated family history of thyroid disease
- No prior history of neck radiation
- Thyroid function tests are not affected

Treatment

- Surgical approaches
  - Thyroidectomy should always be performed
  - Partial or total thyroidectomy depends on involvement of 1 lobe or both lobes by nodular disease
  - Resection of metastases achieves longer overall survival and longer disease-free period
  - Lymph node dissection may improve outcome
- Adjuvant therapy
  - Chemotherapy is indicated for metastatic disease
  - No therapy is advised at initial diagnosis
- Radiation
  - Also used for metastatic disease

Prognosis

- Tumor has indolent course

- Regional lymph node metastases may be seen initially at presentation
- Significant metastatic disease is present in 70% of cases
  - Overall metastatic rate increased from 33% with follow-up < 5 years to 71% if patient is followed > 5 years
  - Late metastases obligates long-term follow-up and removal of metastases
  - Delayed blood-borne metastases up to 20 years post initial diagnosis
  - Metastases usually to lung, lymph nodes, kidney, and soft tissues
  - Removal of metastases prolongs clinical course
- 5-year survival approaches 90%

IMAGING

General Features

- Appears cold on thyroid scan
- Displays heterogeneous solid and cystic densities on CT scan

Ultrasonographic Findings

- Clearly demarcated, solid nodule
- Rare cases may have diffusely hypoechoic structure mimicking Riedel thyroiditis

MACROSCOPIC

General Features

- Grossly encapsulated, partially circumscribed, or infiltrative
- Cut surface shows lobulated grayish-white to tan firm mass with small cysts

Size

- Average: 4.2 cm

MICROSCOPIC

Histologic Features

- Highly cellular lobulated tumor imparted by fibrous septa
- Most tumors are biphasic, spindled, and glandular
- Rare cases may be monophasic, composed exclusively of spindle cells or glandular structures
- Interlacing to reticulated compact fascicles of spindle cells merge almost imperceptibly with tubuloglandular structures
- Spindle cells with elongated nuclei, fine chromatin, and inconspicuous nucleoli
- Glandular component is usually in form of tubules, papillae, cords, epithelium-lined cysts, or small pale-staining cellular islands
- Glandular cells are columnar or cuboidal and may be mucinous and ciliated with oval or round nuclei with fine chromatin
- Mitoses are rare
- Cases with high mitotic activity associated with necrosis behave more aggressively
- Scanty lymphocytes may be present
- Vascular invasion may be present

ANCILLARY TESTS

Cytology

- Smears are cellular, with cohesive clusters of spindle cells with scant fibrillar cytoplasm and bland uniform nuclei
- Glandular structures may be recognized
- Background of extracellular red homogeneous material
  - Fine dust-like granules
  - Irregular clumps of material
- FNA biopsy is seldom diagnostic of SETTLE
- Spindle cells may be confused with other tumors

Immunohistochemistry

- Both spindle cells and glandular component have similar immunophenotype with strong positivity for cytokeratin
  - Both spindle and glandular cells extensively express high molecular weight cytokeratin and CK7
  - Positive: CAM5.2, EMA, AE1/AE3, CD117, INI1, vimentin, p63
  - Negative: TTF-1, thyroglobulin, calcitonin, CEA, CD5, CK20, S100, synaptophysin, chromogranin
  - Rarely spindled cells may demonstrate myoepithelial differentiation

Genetic Testing

- One case revealed somatic mutations in *KRAS* without mutation in *TP53* gene
- Tumor lacks *SS18* gene translocation that characterizes synovial sarcoma

Electron Microscopy

- Spindle cells have features of epithelial cell origin with prominent cytoplasmic tonofilaments, desmosomes, and basal lamina

DIFFERENTIAL DIAGNOSIS

Synovial Sarcoma

- SETTLE and synovial sarcoma are seen in young patients
- Both SETTLE and synovial sarcoma tumors are often biphasic
- Characterized by specific chromosomal translocation t(X;18), *SS18* gene
- SETTLE has lower overall nuclear grade, absence of nuclear debris, glomeruloid glandular structures, and expression of high molecular weight cytokeratin

Solitary Fibrous Tumor

- So-called patternless pattern
- Diffuse or focal collagenization
- Characteristically CD34(+)

Anaplastic Thyroid Carcinoma

- Rapidly enlarging tumor in older patients
- Spindle cell/sarcomatoid variant with numerous mitosis, pleomorphism, necrosis
  - Negative for cytokeratin

Ectopic Thymoma

- Jigsaw-puzzle-like lobulation with numerous T cells

DIAGNOSTIC CHECKLIST

Pathologic Interpretation Pearls

- Lobulated architecture and biphasic growth pattern featuring spindle-shaped epithelial cells that blend with scattered glandular structures, which have primitive thymic differentiation

SELECTED REFERENCES

1. Tavusbay C et al: Spindle epithelial tumor with thymus-like element (Settle): a case report. Indian J Surg Oncol. 8(2):231-233, 2017
2. Ippolito S et al: Spindle epithelial tumor with thymus-like differentiation (SETTLE): clinical-pathological features, differential pathological diagnosis and therapy. Endocrine. 51(3):402-12, 2016
3. Yi K et al: Review of the touch preparation cytology of spindle epithelial tumor with thymus-like differentiation. J Cytol. 33(1):27-9, 2016
4. Llamas-Gutierrez FJ et al: Spindle epithelial tumor with thymus-like differentiation of the thyroid (SETTLE): Report of two cases (one associated with a parathyroid adenoma). Ann Diagn Pathol. 17(2):217-21, 2013
5. Misra RK et al: Spindle epithelial tumor with thymus-like differentiation: a case report and review of literature. Acta Cytol. 57(3):303-8, 2013
6. Hirokawa M et al: Cytological findings of intrathyroidal epithelial thymoma/carcinoma showing thymus-like differentiation: a study of eight cases. Diagn Cytopathol. 40 Suppl 1:E16-20, 2012
7. Kaur J et al: Fine needle aspiration cytology of a spindle epithelial tumour with thymus-like differentiation (SETTLE) occurring in the thyroid. Cytopathology. 23(6):413-5, 2012
8. Rastogi A et al: Recurrent thyroid nodule: spindle epithelial tumor with thymus like differentiation (SETTLE). Indian Pediatr. 49(6):482-4, 2012
9. Folpe AL et al: Spindle epithelial tumor with thymus-like differentiation: a morphologic, immunohistochemical, and molecular genetic study of 11 cases. Am J Surg Pathol. 33(8):1179-86, 2009
10. Grushka JR et al: Spindle epithelial tumor with thymus-like elements of the thyroid: a multi-institutional case series and review of the literature. J Pediatr Surg. 44(5):944-8, 2009
11. Haberal AN et al: Unusual spindle cell tumor of thyroid (SETTLE). Thyroid. 18(1):85-7, 2008
12. Satoh S et al: Spindle epithelial tumor with thymus-like differentiation (SETTLE): youngest reported patient. Pathol Int. 2006 Sep;56(9):563-7. Erratum in: Pathol Int. 57(1):52, 2007
13. Tong GX et al: Fine-needle aspiration biopsy of monophasic variant of spindle epithelial tumor with thymus-like differentiation of the thyroid: report of one case and review of the literature. Diagn Cytopathol. 35(2):113-9, 2007
14. Papi G et al: Primary spindle cell lesions of the thyroid gland; an overview. Am J Clin Pathol. 125 Suppl:S95-123, 2006
15. Reimann JD et al: Carcinoma showing thymus-like differentiation of the thyroid (CASTLE): a comparative study: evidence of thymic differentiation and solid cell nest origin. Am J Surg Pathol. 30(8):994-1001, 2006
16. Abrosimov AY et al: Spindle epithelial tumor with thymus-like differentiation (SETTLE) of the thyroid with neck lymph node metastasis: a case report. Endocr Pathol. 16(2):139-43, 2005
17. Xu B et al: Spindle epithelial tumor with thymus-like differentiation of the thyroid: a case report with pathological and molecular genetics study. Hum Pathol. 34(2):190-3, 2003
18. Iwasa K et al: Spindle epithelial tumor with thymus-like differentiation (SETTLE) of the thyroid. Head Neck. 24(9):888-93, 2002
19. Kloboves-Prevodnik V et al: Thyroid spindle epithelial tumor with thymus-like differentiation (SETTLE): is cytopathological diagnosis possible? Diagn Cytopathol. 26(5):314-9, 2002
20. Rodriguez I et al: Solitary fibrous tumor of the thyroid gland: report of seven cases. Am J Surg Pathol. 25(11):1424-8, 2001
21. Cheuk W et al: Spindle epithelial tumor with thymus-like differentiation (SETTLE): a distinctive malignant thyroid neoplasm with significant metastatic potential. Mod Pathol. 13(10):1150-5, 2000
22. Kirby PA et al: Spindle epithelial tumor with thymus-like differentiation (SETTLE) of the thyroid with prominent mitotic activity and focal necrosis. Am J Surg Pathol. 23(6):712-6, 1999
23. Su L et al: Spindle epithelial tumor with thymus-like differentiation: a case report with cytologic, histologic, immunohistologic, and ultrastructural findings. Mod Pathol. 10(5):510-4, 1997
24. Chan JK et al: Tumors of the neck showing thymic or related branchial pouch differentiation: a unifying concept. Hum Pathol. 22(4):349-67, 1991

Immunohistochemistry

Antibody	Reactivity	Staining Pattern	Comment
34bE12	Positive	Cell membrane & cytoplasm	All tumor cells, both spindle and glandular elements, are positive
AE1/AE3	Positive	Cell membrane & cytoplasm	Nearly all tumor cells, both spindle and glandular elements, are positive
EMA	Positive	Cell membrane	Both spindle and glandular elements are positive
CK7	Positive	Cell membrane & cytoplasm	
Vimentin	Positive	Cell membrane & cytoplasm	
CD99	Positive	Cell membrane	Some cells are positive
p63	Positive	Nuclear	
TTF-1	Negative		
Thyroglobulin	Negative		
Calcitonin	Negative		
CEA-M	Negative		
CD5	Negative		
S100	Negative		
Chromogranin-A	Negative		
Synaptophysin	Negative		
CK20	Negative		
p53	Negative		

Distinguishing Characteristics of Spindle Cell Neoplasms of Thyroid

Feature	SETTLE	Solitary Fibrous Tumor	Anaplastic Thyroid Carcinoma	Synovial Sarcoma
Gross	Variable appearance; vaguely lobular; mean size: 3.6 cm	Lobulated circumscribed mass with gray-white cut surface	Infiltrative tumor	Circumscribed tan soft mass
Cytology	Cellular smears with dissociated or cohesive clusters of bland spindle cells	Spindle-shaped cells with scanty cytoplasm and uniform small nuclei	Marked pleomorphism with extensive necrosis	Sheets of uniform small spindle cells with ovoid nuclei
Histologic characteristics	Biphasic tumor composed of spindle cell component and glandular structures	Alternating cellularity, from highly cellular areas to sparsely cellular areas	Diffuse growth pattern	Small spindle-shaped cells that have scanty cytoplasm with ovoid nuclei with focal glandular differentiation
Immunohistochemistry	Positive for cytokeratin, p63 and CD5; negative for TTF-1 and thyroglobulin	Positive for CD34	Positive for p53; negative for TTF-1 and thyroglobulin	Positive for CD99, CD56, keratin, EMA, calretinin, β-catenin, FLI-1, and TLE1; negative for CD34
Clinical characteristics	Occur in children and adolescents	Occurs in adults with equal gender distribution	Tumor of elderly patients	Occur in young adults (15-35 years)
Other	Males more affected than females		Highly aggressive tumor	Characteristic t(X;18)(p11;q11)

Spindle epithelial tumor with thymus-like differentiation = SETTLE.

(Left) *This photomicrograph demonstrates a cellular spindle cell tumor formed by short intersecting and streaming fascicles. The tumor is composed of long spindle cells with scant cytoplasm.* **(Right)** *Most SETTLE are biphasic, where intersecting bundles of spindle-shaped cells blend with glandular and tubulopapillary structures. These glandular structures form cystic spaces ⊷ that may contain scanty fluid or mucin within the lumen.*

Spindle Cell Component

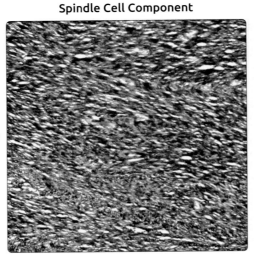

Glandular Arrangements

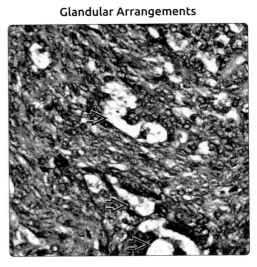

(Left) *This H&E highlights an area of SETTLE formed by compact reticulated fascicles of spindle cells with scant cytoplasm ⊷. This area is separated from an area of epithelioid component ⊷ and microcysts ⊷ with a primitive appearance.* **(Right)** *This figure highlights the cellular spindle cell tumor ⊷ that blends with an epithelioid tubuloglandular structure ⊷ that can contain clear fluid or mucin. In some areas, acellular fibrous septa ⊷ blend with the tumor.*

Spindle Cells

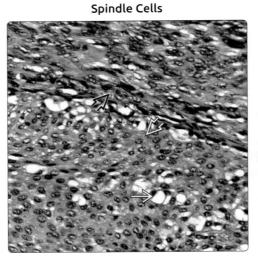

Biphasic Growth Pattern

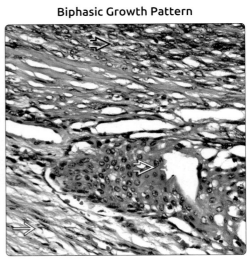

(Left) *This image demonstrates a biphasic cellular tumor formed by short intersecting and streaming spindle cell fascicles ⊷ that blend with the glandular ⊷, tubular ⊷, and epithelioid components ⊷.* **(Right)** *This photomicrograph demonstrates a cellular tumor formed by epithelioid cells with glandular ⊷, tubular ⊷, and solid epithelioid components ⊷, characteristic of a biphasic SETTLE. Both glandular and tubular structures have scant luminal fluid.*

Biphasic Tumor Cells

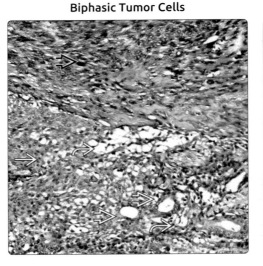

Epithelioid Cells

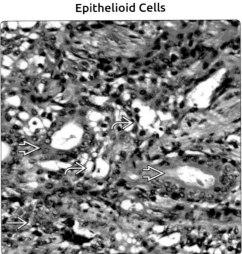

Biphasic Growth Pattern

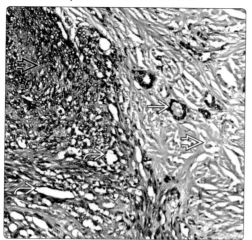

Glandular and Tubulopapillary Pattern

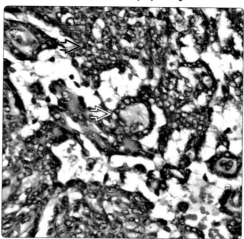

(Left) *A biphasic growth pattern is evident as lobules formed by a spindle cell component* ⊡ *are separated by acellular fibrous septa* ⊡ *that contain scattered glandular elements* ⊡. *In this field, there are also tubular structures* ⊡. **(Right)** *These glandular and tubulopapillary structures are intermixed and located within cystic spaces and nests of epithelioid cells* ⊡. *The glandular-like structures contain mucin-like material within their lumina* ⊡.

Diffuse Nuclear Staining for p63

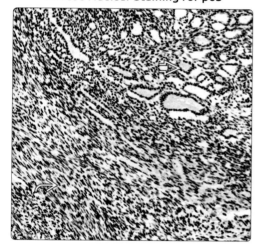

Glandular Arrangements

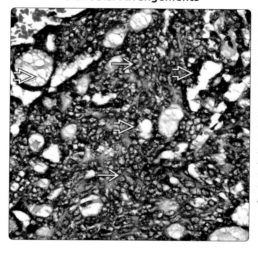

(Left) *Immunohistochemistry for p63 shows intense and diffuse nuclear positivity in both spindle cell* ⊡ *and glandular* ⊡ *components of this biphasic tumor.* **(Right)** *This picture illustrates the epithelioid component with glandular-like structures showing mucin-like material within their lumina. The glandular and tubulopapillary structures* ⊡ *merge into and are located within nests of epithelioid cells in a syncytial pattern* ⊡.

Lack of Thyroid Markers

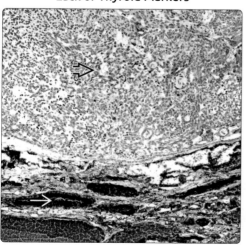

Diffuse HMW Cytokeratin Reactivity

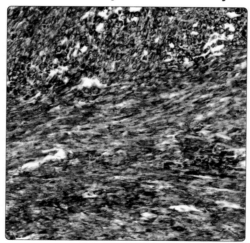

(Left) *SETTLE is characteristically negative for thyroid cell markers, such as thyroglobulin, TTF-1, and calcitonin. The spindle cells and epithelioid cells* ⊡ *above are negative for thyroglobulin, while the compressed thyroid* ⊡ *below is positive.* **(Right)** *SETTLE is characterized by diffuse and intense positivity for high molecular weight cytokeratin (HMW) in both the spindle cell component and the glandular component. This micrograph highlights the positivity in the spindle cell component.*

Intrathyroid Epithelial Thymoma

TERMINOLOGY

- Primary thyroid gland malignant epithelial tumor with thymic epithelial differentiation
- Synonyms
  - Carcinoma showing thymus-like element (CASTLE)
  - Intrathyroid thymic carcinoma

ETIOLOGY/PATHOGENESIS

- Etiology is unknown
  - As it is prevalent in Asia population, that may suggest genetic, ethnic, &/or environmental background
  - May arise from remnants of branchial pouch capable of thymic differentiation

MACROSCOPIC

- Tumor is solid, well circumscribed, and has lobulated surface
- Calcification and cystic changes are absent

MICROSCOPIC

- Morphologically similar to thymic carcinoma
- Composed by multiple interlacing islands of cells separated by fibrous stroma
- Composed by squamoid and focally spindle-shaped cells with lightly eosinophilic cytoplasm and oval, pale to vesicular nuclei
- Histological subtypes
  - Squamous cell carcinoma type
  - Lymphoepithelioma or basaloid type
  - Neuroendocrine carcinoma type similar to mediastinal thymic carcinoma
- Histological grade is low

ANCILLARY TESTS

- Neoplastic cells within islands of tumor are positive for HMWK (34bE12), CD5, p63, CD117, Bcl-2, calretinin, CEA
- Tumor cells are negative for TTF-1, thyroglobulin, calcitonin, chromogranin

---

(Left) Lobules of tumor cells are separated by a lymphocyte-rich fibrous stroma. The tumor cells are squamoid and spindle-shaped with light eosinophilic cytoplasm and oval, pale nuclei with small nucleoli. (Right) Low-power appearance of carcinoma showing thymus-like element (CASTLE) demonstrates a lobular architecture separated by a dense, fibrous, lymphocyte-rich stroma. HMWK staining highlights the lobular architecture, similar to thymic carcinoma.

Lymphoepithelioma-Type CASTLE

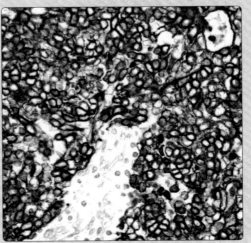

Keratin Highlights Epithelial Islands

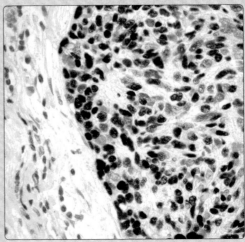

(Left) CD5 immunostain highlights the strong membranous staining characteristic of CASTLE and thymic carcinoma. CD5 shows cytoplasmic immunoreactivity in scattered T lymphocytes. (Right) There is a diffuse immunoreactivity for p63 in the epithelial cells within islands of tumor. The staining is similar to that seen in thyroid solid cell nests, providing further evidence intrathyroid epithelial thymoma may arise from remnants of the branchial pouch and ultimobranchial body.

CD5 Membranous Staining

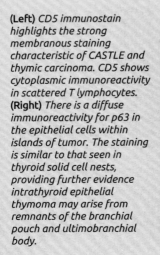

p63 Immunopositivity

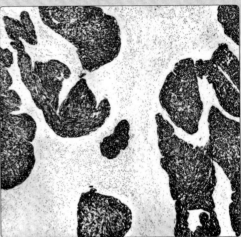

TERMINOLOGY

Synonyms

- Carcinoma showing thymus-like differentiation
- Carcinoma showing thymus-like element (CASTLE)
- Carcinoma showing thymus-like features
- Intrathyroid thymic carcinoma
- Lymphoepithelioma-like carcinoma of thyroid
- Primary thyroid thymoma
- Thymic carcinoma of thyroid

Definitions

- Malignant epithelial tumor of thyroid gland with thymic epithelial differentiation
- Primary thyroid gland malignant neoplasm cytologically and architecturally similar to thymic epithelial neoplasms
  - It is malignant counterpart of ectopic thymoma of thyroid gland

ETIOLOGY/PATHOGENESIS

Developmental Anomaly

- Etiology is unknown
  - As it is prevalent in Asia population, this may suggest genetic, ethnic, &/or environmental background
- Arises from intrathyroidal thymic rests or from thymic rests adjacent to thyroid gland
  - Embryological persistence of cervical thymic tissue
  - Branchial pouch remnants, including solid cell nests, that can differentiate along thymic epithelial cell lines
- Arises from remnants of branchial pouch capable of thymic differentiation
  - Presence of thymic tissue adjacent to CASTLE supports this theory
  - Neoplasm or surrounding areas may have true thymic differentiation
  - Positive staining of tumor cells with markers associated with thymic carcinoma
    - CD5
    - Bcl-2
    - Mcl-1
    - p63

CLINICAL ISSUES

Epidemiology

- Incidence
  - Very rare, representing 0.083% of all thyroid tumors in Japan and 0.15% in China
- Age
  - Affects middle-aged adults
- Sex
  - Female:Male ratio is nearly equal with slight female preponderance (1.3:1)

Site

- Vast majority in lower poles of thyroid gland
  - Rare cases may be present in mid to lower poles
  - Rare cases may arise in perithyroidal soft tissues of neck

Presentation

- Usual presentation is painless, slow-growing thyroid mass
- Patients usually complain of pressure symptoms, like hoarseness and dysphagia
- Less frequently, patients may have tracheal compression
- In ~ 1/2 of cases present with lymph node metastasis at time of initial diagnosis
- Metastases to other sites is very rare
  - Metastases are most common to lung
- No clinical findings associated with thymoma

Laboratory Tests

- No alterations in thyroid function laboratory values

Treatment

- Options, risks, complications
  - Need of long-term follow-up due to protracted clinical course
- Surgical approaches
  - Total thyroidectomy is treatment of choice
  - Lymph node dissection in case of clinically evident metastatic disease
  - Removal of local recurrence
- Adjuvant therapy
  - Neoadjuvant chemotherapy may be used to decrease tumor size allowing surgery with good results
    - Chemotherapy will decrease local symptoms as tumor size decreases
- Drugs
  - Chemotherapy may be used to decrease symptoms
  - Chemotherapy may be used with radiotherapy when recurrences occur
- Radiation
  - Usually used postoperatively, as patients tend not to develop locoregional recurrences
  - Radiation in conjunction with chemotherapy in patients with recurrence improves survival

Prognosis

- Patients with CASTLE have relatively favorable prognosis
- Local recurrences may be present in ~ 30% of patients
- Cervical lymph node metastases are associated with worse prognosis
- Long-term prognosis is good with 10-year survival reaching 80%
- Rare cases may have rapid fatal outcome

IMAGING

General Features

- Location
  - Neck, occupying thyroid gland area
- Morphology
  - Lobulated outline with irregular pattern

Radiographic Findings

- Usually has lobulated appearance with heterogeneous echo pattern
- May display moderate vascularity on color flow images
- Scintigraphy shows "cold" nodule

MR Findings

- Appears as iso- or hypointense mass on T1-weighted MR
- Appears hyperintense on T2-weighted MR

CT Findings

- Shows enhancement after contrast with clear plane between tumor and adjacent thyroid gland
- Shows solid, noncalcified soft tissue density

Thyroid Scan

- Tumor appears as "cold" nodule

MACROSCOPIC

General Features

- Tumor is solid and has lobulated surface
- Cut surface is firm to fleshy, ivory-white
- Tumor has well-demarcated borders

Size

- Tumor may be large with mean diameter around 4 cm

MICROSCOPIC

Histologic Features

- Morphologically similar to thymic carcinoma
- Tumor is basically squamous cell carcinoma with lymphocyte-rich stroma
- Tumor has broad, smooth, and pushing borders
- Composed by multiple interlacing islands of cells separated by fibrous stroma
  - Separated into lobules by scattered lymphocyte-rich fibrous trabecula
  - Tumor islands and stroma are infiltrated by numerous plasma cells and small lymphocytes
- Islands of tumor cells are variably sized and contain delicate vessels
- Composed by squamoid and focally spindle-shaped cells with lightly eosinophilic cytoplasm
- Nuclei are oval, pale to vesicular, containing small to medium-sized nucleoli, easily identified
- Single cell keratinization or stratification of keratinizing tumor cells may be present
- Thymus-like tissue with Hassall corpuscles may be found adjacent to tumor cells
- Mitoses are present and may approach 5/10 HPF
- Histological grade is low compared with that of primary squamous cell carcinoma

Lymphatic/Vascular Invasion

- May be present but is difficult to identify

Margins

- Tumors tend to have circumscribed borders, and some may be infiltrative involving margins

Lymph Nodes

- ~ 2/3 of patients have lymph node metastases at time of presentation

Predominant Pattern/Injury Type

- Circumscribed
- Cords and ribbons
- Lobulated
- Small islands/nested

Predominant Cell/Compartment Type

- Epithelial

Histological Subtypes

- Squamous cell carcinoma type
- Lymphoepithelioma or basaloid type
- Neuroendocrine carcinoma type similar to mediastinal thymic carcinoma

ANCILLARY TESTS

Cytology

- Neoplasm is often misinterpreted as other neoplasms (anaplastic thyroid carcinoma or medullary thyroid carcinoma)
- Cytology of these tumors is characterized by hypercellularity, large cell clusters with round to oval nuclei and distinct nucleoli, and few keratinized cells with intracytoplasmic lumina
- Cellular smears with atypical epithelial cells
  - Cells may be arranged in sheets or are present as single cells
- Nuclei are large, irregular, have vesicular chromatin and prominent nucleoli
- Lymphoid elements are present in background

Frozen Sections

- Very difficult diagnosis on frozen section as immunohistochemistry is needed for diagnosis

Immunohistochemistry

- Neoplastic cells (islands of tumor) are positive for
  - High-molecular-weight keratin (34bE12)
  - Wide-spectrum keratin (AE1/AE3)
  - CD5 (in cell membranes of tumor cells)
  - p63 (positive in all cells)
  - Bcl-2
  - p53
  - CEA
  - CD117 (c-KIT)
  - S100-A9
  - Calretinin
- Tumor cells are negative for TTF-1, thyroglobulin, calcitonin, chromogranin
- Ki-67 proliferative index is ~ 10-30%

Genetic Testing

- No reported cytogenetic studies on CASTLE

Electron Microscopy

- Elongated or oval epithelial cells with prominent desmosomes
- Cytoplasm with bundles of tonofilaments without secretory granules
- Presence of prominent nucleoli
- Presence of desmoplasia and lymphocytes

DIFFERENTIAL DIAGNOSIS

Anaplastic Thyroid Carcinoma

- Large tumor with necrosis and poorly defined borders with significant invasion
- This tumor may have significant cellular pleomorphism, necrosis, numerous mitotic figures
- Usually with limited immunoreactivity: Positive for p53 and high Ki-67 proliferative index

- Negative for CD5, p63, CEA, and HMWK
- Aggressive behavior

Ectopic Thymoma

- Thymomas can be found in ectopic locations, as in thyroid
- Thymomas are noninvasive, encapsulated, and well circumscribed
- Usually positive for CD5 and HMWK; negative for Bcl-2 and Mcl-1

Ectopic Hamartomatous Thymoma

- Usually arises in anterior and lower aspect of neck and sometimes appear to be in thyroid
- Has unique histopathological features with thymic tissue intermixed with adipose tissue

Follicular Dendritic Cell Sarcoma

- Also has lobular pattern and infiltrates into thyroid tissue
- Syncytial arrangements of spindled and epithelioid cells with vesicular nuclei and prominent nucleoli
- Usually immunoreactive for CD21, CD23, and CD35 and negative for CD5 and HMWK

Medullary Thyroid Carcinoma

- Variable morphology, including epithelioid, spindled, and syncytial-shaped cells
- Usually has infiltrative characteristics with islands of tumor cells, separated by amyloid
- Immunoreactive for chromogranin, synaptophysin, calcitonin, CD56, and CEA; negative for CD5

Metastatic Lymphoepithelioma-Like Carcinoma

- Metastases to thyroid from nasopharynx (usual primary location)
- Lacks squamous differentiation, has epithelioid cellular features with prominent nucleoli
- Strong reactivity with Epstein-Barr virus-encoded RNA
- Aggressive behavior

Squamous Cell Carcinoma

- Well-differentiated tumors have significant keratinization, pearl formation, and intercellular bridges
- Immunoreactive for p63 and S100-A9 but negative for CD5 and CEA
- Aggressive behavior

Thymic Carcinoma, Primary

- Thyroid involved by direct invasion from thymic tumor primary
- Morphologically and immunophenotypically same as CASTLE
- Imaging and intraoperative findings should confirm origin

DIAGNOSTIC CHECKLIST

Clinically Relevant Pathologic Features

- Invasive pattern
- Metastatic distribution

Pathologic Interpretation Pearls

- Well circumscribed, lobulated, well demarcated
- Broad, pushing, smooth-bordered cellular islands separated into lobules by fibrous trabeculae

- Squamoid and focal spindle cells with slightly eosinophilic cytoplasm and oval vesicular nuclei with prominent nucleoli
- Characteristic immunophenotype: 34bE12, CD5, p63, Bcl-2, CEA

SELECTED REFERENCES

1. Lloyd RV et al: WHO Classification of Tumours of Endocrine Organs. Lyon, France: IARC Press, 2017
2. Collins JA et al: Carcinoma showing thymus-like differentiation (CASTLE): cytopathological features and differential diagnosis. Acta Cytol. 60(5):421-428, 2016
3. Ge W et al: Clinical analysis of 82 cases of carcinoma showing thymus-like differentiation of the thyroid. Oncol Lett. 11(2):1321-1326, 2016
4. Wu B et al: CT and MR imaging of thyroid carcinoma showing thymus-like differentiation (CASTLE): a report of ten cases. Br J Radiol. 89(1060):20150726, 2016
5. Ebina A et al: Intrathyroid epithelial thymoma: carcinoma showing thymus-like differentiation mimicking squamous cell carcinoma of the thyroid. J Nippon Med Sch. 82(1):2-3, 2015
6. Hirokawa M et al: Intrathyroidal epithelial thymoma/carcinoma showing thymus-like differentiation; comparison with thymic lymphoepithelioma-like carcinoma and a possibility of development from a multipotential stem cell. APMIS. 121(6):523-30, 2013
7. Huang C et al: Carcinoma showing thymus-like differentiation of the thyroid (CASTLE). Pathol Res Pract. 209(10):662-5, 2013
8. Kakudo K et al: Intrathyroid epithelial thymoma (ITET) and carcinoma showing thymus-like differentiation (CASTLE): CD5-positive neoplasms mimicking squamous cell carcinoma of the thyroid. Histol Histopathol. 28(5):543-56, 2013
9. Liu Z et al: Clinical analysis of thyroid carcinoma showing thymus-like differentiation: report of 8 cases. Int Surg. 98(2):95-100, 2013
10. Hirokawa M et al: Cytological findings of intrathyroidal epithelial thymoma/carcinoma showing thymus-like differentiation: a study of eight cases. Diagn Cytopathol. 40 Suppl 1:E16-20, 2012
11. Liu X et al: [Thyroid carcinoma showing thymus-like differentiation: a clinicopathologic study of 8 cases.] Zhonghua Bing Li Xue Za Zhi. 40(2):89-93, 2011
12. Folpe AL et al: Spindle epithelial tumor with thymus-like differentiation: a morphologic, immunohistochemical, and molecular genetic study of 11 cases. Am J Surg Pathol. 33(8):1179-86, 2009
13. Yamazaki M et al: Carcinoma showing thymus-like differentiation (CASTLE) with neuroendocrine differentiation. Pathol Int. 58(12):775-9, 2008
14. Ito Y et al: Clinicopathologic significance of intrathyroidal epithelial thymoma/carcinoma showing thymus-like differentiation: a collaborative study with Member Institutes of The Japanese Society of Thyroid Surgery. Am J Clin Pathol. 127(2):230-6, 2007
15. Ito Y et al: Usefulness of S100A9 for diagnosis of intrathyroid epithelial thymoma (ITET)/carcinoma showing thymus-like differentiation (CASTLE). Pathology. 38(6):541-4, 2006
16. Reimann JD et al: Carcinoma showing thymus-like differentiation of the thyroid (CASTLE): a comparative study: evidence of thymic differentiation and solid cell nest origin. Am J Surg Pathol. 30(8):994-1001, 2006
17. Kusada N et al: A case of aggressive carcinoma showing thymus-like differentiation with distant metastases. Thyroid. 15(12):1383-8, 2005
18. Da J et al: [Thyroid squamous-cell carcinoma showing thymus-like element (CASTLE): a report of eight cases.] Zhonghua Zhong Liu Za Zhi. 21(4):303-4, 1999
19. Dorfman DM et al: Intrathyroidal epithelial thymoma (ITET)/carcinoma showing thymus-like differentiation (CASTLE) exhibits CD5 immunoreactivity: new evidence for thymic differentiation. Histopathology. 32(2):104-9, 1998
20. Chan JK et al: Tumors of the neck showing thymic or related branchial pouch differentiation: a unifying concept. Hum Pathol. 22(4):349-67, 1991

Immunohistochemistry

Antibody	Reactivity	Staining Pattern	Comment
34bE12	Positive	Cell membrane & cytoplasm	All tumor cells are strongly positive
CK-HMW-NOS	Positive	Cell membrane & cytoplasm	All tumor cells are positive
CD5	Positive	Cytoplasmic	All tumor cells have positivity in cytoplasm; adjacent T lymphocytes have nuclear positivity and serve as control
p63	Positive	Nuclear	All tumors cells have strong immunoreactivity
CEA-M	Positive	Cell membrane & cytoplasm	
p53	Positive	Nuclear	
S100-A9	Positive	Nuclear & cytoplasmic	
Bcl-1	Positive	Nuclear	
TTF-1	Negative		
Thyroglobulin	Negative		
Chromogranin-A	Negative		
Synaptophysin	Negative		
Calcitonin	Negative		
CD1a	Negative		

Differential Diagnosis of CASTLE

Feature	CASTLE	MTC	TC	LLC	ATC	SCC
Morphology	Similar to thymic carcinoma, broad and pushing island of tumor cells with smooth borders and desmoplastic stroma	Variable morphology	Similar to CASTLE	Large epithelioid cells lacking squamoid differentiation and with prominent nucleoli	Variable morphology	May have keratinization, pearl formation, intercellular bridges
Necrosis	Rare	Rare	Rare	Present	Characteristically has extensive necrosis	May be present
Mitosis	Present, but not high (< 3/10 HPF)	Present, but not high	Present, but not high	Numerous	Numerous mitoses (> 10/10 HPF)	Present, depending on tumor differentiation
Pleomorphism	Present	Minimal	Present	Present	Marked pleomorphism	May be present
Characteristic features	Tumor lobules separated by desmoplastic stroma containing lymphocytes	Amyloid	Similar to CASTLE	Poorly differentiated neoplasm	Presence of heterologous elements	Keratinization
IHC	Positive for HMWCK, CD5, CEA, p63; negative for TTF-1, chromogranin, calcitonin	Positive for chromogranin, calcitonin, CEA, synaptophysin; negative for CD5	Similar to CASTLE	Strong reactivity for Epstein-Barr virus-encoded RNA	Positive for p53; negative for p63, TTF-1, thyroglobulin, CD5, chromogranin	Positive for cytokeratin, p63, S100-A9; negative for CD5, TTF-1, thyroglobulin

CASTLE = intrathyroid epithelial thymoma; MTC = medullary thyroid carcinoma; TC = thymic carcinoma; LLC = lymphoepithelioma-like carcinoma; ATC = anaplastic carcinoma; SCC = squamous cell carcinoma.

Lymphoepithelioma or Basaloid-Type Tumor

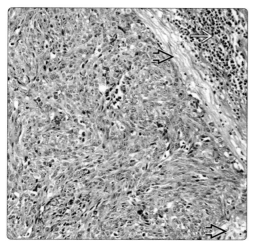

Islands of Epithelioid Cells

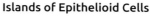
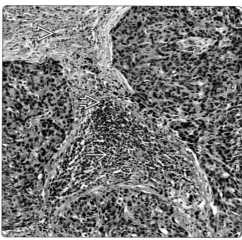

(Left) *Light microscopy reveals that the neoplasm is separated into lobules by scattered fibrous trabeculae ⮞, infiltrated by numerous small lymphocytes and plasma cells ➡. (Right) The tumor lobules are composed of squamoid and spindle-shaped cells with lightly eosinophilic cytoplasm. These cells are separated by fibrous stroma ⮞ containing numerous lymphocytes and plasma cells ➡.*

High Power of Lymphoepithelioid-Type Tumor

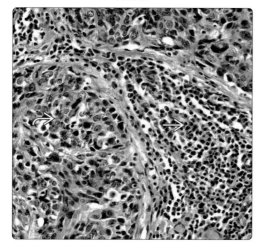

Lymphocyte-Rich Stroma

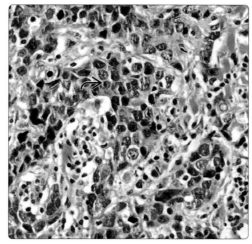

(Left) *The lobules of neoplastic cells show a syncytial appearance ⮞. The cells have a high nuclear:cytoplasmic ratio, vesicular chromatin, and small nucleoli. The stroma contains numerous lymphocytes ➡. (Right) The tumor cells in CASTLE are present in well-demarcated islands separated by dense and hyalinized fibrous stroma, rich in plasma cells and small lymphocytes. The tumor cells may have a predominant epithelioid and spindle-shaped appearance focally.*

High Power of Malignant Cells

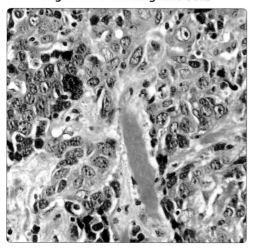

Large Squamoid Cells

(Left) *Microscopic field highlights the syncytial and squamoid appearance of the tumor cells. The neoplastic cells have a lightly eosinophilic cytoplasm and vesicular nuclei containing small distinct nucleoli. (Right) There is a vague squamoid and epithelioid appearance to tumor cells arranged in a syncytial appearance. The cells have a vesicular nuclear chromatin and small nucleoli ⮞. The tumor cells are infiltrated by lymphocytes and separated by fibrous stroma.*

p63 Highlights Tumor Cells

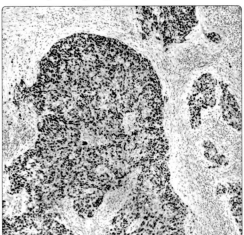

High-Power View of p63(+) Tumor Cells

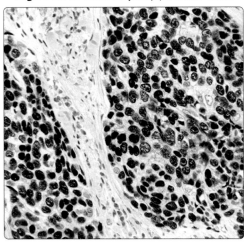

(Left) *The thyroid is infiltrated by lobules of neoplastic cells with strong nuclear positivity for p63. The tumor cells are present in well-demarcated islands separated by fibrous stroma. The stroma is negative for p63.* (Right) *There is a diffuse immunoreactivity for p63 throughout the tumor cells. The pattern of staining is similar to that identified in the solid cell nests of the thyroid in thymic tissue and in thymic carcinomas. p63 is negative in thyroid C cells and follicular cells.*

Focal CEA Immunoreactivity

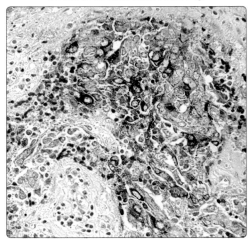

Keratin (+) Island of Tumor

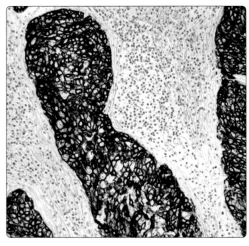

(Left) *Tumor cells in CASTLE show positivity for CEA, a characteristic finding of thymic carcinomas and CASTLE. The immunopositivity is usually patchy, cytoplasmic, and focal in cell membranes. CEA is present in the majority of solid cell nests and only in a minority of thymoma. It is negative in normal thymus.* (Right) *High-molecular-weight keratin (34bE12) is strongly and diffusely positive in CASTLE. This immunostain highlights the lobular appearance of these tumors, separated by lymphocyte-rich fibrous stroma.*

CD5 in Tumor Cells and in T Lymphocytes

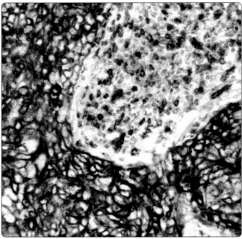

CD5 Stain in Tumor and Cytoplasmic in T Cells

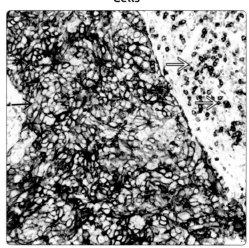

(Left) *Immunohistochemistry for CD5 highlights a strong & diffusely positive membranous staining, characteristic of CASTLE & thymic carcinoma. Staining separates CASTLE from other thyroid tumors. Adjacent T lymphocytes are also positive for CD5.* (Right) *CD5 immunostaining shows a characteristic strong & diffuse membranous immunoreactivity of epithelioid & spindle-shaped tumor cells ➡ in CASTLE. The positively staining T lymphocytes ➡ infiltrating the stroma serve as an internal control.*

Membranous Staining in Tumor Cells

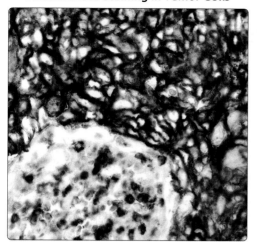

Nuclear Immunopositivity for p63

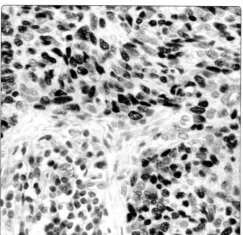

(Left) Immunohistochemistry for CD5 highlights a strong and diffusely positive membranous staining, characteristic of CASTLE and thymic carcinoma. CD5 has the characteristic membranous staining pattern in the tumor cells. (Right) Immunohistochemistry for p63 highlights a strong and diffusely positive nuclear staining, characteristic of CASTLE, thymic carcinoma, and their benign counterparts, solid cell nests and thymus. Solid cell nests are also positive for HMWK and CEA.

Solid Cell Nests

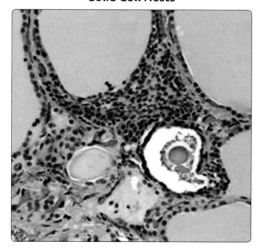

Solid Cell Nests

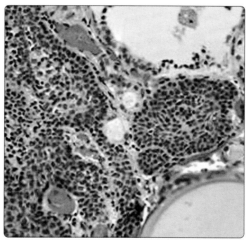

(Left) Solid cell nests are composed of solid nests of small cells with spindle-shaped nuclei; occasionally, central cystic spaces with mucin may be seen. These cells are found in normal thyroid and may be seen in close association with ectopic thymic tissue. (Right) Thyroid solid cell nest, typically found in the posterior lateral and medial portions of the thyroid lobes, are composed of small cells with spindle-shaped bland nuclei with occasional intraepithelial lymphocytes.

p63 in Tumor Cells

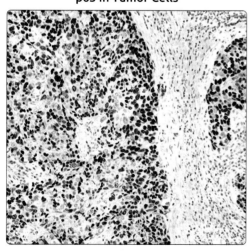

p63 Nuclear Immunopositivity

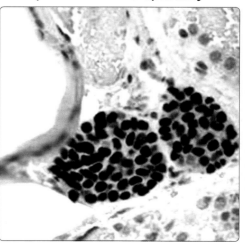

(Left) There is a diffuse immunoreactivity for p63 in CASTLE. The staining is similar to that seen in thyroid solid cell nests, providing further evidence CASTLE may arise from remnants of the branchial pouch and ultimobranchial body (thyroid solid cell nests). (Right) Thyroid solid cell nest displays strong diffuse nuclear positivity for p63 and is positive for HMWK and CD5, providing evidence that CASTLE is likely of ectopic thymic/branchial pouch origin and may arise from solid cell nests.

Sclerosing Mucoepidermoid Carcinoma With Eosinophilia

TERMINOLOGY

- Sclerosing mucoepidermoid carcinoma with eosinophilia: Malignant epithelial neoplasm showing epidermoid and glandular differentiation and displaying sclerotic stroma with eosinophilic and lymphocytic infiltration (WHO 2017)

CLINICAL ISSUES

- Extrathyroidal extension seen in ~ 40% of patients at presentation
- Regional lymph node metastasis also common (~ 35%)
- Distant metastases to lung, liver, and bone in ~ 20%

MACROSCOPIC

- Tumors usually appear as ill-defined, white to yellow, firm, solid masses
- Size range: 1-13 cm

MICROSCOPIC

- Circumscribed (but unencapsulated) to infiltrative

- Anastomosing cords and islands of tumor cells infiltrating sclerotic stroma
- Sclerotic stroma richly infiltrated by eosinophils, lymphocytes, and plasma cells
- Tumor formed by squamous cells and mucous cells
- Associated with lymphocytic thyroiditis in surrounding nonneoplastic thyroid gland

ANCILLARY TESTS

- Intracytoplasmic and intraluminal mucin-positive material
  - Cystic spaces show mucicarminophilic material
- Cytokeratin positive in all cases
- p63, pax-8, and TTF-1 usually positive
- Thyroglobulin negative or focally positive
- Calcitonin, synaptophysin, and chromogranin negative
- *BRAF* mutations not identified

Strands of Epithelial Cells Within Fibrosis

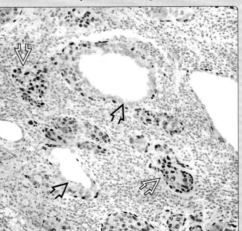

Solid and Glandular Components

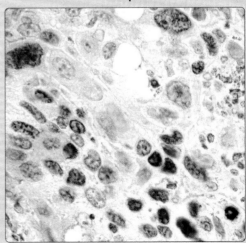

(Left) *Sclerosing mucoepidermoid carcinoma with eosinophilia (SMECE) shows tumor nests ⇨ with an associated sclerotic stroma ⇨ adjacent to scattered residual thyroid follicles ⇨. (Right) The cellular infiltrate in SMECE shows solid ⇨ and glandular growth composed of squamous cells and mucocytes ⇨ with associated sclerosis and numerous eosinophils.*

p63 Positivity

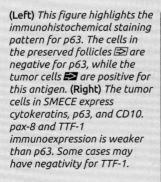

Weak and Focal Expression of TTF-1

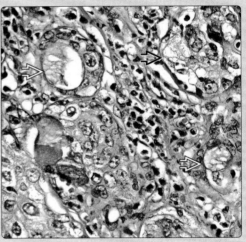

(Left) *This figure highlights the immunohistochemical staining pattern for p63. The cells in the preserved follicles ⇨ are negative for p63, while the tumor cells ⇨ are positive for this antigen. (Right) The tumor cells in SMECE express cytokeratins, p63, and CD10. pax-8 and TTF-1 immunoexpression is weaker than p63. Some cases may have negativity for TTF-1.*

TERMINOLOGY

Abbreviations

- Sclerosing mucoepidermoid carcinoma with eosinophilia (SMECE) of thyroid gland

Synonyms

- Squamous cell carcinoma of thyroid
- Epidermoid carcinoma with eosinophilia (ECE)

Definitions

- SMECE: Malignant epithelial neoplasm showing epidermoid and glandular differentiation and displaying sclerotic stroma with eosinophilic and lymphocytic infiltration (WHO 2017)
  - Characterized by nests or strands of epidermoid tumor cells with squamous differentiation, rare mucous cells, prominent sclerotic stroma, eosinophilic and lymphoplasmacytic infiltration, and background of chronic lymphocytic (Hashimoto) thyroiditis in nonneoplastic thyroid gland
  - Presence of prominent sclerotic stroma with eosinophil-rich and lymphocytic inflammatory cell component
  - Variable numbers of squamous cells and cells with mucous differentiation

ETIOLOGY/PATHOGENESIS

Idiopathic

- No known etiologic agent

Histogenesis

- SMECE consistently associated with and in setting of fibrosing Hashimoto thyroiditis
- Presumed to arise from squamous metaplasia of thyroid follicular epithelium
  - Presence of thyroid-specific mRNAs by RT-PCR in thyroid mucoepidermoid carcinoma
    - TTF-1, TTF-2, pax-8, Na-I symporter, and thyroid peroxidase mRNA support origin from thyroid follicular epithelium
- Origin from ultimobranchial body (solid cell nests) suggested as possible origin for SMECE
  - Some histologic, histochemical, and immunohistochemical features suggest possible origin from SCN
    - p63 positive
- Origin from follicular epithelial cell origin supported by
  - Presence of keratinization, intercellular bridges, and thyroglobulin reactivity
  - Absence of calcitonin and chromogranin reactivity

CLINICAL ISSUES

Epidemiology

- Incidence
  - Rare
- Age
  - Wide range (2nd-8th decades)
- Sex
  - Occurs almost exclusively in females (F:M ~ 7:1)

Presentation

- Slowly growing, painless neck mass
- Rarely presents with rapid enlargement
- Extrathyroidal extension seen in ~ 40% of patients at presentation
  - With symptoms of extrathyroidal extension
    - Hoarseness, dyspnea, or vocal cord paralysis
- Regional lymph node metastasis also common (~ 35%)
- Distant metastases to lung, liver and bone in ~ 20%

Laboratory Tests

- Euthyroid

Treatment

- Surgical approaches
  - Surgery treatment of choice
    - Total thyroidectomy, especially since extrathyroidal extension is frequent
    - Conservative therapy (lobectomy or subtotal thyroidectomy) can be performed
  - Selected cervical lymph node sampling recommended in presence of clinically enlarged nodes

Prognosis

- Excellent
  - Generally follows indolent course
- Extrathyroidal extension in 1/2 of cases
- Metastatic tumor to cervical lymph nodes may be present
  - Occurs in up to 30% of cases at presentation
- Distant metastases uncommon but may occur (lung, liver, and bone)
- Specific prognostic factors unknown

IMAGING

Radiographic Findings

- Hypoactive ("cold") nodule in thyroid imaging

MACROSCOPIC

General Features

- Tumors usually appear as white to yellow, firm, solid masses with ill-defined borders
- Cut surface white-yellow, firm, and solid
- Cystic change may occur but uncommon

Size

- Range: 1-13 cm

MICROSCOPIC

Histologic Features

- Circumscribed (unencapsulated) to infiltrative
- Majority of epidermoid tumor cells arranged in thin strands and small nests with mild to moderate nuclear pleomorphism, distinct nucleoli, and eosinophilic or pale cytoplasm infiltrated in abundant dense fibrohyaline stroma
- Lymphoplasmacytic infiltration with abundant eosinophils seen in sclerosing stroma and epidermoid tumor nests
  - Sclerotic stroma richly infiltrated by eosinophils, lymphocytes, and plasma cells

- Anastomosing cords and narrow strands of tumor cells infiltrating sclerotic stroma
- Neoplastic cells include
  - Foci of squamous differentiation including intercellular bridges, keratinocyte, keratin pearls, and keratinolysis forming pseudovascular appearance could be seen
    - Squamous or epidermoid cells
  - Rare, single or small aggregates of mucous cells and small mucin pools can be identified
    - Occasional mucocyte &/or mucin pools
  - Pseudoangiomatous appearance may be present (loss of tumor cell cohesion)
- Clear cells may be seen
  - Represent minor component (10-30%)
  - Appear to be glycogen-rich squamous cells
- Perineural invasion and obliteration of blood vessels common
- Lymphocytic thyroiditis commonly present in surrounding nonneoplastic thyroid gland
  - Arises in thyroid glands affected by Hashimoto thyroiditis, particularly fibrous variant
  - May include foci of squamous metaplasia
- Papillary carcinoma may be identified
  - Transition between SMECE and papillary carcinoma less common than in mucoepidermoid carcinoma of thyroid gland
- Perineural and vascular invasion may be present
- Neoplastic infiltrate generally confined to thyroid gland
  - Extrathyroidal extension occurs in 1/2 of cases
- Nontumor thyroid always presents Hashimoto thyroiditis or lymphocytic thyroiditis

ANCILLARY TESTS

Cytology

- Definitive diagnosis by fine-needle aspiration cytology difficult due to nonspecific nature of findings
  - Combination of malignant epithelial cells set in mucinous stroma with eosinophils
  - Cohesive clusters of cells with features of epidermoid or glandular differentiation
- Findings suggest malignancy but may also raise possibility of metastatic tumor or Hashimoto thyroiditis

Histochemistry

- Mucin stains (mucicarmine and periodic acid-Schiff with diastase)
  - Intracytoplasmic and intraluminal mucin positive material
  - Cystic spaces show mucicarminophilic material

Immunohistochemistry

- Cytokeratin and p63 positive
  - CK19
  - p63 strongly stains squamous/epidermoid cells
- Carcinoembryonic antigen positive in majority of cases
  - Sometimes express mucocyte
- TTF-1 positive in > 1/2 of cases
- Thyroglobulin usually negative or focally positive
- Galectin-3 positive
- Calcitonin, synaptophysin, chromogranin, calponin, S100, and smooth muscle actin negative
- p53 staining occasionally seen in squamous cells

Genetic Testing

- *BRAF* mutations not identified

DIFFERENTIAL DIAGNOSIS

Conventional Mucoepidermoid Carcinoma

- Lack of sclerotic stroma and prominent eosinophilic infiltrate
- Thyroglobulin almost always positive
- TTF-1 usually positive

Lymphocytic Thyroiditis With Squamous Metaplasia

- Diffuse and tends not to form mass
- Lacks mucocytes, mucin pools, and significant eosinophilic infiltrate

Anaplastic Thyroid Carcinoma

- Characteristic demographics and clinical presentation
  - Most often occurs in older adults
  - Typically occurs as rapidly enlarging neck mass in presence of longstanding history of thyroid lesion
- Histology characterized by presence of
  - Sheet-like growth
  - Marked pleomorphism
  - Increased mitotic activity, atypical mitoses
  - Apoptosis and necrosis
  - Lymphovascular invasion
  - Extensively infiltrative, including
    - Intrathyroidal &/or extrathyroidal extension
- Lacks mucocytes, mucin pools, significant eosinophil cell component

Intrathyroid Thymic Carcinoma (CASTLE)

- Architecture shows some resemblance to lobulated appearance seen in thymic tumors (thymoma or thymic carcinoma), including
  - Solid nests or lobules with expansile or infiltrative growth into thyroid tissue in broad fronts
  - Dense fibrous bands creating lobulated or septated appearance
- Cellular composition similar to nasopharyngeal carcinoma, nonkeratinizing undifferentiated type, including
  - Epithelioid cells with large, pleomorphic nuclei with vesicular chromatin and small, distinct nucleoli, abundant eosinophilic cytoplasm with indistinct cell borders
- Mitotic activity seen on order of 1-2 mitoses per 10 HPF
- Squamous differentiation may be present, including
  - Keratinization, intercellular bridges, foci of abrupt keratinization (resembling Hassall corpuscle)
- May have mucinous material
- Lacks mucocyte, mucin pools, and significant eosinophilic component
- Unique immunohistochemical profile, including
  - Cytokeratin positive
  - Thyroglobulin, TTF-1, and calcitonin negative
  - Immunoreactivity for markers associated with thymic carcinoma, including
    - CD5, p63, HMWK, CEA, Bcl-2, and Mcl-1
    - CD117 (C-kit) reactivity also present
  - EBV negative

Clinical and Pathological Features of Sclerosing Mucoepidermoid Carcinoma With Eosinophilia and Mucoepidermoid Carcinoma

	SMECE	MEC
F:M ratio	7:1	2:1
Extrathyroidal extension	~ 40%	~ 25%
Distant metastases	~ 22%	< 10%
Perineural invasion	Common	Rare
Associated with Hashimoto thyroiditis	Most	~ 40%
Associated with papillary thyroid carcinoma	Rare	~ 50%
Thyroglobulin	Negative of minimal	Positive
TTF-1	~ 50%, weak	Positive

Sclerosing mucoepidermoid carcinoma with eosinophilia (SMECE); mucoepidermoid carcinoma (MEC).

Direct Extension of Carcinoma From Adjacent Organ

- Primary squamous cell carcinomas of larynx and esophagus can invade thyroid gland
- In general, clinical &/or radiographic evidence confirms presence of extrathyroidal cancer invading thyroid gland
- Absence of mucocyte &/or glandular differentiation

Squamous Cell Carcinoma

- Rare type of primary thyroid carcinoma
- SMECE of thyroid gland should be differentiated from primary or secondary squamous cell carcinoma (SCC)
- SCC usually has more prominent pleomorphism and atypia, frequent mitosis, and rarely shows stromal sclerosis
- Lacks mucocyte, mucin pools, or significant eosinophil cell component

Hodgkin Lymphoma

- Rarely, primary Hodgkin disease of thyroid may occur
  - Hodgkin disease involving thyroid usually occurs secondary to cervical or mediastinal nodal disease
- Nodular sclerosing most common histologic type

SELECTED REFERENCES

1. Lloyd RV et al: WHO classification of tumours of endocrine organs. Lyon, France: IARC Press, 2017
2. Shah AA et al: Thyroid sclerosing mucoepidermoid carcinoma with eosinophilia: a clinicopathologic and molecular analysis of a distinct entity. Mod Pathol. 30(3):329-339, 2017
3. Pantola C et al: Sclerosing mucoepidermoid carcinoma with eosinophilia of the thyroid: A cytological dilemma. J Cytol. 33(1):37-9, 2016
4. Kobayashi Y et al: Local recurrence of sclerosing mucoepidermoid carcinoma with eosinophilia in the upper lip: a case report. J Med Case Rep. 9:41, 2015
5. Lai CY et al: Sclerosing mucoepidermoid carcinoma with eosinophilia of thyroid gland in a male patient: a case report and literature review. Int J Clin Exp Pathol. 8(5):5947-51, 2015
6. Geisinger KR et al: Eosinophilic replacement infiltrates in cystic Hashimoto's thyroiditis: a potential diagnostic pitfall. Endocr Pathol. 25(3):332-8, 2014
7. Musso-Lassalle S et al: A diagnostic pitfall: nodular tumor-like squamous metaplasia with Hashimoto's thyroiditis mimicking a sclerosing mucoepidermoid carcinoma with eosinophilia. Pathol Res Pract. 202(5):379-83, 2006
8. Hunt JL et al: p63 expression in sclerosing mucoepidermoid carcinomas with eosinophilia arising in the thyroid. Mod Pathol. 17(5):526-9, 2004
9. Albores-Saavedra J et al: Clear cells and thyroid transcription factor I reactivity in sclerosing mucoepidermoid carcinoma of the thyroid gland. Ann Diagn Pathol. 7(6):348-53, 2003
10. Baloch ZW et al: Primary mucoepidermoid carcinoma and sclerosing mucoepidermoid carcinoma with eosinophilia of the thyroid gland: a report of nine cases. Mod Pathol. 13(7):802-7, 2000
11. Solomon AC et al: Thyroid sclerosing mucoepidermoid carcinoma with eosinophilia: mimic of Hodgkin disease in nodal metastases. Arch Pathol Lab Med. 124(3):446-9, 2000
12. Geisinger KR et al: The cytomorphologic features of sclerosing mucoepidermoid carcinoma of the thyroid gland with eosinophilia. Am J Clin Pathol. 109(3):294-301, 1998
13. Sim SJ et al: Sclerosing mucoepidermoid carcinoma with eosinophilia of the thyroid: report of two patients, one with distant metastasis, and review of the literature. Hum Pathol. 28(9):1091-6, 1997
14. Bondeson L et al: Cytologic features in fine-needle aspirates from a sclerosing mucoepidermoid thyroid carcinoma with eosinophilia. Diagn Cytopathol. 15(4):301-5, 1996
15. Chan JK et al: Sclerosing mucoepidermoid thyroid carcinoma with eosinophilia. A distinctive low-grade malignancy arising from the metaplastic follicles of Hashimoto's thyroiditis. Am J Surg Pathol. 15(5):438-48, 1991

Tumor Nests and Thyroid Follicles

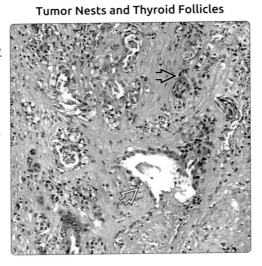

Necrosis

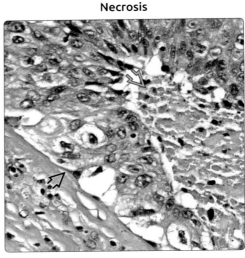

(Left) *Infiltrative SMECE shows tumor nests* ⇒ *infiltrating thyroid follicles* ⇒. *The neoplastic cellular infiltrate shows solid and cystic nests with associated sclerotic stroma and inflammatory infiltrate.* (Right) *This infiltrative tumor is predominantly composed of solid tumor nests* ⇒ *of epidermoid cells surrounded by eosinophil-rich stroma. Necrosis* ⇒ *may be present in the center of larger nests.*

Presence of Mucocytes

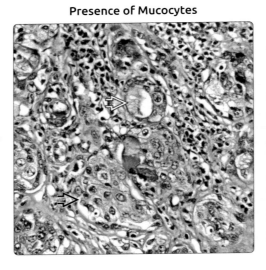

Lymph Node Metastases

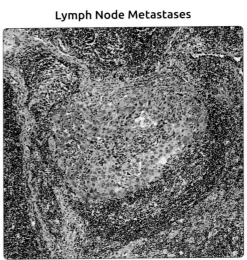

(Left) *The neoplastic cellular infiltrate in SMECE shows a solid and glandular growth pattern. The tumor is composed of squamous cells* ⇒ *and mucocytes* ⇒ *with associated sclerosis and inflammatory infiltrate including eosinophils.* (Right) *Metastatic SMECE to a lymph node shows nests of tumor cells with an associated stroma rich in eosinophilic inflammatory infiltrate.*

Residual Thyroid Follicles

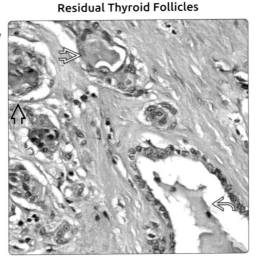

p63 Immunoexpression

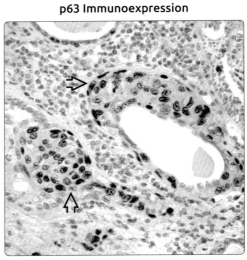

(Left) *The neoplastic cellular infiltrate in SMECE shows solid* ⇒ *and cystic* ⇒ *tumor nests infiltrating thyroid parenchyma with residual colloid within preserved follicles* ⇒. (Right) *Immunohistochemistry for p63 in SMECE shows positive tumor cells* ⇒ *within and around thyroid follicles and mostly in the nests of tumor cells.*

Metastases to Lymph Node

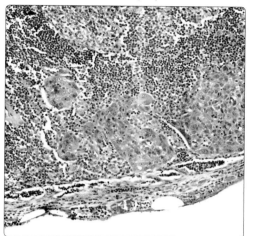

Numerous Eosinophils

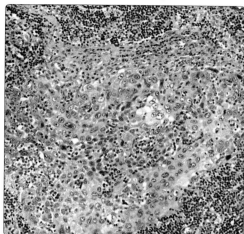

(Left) A small metastatic focus was present in one cervical lymph node in a patient with SMECE. (Right) Metastatic SMECE to a lymph node shows an associated sclerotic stroma and eosinophilic inflammatory infiltrate.

Large Pleomorphic Tumor Cells

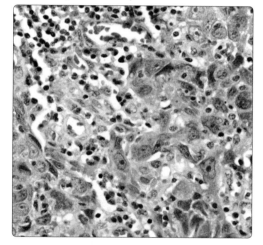

Scattered Mucocytes

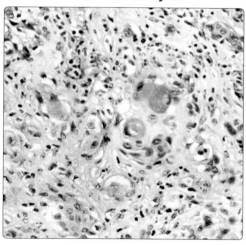

(Left) High-power view shows that the tumor cells are polygonal, with mild to moderate nuclear pleomorphism, and the presence of distinct nucleoli. Interspersed with the epidermoid nests are numerous eosinophils. (Right) In SMECE, there are mucous-secreting cells with squashed nuclei and small pools of mucin interspersed with the epidermoid nests. Mucicarmine stain highlights the presence of scattered mucocytes within the tumor cell nests.

p63(+) Tumor Cells

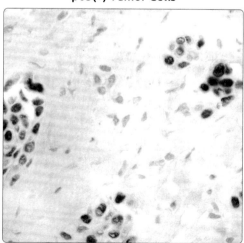

Weak Positivity for pax-8

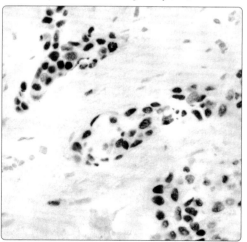

(Left) The nests of tumor cells are strongly positive for p63, and the fibrous stroma is negative for this marker. The positivity for this marker has raised the hypothesis that this tumor may arise from solid cell nests. The positivity for TTF-1 and pax-8 makes this hypothesis unlikely. (Right) Immunohistochemistry for pax-8 in SMECE shows some groups of tumor cells with weak nuclear positivity.

Lymphoma, Thyroid

CLINICAL ISSUES

- Mostly associated with lymphocytic thyroiditis
- Mean age: 65 years
- F:M = 3-4:1
- ~ 5% of all thyroid malignancies
- ~ 2% of extranodal lymphomas
- 60-80% of cases: Diffuse large B-cell lymphoma (DLBCL), germinal center origin
- 10-23% of cases: Mucosa-associated lymphoid tissue (MALT) lymphoma

MICROSCOPIC

- Lymphomas of thyroid include extranodal marginal zone B-cell lymphoma (EMZBCL), DLBCL, and transitions between
- **DLBCL**
  o Obliteration of thyroid tissue by large cells with distinct nucleoli and amphophilic cytoplasm
  o Spectrum of cytologic features resembling centroblasts, immunoblasts, monocytoid B cells, and plasmacytoid cells
  o Increased mitotic figures
  o Perithyroidal extension into fat &/or skeletal muscle commonly seen
- **EMZBCL**
  o Nodular to diffuse heterogeneous B-cell infiltrate (atypical small lymphocytes, centrocyte-like cells, monocytoid B-cells, immunoblasts, and plasma cells)
  o Characteristic lymphoepithelial lesions: Rounded balls filling and distending lumen of thyroid follicle ("MALT balls")
  o 50% of cases have perithyroidal extension

ANCILLARY TESTS

- B-cell immunophenotype of EMZBCL and DLBCL confirmed with positivity for CD20 and CD79a

Lymphoma, Thyroid

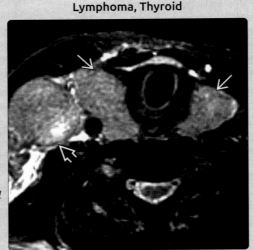

Lymphoma, Thyroid

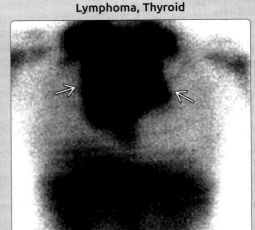

(Left) Axial T2 MR reveals diffuse non-Hodgkin lymphoma replacing the majority of both thyroid lobes (hyperintense soft tissue ➡). On the right, there is also a large, solid, deep right cervical lymph node ➡ involved by non-Hodgkin lymphoma. (Right) Anterior planar gallium scan shows intense uptake in the low neck and mediastinum ➡, typical of thyroid non-Hodgkin lymphoma. Follow-up gallium scans may be useful for differentiating active disease from scar tissue.

Lymphoepithelial Lesion

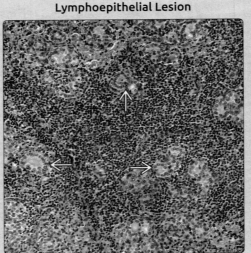

Large Atypical Lymphocytes

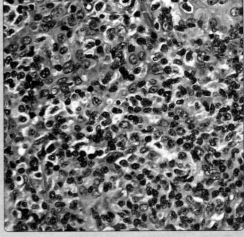

(Left) Extranodal marginal zone B-cell lymphoma of the thyroid gland shows lymphoepithelial lesions (atypical lymphocytes destroying thyroid follicles) ➡ that are characteristic of thyroid lymphomas. (Right) High-power magnification of a diffuse large B-cell lymphoma of the thyroid highlights the infiltrate of large atypical lymphocytes replacing the thyroid follicular architecture.

TERMINOLOGY

Definitions

- Primary thyroid lymphoma: Malignant lymphoma arising in thyroid gland

ETIOLOGY/PATHOGENESIS

Etiology

- Thyroid lymphomas almost always associated with chronic lymphocytic thyroiditis (Hashimoto thyroiditis)
  - Patients with Hashimoto thyroiditis have significantly increased risk of developing thyroid lymphoma
    - In Japanese patients with thyroiditis, increased risk of developing lymphoma 80x > general population
  - Hashimoto thyroiditis was recently divided into IgG4-plasma cell-rich and IgG4-plasma cell-poor subtypes
    - Former (a.k.a. IgG4 thyroiditis) associated with clinical, serological, sonographic, and morphological features distinctive from non-IgG4 subgroup
    - IgG4-positive primary thyroid mucosa-associated lymphoid tissue (MALT) lymphoma arising in background of IgG4 thyroiditis has been reported
- Thyroid lymphomas often exhibit common homologous germline VH genes used by antithyroid antibodies
  - Implicating derivation from chronic lymphocytic thyroiditis

CLINICAL ISSUES

Epidemiology

- Incidence
  - ~ 5% of all thyroid malignancies
  - ~ 2% of extranodal lymphomas
  - Lymphomas of thyroid almost exclusively of non-Hodgkin, almost always of B-cell lineage
  - Most common subtype of primary thyroid lymphoma is diffuse large B-cell lymphoma (DLBCL), germinal center origin (60-80% of cases)
  - 2nd most common thyroid lymphoma is MALT lymphoma (10-23% of cases)
  - Rarer subtypes of primary thyroid lymphoma include follicular (10%), small lymphocytic (3%), and Hodgkin lymphoma (2%)
  - Burkitt, T-cell, mantle cell, and lymphoblastic lymphomas, each accounting for < 1% of cases
    - Occasional T-cell lymphomas have been reported, often in areas endemic for HTLV-I
  - Follicular lymphoma very rare in thyroid
- Age
  - Mean: 65 years
- Sex
  - F:M = 3-4:1

Presentation

- Usually associated with lymphocytic thyroiditis
- Present with mass in thyroid, ± cervical lymphadenopathy
- Rapid enlargement of mass with pain, dyspnea, dysphagia, hemoptysis, hoarseness, and cough
- Can be associated with hypothyroidism (particularly due to association with Hashimoto thyroiditis)

Prognosis

- Generally favorable
- Dependent on clinical stage and histology
  - Localized and low-grade histology: Excellent prognosis
  - Large cell component: Worse prognosis
- Adverse prognostic features
  - Perithyroidal extension, vascular invasion, high mitotic rate and apoptosis

IMAGING

Gallium-67 Scintigraphy

- Only thyroid malignancy in which intense uptake of gallium reported

Ultrasound

- Well-defined, homogeneous, markedly hypoechoic mass, pseudocystic

CT Findings

- Homogeneous, solid, hypodense mass

FDG/PET

- Fluorodeoxyglucose (FDG) positron emission tomography (PET) useful at initial diagnosis and in monitoring therapeutic response
  - Shows FDG-avid uptake

MACROSCOPIC

General Features

- May be unilateral or bilateral
- Variable presentation
  - Soft or firm consistency, lobulation, multinodular or diffuse; can also have solid and cystic areas
- Cut surface: Smooth, bulging, pale tan, white-gray or red with fish-flesh appearance
- Extension into perithyroidal adipose tissue or skeletal muscle common

Size

- Wide range (measuring up to 20 cm)

MICROSCOPIC

Histologic Features

- Lymphomas of thyroid usually occur in setting of lymphocytic thyroiditis
  - Includes extranodal marginal zone B-cell lymphoma (EMZBCL), DLBCL, and transitions between
- DLBCL
  - Obliteration of thyroid tissue by large cells with distinct nucleoli and amphophilic cytoplasm
  - Spectrum of cytologic features resembling centroblasts, immunoblasts, monocytoid B cells, and plasmacytoid cells
  - Increased mitotic figures
  - Perithyroidal extension into fat &/or skeletal muscle commonly seen
  - Vascular invasion common as well
  - Burkitt-like with brisk mitotic activity, apoptosis, and starry-sky pattern can be seen

- Atrophy of residual thyroid parenchyma and fibrosis often present
- **EMZBCL of MALT lymphoma**
  - Nodular to diffuse heterogeneous B-cell infiltrate (atypical small lymphocytes, centrocyte-like cells, monocytoid B cells, immunoblasts, and plasma cells)
  - Reactive germinal centers can be present
  - Characteristic lymphoepithelial lesions: Rounded balls filling and distending lumen of thyroid follicle ("MALT balls")
  - Plasma cells with Dutcher bodies or cytoplasmic immunoglobulin can be seen as well
  - 50% of cases have perithyroidal extension

ANCILLARY TESTS

Cytology

- FNA from DLBCL
  - Hypercellular
  - Noncohesive cells
  - Similar cytology to DLBCL in other sites
- FNA from EMZBCL
  - Mix of small atypical lymphocytes, centrocytes, monocytoid B cells, immunoblasts, and plasma cells
  - Distinction from reactive process not always easy
  - Molecular studies needed for diagnosis generally

Immunohistochemistry

- B-cell immunophenotype of EMZBCL confirmed with positivity for
  - CD20
  - CD79a
  - CD19
  - CD22
  - pax-5
  - Monotypic immunoglobulin light chain best seen in plasmacytoid cells
  - IgM(+) > IgA(+) > IgG(+)
  - CD21 highlights follicular dendritic cell (FDC) meshworks in follicles
  - Bcl-2 reactivity in neoplastic cells present (not in reactive germinal center)
  - Ki-67 low
- These tumors show negativity for
  - CD10
  - BCL6
  - Cyclin-D1
  - T-cell antigens
  - EBV-LMP1
  - Cytokeratin highlights epithelial component in lymphoepithelial lesions
- Immunophenotype of DLBCL
  - Immunopositivity for
    - CD20
    - CD79a
    - pax-5
    - IRF-4/MUM1
    - CD43 usually positive
    - Evidence of EBV infection seen
    - Ki-67 usually high

- DLBCL further classified, for prognostic purposes, into germinal center B-cell-like (GCB) and non-GCB by use of CD10, Bcl-6, and MUM1 (IRF-4)
- Negative for
  - CD5
  - CD10
  - Bcl-6
  - Cases with plasmacytoid differentiation can be CD138 positive

Genetic Testing

- MALT lymphoma: Translocation t(3;14)(p14;q32) with FOXP1-IGH fusions found in ~ 1/2
  - Not as extensive cytogenetic and molecular genetic features of thyroid EMZBCL as in other sites
  - EMZBCL can be associated with loss of Bcl-2 expression and increase in p53 inactivation
- DLBCL shows genetic features similar to those of their nodal counterparts
  - Some cases exhibiting translocation involving *BCL6* or *MYC*

DIFFERENTIAL DIAGNOSIS

Lymphocytic Thyroiditis (Hashimoto Thyroiditis)

- Crucial differential diagnosis; tends to be confused with lymphoma
- No germinal center colonization
- No cytologic atypia
- Lymphoepithelial lesions common in both MALT lymphoma and Hashimoto thyroiditis
- "MALT balls" not present
- No light chain restriction

IgG4 Thyroiditis

- Immunoglobulin G4-related disease (IgG4-RD): New category involving many organ systems, including endocrine system in general and thyroid in particular
- 4 subcategories of IgG4-RTD identified so far
  - Riedel thyroiditis (RT)
  - Fibrosing variant of Hashimoto thyroiditis (FVHT)
  - IgG4-related Hashimoto thyroiditis
  - Graves disease with elevated IgG4 levels
- Histology mainstay of diagnosis with IgG4 immunostaining
  - Thyroid gland shows typical features of IgG4 thyroiditis, including characteristic patterns of storiform fibrosis, increased IgG4-positive plasma cells, and obliterative phlebitis
  - Dense lymphoplasmacytic infiltrate diffusely involves entire gland
  - Abundant IgG4-positive plasma cells with IgG4:IgG ratio exceeding 40%
  - IgG4-positive plasma cells polytypic for lambda and kappa light chain

Reactive Lymphoid Hyperplasia

- Florid thyroiditis can show lymphoepithelial lesions
- Does not form expansile destructive mass as observed in MALT lymphoma
- Plasma cells polytypic
  - No evidence of monotypic B-cell population

Plasmocytoma

- Primary thyroid plasmocytomas rare
- Plasmocytomas at extranodal sites may be closely related to MALT lymphoma
- Results of ancillary tests helpful
  - No component of neoplastic/monotypic B lymphocytes

Anaplastic/Undifferentiated Thyroid Carcinoma

- Usually composed by large pleomorphic cells
- Lymphoid component is usually not prominent
- Usually positive for p53
- May be positive for cytokeratin, pax-8, and TTF-1
- Ki-67 proliferative index very high
- Negative for CD45 and CD20

Melanoma

- Larger pleomorphic cells with prominent nucleoli
- Multifocal areas with block pigment deposition
- Positive for S100, HMB-45, MART-1, and melan-A
- Negative for CD45 and CD20

SELECTED REFERENCES

1. Hirokawa M et al: Preoperative diagnostic algorithm of primary thyroid lymphoma using ultrasound, aspiration cytology, and flow cytometry. Endocr J. ePub, 2017
2. Hirsch MS et al: PAX8 Distinguishes diffuse large B-cell lymphoma mimicking sarcoma. Case Rep Pathol. 2017:6714549, 2017
3. Mengoli MC et al: Mantle cell lymphoma of the thyroid: The helpful role of cell-blocks. Cytopathology. ePub, 2017
4. Nishi Y et al: Primary type3 (non-ABC, non-GCB) subtype of extranodal diffuse large B-cell lymphoma of the thyroid bearing no MYD88 mutation by padlock probe hybridization. Case Rep Oncol. 10(2):508-514, 2017
5. Spielman DB et al: Rare thyroid malignancies: An overview for the oncologist. Clin Oncol (R Coll Radiol). 29(5):298-306, 2017
6. Allaoui M et al: Primary Burkitt lymphoma of the thyroid gland: case report of an exceptional type of thyroid neoplasm and review of the literature. BMC Clin Pathol. 16:6, 2016
7. Fujii H et al: Residual FDG uptake of primary thyroid lymphoma after treatment may overestimate residual lymphoma. Ann Nucl Med. 30(10):756-759, 2016
8. Jeon EJ et al: Primary mucosa-associated lymphoid tissue lymphoma of thyroid with the serial ultrasound findings. Case Rep Endocrinol. 2016:5608518, 2016
9. Kottahachchi D et al: Immunoglobulin G4-related thyroid diseases. Eur Thyroid J. 5(4):231-239, 2016
10. Nan X et al: Primary thyroid lymphoma presenting as dermatomyositis: A first case and review of the literature. BMJ Case Rep. 2016, 2016
11. Quesada AE et al: Burkitt lymphoma presenting as a mass in the thyroid gland: a clinicopathologic study of 7 cases and review of the literature. Hum Pathol. 56:101-8, 2016
12. Tan CL et al: IgG4-positive extranodal marginal zone lymphoma arising in Hashimoto's thyroiditis: clinicopathological and cytogenetic features of a hitherto undescribed condition. Histopathology. 68(6):931-7, 2016
13. Hengjeerajarus N et al: Mucosa-associated lymphoid tissue lymphoma with large cell transformation on the background of Hashimoto's thyroiditis: a case report and review literature. J Med Assoc Thai. 98(5):514-9, 2015
14. Thakral B et al: Extranodal hematopoietic neoplasms and mimics in the head and neck: an update. Hum Pathol. 46(8):1079-100, 2015
15. Troppan K et al: Molecular pathogenesis of MALT lymphoma. Gastroenterol Res Pract. 2015:102656, 2015
16. Yang L et al: 12 cases of primary thyroid lymphoma in China. J Endocrinol Invest. 38(7):739-44, 2015
17. Fatima S et al: Primary thyroid lymphoma: case series with review of literature. Indian J Hematol Blood Transfus. 30(Suppl 1):346-8, 2014
18. Nobuoka Y et al: Cytologic findings and differential diagnoses of primary thyroid MALT lymphoma with striking plasma cell differentiation and amyloid deposition. Diagn Cytopathol. 42(1):73-7, 2014
19. Latheef N et al: Maltoma of thyroid: a rare thyroid tumour. Case Rep Otolaryngol. 2013:740241, 2013
20. Stein SA et al: Primary thyroid lymphoma: a clinical review. J Clin Endocrinol Metab. 98(8):3131-8, 2013
21. Walsh S et al: Thyroid lymphoma: recent advances in diagnosis and optimal management strategies. Oncologist. 18(9):994-1003, 2013
22. Yoshida N et al: Primary peripheral T-cell lymphoma, not otherwise specified of the thyroid with autoimmune thyroiditis. Br J Haematol. 161(2):214-23, 2013
23. Aggarwal N et al: Thyroid carcinoma-associated genetic mutations also occur in thyroid lymphomas. Mod Pathol. 25(9):1203-11, 2012
24. Alzouebi M et al: Primary thyroid lymphoma: the 40 year experience of a UK lymphoma treatment centre. Int J Oncol. 40(6):2075-80, 2012
25. Cheng V et al: Co-occurrence of papillary thyroid carcinoma and primary lymphoma of the thyroid in a patient with long-standing Hashimoto's thyroiditis. Thyroid. 22(6):647-50, 2012
26. Peppa M et al: Primary mucosa-associated lymphoid tissue thyroid lymphoma: a rare thyroid neoplasm of extrathyroid origin. Rare Tumors. 4(1):e2, 2012
27. Kikuchi M et al: [Clinical evaluation of 24 cases of primary thyroid malignant lymphoma.] Nihon Jibiinkoka Gakkai Kaiho. 114(11):855-63, 2011
28. Lee SC et al: Primary thyroid mucosa-associated lymphoid tissue lymphoma; a clinicopathological study of seven cases. J Korean Surg Soc. 81(6):374-9, 2011
29. Graff-Baker A et al: Primary thyroid lymphoma: a review of recent developments in diagnosis and histology-driven treatment. Curr Opin Oncol. 22(1):17-22, 2010
30. Hans CP et al: Confirmation of the molecular classification of diffuse large B-cell lymphoma by immunohistochemistry using a tissue microarray. Blood. 103(1):275-82, 2004
31. Thieblemont C et al: Primary thyroid lymphoma is a heterogeneous disease. J Clin Endocrinol Metab. 87(1):105-11, 2002
32. Jaffe ES et al: World Health Organization Classification of Tumours of Hematopoietic and Lymphoid tissues. Lyon, France: IARC Press, 2001
33. Wirtzfeld DA et al: Clinical presentation and treatment of non-Hodgkin's lymphoma of the thyroid gland. Ann Surg Oncol. 8(4):338-41, 2001
34. Derringer GA et al: Malignant lymphoma of the thyroid gland: a clinicopathologic study of 108 cases. Am J Surg Pathol. 24(5):623-39, 2000
35. Higgins JP et al: Large B-cell lymphoma of thyroid. Two cases with a marginal zone distribution of the neoplastic cells. Am J Clin Pathol. 114(2):264-70, 2000
36. Pedersen RK et al: Primary non-Hodgkin's lymphoma of the thyroid gland: a population based study. Histopathology. 28(1):25-32, 1996
37. Aozasa K et al: Non-Hodgkin's lymphomas in Osaka, Japan. Eur J Cancer Clin Oncol. 21(4):487-92, 1985
38. Staunton MD et al: Clinical diagnosis of thyroid cancer. Br Med J. 4(5891):532-5, 1973
39. Freeman C et al: Occurrence and prognosis of extranodal lymphomas. Cancer. 29(1):252-60, 1972

Thyroid Lymphoma

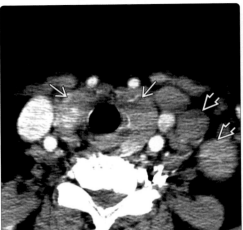

Lymphoepithelial Lesions

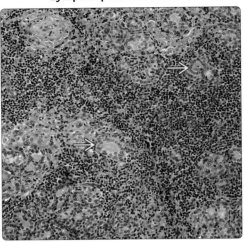

(Left) *Axial contrast-enhanced CT shows a heterogeneous, enlarged thyroid gland ➡ due to diffuse non-Hodgkin lymphoma infiltration and large, nonnecrotic, left-sided, deep cervical and spinal accessory lymph nodes ➡.* **(Right)** *H&E shows an extranodal marginal zone B-cell lymphoma of the thyroid gland with a diffuse infiltrate of small atypical lymphocytes replacing the thyroid parenchyma. Note the lymphoepithelial lesions ➡ present throughout.*

Low-Power View of Thyroid Lymphoma

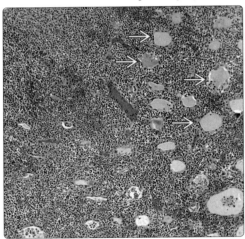

Residual Thyroid Follicles

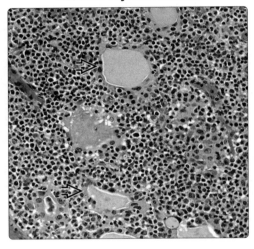

(Left) *H&E shows an extranodal marginal zone B-cell lymphoma of the thyroid with a few residual follicles ➡ being surrounded and replaced by a diffuse infiltrate of atypical small lymphocytes.* **(Right)** *There is a mixture of monocytoid B cells, centrocyte-like cells, and immunoblasts infiltrating and destroying thyroid follicles ➡, making the distinction of thyroid extranodal marginal zone B-cell lymphoma from a reactive process difficult to assess.*

Low-Power View of Thyroid Lymphoma

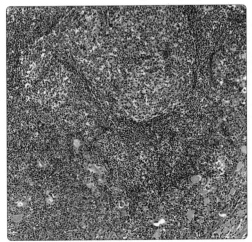

High-Power View of Germinal Center

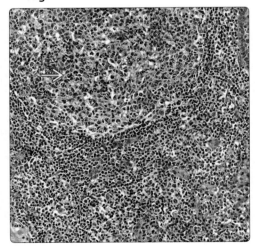

(Left) *Low-power view of extranodal marginal zone B-cell lymphoma of thyroid highlights a component of lymphocytic thyroiditis with germinal center formation in the background of marginal B-cell lymphoma of the thyroid.* **(Right)** *Although not always easily identified, there is nearly always a component of lymphocytic thyroiditis with germinal center formation ➡ in the background of extranodal marginal zone B-cell lymphoma of the thyroid.*

Diffuse Lymphoma Compressing Thyroid Follicles

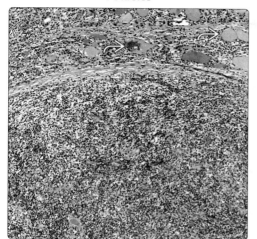

Atypical Lymphocytes

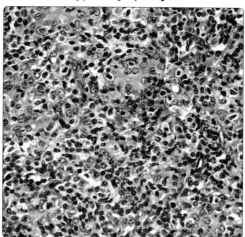

(Left) Low-power view of diffuse large B-cell lymphoma of the thyroid shows sheets of cells surrounding and compressing remaining thyroid follicles ➦. (Right) High-power view of diffuse large B-cell lymphoma of the thyroid shows a diffuse infiltrate of large, atypical lymphocytes replacing the thyroid architecture. There is a spectrum of features with centroblasts, immunoblasts, plasmacytoid cells, and monocytoid B cells.

CD20 Immunoreactivity

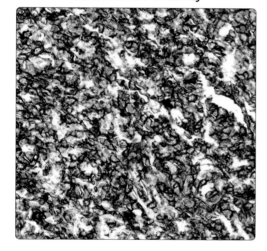

Rare CD3-Positive Cells

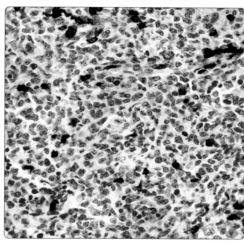

(Left) CD20 immunohistochemical stain shows a strong cytoplasmic positivity throughout this diffuse large B-cell lymphoma of the thyroid gland, confirming the B-cell nature of this tumor. CD79a has a similar staining pattern (although it also stains plasma cells). (Right) CD3 immunohistochemical stain highlights the presence of a few scattered T cells interspersed throughout this diffuse large B-cell lymphoma of the thyroid gland.

Lymphoma, Thyroid

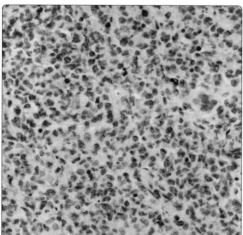

MUM1 Immunoreactivity

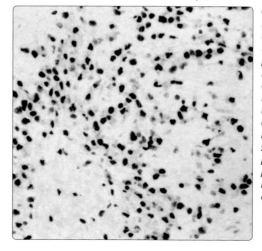

(Left) CD10 immunohistochemical stain of a diffuse large B-cell lymphoma is negative in this particular case. CD10 negativity in DLBCL forecasts a worse overall survival, and it is one of the markers whose negativity implies nongerminal center B-cell origin. (Right) MUM1 immunohistochemical stain shows strong nuclear positivity in DLBCL. MUM1 positivity is a marker of nongerminal center origin and of worse overall survival.

Follicular Dendritic Cell Sarcoma, Thyroid

TERMINOLOGY

- Neoplastic proliferation of cells exhibiting morphological and immunophenotypical features of follicular dendritic cells (FDCs)

ETIOLOGY/PATHOGENESIS

- FDC sarcomas typically arise in sites that are rich in lymphoid tissue

CLINICAL ISSUES

- Primary thyroid FDCS are rare and occurs in adult women
- Slow-growing, painless mass
- Often with cervical lymph node metastasis
- Important prognostic factors include tumor size, mitotic count, necrosis, and cellular atypia

MACROSCOPIC

- White-tan well circumscribed, can be encapsulated

MICROSCOPIC

- Syncytial spindled to ovoid cell proliferation arranged in varied architectural patterns, several growth patterns seen in same tumor
  - Storiform: Most common
- Most cases are cytologically bland
- There is variable numbers of admixed small lymphocytes

ANCILLARY TESTS

- Positive: CD21, CD23, &/or CD35, clusterin, podoplanin
- Recent markers: FDC secreted protein (FDCSP) and serglycin (SRGN) are considered specific markers of FDC
- Negative for cytokeratin, TTF1, pax-8
- Clonal immunoglobulin gene rearrangements and mutations of *PTEN*, *RET*, *BRAF*, and *TP53*
- Frameshift mutations in *NFKBIA*, biallelic loss of *CYLD*, biallelic loss of *CDKN2A*, biallelic loss of *RB1*

Architecture in FDCS

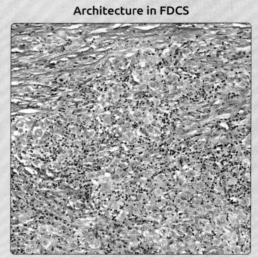

Composition of Cells of FDCS

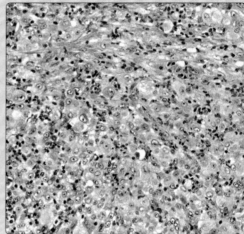

(Left) *Follicular dendritic cell sarcoma (FDCS) usually demonstrates a storiform, whorled, or fascicular architecture composed of spindled or epithelioid cells.* (Right) *The neoplastic cells in FDCS are often ovoid to spindled, but some tumors are composed of predominantly epithelioid cells. Note scattered lymphocytes.*

High-Power View of FDCS

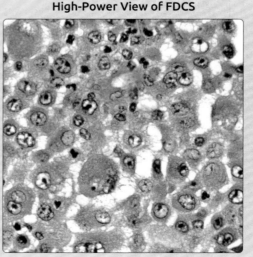

CD23 in FDCS

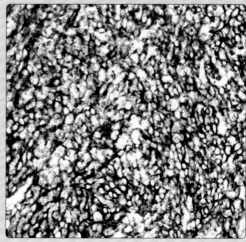

(Left) *The tumor cells in this field have an epithelioid and plasmacytoid appearance, with indistinct cytoplasmic borders. (Courtesy R. Lloyd, MD, PhD.)* (Right) *Follicular dendritic cell sarcoma demonstrates characteristic cytoplasmic positivity for the follicular dendritic cell marker CD23. Staining is uniform throughout all the tumor cells.*

TERMINOLOGY

Abbreviations

- Follicular dendritic cell sarcoma (FDCS)

Synonyms

- Follicular dendritic cell (FDC) tumor

Definitions

- Neoplasm showing morphological and immunophenotypical features of FDCs

ETIOLOGY/PATHOGENESIS

Histogenesis

- FDCs reside in lymphoid follicles and are antigen-presenting cells
- FDCS typically arise in sites that are rich in lymphoid tissue
  - Rarely arise in background of Castleman disease
  - Few reported cases with concurrent myasthenia gravis
- Inflammatory pseudotumor-like variant of FDCS is consistently associated with Epstein-Barr virus

CLINICAL ISSUES

Epidemiology

- Incidence
  - Exceptionally rare in thyroid: Only few reported cases of primary thyroid FDCS
- Sex
  - Adult women

Presentation

- Slow-growing painless thyroid mass; up to 1/3 present at extranodal sites, often in head and neck
- Head and neck
  - Most common primary tumor site: Cervical lymph nodes, followed by oropharynx
  - Tumors in thyroid presented at most advanced age
- Painless, slowly growing mass in thyroid
  - All cases involving thyroid were reported to have arisen in background of Hashimoto thyroiditis
  - Out of analyzed head and neck cases: Tumors of thyroid presented with smallest size (~ 1.8 cm)

Treatment

- Surgical approaches
  - Complete surgical resection
    - No consensus regarding neck dissection
      - Has been shown to confer lower local recurrence rate
- Adjuvant therapy
  - Adjuvant chemotherapy and radiotherapy have been used for large tumors or those with high-grade features
    - Adjuvant or neoadjuvant treatment in FDCS has not been shown to affect overall survival
    - Possible benefit for reducing local recurrence rate

Prognosis

- Variable clinical course with no uniform treatment strategy
  - Local recurrences are common
    - 40-50% of cases
    - In head and neck

  - Tumors of oropharynx more likely to present with local metastases
  - Important prognostic factors include
    - Tumor size (> 6 cm)
    - Mitotic rate (> 10/10 HPF)
    - Coagulative necrosis
    - Significant pleomorphism
  - Mortality rate is 20%

MACROSCOPIC

General Features

- Well circumscribed, can be encapsulated
- White to tan-gray cut surface
- Median size: 5 cm (range: 1-15 cm)
- Necrosis and hemorrhage can be present in large tumors

MICROSCOPIC

Histologic Features

- Spindled or ovoid cells with indistinct cell borders with syncytial appearance
  - Can also be epithelioid
- Syncytial-appearing cell proliferation arranged in varied architectural patterns, several growth patterns seen in same tumor
  - Storiform: Most common pattern
  - Whorled (meningioma-like) bundles
  - Fascicular
  - Diffuse sheets
- Moderate amount of pale eosinophilic cytoplasm
- Vesicular chromatin with small nucleoli
- Prominent admixed lymphocytes
- Occasional scattered multinucleated cells can be seen
- Mitotic count is low
  - 0-10/10 HPF
- Most cases are cytologically bland but pleomorphic cells may be seen in some cases
- Inflammatory pseudotumor-like variant is described
  - Shows loose fascicular and sheet-like growth in background of prominent inflammatory infiltrate, which may obscure neoplastic cells

ANCILLARY TESTS

Cytology

- Large spindled to ovoid cells arranged singly and in small clusters with indistinct cell borders
- Moderate pale eosinophilic cytoplasm and vesicular chromatin
- Characteristic but challenging on cytology; often requires IHC confirmation

Immunohistochemistry

- Nodal and extranodal FDCS have similar immunophenotypes
- Positive: CD21, CD23, &/or CD35, clusterin, podoplanin
- Recent markers
  - FDC secreted protein (FDCSP) and serglycin (SRGN) are considered specific markers of FDC
  - γ-synuclein
- Variably positive

Immunohistochemistry

Antibody	Reactivity	Staining Pattern	Comment
CD21	Positive	Cell membrane	All tumor cells
CD23	Positive	Cell membrane	All tumor cells
CD35	Positive	Cell membrane	All tumor cells
Clusterin	Positive	Cytoplasmic	All tumor cells
Podoplanin	Positive	Cell membrane	All tumor cells
Synuclein	Positive	Nuclear & cytoplasmic	All tumor cells
Vimentin	Positive	Cytoplasmic	All tumor cells
EMA	Positive	Cell membrane	At least focal, 50% of cases
S100	Positive	Nuclear & cytoplasmic	Variably positive, weak, 10% of cases
CD68	Positive	Cytoplasmic	Variably positive
EBER	Positive	Nuclear	All tumor cells; consistently associated with inflammatory pseudotumor-like variant
AE1/AE3	Negative		
CK-PAN	Negative		

- o Epithelial membrane antigen (EMA): At least focally positive in 50% of cases
  - o S100: Weakly positive in 10% of cases
  - o CD68: Variable
  - o BRAF
- Cytokeratin is negative

Electron Microscopy

- Long, slender, well-developed interdigitating cytoplasmic processes, sometimes producing labyrinth-like pattern and desmosome-like junctions

Molecular

- Recent study reports *BRAF* V600E mutation in ~ 20% of FDCS cases
- Clonal immunoglobulin gene rearrangements and mutations of *PTEN*, *RET*, and *TP53* have been reported
- Frameshift mutations in *NFKBIA*, biallelic loss of *CYLD*, biallelic loss of *CDKN2A*, biallelic loss of *RB1*
- Copy-number gain of chromosome 9p24 including genes *CD274* (PD-L1) and *PDCD1LG2* (PD-L2)
- Cases of FDCS reported with complex cytogenetic abnormalities

DIFFERENTIAL DIAGNOSIS

Undifferentiated or Sarcomatoid Carcinoma

- EMA positivity is pitfall but FDSC are nearly always keratin negative
- IHC for CD21, CD23, and CD35, although very useful, are not usually included in typical panel
  - o High index of suspicion is required

Interdigitating Dendritic Cell Sarcoma

- Lacks storiform and whorled growth pattern
- Diffusely positive for S100 protein
- Negative for CD21 and CD35

Langerhans Cell Histiocytosis

- Positive for CD1a, langerin, S100 protein
- Negative for FDC markers

- EM: Birbeck granules

Inflammatory Myofibroblastic Tumor

- Resembles inflammatory pseudotumor-like variant of FDCS
- Often positive for SMA and desmin; ALK1 useful if positive
- Negative for FDC markers

SELECTED REFERENCES

1. Andersen EF et al: Genomic analysis of follicular dendritic cell sarcoma by molecular inversion probe array reveals tumor suppressor-driven biology. Mod Pathol. ePub, 2017
2. Chen T et al: Follicular dendritic cell sarcoma. Arch Pathol Lab Med. 141(4):596-599, 2017
3. Lorenzi L et al: Identification of novel follicular dendritic cell sarcoma markers, FDCSP and SRGN, by whole transcriptome sequencing. Oncotarget. 8(10):16463-16472, 2017
4. Griffin GK et al: Targeted genomic sequencing of follicular dendritic cell sarcoma reveals recurrent alterations in NF-κB regulatory genes. Mod Pathol. 29(1):67-74, 2016
5. Huang W et al: High frequency of clonal IG and T-cell receptor gene rearrangements in histiocytic and dendritic cell neoplasms. Oncotarget. 7(48):78355-78362, 2016
6. Wu A et al: Follicular dendritic cell sarcoma. Arch Pathol Lab Med. 140(2):186-90, 2016
7. Pang J et al: Follicular dendritic cell sarcoma of the head and neck: Case report, literature review, and pooled analysis of 97 cases. Head Neck. ePub, 2015
8. Starr JS et al: Follicular dendritic cell sarcoma presenting as a thyroid mass. J Clin Oncol. 33(17):e74-6, 2015
9. Yu L et al: Primary follicular dendritic cell sarcoma of the thyroid gland coexisting with Hashimoto's thyroiditis. Int J Surg Pathol. 19(4):502-5, 2011
10. Zhang H et al: γ-Synuclein is a promising new marker for staining reactive follicular dendritic cells, follicular dendritic cell sarcoma, Kaposi sarcoma, and benign and malignant vascular tumors. Am J Surg Pathol. 35(12):1857-65, 2011
11. Biddle DA et al: Extranodal follicular dendritic cell sarcoma of the head and neck region: three new cases, with a review of the literature. Mod Pathol. 15(1):50-8, 2002
12. Galati LT et al: Dendritic cell sarcoma of the thyroid. Head Neck. 21(3):273-5, 1999
13. Chan JK et al: Follicular dendritic cell sarcoma. Clinicopathologic analysis of 17 cases suggesting a malignant potential higher than currently recognized. Cancer. 79(2):294-313, 1997
14. Perez-Ordonez B et al: Follicular dendritic cell tumor: report of 13 additional cases of a distinctive entity. Am J Surg Pathol. 20(8):944-55, 1996

Microscopic Characteristics in FDCS

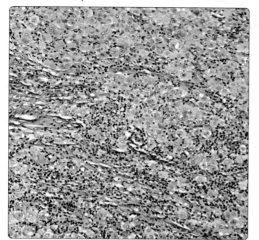

Low-Power View of FDCS

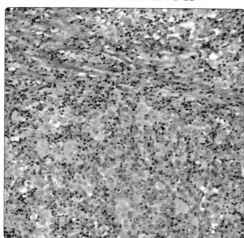

(Left) *The neoplastic cells of FDCS are composed of spindled or epithelioid cells that have vesicular chromatin, pale, eosinophilic cytoplasm, with ill-defined cell borders. Scattered lymphocytes and plasma cells are present.* **(Right)** *One of the characteristic finding in FDCS is a prominent admixed inflammatory cells composed of lymphocytes and scattered plasma cells intermixed with the tumor cells.*

Inflammatory Cells in FDCS

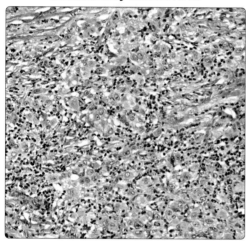

Cellular Characteristics in FDCS

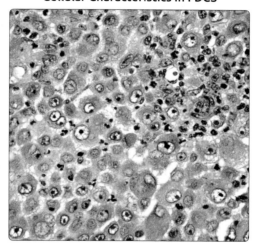

(Left) *In FDCS, prominent admixed inflammatory cells composed of lymphocytes and scattered plasma cells is characteristic.* **(Right)** *High-power photomicrograph showing epithelioid-shaped cells, with abundant eosinophilic cytoplasm, open vesicular nuclei with conspicuous nucleoli, intermixed with inflammatory cells.*

Occasional Pleomorphism in FDCS

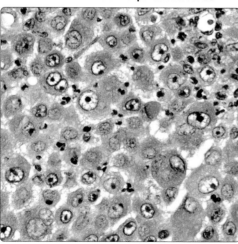

Inflammatory Cells in FDCS

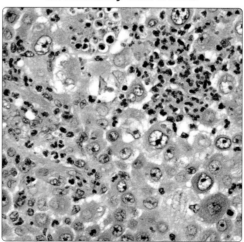

(Left) *Although most cases of FDCS have relatively bland, uniform cytomorphology, this example highlights scattered larger cells with prominent nucleoli.* **(Right)** *Follicular dendritic cell tumor shows classic cytologic features with cells having open vesicular nuclei and well-defined nucleoli. There are multiple inflammatory cells throughout.*

Langerhans Cell Histiocytosis, Thyroid

TERMINOLOGY

- Clonal neoplastic disorder characterized by proliferation of Langerhans dendritic cells

CLINICAL ISSUES

- Cases limited to thyroid exceedingly rare
  o Some associated with Hashimoto thyroiditis
- Most cases involving thyroid occur in patients with multifocal disease
- Present with diffuse or nodular thyroid enlargement
- Isolated thyroid disease does not show progression after surgery
- Cases with thyroid involvement associated with systemic disease have aggressive course
- Pediatric cases receive combined surgical and chemoradiation therapy

MACROSCOPIC

- Nodules indistinguishable grossly from other thyroid nodules

MICROSCOPIC

- Clusters of Langerhans cells infiltrate thyroid follicles and efface thyroid parenchyma; can extend into surrounding soft tissue
- Langerhans histiocyte: Large cell with pale or eosinophilic cytoplasm and vesicular, notched, and grooved nuclei
- Inflammatory infiltrate varies, but includes lymphocytes and eosinophils

ANCILLARY TESTS

- Positive for CD1a, langerin/CD207, S100, CD68, BRAF, cyclin-D1 and p-ERK
- Frequent activating mutations in *BRAF* and *MAP2K1*
- Rare mutations in *ARAF*, *MAP3K1*, *PIK3CA*

LCH of Thyroid

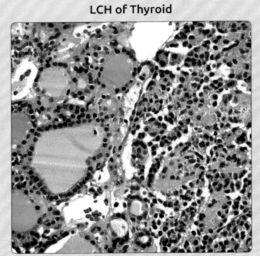

Primary Thyroid LCH

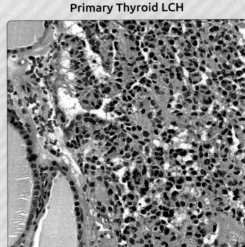

(Left) *In this Langerhans cell histiocytosis (LCH) of the thyroid, loose clusters of neoplastic cells are observed on the right, pushing toward the adjacent thyroid follicles on the left.* **(Right)** *Thyroid involvement by LCH shows clusters of neoplastic cells with eosinophilic cytoplasm and lobulated nuclei infiltrating thyroid follicles.*

Cytological Features of LCH

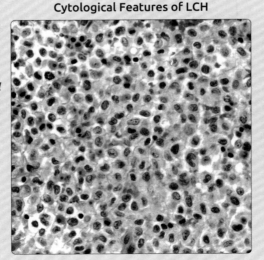

Langerin in LCH

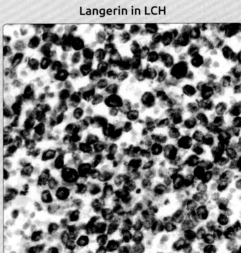

(Left) *High power of LCH reveals large cells with pale, eosinophilic, folded and lobulated nuclei with open chromatin and grooves.* **(Right)** *Langerin stains the cell membranes and Golgi apparatus of Langerhans cells in LCH. The expression is strong and diffuse in all neoplastic cells.*

TERMINOLOGY

Abbreviations

- Langerhans cell histiocytosis (LCH)

Synonyms

- Histiocytosis X
- Eosinophilic granuloma
  - Solitary or few indolent lesions
- Hand-Schüller-Christian syndrome
  - Multifocal, chronic involvement
- Letterer-Siwe disease
  - Acute, fulminant, disseminated disease

Definitions

- Clonal proliferation of Langerhans dendritic cells in single or multiple organs

CLINICAL ISSUES

Epidemiology

- Incidence
  - Rare: ~ 100 reported cases of LCH involving thyroid
    - ~ 1/3 have isolated thyroid involvement
- Age
  - Wide range
    - Median: 28 years
  - Greater number of isolated thyroid cases in adults, pediatric cases present with systemic disease
- Sex
  - Very slight female predilection

Presentation

- LCH is stratified into single system or multisystem disease and varies with degree of involvement
  - Cases involving thyroid present with diffuse or nodular thyroid enlargement
  - Patients are euthyroid
    - Less commonly: Hypothyroid

Treatment

- Treatment tailored to extent of disease
  - Adults often receive only surgical resection for isolated thyroid disease
  - Pediatric cases receive combined surgical and chemoradiation therapy
- Discovery of genomic alterations (particularly in *BRAF* and *MAP2K1*) driving trials for targeted therapy
  - RAF pathway inhibitors: Clinical trials of dabrafenib (BRAF inhibitor) in combination with trametinib (MEK1 inhibitor) are underway

Prognosis

- Single system disease has high chance of spontaneous remission and favorable outcome
- Multisystem disease divided into low-risk and high-risk (defined as involvement of risk organs, which include liver, spleen, and hematopoietic system)
  - Patients with low-risk, multisystem disease have excellent prognosis
  - Patients with multisystem disease with risk-organ involvement have high mortality rate
- Refractory/relapsed LCH has very poor outcome

IMAGING

Ultrasonographic Findings

- Hypoechoic nodules with heterogeneous internal acoustic features

Radioactive I-131 Scan

- Cold nodules

MACROSCOPIC

General Features

- Most frequent presentation in form of small nodules
- Nodules indistinguishable grossly from other thyroid nodules
- Gland can be diffusely involved

MOLECULAR

Mutations

- LCH characterized by frequent activating mutations involving mitogen-activated protein kinase (MAPK) pathway
  - Activating mutations in *MAP2K1* in 10-28% of reported cases; found in cases with *BRAF* wild-type alleles
    - Mutations found in N-terminal negative regulatory domain and N-terminal portion of kinase domain
    - Rare cases identified with mutations in *MAP3K1*
- Activating mutations in *BRAF* in 45-65% of reported cases of LCH; V600E most common
  - Rare cases harbor activating mutations in *ARAF*
  - Case reports of vemurafenib have described good clinical response
- Rare mutations in *PIK3CA*
- All LCH cases show evidence of ERK family activation

MICROSCOPIC

Histologic Features

- Clusters of Langerhans cells infiltrate thyroid follicles
  - Frequently destroys thyroid parenchyma with effacement of architecture
  - Can extend into surrounding soft tissue
- Langerhans histiocyte
  - Large cell with pale or eosinophilic cytoplasm and vesicular, notched, grooved, lobulated, or "coffee bean" nuclei
- Langerhans cell proliferation accompanied by inflammatory infiltrate
  - Varies in composition and distribution
  - Usually includes lymphocytes and eosinophils
  - Abundant eosinophils often cluster around areas of necrosis
  - Foamy histiocytes or multinucleated giant cells can be seen
- Can occur in background of chronic lymphocytic thyroiditis

ANCILLARY TESTS

Cytology

- FNA diagnosis of LCH challenging; requires high index of suspicion
- In rare cases, diagnosis of LCH proposed at FNA with following features has been confirmed on resection

- o Diagnostic clues: Highly cellular smear of cells lacking cohesion with background lymphocytes and eosinophils
- o Cells with abundant, pale cytoplasm, large nuclei with frequent prominent nuclear grooves
- o Cells can be mono- and multinucleated

Immunohistochemistry

- Positive staining with following patterns
  - o CD1a: Membranous
  - o Langerin: Membranous and stains Golgi apparatus
  - o S100: Nuclear and cytoplasmic
  - o CD68: Cytoplasmic, variable
  - o Cyclin-D1: Downstream markers of MAPK pathway activation useful as novel diagnostic markers of LCH
  - o p-ERK expression
- BRAF V600E stain
  - o Potential to be useful if positive
    - − High percentage of LCH cases harbor mutation
  - o IHC has shown good correlation with V600E mutational status in LCH
- Negative for CD163, cytokeratin, thyroglobulin, TTF-1

Electron Microscopy

- Cytoplasmic invaginations of cell membranes, rod-shaped on cross section
  - o Birbeck granules (tennis racquet shape)

DIFFERENTIAL DIAGNOSIS

Papillary Thyroid Carcinoma

- Cohesive epithelial cells with characteristic papillary thyroid carcinoma nuclear features
  - o Nuclear enlargement and clearing, nuclear grooves, intranuclear cytoplasmic inclusions
- S100(-)
- No histiocytes or eosinophils; lymphocytes may be present

Undifferentiated Carcinoma

- Significant pleomorphism with easily identified mitotic forms, often atypical
- Extensive necrosis, hemorrhage, and degeneration
- Evidence of epithelial differentiation
  - o Cytokeratin useful when positive
  - o S100(-)
- Can have acute inflammatory infiltrate

Rosai-Dorfman Disease

- Usually in lymph nodes
  - o Extranodal Rosai-Dorfman disease present in subset
- Extremely rare involvement of thyroid
- Histiocytes exhibit characteristic emperipolesis
  - o Cytoplasmic evidence of phagocytosis of cells
- Histiocytes are S100(+)

Langerhans Cell Sarcoma

- Large, highly pleomorphic neoplastic cells
  - o Prominent nucleoli with numerous mitoses (often atypical)
- If neoplastic cells overtly malignant, these features should exclude LCH and raise suspicion for Langerhans cell sarcoma

DIAGNOSTIC CHECKLIST

Pathologic Interpretation Pearls

- Clusters of Langerhans cell accompanied by inflammatory infiltrate
- Positive for CD1a, langerin/CD207, S100, CD68, BRAF

SELECTED REFERENCES

1. Facchetti F et al: Histiocytic and dendritic cell neoplasms: what have we learnt by studying 67 cases. Virchows Arch. ePub, 2017
2. Héritier S et al: New somatic BRAF splicing mutation in Langerhans cell histiocytosis. Mol Cancer. 16(1):115, 2017
3. Héritier S et al: Circulating cell-free BRAFV600E as a biomarker in children with Langerhans cell histiocytosis. Br J Haematol. ePub, 2017
4. Shanmugam V et al: Cyclin D1 is expressed in neoplastic cells of Langerhans cell histiocytosis but not reactive Langerhans cell proliferations. Am J Surg Pathol. ePub, 2017
5. Demellawy DE et al: Langerhans cell histiocytosis: a comprehensive review. Pathology. 47(4):294-301, 2015
6. Nelson DS et al: MAP2K1 and MAP3K1 mutations in Langerhans cell histiocytosis. Genes Chromosomes Cancer. 54(6):361-8, 2015
7. Rollins BJ: Genomic alterations in Langerhans cell histiocytosis. Hematol Oncol Clin North Am. 29(5):839-51, 2015
8. Saqi A et al: Langerhans cell histiocytosis: Diagnosis on thyroid aspirate and review of the literature. Head Neck Pathol. 9(4):496-502, 2015
9. DiCaprio MR et al: Diagnosis and management of Langerhans cell histiocytosis. J Am Acad Orthop Surg. 22(10):643-652, 2014
10. Roden AC et al: BRAF V600E expression in Langerhans cell histiocytosis: clinical and immunohistochemical study on 25 pulmonary and 54 extrapulmonary cases. Am J Surg Pathol. 38(4):548-51, 2014
11. Girschikofsky M et al: Management of adult patients with Langerhans cell histiocytosis: recommendations from an expert panel on behalf of Euro-Histio-Net. Orphanet J Rare Dis. 8:72, 2013
12. Patten DK et al: Solitary langerhans histiocytosis of the thyroid gland: a case report and literature review. Head Neck Pathol. 6(2):279-89, 2012
13. Vujhini SK et al: Fine needle aspiration diagnosis of Rosai-Dorfman Disease involving thyroid. J Cytol. 29(1):83-5, 2012
14. Abla O et al: Langerhans cell histiocytosis: current concepts and treatments. Cancer Treat Rev. 36(4):354-9, 2010
15. Badalian-Very G et al: Recurrent BRAF mutations in Langerhans cell histiocytosis. Blood. 116(11):1919-23, 2010
16. Behrens RJ et al: Langerhans cell histiocytosis of the thyroid: a report of two cases and review of the literature. Thyroid. 11(7):697-705, 2001
17. Yap WM et al: Langerhans cell histiocytosis involving the thyroid and parathyroid glands. Mod Pathol. 14(2):111-5, 2001
18. el-Halabi DA et al: Langerhans cell histiocytosis of the thyroid gland. A case report. Acta Cytol. 44(5):805-8, 2000
19. Saiz E et al: Isolated Langerhans cell histiocytosis of the thyroid: a report of two cases with nuclear imaging-pathologic correlation. Ann Diagn Pathol. 4(1):23-8, 2000
20. Dey P et al: Fine needle aspiration cytology of Langerhans cell histiocytosis of the thyroid. A case report. Acta Cytol. 43(3):429-31, 1999
21. Sahoo M et al: Fine-needle aspiration cytology in a case of isolated involvement of thyroid with Langerhans cell histiocytosis. Diagn Cytopathol. 19(1):33-7, 1998
22. Wang WS et al: Langerhans' cell histiocytosis with thyroid involvement masquerading as thyroid carcinoma. Jpn J Clin Oncol. 27(3):180-4, 1997
23. Kitahama S et al: Thyroid involvement by malignant histiocytosis of Langerhans' cell type. Clin Endocrinol (Oxf). 45(3):357-63, 1996
24. Thompson LD et al: Langerhans cell histiocytosis of the thyroid: a series of seven cases and a review of the literature. Mod Pathol. 9(2):145-9, 1996

Diffuse Growth Pattern of LCH

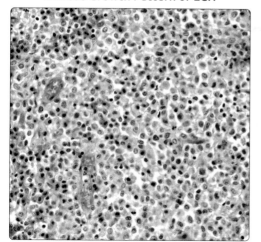

Langerhans Cells

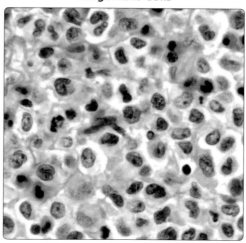

(Left) *H&E depicts the neoplastic cells of LCH exhibiting a sheet-like growth pattern with a relatively sparse inflammatory infiltrate composed of eosinophils and scattered plasma cells.* (Right) *The thyroid shows infiltration by Langerhans cells with deeply grooved nuclei and a moderate amount of pale cytoplasm with scattered eosinophils admixed.*

CD1a in LCH

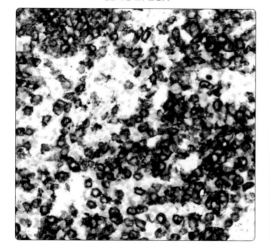

CD1a in LCH of Thyroid

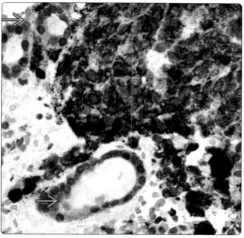

(Left) *CD1a stains Langerhans cells strongly and diffusely in a membranous pattern, supporting the diagnosis.* (Right) *There is strong positivity for CD1a in the Langerhans cells of LCH. Note the negative thyroid follicles at the periphery ⇥. (Courtesy R. Lloyd, MD, PhD.)*

BRAF in LCH

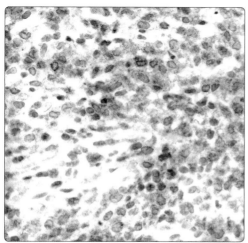

Variable Staining for CD68 in LCH

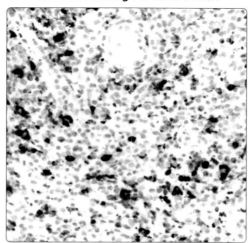

(Left) *BRAF stain for mutant V600E exhibits cytoplasmic positivity in a large subset of LCH cases. Note that negative staining for BRAF is not informative in the diagnosis of LCH.* (Right) *CD68 demonstrates variable cytoplasmic staining in the neoplastic cells of LCH and can be patchy and weak. Macrophages are strongly positive for CD68.*

TERMINOLOGY

- Extremely rare benign or malignant neoplasm showing Schwann cell or perineurial differentiation arising from peripheral nerves within thyroid
- Schwannoma (neurilemmoma) and malignant peripheral nerve sheath tumor (MPNST)

MACROSCOPIC

- Schwannomas encapsulated, firm, and may show cystic foci
- MPNSTs usually larger than schwannomas with infiltrative growth pattern

MICROSCOPIC

- Schwannoma: Typical Antoni A and Antoni B areas
- MPNST: Invasive tumor effacing thyroid parenchyma with fascicular growth, mitosis, pleomorphism, and focal necrosis
- Nuclear palisading (Verocay bodies) may be present

ANCILLARY TESTS

- S100: Strongly positive in schwannomas, less staining in MPNST
  - S100 may be patchy and less intense in MPNST
- SOX10: Diffusely and strongly positive
- Negative for keratin and thyroid markers (pax-8, thyroglobulin, and calcitonin)
  - TTF-1 may be seen in MPNSTs

TOP DIFFERENTIAL DIAGNOSES

- Malignant peripheral nerve sheath tumor
  - Anaplastic thyroid carcinoma
  - Other sarcomas: Vascular, muscle, fibroblastic, and adipose
- DDx of benign peripheral nerve sheath tumors
  - Neurofibroma
  - Perineurioma
  - Schwannoma

Primary Thyroid MPNST

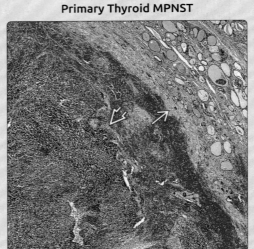

Variable Cellularity

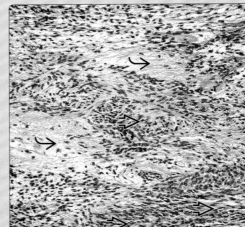

(Left) *Primary thyroid malignant peripheral nerve sheath tumor (MPNST) ➡ is seen within thyroid forming a well-circumscribed nodule and compressing and replacing the adjacent thyroid follicles ➡.* (Right) *Intrathyroid schwannoma shows characteristic alternating densely packed spindle cell hypercellular (Antoni A ➡) and loosely arranged hypocellular myxoid-degenerated (Antoni B ➡) areas.*

Invasive Tumor

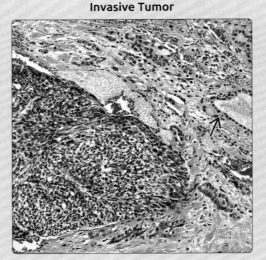

Highly Cellular MPNST With Necrosis

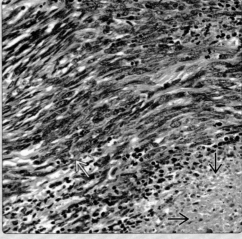

(Left) *In this example of MPNST, a highly cellular tumor is seen destroying, invading, and replacing the adjacent thyroid follicles ➡.* (Right) *High-power view of a thyroid MPNST shows markedly high cellularity ➡ and focal necrosis ➡.*

TERMINOLOGY

Abbreviations
- Peripheral nerve sheath tumor (PNST)

Synonyms
- Schwannoma (neurilemmoma), malignant peripheral nerve sheath tumor (MPNST)
- Neurilemmoma, neurofibrosarcoma

Definitions
- Benign or malignant neoplasm arising within thyroid parenchyma from peripheral nerves or displaying differentiation toward Schwann or perineurial cells

ETIOLOGY/PATHOGENESIS

Etiology
- Postulated hypothesis: Origin sympathetic/parasympathetic innervation of thyroid or sensory nerves
- Rare thyroid neurofibroma (plexiform) in neurofibromatosis
  - Biallelic inactivation NF1 gene (encodes neurofibromin)

CLINICAL ISSUES

Epidemiology
- Incidence
  - Extremely rare; < 0.01% of all primary thyroid gland tumors
  - Any age; highest incidence 40-60 years (20-50 MPNST)

Presentation
- Painless nodule, gradually enlarging mass, may compress upper airways
- MPNST: Difficulty breathing, infiltration soft tissues, destruction of thyroid, weight loss

Treatment
- Surgical excision
- Radiation therapy in selected cases of MPNST

Prognosis
- Schwannomas have benign course, and patients usually curable with surgical resection
  - Rarely undergo malignant transformation
- Thyroid gland MPNSTs have very poor prognosis, irrespective of
  - Clinical features
  - Tumor size
  - Grade
  - Stage
- All patients with primary thyroid MPNST have died from their disease

IMAGING

Radiographic Findings
- US and CT: Solid, well-delineated nodule

MACROSCOPIC

General Features
- Firm, tan-white tumors with neural appearance
- Schwannomas encapsulated and may show cystic foci
- MPNSTs usually larger than schwannomas with infiltrative growth pattern
- Globoid, homogeneously firm

MICROSCOPIC

Histologic Features
- Same histological features as those in other anatomic sites
- **Schwannoma**: Typical Antoni A and Antoni B areas
  - Antoni A: Densely packed, palisading spindle cells areas in cellular fascicles
  - Antoni B: Loosely arranged, hypocellular degenerated areas, thick blood vessels; may show cystic degeneration
  - Slender, fusiform cells have wavy, elongated cytoplasmic extensions
  - Nuclear palisading (Verocay bodies) may be present
- **Neurofibroma**: Bundles of cells in fibromyxoid background
  - Mast cells frequently present
- **Perineurioma**: Predominantly storiform and focally whorled
- **MPNST**: Invasive tumor with infiltrative growth pattern effacing thyroid parenchyma
  - With highly cellular, spindled, neural-appearing cells forming tightly packed fascicular growth pattern
  - Myxoid areas, increased mitotic activity, cellular pleomorphism, and focal necrosis common
  - Grading system specific for primary thyroid MPNST has not been proposed, but general grading system includes
    - Nuclear pleomorphism with anaplasia
    - Increased mitosis
    - Tumor necrosis

Cytologic Features
- **Schwannoma**: Spindle cells with nuclear palisading forming Verocay bodies
  - Few typical mitotic figures can be present
- **Neurofibroma**: Elongated cells with eosinophilic cytoplasm and wavy nuclei
- **Perineurioma**: Very thin spindle cells with wavy nuclei and delicate, elongated, bipolar cytoplasmic processes
- **MPNST**: Neural-appearing cells with increased cellularity, marked atypia, and increased mitotic activity
- Fine-needle aspiration not very successful in reaching definitive diagnosis prior to surgical removal

ANCILLARY TESTS

Immunohistochemistry
- Diffusely and strongly positive for S100
  - MPNST may lose some S100 reactivity depending on degree of dedifferentiation (high-grade tumors)
    - S100 may be patchy and less intense
    - TTF-1 may be seen in MPNSTs
  - Neurofibromas have partial S100 positivity (composed perineural cells, Schwann cells, and fibroblasts)
  - Perineuriomas usually negative for S100
  - Schwannomas strongly and diffusely S100 positive

- Strongly positive for SOX10
  - Consistently expressed in benign Schwann cell tumors, in metastatic melanoma, and variably present in MPNSTs
  - Absent in many mimics of nerve sheath tumors: Cellular neurothekeoma, meningioma, gastrointestinal stromal tumors, perivascular epithelioid cell tumor, and fibroblastic-myofibroblastic tumors
- Negative for keratin, pax-8, thyroglobulin, HMB45, and Melan A

Genetic Testing

- PNST increased in frequency in NF1
  - However, neurofibromin gene mutations not documented in primary thyroid gland tumors

DIFFERENTIAL DIAGNOSIS

DDx of Malignant Peripheral Nerve Sheath Tumors

- **Undifferentiated (anaplastic) thyroid carcinoma**
  - Positive for keratin and p53; negative for S100 and SOX10
- **Other sarcomas**
  - Vascular, muscle, fibroblastic, and adipose markers
- **Malignant melanoma**
  - SOX10 consistently expressed in schwannomas and metastatic melanoma, variably present in MPNST
  - MPNST tumor cells negative for HMB45 and Melan-A

DDx of Benign Peripheral Nerve Sheath Tumors

- **Neurofibroma**
  - Focal (30-50%) S100 positivity
  - Negative: TTF-1, thyroglobulin, chromogranin, calcitonin
- **Perineurioma**
  - Usually nonencapsulated; negative for S100, TTF-1, thyroglobulin, chromogranin, calcitonin
- **Schwannoma**
  - Usually encapsulated
  - Strong diffuse S100 and SOX10 positivity; negative for TTF-1, thyroglobulin, chromogranin

Psammomatous Melanotic Schwannoma

- Despite term "melanotic schwannoma" suggesting benign process, metastases have been reported to occur in up to 15% of patients
  - In 18% of those with Carney complex-associated melanotic schwannoma

DIAGNOSTIC CHECKLIST

Clinically Relevant Pathologic Features

- Neurofibromas can be associated with NF1

Pathologic Interpretation Pearls

- Extremely rare and usually benign asymptomatic tumors

SELECTED REFERENCES

1. Chen G et al: Primary peripheral nerve sheath tumors of the thyroid gland: A case report and literature review. Mol Clin Oncol. 4(2):209-210, 2016
2. Lee YS et al: Primary neurilemmoma of the thyroid gland clinically mimicking malignant thyroid nodule. J Pathol Transl Med. 50(2):168-71, 2016
3. Vázquez-Benítez G et al: Unexpected tumor: Primary asymptomatic schwannoma in thyroid gland. Endocr Pathol. 27(1):46-9, 2016
4. Ye DM et al: [Schwannoma of the thyroid gland: report of a case.] Zhonghua Bing Li Xue Za Zhi. 45(6):419-20, 2016
5. De Simone B et al: Schwannoma mimicking a neoplastic thyroid nodule. Updates Surg. 66(1):85-7, 2014
6. Dhar H et al: Primary thyroid schwannoma masquerading as a thyroid nodule. J Surg Case Rep. 2014(9), 2014
7. Doulias T et al: Thyroid neurofibroma in a female patient with neurofibromatosis type I: report of a case. BMJ Case Rep. 2013, 2013
8. Graceffa G et al: Primary schwannoma of the thyroid gland involving the isthmus: report of a case. Surg Today. 43(1):106-9, 2013
9. Murata T et al: Subglottic Schwannoma: a report of a rare case that was treated with medial thyrotomy. Am J Otolaryngol. 34(5):569-73, 2013
10. Scherl S et al: Rare tracheal tumors and lesions initially diagnosed as isolated differentiated thyroid cancers. Thyroid. 23(1):79-83, 2013
11. Jong YN et al: Neurilemmoma of the thyroid gland. Intern Med. 51(12):1641, 2012
12. Gamal WL et al: Hoarseness due to a thyroid mass. Symptomatic thyroid schwannoma. Neth J Med. 69(1):39-40, 2011
13. An J et al: Primary schwannoma of the thyroid gland: a case report. Acta Cytol. 54(5 Suppl):857-62, 2010
14. Kandil E et al: Primary peripheral nerve sheath tumors of the thyroid gland. Thyroid. 20(6):583-6, 2010
15. Murali R et al: Melanotic schwannoma mimicking metastatic pigmented melanoma: a pitfall in cytological diagnosis. Pathology. 42(3):287-9, 2010
16. Gaud U et al: Isolated intrathyroidal neurofibroma. Otolaryngol Head Neck Surg. 141(2):300-1, 2009
17. Hornick JL et al: Soft tissue perineurioma: clinicopathologic analysis of 81 cases including those with atypical histologic features. Am J Surg Pathol. 29(7):845-58, 2005
18. Kurtkaya-Yapicier O et al: The pathobiologic spectrum of schwannomas. Histol Histopathol. 18(3):925-34, 2003
19. Al-Ghamdi S et al: Malignant schwannoma of the thyroid gland. Otolaryngol Head Neck Surg. 122(1):143-4, 2000
20. Sugita R et al: Primary schwannoma of the thyroid gland: CT findings. AJR Am J Roentgenol. 171(2):528-9, 1998
21. Thompson LD et al: Peripheral nerve sheath tumors of the thyroid gland: a series of four cases and a review of the literature. Endocr Pathol. 7(4):309-318, 1996

Primary Thyroid MPNST

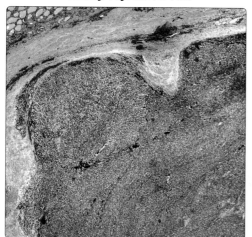

Schwannoma With Variable Cellularity

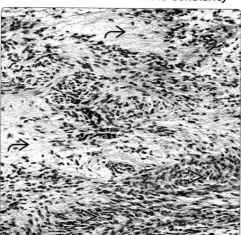

(Left) *There is the presence of a thick, fibrous capsule in one area of the tumor. This primary thyroid MPNST had mostly invasive component with focal areas of fibrosis.* (Right) *In this example of an intrathyroid schwannoma, the typical intermittent hypercellular (Antoni A ⇲) and loosely arranged hypocellular myxoid (Antoni B ⇲) areas of this tumor are evident.*

Thyroid Perineurioma

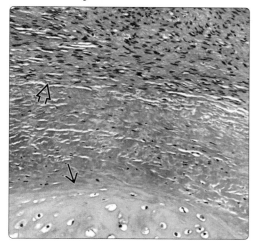

Slender Fusiform Spindle Cells

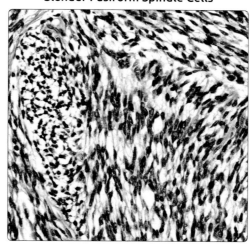

(Left) *H&E of perineurioma involving thyroid gland with extensive extrathyroidal extension shows the tumor ⇲ surrounding the cricoid cartilage ⇲.* (Right) *In this intrathyroid schwannoma, the typical densely packed spindle cell hypercellular areas are evident. The fusiform cells have elongated cytoplasmic extensions and are arranged in interlacing fascicles. Nuclear palisading may be seen.*

Nuclear Positivity for SOX10

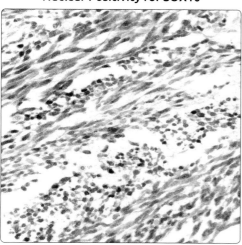

S100 Negativity

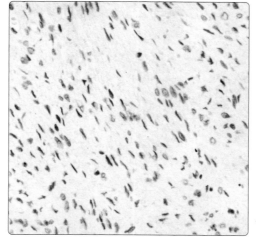

(Left) *SOX10 transcription factor is expressed in schwannian and melanocytic lineages and can be used as a marker for corresponding tumors. SOX10 was consistently expressed in benign Schwann cell tumors and in metastatic melanoma and was variably present in MPNST.* (Right) *Immunohistochemistry for S100 can be useful in distinguishing some of these neoplasms. In this example of an intrathyroid perineurioma, the tumor cells are negative for this marker.*

Solitary Fibrous Tumor, Thyroid

TERMINOLOGY

- Solitary fibrous tumor (SFT): Mesenchymal neoplasm with prominent branching ectatic vascular pattern

CLINICAL ISSUES

- Extremely rare in thyroid
- Most tumors are benign
- Slow-growing, painless neck mass, present for years
- Total thyroidectomy or lobectomy with clear margins is sufficient if no malignant features are identified
- Behavior can be unpredictable; therefore, close follow-up is advised

MACROSCOPIC

- Well-circumscribed, may be partially encapsulated
- Firm, solid mass with gray-white, often multinodular cut surfaces

MICROSCOPIC

- Histologically indistinguishable from pleural/extrapleural SFTs
- Alternating hypercellular and hypocellular areas with bundles of hyalinized keloid-like collagen
- Hypercellular areas composed of bland, uniform, ovoid to spindle-shaped cells with indistinct cell borders
- Numerous thin-walled staghorn branching vessels

ANCILLARY TESTS

- Positive for STAT6 (nuclear), CD34, CD99, Bcl-2, vimentin
- Gene fusion of *NAB2-STAT6*

TOP DIFFERENTIAL DIAGNOSES

- Undifferentiated thyroid carcinoma, paucicellular variant
- Medullary thyroid carcinoma
- Peripheral nerve sheath tumors
- Smooth muscle tumors
- Invasive fibrous thyroiditis

Primary SFT of Thyroid

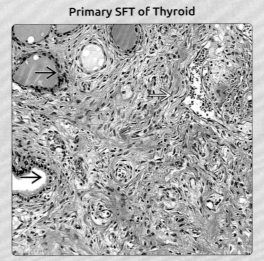

STAT6 in SFT

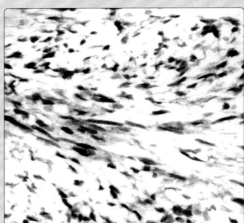

(Left) The lesion is composed of bland spindle cells with bundles of thick collagen. Thyroid follicles ➡ are observed at the periphery of the lesion, with no clear demarcation. Thin-walled branching vessels are characteristic ➡. (Courtesy C. Fletcher, MD.) (Right) STAT6 shows strong and diffuse nuclear staining of lesional cells in solitary fibrous tumor (SFT).

Characteristic SFT Architecture

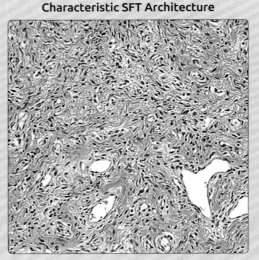

CD34 Immunopositivity in SFT

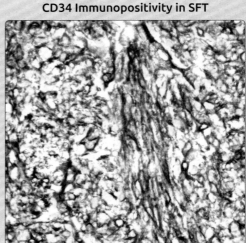

(Left) Bland, monotonous spindle cells are arranged in a haphazard fashion intermixed with bundles of thick collagen. Numerous thin-walled vessels are observed. (Courtesy C. Fletcher, MD.) (Right) In a majority of cases, the lesional cells show characteristic diffuse and strong cytoplasmic and membranous staining for CD34.

TERMINOLOGY

Abbreviations

- Solitary fibrous tumor (SFT)

Synonyms

- Not recommended: Fibroma or fibrosarcoma
- Hemangiopericytoma (HPC)

Definitions

- SFT of thyroid is mesenchymal neoplasm indistinguishable from pleural and other extrapleural SFTs
  - Historically designated as hemangiopericytoma, umbrella term encompassing many other tumor types exhibiting HPC-like vessels
    - HPC now term of limited value
  - Initially described in pleura, now frequently found in diverse anatomic locations

ETIOLOGY/PATHOGENESIS

Unknown

- Possibly arising from uncommitted mesenchymal cell
- Ultrastructural evidence for fibroblastic and myofibroblastic differentiation

CLINICAL ISSUES

Epidemiology

- Incidence
  - Extremely rare in thyroid
  - SFT is most frequent spindle cell mesenchymal tumor of thyroid
- Age
  - Middle aged (median: 56 years)
- Sex
  - M = F

Presentation

- Slow-growing, painless neck mass, present for years
  - Isolated cases of rapidly growing nodules
- May occur in association with longstanding goiter
- Patients are euthyroid
- Hoarseness and dysphagia may be present

Treatment

- Surgical approaches
  - Total thyroidectomy or lobectomy with clear margins sufficient if no malignant features identified
- Adjuvant therapy
  - Combination radiation/chemotherapy have been used in malignant SFT with no clear benefits

Prognosis

- Most tumors are benign
- Behavior can be unpredictable; therefore, close follow-up is advised
- Local recurrence can develop; tied to positive surgical margins
- Most tumors with benign morphology do not recur/metastasize; rare exceptions are documented
- Certain features portend more aggressive behavior
  - Large tumor size and high mitotic rate (> 4/10 HPF)
    - Most reliably predict metastasis
  - Nuclear pleomorphism
  - Increased cellularity
  - Tumor necrosis
- Rare cases of malignant SFT of thyroid gland have been reported with recurrence and metastasis

IMAGING

Radiographic Findings

- Ultrasonography and CT demonstrate solid mass
- Assessment of radioactive iodine uptake reveals cold nodule

MACROSCOPIC

General Features

- Well-circumscribed, usually unencapsulated
- Firm, solid mass with gray-white, often multinodular cut surfaces
  - Cystic foci are rare

Size

- Range: 1.5-13.8 cm

MOLECULAR

Gene Fusion

- Intrachromosomal inversion-derived gene fusion of *NAB2-STAT6* on 12q13
  - ~ 90% harbor fusions
  - Several fusion variants with heterogeneous exon compositions
  - Most fusion-negative cases are positive for STAT6 IHC; these likely represent as yet undetected rearrangements

MICROSCOPIC

Histologic Features

- Histologically indistinguishable from pleural/extrapleural SFTs
- Wide spectrum of appearances ranging from cellular to predominantly fibrous lesions
- Alternating hypercellular and hypocellular areas with bundles of hyalinized collagen (may be keloid-like)
- Hypercellular areas composed of bland, uniform, ovoid to spindle-shaped cells with indistinct cell borders arranged haphazardly
  - Patternless architecture
- Numerous thin-walled staghorn branching vessels
  - Fibrous lesions may have thickened vessels with hyalinized walls
- Entrapped thyroid follicles may be seen at margin of tumor
- Foci of lymphocytes and scattered mast cells are common
- Necrosis is absent and mitoses are rare
- May have giant cells
- May be fat forming

Cytologic Features

- Spindled cells are bland with vesicular nuclei with finely dispersed chromatin, scant cytoplasm, and indistinct borders

ANCILLARY TESTS

Immunohistochemistry

- Positive for STAT6 (nuclear)
  - Most sensitive and specific marker
  - Identifies CD34(-) subset
- Positive for CD34 (90%) and CD99 (70%)
  - Small subset positive for EMA, SMA, Bcl-2
  - May show positivity for factor VIII, PR, ER
- Negative for cytokeratin, TTF-1, thyroglobulin, pax-8, and calcitonin
- Negative for cytokeratin, desmin, CD117 (C-kit), S100, and CD31

Cytology

- Smears tend to be paucicellular, limiting their utility for definitive diagnosis
- Small cells with spindled, vesicular nuclei with finely dispersed chromatin, scant cytoplasm with indistinct borders
- Fragments of interspersed collagen can be seen
- No nuclear atypia

Electron Microscopy

- Neoplastic cells demonstrate fibroblastic differentiation
  - Cells with well-formed branching RER (rough endoplasmic reticulum), embedded within collagen fibers

DIFFERENTIAL DIAGNOSIS

Undifferentiated Thyroid Carcinoma, Paucicellular Variant

- Hypocellular proliferation with extensive fibrosis and keloid-like hyalinization
  - Hypocellular areas composed of scattered spindle cells with marked nuclear atypia and increased mitotic activity
- Majority of cases are positive for cytokeratin, EMA, and pax-8 (nuclear)
  - Array of cytokeratins recommended; often focal
- Immunoreactive for p53

Medullary Thyroid Carcinoma

- Spindle cell variant of MTC
- Tumor cells are immunoreactive for calcitonin, chromogranin, TTF-1, CEA, and cytokeratin

Peripheral Nerve Sheath Tumors

- Hypocellular and hypercellular areas with hyalinized vessels
- Strong S100 positivity in schwannoma, MPNST can be positive for CD34
- Both tumors are negative for STAT6

Smooth Muscle Tumors

- Intersecting fascicles of blunt-ended spindled cells with abundant eosinophilic cytoplasm
- Tend to lack collagen deposition
- Positive for SMA, MSA, desmin, and HCAD
- Leiomyosarcomas can be positive for CD34 but are negative for STAT6

Invasive Fibrous Thyroiditis

- Belongs to spectrum of IgG4-related diseases

- Replacement of thyroid parenchyma by
  - Dense keloid-like collagen (storiform fibrosis)
  - Inflammatory infiltrate composed of plasma cells and lymphocytes
- Fibrosing process infiltrates surrounding tissue whereas SFT is well-demarcated without prominent inflammatory infiltrate

Hyalinizing Trabecular Tumor

- Prominent nuclear pseudo-inclusions

Post Fine-Needle Aspiration Biopsy Site

- Localized reactive spindle cell proliferation with hemosiderin-laden macrophages

Intrathyroid Thymic Carcinoma (CASTLE)

- Epithelioid neoplastic cells

Spindle Epithelial Tumor With Thymus-Like Differentiation (SETTLE)

- Biphasic tumor

DIAGNOSTIC CHECKLIST

Pathologic Interpretation Pearls

- Alternating hypercellular and hypocellular areas with bundles of hyalinized collagen
- Hypercellular areas composed of bland, uniform, ovoid to spindle shaped cells with indistinct cell borders arranged haphazardly
- Numerous thin-walled staghorn branching vessels
- Immunopositive for STAT6 (nuclear), CD34, and CD99
- Gene fusion of *NAB2-STAT6*

SELECTED REFERENCES

1. Agaimy A et al: Phosphaturic Mesenchymal Tumors: Clinicopathologic, Immunohistochemical and Molecular Analysis of 22 Cases Expanding their Morphologic and Immunophenotypic Spectrum. Am J Surg Pathol. ePub, 2017
2. Fusco N et al: Recurrent NAB2-STAT6 gene fusions and oestrogen receptor-α expression in pulmonary adenofibromas. Histopathology. 70(6):906-917, 2017
3. Oda Y et al: Soft tissue sarcomas: From a morphological to a molecular biological approach. Pathol Int. 67(9):435-446, 2017
4. Rekhi B et al: Molecular characterization of a series of solitary fibrous tumors, including immunohistochemical expression of STAT6 and NATB2-STAT6 fusion transcripts, using Reverse Transcriptase(RT)-Polymerase chain reaction(PCR) technique: An Indian experience. Pathol Res Pract. ePub, 2017
5. Salas S et al: Prediction of local and metastatic recurrence in solitary fibrous tumor: construction of a risk calculator in a multicenter cohort from the French Sarcoma Group (FSG) database. Ann Oncol. 28(8):1979-1987, 2017
6. Smith MH et al: STAT6 Reliably Distinguishes Solitary Fibrous Tumors from Myofibromas. Head Neck Pathol. ePub, 2017
7. Uehara K et al: Molecular Signature of Tumors with Monoallelic 13q14 Deletion: a Case Series of Spindle Cell Lipoma and Genetically-Related Tumors Demonstrating a Link Between FOXO1 Status and p38 MAPK Pathway. Pathol Oncol Res. ePub, 2017
8. Ullman D et al: PAX8 Expression in Solitary Fibrous Tumor: A Potential Diagnostic Pitfall. Appl Immunohistochem Mol Morphol. ePub, 2017
9. Luo Q et al: [A case of large solitary fibrous tumor originated from the neck.] Lin Chung Er Bi Yan Hou Tou Jing Wai Ke Za Zhi. 30(2):153-4, 2016
10. Ricciuti B et al: Malignant giant solitary fibrous tumor of the pleura metastatic to the thyroid gland. Tumori. 102(Suppl. 2), 2016
11. DeVito N et al: Clinical characteristics and outcomes for solitary fibrous tumor (SFT): a single center experience. PLoS One. 10(10):e0140362, 2015
12. Kao YC et al: Clinicopathological and genetic heterogeneity of the head and neck solitary fibrous tumours: a comparative histological, immunohistochemical and molecular study of 36 cases. Histopathology. 68(4):492-501, 2015
13. Tai HC et al: NAB2-STAT6 fusion types account for clinicopathological variations in solitary fibrous tumors. Mod Pathol. 28(10):1324-35, 2015

Main Differential Diagnosis of Solitary Fibrous Tumor of Thyroid

Tumor	Characteristics
Paucicellular variant of anaplastic thyroid carcinoma	Hypocellular proliferation with hypocellular areas composed of scattered spindle cells with marked nuclear atypia and increased mitotic activity Majority of cases are positive for cytokeratin, EMA, and nuclear pax-8; often focal immunoreactivity for p53
Medullary thyroid carcinoma, spindle cell variant	Tumor cells are immunoreactive for calcitonin, chromogranin, TTF-1, PAX-8, cytokeratin, and CEA
Peripheral nerve sheath tumors	Mixed hypocellular and hypercellular areas with hyalinized vessels, and strong S100 positivity in schwannoma MPNST can be positive for CD34
Smooth muscle tumors	Positive for SMA, MSA, desmin, and HCAD Leiomyosarcomas can be positive for CD34 but are negative for STAT6
Fibrosing thyroiditis	Fibrosing process infiltrates surrounding tissue; SFT is well-demarcated without prominent inflammatory infiltrate
Hyalinizing trabecular adenoma/tumor	Trabecular/organoid growth pattern of elongated cells oriented perpendicular to stroma with extracellular and intracellular hyalinization; prominent nuclear pseudoinclusions; immunoreactive for TTF-1, thyroglobulin, and keratin
Post fine-needle aspiration	Localized reactive spindle cell proliferation in close proximity to thyroid nodule with hemosiderin-laden macrophages, reactive vascular pattern, and extravasated erythrocytes
Intrathyroid thymic carcinoma (CASTLE)	Solid nests with infiltrative growth pattern separated by dense fibrous bands; neoplastic cells are epithelioid with large pleomorphic nuclei but can be spindle-shaped; immunoreactive for p63, CD5, and CD117
SETTLE	Biphasic histology: Spindle-shaped cells blending with epithelial structures; sclerotic stroma; tends to occur in 1st and 2nd decades of life; wide expression of cytokeratins
Follicular adenoma with spindle cell metaplasia	Short fascicles of spindled cells with bland cytomorphology, lacks collagen deposition; immunoreactive for TTF-1, pax-8, and cytokeratin

Carcinoma showing thymus-like differentiation = CASTLE; spindle epithelial tumor with thymus-like differentiation = SETTLE.

14. Alves Filho W et al: Malignant solitary fibrous tumor of the thyroid: a case-report and review of the literature. Arq Bras Endocrinol Metabol. 58(4):402-6, 2014
15. Mizuuchi Y et al: Solitary fibrous tumor of the thyroid gland. Med Mol Morphol. 47(2):117-22, 2014
16. Mohammedi K et al: Paraneoplastic hypoglycemia in a patient with a malignant solitary fibrous tumor. Endocrinol Diabetes Metab Case Rep. 2014:140026, 2014
17. Vaziri M et al: Solitary fibrous tumor of the intrathoracic goiter. Med J Islam Repub Iran. 28:51, 2014
18. Boleko Á et al: [Solitary fibrous tumour associated with papillary thyroid carcinoma and pituitary macroadenoma.] Cir Esp. 91(9):606-7, 2013
19. Chmielecki J et al: Whole-exome sequencing identifies a recurrent NAB2-STAT6 fusion in solitary fibrous tumors. Nat Genet. 45(2):131-2, 2013
20. Topaloglu O et al: Solitary fibrous tumor of neck mimicking cold thyroid nodule in 99m tc thyroid scintigraphy. Case Rep Endocrinol. 2013:805745, 2013
21. van Houdt WJ et al: Prognosis of solitary fibrous tumors: a multicenter study. Ann Surg Oncol. 20(13):4090-5, 2013
22. Ning S et al: Malignant solitary fibrous tumor of the thyroid gland: report of a case and review of the literature. Diagn Cytopathol. 39(9):694-9, 2011
23. Verdi D et al: Solitary fibrous tumor of the thyroid gland: a report of two cases with an analysis of their clinical and pathological features. Endocr Pathol. 22(3):165-9, 2011
24. Cameselle-Teijeiro J: Uncommon tumors of the thyroid gland. Int J Surg Pathol. 18(3 Suppl):205S-208S, 2010
25. Larsen SR et al: Solitary fibrous tumor arising in an intrathoracic goiter. Thyroid. 20(4):435-7, 2010
26. Sevinc AI et al: Clinical images. Solitary fibrous tumor of the perithyroidal soft tissue mimicking substernal goiter. Am J Surg. 199(6):e82-3, 2010
27. Kojima M et al: Inflammatory pseudotumor of the thyroid gland showing prominent fibrohistiocytic proliferation. A case report. Endocr Pathol. 20(3):186-90, 2009

28. Santeusanio G et al: Solitary fibrous tumour of thyroid: report of two cases with immunohistochemical features and literature review. Head Neck Pathol. 2(3):231-5, 2008
29. Papi G et al: Solitary fibrous tumor of the thyroid gland. Thyroid. 17(2):119-26, 2007
30. Papi G et al: Primary spindle cell lesions of the thyroid gland; an overview. Am J Clin Pathol. 125 Suppl:S95-123, 2006
31. Tanahashi J et al: Solitary fibrous tumor of the thyroid gland: report of two cases and review of the literature. Pathol Int. 56(8):471-7, 2006
32. Rodriguez I et al: Solitary fibrous tumor of the thyroid gland: report of seven cases. Am J Surg Pathol. 25(11):1424-8, 2001
33. Cameselle-Teijeiro J et al: Solitary fibrous tumor of the thyroid. Am J Clin Pathol. 101(4):535-8, 1994
34. Taccagni G et al: Solitary fibrous tumour of the thyroid: clinicopathological, immunohistochemical and ultrastructural study of three cases. Virchows Arch A Pathol Anat Histopathol. 422(6):491-7, 1993

(Left) *Spindle cells are observed infiltrating thyroid follicles at the periphery of the lesion* ➡. *Ectatic branching vessels are common* ➡. *(Courtesy C. Fletcher, MD.)* **(Right)** *Haphazard arrangement of spindle cells with variable cellularity with a patternless architecture and collagenous stroma are characteristic features. Prominent staghorn branching vessels are characteristic and scattered lymphocytes are common.*

SFT Infiltrating Thyroid

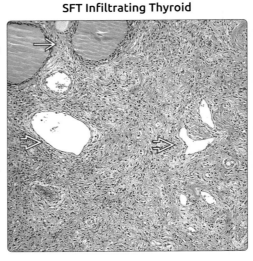

Branching Vessels in SFT

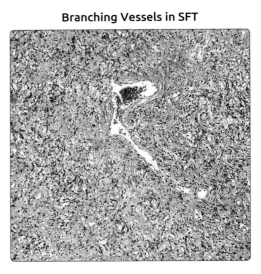

(Left) *Haphazard architecture of bland spindle cells with indistinct cell borders is characteristic of solitary fibrous tumor. No cytologic atypia is observed. (Courtesy C. Fletcher, MD.)* **(Right)** *The spindled cells have vesicular nuclei with finely dispersed chromatin, scant cytoplasm, and indistinct borders. Scattered lymphocytes and mast cells are observed.*

SFT Haphazard Architecture

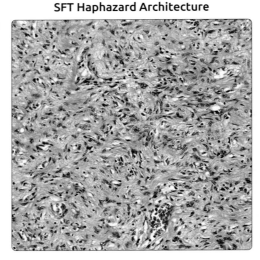

SFT Cytology

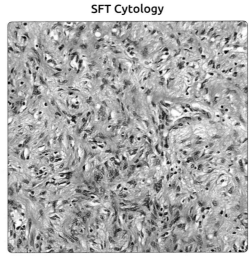

(Left) *SFTs display a variegated, wavy, storiform, hemangiopericytic or desmoid-like arrangement of spindle cells. Collagenous stroma with thick, keloid-like areas are characteristic of SFT.* **(Right)** *SFTs characteristically have alternation of hypocellular, keloid-like areas and hypercellular areas. A transition between a hypercellular region to a hypocellular region is observed. The hypocellular regions are often characterized by thick, collagenous bands* ➡.

Collagen in Primary Thyroid SFT

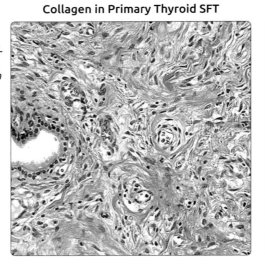

Keloid-Like Bands in SFT

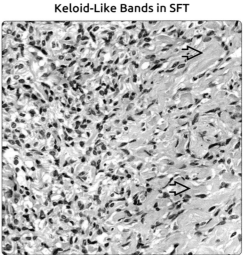

Collagenous Areas in SFT

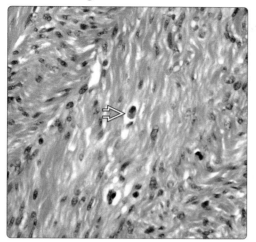

Bundles of Collagen in SFT

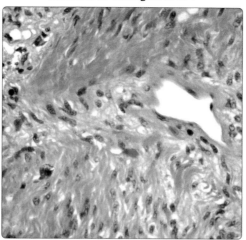

(Left) *Bland, uniform spindle cells are interspersed with collagen fibers in SFT. Myxoid changes and the presence of interstitial inflammatory cells, as mast cells ⇒ are commonly observed.* (Right) *The tumor cells have scant cytoplasm and indistinct cell borders. Bland spindle cells with adjacent bundles of thick collagen fibers are characteristic of these lesions.*

Keloid-Like Collagen in SFT

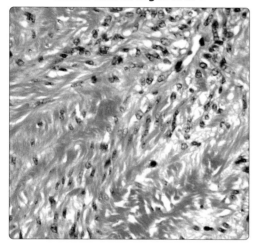

Cytoplasmic/Membranous CD34

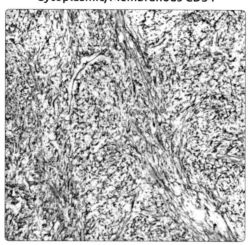

(Left) *Hypocellular areas of SFT can often have keloid-like bundles of collagen. The spindle cells present are typical, and no mitosis are usually identified.* (Right) *Immunohistochemistry for CD34 highlights the characteristic patternless architecture of SFT. This photomicrography highlights the storiform arrangement of the spindle cells.*

STAT6 Immunostaining in SFT

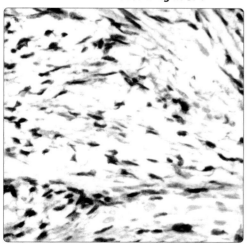

Characteristic Nuclear Positivity for STAT6

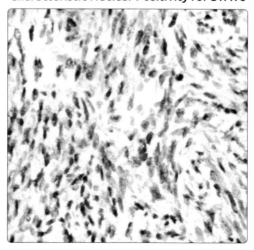

(Left) *Nuclear staining of STAT6 highlights the spindle-shaped lesional cells. Endothelial cells of vessels within the lesion are negative.* (Right) *STAT6 staining in a cellular area of SFT demonstrates strong immunopositivity in the nuclei of the majority of cells.*

TERMINOLOGY

- Paragangliomas are slow-growing, benign neuroendocrine tumors that derive from extraadrenal paraganglia of autonomic nervous system
- Paragangliomas adjacent to or inside thyroid gland are likely subset of laryngeal paragangliomas

CLINICAL ISSUES

- Paragangliomas of head and neck region comprise only 0.6% of all head and neck tumors
- Asymptomatic neck mass
- If multiple tumors found, familial syndrome should be considered
- Recommended that all patients with newly diagnosed paraganglioma should undergo biochemical work-up for catecholamine excess

MICROSCOPIC

- Well-circumscribed or encapsulated intrathyroidal mass

- Usually form loose cell nests called zellballen, surrounded by extensive fibrovascular network
- Predominant cell of paragangliomas: Chief cell, a polygonal cell with delicate oncocytic cytoplasm, round nucleus, and granular chromatin

TOP DIFFERENTIAL DIAGNOSES

- Medullary thyroid carcinoma
- Hyalinizing trabecular tumor
- Poorly differentiated carcinoma (insular carcinoma)
- Parathyroid neoplasia
- Metastatic neuroendocrine tumors to thyroid

DIAGNOSTIC CHECKLIST

- Well-circumscribed or encapsulated intrathyroidal mass
- Formed by cell nests (zellballen) surrounded by fibrovascular network
- Paragangliomas chief cells positive for NSE, CD56, chromogranin-A, and synaptophysin

Head and Neck Paraganglia

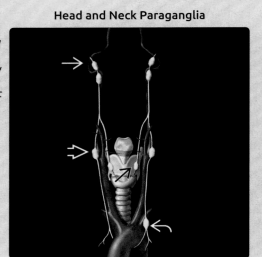

Thyroid Paraganglioma

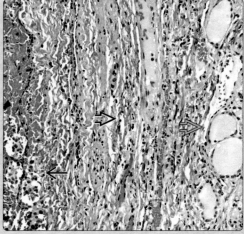

(Left) Graphic shows paraganglia in head, neck, and upper thorax associated with arteries or cranial nerves. They include aortic ➡ and carotid ➡ bodies, and jugulotympanic ➡, vagal, and laryngeal ➡ paraganglia. (Right) This well-encapsulated thyroid paraganglioma ➡ is separated from the thyroid tissue ➡ by a focally thick, highly vascularized fibrous capsule ➡. The tumor is highly vascularized.

Preserved SDHB Expression

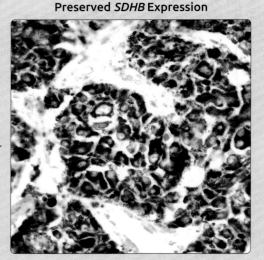

Paraganglioma With SDHB Loss

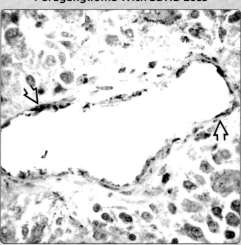

(Left) This thyroid paraganglioma without mutation of SDHx genes shows preserved SDHB immunoreactivity. The stain is coarsely granular, as the protein is localized in the mitochondria. (Right) The tumor cells in this paraganglioma with mutation of SDHB gene are negative for SDHB protein, while the endothelial cells ➡ show preserved immunoexpression and serve as intrinsic positive control.

TERMINOLOGY

Abbreviations

- Paraganglioma (PGL)

Synonyms

- Thyroid-associated paraganglioma
  - Previously termed chemodectoma or glomus tumor

Definitions

- Slow-growing, benign neuroendocrine tumors that derive from extraadrenal paraganglia of autonomic nervous system
  - Paragangliomas adjacent to or inside thyroid gland are likely subset of laryngeal paragangliomas

ETIOLOGY/PATHOGENESIS

Head and Neck Paraganglioma

- Paragangliomas may be found throughout embryologic migration routes of neural crest tissue
- Virtually all head and neck paragangliomas derive from parasympathetic nervous system
  - Carotid body (carotid body tumor) is most common head and neck location
  - Other rare head and neck locations include nasal cavity, orbit, larynx, aortic arch, and those associated with thyroid gland
  - Rare sites: Jugular bulb, Jacobsen tympanic plexus in middle ear, and vagal nerve

Thyroid Paraganglioma

- Paragangliomas adjacent to or inside thyroid gland are likely subset of laryngeal paragangliomas
  - Laryngeal paraganglia are branchiomeric, consist of 2 paired structures, and reside between superior edge of thyroid cartilage and 1st tracheal ring
  - Thyroid paragangliomas are thought to arise from inferior laryngeal paraganglia
  - Normal inferior laryngeal paraganglia measure 0.4 mm and are located at lateral margin of cricoid cartilage in cricothyroid membrane
    - One possibility: Inferior laryngeal paraganglia may form within thyroid capsule itself, which could ultimately create intrathyroidal paraganglioma
- Registry-based study of thyroid paraganglioma: 5 cases
  - Multinational population-based study on thyroid paraganglioma and analyzed prevalence, immunohistochemistry, and molecular genetics
  - Patients with thyroid paraganglioma recruited from European American Head and Neck Paraganglioma Registry
  - All patients underwent molecular genetic analyses of SDHA, SDHB, SDHC, SDHD, SDHAF2, VHL, RET, TMEM127, and MAX genes
  - Germline variants were found in 4 of 5 confirmed thyroid paraganglioma cases, 2 each in SDHA and SDHB
    - ~ 80% of thyroid paragangliomas are associated with germline variants
    - With implications for additional tumors and potential risk for family

CLINICAL ISSUES

Epidemiology

- Incidence
  - Paragangliomas of head and neck region comprise only 0.6% of all head and neck tumors
    - Thyroid paragangliomas are exceedingly rare
- Age
  - Epidemiologically, paragangliomas typically present in younger adult patients
  - Intrathyroidal paragangliomas are tumors affecting women 40-50 years of age
- Sex
  - Paragangliomas are up to 3x more common in women than men

Presentation

- Most of time, intrathyroidal paragangliomas appear as asymptomatic thyroid nodule
- Asymptomatic neck mass
  - Incidence of hyperfunctioning paragangliomas is only 1-3% in head and neck
    - No reported patients with hyperfunctioning thyroid-associated paragangliomas
- If multiple tumors found, familial syndrome should be considered

Laboratory Tests

- Recommended that all patients with newly diagnosed paraganglioma should go through biochemical work-up for catecholamine excess

Treatment

- Surgical excision is treatment of choice

Prognosis

- < 10% of all paragangliomas are malignant
- No unequivocal histologic or immunohistochemical markers that distinguish benign from malignant paragangliomas
  - Paraganglioma is considered malignant only if it metastasizes to nonneuroendocrine tissues
    - Sites include regional spread to cervical lymph nodes and distant spread to lung, liver, bone, and skin
- No description in medical literature of patients with malignant paragangliomas adjacent to or inside thyroid gland
  - Reported follow-up times have been relatively short (2 months to 8 years)
- Local tissue extension of paragangliomas near or in thyroid does not correspond to malignant disease and is usually treated with limited resection
- ~ 14% of patients who presented with thyroid-associated paraganglioma also had disease in either carotid body or glomus vagale

IMAGING

General Features

- Hypervascular thyroid nodule
  - Although paragangliomas of head and neck and particularly those associated with thyroid gland are rare, these should be considered in differential diagnosis of hypervascular thyroid nodule

MACROSCOPIC

General Features

- Large, well-circumscribed nodule with gray-brown cut surface
- Most thyroid paragangliomas are solitary nodules
- They can be partially to completely encapsulated solid tumors
- Rare cases have described infiltrating growth pattern with direct extension into cricoid cartilage, trachea, subglottic larynx, and esophagus

Size

- Usually measures ~ 3 cm

MICROSCOPIC

Histologic Features

- Well-circumscribed or encapsulated intrathyroidal mass
- Highly vascular with rich fibrovascular plexus
- Usually form loose cell nests called zellballen, surrounded by extensive fibrovascular network
- Other tumor architecture: Lobular, alveolar, sheath
- Paragangliomas are composed of 2 different cell types: Chief cells and sustentacular cells
  - Predominant cell: Chief cell, a polygonal cell with delicate oncocytic cytoplasm, round nucleus, and granular chromatin
  - Sustentacular cells are better identified by immunohistochemistry
  - Nuclei are usually round to oval with occasional isolated pleomorphic nuclei
- Microscopic features of paraganglioma overlap with those of other neuroendocrine tumors, especially medullary thyroid carcinoma
  - Immunohistochemical studies can be used to distinguish paraganglioma from other entities

ANCILLARY TESTS

Immunohistochemistry

- Chief cells of paragangliomas are positive for NSE, CD56, chromogranin-A, and synaptophysin
- Sustentacular cells are positive for S100 and GFAP
- Paragangliomas are negative for calcitonin, CEA, thyroglobulin, TTF-1, EMA, and cytokeratin
- Some rare subsets of laryngeal paragangliomas have been described that are positive for calcitonin
  - Medullary thyroid carcinomas that contain S100(+) sustentacular cells have also been reported
- Loss of SDHB immunoexpression in some familial thyroid paragangliomas

Genetic Testing

- Although most of these tumors are considered sporadic, ~ 30-40% are associated with at least 14 known susceptibility genes
  - *MEN1, NF1, RET, VHL, SDHA, SDHB, SDHC, SDHD, SDHAF2, TMEM127, EGLN1, HIF2A, KIF1Bβ*, and *MAX*
- Occasional *VHL, TMEM127*, and *SDHA*-related head and neck paragangliomas have been described in literature
- Most familial disease in head and neck paraganglioma is associated with *SDHD, SDHC, SDHB*, and *SDHAF2* mutations

- Biochemical phenotype of most of genes are either nonsecreting or secrete dopamine, epinephrine, norepinephrine, metanephrine, normetanephrine, and methoxytyramine
- Up to 30% of all apparently sporadic head and neck paragangliomas are caused by germline mutation and are part of paraganglioma syndrome
- Paraganglioma syndromes have been classified into 4 types, each with corresponding gene mutation in succinate dehydrogenase
  - Succinate dehydrogenase normally encodes for protein subunits of complex II in mitochondrial electron transport chain
  - Mutations in succinate dehydrogenase may activate angiogenic pathway that ultimately leads to tumorigenesis
  - Because of important implications of germline mutations in succinate dehydrogenase genes, all patients with these rare tumors should undergo genetic counseling and possibly genetic testing

DIFFERENTIAL DIAGNOSIS

Medullary Thyroid Carcinoma

- Poorly circumscribed and invasive tumor
- Presence of amyloid deposition
- Positive for TTF-1, chromogranin, calcitonin, cytokeratin, and CEA

Hyalinizing Trabecular Tumor

- Usually small, well circumscribed, and present as incidental finding
- Inter- and intratrabecular fibrosis
- Characteristic MIB-1 membranous staining
- Positive for TTF-1 and thyroglobulin

Poorly Differentiated Carcinoma (Insular Carcinoma)

- Infiltrative tumor
- Presence of mitosis and necrosis
- Positive for TTF-1 and thyroglobulin

Parathyroid Neoplasia

- Immunohistochemistry positive for PTH and chromogranin

Metastatic Renal Cell Carcinoma

- Positive for RCA, CD10

Metastatic Neuroendocrine Tumors to Thyroid

- Usually multifocal tumors with infiltrative growth pattern, cytological atypia, and mitosis
- Nuclei are large with salt and pepper chromatin

Atypical Follicular Adenoma

- Negative for neuroendocrine markers

DIAGNOSTIC CHECKLIST

Pathologic Interpretation Pearls

- Cytologic and histologic features overlap with more common primary thyroid neoplasms, but immunohistochemical studies can be used to aid in diagnosis

Major Familial Paraganglioma Syndromes

Syndrome	Gene (Chromosome)	Associated With Head and Neck Tumors	Associated Tumors
MEN2A and 2B	*RET* (10q11)	(+/-)	Medullary thyroid carcinoma, parathyroid adenoma, other endocrine tumors
NF1	*NF1* (17q11.2)	(+/-)	Neurofibroma, GIST, neuroendocrine tumors
VHL	*VHL* (3p25-26)	(+/-)	RCC, hemangioblastoma, endolymphatic sac tumor, pancreatic endocrine tumor, neuroendocrine tumor
PGL1	*SDHD*	(+++)	
PGL2	*SDHAF2*	(+++)	
PGL3	*SDHC*	(+++)	GIST
PGL4	*SDHB*	(++)	RCC, GIST
SDHA related	*SDHA*	(+)	GIST
Carney-Stratakis dyad	*SDHx*	(+)	GIST
MAX related	*MAX*		
KIF1Bβ related	KIF1Bβ		Neuroblastoma, medulloblastoma
Familial pho/paraganglioma	TMEM127	(+/-)	

SELECTED REFERENCES

1. Lee SM et al: Thyroid paraganglioma. Arch Pathol Lab Med. 139(8):1062-7, 2015
2. Taweevisit M et al: Thyroid paraganglioma: "naked" nuclei as a clue to diagnosis on imprint cytology. Endocr Pathol. 26(3):232-8, 2015
3. von Dobschuetz E et al: A registry-based study of thyroid paraganglioma: histological and genetic characteristics. Endocr Relat Cancer. 22(2):191-204, 2015
4. Yu X et al: Primary thyroid paraganglioma mimicking medullary thyroid carcinoma: a case report. Oncol Lett. 10(2):1000-1002, 2015
5. Zhang W et al: Aspiration cytology of primary thyroid paraganglioma. Diagn Cytopathol. 43(10):838-43, 2015
6. Boedeker CC et al: Genetics of hereditary head and neck paragangliomas. Head Neck. 36(6):907-16, 2014
7. Filipović A et al: Paraganglioma of the thyroid gland: a case report. Vojnosanit Pregl. 71(9):875-8, 2014
8. Huang D et al: Primary paraganglioma located between the thyroid gland and the left common carotid artery: a case report. Oncol Lett. 8(5):1925-1928, 2014
9. Treglia G et al: A rare case of thyroid paraganglioma detected by ¹⁸F-FDG PET/CT. Rev Esp Med Nucl Imagen Mol. 33(5):320-1, 2014
10. Papaspyrou K et al: Head and neck paragangliomas: report of 175 patients (1989-2010). Head Neck. 34(5):632-7, 2012
11. Bargellini T et al: [Left laparoscopic adrenalectomy for pheochromocytoma in MEN 2B: case report.] G Chir. 32(3):132-4, 2011
12. Phitayakorn R et al: Thyroid-associated paragangliomas. Thyroid. 21(7):725-33, 2011
13. Raygada M et al: Hereditary paragangliomas. Adv Otorhinolaryngol. 70:99-106, 2011
14. Zhang Y et al: Endocrine tumors as part of inherited tumor syndromes. Adv Anat Pathol. 18(3):206-18, 2011
15. Almeida MQ et al: Solid tumors associated with multiple endocrine neoplasias. Cancer Genet Cytogenet. 203(1):30-6, 2010
16. Ye L et al: The evolving field of tyrosine kinase inhibitors in the treatment of endocrine tumors. Endocr Rev. 31(4):578-99, 2010
17. Donatini G et al: Neck lesions mimicking thyroid pathology. Langenbecks Arch Surg. 394(3):435-40, 2009
18. Erem C et al: Primary thyroid paraganglioma presenting with double thyroid nodule: a case report. Endocrine. 36(3):368-71, 2009
19. Ferri E et al: Primary paraganglioma of thyroid gland: a clinicopathologic and immunohistochemical study with review of the literature. Acta Otorhinolaryngol Ital. 29(2):97-102, 2009
20. Garrel R et al: An unusual succinate dehydrogenase gene mutation C in a case of laryngeal paraganglioma. J Laryngol Otol. 123(1):141-4, 2009
21. González Poggioli N et al: Paraganglioma of the thyroid gland: a rare entity. Endocr Pathol. 20(1):62-5, 2009
22. Henderson A et al: SDHB-associated renal oncocytoma suggests a broadening of the renal phenotype in hereditary paragangliomatosis. Fam Cancer. 8(3):257-60, 2009
23. Mun KS et al: Extra-adrenal paraganglioma: presentation in three uncommon locations. Malays J Pathol. 31(1):57-61, 2009
24. Ryska A et al: Paraganglioma-like medullary thyroid carcinoma: fine needle aspiration cytology features with histological correlation. Cytopathology. 20(3):188-94, 2009
25. Ashraf MJ et al: Thyroid paraganglioma: diagnostic pitfall in fine needle aspiration biopsy. Acta Cytol. 52(6):745-7, 2008
26. Callender GG et al: Multiple endocrine neoplasia syndromes. Surg Clin North Am. 88(4):863-95, viii, 2008
27. Malek R et al: A gastrointestinal stromal tumor in a patient with multiple endocrine neoplasia type 2A and metastatic medullary thyroid cancer to the ovaries. Endocr Pract. 14(7):898-901, 2008
28. Ni Y et al: Germline mutations and variants in the succinate dehydrogenase genes in Cowden and Cowden-like syndromes. Am J Hum Genet. 83(2):261-8, 2008
29. Nosé V et al: Hyalinizing trabecular tumor of the thyroid: an update. Endocr Pathol. 19(1):1-8, 2008
30. Pinto FR et al: Unusual location of a cervical paraganglioma between the thyroid gland and the common carotid artery: case report. Clinics (Sao Paulo). 63(6):845-8, 2008
31. Volante M et al: A practical diagnostic approach to solid/trabecular nodules in the thyroid. Endocr Pathol. 19(2):75-81, 2008
32. Papacharalampous GX et al: Paraganglioma of the larynx: a case report. Med Sci Monit. 13(12):CS145-8, 2007
33. Zantour B et al: A thyroid nodule revealing a paraganglioma in a patient with a new germline mutation in the succinate dehydrogenase B gene. Eur J Endocrinol. 151(4):433-8, 2004

(Left) *A low-power view of an intrathyroid paraganglioma* ➡ *shows an encapsulated tumor separated from the adjacent thyroid* ➡ *by an irregular fibrous capsule* ➡. *There is a characteristic nesting pattern of this tumor.* (Right) *The thyroid paraganglioma is present within the capsule* ➡ *and is separated from the thyroid tissue* ➡ *by a focally thick fibrous capsule* ➡.

Intrathyroid Paraganglioma

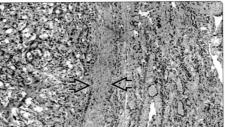

Thyroid and Paraganglioma

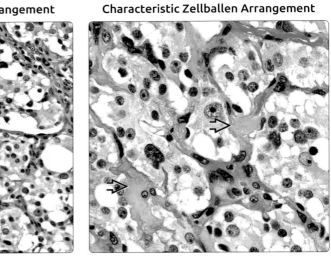

(Left) *This high-power view of a thyroid paraganglioma shows the characteristic alveolar nesting pattern (zellballen) with variably sized nests of tumor cells surrounded by thin-walled vessels* ➡. (Right) *A thick fibrovascular stroma* ➡ *surrounds the variably sized nests of tumor cells in this thyroid paraganglioma. The chief cells have a large amount of amphophilic cytoplasm and round to elongated nuclei with prominent nucleoli.*

Characteristic Alveolar Arrangement

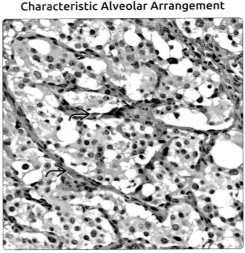

Characteristic Zellballen Arrangement

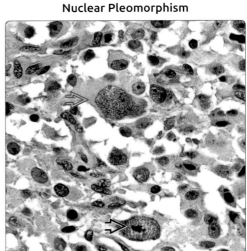

(Left) *This thyroid paraganglioma has a patternless architecture lacking the characteristic zellballen arrangement of cells. Note the atypical cells with an amphophilic cytoplasm and focally pleomorphic nuclei* ➡. (Right) *Paragangliomas are usually composed of a monotonous population of uniform chief cells. In this photomicrograph, the tumor cells show abundant granular cytoplasm with marked nuclear pleomorphism* ➡ *with focally prominent nucleoli* ➡.

Diffuse Architecture

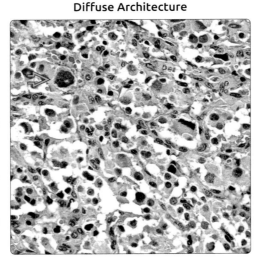

Nuclear Pleomorphism

Fibrous Capsule

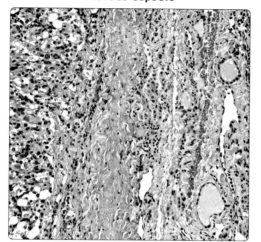

Thyroid and Paraganglioma Edge

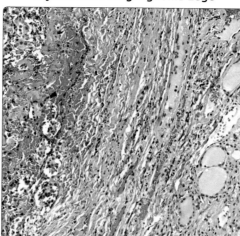

(Left) *This well-encapsulated thyroid paraganglioma (left) is well separated from the compressed thyroid tissue (right) by a prominent thick fibrous capsule with scattered lymphocytic infiltration.* **(Right)** *This thyroid paraganglioma is separated from the thyroid tissue by a focally and highly vascularized fibrous capsule. The tumor is also highly vascularized and shows area of hemorrhage.*

Characteristic Alveolar Pattern

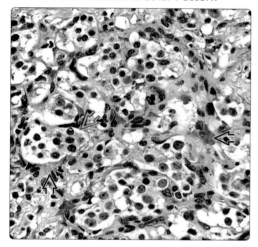

Large Cells in Paraganglioma

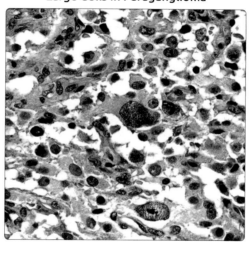

(Left) *H&E shows the characteristic alveolar pattern (zellballen) of thyroid paraganglioma. Small nests of cells ⇲ are surrounded by a fibrovascular stroma ⇲.* **(Right)** *An individual paraganglioma may contain populations of both large cells with prominent nucleoli and small cells. Some cases may also contain spindle cells.*

SDHB Immunoreactivity

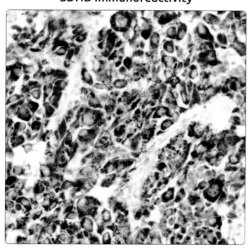

S100-Positive Sustentacular Cells

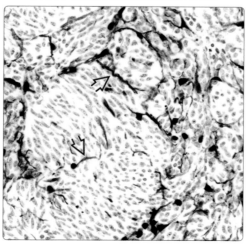

(Left) *This thyroid paraganglioma shows preserved SDHB immunoreactivity, indicative that this paraganglioma has no mutation of SDHx genes. The stain is cytoplasmic and coarsely granular.* **(Right)** *S100 immunostain in this paraganglioma shows nuclear and cytoplasmic staining of sustentacular cells. Some of these cells have long cytoplasmic processes ⇲.*

TERMINOLOGY

- **Leiomyoma (LM)**: Benign neoplasm with smooth muscle differentiation
- **Leiomyosarcoma (LMS)**: Malignant neoplasm with pure smooth muscle differentiation
  - Both arising from thyroid gland vascular smooth muscle

CLINICAL ISSUES

- Exceedingly rare; < 0.01% of all thyroid tumors
- **LMS**
  - Painless, rapidly enlarging mass
  - Extremely poor prognosis
- **LM**: Surgical excision is curative

MACROSCOPIC

- **LM**: Well-circumscribed, rubbery nodules
- **LMS**: Gray-white, fleshy cut surfaces with areas of necrosis and hemorrhage

MICROSCOPIC

- **LM**: Intersecting fascicles of spindled cells resembling smooth muscle cells
- **LMS**: Spindled to epithelioid cells arranged in intersecting fascicles with sharp margination
  - Grading primary thyroid LMS is not performed, but general grading criteria includes: Anaplasia, increased mitoses, and necrosis

ANCILLARY TESTS

- Positive for smooth muscle actin, muscle-specific actin, desmin, calponin, and h-caldesmon
- Neoplastic cells negative for TTF-1, thyroglobulin, S100, SOX10, calcitonin

TOP DIFFERENTIAL DIAGNOSES

- Metastatic LMS
- Anaplastic/undifferentiated carcinoma
- Medullary thyroid carcinoma

Primary LMS of Thyroid

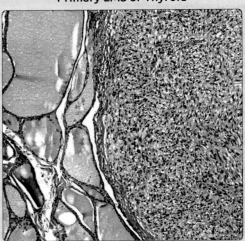

LMS in Vessel Wall

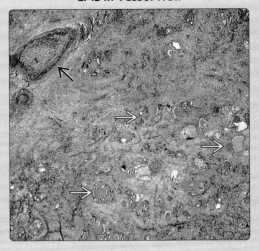

(Left) Medium-power H&E of a primary LMS of the thyroid demonstrates a highly cellular neoplasm composed of spindle cells arranged in distinct fascicles with a fairly circumscribed border with adjacent thyroid follicles. (Right) LMS of the thyroid are hypothesized to originate from the wall of of intrathyroidal blood vessels. Depicted in this image is one such example of an LMS in a blood vessel at the periphery of the thyroid ⭢. Note the poor circumscription of the lesion and the adjacent thyroid follicles ⭢.

H-Caldesmon in Smooth Muscle Tumors

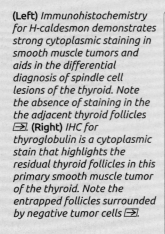
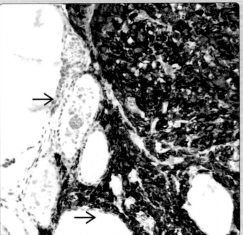

Thyroglobulin in Smooth Muscle Tumors

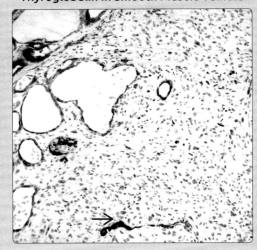

(Left) Immunohistochemistry for H-caldesmon demonstrates strong cytoplasmic staining in smooth muscle tumors and aids in the differential diagnosis of spindle cell lesions of the thyroid. Note the absence of staining in the the adjacent thyroid follicles ⭢. (Right) IHC for thyroglobulin is a cytoplasmic stain that highlights the residual thyroid follicles in this primary smooth muscle tumor of the thyroid. Note the entrapped follicles surrounded by negative tumor cells ⭢.

TERMINOLOGY

Abbreviations

- Leiomyoma (LM)
- Leiomyosarcoma (LMS)

Definitions

- **LM**: Benign neoplasm with smooth muscle differentiation arising from thyroid gland vascular smooth muscle
- **LMS**: Malignant neoplasm with pure smooth muscle differentiation arising from thyroid gland vascular smooth muscle

ETIOLOGY/PATHOGENESIS

Histogenesis

- Postulated to arise from smooth muscle cells of vessels within thyroid gland

CLINICAL ISSUES

Epidemiology

- Incidence
  - Exceedingly rare; < 0.01% of all thyroid tumors; ~ 20 cases of LMS reported in literature
    - LMS represents ~ 11% of primary thyroid sarcomas reported in literature
- Age
  - 6th and 7th decades
- Sex
  - Female predilection for LMS; 1.5:1

Site

- Often at periphery of thyroid

Presentation

- LMS: Painless, rapidly enlarging mass
  - Local, compressive symptoms; occasionally present with hoarseness, dysphagia

Treatment

- Surgical approaches
  - **LM**: Surgical excision is curative; subtotal thyroidectomy may also be performed
  - **LMS**: Complete, radical surgical removal
- Other treatment modalities
  - Chemotherapy and radiotherapy have been administered in subset of cases with no clear benefit

Prognosis

- **LM**: Excellent
- **LMS**: Extremely poor
  - 1-year survival rate of < 20%

IMAGING

Radiographic Findings

- **LM**
  - Usually well-circumscribed and homogeneous density
- **LMS**
  - Radiographic features are nonspecific but can be suggestive of malignancy

- Compression of upper airway, infiltration into soft tissues or thyroid cartilage, thyroid destruction, and necrosis
- Hypoechoic nodular lesion on ultrasound
- Nonhomogeneous hypo- to hyperdense lesion with irregular margins on CT

MACROSCOPIC

General Features

- **LM**: Well-circumscribed, rubbery nodules
- **LMS**: Gray-white, fleshy cut surfaces with areas of necrosis and hemorrhage
  - Can be well circumscribed, but infiltrative borders are also observed

Size

- LM tends to be smaller than its malignant counterpart
  - Average: 2 cm
- LMS > LM
  - Average: 6 cm

MICROSCOPIC

Histologic Features

- **LM**
  - Well circumscribed
  - Intersecting fascicles of spindled cells resembling smooth muscle cells
    - Cells are eosinophilic and uniform
    - Nuclei are described as blunt ended and cigar-shaped
- **LMS**
  - Low-grade tumors can be well circumscribed, mimicking LMs
  - Infiltrative margins can be seen with invasion into peripheral soft tissues
    - Entrapment of thyroid follicles and destruction of thyroid parenchyma observed in primary LMS
  - Origin from smooth muscle-walled vessels may be seen
  - Highly cellular neoplasm
    - Spindled to epithelioid cells arranged in intersecting fascicles with sharp margination
    - Can have areas that are less well defined with storiform or palisading
  - Cells are elongated and large with brightly eosinophilic (often fibrillar) to pale cytoplasm
  - Nuclei are variably blunt ended and may be indented
    - Higher grade tumors may show more variable nuclear features with pleomorphism
      - □ Identification of cells with more typical nuclear features is important for diagnosis
      - □ Ancillary IHC may be necessary for proper diagnosis
  - Coagulative tumor necrosis is frequently observed in larger tumors: Presence indicates malignancy
  - Mitoses are usually present and found readily but can be variable
    - > 5/10 HPF usually indicates LMS
    - Mitotic activity contributes to grading of tumor

Cytologic Features

- **LM**
  - Bland-looking, uniform, blunt-ended spindle cells

- - No nuclear pleomorphism; degenerative atypia may be seen
- **LMS**
  - Centrally placed, hyperchromatic, blunt-ended nuclei
    - Perinuclear cytoplasmic vacuoles or clear halos may be seen
  - Nuclear pleomorphism is present

ANCILLARY TESTS

Cytology

- FNA: While distinction between smooth muscle tumors and other spindle cell tumors is challenging, few features are suggestive of diagnosis
  - Fascicular architecture
  - Cells with brightly eosinophilic cytoplasm, blunt-ended nuclei, and intranuclear vacuoles

Immunohistochemistry

- Diffusely positive for smooth muscle actin, vimentin, muscle-specific actin, desmin, calponin, and h-caldesmon
  - MYOD1 and myogenin can be focally positive
  - Neoplastic cells negative for TTF-1, thyroglobulin, pankeratin, S100, calcitonin

Genetic Testing

- **LM**
  - Molecular alterations of soft tissue LMs remain to be demonstrated
- **LMS**
  - Gene expression profiling has identified 3 distinct, potentially clinically relevant molecular subtypes
    - Subtype I associated with good prognosis, subtype II associated with poor outcome
    - Subtype III with anatomical preference for uterus
    - Potentially new IHC markers to identify subtypes: LMOD1 and ARL4C
  - Complex karyotypes without recurrent chromosomal aberrations
  - Mutations: *TP53*, *RB1*, *ATRX*
  - Copy number alterations in regions of known tumor suppressor genes: *PTEN*, *RB1*, and *TP53*

Electron Microscopy

- Cytoplasmic thin myofilaments with dense bodies and discontinuous basal lamina

DIFFERENTIAL DIAGNOSIS

Metastatic Leiomyosarcoma

- Direct extension and metastatic LMS to thyroid gland must be excluded
  - Given extremely rare possibility of primary thyroid LMS, lesion in thyroid in patient with known primary tumor should be considered metastatic
- Clinical and radiographic correlation required

Anaplastic/Undifferentiated Carcinoma

- Significant overlap clinically, radiographically, and histologically between LMS and anaplastic thyroid carcinoma (ATC)
- ATC is usually associated with longstanding history of preexisting thyroid lesion that is rapidly enlarging

- Presence of residual well-differentiated thyroid carcinoma strongly favors ATC
- May show epithelial differentiation (histologic, immunophenotypic, ultrastructural) and lacks myogenic markers

Medullary Thyroid Carcinoma

- Spindled cell morphology can be seen in medullary thyroid carcinoma (MTC)
- Characteristic salt and pepper nuclear quality, presence of amyloid, and background of C-cell hyperplasia are distinguishing features of MTC
- MTC is positive for TTF-1, calcitonin, chromogranin, CD56, and CEA

Malignant Peripheral Nerve Sheath Tumors

- Causes more of problem in poorly differentiated LMS lacking distinct cytological features
- Combination of SMA, desmin, and h-caldesmon should support LMS
- Loss of H3K27me3 can be useful to support diagnosis of MPNST

DIAGNOSTIC CHECKLIST

Clinically Relevant Pathologic Features

- Exceedingly rare thyroid tumors
  - Metastatic LMS should always be 1st consideration

Pathologic Interpretation Pearls

- Spindle cell neoplasms with fascicular architecture, brightly eosinophilic cytoplasm, and cigar-shaped nuclei
  - Pleomorphism, necrosis, and mitoses should favor diagnosis of LMS

SELECTED REFERENCES

1. Ayadi M et al: Primary leiomyosarcoma of thyroid gland: the youngest case. Pan Afr Med J. 26:113, 2017
2. Gupta AJ et al: Primary sarcomas of thyroid gland-series of three cases with brief review of spindle cell lesions of thyroid. J Clin Diagn Res. 11(2):ER01-ER04, 2017
3. Guo X et al: Clinically relevant molecular subtypes in leiomyosarcoma. Clin Cancer Res. 21(15):3501-11, 2015
4. Surov A et al: Primary thyroid sarcoma: a systematic review. Anticancer Res. 35(10):5185-91, 2015
5. Conzo G et al: Leiomyosarcoma of the thyroid gland: a case report and literature review. Oncol Lett. 7(4):1011-1014, 2014
6. Amal B et al: A rare primary tumor of the thyroid gland: report a new case of leiomyosarcoma and literature review. Diagn Pathol. 8:36, 2013
7. Tanboon J et al: Leiomyosarcoma: a rare tumor of the thyroid. Endocr Pathol. 24(3):136-43, 2013
8. Piana S et al: Thyroid leiomyosarcoma: primary or metastasis? that's the question! Endocr Pathol. 22(4):226-8, 2011
9. Nemenqani D et al: Leiomyosarcoma metastatic to the thyroid diagnosed by fine needle aspiration cytology. J Pak Med Assoc. 60(4):307-9, 2010
10. Mansouri H et al: Leiomyosarcoma of the thyroid gland. Acta Otolaryngol. 128(3):335-6, 2008
11. Wang TS et al: Primary leiomyosarcoma of the thyroid gland. Thyroid. 18(4):425-8, 2008
12. Papi G et al: Primary spindle cell lesions of the thyroid gland; an overview. Am J Clin Pathol. 125 Suppl:S95-123, 2006
13. Erkiliç S et al: Primary leiomyoma of the thyroid gland. J Laryngol Otol. 117(10):832-4, 2003
14. Ozaki O et al: Primary leiomyosarcoma of the thyroid gland. Surg Today. 27(2):177-80, 1997
15. Thompson LD et al: Primary smooth muscle tumors of the thyroid gland. Cancer. 79(3):579-87, 1997

Nuclear Features of Leiomyoma

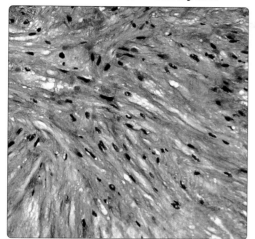

Cytology of LMS

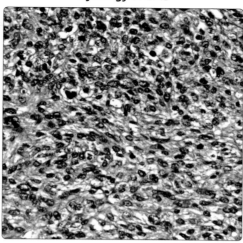

(Left) *High-power H&E of a leiomyoma demonstrates characteristic features of smooth muscle tumors: Bland cells with brightly eosinophilic cytoplasm, blunt-ended nuclei, and fascicular architecture.* **(Right)** *High-power H&E of a LMS is highly cellular, arranged in fascicles, and demonstrates malignant features: Frequent mitoses and hyperchromatic, pleomorphic nuclei.*

Infiltration of Thyroid

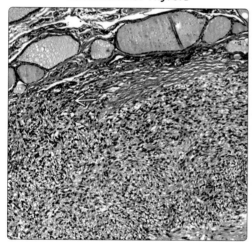

Tumor Necrosis in LMS

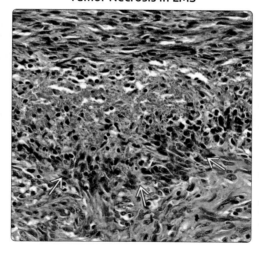

(Left) *Although at this power, the distinction between an leiomyoma and a LMS is not immediately evident, the poorly circumscribed nature of the tumor and the infiltrative pattern observed at the periphery, extending into the thyroid follicles ➡, are suggestive of malignancy.* **(Right)** *High-power H&E of a LMS demonstrates tumor necrosis, which is suggestive of malignancy in smooth muscle tumors. Hyperchromatic, pleomorphic nuclei are observed at the periphery of the necrosis ➡.*

Desmin in Smooth Muscle Tumors

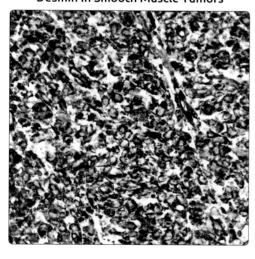

Infiltrative Nature of LMS

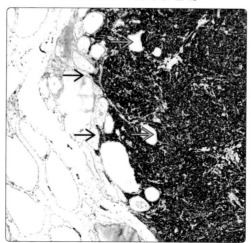

(Left) *Smooth muscle tumors show strong and diffuse cytoplasmic staining for desmin. Although desmin is usually positive in LMS, some poorly differentiated tumors might only be focally positive or even absent.* **(Right)** *Medium-power H&E of IHC for smooth muscle actin demonstrates the infiltrative nature of the LMS. The neoplastic cells are observed trickling through the thyroid parenchyma ➡, leaving few entrapped follicles along the way ➡.*

TERMINOLOGY

- Primary angiosarcoma of thyroid: Malignant neoplasm with endothelial cell differentiation

CLINICAL ISSUES

- Extremely rare
- Predilection for European alpine regions; 2% of malignant thyroid tumors in this population
- Poor prognosis
- Treatment: Total thyroidectomy
- Local recurrences and metastases are common despite complete resection

MACROSCOPIC

- Circumscribed nodule with necrosis and hemorrhage; less commonly multinodular

MICROSCOPIC

- Similar to high-grade angiosarcomas of soft tissue

- Invasive growth pattern with irregular periphery, destruction of thyroid parenchyma, often with extrathyroidal extension
- Irregular anastomosing endothelial-lined vascular spaces

ANCILLARY TESTS

- Positive for endothelial markers: CD31, CD34 (both membranous), ERG, FLI-1 (both nuclear), factor VIII-related protein (cytoplasmic)
- Negative: TTF-1, thyroglobulin, pax-8, calcitonin, neuroendocrine markers

TOP DIFFERENTIAL DIAGNOSES

- Anaplastic thyroid carcinoma
- Metastatic angiosarcoma
- Degenerative adenomatoid nodules
- Post fine-needle aspiration
- Other sarcomas

Destruction of Thyroid Follicles by Tumor

Infiltration of Thyroid by Malignant Cells

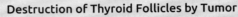

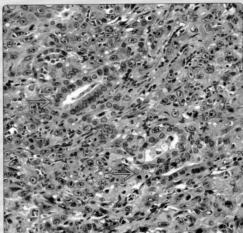

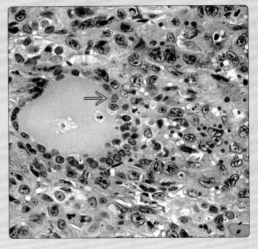

(Left) An infiltrative vascular proliferation composed of enlarged, pleomorphic nuclei surrounds individual thyroid follicles ➡. (Right) The malignant endothelial proliferation is infiltrating the thyroid parenchyma. Note the thyroid follicle ➡ surrounded by the enlarged, highly pleomorphic tumor cells.

CD31 in Thyroid Angiosarcoma

ERG Immunostain in Angiosarcoma

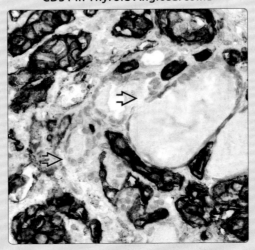

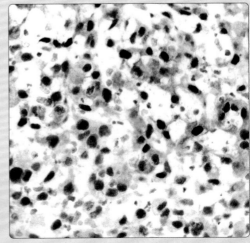

(Left) CD31 shows membranous positivity of the malignant endothelial cells. Note the entrapped thyroid follicles that are negative for CD31 ➡. (Right) ERG immunostaining shows strong nuclear positivity by the angiosarcoma cells. FLI-1 is also proactive in these tumors.

TERMINOLOGY

Definitions

- Primary angiosarcoma of thyroid: Malignant neoplasm of thyroid with endothelial cell differentiation

ETIOLOGY/PATHOGENESIS

Environmental Exposure

- Likely multifactorial but may be related to iodine deficiency resulting in endemic goiters
  - Prevalence reduced with iodized salt prophylaxis

Pathogenesis

- Endothelial rather than follicular origin seems supported: Absence of thyroglobulin mRNA expression in angiosarcomas

CLINICAL ISSUES

Epidemiology

- Incidence
  - Extremely rare
  - Predilection for European alpine regions; 2% of malignant thyroid tumors in this population
- Age
  - 5th-8th decades
- Sex
  - Female preponderance

Presentation

- Rapidly increasing painless neck mass
  - Often in setting of longstanding goiter
- May have dyspnea, dysphagia
- Onset of symptoms: Weeks to months
- Hyperthyroidism is rare

Treatment

- Options, risks, complications
  - Severe bleeding at primary or metastatic sites may complicate surgery
- Surgical approaches
  - Total thyroidectomy
- Drugs
  - Role of chemotherapy is unclear; minority of patients have shown good response
  - Studies of targeted therapy to include VEGF/VEGFR pathway are underway
- Radiation
  - Adjuvant radiotherapy, frequently administered as brachytherapy, shown to improve outcome

Prognosis

- Poor
  - Median survival: < 4 months
- Local recurrences and metastases are common despite complete resection
  - Most common site of metastasis: Lung
  - Uncommon sites: Brain, gastrointestinal tract, bone
  - Local extension common: Lymph nodes, mediastinum, neck muscles, or trachea
- Small tumors confined to gland may have more favorable prognosis

IMAGING

Radiographic Findings

- Radioactive iodine uptake studies usually demonstrate cold nodules

MACROSCOPIC

General Features

- Circumscribed nodule with necrosis and hemorrhage; less commonly multinodular
- Variegated cut surfaces with solid and cystic areas

Size

- Often > 5 cm; range: 2-15 cm

MICROSCOPIC

Histologic Features

- Similar to high-grade angiosarcomas of soft tissue
- Invasive growth pattern with irregular periphery, destruction of thyroid parenchyma, often with extrathyroidal extension
- Irregular anastomosing endothelial-lined vascular spaces
  - Many patterns: Solid, spindled, papillary, pseudoglandular
  - Irregular, cleft-like to patulous vascular channels
- Endothelial cells are atypical or overtly malignant and have spindled or epithelioid morphology
  - Large pleomorphic, vesicular nuclei with prominent nucleoli
  - Abundant eosinophilic to vacuolated cytoplasm
- Increased mitotic figures, including atypical forms
- Tumor necrosis and hemorrhage with hemosiderin-laden macrophages throughout
- Other findings include
  - Multinucleated giant cells or bizarre cells
  - Intracytoplasmic vacuoles representing early neolumen

ANCILLARY TESTS

Cytology

- Fine-needle aspiration difficult to interpret and often inconclusive; diagnosis can be made in minority of cases
- Single cells or small clusters of round/oval cells with prominent nucleoli, vacuolated cytoplasm, indistinct cell borders
- Features of intracytoplasmic lumina may be seen

Immunohistochemistry

- Positive for endothelial markers: CD31, CD34 (both membranous), ERG, FLI-1 (both nuclear), factor VIII-related protein (cytoplasmic)
- Keratins may be positive, particularly in epithelioid angiosarcoma
- Negative: TTF-1, thyroglobulin, pax-8, calcitonin, neuroendocrine markers

Electron Microscopy

- Weibel-Palade bodies: Membrane-bound, intracytoplasmic rod-shaped structures; storage site for factor VIII-related protein; difficult to identify in poorly differentiated vascular tumors

Immunohistochemistry

Antibody	Reactivity	Staining Pattern	Comment
CD31	Positive	Cell membrane	Most sensitive and specific endothelial marker
CD34	Positive	Cell membrane	
FLI-1	Positive	Nuclear	Sensitive marker but not specific; particularly useful in setting of crushed or poorly preserved specimen
ERG	Positive	Nuclear	
TTF-1	Negative		
Thyroglobulin	Negative		
pax-8	Negative		

DIFFERENTIAL DIAGNOSIS

Anaplastic Thyroid Carcinoma

- Angiosarcomatous features can be seen in anaplastic thyroid carcinoma
- Undifferentiated carcinoma frequently has coexisting thyroid gland disease
- Negative thyroglobulin and pax-8 and positive vascular markers support diagnosis of angiosarcoma
- Distinction is academic as both malignancies have similar prognoses and treatment

Metastatic Angiosarcoma

- Important to exclude metastasis with history, clinical exam, and radiology
- Direct invasion (soft tissue or skin) into thyroid is possible

Medullary Thyroid Carcinoma

- Pseudoangiosarcomatous variant of medullary thyroid carcinoma may have prominent cellular dehiscence leading to formation of cleft-like spaces with hemorrhage
- Despite architectural similarity of variant, nuclear features of MTC are retained; although nuclear pleomorphism and mitotic figures may be seen, significant pleomorphism is generally not apparent in MTC
- Presence of amyloid is helpful
- Tumor cells are positive for calcitonin, synaptophysin, and chromogranin; TTF-1 is variable but helpful when positive

Degenerative Adenomatoid Nodules

- Nodules frequently undergo degenerative changes, with hemorrhage followed by organization
    o Granulation-type tissue, blood, hemosiderin-laden macrophages, cyst formation, and calcification
- No cytologic atypia, no freely anastomosing vessels

Post Fine-Needle Aspiration

- Papillary endothelial hyperplasia often observed
- Single area of involvement with breached capsule, hemosiderin-laden macrophages, extravasated erythrocytes, dilated vascular channels with thrombosis and organization
- No cytologic atypia, no freely anastomosing vessels

Other Sarcomas

- Vascular channels in angiosarcomas
- Positive vascular markers (CD31 and CD34) plus FLI-1 and ERG support diagnosis of angiosarcoma

SELECTED REFERENCES

1. Bayır Ö et al: An extremely rare case of thyroid malignancy from the non-Alpine region: Angiosarcoma. Int J Surg Case Rep. 19:92-96, 2015
2. Rotellini M et al: Epithelioid angiosarcoma of the thyroid: report of a case from an italian non-alpine area and review of the literature. Endocr Pathol. 26(2):152-6, 2015
3. Surov A et al: Primary thyroid sarcoma: a systematic review. Anticancer Res. 35(10):5185-91, 2015
4. Kaur A et al: Angiosarcoma of the thyroid: a case report with review of the literature. Endocr Pathol. 24(3):156-61, 2013
5. Petronella P et al: Primary thyroid angiosarcoma: an unusual localization. World J Surg Oncol. 10:73, 2012
6. Hart J et al: Epithelioid angiosarcoma: a brief diagnostic review and differential diagnosis. Arch Pathol Lab Med. 135(2):268-72, 2011
7. Isa NM et al: Primary angiosarcoma of the thyroid gland with recurrence diagnosed by fine needle aspiration: a case report. Diagn Cytopathol. 37(6):427-32, 2009
8. Kalitova P et al: Angiosarcoma of the thyroid. Eur Arch Otorhinolaryngol. 266(6):903-5, 2009
9. Njim L et al: [Angiomatoid tumor of the thyroid gland: primitive angiosarcoma or variant of anaplastic carcinoma?.] Ann Pathol. 28(3):221-4, 2008
10. Ortiz J et al: Primary epithelioid angiosarcoma of the thyroid: an infrequent malignant thyroid tumor. Endocrinol Nutr. 55(4):181-3, 2008
11. Papotti M et al: Diagnostic controversies in vascular proliferations of the thyroid gland. Endocr Pathol. 19(3):175-83, 2008
12. Abraham JA et al: Treatment and outcome of 82 patients with angiosarcoma. Ann Surg Oncol. 14(6):1953-67, 2007
13. Del Rio P et al: A rare case of thyroid haemangiosarcoma. Chir Ital. 59(5):747-9, 2007
14. Eng SP et al: Metastatic angiosarcoma to the thyroid. Rev Laryngol Otol Rhinol (Bord). 126(2):111-4, 2005
15. Yilmazlar T et al: A case of hemangiosarcoma in thyroid with severe anemia due to bone marrow metastasis. Endocr J. 52(1):57-9, 2005
16. Ryska A et al: Epithelioid haemangiosarcoma of the thyroid gland. Report of six cases from a non-Alpine region. Histopathology. 44(1):40-6, 2004
17. Goh SG et al: Two cases of epithelioid angiosarcoma involving the thyroid and a brief review of non-Alpine epithelioid angiosarcoma of the thyroid. Arch Pathol Lab Med. 127(2):E70-3, 2003
18. Lin O et al: Cytologic findings of epithelioid angiosarcoma of the thyroid. A case report. Acta Cytol. 46(4):767-71, 2002
19. Tacheci I et al: Epithelioid hemangiosarcoma of the thyroid gland. Cas Lek Cesk. 141(9):291-3, 2002
20. Yu J et al: Juxtathyroidal neck soft tissue angiosarcoma presenting as an undifferentiated thyroid carcinoma. Thyroid. 12(5):427-32, 2002
21. Astl J et al: Hemangiosarcoma of the thyroid gland. A case report. Neuro Endocrinol Lett. 21(3):213-216, 2000

Infiltration of Thyroid Parenchyma

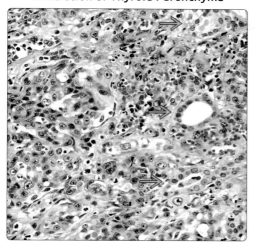

Anastomosing Vascular Channels

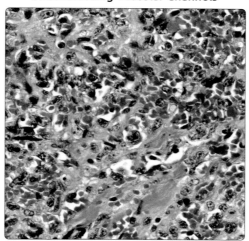

(Left) *Large angiosarcoma cells with pleomorphic nuclei are seen infiltrating and destroying thyroid parenchyma. There are a few thyroid follicles remaining ⇒. Areas of tumor necrosis are common.* (Right) *Angiosarcoma with anastomosing vascular channels lined by large, highly pleomorphic cells infiltrates the thyroid parenchyma. No residual follicular cells are present.*

Growth Patterns in Angiosarcoma

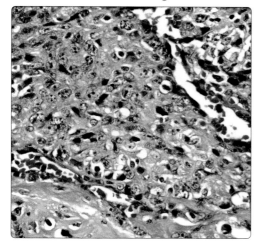

TTF-1 Absent in Angiosarcoma

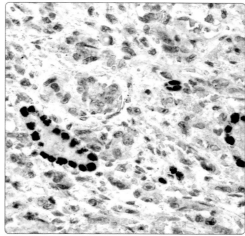

(Left) *Large, highly pleomorphic cells in solid growth pattern and lining vascular channels in angiosarcoma are seen in this image.* (Right) *Nuclear TTF-1 highlights the thyroid follicles entrapped and destroyed by malignant endothelial cells.*

Vascular Spaces Highlighted by CD31

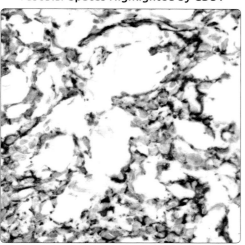

Solid-Patterned Growth Areas

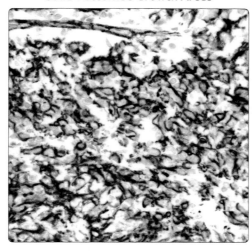

(Left) *In this angiosarcoma, CD31 membranous immunostaining demonstrates the tumor forming vascular spaces.* (Right) *CD31 highlights an area of solid growth pattern in this thyroid angiosarcoma. Note the membranous staining of the tumor cells.*

Squamous Cell Carcinoma, Thyroid

TERMINOLOGY

- Primary thyroid squamous cell carcinoma (SCC) is malignant epithelial tumor composed entirely of cells with squamous cell differentiation
- Apply strict criteria for diagnosis of primary thyroid SCC to exclude invasion/metastases from other primary sites

CLINICAL ISSUES

- 1% of thyroid malignancies
- M > F = 1:2
- Patients present with rapidly enlarging neck mass
- Frequent recurrent laryngeal nerve compression and pressure symptoms
- Many have preexisting thyroid disease
- Nearly all patients present with advanced disease
- Tumor follows rapidly fulminant course

IMAGING

- Large mass, often showing necrosis

MACROSCOPIC

- Usually large, single tumor nodule

MICROSCOPIC

- Widely invasive tumor, destroying thyroid parenchyma
- Cohesive cells arranged in sheets, ribbons, and nests
- Polygonal, polyhedral, and spindle tumor cells

ANCILLARY TESTS

- Positive for p63, keratin, CK5/6, CK19, and pax-8
  - pax-8 staining is useful for distinguishing between primary thyroid SCC and invasion or metastasis
- Negative for thyroglobulin, CEA, calcitonin, and CD5

TOP DIFFERENTIAL DIAGNOSES

- Direct extension of SCC from adjacent organs
- Metastatic SCC
- Extensive squamous metaplasia

(Left) This high-grade primary thyroid squamous cell carcinoma (SCC) is composed of large cells with eosinophilic cytoplasms and large pleomorphic nuclei. No keratinization is present. A remnant thyroid follicle is present ➡. (Right) Neoplastic cells in primary thyroid SCC are strongly and diffusely positive for highlighted CK19 (and also for CK5/6), although in general, immunohistochemistry is not required for the diagnosis.

Malignant Cells Invading Thyroid Follicles

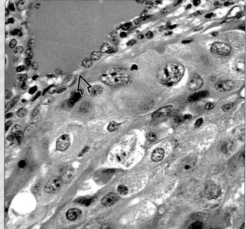

Cytokeratin 19 in Thyroid Squamous Cell Carcinoma

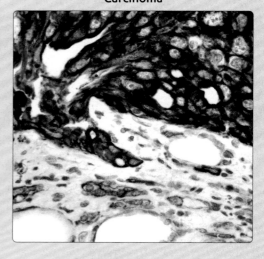

(Left) The thyroid gland is focally replaced by a primary infiltrating poorly differentiated SCC with numerous mitoses ➡ present. There is extensive infiltration and destruction of the thyroid follicles ➡. (Right) As SCC of other origin, the primary thyroid SCC has p63 expression in the majority of tumor cells. These cells also stain for CK19, CK5/6, and EMA.

High-Grade Tumor With Numerous Mitosis

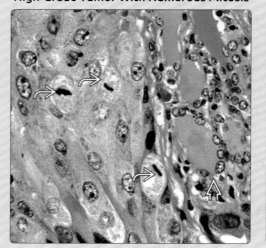

Immunopositivity for p63

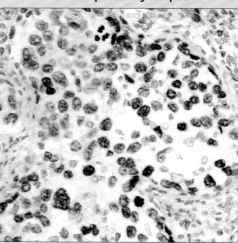

TERMINOLOGY

Abbreviations
- Squamous cell carcinoma (SCC)

Synonyms
- Epidermoid carcinoma

Definitions
- Malignant epithelial tumor composed entirely of cells with squamous cell differentiation
  - Lacks mucocyte and direct invasion from adjacent organs (larynx, esophagus)

ETIOLOGY/PATHOGENESIS

Environmental Exposure
- Radiation history is occasionally present

Pathogenesis
- Derived from thyroid follicular epithelium
  - Directly or via squamous metaplasia, then additional alterations to reach malignant tumor
- Persistence of thyroglossal duct or branchial pouch embryonic remnants

CLINICAL ISSUES

Epidemiology
- Incidence
  - 1% of thyroid malignancies
- Age
  - Mean: 6th and 7th decades
- Sex
  - M > F = 1:2

Site
- Affects 1 or both lobes of thyroid gland

Presentation
- Patients present with rapidly enlarging neck mass
- Frequent recurrent laryngeal nerve compression and pressure symptoms
  - Airway obstruction, dyspnea, and dysphagia
  - Direct involvement of nerves, vessels, and soft tissues
- Many have preexisting thyroid disease
  - Hashimoto thyroiditis is concurrently identified in few patients
    - Hypercalcemia, fever, and leukocytosis
    - Probably develops as result of tumor-derived humoral mediators
- Cervical lymph node enlargement is common
- May present with paraneoplastic syndrome with hypercalcemia and leukocytosis

Endoscopic Findings
- Endoscopic evaluation (laryngoscopy, esophagoscopy, bronchoscopy) to exclude direct extension

Treatment
- Options, risks, complications
  - Airway collapse and esophagotracheal fistula may complicate course
- Primary thyroid SCC is relatively resistant to radiotherapy and poorly responsive to chemotherapy
- Surgical approaches
  - Early radical resection yields best prognosis
- Drugs
  - Thyroid hormone suppression may help
    - Thyroid-stimulating hormone may be growth factor
  - Chemotherapy does not alter disease course
- Radiation
  - Radical dose radiotherapy is part of initial treatment
  - Radiation alone for unresectable tumor &/or poor surgical candidates
  - Radioiodine therapy does not work

Prognosis
- Nearly all patients present with advanced disease
- Tumor follows rapidly fulminant course
  - Prognosis is poor; mean survival: < 1 year; 5-year survival: < 10%
  - Localized disease only; managed aggressively, patients may survive longer
- Local invasion and lymph node metastases are common
- Distant metastasis (lung) is less common (30%)
- Complete resection of disease correlates with improved survival

IMAGING

Radiographic Findings
- Large mass, often showing necrosis
- Radiographic studies exclude direct invasion from contiguous organs

MACROSCOPIC

General Features
- Usually large, single tumor nodule
  - Multiple satellite tumor nodules can be seen
  - Involves 1 or both lobes
- Firm, gray-white mass with areas of necrosis
- Extrathyroidal extension is frequent

Size
- Large; up to 12 cm

MICROSCOPIC

Histologic Features
- Must exclude direct extension from tumor in larynx or esophagus
- Widely invasive tumor, destroying thyroid parenchyma
- Cohesive cells arranged in sheets, ribbons, and nests
- Polygonal, polyhedral, and spindle tumor cells
  - Variable pleomorphism
- Keratinization and keratin pearl formation
  - Classified as keratinizing or nonkeratinizing
- High mitotic index, including atypical forms
- Vascular and perineural invasion is common
- Inflammatory infiltrate and stomal fibroplasia often present
  - Association with Hashimoto thyroiditis is known
- Associated tumors: Papillary carcinoma, follicular carcinoma, and follicular adenoma

- By convention, if another tumor is present, it is diagnosed with "squamous differentiation" incorporated into diagnosis

ANCILLARY TESTS

Cytology

- Confirm site of FNA (thyroid, larynx, lymph node, esophagus, metastasis) before diagnosis
- Cellular smears contain cohesive clusters and isolated cells
- Irregular shapes (tadpole cells), nuclear hyperchromasia, and cytoplasmic organgeophilia and dyskeratosis
- Background filled with necrotic and granular eosinophilic keratin debris

Immunohistochemistry

- Positive for p63, EMA, keratin, CK19, CK5/6, pax-8
  - pax-8 staining is useful for distinguishing between primary thyroid SCC and invasion or metastasis
  - CK7 and CK18 may be focally present
- Negative for thyroglobulin, CEA, calcitonin, CK20, and CD5

Genetic Testing

- Abnormal *TP53* expression and loss of *CDKN1A* expression
  - *TP53* expression is greater in tumors with less squamous differentiation

DIFFERENTIAL DIAGNOSIS

Metastatic SCC

- Different primary site known clinically
  - Usually develops within 3 years of primary site documentation
- Tend to be multifocal with high rate of lymph-vascular invasion

Extensive Squamous Metaplasia

- Squamous differentiation can be seen in lymphocytic thyroiditis, adenomatous nodules, diffuse sclerosing variant of papillary thyroid carcinoma, and anaplastic thyroid carcinoma
- Tends to be focal, does not form mass clinically; lacks "infiltration," cytologic atypia, and necrosis
- Squamous metaplasia does not predispose to developing SCC

Direct Extension From Adjacent Organs

- Much more frequent than primary thyroid SCC
- Tumor or bulk of tumor is centered in larynx, esophagus, or trachea
  - Up to 25% of radical laryngectomies show direct thyroid invasion, especially if true vocal cord fixation present
  - May show cricothyroid membrane, anterior commissure, laryngeal ventricle, and thyroid cartilage invasion
- Confirmed endoscopically, radiographically, or during surgery
- Primary thyroid SCC have much worse prognosis than tumors with direct extension
- Usually, primary malignancy detected before thyroid involvement
- pax-8 staining is useful for distinguishing between primary thyroid SCC and invasion or metastasis from extrathyroidal SCC

Carcinoma Showing Thymus-Like Differentiation

- Greater degree of tumor spindling, more keloid-like collagen disposition, and inflammatory cells
- Positive with CD5, p63, CEA, and HMWK

DIAGNOSTIC CHECKLIST

Pathologic Interpretation Pearls

- Apply strict criteria for diagnosis of primary thyroid SCC
  - Need to exclude invasion/metastases from other primary sites

GRADING

Thyroid SCC

- Classified in 3 grades
  - Well differentiated
  - Moderately differentiated
  - Poorly differentiated
    - Most thyroid tumors are poorly differentiated

STAGING

Same as Anaplastic Thyroid Carcinoma

- By convention, SCC is staged as if it were anaplastic/undifferentiated carcinoma

SELECTED REFERENCES

1. Au JK et al: Primary squamous cell carcinoma of the thyroid: a population-based analysis. Otolaryngol Head Neck Surg. 157(1):25-29, 2017
2. Struller F et al: Primary squamous cell carcinoma of the thyroid: case report and systematic review of the literature. Int J Surg Case Rep. 37:36-40, 2017
3. Yoshihiro T et al: Cardiac metastasis of squamous cell carcinoma of the thyroid gland with severe disseminated intravascular coagulation: a case report. Mol Clin Oncol. 6(1):91-95, 2017
4. Ebina A et al: Intrathyroidal epithelial thymoma: carcinoma showing thymus-like differentiation mimicking squamous cell carcinoma of the thyroid. J Nippon Med Sch. 82(1):2-3, 2015
5. Suzuki A et al: Diagnostic significance of PAX8 in thyroid squamous cell carcinoma. Endocr J. 62(11):991-5, 2015
6. Cai L et al: Primary squamous cell carcinoma of the thyroid on FDG PET/CT. Clin Nucl Med. 39(11):1014-6, 2014
7. Cho JK et al: Primary squamous cell carcinomas in the thyroid gland: an individual participant data meta-analysis. Cancer Med. 3(5):1396-403, 2014
8. Sapalidis K et al: Primary squamous cell carcinoma of the thyroid gland. J Surg Case Rep. 2014(12), 2014
9. Ito Y et al: Biological behavior of papillary carcinoma of the thyroid including squamous cell carcinoma components and prognosis of patients who underwent locally curative surgery. J Thyroid Res. 2012:230283, 2012
10. Gaillardin L et al: Thyroid gland invasion in laryngopharyngeal squamous cell carcinoma: prevalence, endoscopic and CT predictors. Eur Ann Otorhinolaryngol Head Neck Dis. 129(1):1-5, 2011
11. Pusztaszeri M: Fine needle aspiration biopsy of three cases of squamous cell carcinoma presenting as a thyroid mass: cytological findings and differential diagnosis. the differential diagnosis includes CASTLE. Cytopathology. Epub 23(1):67-8, 2011
12. Laury AR et al: A comprehensive analysis of PAX8 expression in human epithelial tumors. Am J Surg Pathol. 35(6):816-26, 2011
13. Syed MI et al: Squamous cell carcinoma of the thyroid gland: primary or secondary disease? J Laryngol Otol. 125(1):3-9, 2011
14. Bonetti LR et al: EGFR polysomy in squamous cell carcinoma of the thyroid. Report of two cases and review of the literature. Tumori. 96(3):503-7, 2010

Thyroid With Adjacent Structures

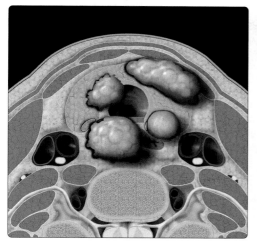

Imaging of Thyroid Squamous Cell Carcinoma

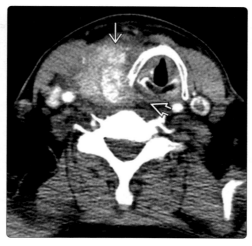

(Left) The thyroid gland is located in close proximity to other structures that are more frequently involved by SCC. To diagnose a primary thyroid carcinoma, it is necessary to apply strict criteria to exclude invasion/metastases from other primary sites. (Right) Radiographs are used to highlight the extent of tumor and specifically to exclude invasion from the adjacent larynx ➡ or esophagus. In this case, there is a large mass ➡ replacing the right thyroid lobe.

Large Tumor Cells With Prominent Nucleoli

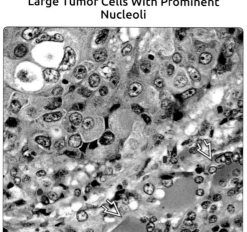

High-Grade Thyroid Squamous Cell Carcinoma

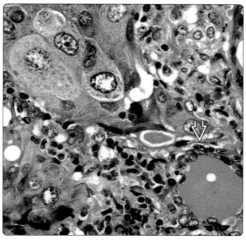

(Left) High-power H&E of a primary thyroid SCC shows groups of tumor cells infiltrating thyroid follicles ➡. The tumor cells are large with eosinophilic cytoplasm, well-defined cytoplasmic membranes, and prominent nucleoli. (Right) High-grade SCC has large cells with eosinophilic cytoplasms and very large pleomorphic nuclei. No keratin pearls are present. A remnant thyroid follicle is present ➡.

High Mitotic Rate in High-Grade Squamous Cell Carcinoma

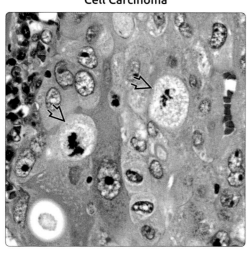

HER2 Membranous Staining in Squamous Cell Carcinoma

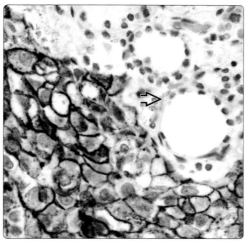

(Left) High-grade SCC has destroyed the thyroid follicles and has numerous mitosis ➡ with a very high mitotic rate. The tumor cells are large with eosinophilic cytoplasms and very large pleomorphic nuclei, some with prominent nucleoli. (Right) Thyroid neoplastic cells in primary SCC may demonstrate diffuse and membranous immunoreactivity for HER2. The residual follicular cells are negative ➡.

Primary Ewing Sarcoma, Thyroid

TERMINOLOGY

- Translocation-associated small round blue cell sarcoma
- Ewing sarcoma (ES) family tumors include intraosseous ES, extraosseous ES, and peripheral primitive neuroectodermal tumors (PNETs)

CLINICAL ISSUES

- Extremely rare primary tumor in thyroid with ~ 15 reported cases
- 5-year overall survival
  - Localized disease: 65-75%
  - Initially metastatic disease: < 30%

MICROSCOPIC

- Sheets and nests of densely cellular, monotonous-appearing cells with indistinct cell borders
- Uniform cells with relatively small round nuclei with finely dispersed chromatin and scant, clear (abundant collagen) to eosinophilic cytoplasm

- Some tumors show varying degrees of neuroectodermal differentiation with rosette-like configuration (peripheral PNET)

ANCILLARY TESTS

- Characterized by translocations that fuse *EWSR1* to gene of ETS family of transcription factors
- 85% of cases have t(11;22)(q24;q12), resulting in *EWSR1-FLI1* gene fusion
- 5-10% of cases have t(21;22)(q22;q12), resulting in *EWSR1-ERG* gene fusion
- Strong and diffuse membranous immunoreactivity for CD99
- Diffuse nuclear staining for FLI-1

TOP DIFFERENTIAL DIAGNOSES

- Neuroblastoma, alveolar rhabdomyosarcoma, small cell carcinoma, lymphoma, and poorly differentiated synovial sarcoma

Ewing Sarcoma Infiltrating Thyroid Follicles

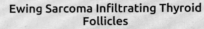
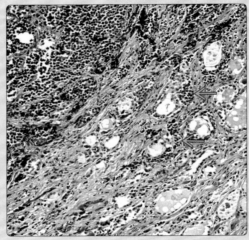

Ewing Sarcoma of Thyroid

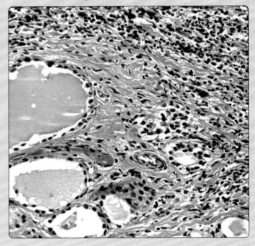

(Left) Monotonous populations of small round blue cells of Ewing sarcoma are observed in this low-power H&E-stained section. The tumor is infiltrating thyroid follicles ➡. (Right) H&E shows a primary thyroid Ewing sarcoma with tumor cells destroying thyroid parenchyma. The tumor cells have scant, often clear cytoplasm and small nuclei.

Conventional Ewing Sarcoma

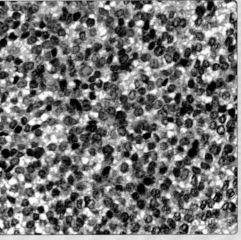

CD99 in Ewing Sarcoma

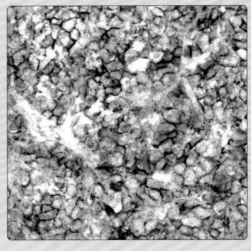

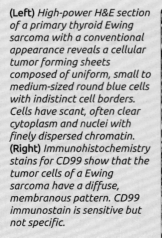

(Left) High-power H&E section of a primary thyroid Ewing sarcoma with a conventional appearance reveals a cellular tumor forming sheets composed of uniform, small to medium-sized round blue cells with indistinct cell borders. Cells have scant, often clear cytoplasm and nuclei with finely dispersed chromatin. (Right) Immunohistochemistry stains for CD99 show that the tumor cells of a Ewing sarcoma have a diffuse, membranous pattern. CD99 immunostain is sensitive but not specific.

TERMINOLOGY

Abbreviations
- Ewing sarcoma (ES)

Synonyms
- Primitive neuroectodermal tumor (PNET)
- Carcinomas of thyroid with Ewing family tumor element

Definitions
- Translocation-associated thyroid small round blue cell tumor
  - ES family tumors include intraosseous ES, extraosseous ES, and peripheral PNETs

CLINICAL ISSUES

Epidemiology
- Incidence
  - Extremely rare primary tumor in thyroid with ~ 15 reported cases

Presentation
- Painless, rapidly enlarging neck mass

Treatment
- Complete surgical resection: Total thyroidectomy
- Risk-tailored treatment
  - Neoadjuvant and adjuvant chemotherapies &/or radiotherapy for control of primary site and possible metastatic disease

Prognosis
- 5-year overall survival
  - Localized disease: 65-75%
  - Initially metastatic disease: < 30%
  - Survival rates are slightly better for head and neck cases
    - Possibly due to earlier detection
- For localized tumors resected after induction chemotherapy
  - Histologic response is strongest independent prognostic factor
- Initial tumor size is strong prognostic factor
- In head and neck, patient age and disease stage have been shown to be important prognostic factors

IMAGING

General Features
- MR shows heterogeneously T2-enhancing mass
- CT shows heterogeneous mass with rim of enhancement
- Limited case reports of thyroid: Ultrasound reveals heterogeneous hypervascular solid nodule

MACROSCOPIC

General Features
- Gray-white, soft, often lobulated, cut surfaces
- Frequent areas of necrosis and hemorrhage
- Treated tumors can show sclerosis and reparative changes

MICROSCOPIC

Histologic Features
- Conventional ES
  - Sheets and nests of densely cellular, monotonous-appearing cells with indistinct cell borders
  - Uniform cells with relatively small round nuclei with finely dispersed chromatin and scant, clear (abundant collagen) to eosinophilic cytoplasm
  - Periodic acid-Schiff stain is often positive
    - Not useful in differential diagnosis
  - Some tumors show varying degrees of neuroectodermal differentiation with rosette-like configuration (peripheral PNET)
    - No consistent prognostic difference from conventional ES
- Atypical variant has been described
  - Similar low-power architecture with larger cells, nuclei with irregular contours and conspicuous nucleoli
  - Immunophenotypic and molecular features similar to those of conventional ES
  - No prognostic importance
- Rare adamantinoma-like ES family of tumors described in head and neck (2 in thyroid)
  - Shares histological features with conventional ES
  - Additional characteristics include
    - Complex epithelial differentiation
    - Histological &/or immunophenotypic evidence of squamous differentiation
  - Round cell malignancies with strong keratin positivity should have CD99 included in panel
    - Diffuse CD99 positivity in these cases should prompt FISH analysis

ANCILLARY TESTS

Immunohistochemistry
- Strong and diffuse membranous immunoreactivity for CD99
  - Sensitive but not specific
  - Many other small round blue cell tumors are positive
- Diffuse nuclear staining for FLI-1
  - Best used in panel
  - Not as sensitive
    - Limited by low level of expression in some cases and those with variant translocations
  - Not specific
    - Can be seen in lymphomas and endothelial-derived neoplasms
- Keratin positivity seen in up to 30% of tumors
  - Can be diffuse or focal
- Areas with neuroectodermal differentiation show higher expression of neuron-specific enolase
- Strong and diffuse nuclear expression of NKX2.2 seen in ~ 80% of ES cases
  - Might be useful in combination with CD99; combination confers high specificity
  - NKX2.2 is transcription factor that is target gene product of *EWSR1-FLI1* fusion

In Situ Hybridization

- FISH with break-apart probe for *EWSR1* gene (22q12) shows rearrangement
  - Caveat
    - Probe does not distinguish from other tumors harboring *EWSR1* fusions
    - Usually nonissue given properties of entities in differential diagnosis
  - Pitfall
    - FISH could be negative for *EWSR1* rearrangement
    - Classic morphology and immunohistochemical profile should prompt addition testing in these cases

Molecular

- Characterized by translocations that fuse *EWSR1* to gene of ETS family of transcription factors
  - 85% of cases have t(11;22)(q24;q12), resulting in *EWSR1-FLI1* gene fusion
  - 5-10% of cases have t(21;22)(q22;q12), resulting in *EWSR1-ERG* gene fusion
  - Less frequently, *EWSR1* is fused with *FEV and ETV1* or *ETV4*
  - Rare case reports have described other fusions
    - *EWSR1* fused to non-ETS partners
    - *FUS* with ETS transcription factors
    - Given possibility of non-*EWSR1* fusion
      - Cases with classic morphology &/or strong CD99 and FLI-1 immunoreactivity that yield negative FISH result should prompt additional targeted molecular testing

DIFFERENTIAL DIAGNOSIS

Neuroblastoma

- 90% of patients are < 5 years
- CD99(-), frequently synaptophysin and chromogranin (+)
- Neuron-specific enolase positive (sensitive, not specific)
  - Can be positive in ES showing neuroectodermal differentiation
  - Histological correlation is important
- Can have *MYC* amplification

Alveolar Rhabdomyosarcoma

- Alveolar architecture except in solid variant
- Desmin and myogenin (+)
- Can be CD99(+)
  - Shows cytoplasmic pattern rather than membranous as seen in ES
- Characteristic t(2;13) and t(1;13) resulting in *PAX3-FOXO1* and *PAX7-FOXO1* fusions

Small Cell Carcinoma

- Nuclear molding and crush artifact
- Paranuclear dot-like positivity of CK20
- CD99(+)

Lymphoma

- Less cohesive population
- Positive for lymphoid markers
- CD99 and FLI-1 can be positive

Poorly Differentiated Synovial Sarcoma

- Primitive epithelial structures are helpful if present
- Transition to spindle cell pattern is sometimes present and can be helpful
- Majority of cases shows diffuse loss of immunohistochemical expression INI1
- CD99 is often positive
- Characteristic t(X;18) resulting in *SYT1-SSX1* and *SYT1-SSX2* fusions

DIAGNOSTIC CHECKLIST

Pathologic Interpretation Pearls

- Strong and diffuse membranous immunoreactivity for CD99
  - Sensitive, not specific
- Diffuse nuclear staining for FLI-1
- Characterized by translocations that fuse *EWSR1* to gene of ETS family of transcription factors
  - FISH with break-apart probe for *EWSR1* gene (22q12) shows rearrangement

SELECTED REFERENCES

1. Oliveira G et al: EWSR1 rearrangement is a frequent event in papillary thyroid carcinoma and in carcinoma of the thyroid with Ewing family tumor elements (CEFTE). Virchows Arch. 470(5):517-525, 2017
2. Bishop JA et al: Adamantinoma-like Ewing family tumors of the head and neck: a pitfall in the differential diagnosis of basaloid and myoepithelial carcinomas. Am J Surg Pathol. 39(9):1267-74, 2015
3. Chen S et al: Ewing sarcoma with ERG gene rearrangements: a molecular study focusing on the prevalence of FUS-ERG and common pitfalls in detecting EWSR1-ERG fusions by FISH. Genes Chromosomes Cancer. 55(4):340-9, 2015
4. Funakoshi T et al: Application of electron microscopic analysis and fluorescent in situ hybridization technique for the successful diagnosis of extraskeletal Ewing's sarcoma. J Dermatol. 42(9):893-6, 2015
5. Grevener K et al: Management and outcome of Ewing sarcoma of the head and neck. Pediatr Blood Cancer. 63(4):604-10, 2015
6. Antonescu C: Round cell sarcomas beyond Ewing: emerging entities. Histopathology. 64(1):26-37, 2014
7. Eloy C et al: Small cell tumors of the thyroid gland: a review. Int J Surg Pathol. 22(3):197-201, 2014
8. Eloy C et al: Carcinoma of the thyroid with Ewing/PNET family tumor elements: a tumor of unknown histogenesis. Int J Surg Pathol. 22(6):579-81, 2014
9. Shibuya R et al: The combination of CD99 and NKX2.2, a transcriptional target of EWSR1-FLI1, is highly specific for the diagnosis of Ewing sarcoma. Virchows Arch. 465(5):599-605, 2014
10. Somarouthu BS et al: Multimodality imaging features, metastatic pattern and clinical outcome in adult extraskeletal Ewing sarcoma: experience in 26 patients. Br J Radiol. 87(1038):20140123, 2014
11. Chan JM et al: Ewing sarcoma of the thyroid: report of 2 cases and review of the literature. Head Neck. 35(11):E346-50, 2013
12. Chirila M et al: Extraosseous Ewing sarcoma and peripheral primitive neuroectodermal tumor of the thyroid gland: case report and review. Ear Nose Throat J. 92(4-5):E3-6, 2013
13. Elbashier SH et al: Cytokeratin immunoreactivity in Ewing sarcoma/primitive neuroectodermal tumour. Malays J Pathol. 35(2):139-45, 2013
14. Yang F et al: [Four cases of extraskeletal Ewing's sarcoma in the head and neck and literature review.] Lin Chung Er Bi Yan Hou Tou Jing Wai Ke Za Zhi. 27(18):1000-2, 1005, 2013
15. Maldi E et al: Extra-osseous Ewing sarcoma of the thyroid gland mimicking lymphoma recurrence: a case report. Pathol Res Pract. 208(6):356-9, 2012
16. Adapa P et al: Extraosseous Ewing sarcoma of the thyroid gland. Pediatr Radiol. 39(12):1365-8, 2009
17. Chung CH et al: Extraskeletal Ewing sarcoma mimicking a thyroid nodule. Thyroid. 16(10):1065-6, 2006
18. Castellino S et al: Ewing's tumor and papillary adenocarcinoma of the thyroid in a 14-year-old girl. J Pediatr Hematol Oncol. 20(2):177-80, 1998
19. Donhuijsen-Ant R et al: [Thyroid tumor as leading symptom in Ewing's sarcoma.] Dtsch Med Wochenschr. 103(21):907, 1978

Ewing Sarcoma in Sheets

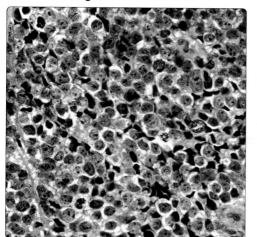

FLI-1 in Ewing Sarcoma

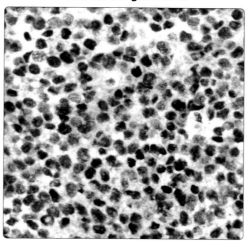

(Left) High-power H&E view of Ewing sarcoma reveals sheets of monotonous blue cells. A small number of darker cells are observed, likely undergoing apoptosis (as evident with electron microscopy studies). (Right) Diffuse nuclear immunostaining of FLI-1 can be seen ~ 80% of cases of Ewing sarcoma with sensitivity limited by occasional low levels of expression and variant translocations.

Ewing Sarcoma Cytology

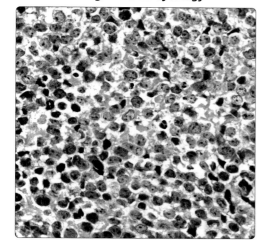

Variation in Cellular Appearance

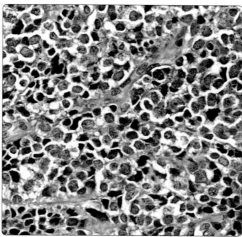

(Left) High-power view of a thyroid Ewing sarcoma shows a finely granular nuclear pattern nuclei with finely dispersed chromatin. Some nuclei have small nucleoli. Apoptotic bodies are often observed. Cells have scant, often clear cytoplasm. (Right) High-power H&E view of Ewing sarcoma reveals sheets of blue cells in a diffuse pattern. Ewing sarcoma cytology can show a spectrum with some cases having larger cells with irregular nuclear contours. Mitoses are readily identified.

Nodular Growth Pattern

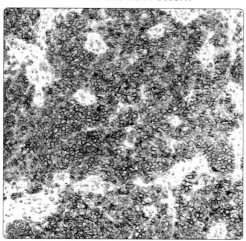

Keratin in Ewing Sarcoma

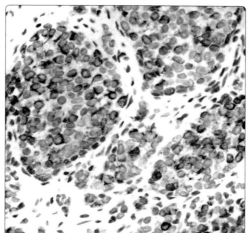

(Left) Low-power view of immunohistochemical stain for CD99 shows a membranous pattern. This immunostain highlights the nodular growth pattern of this Ewing sarcoma. (Right) Ewing sarcoma can occasionally be positive for keratins, as depicted here. The stain is cytoplasmic, in a fibrillary pattern, with focal perinuclear accumulation of keratin.

Secondary Tumors, Thyroid

ETIOLOGY/PATHOGENESIS

- Thyroid identified as site for metastasis in ~ 24% of autopsies
- Metastases to thyroid corresponds to < 0.2% of thyroid malignancies and are most commonly seen
  o Clear cell renal cell carcinoma (RCC)
  o Adenocarcinoma of lung
  o Adenocarcinoma of breast
  o Adenocarcinoma of colon
- Tumor-to-tumor metastases
  o Abnormal thyroid (as seen in adenomas, hyperplasias, and inflammations) have greater predisposition for metastatic seeding
- Head and neck SCC, as direct extension
  o SCC of larynx is most common primary to spread by direct extension

MICROSCOPIC

- Morphology depends on primary source

- Metastatic tumors commonly less differentiated but still retain morphology of original tumor
- On tumor-to-tumor metastases, malignant metastatic glands and single cells (donor tumor) dispersed within thyroid neoplasm (recipient tumor)

ANCILLARY TESTS

- In challenging cases, immunohistochemistry can be useful
- Thyroid-specific antibodies: Thyroglobulin, TTF-1 and pax-8
- Nonthyroidal markers: other primary site-specific markers
  o e.g.: Napsin-A, CDX2, ER/PR/HER2, CD10, HMB45, Melan-A, RCC

TOP DIFFERENTIAL DIAGNOSES

- Primary carcinomas of thyroid
- Primary thyroid lesions with clear cell changes
- Anaplastic thyroid carcinoma
- Direct extension from adjacent tumors

Metastatic Renal Cell Carcinoma

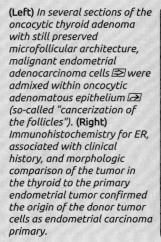
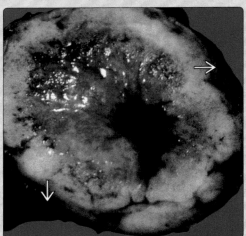

(Left) Cut surface of a metastatic renal cell carcinoma to thyroid shows near-complete replacement of the gland with only a rim of normal thyroid parenchyma ➡ present. (Right) Metastatic poorly differentiated carcinoma to the thyroid shows the interface between tumor ➡ and normal thyroid. There is central comedo-type necrosis ➡.

Metastatic Carcinoma

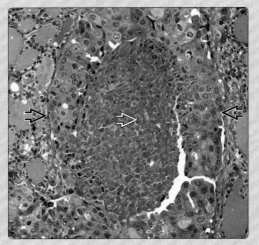

Tumor-to-Tumor Metastasis

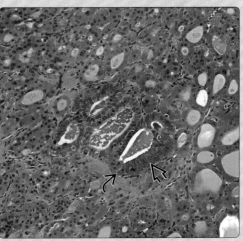

(Left) In several sections of the oncocytic thyroid adenoma with still preserved microfollicular architecture, malignant endometrial adenocarcinoma cells ➡ were admixed within oncocytic adenomatous epithelium ➡ (so-called "cancerization of the follicles"). (Right) Immunohistochemistry for ER, associated with clinical history, and morphologic comparison of the tumor in the thyroid to the primary endometrial tumor confirmed the origin of the donor tumor cells as endometrial carcinoma primary.

ER Positivity in Metastases

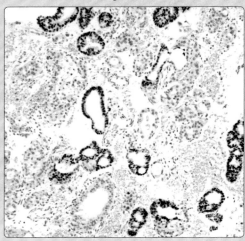

TERMINOLOGY

Synonyms

- Metastatic tumors to thyroid

Definitions

- Secondary tumors of thyroid gland are tumors that arise in thyroid gland by direct extension from adjacent structures or by vascular spread from nonthyroidal sites (WHO 2017)
  - Thyroid tumors resulting from hematogenous or lymphatic spread of distant neoplasm

ETIOLOGY/PATHOGENESIS

Preexisting Thyroid Pathology

- Thyroid gland relatively vascular and may harbor metastases at higher frequency than other organs
- Some studies suggest that abnormal thyroid (as seen in adenomas, hyperplasias, and inflammations) has greater predisposition for metastatic seeding
  - Despite extremely rich vascularization, metastatic tumors to thyroid uncommon

Tumor-to-Tumor Metastasis

- Rare occurrence
  - Unique case of endometrial endometrioid adenocarcinoma metastatic to thyroid Hürthle cell adenoma 9 years after initial diagnosis was reported
    - Histology of thyroid showed malignant endometrioid glands and single cells (donor tumor) were dispersed within Hürthle cell adenoma (recipient tumor)
    - In several sections of adenoma with still preserved microfollicular architecture, malignant endometrial adenocarcinoma cells were admixed within oncocytic adenomatous epithelium (so-called "cancerization of follicles")
    - Molecular analysis of both metastatic and primary endometrial tumors demonstrated PIK3CA and PTEN mutations in both tumors
      - ☐ Characteristic of well-differentiated endometrioid tumors of endometrium
  - Case of malignant phyllodes tumor metastasizing to Hürthle cell adenoma of thyroid was also reported
    - Histologically, thyroid tumor was composed of 2 distinct types of cellular proliferation
    - There were atypical spindle cells were infiltrating between Hürthle cell cords and follicles in fibrosarcomatous pattern
    - Battery of immunohistochemical stains was applied to both thyroid and breast tumors for comparison
  - 2 cases of renal cell carcinoma (RCC) metastatic to Hürthle cell adenoma and follicular adenoma were reported
    - Total thyroidectomy revealed Hürthle cell adenoma containing clusters of cytologically atypical cells with clear cytoplasm
    - Although carcinoma of kidney is responsible in most instances of metastatic disease to thyroid, metastatic RCC to thyroid neoplasm extremely rare

Primary Sources (Carcinomas)

- Thyroid identified as site for metastasis in ~ 24% of autopsies

- Metastases to thyroid corresponds to < 0.2% of thyroid malignancies
- Most common primary tumors are
  - Clear cell RCC
  - Adenocarcinoma of lung
  - Adenocarcinoma of breast
  - Adenocarcinoma of colon
  - Head and neck SCC, as direct extension
    - SCC of larynx is most common primary to spread by direct extension
- Less common are metastases from
  - Esophagus [adenocarcinoma and squamous cell carcinoma (SCC)]
  - Uterine SCC
  - Pancreas
  - Prostate
  - Stomach
- Tumor-to-tumor metastases

Noncarcinoma Sources

- < 15%
  - Melanoma
    - Thyroid metastasis is rare occurrence with cutaneous melanoma and even more uncommon with uveal melanoma
  - Leiomyosarcoma
  - Secondary lymphoma

CLINICAL ISSUES

Epidemiology

- Incidence
  - Data in literature shows ~ 24% of autopsy patients who died of widespread metastatic disease
  - Clinically detectable lesions much less frequent
- Age
  - Tend to occur with advancing age (> 60 years old)
- Sex
  - Thyroid metastases more common in females (F:M = 1.2:1)

Site

- Predominantly seen in larger vessels at periphery of thyroid

Presentation

- Most patients asymptomatic
- Palpable mass
- Compressive signs (dyspnea, dysphagia, hoarseness)
- Rarely, symptoms of transitional hyperthyroidism due to destruction of gland and hormonal release can be seen

Natural History

- Some lesions (especially when kidney is primary source) may occur long time after primary diagnosis
  - Cases occurring up to 26 years after discovery of original tumor have been reported
- As in any thyroid nodule, FNA diagnostic procedure of choice

Treatment

- Thyroidectomy shown to have potential benefit in select patients

○ Solitary lesions usually treated with surgical approach

Prognosis

- When thyroid metastases clinically recognized, long-term survival reported to be dismal

MACROSCOPIC

General Features

- In clinical series, usually solitary masses
- In autopsy series, usually multifocal lesions
- Multinodular metastases may be mistaken by multinodular hyperplasia
- If primary is from adjacent structure, gross extension from primary site

Size

- Up to 15 cm in diameter

MICROSCOPIC

Histologic Features

- Morphology depends on primary source
- Metastatic tumors commonly less differentiated but still retain morphology of original tumor
- When metastases mimic follicular structures, it may be difficult to differentiate from primary neoplasm
- Tumors with clear cell changes most challenging to identify as metastases
  ○ RCCs and some breast carcinomas
- Correlation with clinical history crucial
- Immunohistochemistry will enable correct diagnosis
- On tumor-to-tumor metastases, malignant metastatic glands and single cells (donor tumor) are dispersed within thyroid neoplasm (recipient tumor)

ANCILLARY TESTS

Immunohistochemistry

- In challenging cases, immunohistochemistry can be useful with thyroid-specific markers and nonthyroidal markers
- Thyroid-specific antibodies
  ○ pax-8
  ○ TTF-1
- Nonthyroidal markers
  ○ Napsin-A for lung
  ○ Renal cell antigens and other markers for kidney
  ○ ER/PR for breast
  ○ HMB45 and others for melanoma
  ○ CDX2 for colonic and other GI tumors

DIFFERENTIAL DIAGNOSIS

Primary Carcinomas of Thyroid

- Immunoreactivity for pax-8, TTF-1, and thyroglobulin expected
  ○ If metastatic lung cancer suspected, thyroglobulin should always be used due to positivity of TTF-1 in pulmonary adenocarcinomas and some small cell carcinomas

Primary Thyroid Lesions With Clear Cell Changes

- Follicular neoplasms, papillary carcinoma, medullary carcinoma, and paraganglioma presenting with clear cells should be distinguished from metastatic RCC
- Features like rich vascularity and glandular lumina filled with red blood cells favor diagnosis of metastatic RCC

Direct Extension from Adjacent Tumors

- Clinical and radiological correlation necessary to exclude invasion of thyroid from contiguous neoplasms

Anaplastic Thyroid Carcinoma

- Usually weakly positive for TTF-1
- pax-8 positive: May rule out malignancy from lung or larynx

DIAGNOSTIC CHECKLIST

Clinically Relevant Pathologic Features

- Metastatic carcinoma to thyroid should be always considered in patients with known primary tumor, particularly in cases of widespread disease

Pathologic Interpretation Pearls

- Immunohistochemistry studies key in these cases

SELECTED REFERENCES

1. Bayraktar Z et al: Metastasis of renal cell carcinoma to the thyroid gland 9 years after nephrectomy: A case report and literature review. Arch Ital Urol Androl. 89(2):151-153, 2017
2. Kim YJ et al: Multiple metastasis of follicular variant of papillary thyroid carcinoma coexistent with malignant melanoma. Korean J Intern Med. ePub, 2017
3. Valero-Torres A et al: Metastatic melanoma with papillary features: A mimic and possible diagnostic pitfall. Am J Dermatopathol. 39(6):468-470, 2017
4. Afrogheh AH et al: Molecular characterization of an endometrioid endometrioid adenocarcinoma metastatic to a thyroid Hürthle cell adenoma showing cancerization of follicles. Endocr Pathol. 27(3):213-9, 2016
5. Collins DC et al: A rare thyroid metastasis from uveal melanoma and response to immunotherapy agents. Case Rep Oncol Med. 2016:6564094, 2016
6. McDonnell KJ et al: A novel BAP1 mutation is associated with melanocytic neoplasms and thyroid cancer. Cancer Genet. 209(3):75-81, 2016
7. Stevens TM et al: Tumors metastatic to thyroid neoplasms: a case report and review of the literature. Patholog Res Int. 2011:238693, 2011
8. DeLellis R et al: Pathology and Genetics of Tumours of Endocrine Organs. 1st ed. World Health Organization Classification of Tumours. Lyon, France: IARC Press, 2004
9. Koo HL et al: Renal cell carcinoma metastatic to follicular adenoma of the thyroid gland. A case report. Acta Cytol. 48(1):64-8, 2004
10. Qian L et al: Renal cell carcinoma metastatic to Hurthle cell adenoma of thyroid. Ann Diagn Pathol. 8(5):305-8, 2004
11. Giorgadze T et al: Phyllodes tumor metastatic to thyroid Hürthle cell adenoma. Arch Pathol Lab Med. 126(10):1233-6, 2002
12. Chen H et al: Clinically significant, isolated metastatic disease to the thyroid gland. World J Surg. 23(2):177-80; discussion 181, 1999
13. Lam KY et al: Metastatic tumors of the thyroid gland: a study of 79 cases in Chinese patients. Arch Pathol Lab Med. 122(1):37-41, 1998
14. Nakhjavani MK et al: Metastasis to the thyroid gland. A report of 43 cases. Cancer. 79(3):574-8, 1997

Renal Cell Carcinoma

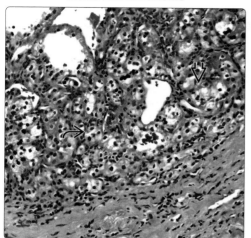

RCA in Metastatic Clear Cell RCC

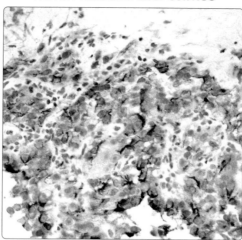

(Left) *Metastatic renal cell carcinoma to the thyroid shows clear cells* ⇗ *and prominent vasculature* ⇗. *Primary thyroid tumors with clear cell features should be considered in the differential diagnosis.* (Right) *Clear cell neoplasms of the thyroid include primary thyroid carcinoma and metastatic clear cell tumors from other sites, including clear cell renal cell carcinoma (RCC) of the kidney. Immunoreactivity for renal cell antigen (RCA) by the tumoral cells is seen in this example of metastatic RCC.*

Thyroglobulin-Negative Tumor

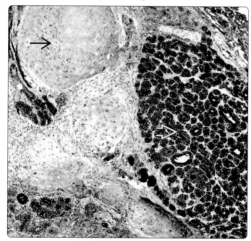

Breast Carcinoma

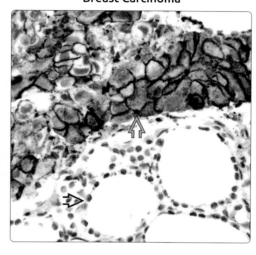

(Left) *Low-power view of a metastatic, poorly differentiated adenocarcinoma shows negativity of the tumor cells for thyroglobulin. Tireoglobulin highlights the normal thyroid follicles* ⇗, *whereas the neoplastic cells* ⇗ *are negative.* (Right) *A tumor embolus* ⇗ *within thyroid parenchyma* ⇗ *is shown in this example of metastatic breast carcinoma, highlighted by HER2 immunohistochemistry.*

Tumor-to-Tumor Metastasis

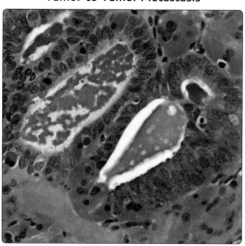

Tumor-to-Tumor Metastasis

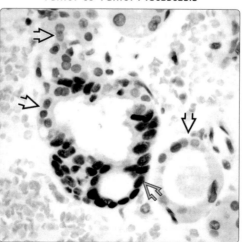

(Left) *Tumor-to-tumor metastasis is rare. H&E shows a unique case of endometrial endometrioid adenocarcinoma metastatic to a thyroid Hürthle cell adenoma. On histologic examination of the thyroid, the malignant endometrioid glands (donor tumor) were dispersed within the adenoma (recipient tumor).* (Right) *Oncocytic follicular adenoma* ⇗ *with endometrial carcinoma is better seen on estrogen receptor (ER) immunohistochemical stain. The endometrioid cells* ⇗ *are positive for ER.*

TERMINOLOGY

Abbreviations

- Protein kinase B (AKT)
- Extracellular signal-regulated kinase (ERK)
- Hereditary medullary thyroid carcinoma (hMTC)
- Mitogen-activated protein kinase (MAPK)
- Multiple endocrine neoplasia (MEN) syndromes (MEN2, including MEN2A and MEN2B)
- Mammalian target of rapamycin (mTOR)
- Papillary thyroid carcinoma (PTC)
- Phosphatidylinositol 3-kinase protein (P13K)
- Receptor tyrosine kinase (RTK)
- Differentiated thyroid carcinoma (DTC)

Genes Discussed

- *BRAF*: v-raf murine sarcoma viral oncogene homolog B1
- *CTNNB1*: Gene that codes for β-catenin protein
- *PAX8/PPARG* (PPARγ): Rearrangement generating fusion product involving **pa**ired bo**x8** transcription factor and **p**eroxisome **p**roliferator-**a**ctivated **r**eceptor **g**amma 1 genes
- *PIK3CA*: Oncogene that codes for PI3K protein
- *PTEN*: Phosphatase and tensin homolog
- *RAF*: Rapidly accelerated fibrosarcoma
- *RET*: Rearranged during transfection proto-oncogene
- *RAS*: Rat sarcoma oncogene
- *RET/TAS2R38* (PTC): Fusion genes containing intact tyrosine kinase domain of *RET* fused to several unrelated genes
- *TP53*: Tumor suppressor gene that encodes p53 protein
- *NTRK1*: Encodes high-affinity nerve growth factor (NGF) receptor and is activated through MAPK pathway

COMMON MOLECULAR CHANGES IN THYROID ONCOGENESIS

Overview of Pathways to Thyroid Carcinogenesis

- Current understanding of thyroid oncogenesis suggests at least 3 major pathways leading to thyroid cancer

- o *BRAF* mutations, *RET/TAS2R38* translocations, and, to lesser extent, *RAS* mutations are thought to be early events in PTC oncogenesis
  - o Mutations in *RAS*, *PTEN*, and *PAX8/PPARG* rearrangements are associated with follicular carcinoma tumorigenesis
  - o Changes in β-catenin and p53 are often present in poorly differentiated &/or anaplastic carcinomas and are thought to represent late events in oncogenesis and tumor progression of thyroid carcinomas
- Aberrant activation of MAPK pathway due to mutations or gene rearrangements is most common genetic event in PTC
- Point mutations in *BRAF* or *RAS* genes and *RET/TAS2R38* or *NTRK1* rearrangements are mutually exclusive and identified in > 70% of PTCs
- *NTRK1* rearrangements are found in < 10% of PTCs and result from *NTRK1* gene fusion with different partners
- Genetic changes are found in > 90% of PTC and FTC
- Most thyroid carcinomas carry mutations or gene rearrangements (deletions and translocations) that lead to activation of MAPK or PI3K/AKT cascades and downstream effectors
- Mutations identified in thyroid cancers thought to be mutually exclusive (each tumor carries only 1 of described mutations)

Mitogen-Activated Protein Kinase/Extracellular Signal-Regulated Kinase Pathway

- Most common recurrent molecular events involve point mutations and gene rearrangements that activate MAPK/ERK pathway
- MAPK/ERK cascade integrates extracellular stimuli and intracellular signals from other pathways and modulates gene expression
- MAPK/ERK influences various tumorigenic events, such as cell proliferation, mitosis, survival, apoptosis, motility, and differentiation
- Activation of MAPK/ERK occurs in series by sequential phosphorylation of downstream effectors (e.g., *RET* → *RAS* → *RAF* → *MEK* → *MAPK/ERK*)

(Left) *Genes involved in thyroid carcinogenesis are diverse. In PTC, there is a high frequency of activating somatic alterations of genes encoding effectors in the MAPK pathways (BRAF, RAS, RET, NTRK1). Mutations in members of the PI3K pathways occurs at a lower frequency (PTEN, PIK3CA, AKT1).* **(Right)** *Mutations and rearrangements that activate MAPK/ERK are the most common molecular events in thyroid oncogenesis. The MAPK/ERK and P13K/AKT cascades integrate multiple signals leading to cell growth.*

Genes Involved in Thyroid Tumors

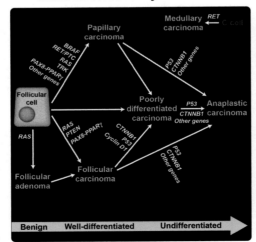

MAPK Pathway

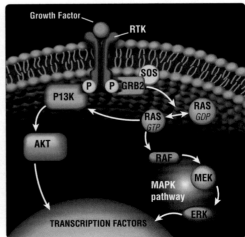

- Diagnostically important molecular markers in MAPK/ERK pathway include *RET*, *RAS*, and *RAF* genes

Phosphatidylinositol 3-Kinase Protein/Protein Kinase B Pathway

- Overactive in many cancers leading to cell proliferation and loss of apoptosis
- PI3K is activated through coupled G protein and growth factor receptors leading to production of phosphatidylinositol-triphosphate (PIP3)
- PIP3 recruits and activates AKT, which in turn stimulates mTOR to block apoptosis and promote protein synthesis and cell growth
- *PI3K* activation of AKT is inhibited by tumor suppressor gene, *PTEN*
- *PI3K* and *MAPK* can both be regulated by *RAS*, which is common activator of these parallel cascades

RET

- *RET* proto-oncogene, located on chromosome 10q11.2, encodes tyrosine kinase receptor
- *RET* protein is usually expressed in cells derived from neural crest, and gain-of-function mutations are associated with MTC
- *RET* is receptor tyrosine kinase (RTK) that activates multiple signaling pathways, including MAPK/ERK, PI3K/AKT, and phosphorylation of β-catenin
- Most commonly mutated RTK in thyroid tumors
- *RET* normally expressed in parafollicular cells or C cells
- Clinically relevant *RET* mutations tend to cluster in 2 hotspots
  - Extracellular cysteine-rich region
    - Mutations lead to ligand-independent constitutive activation of *RET*
  - Intracellular tyrosine kinase domain
    - Mutations lead to increased catalytic activity
- Mutations in *RET* can be somatic or represent germline inherited diseases, such as MEN2 and hMTC
- Germline *RET* mutations
  - MEN2A
    - Extracellular mutations in cysteine-rich region
    - Exon 10 codons 609, 611, 618, and 620
    - Exon 11 codons 630 and 634
  - MEN2B
    - Mutations in tyrosine kinase domain
    - Met918Thr in 95% of cases
    - Ala883Phe and mutations in codons 804, 805, and 806 reported
  - hMTC
    - Common mutations involve codons 321, 533, 768, 790, 791, 804, and 891
  - Timing of prophylactic thyroidectomy is guided by specific mutations present
- Somatic *RET* mutations
  - Present in up to 60% of sporadic MTC
  - Met918Thr is most common mutation

RET/TAS2R38

- Fusion transcripts that arise from translocations that juxtapose promoter from unrelated gene with kinase domain of *RET*
  - Resulting fusion proteins have constitutive ligand-independent activation of RET kinase activity and its downstream effectors
- *RET* is prone to rearrangements with multiple partner genes (13 identified to date)
- *RET/PTC1*, *RET/PTC2*, and *RET/PTC3* account for > 80% of rearrangements seen in PTC
- Observed in ~ 13-43% of cases
  - *RET/PTC1* comprises up to 60% of rearrangements and is derived from intrachromosomal rearrangement (10q), leading to fusion of RET tyrosine kinase domain to *H1ST1H4F* (H4) gene
  - *RET/PTC3* accounts for 20-30% of rearrangements and is formed by *RET* gene fusion with nuclear receptor coactivator 4 (*NCOA4* or ELE1) gene
  - *RET/TAS2R38* rearrangements occur most frequently in pediatric population and may confer increased susceptibility to cancer upon radiation exposure
- Translocations of *RET/TAS2R38* are thought to be early oncogenic events in thyroid carcinoma
- Tumors harboring *RET/TAS2R38* rearrangements rarely associated with progression to poorly differentiated or anaplastic carcinomas

PTEN

- Tumor suppressor gene that antagonizes PI3K by converting PIP3 back to its diphosphate form
- Loss of function mutations and deletions of *PTEN* are commonly seen in glioblastomas and prostate, lung, breast, and endometrial cancers
- Causes of *PTEN*-hamartoma tumor syndromes
  - Cowden syndrome (hamartomas and increased propensity to breast, thyroid, endometrial, and renal cancers)
  - Bannayan-Riley-Ruvalcaba syndrome, Proteus syndrome, and Proteus-like syndrome
- Several genetic alterations have been described in thyroid tumorigenesis and progression

β-catenin

- Pathway that regulates cell adhesion, division, growth, and differentiation
- Point of convergence that integrates multiple signals downstream of *RET*, MAPK/ERK, and PI3K/AKT cascades to promote cell proliferation
- *RET/TAS2R38* fusion proteins stimulate β-catenin by direct interaction and indirectly via RAS/MAPK and PI3K/AKT stimulation
- Mutations in *CTNNB1* seen in advanced thyroid tumors correlate with β-catenin nuclear localization and poor prognosis

PAX8/PPARG

- *PPARG* is ligand-dependent nuclear transcription factor highly expressed in adipose tissue, where it plays critical role in adipocyte differentiation and fat metabolism regulation
- Thyroid-specific transcription factor (*PAX8*) gene is involved in regulation of important thyroid iodine transporter and may play role in acquired resistance to iodine therapy
- *PAX8* gene is critical regulator of thyroid differentiation and growth

- Fusion gene results from translocation between chromosomes 2 and 3, t(2;3)(q13;p25)
- Follicular adenomas and carcinomas have been shown to have lower frequency rates of *PAX8/PPARG* rearrangements
  o Suggests that this chromosomal translocation may be involved in early phases of neoplastic process of FTC and PTC, possibly even in premalignant lesions
- Transfection studies of *PAX8/PPARG* in thyroid follicular epithelial cells have demonstrated accelerated growth rates and lower number of cells in G0/G1 resting state

TP53

- Tumor suppressor gene that encodes p53 protein and controls cell cycle, apoptosis, and DNA repair
- Mutations of *TP53* are considered late events in thyroid carcinogenesis associated with loss of differentiation markers and accelerated growth
- Point mutations in *TP53* are present in 15-30% of poorly differentiated carcinomas and up to 80% of anaplastic carcinomas
- Exons 5-8 most commonly involved

NTRK1

- Neurotrophic tyrosine kinase receptor, type 1 (*NTRK1*) gene, located on chromosome 1, encodes high-affinity nerve growth factor (NGF) receptor and is activated through MAPK pathway
- *NTRK1* rearrangements are found in < 10% of PTCs and result from *NTRK1* gene fusion with different partners
- *NTRK1* rearrangements are associated with younger age at diagnosis and less favorable outcome
- Experimental evidence suggests that *NTRK1* oncogene represents early event in process of thyroid carcinogenesis

Distribution of Genetic Changes in Thyroid Carcinomas

- Genetic changes in PTC
  o *BRAF* mutations: 45%
    – BRAFV600E is oncogenic protein with markedly elevated kinase activity that overactivates MAPK pathway
    – Presence of *BRAF* mutations in micro-PTC (~ 40%) and some benign tumors suggests role of this alteration in early stages of PTC development
    – *BRAF* mutations are typically identified in classic and tall cell variant of PTC
    – Associated with more aggressive tumor behavior
  o *RAS* mutations: ~ 15%
    – *RAS* gene mutations are found in 10-43% of PTCs, particularly in follicular variant
    – *RAS*-mutated PTC is usually encapsulated with low rate of lymph node metastasis
  o *RET/TAS2R38* translocation: 13-43%
    – *RET/TAS2R38* rearrangements are 2nd most common genetic alteration described in PTC
    – Observed in up to 43% of cases
    – Mostly identified in pediatric tumors or in individuals exposed to ionizing radiation from nuclear accidents
    – Over 12 types of *RET/TAS2R38* rearrangements have been reported

- *RET/PTC1* comprises up to 60% of rearrangements and exhibits classic papillary morphology
- *RET/PTC3* accounts for 20-30% of rearrangements; *RET/PTC3* tumors normally present as solid variant
  o *NTKR1* rearrangement: < 10%
    – *NTRK1* rearrangements are result from *NTRK1* gene fusion with different partners
    – *NTRK1* rearrangements are associated with classic or tall cell variant
  o *PAX8/PPARG* translocation: < 5%
    – *PAX8/PPARG* rearrangement are found in follicular variant of PTC, follicular adenomas, and carcinomas
  o Uncharacterized changes: 10%
- *NTRK1* translocations and fusion
  o *NTRK1* rearrangements are found in < 10% of PTCs: Classic and tall cell variant
- Genetic changes in FC
  o *RAS* mutations
    – Early event in follicular thyroid tumorigenesis
      □ Identified in up to 50% of benign follicular tumors
    – Activating mutations in *RAS* gene are observed in 18-52% of follicular carcinomas and on encapsulated follicular variant of PTCs
    – Associated with tumor dedifferentiation and less favorable prognosis
  o *PAX8/PPARG* translocation: < 10%
    – Patients with FTC harboring *PAX8/PPARG* rearrangement are usually diagnosed at young age
    – Tumors are usually small and may have invasive at presentation
  o Uncharacterized changes: < 10%
- Genetic changes in ATC
  o ATC tumors present significant prevalence of *RAS* (6-55%) and *BRAF* mutations (24-50%)
  o *BRAF* V600E mutation is typically found in ATC tumors, which contain areas of well-differentiated PTC
    – Also identified in poorly differentiated and anaplastic tumor areas
    – *BRAF* mutations may predispose to additional genetic alterations, which in turn activate more aggressive pathways and lead to dedifferentiation
    – Patients with ATCs harboring *BRAF* mutations have higher mortality rate than those with *RAS* or with no identified mutation
  o *RAS* mutations are found in high prevalence in ATCs (6-55%)
  o Several genetic alterations in *PTEN* suppressor gene have been described in ATCs
    – 12% present mutated form, 28% gene silencing, and 69% hypermethylated *PTEN* gene
    – These alterations lead to *PTEN* inactivation by different mechanisms, with role in pathogenesis of follicular, epithelium-derived thyroid carcinomas
      □ Present in most aggressive or undifferentiated tumors and correlate with regions of tumor invasion and metastasis
  o *TP53* mutations are commonly observed in anaplastic carcinomas (~ 70%) and are rarely described in well-differentiated thyroid carcinomas

- *TP53* mutations are late event in tumor progression, and this gene may play critical role in transformation of DTC into anaplastic form
  - Genetic alterations in β-catenin (*CTNNB1*) gene are observed in ~ 65% of thyroid anaplastic tumors
    - Gain-of-function mutations can promote β-catenin nuclear translocation
    - Expression of E-cadherin (component of β-catenin pathway) normally expressed in thyroid tissue is usually absent in ATC
    - Plays pathogenic role in thyroid tumor invasion and regional lymph node metastasis
  - *RET/TAS2R38*, *NTRK*, and *PPARG-PAX8* rearrangements are rarely observed in these undifferentiated tumors

DIAGNOSTIC AND PROGNOSTIC MOLECULAR MARKERS IN THYROID CANCER

BRAF

- Mutations in *BRAF* gene are most common genetic alteration in PTC, occurring in ~ 45% of cases
  - Up to 70% (40-70%) of PTCs carry *BRAF* mutations
- Thymine to adenine transversion at position 1799 (T1799A) leading to valine to glutamic acid substitution at residue 600 (V600E) accounts for > 95% of *BRAF* mutations
- *V600E* mutation renders *BRAF* kinase constitutively active leading to upregulation of MAPK/ERK cascade and its oncogenic effects
- Less common *BRAF* genetic alterations include insertions, deletions, and point mutations
  - Other described alterations include A > G transversion at gene position 1801 (K601E) near 600 residue, fusion with A-kinase anchor protein 9 (*AKAP9*) gene, and small in-frame insertions or deletions around codon 600
  - Rearrangement of *BRAF/AKAP9* has been associated with radiation-induced PTCs
- Prevalence of *BRAF* mutation in PTCs correlates with histological variant
  - Tall cell variant: 80%
  - Classic papillary: 60%
  - Hobnail variant: 57%
  - Columnar cell variant: 33%
  - Follicular variant: 10%
- V600E is also present in poorly differentiated and anaplastic carcinomas arising from PTC
- Present in malignant struma ovarii (67%)
- *BRAF* mutant tumors tend to show aggressive behavior, including invasive borders, extrathyroidal extension, advanced stage at presentation, and node or distant metastasis
- V600E not found in follicular carcinomas and benign thyroid nodules

RAS

- *RAS* genes encode highly related G-proteins, which play central role in intracellular signal transduction by activation of MAPK and other signaling pathways, such as PI3K/AKT
  - 3 members constitute human *RAS* gene family: *HRAS*, *KRAS*, and *NRAS*
- *RAS* activates MAPK/ERK via stimulation of *BRAF*
- Mutations that lead to constitutional activation of *RAS* deregulate certain functions, such as cell proliferation, adhesion, migration, differentiation, and apoptosis leading to cancer and metastasis
- Mutations involving codon 61 of *NRAS* and *HRAS* are most common in thyroid tumors
- Distribution of *RAS* mutations in thyroid neoplasms
  - Conventional-type follicular carcinomas: 40-50%
  - Conventional-type follicular adenomas: 20-40%
  - Oncocytic carcinomas: 15-20%
  - Oncocytic adenomas: Up to 4%
  - Papillary carcinoma: 15-20%
    - PTCs carrying *RAS* mutations show follicular variant histology with less prominent nuclear features and low rate of lymph node metastases
    - *RAS*-mutated PTC tends to be encapsulated and exhibits low rate of lymph node metastasis
- *RAS* mutations in follicular carcinomas may be associated with tumor dedifferentiation, metastases, and poor prognosis

RET/TAS2R38

- *RET* protein is usually expressed in cells derived from neural crest
- Gain-of-function mutations are associated with MTC
- In PTC, genomic rearrangements juxtapose *RET* tyrosine kinase domain to unrelated genes, thereby creating dominantly transforming oncogenes, so-called *RET/TAS2R38*
- *RET/TAS2R38* rearrangements are 2nd most common genetic alteration described in PTC
- Characteristics of *RET/PTC*(+) cancers
  - Present at young age
  - Papillary tumors harboring *RET/PTC1* rearrangement commonly exhibit classic papillary histology, whereas *RET/PTC3* tumors normally present solid variant
    - *RET/PTC1* tumors: Associated with classic PTC morphology and benign clinical course
    - *RET/PTC3* tumors: Correlated with solid variant morphology and aggressive behavior
  - Frequent metastasis to lymph nodes
- *RET/TAS2R38* distribution in PTC
  - 10-20% of sporadic adult cases
  - Up to 80% of PTC associated with radiation exposure
  - Up to 70% in young adults and children
  - Specificity of *RET/TAS2R38* to diagnose PTC remains controversial in part due to differences in sensitivity of detection methods and variations in amount and distribution of *RET/TAS2R38* rearrangements within tumor
- *RET/TAS2R38* is commonly detected by RT-PCR and FISH analysis

PAX8/PPARG

- Present in < 10% of follicular carcinomas
- Also present in follicular variants of PTC and follicular adenomas
- Not diagnostic of malignancy but warrants exhaustive search for capsular invasion
- Characteristics of *PAX8/PPARG*(+) tumors
  - Present at younger age
  - Small size

Common Molecular Changes in Thyroid Tumors

	Follicular Adenoma	Follicular Carcinoma	PTC, Follicular Variant	PTC, Classic and Tall Cell	Poorly Differentiated Carcinoma	Anaplastic Thyroid Carcinoma
BRAF V600E				(+++)	(+)	(+)
BRAF K601E	(+)	(+)	(+++)			
NRAS	(++)	(++)	(+++)		(+)	(+)
HRAS	(+)	(+)	(++)			
KRAS	(++)	(+)	(++)	(+)		
PTEN	(++)	(+)				
TSHR	(++)					
GNAS	(++)					
RET/PTC				(+++)		
PAX8/PPRγ		(++)	(++)			
ALK fusions			(+)	(+)	(++)	(++)
BRAF fusions			(+)	(+)		
ETV6/NTRK				(++)		
NTRK fusions				(++)		

PTC = papillary thyroid carcinoma.

- o Often show vascular invasion

Other

- Markers of aggressive thyroid cancer includes
  - o TP53 mutations: 25-30%
  - o PIK3CA mutation: 10-20%
  - o CTNNB1 mutation: 10-20%
  - o AKT1 mutation: 5-10%
  - o TERT promoter mutations: 7-22% PTC and 35% FTC

SELECTED REFERENCES

1. Seethala RR et al: Clinical and morphologic features of ETV6-NTRK3 translocated papillary thyroid carcinoma in an adult population without radiation exposure. Am J Surg Pathol. ePub, 2017
2. Gertz RJ et al: Mutation in BRAF and other members of the MAPK pathway in papillary thyroid carcinoma in the pediatric population. Arch Pathol Lab Med. 140(2):134-9, 2016
3. Giordano TJ: Follicular cell thyroid neoplasia: insights from genomics and The Cancer Genome Atlas research network. Curr Opin Oncol. 28(1):1-4, 2016
4. Haugen BR et al: 2015 American Thyroid Association Management Guidelines for adult patients with thyroid nodules and differentiated thyroid cancer: The American Thyroid Association Guidelines Task Force on Thyroid Nodules and Differentiated Thyroid Cancer. Thyroid. 26(1):1-133, 2016
5. Nikiforov YE et al: Nomenclature revision for encapsulated follicular variant of papillary thyroid carcinoma: a paradigm shift to reduce overtreatment of indolent tumors. JAMA Oncol. 2(8):1023-9, 2016
6. Poller DN et al: Non-invasive follicular thyroid neoplasm with papillary-like nuclei: reducing overtreatment by reclassifying an indolent variant of papillary thyroid cancer. J Clin Pathol. ePub, 2016
7. Tong GX et al: Targeted next-generation sequencing analysis of a pendred syndrome-associated thyroid carcinoma. Endocr Pathol. 27(1):70-5, 2016
8. Graham ME et al: Serum microRNA profiling to distinguish papillary thyroid cancer from benign thyroid masses. J Otolaryngol Head Neck Surg. 44:33, 2015
9. Johnson JM et al: Mitochondrial metabolism as a treatment target in anaplastic thyroid cancer. Semin Oncol. 42(6):915-22, 2015
10. Lin Z et al: Association of cancer stem cell markers with aggressive tumor features in papillary thyroid carcinoma. Cancer Control. 22(4):508-14, 2015
11. Nikiforov YE et al: Impact of the multi-gene thyroSeq next-generation sequencing assay on cancer diagnosis in thyroid nodules with atypia of undetermined significance/follicular lesion of undetermined significance cytology. Thyroid. 25(11):1217-23, 2015
12. Werner RA et al: Prognostic value of serum tumor markers in medullary thyroid cancer patients undergoing vandetanib treatment. Medicine (Baltimore). 94(45):e2016, 2015
13. Zhou GJ et al: MicroRNAs as novel biomarkers for the differentiation of malignant versus benign thyroid lesions: a meta-analysis. Genet Mol Res. 14(3):7279-89, 2015
14. Cancer Genome Atlas Research Network: integrated genomic characterization of papillary thyroid carcinoma. Cell. 159(3):676-90, 2014
15. Romitti M et al: Signaling pathways in follicular cell-derived thyroid carcinomas (review). Int J Oncol. 42(1):19-28, 2013
16. Chen JH et al: Clinicopathological and molecular characterization of nine cases of columnar cell variant of papillary thyroid carcinoma. Mod Pathol. 24(5):739-49, 2011
17. Laury AR et al: Thyroid pathology in PTEN-hamartoma tumor syndrome: characteristic findings of a distinct entity. Thyroid. 21(2):135-44, 2011
18. Nosé V: Familial thyroid cancer: a review. Mod Pathol. 24 Suppl 2:S19-33, 2011
19. Smith JR et al: Thyroid nodules and cancer in children with PTEN hamartoma tumor syndrome. J Clin Endocrinol Metab. 96(1):34-7, 2011
20. Zhang Y et al: Endocrine tumors as part of inherited tumor syndromes. Adv Anat Pathol. 18(3):206-18, 2011
21. Nosé V: Thyroid cancer of follicular cell origin in inherited tumor syndromes. Adv Anat Pathol. 17(6):428-36, 2010
22. Nucera C et al: B-Raf(V600E) and thrombospondin-1 promote thyroid cancer progression. Proc Natl Acad Sci U S A. 107(23):10649-54, 2010
23. Sadow PM et al: Absence of BRAF, NRAS, KRAS, HRAS mutations, and RET/PTC gene rearrangements distinguishes dominant nodules in Hashimoto thyroiditis from papillary thyroid carcinomas. Endocr Pathol. 21(2):73-9, 2010
24. Nucera C et al: A novel orthotopic mouse model of human anaplastic thyroid carcinoma. Thyroid. 19(10):1077-84, 2009
25. Nucera C et al: FOXA1 is a potential oncogene in anaplastic thyroid carcinoma. Clin Cancer Res. 15(11):3680-9, 2009
26. Nikiforova MN et al: MicroRNA expression profiling of thyroid tumors: biological significance and diagnostic utility. J Clin Endocrinol Metab. 93(5):1600-8, 2008
27. Xing M: Recent advances in molecular biology of thyroid cancer and their clinical implications. Otolaryngol Clin North Am. 41(6):1135-46, ix, 2008
28. Schmidt J et al: BRAF in papillary thyroid carcinoma of ovary (struma ovarii). Am J Surg Pathol. 31(9):1337-43, 2007
29. Ciampi R et al: Oncogenic AKAP9-BRAF fusion is a novel mechanism of MAPK pathway activation in thyroid cancer. J Clin Invest. 115(1):94-101, 2005
30. French CA et al: Genetic and biological subgroups of low-stage follicular thyroid cancer. Am J Pathol. 162(4):1053-60, 2003

FISH for *PAX8/PPARG* Rearrangement

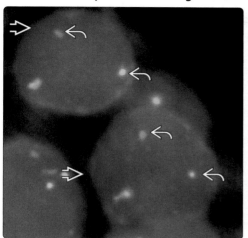

β-Catenin Accumulation

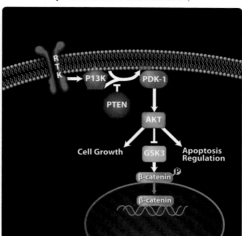

(Left) *Two cells* ⇛ *in this thyroid specimen show PAX8/PPARG rearrangement, seen in < 15% of FTC and in follicular variant of papillary carcinoma. A FISH break-apart probe was used. Rearrangement is shown as separate red and green signals* ⇗. (Right) *Ligand binding to RTK activates PI3K, which causes phosphorylation of AKT, stimulating cell growth. PTEN inhibits PI3K signaling. AKT inhibits GSK3, leading to decreased β-catenin turnover. β-catenin accumulation leads to further cell growth and resistance to apoptosis.*

RET Mutations in Medullary Carcinoma

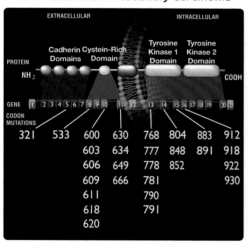

Pathways in Papillary Carcinoma

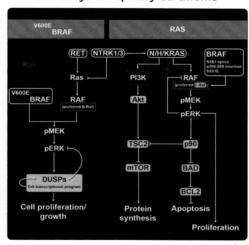

(Left) *RET is a tyrosine kinase receptor often mutated in MTC. Activating point mutations are in 2 hotspots: The extracellular cysteine-rich domain (MEN2A) and the intracellular tyrosine kinase domain (MEN2B). Guidelines for treatment and prophylactic thyroidectomy are dictated by the specific mutation.* (Right) *This graphic shows 2 distinct pathways in PTC and the downstream signaling of BRAF-like and RAS-like pathways. MAPK and PI3K pathways are differentially activated in the BRAF-like and RAS-like PTC.*

RET/PTC Fusion in Papillary Carcinoma

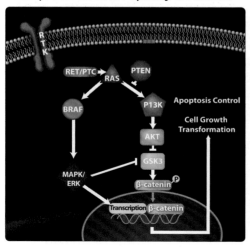

Progress in Discovery of Mutations

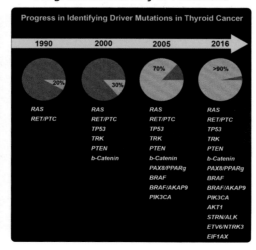

(Left) *RET/PTC fusion proteins are constitutively active independently of RTK ligand binding. RET/PTCs activate RAS, which, in turn, can cause parallel activation of MAPK, PI3K, and β-catenin signaling.* (Right) *In PTC, there is a high frequency of activating somatic alterations of genes encoding effectors in the MAPK signaling pathways and phosphoinositide 3-kinase (PI3K) pathways. Today, with the new discoveries, over 90% of the PTC have driving somatic genetic alterations.*

TERMINOLOGY FOR DEFINITIONS, STAGING, AND CANCER PROTOCOLS

- Thyroid carcinomas are malignant neoplasms that can arise from either follicular or calcitonin-producing C cells
- 2017 WHO classification of thyroid carcinomas divides these tumors based on their histologic types
  - Papillary thyroid carcinoma (PTC) and its variants
  - Follicular thyroid carcinoma (FTC) and its variants
  - Poorly differentiated thyroid carcinoma
  - Undifferentiated (anaplastic) thyroid carcinoma
  - Medullary thyroid carcinoma
- Use of cancer protocol for incidental papillary thyroid microcarcinoma ≤ 1 cm is recommended
- For resection specimens, TNM stage is based on macroscopic assessment of size, presence, or absence of extrathyroidal extension and metastases
  - T1: Tumor ≤ 2 cm in greatest dimension, intrathyroidal
    - T1a: Tumor ≤ 1 cm in greatest dimension, intrathyroidal
    - T1b: Tumor > 1 cm, but ≤ 2 cm in greatest dimension, intrathyroidal
  - T2: Tumor > 2 cm, but ≤ 4 cm in greatest dimension, intrathyroidal
  - T3: Tumor > 4 cm intrathyroidal or gross extrathyroidal extension invading only strap muscles
    - T3a: Tumor > 4 cm intrathyroidal
    - T3b: Gross extrathyroidal extension invading only strap muscles (sternohyoid, sternothyroid, thyrohyoid, or omohyoid muscles) from tumor of any size
  - T4: Includes gross extrathyroidal extension beyond strap muscles
    - T4a: Gross extrathyroidal extension invading subcutaneous soft tissues, larynx, trachea, esophagus, or recurrent laryngeal nerve from tumor of any size
    - T4b: Gross extrathyroidal extension invading prevertebral fascia or encasing carotid artery or mediastinal vessels from tumor of any size

Thyroid Carcinoma, pT1a and pT1b

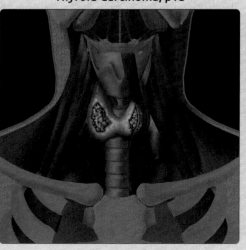

Thyroid Carcinoma, pT2

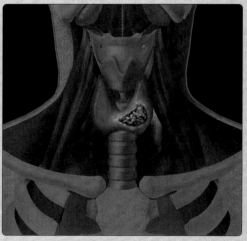

(Left) Coronal graphic shows T1 bilateral thyroid carcinomas, which are confined to the thyroid gland. One tumor is called microcarcinoma because it is < 1 cm (L) (T1a). The presence of bilateral disease is given an "m" designation in the staging system to represent multiple tumors. (Right) Coronal graphic shows a T2 thyroid carcinoma defined as > 2 cm but ≤ 4 cm and confined to the thyroid gland.

Thyroid Carcinoma, pT3

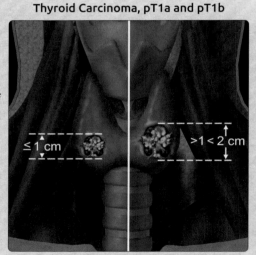

Thyroid Carcinoma, pT4a

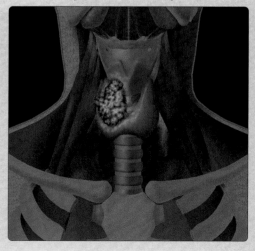

(Left) Coronal graphic shows a T3 thyroid carcinoma, > 4 cm and limited to the thyroid (T3a) or any tumor with minimal extrathyroid extension (e.g., extension to sternothyroid muscle or perithyroid soft tissues) (T3b). The lesion in the left lobe involves the muscle (T3b). (Right) Coronal graphic shows a T4a thyroid carcinoma. These lesions can be any size, extending beyond the thyroid gland macroscopically to invade into subcutaneous soft tissues, larynx, trachea, esophagus, or recurrent laryngeal nerve.

Thyroid Carcinoma, pT4b

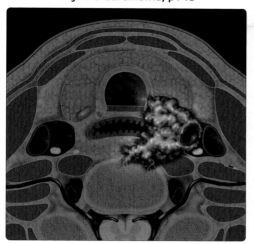

Thyroid Tumors With Invasion Into Adjacent Structures

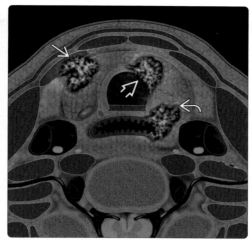

(Left) *Axial graphic shows a T4b thyroid carcinoma, which is defined as any size tumor invading the prevertebral fascia or encasing the carotid artery or mediastinal vessels.* (Right) *Axial graphic shows 3 separate tumors within the thyroid gland. The right lobe tumor ➡ shows extrathyroidal soft tissue invasion. The anterior left lobe tumor ➡ shows larynx invasion. The posterior left lobe tumor ➡ shows esophagus involvement.*

Thyroid Tumors at Different Tumor Stages

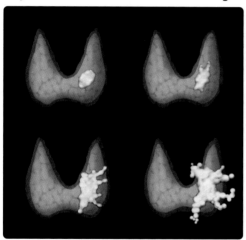

Left Thyroid Lobe Tumor With Metastases to Lymph Nodes

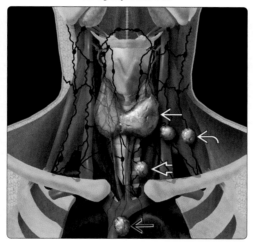

(Left) *Coronal graphics (top row) show T1a (≤ 1 cm) and T1b (> 1 cm but not > 2 cm) thyroid carcinomas, which are confined to the thyroid gland. Bottom row shows T2 (> 2 cm but not > 4 cm and confined to the thyroid) and T3 (> 4 cm and limited to the thyroid or any tumor with minimal extrathyroid extension).* (Right) *Coronal graphic shows a left lobe thyroid carcinoma ➡ with multiple paratracheal ➡, low jugular ➡, and superior mediastinal ➡ lymph node metastases.*

Thyroid Gland Location and Relationship With Adjacent Structures

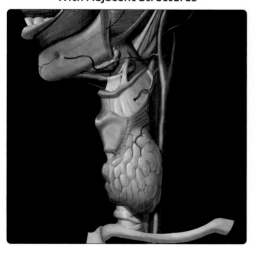

Thyroid Gland and Parathyroid Gland Anatomic Location

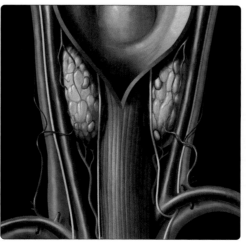

(Left) *Sagittal graphic highlights the left lobe of the thyroid gland and its relationship to the tracheal cartilages, membranes, and vessels of the neck. These anatomic landmarks are helpful in the staging of tumors.* (Right) *Coronal posterior graphic demonstrates the anatomic position of the thyroid gland lobes along with the embedded parathyroid glands. The relationship to the larynx and vessels, along with the nerves, is illustrated.*

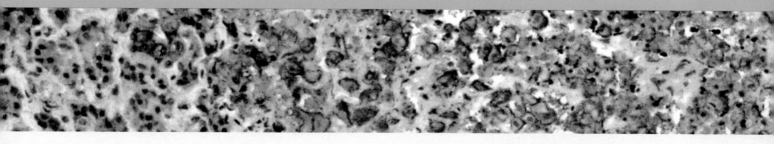

SECTION 2
Parathyroid Gland

Primary Chief Cell Hyperplasia

TERMINOLOGY

- Absolute increase in parathyroid parenchymal mass resulting from proliferation of chief cells, oncocytes, and transitional cells in multiple parathyroid glands in absence of recognized stimulus for parathyroid hormone secretion

CLINICAL ISSUES

- 20% of primary parathyroid hyperplasia associated with multiple endocrine neoplasia type 1 (MEN1) (consider genetic testing)

MACROSCOPIC

- At least 2 enlarged glands; only subset of cases show diffuse enlargement of all 4 glands

MICROSCOPIC

- Nodular (most) or diffuse increase in parathyroid parenchymal cells
- Chief cells most prominent but can have mix of oncocytic, transitional, and clear cells

- Nodular areas composed of pure populations of cells
- Decrease in adipocytes, more adipocytes in internodular and diffuse areas
- Rim of normal compressed parathyroid tissue can be seen in hyperplasia
- Occasional mitosis, fibrosis, and hemosiderin but lacks invasive growth

ANCILLARY TESTS

- Positive for parathyroid hormone (PTH), chromogranin, synaptophysin, keratin (CAM5.2)
- Negative for TTF-1 and thyroglobulin

TOP DIFFERENTIAL DIAGNOSES

- Normal parathyroid
- Parathyroid adenoma
- Secondary or tertiary parathyroid hyperplasia
- Primary clear cell hyperplasia
- Parathyroid carcinoma

Parathyroid Hyperplasia

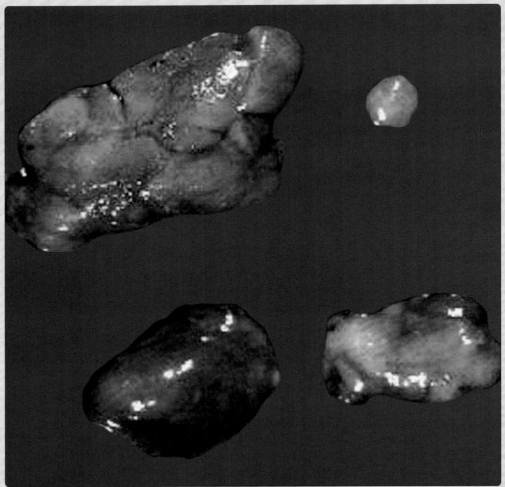

Asymmetric hyperplasia or pseudoadenomatous variant shows marked variation in extent of glandular involvement, easily confused with adenoma or multiple adenomas. This gross photograph of 4 parathyroid glands in a case of parathyroid hyperplasia shows marked asymmetry in size in a patient with multiple endocrine neoplasia type 1 (MEN1).

TERMINOLOGY

Synonyms

- Nodular hyperplasia
- Diffuse hyperplasia
- Multiple adenomatosis
- Multiglandular parathyroid tumors

Definitions

- Absolute increase in parathyroid parenchymal mass resulting from proliferation of chief, oxyphil, and transitional cells in multiple parathyroid glands in absence of recognized stimulus for parathyroid hormone (PTH) secretion

ETIOLOGY/PATHOGENESIS

Sporadic

- Etiology of sporadic primary hyperplasia is unclear

Familial

- Hereditary hyperparathyroidism is less common than primary sporadic hyperparathyroidism
  o 5-25% of cases
- Most common hereditary hyperparathyroidism includes
  o Multiple endocrine neoplasia type 1 (MEN1), MEN2A, familial hypocalciuric hypercalcemia (FHH), neonatal severe primary hyperparathyroidism, hyperparathyroidism-jaw tumor (HPT-JT) syndrome, and familial isolated hyperparathyroidism
- **MEN1**
  o Autosomal dominant, high penetrance, germline mutation *MEN1* tumor suppressor gene (11q13)
    – *MEN1* encodes menin protein (truncated with *MEN1* mutation)
    – Sporadic MEN1 cases due to new mutations
    – > 400 distinct germline mutations in *MEN1*
    – Germline inactivation of one allele of *MEN1* gene confers tumor susceptibility
    – Most syndromic tumors have somatic mutation or deletion of 2nd wild-type *MEN1* allele
  o MEN1 equally affects females and males; no ethnic or geographic differences
  o MEN1 most common familial cause of primary hyperparathyroidism
  o Primary parathyroid hyperplasia (multiglandular parathyroid tumors) is most common manifestation of MEN1
    – 90% with MEN1 have parathyroid hyperplasia
    – In 1-18% of all primary hyperparathyroidism, patients are found to be MEN1
    – MEN1-associated hyperparathyroidism has onset of 20-25 years of age and affects males and females equally
      □ Sporadic primary hyperparathyroidism typical age of onset ~ 30 years later
    – Parathyroid adenomas and rare report of carcinoma in MEN1 but much less common than hyperplasia
  o Other MEN1 features

    – Endocrine: Pituitary adenomas, neuroendocrine tumor of pancreas, duodenum, thymus, and lung; gastrinomas; adrenal cortical adenomas and hyperplasia
    – Nonendocrine: Angiofibromas, collagenomas, café au lait macules, lipomas, gingival papules, meningiomas, ependymomas, leiomyomas
- **MEN2A**
  o 20-30% associated with parathyroid hyperplasia (or adenomas, rare report of carcinoma)
  o Diagnosed clinically by occurrence of at least 2 specific endocrine tumors (medullary thyroid carcinoma, pheochromocytoma, or parathyroid hyperplasia/adenoma) in individual or close relatives
  o Autosomal dominant, high penetrance, germline *RET* activating protooncogene mutation (10q11.2)
- **Familial isolated hyperparathyroidism**
  o Autosomal dominant
  o 1% of primary hyperparathyroidism
    – Parathyroid is only endocrine organ involved
      □ Parathyroid adenoma or hyperplasia and suggested increased risk of parathyroid carcinoma (but may be due to inclusion of HPT-JT cases)
  o Cause unknown in most families, but *CDC73* (HRPT2), *MEN1*, and area on chromosome 2 implicated
  o Minority of kindreds have germline mutations in *MEN1*, *CDC73* (HRPT2), or *CASR*
  o Clinically defined diagnosis of exclusion in kindred with 2 or more persons with hyperparathyroidism but lacking specific features of MEN1, MEN2A, HPT-JT, or FHH
- **Calcium-sensing receptor (*CASR*) mutation**
  o Calcium-sensing receptors present in parathyroid, kidney, thyroid C cells, intestine, and bone and detect extracellular calcium levels that regulate PTH release
  o Inactivating *CASR* (3q13.3-21) mutation causes decreased calcium sensitivity of parathyroid and kidney and results in PTH-dependent hypercalcemia
  o Homozygous inactivating *CASR* mutations in neonatal severe hyperparathyroidism, a life-threatening disorder with markedly hypercellular, hyperplastic parathyroid glands
  o Activating *CASR* mutations in familial autosomal dominant hypoparathyroidism and familial hypocalcemia
  o Heterozygous inactivating *CASR* mutations in FHH
  o Hypocalciuric hypercalcemia is caused by autoantibodies directed at *CASR* and can simulate FHH
- **HPT-JT**
  o Autosomal dominant, inactivating mutations in putative tumor suppressor gene *CDC73* (HRPT2) (1q21-q31)
    – 80% mutations are truncating (frameshift and nonsense), most involve exon 1
  o *CDC73* (HRPT2) encodes parafibromin/CDC73 protein
  o Disorder of hyperparathyroidism, fibroosseous jaw tumors, kidney cysts, hamartomas, and Wilms tumors
  o 80% of HPT-JT patients present with hyperparathyroidism
  o Penetrance of hyperparathyroidism is 80%
  o Parathyroid adenoma or hyperplasia and increased risk of parathyroid carcinoma
  o Hyperparathyroidism usually develops by late adolescence

- *CDC73*-**Related Disorders**
  - Inactivating mutation tumor suppressor gene *CDC73* (HRPT2) on 1q21-q31
    - CDC73 transcript spans 2.7 kb
    - CDC73 protein binds RNA polymerase II as part of PAF1 transcriptional regulatory complex, mediates H3K9 methylation that silences expression of cyclin-D1
    - CDC73 protein regulates gene expression and inhibits cell proliferation

CLINICAL ISSUES

Epidemiology

- Incidence
  - Primary parathyroid hyperplasia accounts for 15% of primary hyperparathyroidism (parathyroid adenomas = 80-85%; carcinomas = 1%)
  - Incidence increased in past 3 decades with increased calcium screening with multichannel autoanalyzer
  - Parathyroid hyperplasia occurs in 90% of patients with MEN1 and 30% with MEN2A
  - 20% of patients with primary parathyroid hyperplasia have MEN
  - Prevalence of 7% in autopsy study (patients did have elevated serum calcium but no bone disease)
- Age
  - 5th decade but wide range
  - Familial cases occur earlier (often 25 years of age)
- Sex
  - F:M = 2:1
  - Females and males equally affected in familial cases

Site

- In 50% of cases, all 4 parathyroid glands symmetrically enlarged
  - Caution with asymmetric hyperplasia as it can be mistaken for adenoma or double adenomas

Presentation

- Clinical presentation changed from patients presenting with nephrocalcinosis and osteopenia to those presenting today with weakness and lethargy or asymptomatic with elevated screening serum calcium
- Clinically similar to parathyroid adenoma
- During pregnancy may cause
  - Nephrolithiasis, hypertension, preeclampsia, decreased bone mineral density

Laboratory Tests

- Serum calcium elevated but < in parathyroid carcinoma in which calcium often > 13 mg/dL
- Hypophosphatemia

Treatment

- Surgical approaches
  - Subtotal parathyroidectomy with 3 glands removed, leaving vascularized remnant of 4th gland
    - Or total parathyroidectomy with autotransplantation of portion of parathyroid gland into neck or forearm
  - Difficult or impossible to differentiate primary hyperplasia from adenoma based only on histologic examination of 1 gland

  - Rapid intraoperative PTH measurements decrease risk of missing multiglandular disease and help confirm removal of diseased parathyroid gland(s)
  - Residual tissue may become hyperplastic, requiring additional surgery

MACROSCOPIC

Normal Parathyroid Gland

- Size and shape of kidney bean (4-6 mm x 2-4 mm), 20-40 mg each
- Most people have 4 parathyroid glands, 10% have ≥ 5, and 3% have < 4 parathyroid glands

Primary Parathyroid Hyperplasia

- 50% show symmetric enlargement of all 4 glands, although others report that in 2/3 of cases, only 2 glands appeared enlarged
- Asymmetric hyperplasia or pseudoadenomatous variant of hyperplasia with marked variation in extent of glandular involvement is easily confused with adenoma or multiple adenomas
- MEN1-associated hyperplasia/multiglandular disease often asymmetric
- Surgeons and pathologists must be cautious in evaluating parathyroid glands in relation to size and cellularity, as these parameters can vary greatly within single patient with parathyroid hyperplasia
  - Asymmetrically enlarged gland can be misinterpreted as parathyroid adenoma
- Occult pattern of involvement may show subtle enlargement and subtle microscopic features of hyperplasia (difficult to differentiate from normal)
- Cystic change not uncommon

MICROSCOPIC

Histologic Features

- **Normal parathyroid gland**
  - Can show significant variation in cellularity even in single individual
  - Normal parathyroid cellularity variable, distributed unevenly, high in infants and children, decreases with age
  - Age, gender, constitutional factors (body fat), etc. affect cellularity of normal parathyroid glands
  - Stromal fat constitutes 10-30% of parathyroid, increases with age
  - More stromal fat in polar regions of parathyroid than centrally
- **Constituent cells of parathyroid gland**
  - Parathyroid glands composed of chief, transitional, and oxyphil cells and adipose tissue
  - Chief cells: 10 μm, polyhedral, round central nuclei, eosinophilic to amphophilic cytoplasm, fat droplets (adults), well-defined cytoplasmic membranes
  - Oxyphil cells: 10-20 μm, abundant eosinophilic cytoplasm, appear at puberty, increase with age, and may form nodules
  - Transitional cells: Smaller parenchymal cells with less cytoplasm

- Clear/water-clear cells: Parenchymal cells with clear cytoplasm (may be due to increased vacuolization in chief or oxyphilic cells)
- **Primary parathyroid hyperplasia histology**
  - Increase in parenchymal cell mass of multiple parathyroid glands
  - Chief cell is predominant, but oxyphil, transitional, and clear cells may be present
  - Sporadic and hereditary forms of primary hyperplasia histologically indistinguishable
    - Parathyroid hyperplasia in MEN1 usually involves increased numbers of chief cells that may have nodular or diffuse pattern
    - MEN1-associated hyperplasia often asymmetric
  - Hyperplastic chief cells arranged in cords, nests, sheets, or follicular structures
  - Cystic change can be seen
  - Nodular or diffuse growth (nodular is most common pattern in primary hyperplasia)
    - Nodules usually pure populations of chief, oxyphil, or clear cells (less fat in nodules than internodular or diffuse areas)
    - Caution: As oxyphil cells increase with age, may form nodules (do not confuse with hyperplastic gland)
    - Study of sporadic hyperplasia found diffuse growth more prevalent in young with moderate hypercalcemia and moderately enlarged glands with little variability in gland size or morphologic patterns
    - Nodular hyperplasia more frequent in elderly and asymmetric, variable cellularity with more oxyphil cells
    - MEN1 cases usually show increase in chief cells and may have nodular or diffuse growth pattern (often asymmetric hyperplasia)
    - Primary water-clear cell hyperplasia shows increase in clear cells and diffuse rather than nodular growth
  - Stromal fat is decreased, but regional variations in stromal fat even among glands in single individual (pitfall in evaluating small biopsies)
  - Scattered mitotic figures may be seen, but more mitoses and atypical mitoses in carcinoma
  - Cells show slight variation in size and shape
  - Foci of endocrine atypia with pleomorphism and hyperchromasia (more common in adenomas)
  - Rim of normal parathyroid tissue can be seen, although less common than in adenoma
  - Fibrosis and hemosiderin, especially in markedly enlarged glands or glands with cystic degeneration
  - Cystic change uncommon but can be seen in markedly enlarged glands
  - No capsular, vascular, or perineural invasion or invasion into adjacent structures
  - Histologic features in HPT-JT-associated cases similar to sporadic lesions, but HPT-JT cases often cystic
- **Primary parathyroid hyperplasia variants**
  - **Clear (water-clear) cell hyperplasia**
    - Multiple enlarged parathyroid glands associated with hyperplasia with parenchymal cells having abundant vacuolated, clear cytoplasm
    - Not known to be associated with multiple endocrine neoplasia syndromes
    - No malignant potential
  - **Lipohyperplasia**
    - Enlarged parathyroid glands with hyperparathyroidism, but abundant stromal fat of lipohyperplasia (or lipoadenoma) can be confused with normal parathyroid tissue

ANCILLARY TESTS
Frozen Sections
- **Assessing cellularity in small biopsies**
  - Cellularity variable within parathyroid gland and among glands in single individual
  - Polar regions of parathyroid more cellular than central
  - Cellularity increases with age, varies with gender, ethnicity, and body habitus
- **Differentiating parathyroid from thyroid on small biopsies**
  - Parathyroid has well-defined cytoplasmic membranes
  - Cytoplasmic lipid (fat droplets) common in parathyroid parenchymal cytoplasm (not thyroid)
  - Parathyroid cells generally smaller and more vacuolated than thyroid
  - Parathyroid nuclei rounder with denser chromatin than thyroid
  - Parathyroid lacks calcium oxalate crystals of thyroid

Immunohistochemistry
- Positive for chromogranin and synaptophysin
- Positive for keratin (CAM5.2 most helpful keratin for neuroendocrine tumors)
- Positive for parathyroid hormone
- Negative for TTF-1, thyroglobulin, variable calcitonin
- p27, cyclin-dependent kinase inhibitor that helps regulate transition from G1 to S phase of cell cycle, is highest normal parathyroid, followed by hyperplasia, adenoma, and carcinoma
- Ki-67 lower in hyperplasia and adenomas than carcinomas

Genetic Testing
- Parathyroid hyperplasia often polyclonal but monoclonality identified, particularly in nodular areas and in MEN1 (multiglandular parathyroid tumors)
- Specific genetic abnormalities in idiopathic primary parathyroid hyperplasia not as well defined as in hereditary forms of hyperparathyroidism
- *MEN1* **mutation (tumor suppressor gene, 11q13, results in truncated menin protein)**
  - Primary parathyroid hyperplasia (multiglandular parathyroid tumors) is most common manifestation of MEN1 (90% of MEN1 have hyperplasia)
    - Autosomal dominant, high penetrance, germline mutation in *MEN1* tumor suppressor gene (11q13) encodes menin (truncated with *MEN1* mutation)
    - Sporadic MEN1 cases due to new mutations
    - Although classically referred to as parathyroid hyperplasia, recent studies demonstrate clonality (multiglandular parathyroid tumors)
  - Somatic *MEN1* mutations occur in 15-20% of sporadic parathyroid adenomas and some sporadic parathyroid carcinomas

- Genetic diagnosis to identify germline *MEN1* mutations has facilitated appropriate targeting of clinical, biochemical, and radiological screening
- *MEN1* mutation detection rate increases with family history of MEN1
- *MEN1* mutation detection rate increases with the number of MEN1-related tumors and in patients with both parathyroid and pancreatic neuroendocrine tumors

- **RET mutation (protooncogene, 10q21)**
  - *RET* germline activating protooncogene mutation in MEN2A (autosomal dominant, with high penetrance, 95% patients have mutation in exon 10 or 11, codon 634)
    - 20-30% of MEN2A associated with parathyroid hyperplasia or adenoma
  - *RET* mutation is generally not identified in sporadic parathyroid disease

- **Cyclin-D1/CCND1**
  - Encodes cyclin-D1, cell cycle regulator from G1 to S phase
  - Cyclin-D1 overexpression has been observed in hyperplastic parathyroid glands, but lack of definitive correlation limits utility

- **Familial isolated hyperparathyroidism**
  - Cause unknown in most, but *CDC73*, *MEN1*, and area on chromosome 2 implicated

- **CASR**
  - Inactivating *CASR* (3q13.3-21) mutation causes decreased calcium sensitivity of parathyroid and kidney, resulting in PTH-dependent hypercalcemia
  - Heterozygous inactivating *CASR* mutations occur in FHH
    - Homozygous inactivating mutations occur in neonatal severe hyperparathyroidism
    - Activating *CASR* mutations occur in familial autosomal-dominant hypoparathyroidism and familial hypocalcemia
  - *CASR* mutations generally not seen in sporadic parathyroid disease

- *CDC73* (HRPT2) mutation (tumor suppressor gene, 1q21-q31, encodes parafibromin)
  - Germline *CDC73* inactivating mutation in HPT-JT-associated hyperplasia, adenoma, and carcinoma
  - Strong association between *CDC73* mutations and familial and sporadic parathyroid cancer
  - Germline *CDC73* mutations identified in subset of patients with mutation-positive carcinomas

DIFFERENTIAL DIAGNOSIS

Parathyroid Adenoma

- Benign neoplasm composed of chief, oxyphil, transitional, and water-clear cells or mixture of cell types affecting single parathyroid gland
- Difficult/impossible to differentiate primary parathyroid hyperplasia from parathyroid adenoma based only on histologic examination of 1 gland
  - Distinguishing parathyroid adenoma from hyperplasia usually requires examination of at least 1 additional gland, which should be normal
  - Hyperplasia shows enlargement of at least 2 glands, while adenoma typically involves single gland

- Rim of normal tissue in 50-60% of parathyroid adenomas but can occasionally be seen in hyperplasia

Double or Triple Parathyroid Adenoma

- Rare; strongly consider asymmetric hyperplasia before diagnosing multiple adenomas
- Occasional glands of parathyroid hyperplasia may show rims of normal parathyroid tissue (rims not specific for adenomas)
- Diagnosis requires resolution of hypercalcemia and hyperparathyroidism and long-term follow-up to be certain no other glands involved

Primary Clear Cell Hyperplasia

- Diffuse increase in clear cells rather than nodular growth of predominantly chief cells in primary chief cell hyperplasia

Lipohyperplasia

- Rare; can occur as sporadic form and with familial benign hypocalciuric hypercalcemia
- Increase in adipose tissue and myxoid change in parathyroid glands associated with hyperfunction
- Enlarged parathyroid glands with abundant stromal fat can be microscopically confused with normal parathyroid

Secondary Parathyroid Hyperplasia

- Secondary increase in PTH due to hypocalcemia and hyperphosphatemia (renal failure, vitamin D deficiency, pseudohypoparathyroidism, etc.)
- Increased PTH due to low serum calcium caused by
  - Disorders of vitamin D (rickets, vitamin D deficiency, or malabsorption)
  - Disorders of phosphate metabolism (malnutrition or malabsorption, renal disease, aluminum toxicity)
  - Tissue resistance to vitamin D, hypomagnesemia, pseudohypoparathyroidism, and calcium deficiency
- Often, history of chronic renal failure (most common cause of secondary hyperparathyroidism)
- Parathyroid glands show more diffusely hyperplastic changes than in primary hyperparathyroidism
- Chief cells usually predominate, but chief cells and oxyphil cells can form nodular areas
  - Nodularity may increase with increasing renal failure, making glands indistinguishable from primary or tertiary hyperplasia

Tertiary Hyperplasia

- Rare condition in which patients with secondary hyperparathyroidism develop autonomously functioning parathyroid gland

Parathyroid Carcinoma

- Often symptomatic, high serum calcium (> 13 mg/dL)
- Involves 1 parathyroid gland, not multiple (although rare reports of carcinoma arising in setting of hyperplasia, particularly secondary hyperplasia)
- Unequivocal invasion (capsular, vascular, perineural, or invasion into adjacent structures)

Parathyromatosis

- Recurrent hyperparathyroidism after subtotal parathyroidectomy may result from multiple small nests of parathyroid cells in neck or mediastinum from lesional tissue left behind or from stimulation of embryonic nests of parathyroid cells

DIAGNOSTIC CHECKLIST

Clinically Relevant Pathologic Features

- 20% of primary hyperplasia are associated with MEN1
- Mild, nonspecific symptoms or asymptomatic and identified by screening serum calcium

Pathologic Interpretation Pearls

- Normal parathyroid has significant variation in cellularity in and among glands (caution small biopsies)
- Distinguishing parathyroid tissue from thyroid: Well-demarcated cytoplasmic membranes, lack colloid, cytoplasmic lipid, rounder nuclei, denser chromatin
- Symmetric enlargement of all 4 glands only in subset of cases, many show enlargement of < 4 glands
  - Be very cautious in attempting to diagnose multiple adenomas (most likely asymmetric hyperplasia)
- Rims of normal tissue occasionally seen in parathyroid hyperplasia
- Be aware of parathyroid hyperplasia variants (lipohyperplasia and clear cell hyperplasia)

SELECTED REFERENCES

1. Akpinar G et al: Proteomics analysis of tissue samples reveals changes in mitochondrial protein levels in parathyroid hyperplasia over adenoma. Cancer Genomics Proteomics. 14(3):197-211, 2017
2. Alhefdhi A et al: Intraoperative parathyroid hormone levels at 5 min can identify multigland disease. Ann Surg Oncol. 24(3):733-738, 2017
3. Iacobone M et al: Surgical approaches in hereditary endocrine tumors. Updates Surg. 69(2):181-191, 2017
4. Simonds WF: Genetics of hyperparathyroidism, including parathyroid cancer. Endocrinol Metab Clin North Am. 46(2):405-418, 2017
5. Zanocco KA et al: Primary hyperparathyroidism: effects on bone health. Endocrinol Metab Clin North Am. 46(1):87-104, 2017
6. Wilhelm SM et al: The American Association of Endocrine Surgeons Guidelines for Definitive Management of Primary Hyperparathyroidism. JAMA Surg. 151(10):959-968, 2016
7. Alevizaki M et al: Primary hyperparathyroidism in MEN2 syndromes. Recent Results Cancer Res. 204:179-86, 2015
8. Duan K et al: Clinicopathological correlates of hyperparathyroidism. J Clin Pathol. 68(10):771-87, 2015
9. Lassen T et al: Primary hyperparathyroidism in young people. when should we perform genetic testing for multiple endocrine neoplasia 1 (MEN-1)? J Clin Endocrinol Metab. 99(11):3983-7, 2014
10. Thakker RV: Multiple endocrine neoplasia type 1 (MEN1) and type 4 (MEN4). Mol Cell Endocrinol. Epub ahead of print, 2013
11. Williams BA et al: Surgical management of primary hyperparathyroidism in Canada. J Otolaryngol Head Neck Surg. 43(1):44, 2014
12. Ezzat T et al: Primary hyperparathyroidism with water clear cell content: the impact of histological diagnosis on clinical management and outcome. Ann R Coll Surg Engl. 95(3):e60-2, 2013
13. DeLellis RA: Parathyroid tumors and related disorders. Mod Pathol. 24 Suppl 2:S78-93, 2011
14. Zhang Y et al: Endocrine tumors as part of inherited tumor syndromes. Adv Anat Pathol. 18(3):206-18, 2011
15. DeLellis RA et al: Primary hyperparathyroidism: a current perspective. Arch Pathol Lab Med. 132(8):1251-62, 2008
16. DeLellis RA: Tumors of the Parathyroid Gland. AFIP Atlas of Tumor Pathology Series 3, Fascicle 6. Washington DC: American Registry of Pathology, 1-102, 1991
17. Woolner LB et al: Tumors and hyperplasia of the parathyroid glands; a review of the pathological findings in 140 cases of primary hyperparathyroidism. Cancer. 5(6):1069-88, 1952
18. Albright F et al: Hyperparathyroidism due to diffuse hyperplasia of all parathyroid glands rather than adenoma of one. Clinical studies on three such cases. Arch Intern Med. 45:315-29, 1934

Primary Chief Cell Hyperplasia

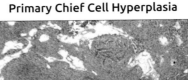

(Left) *Parathyroid hyperplasia shows diffuse increase in chief cells. Diffuse growth can be seen in primary parathyroid hyperplasia but is common in secondary parathyroid hyperplasia.* **(Right)** *Diffuse growth can be seen in primary and secondary parathyroid hyperplasia. Scattered single and small nests of fat cells are identified throughout the gland.*

Diffuse Growth Pattern in Parathyroid Hyperplasia

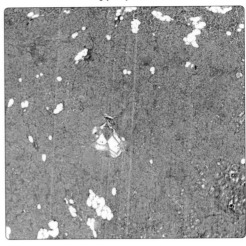

(Left) *Primary parathyroid hyperplasia with a nodular growth pattern is shown. Diffuse growth can also be seen. The nodules are composed of of chief cells ⊡ as well as nodules of oxyphil cells ⊡.* **(Right)** *Primary parathyroid hyperplasia with a nodular pattern of growth is shown.*

Nodular Growth in Parathyroid Hyperplasia

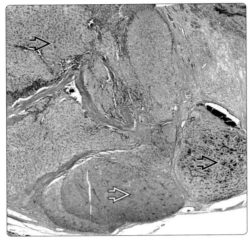

Parathyroid Hyperplasia With Nodular Growth

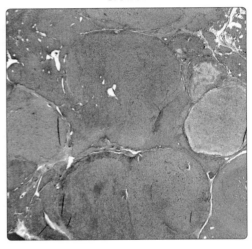

(Left) *A rim of normal-appearing parathyroid tissue ⊡ is frequently seen in parathyroid adenoma; this can occasionally be seen in hyperplastic glands.* **(Right)** *Parathyroid chief cells are the predominant cell type in parathyroid hyperplasia.*

Parathyroid Hyperplasia With Rim-Like Area

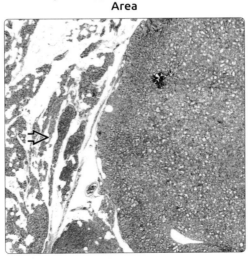

Primary Chief Cell Parathyroid Hyperplasia

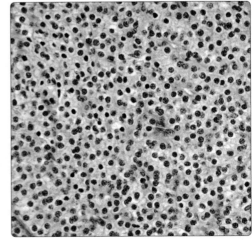

Hyperplastic Parathyroid With Edematous Change

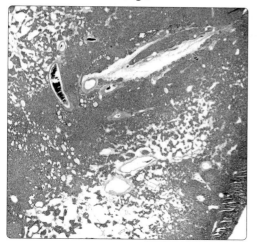

Chief Cell Parathyroid Hyperplasia

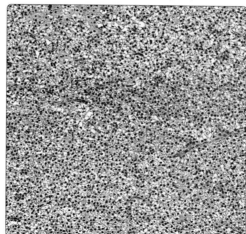

(Left) *Hyperplastic parathyroid with edematous change is shown.* (Right) *This hyperplastic parathyroid gland is composed predominantly of chief cells, but mixtures of chief, oxyphil, transitional, and clear cell types can occur.*

Chief Cell Parathyroid Hyperplasia

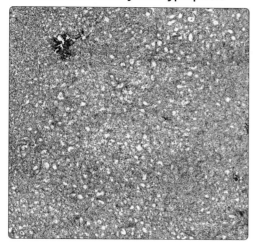

Primary Parathyroid Hyperplasia

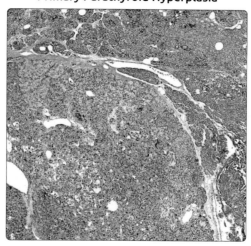

(Left) *Chief cells are the predominant cell in most primary parathyroid hyperplasias, both with a nodular and with a diffuse growth pattern.* (Right) *Primary parathyroid hyperplasia with nodular and diffuse growth is shown.*

Parathyroid Hyperplasia With Fibrosis and Calcification

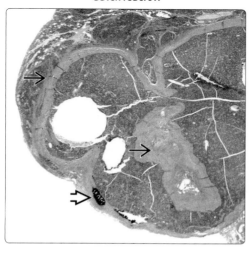

Hemosiderin and Fibrosis in Parathyroid Hyperplasia

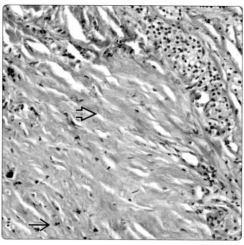

(Left) *Hyperplastic parathyroid gland shows fibrosis ⇨ and calcification ⇨, degenerative features that can be seen in hyperplastic parathyroid glands.* (Right) *Fibrosis ⇨ and hemosiderin ⇨ deposition in parathyroid hyperplasia are shown. Degenerative features can be seen in hyperplastic parathyroid glands, but invasive growth is only seen in parathyroid carcinoma.*

Primary Parathyroid Hyperplasia

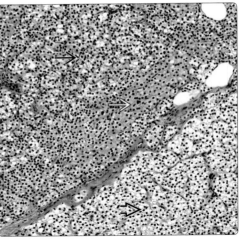

Chief Cells in Parathyroid Hyperplasia

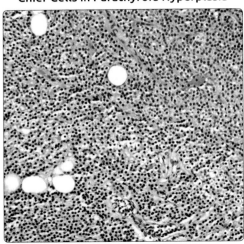

(Left) *Parathyroid gland with a nodular growth pattern shows nodules of chief cells* 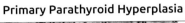, *oxyphil cells* ➡, *and transitional cells* ➨. **(Right)** *Diffuse growth of chief cells in a parathyroid gland involved by primary parathyroid hyperplasia is shown.*

Chief and Oxyphilic Cells in Parathyroid Hyperplasia

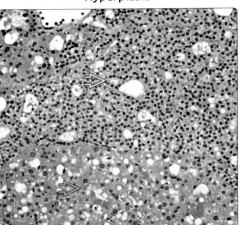

Palisading of Nuclei in Parathyroid Hyperplasia

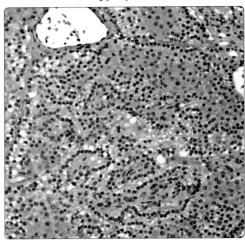

(Left) *Chief* ➨ *and oxyphilic* ➨ *parathyroid cells in a gland involved by primary parathyroid hyperplasia are shown.* **(Right)** *Parathyroid gland shows an area of palisading of nuclei around vascular structures.*

Parathyroid Hyperplasia With Scattered Adipocytes

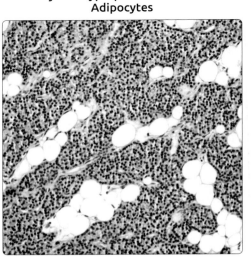

Follicular Structures in Parathyroid Hyperplasia

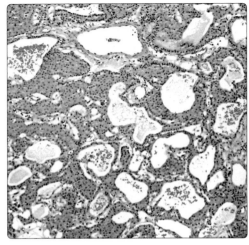

(Left) *Parathyroid hyperplasia shows increase in parathyroid parenchymal cells and scattered single and small groups of adipocytes.* **(Right)** *Parathyroid hyperplasia with follicular/glandular structures is shown.*

Follicular Growth Pattern

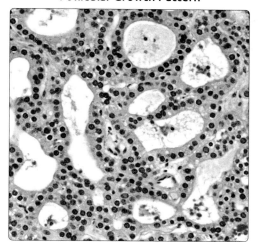

Chief Cells and Oxyphil Cells

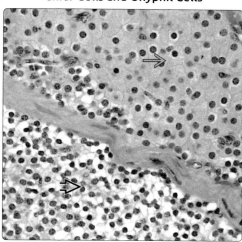

(Left) Follicular/glandular growth pattern is shown in an parathyroid gland in parathyroid hyperplasia. (Right) Chief cells ⇛ and oxyphil cells ⇒ are shown in parathyroid hyperplasia.

Oxyphilic Cells in Parathyroid Hyperplasia

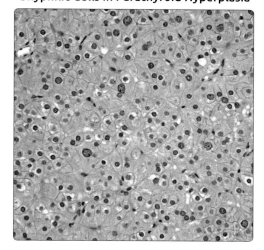

Oxyphilic/Oncocytic Cells

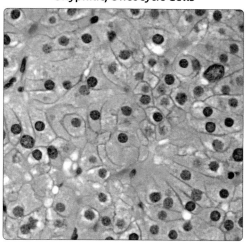

(Left) Hyperplastic parathyroid gland shows predominantly oxyphilic cells. The nuclei are mildly pleomorphic, but markedly increased nuclear:cytoplasmic ratios and mitotic figures are not identified. (Right) High-power view shows oxyphilic cells in parathyroid hyperplasia.

Clear Cell Parathyroid Hyperplasia

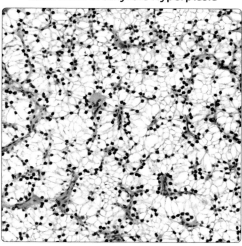

Parathyroid Clear Cells

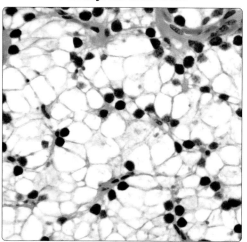

(Left) Clear cell parathyroid hyperplasia shows a diffuse increase in clear (water-clear) cells in multiple parathyroid glands. (Right) Clear cells are identified in this hyperplastic parathyroid gland.

Primary Clear Cell Hyperplasia

TERMINOLOGY

- Absolute increase in parathyroid parenchymal mass resulting from proliferation of clear cells in multiple parathyroid glands in absence of known stimulus for parathyroid hormone secretion

CLINICAL ISSUES

- Extraordinarily rare cause of hyperparathyroidism
- Most cases in historical literature
- No association with multiple endocrine neoplasia
- Patients symptomatic with bone disease and nephrolithiasis (but most cases are generally in historical literature)

MACROSCOPIC

- Usually all 4 glands enlarged, but can be 3 or fewer
- Variation in gland size: Upper glands often larger than lower glands

MICROSCOPIC

- Diffuse growth, can have glandular or tubular pattern
- Well-defined cytoplasmic membranes characteristic feature of parathyroid tissues and helpful in differentiating from thyroid
- Nuclei small, round, hyperchromatic, and may be basally oriented
- Clear cytoplasm composed of numerous small clear vacuoles
- May have cystic structures lined by clear cells
- May show hemorrhage and fibrosis
- Lacks invasive growth

TOP DIFFERENTIAL DIAGNOSES

- Clear cell parathyroid adenoma
- Thyroid tumor with clear cell change
- Metastatic clear cell carcinoma

Diffuse Growth Pattern

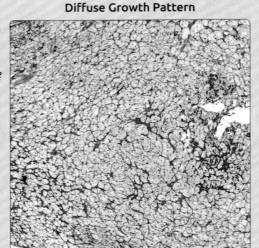

Cells With Clear Cytoplasm

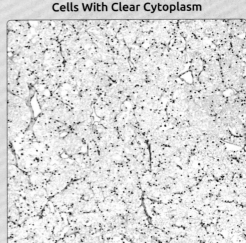

(Left) *Parathyroid gland enlarged with diffuse proliferation of clear cells is shown. Clear cell parathyroid hyperplasia often has a diffuse rather than nodular growth pattern.* (Right) *The glands in primary clear cell parathyroid hyperplasia usually show a diffuse growth pattern, although the cells can show a glandular or tubular growth pattern. This specimen shows sheets of clear cells in a solid diffuse growth pattern.*

Monotonous Cell Proliferation

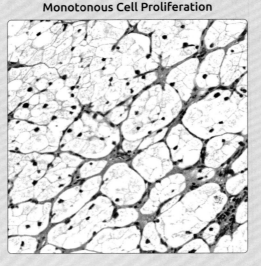

Basally Located Nuclei

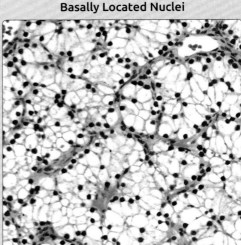

(Left) *Parathyroid gland involved by clear cell parathyroid hyperplasia is shown. Although the cells show clearing on low power, on high power the cytoplasmic appears vacuolated.* (Right) *Clear cell parathyroid adenoma involves only one parathyroid gland, unlike clear cell hyperplasia, which involves multiple glands. In parathyroid lesions, nuclei can be basally located next to stroma and vessels, as demonstrated here.*

TERMINOLOGY

Abbreviations
- Water-clear cell parathyroid hyperplasia (WCCH)

Synonyms
- Water-clear (Wasserhelle) cell parathyroid hyperplasia

Definitions
- Absolute increase in parathyroid parenchymal cells with abundant clear cytoplasm involving multiple parathyroid glands in absence of known stimulus for parathyroid hormone hypersecretion

ETIOLOGY/PATHOGENESIS

Associations
- No familial associations
- Not associated with multiple endocrine neoplasia (MEN)

CLINICAL ISSUES

Epidemiology
- Incidence
  o Extraordinarily rare today (has decreased in incidence)
    – Most described in historical literature
  o Rare cause of hyperparathyroidism

Site
- Multiple parathyroid glands involved

Presentation
- Historically, when most cases were described, patients presented with signs and symptoms of hyperparathyroidism (bone disease, nephrolithiasis)
- Recent case in literature found water-clear cell hyperplasia was not associated with higher biochemical markers or more severe clinical presentations than other types
- Clinical presentation of patients with water-clear cells parathyroid content and hyperparathyroidism is indistinguishable from that of common causes of primary hyperparathyroidism of adenoma or hyperplasia
  o Diagnosis is made only on pathological examination

Treatment
- Surgical approaches
  o Subtotal parathyroidectomy with 3 entire parathyroid glands removed, leaving vascularized remnant of 4th gland
  o Or, total parathyroidectomy with autotransplantation of portion of parathyroid gland into forearm
  o Caution: Difficult to impossible to differentiate hyperplasia from adenoma based on histologic examination of only 1 gland
  o Intraoperative parathyroid hormone (PTH) monitoring
    – Rapid intraoperative PTH measurements have decreased risk of missing multiglandular disease and helped confirm removal of diseased parathyroid glands
  o Clinical follow-up to monitor calcium

IMAGING

General Features
- Ultrasonography shows multilobulated, hypoechoic, well-defined masses
- Technetium sestamibi scanning shows large areas of increased activity

MACROSCOPIC

General Features
- Usually all glands enlarged
- May be variation in size of glands in single patient
- Upper glands may be larger than lower glands
- Pseudopods may extend from glands
- Total gland weights variable (< 10 g to > 100 g)
  o Correlation increased weights with symptoms and calcium levels
- Red-brown or brown; can be cystic, hemorrhagic, fibrosis

MICROSCOPIC

Histologic Features
- In WCCH, individual parathyroids may vary considerably in size and may not all be completely replaced by water-clear cells
- Diffuse growth pattern
- Cells may be in glandular or tubular pattern
- Occasional cystic structures lined by clear cells
- Cells polyhedral, round-ovoid, 15-20 μm (range 10-40 μm)
- Distinct plasma membranes
- Nuclei can be multiple and hyperchromatic
- Nuclei may be at pole of cell (basally located), next to stroma and vessels
- Clear cytoplasm, small cytoplasmic vacuoles (0.8 μm) (likely from Golgi vessels with electron microscopy)
- Lacks invasive growth

ANCILLARY TESTS

Immunohistochemistry
- Positive for chromogranin, synaptophysin, PTH, keratin (CAM5.2)
- Negative for TTF-1 and thyroglobulin

Genetic Testing
- Not extensively studied, not associated with familial hyperparathyroidism (not associated with multiple endocrine neoplasia)

DIFFERENTIAL DIAGNOSIS

Clear Cell Parathyroid Adenoma
- Involves single parathyroid gland, not multiple
- Histologic examination of single parathyroid gland alone not sufficient to differentiate parathyroid adenoma from parathyroid hyperplasia
- May be associated with familial tumor syndromes
  o NF1
  o MEN1

- Distinction between water-clear cell hyperplasia and adenoma may not always be possible owing to incomplete gland replacement by clear cells in hyperplasia or presence of asymmetrical hyperplasia

Parathyroid Lipohyperplasia

- Rare; can occur both as sporadic form and with familial benign hypocalciuric hypercalcemia
- Parathyroid lipohyperplasia shows prominent adipocytes, a feature not seen in clear cell parathyroid hyperplasia

Parathyroid Carcinoma

- Shows invasive growth (capsular, vascular, perineural or invasion into adjacent structures)
- Single parathyroid gland involvement, not multiple

Thyroid Tumor With Clear Cell Change

- Intrathyroidal, positive for TTF-1 and thyroglobulin
- Usually single tumor

Metastatic Clear Cell Carcinoma

- Metastases to parathyroid gland reported, such as from clear cell renal cell carcinoma, but rare and usually involves single gland
- Immunophenotype would be helpful in difficult case

DIAGNOSTIC CHECKLIST

Clinically Relevant Pathologic Features

- Absolute increase in parathyroid parenchymal mass resulting from proliferation of clear cells in multiple parathyroid glands in absence of recognized stimulus for parathyroid hormone secretion
- Extraordinarily rare cause of hyperparathyroidism today
- No association with multiple endocrine neoplasia or other types of familial hyperparathyroidism

Pathologic Interpretation Pearls

- Classic form of WCCH involves all 4 glands
  - Multiple parathyroid glands involved
  - Marked variation in size of glands
    - Usually characterized by increase of upper glands and may reach large sizes before involvement of inferior ones
- Diffuse proliferation of cells with clear cytoplasm, well-defined cell membranes, and often basally oriented nuclei

SELECTED REFERENCES

1. Boutzios G et al: Primary hyperparathyroidism caused by enormous unilateral water-clear cell parathyroid hyperplasia. BMC Endocr Disord. 17(1):57, 2017
2. Caleo A et al: Fine needle cytology pre-surgical differentiation of parathyroid neoplasms: Is it reliable? Cytopathology. ePub, 2017
3. El Hussein S et al: Water clear cell adenoma of the parathyroid gland: A forgotten cause of primary hyperparathyroidism. Int J Surg Pathol. 1066896917701577, 2017
4. Hosny Mohammed K et al: Parafibromin, APC, and MIB-1 are useful markers for distinguishing parathyroid carcinomas from adenomas. Appl Immunohistochem Mol Morphol. ePub, 2016
5. Pirela D et al: Intrathyroidal clear cell tumor of parathyroid origin with review of literature. Case Rep Pathol. 2016:7169564, 2016
6. Murakami K et al: Water-clear cell adenoma associated with primary hyperparathyroidism: report of a case. Surg Today. 44(4):773-7, 2014
7. Ezzat T et al: Primary hyperparathyroidism with water clear cell content: the impact of histological diagnosis on clinical management and outcome. Ann R Coll Surg Engl. 95(3):e60-2, 2013
8. Papanicolau-Sengos A et al: Cytologic findings of a clear cell parathyroid lesion. Diagn Cytopathol. 41(8):725-8, 2013
9. Piggott RP et al: Water-clear cell adenoma: A rare form of hyperparathyroidism. Int J Surg Case Rep. 4(10):911-3, 2013
10. Varshney S et al: Chief cell and clear cell parathyroid adenoma do not influence clinical and biochemical expression of the sporadic primary hyperparathyroidism. Endocrine. 43(2):440-3, 2013
11. Bai S et al: Water-clear parathyroid adenoma: report of two cases and literature review. Endocr Pathol. 23(3):196-200, 2012
12. Kodama H et al: Water-clear cell parathyroid adenoma causing primary hyperparathyroidism in a patient with neurofibromatosis type 1: report of a case. Surg Today. 37(10):884-7, 2007
13. Gill AJ et al: Loss of nuclear expression of parafibromin distinguishes parathyroid carcinomas and hyperparathyroidism-jaw tumor (HPT-JT) syndrome-related adenomas from sporadic parathyroid adenomas and hyperplasias. Am J Surg Pathol. 30(9):1140-9, 2006
14. Prasad KK et al: Water-clear cell adenoma of the parathyroid gland: a rare entity. Indian J Pathol Microbiol. 47(1):39-40, 2004
15. Kuhel WI et al: Synchronous water-clear cell double parathyroid adenomas a hitherto uncharacterized entity? Arch Pathol Lab Med. 125(2):256-9, 2001
16. Bégueret H et al: [Clear cell adenoma of the parathyroid gland: a rare and misleading lesion.] Ann Pathol. 19(4):316-9, 1999
17. Roth SI: Water-clear cell 'adenoma'. A new entity in the pathology of primary hyperparathyroidism. Arch Pathol Lab Med. 119(11):996-7, 1995
18. Hedbäck G et al: Parathyroid water clear cell hyperplasia, an O-allele associated condition. Hum Genet. 94(2):195-7, 1994
19. Kovacs K et al: Large clear cell adenoma of the parathyroid in a patient with MEN-1 syndrome. Ultrastructural study of the tumour exhibiting unusual RER formations. Acta Biol Hung. 45(2-4):275-84, 1994
20. Tominaga Y et al: Histological and clinical features of non-familial primary parathyroid hyperplasia. Pathol Res Pract. 188(1-2):115-22, 1992
21. DeLellis RA: Tumors of the Parathyroid Gland. AFIP Atlas of Tumor Pathology Series 3, Fascicle 6. Washington DC: American Registry of Pathology. 1-102, 1991
22. Persson S et al: Primary parathyroid hyperplasia of water-clear cell type. Transformation of water-clear cells into chief cells. Acta Pathol Microbiol Immunol Scand A. 94(6):391-5, 1986
23. Cheron G et al: [Neonatal primary hyperparathyroidism caused by clear cell hyperplasia.] Pediatrie. 40(1):35-9, 1985
24. Stout LC Jr: Water-clear-cell hyperplasia mimicking parathyroid adenoma. Hum Pathol. 16(10):1075-6, 1985
25. Tisell LE et al: Clinical characteristics and surgical results in hyperparathyroidism caused by water-clear cell hyperplasia. World J Surg. 5(4):565-71, 1981
26. Castleman B et al: Parathyroid hyperplasia in primary hyperparathyroidism: a review of 85 cases. Cancer. 38(4):1668-75, 1976
27. Dorado AE et al: Water clear cell hyperplasia of parathyroid: autopsy report of a case with supernumerary glands. Cancer. 38(4):1676-83, 1976
28. Roth SI: The ultrastructure of primary water-clear cell hyperplasia of the parathyroid glands. Am J Pathol. 61(2):233-48, 1970

Large Clear Cytoplasm

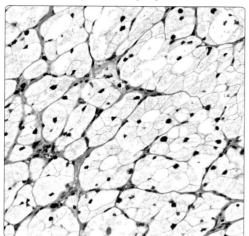

Peripheral Nuclei

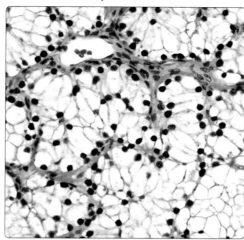

(Left) *This primary clear cell parathyroid hyperplasia is composed of cells with prominent clear cytoplasm and small, pyknotic nuclei. Note the well-defined cytoplasmic membranes characteristic of parathyroid tissue.* (Right) *Parathyroid gland involved by clear cell parathyroid hyperplasia is shown. The cells show cytoplasmic clearing and peripheral localization of nuclei.*

Proliferation and Clear Cells

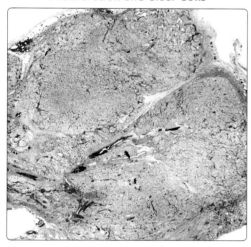

Irregular Proliferation of Cells

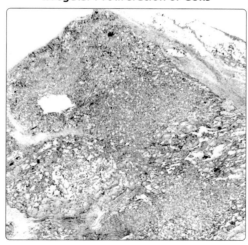

(Left) *Right superior parathyroid gland shows hypercellular parathyroid in a patient with primary clear cell hyperplasia. Unlike clear cell parathyroid adenoma, in which only a single parathyroid gland is involved, clear cell primary parathyroid hyperplasia affects multiple parathyroid glands.* (Right) *Left superior parathyroid gland shows primary clear cell parathyroid hyperplasia. In this patient, all 4 parathyroid glands were involved.*

Homogeneous Clear Cell Proliferations

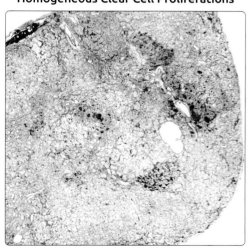

Clear Cells Present

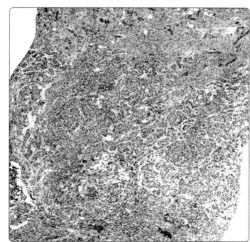

(Left) *Right inferior parathyroid gland shows primary clear cell parathyroid hyperplasia. Unlike conventional primary parathyroid hyperplasia, primary clear cell hyperplasia is not known to have a familial association.* (Right) *Portion of left inferior parathyroid gland shows primary clear cell parathyroid hyperplasia. The remainder of the left inferior parathyroid was transplanted into the forearm.*

TERMINOLOGY

- Secondary increase in PTH due to hypocalcemia and hyperphosphatemia (renal failure, vitamin D deficiency, pseudohypoparathyroidism, etc.)

ETIOLOGY/PATHOGENESIS

- Increased PTH due to low serum calcium caused by disorders of vitamin D, disorders of phosphate metabolism, pseudohypoparathyroidism, hypomagnesemia, and calcium deficiency

CLINICAL ISSUES

- Often history of chronic renal failure (most common cause of secondary hyperparathyroidism)

MACROSCOPIC

- Symmetric enlargement of all 4 glands only in subset of cases; many show enlargement of < 4 glands

MICROSCOPIC

- Parathyroid glands show more diffusely hyperplastic changes than in primary hyperparathyroidism
- Chief cells usually predominate, but chief cells and oxyphil cells can form nodular areas
- Nodularity may increase with progressive renal failure, making glands indistinguishable from primary or tertiary hyperplasia
- No invasive growth

ANCILLARY TESTS

- Positive for neuroendocrine markers chromogranin and synaptophysin

TOP DIFFERENTIAL DIAGNOSES

- Parathyroid adenoma, primary parathyroid hyperplasia, and parathyroid carcinoma

Secondary Parathyroid Hyperplasia

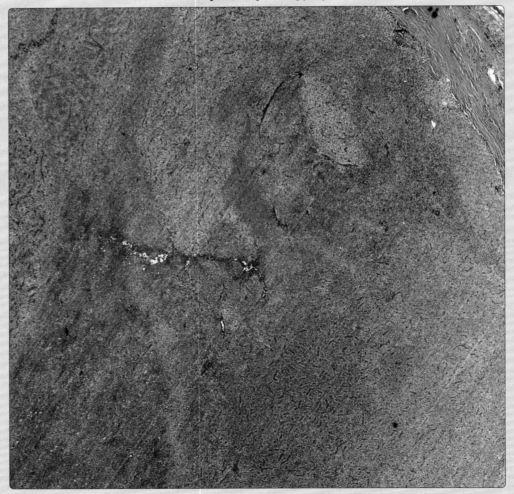

Parathyroid gland involved by secondary parathyroid hyperplasia is shown. Glands often show diffuse hyperplasia early in disease, but with disease progression, the parathyroid glands may become more nodular.

TERMINOLOGY

Definitions

- Adaptive increase in parathyroid parenchymal mass resulting from proliferation of chief, oncocytic/oxyphilic, and transitional cells in multiple glands in presence of known stimulus for parathyroid hormone (PTH) secretion

ETIOLOGY/PATHOGENESIS

Underlying Causes

- Chronic renal failure (# 1 cause)
- Vitamin D disorders (deficiency or malabsorption, tissue resistance to)
- Phosphate metabolism disorders (malnutrition, malabsorption, renal disease, aluminum toxicity)
- Pseudohypoparathyroidism
- Hypomagnesemia
- Calcium deficiency

CLINICAL ISSUES

Presentation

- Bone (pain, osteitis fibrosa cystica, osteomalacia)
- Soft tissue and visceral calcifications
- Paraarticular calcifications with associated arthritis
- Calciphylaxis: Rare, life-threatening, necrosis of skin and soft tissue
- Elevated serum calcium
- Severity of parathyroid hyperplasia often correlates with severity of underlying disease

Treatment

- Surgical approaches
  - Subtotal parathyroidectomy with 3 entire glands removed, leaving vascularized remnant of 4th gland
    - Or total parathyroidectomy with autotransplantation of portion of parathyroid gland into neck or forearm
  - Residual tissue may become hyperplastic, requiring additional surgery
  - Often difficult to impossible to differentiate primary parathyroid hyperplasia from parathyroid adenoma based only on histologic examination of 1 gland
  - Rapid intraoperative PTH measurements have decreased risk of missing multiglandular disease and help confirm removal of diseased gland(s)

Prognosis

- Complications: Bone disease, calcifications, calciphylaxis

IMAGING

General

- Technetium (Tc-99m) sestamibi is particularly helpful in localizing parathyroids
  - Also may use ultrasound, computed tomography, magnetic resonance imaging, nuclear scintigraphy

MACROSCOPIC

Normal Parathyroid Gland

- Size and shape of kidney bean (4-6 mm x 2-4 mm), 20-40 mg each

- Most have 4 parathyroid glands; 10% ≥ 5; 3% < 4 glands

Secondary Parathyroid Hyperplasia

- Multiple enlarged parathyroid glands
- Vary in size and weight (120-6,000 mg)
- Yellow to gray in color
- Glands more uniformly increased in size early in disease than those of primary parathyroid hyperplasia
- Size more variable and multinodular later in disease
- Hemorrhage, cystic change, chronic inflammation, and fibrosis more prominent with time

MICROSCOPIC

Normal Parathyroid Gland Histology

- Can show significant variation in cellularity even in single individual
- Cellularity variable, distributed unevenly, high in infants/children, decreases with age
- Age, gender, and constitutional factors (body fat, etc.) affect cellularity of normal parathyroid glands
- Stromal fat constitutes 10-30% of parathyroid, increases with age, more fat in poles of parathyroid than center

Constituent Cells of Parathyroid Gland

- Composed of chief cells, transitional cells, oxyphil cells, clear/water-clear cells, and adipose tissue
- Chief cells: 10 μm, polyhedral, round central nuclei, eosinophilic to amphophilic cytoplasm, fat droplets (adults), well-defined cytoplasmic membranes
- Oxyphil cells: 10-20 μm, abundant eosinophilic cytoplasm; appear at puberty, increase with age, may form nodules
- Transitional cells: Smaller cells with less cytoplasm
- Clear/water-clear cells: Parenchymal cells with clear cytoplasm (may be due to increased vacuolization in chief or oxyphilic cells)

Secondary Parathyroid Hyperplasia Histology

- Earliest change is decrease in adipocytes and diffuse increase in parathyroid parenchymal chief cells
- Chief cells measure 6-8 μm, cytoplasmic vacuolization, eccentric small nuclei
- Chief cells predominate early, and oxyphil cells increase over time and may predominate later
- Chief cells in sheets, cords, follicular/acinar patterns
- More diffusely hyperplastic changes identified early in secondary hyperplasia than in primary hyperplasia
- Later, nodules of chief, oncocytic, and transitional cells become more prominent
- Fibrosis, inflammation, cystic change, hemosiderin

Cytologic Features

- Round to oval cells with stippled nuclear chromatin
  - Lack significant pleomorphism, but occasional cells with enlarged hyperchromatic nuclei can be seen
  - Lack mitotic activity
- Single cells with naked nuclei and clusters of cells
- Prominent vascularity with attached epithelial cells
- Distinguishing among adenoma, hyperplasia, and carcinoma generally not possible on cytology
- Follicular pattern can mimic thyroid parenchyma, and oxyphil cells can mimic thyroid Hürthle cells

ANCILLARY TESTS

Cytology

- Follicular, cord-like, rosette patterns of chief, oxyphilic, transitional, or clear cells
- Can have intranuclear inclusions
- In fine needle aspirate samples, cells may appear in clusters and many nuclei appear naked
- Occasional cells with enlarged hyperchromatic nuclei, but prominent nuclear pleomorphism is generally absent

Frozen Sections

- **Assessing cellularity in small biopsy specimens can be difficult**
  - Cellularity increases with age and varies with gender, ethnicity, and body habitus
  - Cellularity is variable within parathyroid gland and among glands in individual
  - Poles of parathyroid more cellular than central
- **Differentiating parathyroid from thyroid on small biopsy specimens can be difficult**
  - Parathyroid cells: Well-defined cytoplasmic membranes
  - Cytoplasmic lipid (fat droplets) common in parathyroid cell cytoplasm (not in thyroid)
  - Parathyroid cells generally smaller and more vacuolated than thyroid
  - Parathyroid nuclei are rounder with denser chromatin than thyroid nuclei
  - Parathyroid lacks birefringent calcium oxalate crystals seen in thyroid
  - Parathyroid lacks colloid

Immunohistochemistry

- Positive for neuroendocrine markers chromogranin and synaptophysin
- Positive for keratin (CAM5.2 most helpful keratin for neuroendocrine tumors)
- Negative for TTF-1, thyroglobulin, variable calcitonin
- Positive for PTH

Genetic Testing

- Aneuploid populations of cells can be identified

DIFFERENTIAL DIAGNOSIS

Primary Parathyroid Hyperplasia

- Absolute increase in parathyroid parenchymal mass resulting from proliferation of chief cells, oncocytes, and transitional cells in multiple parathyroid glands in **absence** of recognized stimulus for PTH secretion
- More often has nodular growth but can be diffuse
- Parathyroid glands in secondary hyperplasia usually show more diffusely hyperplastic changes than in primary hyperparathyroidism

Tertiary Hyperparathyroidism

- Rare; patients with secondary hyperparathyroidism develop autonomously functioning parathyroid gland

Parathyroid Adenoma

- Benign neoplasm composed of chief cells, oxyphil cells, transitional cells, water clear cells, or mixture of cell types affecting single parathyroid gland
- Difficult to impossible to differentiate parathyroid adenoma from primary parathyroid hyperplasia based only on histologic examination of 1 gland
- Distinguishing parathyroid adenoma from hyperplasia usually requires examination of at least 1 additional gland, which should be normal
- Hyperplasia shows enlargement of at least 2 glands, while adenoma typically involves single gland
- Rim of normal tissue in 50-60% of parathyroid adenomas but can occasionally be seen in hyperplasia

Parathyroid Carcinoma

- Malignant neoplasm of parathyroid parenchymal cells (chief cells, oxyphilic cells, transitional cells, water/clear cells, or mixtures of cell types)
- Often symptomatic, high serum calcium (> 13 mg/dL)
- Involves 1 parathyroid gland, not multiple
  - Rare reports of carcinoma arising in setting of hyperplasia, particularly secondary hyperplasia
- Unequivocal invasion (capsular, vascular, perineural, or invasion into adjacent structures)

Parathyromatosis

- Recurrent hyperparathyroidism after subtotal parathyroidectomy may result
  - From multiple small nests of parathyroid cells in neck or mediastinum from lesional tissue left behind
  - Stimulation of embryonic nests of parathyroid cells

DIAGNOSTIC CHECKLIST

Clinically Relevant Pathologic Features

- Secondary increase in PTH due to hypocalcemia and hyperphosphatemia (renal failure, vitamin D deficiency, pseudohypoparathyroidism, etc.)

Pathologic Interpretation Pearls

- Normal parathyroid has significant variation in cellularity (use caution in assessing small biopsies)
- Distinguishing parathyroid tissue from thyroid: Well-demarcated cytoplasmic membranes, cytoplasmic lipid, rounder nuclei, denser chromatin, and lack colloid
- Symmetric enlargement of all 4 glands only in subset of cases; many show enlargement of < 4 glands
- Be very cautious in attempting to diagnose multiple adenomas (most likely asymmetric hyperplasia)
- Rim of normal parathyroid occasionally present in parathyroid hyperplasia

SELECTED REFERENCES

1. Cocchiara G et al: The medical and surgical treatment in secondary and tertiary hyperparathyroidism. Review. Clin Ter. 168(2):e158-e167, 2017
2. Portillo MR et al: Secondary hyperparthyroidism: pathogenesis, diagnosis, preventive and therapeutic strategies. Rev Endocr Metab Disord. 18(1):79-95, 2017
3. DeLellis RA: Parathyroid tumors and related disorders. Mod Pathol. 24 Suppl 2:S78-93, 2011
4. DeLellis RA et al: Primary hyperparathyroidism: a current perspective. Arch Pathol Lab Med. 132(8):1251-62, 2008
5. Erickson LA et al: Parathyroid hyperplasia, adenomas, and carcinomas: differential expression of p27Kip1 protein. Am J Surg Pathol. 23(3):288-95, 1999
6. DeLellis RA: Tumors of the Parathyroid Gland. AFIP Atlas of Tumor Pathology Series 4, Fascicle 21. Washington DC: American Registry of Pathology, 1-102, 2014

Secondary Parathyroid Hyperplasia

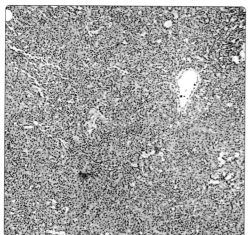

Hypercellular Parathyroid Involved By Secondary Hyperplasia

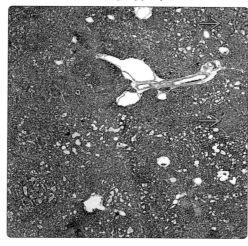

(Left) *Diffuse growth pattern in a parathyroid gland involved by secondary parathyroid hyperplasia is shown.* (Right) *Hypercellular parathyroid gland is composed predominantly of chief cells, but a few small groups of oxyphilic ⇨ cells are shown.*

Secondary Parathyroid Hyperplasia With Small Clusters of Adipocytes

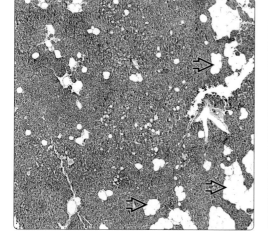

Diffuse Hyperplasia in Case of Secondary Parathyroid Hyperplasia

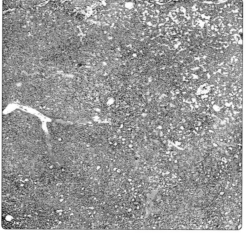

(Left) *Secondary parathyroid hyperplasia with hypercellular parathyroid gland composed predominantly of chief cells. Single adipocytes and small clusters of adipocytes ⇨ are present.* (Right) *Secondary parathyroid hyperplasia usually shows diffuse architectural pattern but can become more nodular in long-standing disease.*

Primary Parathyroid Hyperplasia

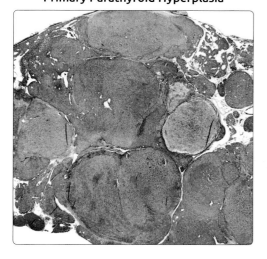

Nodular Growth in Secondary Parathyroid Hyperplasia

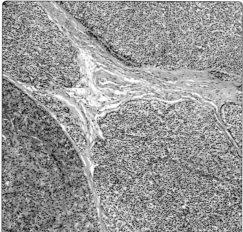

(Left) *This gland from a patient with primary parathyroid hyperplasia shows a more nodular growth, but nodular and diffuse growth can be seen in both primary and secondary hyperplasia.* (Right) *Parathyroid gland in patient with long-standing chronic renal failure and secondary parathyroid hyperplasia shows nodular growth pattern.*

(Left) *Diffuse pattern of growth in this parathyroid gland involved by secondary parathyroid hyperplasia is shown. Chief cells are thought to be more prominent early with oxyphil cells increasing over time.* **(Right)** *Oxyphilic/oncocytic parathyroid cells have prominent eosinophilic cytoplasm (mitochondria) and small, round, hyperchromatic nuclei.*

Diffuse Pattern of Growth of Chief Cells in Secondary Parathyroid Hyperplasia

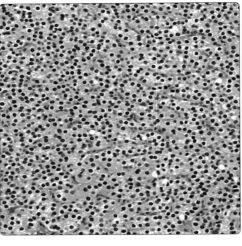

Oxyphilic/Oncocytic Cells

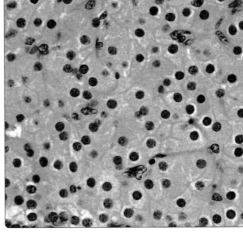

(Left) *Various growth patterns can be seen, including follicular, acinar, solid, or nested. The nuclei show little variation in size or shape.* **(Right)** *Various growth patterns can be seen, including follicular, acinar, solid, or nested. This picture illustrates the classic follicular pattern arrangement. This pattern may mimic thyroid during frozen section examination.*

Follicular Growth Pattern in Parathyroid Hyperplasia

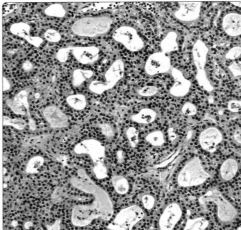

Follicular Growth Pattern in Parathyroid Hyperplasia

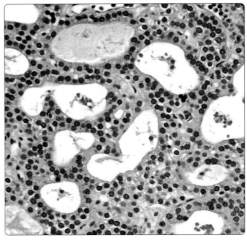

(Left) *Adipocytes in a background of increased numbers of parathyroid chief cells are seen in this parathyroid gland involved by secondary parathyroid hyperplasia.* **(Right)** *Foci of pleomorphic cells "endocrine atypia" can be seen in many endocrine lesions, including hyperplastic parathyroid glands.*

Scattered Adipocytes in Hypercellular Parathyroid in Secondary Hyperplasia

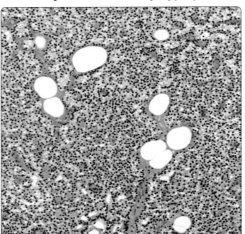

Endocrine Atypia

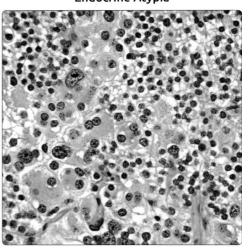

Basal Nuclei Around Vessels

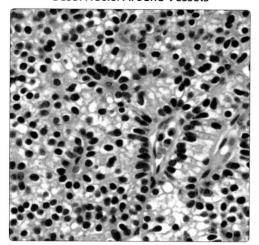

Rim-Like Area in Parathyroid Hyperplasia

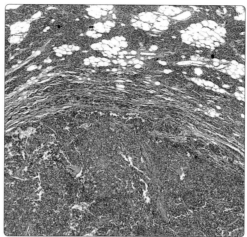

(Left) *Hyperplastic parathyroid gland shows nuclei basally located (polar) around vessels, a pattern often seen in parathyroid lesions. Note the well-defined cytoplasmic membranes of parathyroid cells, a feature helpful in differentiating parathyroid from thyroid.* (Right) *Although rims of normal appearing parathyroid tissue are often identified in parathyroid adenoma, they can also be seen in parathyroid hyperplasia.*

Fibrous Bands in Parathyroid Hyperplasia

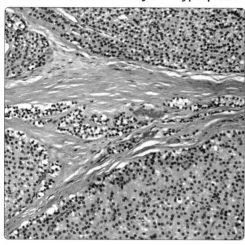

Fibrous Bands in Longstanding Secondary Parathyroid Hyperplasia

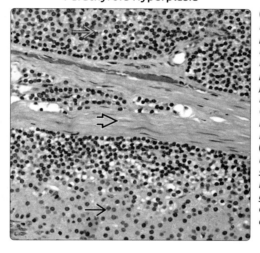

(Left) *Fibrous bands are seen in this case of secondary parathyroid hyperplasia. Fibrous bands can be seen in both benign and malignant parathyroid glands. Mitotic figures can also be seen in benign parathyroid tissue. Generally a diagnosis of malignancy in parathyroid requires invasive growth.* (Right) *Fibrous bands ⇨ in a longstanding case of secondary parathyroid hyperplasia with a nodular growth pattern is shown. Chief cells ⇨ and oxyphil cells ⇨ are present.*

Entrapped Cells in Parathyroid Hyperplasia

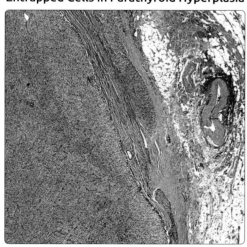

Fibrosis and Calcification in Secondary Parathyroid Hyperplasia

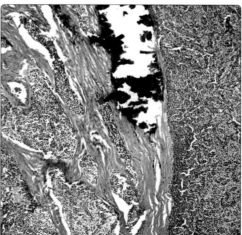

(Left) *Entrapped cells in capsule in parathyroid hyperplasia are shown. Importantly, invasion (capsular, vascular, or perineural) is not identified as would be required for a diagnosis of parathyroid carcinoma.* (Right) *Parathyroid gland involved by secondary parathyroid hyperplasia with fibrous bands and calcification is shown.*

Tertiary Parathyroid Hyperplasia

TERMINOLOGY

- Tertiary hyperparathyroidism: Rare condition in which patients with secondary hyperparathyroidism develop autonomously functioning parathyroid gland(s) and hypersecretion of parathyroid hormone (PTH)

ETIOLOGY/PATHOGENESIS

- Etiology unclear, but may be due to resetting of set point of PTH or calcium
- Development of autonomous parathyroid function with hypersecretion of PTH resulting in hypercalcemia

CLINICAL ISSUES

- Parathyroid glands of patients with secondary hyperparathyroidism after renal transplantation do not return to normal and continue oversecreting PTH
  - In tertiary hyperplasia, parathyroid hyperfunction is autonomous and not due to stimulus for PTH secretion
- Occurs in 6-8% with secondary hyperparathyroidism

MACROSCOPIC

- Usually multiple (≥ 4) parathyroid glands involved and enlarged, but can be only 1 gland

MICROSCOPIC

- Hypercellular parathyroid tissue with increase in parathyroid parenchymal chief, oxyphil, and transitional cells and decrease in adipocytes
- Can be impossible to distinguish primary, secondary, and tertiary hyperparathyroidism on histologic features alone
- Morphologic features may be identical to primary and secondary hyperplasia

TOP DIFFERENTIAL DIAGNOSES

- Parathyroid adenoma
- Primary parathyroid hyperplasia
- Secondary parathyroid hyperplasia
- Parathyroid carcinoma

Nodular Growth Pattern in Hypercellular Parathyroid Gland

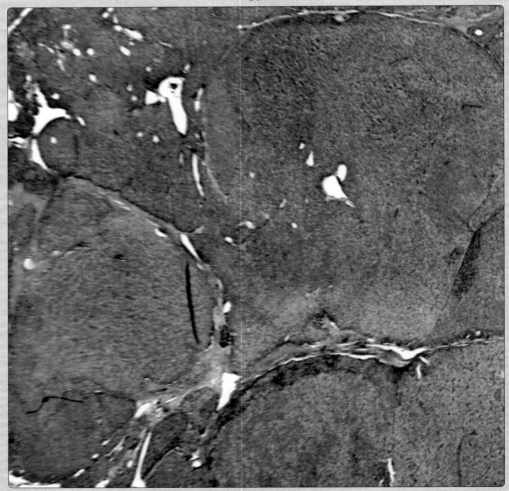

Hyperplastic parathyroid glands, including tertiary hyperplasia, can have a nodular growth pattern. Generally, types of hyperplasia (primary, secondary, or tertiary) cannot be separated based on histologic features alone.

TERMINOLOGY

Definitions

- Rare condition in which patients with secondary hyperparathyroidism develop autonomously functioning parathyroid gland(s) and hypersecretion of parathyroid hormone (PTH)

ETIOLOGY/PATHOGENESIS

Unknown

- Development of autonomous parathyroid function with hypersecretion of PTH resulting in hypercalcemia
- Change set point of calcium-sensing mechanism
- In patients with secondary hyperparathyroidism, parathyroid glands do not return to normal and continue oversecreting PTH after renal transplant
- Glands may become resistant to calcimimetic agents despite normalized serum calcium

CLINICAL ISSUES

Presentation

- Patient with history of secondary hyperparathyroidism, often due to chronic renal failure and after renal transplantation, develops excess secretion of PTH and hypercalcemia
- Occurs in 6-8% with secondary hyperparathyroidism
- Persistent hyperparathyroidism after renal transplantation or new hypercalcemia in setting of chronic secondary hyperparathyroidism

Treatment

- Total parathyroidectomy with autotransplantation or subtotal parathyroidectomy

Prognosis

- Most patients with renal failure-associated hyperparathyroidism will have progressive normalization of serum calcium after renal transplant
  - In some patients, hyperparathyroidism persists or develops after transplant
- This type of hyperparathyroidism can be detrimental to renal allograft and is associated with other complications due to hypercalcemia

MACROSCOPIC

General Features

- Usually multiple glands enlarged, but can be only 1 gland
- Ectopic glands reported in up to 1/3
- Superior glands may be larger than inferior

MICROSCOPIC

Histologic Features

- Morphologic features may be identical to primary and secondary hyperplasia
- More prominent internodular diffuse changes may be seen in secondary and tertiary hyperplasia compared to primary hyperplasia
- Hypercellular parathyroid gland(s) with increase in chief and oxyphil cells and decrease in adipocytes

ANCILLARY TESTS

Immunohistochemistry

- Parathyroid cells are positive for chromogranin, synaptophysin, keratin (CAM5.2), and parathyroid hormone, while negative for TTF-1 and thyroglobulin

DIFFERENTIAL DIAGNOSIS

Parathyroid Adenoma

- Generally involves only 1 parathyroid gland, while tertiary hyperplasia develops in setting of secondary parathyroid hyperplasia with multiglandular disease
- Occasionally, rather than multiglandular involvement in tertiary hyperplasia, single gland may be involved, but usually still in setting of secondary hyperplasia history

Parathyroid Carcinoma

- Rare, may occur in setting of tertiary hyperparathyroidism
- Requires invasive growth (capsular, vascular, perineural, or invasion into adjacent structures) or metastases
- Atypical features (fibrosis, occasional mitoses) can be seen in parathyroid adenoma and parathyroid hyperplasias, but invasive growth is required for diagnosis of parathyroid carcinoma

Primary Parathyroid Hyperplasia

- Absolute increase in parathyroid parenchymal mass resulting from proliferation of chief cells, oncocytes, and transitional cells in multiple parathyroid glands in absence of recognized stimulus for PTH secretion
- Morphologic features may be identical to primary and secondary hyperplasia

Secondary Parathyroid Hyperplasia

- Increase in parathyroid parenchymal mass resulting from proliferation of chief cells, oncocytes, and transitional cells in multiple glands in presence of known stimulus for PTH secretion, most commonly renal failure
- Tertiary hyperplasia generally develops in patients with history of secondary hyperplasia
  - In tertiary hyperplasia, parathyroid hyperfunction is autonomous and not due to stimulus for PTH secretion
  - e.g., tertiary hyperplasia may be continual hyperparathyroidism or development of hyperparathyroidism after renal transplant

SELECTED REFERENCES

1. Cocchiara G et al: The medical and surgical treatment in secondary and tertiary hyperparathyroidism. Review. Clin Ter. 168(2):e158-e167, 2017
2. Dulfer RR et al: Systematic review of surgical and medical treatment for tertiary hyperparathyroidism. Br J Surg. 104(7):804-813, 2017
3. Shindo M et al: The changing landscape of primary, secondary, and tertiary hyperparathyroidism: highlights from the American College of Surgeons Panel, "What's New for the Surgeon Caring for Patients with Hyperparathyroidism". J Am Coll Surg. 222(6):1240-50, 2016
4. Yamamoto T et al: Characteristics of persistent hyperparathyroidism after renal transplantation. World J Surg. 40(3):600-6, 2016
5. Lorenz K et al: Surgical management of secondary hyperparathyroidism in chronic kidney disease–a consensus report of the European Society of Endocrine Surgeons. Langenbecks Arch Surg. 400(8):907-27, 2015
6. DeLellis R: Tumors of the Parathyroid Gland. AFIP Atlas of Tumor Pathology Series 4. Fascicle 21. Washington DC: American Registry of Pathology, 2014

(Left) This figure illustrates a hypercellular parathyroid with a solid growth pattern and bands of fibrosis. Fibrosis can be seen in tertiary parathyroid hyperplasia, but parathyroid adenoma, hyperplasia, and carcinoma can all show fibrosis. **(Right)** This low-power picture shows a hypercellular parathyroid gland composed predominantly of chief cells with foci of oxyphilic cells and a decrease in adipocytes.

Fibrosis in Hypercellular Parathyroid Gland

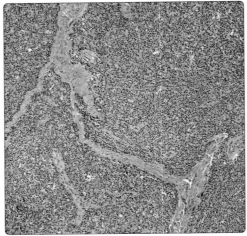

Hypercellular Parathyroid

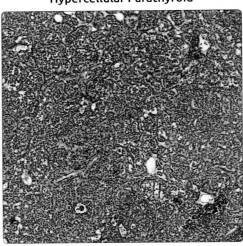

(Left) This hypercellular parathyroid has a nodular growth pattern with nodules of oxyphilic cells ⇨ and nodules of chief cells ⇨. This illustration also shows absence of adipocytes within both oxyphilic and chief cells nodules. **(Right)** This low-power histopathologic figure of a parathyroid gland shows a proliferation of small cells in a diffuse pattern with increased cellularity. The cells are predominantly chief cells.

Nodular Growth Pattern

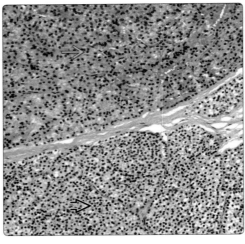
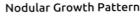

Diffuse Growth Pattern

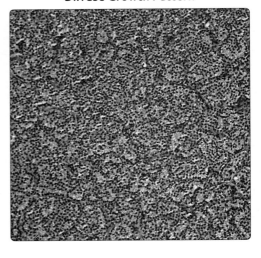

(Left) The parathyroid shown in this figure has a proliferation of small chief cells in a diffuse pattern of growth. This hypercellular parathyroid is composed exclusively of chief cells. **(Right)** This photomicrograph of a parathyroid gland shows groups of oxyphilic cells ⇨ intermixed with chief cells ⇨. This finding is one of the characteristic features seen in hyperplastic parathyroid glands.

Chief Cells in Diffuse Pattern

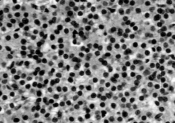

Oxyphilic Cells and Chief Cells

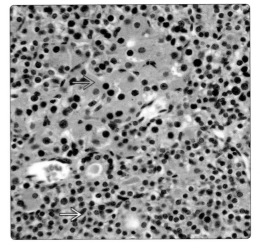

Hypercellular Parathyroid Gland

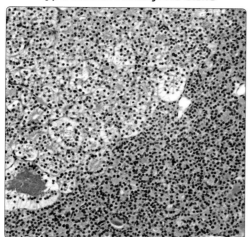

Predominant Chief Cells

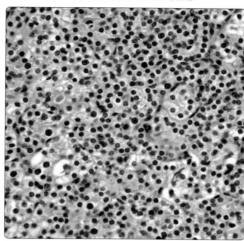

(Left) *This hypercellular parathyroid gland shows 2 distinct populations of areas composed by cells with distinct morphology in a low-power examination. This figure shows chief cells and transitional cells.* (Right) *This medium-power view of a hypercellular parathyroid gland shows a predominant chief cell population with areas of intermixture of chief cells and scattered oxyphilic cells.*

Oxyphilic Cells

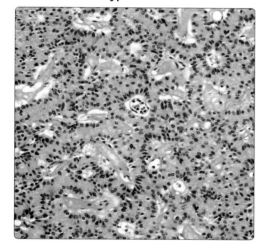

Oxyphilic Cells

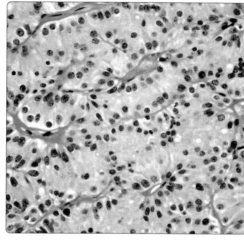

(Left) *Medium-power photomicrograph shows a hypercellular parathyroid gland with a trabecular/sinusoidal growth pattern, composed by predominantly oxyphilic cells with peripheral nuclei. This nuclear palisading is often around vascular structures.* (Right) *Oxyphilic (oncocytic) cells in a hypercellular parathyroid gland are shown. The cytoplasm of the oncocytic cells is ample and eosinophilic, and the nuclei are round with delicate stippled chromatin.*

Stippled Neuroendocrine Chromatin

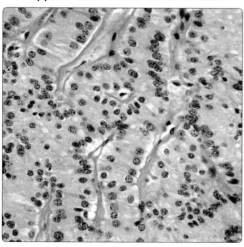

Endocrine Atypia

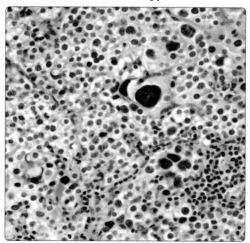

(Left) *Parathyroid cells have stippled neuroendocrine chromatin pattern, as is demonstrated in this photomicrograph of an area of oxyphilic cells. Other parathyroid cell types also show neuroendocrine stippled chromatin.* (Right) *This focus of cells with pleomorphic, large, hyperchromatic nuclei are characteristic of an area that is referred to as "endocrine atypia."*

Chronic Parathyroiditis

TERMINOLOGY

- Thought to represent rare autoimmune process, with lymphocytic infiltration, atrophy of parathyroid parenchyma and replacement with fibrosis that can be associated with hypoparathyroidism or hyperparathyroidism

ETIOLOGY/PATHOGENESIS

- Unknown, poorly understood; possibly autoimmune
- Few patients reported to have antibodies to parathyroid

CLINICAL ISSUES

- Most asymptomatic, but may be associated with hypoparathyroidism or hyperparathyroidism
- Up to 10% of autopsies show focal lymphocytic infiltration of parathyroid in patients without known parathyroid disease (significance uncertain)

MICROSCOPIC

- Infiltration of lymphocytes and lymphoid aggregates in parathyroid parenchyma

- o May have prominent lymphoid follicles with germinal center formation
- Parathyroid parenchyma may be replaced by fibrous and adipose tissue
- Multiple parathyroid glands may be involved, particularly with autoimmune disorders, such as Sjögren
- 2 patterns suggested
  - o Nonspecific: Diffuse lymphocytic infiltrates in vicinity of venules without fibrosis or epithelial degeneration is nonspecific pattern
  - o Lymphocytic parathyroiditis:Interstitial lymphocytes away from vessels with plasma cells or germinal centers and features of epithelial reaction (degenerative or proliferative)

TOP DIFFERENTIAL DIAGNOSES

- Nonspecific finding of unknown significance
- Malignant lymphoma
- Infection

Chronic Parathyroiditis

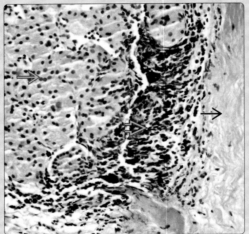

Fibrosis in Chronic Parathyroiditis

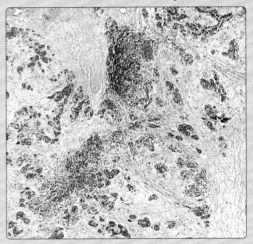

(Left) Photomicrograph of a parathyroid with chronic parathyroiditis shows parathyroid cells ➡, infiltrating small lymphocytes ➡, and fibrosis ➡. (Right) Aggregates of lymphoid cells are seen in association with nests of parathyroid cells and marked fibrosis in this parathyroid involved by chronic parathyroiditis.

Lymphoid Infiltrate in Chronic Parathyroiditis

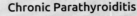
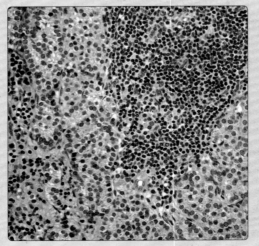

Lymphoid Follicle With Germinal Center

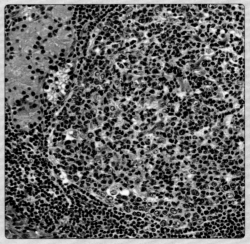

(Left) Photomicrograph shows dense aggregate of lymphoid cells in parathyroid parenchyma. Histologic changes vary from focal lymphocytic infiltration of parathyroid gland to extensive involvement. (Right) Histologic changes vary from focal lymphocytic infiltration with formation of lymphoid follicles with germinal center formation. Photomicrograph shows lymphoid infiltrate with germinal center formation in a case of chronic parathyroiditis.

TERMINOLOGY

Definitions

- Thought to represent rare autoimmune process with lymphocytic infiltration, atrophy of parathyroid parenchyma, and replacement with fibrosis
  - Can be associated with hypoparathyroidism or hyperparathyroidism
- Variable descriptive terminology
  - Lymphocytic infiltrate
  - Parathyroidtitis
  - Lymphocytic parathyroiditis
  - Chronic parathyroiditis

ETIOLOGY/PATHOGENESIS

Poorly Understood

- Possibly autoimmune
  - Antibody to parathyroid tissue found in few patients with idiopathic hypoparathyroidism, some with other autoimmune disorders (e.g., Addison disease, pernicious anemia, thyroid disease)
    - Other studies do not identify antibody
  - Autoimmune destruction of parathyroid glands may account for some cases of primary idiopathic hypoparathyroidism
    - Few parathyroid glands identified at autopsy in patients with primary hypoparathyroidism showed parenchymal atrophy, lymphocytic infiltration reminiscent of diffuse atrophic changes in autoimmune thyroiditis
- Terminological variation and lack of studies confound classification difficulty
  - No well-defined, agreed upon classification
  - Descriptive terminology
    - Lymphocytic infiltrate, parathyroiditis, chronic parathyroiditis, and lymphocytic parathyroiditis are terms that have been used to describe lymphoid infiltrates in parathyroid gland(s)
  - Lacks well-defined classification scheme
  - Lack of well-defined association between histologic parathyroiditis and parathyroid disease
  - Lack well-defined entity/entities
- Acquired hypocalciuric hypercalcemia
  - Autoimmune lymphocytic parathyroiditis and acquired hypocalciuric hypercalcemia associated with autoantibodies against calcium-sensing receptor (anti-CaSR) are rare and poorly understood conditions
  - Recent report on autoimmune lymphocytic parathyroiditis and acquired hypocalciuric hypercalcemia described as associated with anti-CaSR antibodies
    - Although very rare condition, should be considered
    - Subtotal parathyroidectomy unlikely to correct hypercalcemia; may respond to short course of prednisone therapy

CLINICAL ISSUES

Epidemiology

- Incidence
  - Extremely rare entity in diagnostic surgical pathology

- Few reports of lymphocytic infiltrate of parathyroid glands in primary hyperparathyroidism
  - Lymphocytic infiltration of parathyroid glands found at autopsy in up to 10% without known parathyroid dysfunction in life or organ damage related to parathyroid dysfunction

Presentation

- Most asymptomatic but can occur with hypoparathyroidism and hyperparathyroidism
  - Few patients have antibodies to parathyroid tissue
  - Focal lymphocytic infiltration of parathyroid gland(s) in up to 10% at autopsy without known parathyroid disorder in life
  - Signficance of finding of lymphoid infiltration in parathyroid gland or glands remains unclear
- Hyperparathyroidism
  - Chronic parathyroiditis can be associated with primary hyperplasia and hyperparathyroidism
    - Reported in patient with MEN1 (multiple endocrine neoplasia type 1)
    - Reports involving parathyroid adenomas
- Hypoparathyroidism
  - Autoimmune chronic parathyroiditis with destruction of parathyroid glands may account for some forms of primary idiopathic hypoparathyroidism

Treatment

- Supportive, if necessary

MACROSCOPIC

General Features

- Mild enlargement of parathyroid gland(s)

MICROSCOPIC

Histologic Features

- Histologic changes vary from focal lymphocytic infiltration of parathyroid gland(s) to extensive involvement with changes similar to Hashimoto thyroiditis
- Lymphoid follicles and lymphocytes infiltrating parathyroid parenchyma
- Lymphoid infiltrate may be focal or diffuse
- May have prominent lymphoid follicles with germinal center formation
- Parathyroid parenchyma may be replaced by fibrous and adipose tissue
- Remaining parathyroid parenchyma may be as small nests and islands of parathyroid parenchymal cells (chief or oncocytic/oxyphilic cells) in background of fibrous tissue
- Residual parathyroid parenchymal tissue may become atrophic
- Multiple parathyroid glands may be involved, particularly with autoimmune disorders, such as Sjögren syndrome and other autoimmune disorders
- Recently, 2 patterns described
  - Nonspecific
    - Diffuse lymphocytic infiltrates in vicinity of venules
    - Lacks fibrosis or epithelial degeneration
  - Lymphocytic parathyroiditis
    - Interstitial lymphocytes away from vessels with plasma cells or germinal centers

— Features of epithelial reaction (degenerative or proliferative)

ANCILLARY TESTS

Immunohistochemistry

- Parathyroid parenchymal tissue positive for keratin (CAM5.2), chromogranin, synaptophysin, and parathyroid hormone
- Parathyroid parenchymal tissue negative for TTF-1 (thyroid transcription factor-1) and thyroglobulin
- Immunohistochemical studies can be used to demonstrate reactive immunophenotype in lymphoid infiltrate in chronic parathyroiditis
- Immunohistochemical studies may help differentiate reactive lymphoid infiltrate from malignant lymphoma

Serologic Testing

- Reports of few patients with antibodies against parathyroid, but many studies show serology is negative

DIFFERENTIAL DIAGNOSIS

Nonspecific Finding of Unknown Significance

- Up to 10% of autopsies show focal lymphocytic infiltration of parathyroid(s) in patients without known abnormality in parathyroid function
- Significance of this finding in autopsy cases remains unknown and may be nonspecific
- Significance of finding in clinical cases remains unclear
- Desciptive terminology (lymphocytic infiltrate, parathyroiditis, chronic parathyroiditis, and lymphocytic parathyroiditis) have been used to describe lymphoid infiltrates in parathyroid gland(s) complicates the interpretation and classification of an entity versus a nonspecific finding of unknown significance

Malignant Lymphoma

- Malignant lymphoma involving parathyroid gland(s) is extremely rare, but reports exist
- Cytologic and architectural atypia in keeping with diagnosis of malignant lymphoma and abnormal immunophenotype and other studies if appropriate
- Immunohistochemical studies may help differentiate reactive lymphoid infiltrate from malignant lymphoma in difficult cases or if malignant lympoma suspected

Infection

- Lymphocytic infiltrate may occur in patients with various infectious diseases
- Lymphocytic infiltrate in infectious disease may be sparse and predominantly perivascular
- Little is known about infectious etiologies in parathyroid lymphoid infiltrates

DIAGNOSTIC CHECKLIST

Clinically Relevant Pathologic Features

- Usually asymptomatic
- Few reports of antibodies against parathyroid
- Can be associated with hyperparathyroidism or hypoparathyroidism

- Focal lymphocytic infiltrate identified in up to 10% of autopsies in patients without known parathyroid disease, thus significance is unknown in some cases

Pathologic Interpretation Pearls

- Infiltration of lymphocytes and lymphoid aggregates in parathyroid parenchyma
- Parathyroid parenchyma may become replaced by fibrosis
- Remaining parathyroid parenchyma may become atrophic

SELECTED REFERENCES

1. Song L et al: Glucocorticoid-responsive lymphocytic parathyroiditis and hypocalciuric hypercalcemia due to autoantibodies against the calcium-sensing receptor: a case report and literature review. Eur J Endocrinol. 177(1):K1-K6, 2017
2. Ting S et al: [Inflammation of the parathyroid glands.] Pathologe. 37(3):224-9, 2016
3. Talat N et al: Inflammatory diseases of the parathyroid gland. Histopathology. 59(5):897-908, 2011
4. Kovacs K et al: Parathyroid chief cell adenoma associated with massive chronic parathyroiditis in a woman with hyperparathyroidism. Endocr Pathol. 18(1):42-5, 2007
5. Furuto-Kato S et al: Primary hyperparathyroidism presumably caused by chronic parathyroiditis manifesting from hypocalcemia to severe hypercalcemia. Intern Med. 44(1):60-4, 2005
6. Thompson L: Parathyroiditis. Ear Nose Throat J. 84(10):636, 2005
7. Vaizey CJ et al: Chronic parathyroiditis associated with primary hyperplastic hyperparathyroidism. J R Soc Med. 90(6):336-7, 1997
8. Sinha SN et al: Hyperparathyroidism with chronic parathyroiditis in a multiple endocrine neoplasia patient. Aust N Z J Surg. 63(12):981-2, 1993
9. DeLellis RA: Tumors of the parathyroid gland. AFIP Atlas of Tumor Pathology Series 3, Fascicle 6. Washington DC: American Registry of Pathology, 1-102, 1991
10. Chetty R et al: Parathyroiditis associated with hyperparathyroidism and branchial cysts. Am J Clin Pathol. 96(3):348-50, 1991
11. Pizzolitto S et al: [Chronic hyperplastic parathyroiditis: the anatomico-clinical and pathogenetic aspects.] Acta Otorhinolaryngol Ital. 11(5):505-9, 1991
12. Bondeson AG et al: Chronic parathyroiditis associated with parathyroid hyperplasia and hyperparathyroidism. Am J Surg Pathol. 8(3):211-5, 1984
13. Boyce BF et al: Hyperplastic parathyroiditis--a new autoimmune disease? J Clin Pathol. 35(8):812-4, 1982
14. Atwal OS: Ultrastructural pathology of ozone-induced experimental parathyroiditis. IV. Biphasic activity in the chief cells of regenerating parathyroid glands. Am J Pathol. 95(3):611-32, 1979
15. Atwal OS et al: A possible autoimmune parathyroiditis following ozone inhalation. II. A histopathologic, ultrastructural, and immunofluorescent study. Am J Pathol. 80(1):53-68, 1975
16. Van de Casseye M et al: Case report: primary (autoimmune?) parathyroiditis. Virchows Arch A Pathol Pathol Anat. 361(3):257-61, 1973
17. MOSCA L: [Parathyroiditis in the human newborn.] Biol Lat. 8(4 Pt 2):1331-85, 1955
18. Thompson RL et al: The results of chronic parathyroiditis as obtained by ligation of the parathyroid glandules in the Dog. J Med Res. 19(1):121-134.3, 1908

Parathyroid Gland With Lymphoid Aggregates

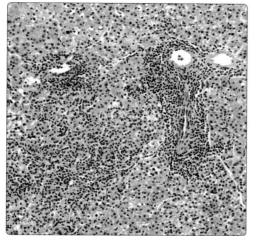

Hyperplastic Parathyroid With Chronic Parathyroiditis

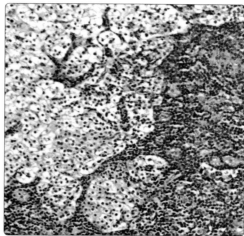

(Left) *Aggregates of lymphocytes are shown in a hypercellular parathyroid gland. The parathyroid cells have oncocytic cytoplasm.* **(Right)** *Hyperplastic parathyroid gland involved by chronic parathyroiditis is shown. In this case, the lymphoid infiltrate formed nodular aggregates in areas, with other areas showing lymphoid aggregates.*

Diffuse Lymphoid Infiltrate in Chronic Parathyroiditis

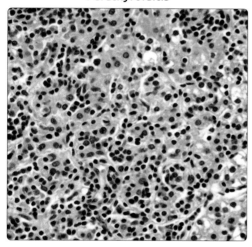

Atrophy of Parathyroid Parenchyma in Chronic Parathyroiditis

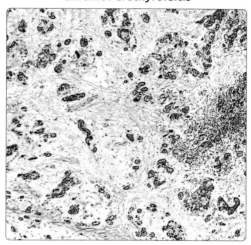

(Left) *Diffuse infiltrate of lymphocytes is present in chronic parathyroiditis. The histologic changes can be variable. Interestingly, up to 10% of autopsies show focal lymphocytic infiltrate of parathyroid tissue.* **(Right)** *Atrophy of remaining parathyroid parenchymal cells is shown in a parathyroid gland involved by chronic parathyroiditis. Note the extensive replacement of the parathyroid parenchymal cells by fibrosis with small nests of parathyroid parenchymal cells remaining in the background of fibrosis.*

Chronic Parathyroiditis

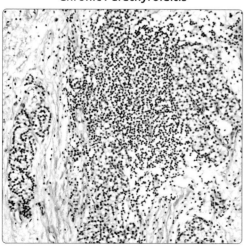

Lymphoid Infiltrate

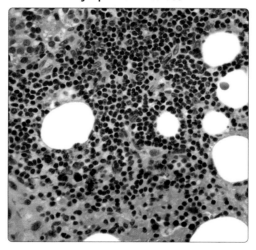

(Left) *Nests of remaining parathyroid parenchymal chief cells with lymphocytic inflammation are present in chronic parathyroiditis. Some cases of idiopathic hypoparathyroidism may be due to autoimmune destruction of parenchyma by chronic parathyroiditis.* **(Right)** *Prominent lymphoid aggregate is seen in a parathyroid involved by chronic parathyroiditis with extensive lymphocytic infiltrate. Dense lymphoid infiltrates need to be differentiated from malignant lymphoma.*

Parathyroid Adenoma

TERMINOLOGY

- Benign neoplasm of chief, oncocytic, transitional, water-clear, or mixture of cells

ETIOLOGY/PATHOGENESIS

- Most are sporadic
- ~ 5-10% of cases of primary hyperparathyroidism are associated with familial syndromes
- Most common genetic syndromes
  o Hyperparathyroidism-jaw tumor syndrome
  o Familial isolated hyperparathyroidism
  o Multiple endocrine neoplasia types 1 and 2A
  o Familial hypocalciuric hypercalcemia

CLINICAL ISSUES

- Often asymptomatic or vague symptoms, identified with serum calcium screening

MACROSCOPIC

- Single enlarged hypercellular parathyroid gland (if multiple, likely hyperplasia or asymmetric hyperplasia)

MICROSCOPIC

- Parathyroid adenoma is composed of chief, oxyphilic, transitional, clear cells, or mixtures of cell types

ANCILLARY TESTS

- Positive for chromogranin, synaptophysin, CAM5.2, and PTH; negative for TTF-1 and thyroglobulin
- Complete loss of nuclear or nucleolar parafibromin expression in parathyroid carcinoma is helpful differentiating from parathyroid adenoma, which usually shows intact nuclear and nucleolar parafibromin expression

TOP DIFFERENTIAL DIAGNOSES

- Parathyroid hyperplasia, parathyroid carcinoma, thyroid tumor

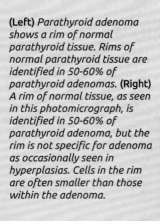

(Left) *Parathyroid adenoma is a single enlarged parathyroid gland, usually 0.2 to > 1 g. The cut surface of a parathyroid adenoma is usually homogeneous tan-yellow to tan-red with focal areas of hemorrhage.* (Right) *This chief cell parathyroid adenoma has a nested growth pattern and prominent vascularity. The nuclei are round and dense. The cytoplasm of the chief cells is eosinophilic to amphophilic. The cells do not show significant nuclear pleomorphism or mitotic activity.*

Cut Surface of Parathyroid Adenoma

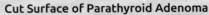
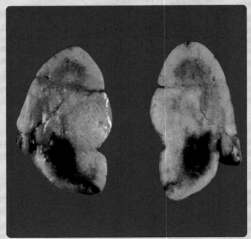

Parathyroid Chief Cell Adenoma

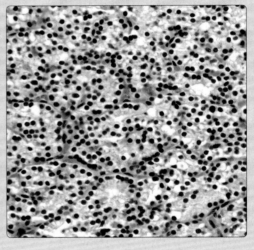

(Left) *Parathyroid adenoma shows a rim of normal parathyroid tissue. Rims of normal parathyroid tissue are identified in 50-60% of parathyroid adenomas.* (Right) *A rim of normal tissue, as seen in this photomicrograph, is identified in 50-60% of parathyroid adenoma, but the rim is not specific for adenoma as occasionally seen in hyperplasias. Cells in the rim are often smaller than those within the adenoma.*

Rim of Normocellular Parathyroid

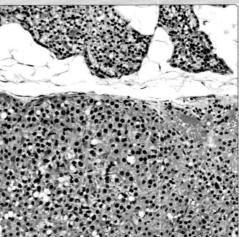

Rim in Parathyroid Adenoma

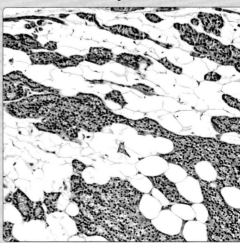

TERMINOLOGY

Abbreviations

- Parathyroid adenoma (PTA)

Definitions

- Benign parathyroid neoplasm composed of chief cells, oncocytic cells, transitional cells, water-clear cells, or mixture of these cell types (WHO 2017)

ETIOLOGY/PATHOGENESIS

Sporadic Parathyroid Adenomas

- Predisposing factors poorly understood
- Possible association with prior ionizing radiation
  - Particularly external ionizing radiation in childhood
  - Persons exposed to nuclear events
  - Diagnostic or therapeutic doses of radioactive iodine does not appear to be significant risk factor
- Long-term lithium therapy

Hereditary Parathyroid Adenomas

- Hereditary hyperparathyroidism is less common than sporadic hyperparathyroidism
- ~ 5-10% of cases of primary hyperparathyroidism are associated with familial syndromes
  - Study of this group has provided insight into genetic and molecular changes that underlie neoplastic transformation of parathyroid tissue
- Most common genetic syndromes associated with primary hyperparathyroidism are multiple endocrine neoplasia types 1 and 2A (MEN1, MEN2A), hyperparathyroidism-jaw tumor syndrome (HPT-JT), familial isolated hyperparathyroidism (FIHP), and familial hypocalciuric hypercalcemia
- HPT-JT
  - Autosomal dominant
  - Inactivating mutations in *CDC73* (HRPT2) (1q21-q31) tumor suppressor gene
    - 80% mutations are truncating (frameshift and nonsense), and most involve exon 1
  - *CDC73* (HRPT2) gene encodes parafibromin/CDC73 protein
  - HPT-JT is disorder of hyperparathyroidism, fibroosseous jaw tumors, kidney cysts, hamartomas, and Wilms tumors
  - Parathyroid hyperplasia or adenoma and increased risk of parathyroid carcinoma
    - 15% of patients with HPT-JT develop parathyroid carcinoma
  - Germline *CDC73* (HRPT2) mutations identified in subset of patients with mutation-positive carcinomas thought to be sporadic
  - 80% of HPT-JT patients present with hyperparathyroidism
    - Penetrance of hyperparathyroidism is 80%
    - Hyperparathyroidism usually develops by late adolescence
- FIHP
  - Autosomal dominant, 1% of primary hyperparathyroidism
  - Parathyroid gland is only endocrine organ involved
    - Parathyroid adenoma or hyperplasia, and increased risk of parathyroid carcinoma
    - Cause unknown in most families, but *CDC73* (HRPT2) gene involved 15%, *MEN1* gene, and area on chromosome 2 implicated
- MEN1
  - Autosomal dominant, high-penetrance germline mutation in *MEN1* tumor suppressor gene (11q13) encoding menin protein
  - Parathyroid adenomas and carcinomas occur in MEN1 but are less common than hyperplasia (multiglandular parathyroid disease)
  - Somatic *MEN1* mutations occur in 15-20% of sporadic adenomas and occasionally in sporadic carcinomas
  - Other MEN1 features
    - Endocrine: Pituitary adenomas; neuroendocrine tumors of pancreas, duodenum, thymus and lung; gastrinomas; adrenal cortical adenomas and hyperplasia
    - Nonendocrine: Angiofibromas, collagenomas, café au lait macules, lipomas, gingival papules, meningiomas, ependymomas, leiomyomas
- MEN2A
  - Autosomal dominant, high-penetrance germline *RET*-activating protooncogene (10q11.2) mutation
  - 20-30% of MEN2A is associated with parathyroid hyperplasia or adenomas; may also have medullary thyroid carcinoma &/or pheochromocytomas

CLINICAL ISSUES

Epidemiology

- Incidence
  - Most common cause of primary hyperparathyroidism (80-85%)
    - Followed by parathyroid hyperplasia (15%) and carcinoma (1-2%)
  - Incidence has been increasing for 3 decades
    - Attributable to introduction of automatic serum calcium screening
- Age
  - Any age, but most commonly in patients 50-60 years
  - Familial cases occur at younger ages (20-25 years)
- Sex
  - F:M = 3:1 (in patients 50 to 60 years of age)
    - But F:M = 1:1 in patients < 40 years of age; 5:1 in patients > 75 years of age
  - Females and males equally affected in familial cases

Site

- Single parathyroid gland usually involved
  - Lower parathyroid glands involved slightly more often than upper parathyroid glands
  - 10% in other locations: Intrathyroidal, mediastinum, thymus, soft tissue behind esophagus & pharynx
  - Up to 15% have "double adenoma," but asymmetric hyperplasia should be considered
    - "Double adenomas" often involve superior parathyroid glands ("4th pouch disease")

Presentation

- Usually asymptomatic or vague symptoms of fatigue, weakness, gastrointestinal symptoms, cognitive impairment
  - Most identified by abnormal calcium levels
  - 4-15% may present with nephrolithiasis
- Historical symptoms of nephrolithiasis and severe bone disease (osteitis fibrosa cystica) less common today
- Risk of bone fractures increased with primary hyperparathyroidism

Laboratory Tests

- Elevated intact parathyroid hormone (PTH) with elevated albumen adjusted calcium
  - But, some may have normocalcemic primary hyperparathyroidism
- Vast majority of primary hyperparathyroidism, metabolic disease resulting from hypersecretion of hormone from parathyroid tumors, is sporadic
- Serum calcium levels are elevated but less so than in parathyroid carcinoma in which calcium levels are often > 13 mg/dL
- Hypophosphatemia

Natural History

- 25% of asymptomatic patients show disease progression if adenoma is not removed
- Chronic hypercalcemia is associated with increased cardiovascular mortality
- Increased risk bone fractures in primary hyperparathyroidism (4-15%)

Treatment

- Surgical approaches
  - Bilateral neck exploration with excision of adenoma is classic approach
    - Although minimally invasive surgery guided by noninvasive imaging and intraoperative PTH monitoring is gaining favor in nonfamilial cases
  - Subtotal parathyroidectomy is indicated in familial syndromes, such as MEN1 and FIHP
  - Using surgical approach in HPT-JT is controversial because of increased risk of parathyroid cancer
    - But subtotal parathyroidectomy with close postoperative biochemical monitoring for recurrence is currently recommended over prophylactic total parathyroidectomy
  - Resection of single gland (parathyroid adenoma), often with assistance of intraoperative PTH monitoring
    - ≥ 50% drop in intraoperative PTH from baseline at 10 minutes after gland excision is helpful to ensure that abnormal gland(s) has been removed
- Medical therapy with calcimimetics is useful for patients with primary hyperparathyroidism who are poor surgical candidates or have nonlocalizable tumors or inoperable disease
- Clinical follow-up to monitor for recurrent hypercalcemia
  - Asymmetric hyperplasia may present with predominant involvement of 1 gland (mistaken for adenoma) then progress to involve more glands

Prognosis

- Excellent
- Incomplete excision or rupture can result in parathyromatosis

IMAGING

General

- Tc-99m sestamibi and ultrasound are commonly used to localize site of adenoma
- May use computed tomography (CT), magnetic resonance (MR) imaging, etc.

MACROSCOPIC

Normal Parathyroid Gland Macroscopic Features

- Normal parathyroid gland is size and shape of kidney bean (4-6 mm x 2-4 mm), 20-40 mg each
- Most people have 4 parathyroid glands; 10% have ≥ 5 glands, and 3% have < 4 glands

Parathyroid Adenoma Macroscopic Features

- Single enlarged gland: Usually 0.2 to > 1 g, tan to pink-tan, encapsulated, ± rim of normal tissue
- Ovoid, often surrounded by thin capsule
- May have rim of normal (pale tan or yellow)
- Vary in size: < 1 cm to > 10 cm
- Parathyroid adenomas < 0.6 cm and weighing < 100 mg may be referred to as "microadenomas"
- Larger adenomas may show fibrosis, hemosiderin, cystic degeneration, calcification
- Cystic change may occur in adenomas, particularly larger adenomas and in those with HPT-JT syndrome
- Parathyroid adenoma is ectopic in up to 10% (intrathyroidal, mediastinum, thymus, soft tissue behind esophagus and pharynx)
- Double adenomas (also consider asymmetric hyperplasia), which often involves upper parathyroid glands ("4th pouch disease")

MICROSCOPIC

Histologic Features

- **Normal parathyroid gland histology**
  - Normal parathyroid glands can show significant variation in cellularity, even within single individual
  - Normal parathyroid cellularity is distributed unevenly; it is high in infants and children and decreases with age
  - Age, gender, and constitutional factors (body fat, etc.) affect cellularity of normal parathyroid
  - Stromal fat constitutes 10-30% of parathyroid; increases with age
  - More stromal fat in polar regions of parathyroid than central
- **Constituent cells of parathyroid gland**
  - Parathyroid glands are composed of chief cells, transitional cells, oxyphil cells, and adipose tissue
  - Chief cells: 10 μm, polyhedral, round central nuclei, eosinophilic to amphophilic cytoplasm, fat droplets (adults), well-defined cytoplasmic membranes

- o Oxyphil cells: 10-20 μm, abundant eosinophilic cytoplasm (mitochondria), appear at puberty, increase with age, may form nodules
- o Transitional cells: Smaller parenchymal cells with less cytoplasm
- o Clear/water-clear cells: Parenchymal cells with clear cytoplasm (may result from increased vacuolization in chief or oxyphilic cells)
- **Parathyroid adenoma histology**
  - o Proliferation of parathyroid parenchymal chief cells, oxyphil cells, transitional cells, clear cells, or mixtures of cell types
  - o May have thin connective tissue capsule
  - o 50-60% have rim of normal parathyroid tissue
    - Rim more often identified in small adenomas
    - Rim often separated from adenoma by connective tissue capsule, but not always
    - Parathyroid parenchymal cells within rim are typically smaller than those within adenoma
    - Suppressed parathyroid parenchymal cells within rim have larger and more fat droplets than in adenoma cells, which have less lipid and more dispersed lipid than cells in rim
    - Parathyroid hyperplasia can occasionally also have rims of normal tissue
  - o Fat cells sparse (scattered or nested) or absent
  - o Stroma is sparse but vascular, may be fibrotic with hemosiderin deposition in large adenomas or those with cystic change
  - o Adenoma cells may be larger than normal parathyroid cells and have more variably sized nuclei
  - o Often mixture of growth patterns: Solid, follicular, acinar, cords, solid, rosette-like, and rarely papillae
  - o Nuclear palisading around blood vessels is common
  - o Foci of "endocrine atypia" with pleomorphic, hyperchromatic nuclei (up to 25% of cases)
  - o Scattered mitoses in up to 80% of adenomas (more in parathyroid carcinoma)
    - Usually < 1 mitoses/10 high power fields
  - o No atypical mitoses
  - o Cysts and cystic change and degeneration common, especially in large adenomas and HPT-JT cases
  - o May have fibrous bands due to degenerative changes, fibrosis, and hemosiderin
  - o Fibrous bands and fibrosis common in both parathyroid adenoma and carcinoma
  - o No angiolymphatic invasion, perineural invasion, or invasion into adjacent structures
  - o Parathyroid adenomas in MEN1 are histologically similar to sporadic parathyroid adenomas

Parathyroid Adenoma Variants

- **Parathyroid microadenoma**
  - o Parathyroid adenoma weighing < 100 mg; and measuring < 0.6 cm
- **Oncocytic (oxyphilic) parathyroid adenoma**
  - o Benign encapsulated neoplasm composed exclusively or predominantly (> 75%) of mitochondrion-rich oncocytes
  - o 3-6% of parathyroid adenomas
  - o Similar age, female predominance, and serum calcium as conventional parathyroid adenomas but often larger size

- o Originally thought to be nonfunctional but now recognized as cause of hyperparathyroidism
- o Oxyphil cells increase in number and may become nodular in elderly (do not confuse nodular foci of oxyphil cells with oxyphil adenoma)
- o May have less fat in rims of normal tissue than in rims of chief cell adenomas
- o Parathyroid oncocytic (oxyphilic) adenomas cells arranged in sheets, nests, acini, or trabecula
- o Cells are mitochondrion-rich oncocytes with abundant granular eosinophilic cytoplasm, round to oval nuclei with coarse chromatin and may have prominent nucleoli
- o Occasionally may have enlarged nuclei that are irregular and hyperchromatic
- **Water-clear (clear, wasserhelle) cell parathyroid adenoma**
  - o Benign neoplasm of large polyhedral cells with distinct plasma membranes, extensively vacuolated (water-clear) cytoplasm
  - o Exceedingly rare cause of hyperparathyroidism
  - o Must differentiate from clear cell hyperplasia, which is more common than clear cell adenoma
  - o Absence of normalization of PTH suggests that putative clear cell parathyroid adenoma may be normal parathyroid or may be clear cell hyperplasia
  - o Clear cells may be highly glycogenated chief cells or artifact
- **Parathyroid lipoadenoma**
  - o Benign tumor/hamartoma with abundant mature adipose tissue and only scattered nests of parenchymal cells
  - o Rare cause of hyperparathyroidism
  - o Parenchymal chief cells arranged in scattered nests or anastomosing trabeculae or acinar formations amid abundant mature adipose tissue
  - o Must differentiate from normal parathyroid tissue (intraoperative PTH monitoring may be very helpful)
  - o Must differentiate from parathyroid lipohyperplasia since parathyroid adenoma generally affects 1 gland rather than multiple glands in parathyroid hyperplasia
  - o Exceptional cases have oxyphil cells (rather than chief cells) in anastomosing trabeculae or acinar formations (oxyphil lipoadenoma)
  - o Weights are variable: 0.5-420 g
- **Ectopic parathyroid adenoma**
  - o Intrathyroidal, mediastinum, thymus, soft tissue behind esophagus & pharynx
  - o Thymus or mediastinal parathyroid adenomas usually derive from inferior parathyroid glands
  - o Intrathyroidal parathyroid adenomas usually derive from superior parathyroid glands
  - o Intrathyroidal parathyroid adenomas are often partly situated in thyroid capsule or cleft in thyroid surface rather than truly within thyroid

ANCILLARY TESTS

Cytology

- Intermediate cellularity
- Round to oval cells with stippled nuclear chromatic
- Single cells with naked nuclei and groups or clusters of cells
- Prominent vascularity with attached epithelial cells

- Follicular, cord-like, rosette patterns of chief, oxyphilic, transitional, or clear cells
- Can have intranuclear inclusions
- Distinguishing between adenoma, hyperplasia, and carcinoma is generally not possible on fine-needle aspiration specimens
- Occasionally, cells with enlarged hyperchromatic nuclei are seen, but prominent nuclear pleomorphism is generally absent
- Mitotic activity is generally absent
- Follicular pattern can mimic thyroid parenchyma, and oxyphil cells can mimic thyroid Hürthle cells

Frozen Sections

- **Assessing cellularity in small biopsies can be difficult**
  - Cellularity is difficult to assess in small biopsies because it is variable within parathyroid glands and among glands within single individual
  - Polar regions of parathyroid are more cellular than are central regions
  - Cellularity decreases with age and varies with gender, ethnicity, and body habitus
- **Features helpful in differentiating parathyroid from thyroid**
  - Parathyroid cells have well-defined cytoplasmic membranes (very helpful feature in differentiating parathyroid from thyroid)
  - Cytoplasmic lipid (fat droplets) common in parathyroid cell cytoplasm (not in thyroid)
  - Parathyroid cells are smaller and more vacuolated than thyroid cells
  - Parathyroid nuclei have rounder and denser chromatin than thyroid nuclei
  - Parathyroid lacks birefringent calcium oxalate crystals seen in thyroid
  - Parathyroid lacks colloid

Immunohistochemistry

- Positive for neuroendocrine markers chromogranin and synaptophysin
- Positive for keratin (CAM5.2 is most helpful keratin for neuroendocrine tumors)
- Negative for TTF-1, thyroglobulin, calcitonin (usually, but calcitonin can be variable in staining, thus panel of immunostains is often helpful)
- Positive for PTH but less intense staining in adenomas compared to normal parathyroid or rim of normal parathyroid
- Increased p27 (cyclin-dependent kinase inhibitor protein) in parathyroid adenomas compared to carcinomas
- Adenomas are positive for p27, Bcl-2, and MDM2, and have low Ki-67 labeling index (< 4%)
- Carcinomas often low/absent p27, MDM2, and higher Ki-67 labeling index (> 4%)
- Positive for GCM2 (transcription factor) regulatory gene in parathyroid development
- Positive for GATA3 (transcription factor)
- Positive for RB and APC
- Positive for combination of CDKN1B (p27), BCL2, and MDM12
- Negative for galectin-3 and PGP9.5
- Parafibromin/CDC73 (encoded by *CDC73*/HRPT2))

- Loss of nuclear parafibromin in *CDC73* (HRPT2)-associated parathyroid carcinomas and adenomas
- Sporadic adenomas are usually positive for parafibromin, and many carcinomas show loss of parafibromin
- Complete loss of nuclear or nucleolar parafibromin expression in parathyroid carcinoma is helpful differentiating from parathyroid adenoma, which usually shows intact nuclear and nucleolar parafibromin expression
- Caution: Parathyroid carcinomas in hemodialysis patients can show staining in parathyroid carcinomas and metastasis
- Caution: Parafibromin expression may be lost in parathyroid adenomas associated with *CDC73* (HRPT2) germline mutations
- Parafibromin is helpful, but requires rigorously controlled testing as variability exists among laboratories

Genetic Testing

- Study of uncommon familial syndromes has helped to define pathophysiology of both familial and sporadic parathyroid neoplasms
  - Tumor suppressor genes *MEN1* and *CDC73* (HRPT2) were discovered through genetic analysis of kindreds with MEN1 and HPT-JT
  - Somatic mutations in *MEN1* and *CDC73* (HRPT2) are frequent events in clonal development of sporadic parathyroid adenomas and carcinomas, respectively
- *CDC73* (HRPT2) mutation (tumor suppressor gene, 1q21-q31)
  - *CDC73* (HRPT2) gene encodes parafibromin/CDC73 protein
  - Germline *CDC73* (HRPT2)-inactivating mutation in HPT-JT syndrome-associated parathyroid adenoma or hyperplasia and increased risk of parathyroid carcinoma
  - 20% of sporadic cystic adenomas have *CDC73* (HRPT2) mutation; may be HPT-JT related
  - Germline *CDC73* (HRPT2) mutations have been identified in subset of patients with mutation-positive carcinomas (consider genetic testing in patients with parathyroid carcinoma)
  - Somatic *CDC73* (HRPT2) mutations are common in sporadic parathyroid carcinomas and rare in sporadic adenomas
  - Strong association with *CDC73* (HRPT2) mutation and familial and sporadic parathyroid cancer
- Cyclin-D1/*CCND1* oncogene (11q13)
  - 5-8% of parathyroid adenomas have genetic alterations in cyclin-D1/*CCND1* (parathyroid adenoma) gene
  - Cyclin-D1/*CCND1* encodes cyclin-D1, cell cycle regulator from G1 to S phase transition
  - Cyclin-D1 protein overexpression observed in up to 40% of adenomas
- *MEN1* mutation (tumor suppressor gene, 11q13, results in truncated menin protein)
  - Parathyroid adenomas and carcinomas occur in MEN1, but parathyroid hyperplasia occurs more commonly
  - Up to 40% of sporadic parathyroid adenomas have loss of 1 *MEN1* allele, and 1/2 of these have inactivating mutation in 2nd allele
- *RET* mutation (protooncogene, 10q11.2)

○ Germline *RET*-activating mutation in MEN2A (95% mutation in exon 10 or 11, codon 634)

○ 30% of patients with MEN2A have parathyroid hyperplasia, but adenomas can also occur

○ *RET* mutation is generally not identified in sporadic parathyroid disease

- Chromosome 11: Frequent loss in adenomas and frequent gain in carcinomas

DIFFERENTIAL DIAGNOSIS

Parathyroid Carcinoma

- Malignant neoplasm of parathyroid parenchymal cells (chief cells, oxyphilic cells, transitional cells, water-clear cells, or mixture of cell types)
- May be palpable (unusual for adenoma) and larger than adenoma but overlap in size
- Often symptomatic and higher serum calcium levels (> 13 mg/dL) than in adenomas
- Fibrosis and fibrous bands but can be seen in both parathyroid adenoma and carcinoma
- Mitotic figures, but occasional mitoses can also be seen in parathyroid adenoma
  ○ Parathyroid adenomas generally have < 1 mitosis/10 high power fields
- Atypical mitotic figures (usually absent in parathyroid adenoma)
- Parathyroid carcinoma Ki-67 labeling index > 4% (adenomas < 4%)
- Monotonous or trabecular growth, prominent nucleoli, high nuclear to cytoplasmic ratios
- Invasion into adjacent structures, capsular invasion, vascular invasion, perineural invasion
- Complete loss of nuclear or nucleolar parafibromin expression in parathyroid carcinoma is helpful differentiating from parathyroid adenoma, which usually shows intact nuclear and nucleolar parafibromin expression
  ○ But parathyroid carcinomas in hemodialysis patients can show staining in parathyroid carcinomas and metastasis
  ○ Parafibromin expression may be lost in parathyroid adenomas associated with *CDC73* (HRPT2) germline mutations

Atypical Parathyroid Adenoma

- Noninvasive parathyroid neoplasm composed of chief cells with variable oncocytes, transitional cells, and water-clear cells with some features of parathyroid carcinoma
  ○ Adherence to adjacent structures, mitotic activity, fibrosis, trabecular growth, tumor cells in capsule
- No definitive invasion (no invasion into adjacent structures, no capsular invasion, no vascular invasion, no perineural invasion)

Parathyroid Hyperplasia

- Absolute increase in parathyroid parenchymal mass resulting from proliferation of chief, oxyphil, and transitional cells in multiple parathyroid glands
- Distinguishing parathyroid adenoma from hyperplasia classically requires examination of at least 1 additional gland
- Increased utilization of preoperative imaging and localization and intraoperative PTH monitoring assists in identification and removal of diseased parathyroid gland(s)

- Rim of normal tissue seen in 50-60% of parathyroid adenomas and occasionally in parathyroid hyperplasias
- Asymmetric hyperplasia must be strongly considered before diagnosing "double" adenomas

"Double" Parathyroid Adenoma

- May account for up to 15% of adenomas
- Caution: Asymmetric hyperplasia can be easily mistaken for "double" adenoma
- Occasionally, glands of parathyroid hyperplasia may show rims of normal parathyroid tissue
- Diagnosis requires resolution of hypercalcemia and hyperparathyroidism and long-term follow-up to be certain that no other glands are involved

Thyroid Follicular Neoplasm

- Often shows follicular growth, which can be seen in some parathyroid adenomas
- Thyroid tissues and neoplasms often have colloid and calcium oxylate crystals but lack intracytoplasmic lipid and well-defined cytoplasmic membranes of parathyroid tissue
- Oncocytic parathyroid adenomas must be distinguished from Hürthle cell thyroid tumors
- Immunohistochemical studies can be helpful in differentiating thyroid follicular neoplasms from parathyroid in difficult cases
  ○ Thyroid tissues and tumors are positive for TTF-1 and thyroglobulin and negative for PTH, chromogranin, and synaptophysin

Medullary Thyroid Carcinoma

- Both medullary thyroid carcinoma and parathyroid lack colloid and have neuroendocrine-type chromatin
- Both parathyroid cells and medullary thyroid carcinoma cells can have intranuclear inclusions
- Both medullary thyroid carcinoma and parathyroid are positive for neuroendocrine markers chromogranin and synaptophysin and keratin (particularly CAM5.2)
- Medullary thyroid carcinoma is positive for calcitonin and CEA and negative for PTH

DIAGNOSTIC CHECKLIST

Clinically Relevant Pathologic Features

- Often asymptomatic, identified by screening calcium
- Serum calcium elevated, but markedly elevated serum calcium (> 13 mg/dL) worrisome for carcinoma

Pathologic Interpretation Pearls

- Composed of chief, oxyphilic, transitional, clear, or mixtures of cell types
- Parathyroid (unlike thyroid) has well-demarcated cytoplasmic membranes, cytoplasmic lipid, round nuclei, and dense chromatin and lacks colloid and calcium oxylate crystals
- Normal parathyroid tissue shows significant variation in cellularity within and among glands
- Fibrosis, hemosiderin, and occasional mitoses may be seen, but no capsular, vascular, or perineural invasion in adenomas
- Rims of normal tissue in 50-60% of adenomas but can be seen in hyperplasia

- Complete loss of nuclear or nucleolar parafibromin expression in parathyroid carcinoma is helpful differentiating from parathyroid adenoma, which usually shows intact nuclear and nucleolar parafibromin expression

SELECTED REFERENCES

1. Al-Hraishawi H et al: Intact parathyroid hormone levels and primary hyperparathyroidism. Endocr Res. 1-5, 2017
2. Arya AK et al: Promoter hypermethylation inactivates CDKN2A, CDKN2B and RASSF1A genes in sporadic parathyroid adenomas. Sci Rep. 7(1):3123, 2017
3. Clark CM et al: Atypical parathyroid adenoma with diffuse fibrosis. Ear Nose Throat J. 96(2):57-58, 2017
4. El Hussein S et al: Water clear cell adenoma of the parathyroid gland: a forgotten cause of primary hyperparathyroidism. Int J Surg Pathol. 1066896917701577, 2017
5. Jervis L et al: Osteolytic lesions: osteitis fibrosa cystica in the setting of severe primary hyperparathyroidism. BMJ Case Rep. 2017, 2017
6. Krishna Mohan VS et al: Atypical parathyroid adenoma with multiple brown tumors as initial presentation: a rare entity. Indian J Nucl Med. 32(2):133-136, 2017
7. Leere JS et al: Contemporary medical management of primary hyperparathyroidism: a systematic review. Front Endocrinol (Lausanne). 8:79, 2017
8. Marchiori E et al: Specifying the molecular pattern of sporadic parathyroid tumorigenesis-The Y282D variant of the GCM2 gene. Biomed Pharmacother. 92:843-848, 2017
9. Padinhare-Keloth TNTK et al: Sensitive detection of a small parathyroid adenoma using fluorocholine PET/CT: a case report. Nucl Med Mol Imaging. 51(2):186-189, 2017
10. Ruanpeng D et al: Intrathymic parathyroid adenoma. Am J Med Sci. 353(5):506, 2017
11. Silva-Figueroa AM et al: Epigenetic processes in sporadic parathyroid neoplasms. Mol Cell Endocrinol. ePub, 2017
12. Verdelli C et al: Epigenetic alterations in parathyroid cancers. Int J Mol Sci. 18(2), 2017
13. Agarwal C et al: Parathyroid lesions: difficult diagnosis on cytology. Diagn Cytopathol. 44(8):704-9, 2016
14. Christakis I et al: Parathyroid carcinoma and atypical parathyroid neoplasms in MEN1 patients; a clinico-pathologic challenge. The MD Anderson case series and review of the literature. Int J Surg. 31:10-6, 2016
15. Christakis I et al: Differentiating atypical parathyroid neoplasm from parathyroid cancer. Ann Surg Oncol. 23(9):2889-97, 2016
16. Hosny Mohammed K et al: Parafibromin, APC, and MIB-1 are useful markers for distinguishing parathyroid carcinomas from adenomas. Appl Immunohistochem Mol Morphol. ePub, 2016
17. Kumari N et al: Role of histological criteria and immunohistochemical markers in predicting risk of malignancy in parathyroid neoplasms. Endocr Pathol. 27(2):87-96, 2016
18. Mathews JW et al: Hyperparathyroidism-jaw tumor syndrome: an overlooked cause of severe hypercalcemia. Am J Med Sci. 352(3):302-5, 2016
19. Serrano-Gonzalez M et al: A germline mutation of HRPT2/CDC73 (70 G>T) in an adolescent female with parathyroid carcinoma: first case report and a review of the literature. J Pediatr Endocrinol Metab. 29(9):1005-12, 2016
20. Shifrin A et al: Primary and metastatic parathyroid malignancies: a rare or underdiagnosed condition? J Clin Endocrinol Metab. 100(3):E478-81, 2015
21. Forde HE et al: Parathyroid adenoma in a patient with familial hypocalciuric hypercalcaemia. BMJ Case Rep. 2014, 2014
22. Gill AJ: Understanding the genetic basis of parathyroid carcinoma. Endocr Pathol. 25(1):30-4, 2014
23. Kruijff S et al: Negative parafibromin staining predicts malignant behavior in atypical parathyroid adenomas. Ann Surg Oncol. 21(2):426-33, 2014
24. Mishra A et al: An interesting case of life-threatening hypercalcemia secondary to atypical parathyroid adenoma versus parathyroid carcinoma. Case Rep Med. 2014:473814, 2014
25. Sadler C et al: Parathyroid carcinoma in more than 1,000 patients: a population-level analysis. Surgery. 156(6):1622-9; discussion 1629-30, 2014
26. Soong CP et al: Recurrent ZFX mutations in human sporadic parathyroid adenomas. Oncoscience. 1(5):360-6, 2014
27. Thompson LD: Parathyroid adenoma. Ear Nose Throat J. 93(7):246-68, 2014
28. Truran PP et al: Parafibromin, galectin-3, PGP9.5, Ki67, and cyclin D1: using an immunohistochemical panel to aid in the diagnosis of parathyroid cancer. World J Surg. 38(11):2845-54, 2014
29. DeLellis RA: Parathyroid tumors and related disorders. Mod Pathol. 24 Suppl 2:S78-93, 2011
30. Zhang Y et al: Endocrine tumors as part of inherited tumor syndromes. Adv Anat Pathol. 18(3):206-18, 2011
31. Chow LS et al: Parathyroid lipoadenomas: a rare cause of primary hyperparathyroidism. Endocr Pract. 12(2):131-6, 2006
32. Prasad KK et al: Water-clear cell adenoma of the parathyroid gland: a rare entity. Indian J Pathol Microbiol. 47(1):39-40, 2004
33. DeLellis RA et al: Paraneoplastic endocrine syndromes: a review. Endocr Pathol. 14(4):303-17, 2003
34. World Health Organization Tumors of Endocrine Organs. 2017

Parathyroid Adenoma

Parathyroid Adenoma vs. Carcinoma

Feature	Parathyroid Adenoma	Parathyroid Carcinoma
Symptoms	Usually asymptomatic or vague	Often symptomatic
Serum calcium	Elevated	Markedly elevated (> 13 mg/dL)
Palpable mass	Unusual	Yes
Tumor size	Enlarged	Larger but may overlap
Invasion into adjacent structures	No (but can have irregular growth and cells in capsule due to degenerative features)	Yes
Fibrous bands	Can be present due to degenerative features	Yes
Perineural invasion	No	Yes
Vascular invasion	No	Yes
Growth pattern	Patterns of growth (follicular, acinar, etc.)	Monotonous, sheet-like growth
Cellular features	Often mixed cell types, can show endocrine atypia	Often monotonous cytomorphology, prominent nucleoli
Mitoses	Few, scattered	Yes, more numerous mitoses than adenomas
Proliferation markers (Ki-67/MIB-1)	Low	Moderate to high
Parafibromin (CDC73) protein expression	Parathyroid adenoma usually shows intact nuclear and nucleolar parafibromin expression	Complete loss of nuclear or nucleolar parafibromin expression in parathyroid carcinoma

Parathyroid and Thyroid Immunohistochemistry

Tissue	Keratin	TTF-1	PTH	Chro	Syn	Calcitonin
Parathyroid cells and tumors	Positive (particularly low molecular weight keratins, e.g., CAM5.2)	Negative	Positive (but often not an overly robust stain)	Positive	Positive	Negative
Thyroid follicular cells and neoplasms	Positive	Positive (strong nuclear staining)	Negative	Negative	Negative	Negative
Medullary thyroid carcinoma	Positive (particularly low molecular weight keratins, e.g., CAM5.2)	Positive (nuclear staining, may not be as strong as in follicular cells and neoplasms)	Negative	Positive	Positive	Positive

Chro = chromogranin; syn = synaptophysin.

(Left) *Chief cell parathyroid adenoma ⇥ shows adjacent rim of normal ⇥ parathyroid tissue, a feature often identified in smaller rather than larger adenomas. The rim is often separated from the adenoma by connective tissue but not always.* **(Right)** *Chief cell parathyroid adenoma shows an area of cystic change. Cystic change is common in larger parathyroid adenomas and those associated with hyperparathyroidism-jaw tumor syndrome.*

Chief Cell Adenoma With Rim

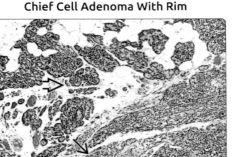

Cystic Change in Parathyroid Adenoma

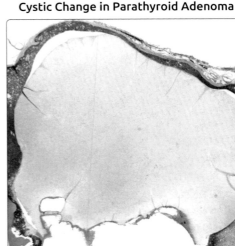

(Left) *This parathyroid chief cell adenoma ⇥ is present within the thymus ⇥. 10% of parathyroid adenomas occur in unusual locations, such as intrathyroidal or within mediastinum, thymus, or soft tissues behind the esophagus and pharynx.* **(Right)** *Benign parathyroid lesions can show foci of "endocrine atypia" with pleomorphism and nuclear hyperchromasia. These foci should not be mistaken for the atypia of parathyroid carcinoma. Often, parathyroid carcinomas will show a markedly monotonous growth pattern and cytomorphology.*

Intrathymic Parathyroid Adenoma

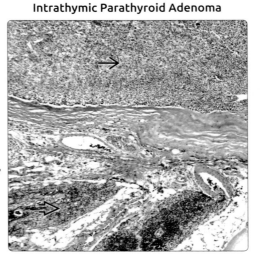

"Endocrine Atypia"

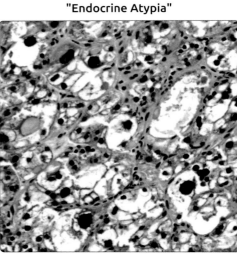

(Left) *Follicular patterns are relatively common in parathyroid adenoma. Occasionally, parathyroid adenomas may show large follicular-like spaces with proteinaceous fluid and can be mistaken for thyroid follicles with colloid.* **(Right)** *This chief cell adenoma has a glandular growth pattern. Parathyroid adenomas may have various growth patterns, while parathyroid carcinomas often have a monotonous or trabecular growth pattern.*

Follicles With Colloid-like Material

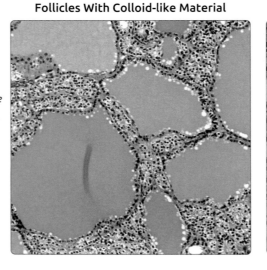

Follicular Growth Pattern

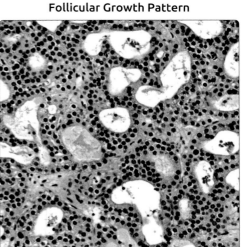

Hemorrhage in Parathyroid Adenoma

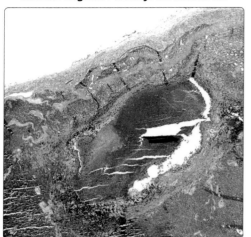

Edematous Change

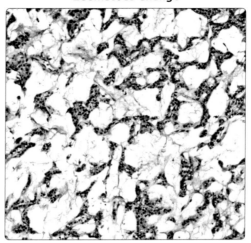

(Left) *Hemorrhage, hemosiderin, and fibrosis can be seen as degenerative features in a parathyroid adenoma, particularly those that are large or show cystic change. These features can also be due to prior trauma, such as fine-needle aspiration.* **(Right)** *This is edematous change in a chief cell adenoma. Various degenerative features can be seen in parathyroid adenomas, particularly in large adenomas.*

Clear Cell Parathyroid Adenoma

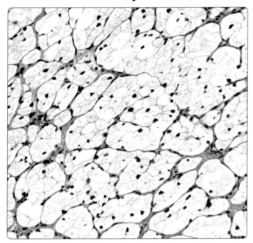

Oxyphil Parathyroid Adenoma With Rim

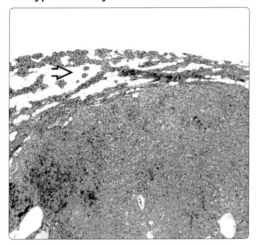

(Left) *This clear (water-clear/wasserhelle) cell parathyroid adenoma is composed of large polyhedral cells with distinct plasma membranes and extensively vacuolated cytoplasm.* **(Right)** *Oxyphil parathyroid adenoma shows a rim of normal parathyroid ⮕. Oxyphil adenomas are usually functional tumors and are associated with levels of serum calcium that are similar to those seen in chief cell adenomas.*

Oxyphil Parathyroid Adenoma

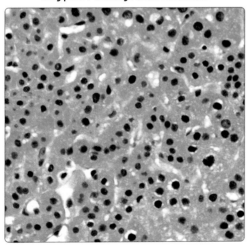

Pleomorphic Cells in Parathyroid Adenoma

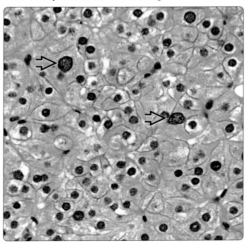

(Left) *Oxyphil cells (10-20 μm) are larger than chief cells (10 μm) and have abundant eosinophilic granular cytoplasm. Oxyphil cell adenomas are uncommon, comprising ~ 3-6% of parathyroid adenomas.* **(Right)** *Foci of nuclear pleomorphism (endocrine atypia) ⮕ can be seen in oxyphil cell adenomas. Well-defined cytoplasmic membranes of parathyroid cells help to differentiate parathyroid from thyroid.*

Parathyroid Lipoadenoma

TERMINOLOGY

- Benign tumor/hamartoma containing abundant mature adipose tissue with only scattered nests of parenchyma involving 1 parathyroid gland
  - In conjunction with primary hyperparathyroidism and resolution of hypercalcemia postoperatively

CLINICAL ISSUES

- Presentation similar to conventional parathyroid adenoma
- Patients usually asymptomatic and identified by screening serum calcium
- Intraoperative parathyroid hormone monitoring important in identifying removal of appropriate gland(s)

IMAGING

- Tc-99m sestamibi parathyroid imaging and ultrasound helpful in locating lesion

MACROSCOPIC

- Enlarged parathyroid gland, yellow-tan in color, soft, may be lobulated

MICROSCOPIC

- Proliferation of stromal and parenchymal elements in 1 parathyroid gland associated with primary hyperparathyroidism
- Abundant adipocytes with scattered nests and cords of parenchymal (usually chief) cells
- Parenchymal cells can be purely oxyphilic (oxyphilic lipoadenoma)
- Myxoid change and fibrosis common

TOP DIFFERENTIAL DIAGNOSES

- Normal parathyroid gland
- Parathyroid lipohyperplasia
- Thymolipoadenoma
- Lipoma

Parathyroid Lipoadenoma

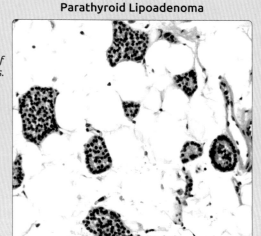

Mature Adipose Tissue and Chief Cells

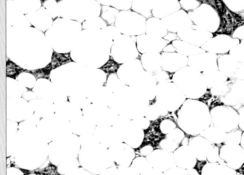

(Left) Parathyroid lipoadenomas are composed of abundant (> 50%) mature fat cells and scattered nests of parathyroid parenchymal cells. Hyperparathyroidism resolves after removal of the involved gland. (Right) Parathyroid lipoadenomas are functional lesions. They are composed predominantly of mature adipose cells with scattered small nests of parathyroid parenchymal chief cells.

Myxoid Change in Lipoadenoma

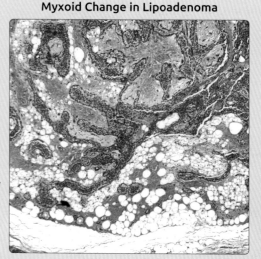

Prominent Myxoid Changes

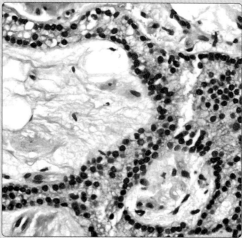

(Left) Parathyroid lipoadenoma with myxoid change is shown. Myxoid changes can be prominent in some cases with less lipomatous components. These tumors may also be called myxoid lipoadenomas. (Right) Myxoid changes can be very prominent in lipoadenomas. Parathyroid adenoma with prominent myxoid change is shown. These areas are surrounded by chief cells.

TERMINOLOGY

Synonyms

- Parathyroid hamartoma

Definitions

- Rare, benign tumor/hamartoma containing abundant mature adipose tissue with only scattered nests of parathyroid parenchyma involving 1 parathyroid gland in conjunction with primary hyperparathyroidism and resolution of hypercalcemia postoperatively
- Recent study defined as single adenoma with > 50% fat on histologic examination in conjunction with primary hyperparathyroidism and resolution of hypercalcemia upon resection of involved parathyroid gland

ETIOLOGY/PATHOGENESIS

Unknown

- No specific underlying etiology known
  - Extremely rare entity

CLINICAL ISSUES

Epidemiology

- Incidence
  - Extraordinarily rare cause of primary hyperparathyroidism
  - Exact incidence unknown
- Age
  - Middle-aged and older individuals, generally appears to occur at similar age as conventional parathyroid adenoma
- Sex
  - Possible female predominance (F:M = 3:2) suggested but unclear since so few cases reported

Site

- Parathyroid tissue, but report supernumerary mediastinal lipoadenoma
- Involves 1 parathyroid gland (if multiple glands, then lipohyperplasia)
  - Rare examples of double lipoadenomas, but asymmetric hyperplasia would need to be considered

Presentation

- Presentation similar to conventional parathyroid adenoma
- Patients usually asymptomatic and identified by screening serum calcium
- Symptomatic cases have been reported

Laboratory Tests

- Serum calcium elevated (mean: 11.1 mg/dL) but < in parathyroid carcinoma in which calcium levels often > 13-14 mg/dL
- Hypophosphatemia
- Elevated serum parathyroid hormone (PTH)

Treatment

- Resection of single gland (parathyroid adenoma), often with assistance of intraoperative PTH monitoring
  - ≥ 50% drop in intraoperative PTH from baseline at 10 minutes after gland excised helpful to ensure abnormal gland(s) removed

- Clinical follow-up to monitor for recurrent hypercalcemia

Prognosis

- All cases thus far behaved in benign manner

IMAGING

General Features

- Can be more difficult to locate with imaging than conventional parathyroid adenomas
- Tc-99m sestamibi parathyroid imaging helpful in locating lesion for surgical purposes
- Ultrasound reportedly also identifies some lesions

MACROSCOPIC

Normal Parathyroid Gland

- Normal parathyroid gland has size and shape of kidney bean (4-6 mm x 2-4 mm), weighs 20-40 mg each
- Most people have 4 parathyroid glands, 3% have > 4, and 10% have ≥ 5

Parathyroid Lipoadenoma

- Single enlarged parathyroid gland, grossly encapsulated and yellow or tan
  - If > 1 enlarged gland, then hyperplasia (lipohyperplasia) most likely
- Weight of involved gland variable: 0.5-420.0 g
- Involvement of supernumerary parathyroid in mediastinum reported
- Round, oval, or lobular tumor with smooth outer surface

MICROSCOPIC

Histologic Features

- **Normal parathyroid gland**
  - Can show significant variation in cellularity even in single individual
  - Cellularity variable, distributed unevenly, high in infants and children, decreases with age
  - Age, gender, constitutional factors, ethnicity, etc. affect cellularity of normal parathyroid glands
  - Stromal fat constitutes 10-30% of normal parathyroid, increases with age
  - More stromal fat in polar regions of parathyroid than centrally
  - **Constituent cells of parathyroid gland**
    - Parathyroid glands are composed of chief cells, transitional cells, oxyphil cells, and adipose tissue
    - Chief cells: 10 μm, polyhedral, round central nuclei, eosinophilic to amphophilic cytoplasm, fat droplets (adults), well-defined cytoplasmic membranes
    - Oxyphil cells: 10-20 μm, abundant eosinophilic cytoplasm (mitochondria), appear at puberty, increase with age, may form nodules
    - Transitional cells: Smaller parenchymal cells with less cytoplasm
    - Clear/water-clear cells: Parenchymal cells with clear cytoplasm (may be due to increased vacuolization in chief or oxyphilic cells)
- **Parathyroid lipoadenoma**

- Proliferation of stromal and parenchymal elements in 1 parathyroid gland associated with primary hyperparathyroidism
- Abundant adipocytes (> 50%) and only scattered nests of parenchymal chief cells (or oxyphilic cells)
- Stroma is abundant adipose tissue, ± myxoid change and fibrosis
- May have foci of lymphoid cells or scattered inflammatory cells
- Stroma may also show calcium deposits
- Parathyroid parenchymal cells usually chief cells but can be mixture of cell types or, in rare cases, purely oxyphil cells
- Parenchymal cells in small nests and thin, branching cords and anastomosing trabeculae or acini
- Lipoadenoma with parenchymal oxyphilic cells (oncocytic/oxyphilic lipoadenoma) reported
- Myxoid change can be prominent in some cases with less lipomatous component (myxoid lipoadenoma)
- Parathyroid lipoadenoma can have thymic elements (thymolipoadenoma)
- Adjacent rim of normocellular parathyroid useful clue when present
- Foci of lipoadenomatous change can be seen in otherwise conventional parathyroid adenomas

DIFFERENTIAL DIAGNOSIS

Normal Parathyroid Gland

- Smaller than lipoadenoma
  - Size and shape of kidney bean (4-6 mm x 2-4 mm), 20-40 mg each
- Not associated with increased serum calcium or PTH
- Caution, as cellularity of normal parathyroid gland is variable, among individuals and within single parathyroid gland
  - Cellularity also varies with age and constitutional factors
- Intraoperative PTH monitoring important in removal of appropriate gland

Parathyroid Lipohyperplasia

- Hyperparathyroidism with > 1 (usually 3 or 4) enlarged parathyroid glands
- Similar to parathyroid lipoadenoma, involved glands of parathyroid lipohyperplasia show admixture of large amounts of mature fat focal myxoid stroma and parenchymal cell nests
- Multiple gland involvement identified in parathyroid lipohyperplasia differentiates it from single gland involvement of parathyroid lipoadenoma

Thymolipoadenoma

- Variant morphology of parathyroid lipoadenoma with thymic elements

Lipoma

- Unlike lipoadenomas, lipomas not associated with hyperparathyroidism
- Lipomas lack nests and cords of parathyroid parenchymal elements present in parathyroid lipoadenoma

DIAGNOSTIC CHECKLIST

Clinically Relevant Pathologic Features

- Extraordinarily rare form of hyperparathyroidism
- No known specific underlying etiology
- Clinical presentation similar to conventional parathyroid adenoma
  - Patients often asymptomatic, identified by screening serum calcium
  - Symptomatic cases have been reported

Pathologic Interpretation Pearls

- Rare, benign tumor/hamartoma containing abundant mature adipose tissue with only scattered nests of parenchyma involving single parathyroid gland in conjunction with primary hyperparathyroidism and resolution of hypercalcemia postoperatively
- Usually occurs at site of normal parathyroid, but supranumerary case in mediastinum reported
- Parenchymal chief cells arranged in scattered nests or anastomosing trabeculae or acinar formations amid abundant mature adipose tissue
  - Exceptional cases may have oxyphil cells (oxyphil/oncocytic lipoadenomas) rather than chief cells
- Must be differentiated from normal parathyroid tissue
- Normal parathyroid gland is smaller than parathyroid adenoma and not associated with hypercalcemia or hyperparathyroidism
- Clinical correlation with imaging studies, intraoperative parathyroid hormone testing, and clinical follow-up can be helpful in confirming that appropriate parathyroid gland(s) removed

SELECTED REFERENCES

1. Cetani F et al: A large functioning parathyroid lipoadenoma. Endocrine. 53(2):615-6, 2016
2. Hyrcza MD et al: Parathyroid lipoadenoma: a clinicopathological diagnosis and possible trap for the unaware pathologist. Endocr Pathol. 27(1):34-41, 2016
3. Ogrin C: A rare case of double parathyroid lipoadenoma with hyperparathyroidism. Am J Med Sci. 346(5):432-4, 2013
4. Sanei MH et al: Ectopic lipoadenoma of parathyroid. J Res Med Sci. 17(10):983-4, 2012
5. Lee AY et al: Importance of intraoperative parathyroid hormone measurement in the diagnosis of parathyroid lipoadenoma. Head Neck. 33(6):917-9, 2011
6. Meng Z et al: Tc-99m sestamibi parathyroid imaging in a rare case of parathyroid lipoadenoma. Ann Nucl Med. 23(3):317-20, 2009
7. Chow LS et al: Parathyroid lipoadenomas: a rare cause of primary hyperparathyroidism. Endocr Pract. 12(2):131-6, 2006
8. DeLellis RA: Tumors of the Parathyroid Gland. AFIP Atlas of Tumor Pathology Series 3, Fascicle 6. Washington DC: American Registry of Pathology. 1-102, 1991
9. Obara T et al: Functioning parathyroid lipoadenoma–report of four cases: clinicopathological and ultrasonographic features. Endocrinol Jpn. 36(1):135-45, 1989
10. Straus FH 2nd et al: Five cases of parathyroid lipohyperplasia. Surgery. 94(6):901-5, 1983
11. Wolff M et al: Functioning lipoadenoma of a supernumerary parathyroid gland in the mediastinum. Head Neck Surg. 2(4):302-7, 1980
12. Abul-Haj SK et al: Functioning lipoadenoma of the parathyroid gland. Report of a unique case. N Engl J Med. 266:121-3, 1962

Lipoadenoma

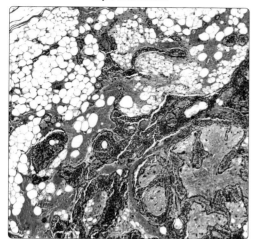

Adipose Tissue and Oxyphil Cells

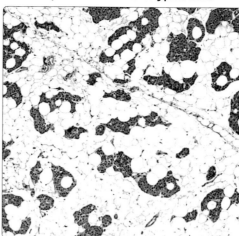

(Left) This low-power view of a parathyroid lipoadenoma (hamartoma) shows parathyroid chief cells intermixed with bands of fibrous tissue, myxoid stroma, and mature adipocytes. (Right) This parathyroid lipoadenoma has evenly distributed nests and cords of chief and oxyphil cells in a background of abundant adipose tissue.

Abundant Adipose Tissue

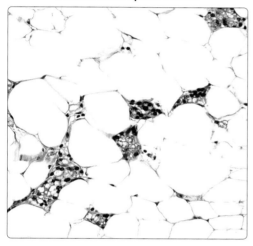

Scattered Parathyroid Chief Cells

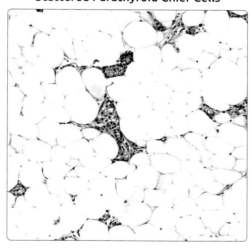

(Left) Parathyroid lipoadenoma with small groups of parathyroid chief cells with abundant adipose tissue is shown. (Right) Parathyroid lipoadenoma shows irregular branching nests of parathyroid parenchymal chief cells and abundant mature adipose tissue (> 50%).

Groups of Oxyphil Cells Within Fat

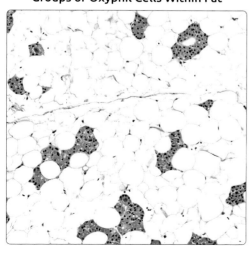

Oxyphil Lipoadenoma

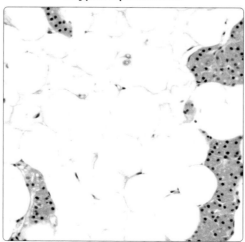

(Left) Oxyphil parathyroid lipoadenoma with parathyroid oxyphil cells amid abundant adipose tissue is shown. Oxyphil lipoadenomas are very rare, but they are functional tumors associated with normalization of serum calcium and parathyroid hormone upon removal. (Right) Oxyphil parathyroid lipoadenoma with irregularly branching nests of oxyphil cells and abundant adipose is shown. Oxyphil lipoadenomas are rare.

Parathyroid Atypical Adenoma

TERMINOLOGY

- Atypical parathyroid adenoma is noninvasive parathyroid neoplasm composed of chief cells with variable amounts of oxyphil and transitional cells
  - Some features of parathyroid carcinoma (adherence to adjacent structures, mitotic activity, fibrosis, cells within capsule) but lacking unequivocal capsular, vascular, or perineural invasion
- Shares features with parathyroid carcinoma, such as adherence to adjacent structures, mitotic activity, fibrosis, trabecular growth pattern, and tumor cells within capsule

CLINICAL ISSUES

- Atypical parathyroid adenoma and parathyroid carcinomas may be clinically indistinguishable
- Intraoperative findings may be similar in atypical parathyroid adenoma and carcinoma as both may show adherence to adjacent structures and thickened capsules

MICROSCOPIC

- Hypercellular parathyroid gland with atypical features (mitoses, fibrosis, tumor cells trapped in capsule)
- No invasive growth (no capsular, vascular, or perineural invasion, and no invasion into adjacent structures)

ANCILLARY TESTS

- Parathyroid tumors positive for chromogranin, synaptophysin, parathyroid hormone, and keratin (CAM5.2), and negative for pax-8, TTF-1 and thyroglobulin
- Parafibromin (CDC73) often absent in parathyroid carcinoma and usually present in parathyroid adenoma, including atypical adenoma
- Parafibromin-positive atypical adenomas usually do not recur
- Parafibromin-negative tumors have 10-20% risk of recurrence and may be considered tumors of low malignant potential

Bands of Fibrosis and Nodular Growth

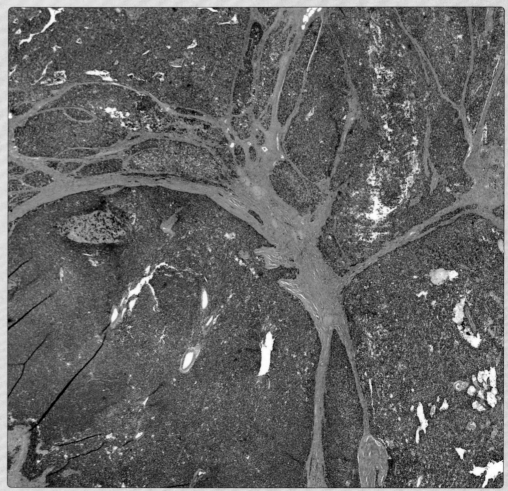

This atypical parathyroid adenoma has nodular growth with associated fibrous bands. Atypical features can be seen in these lesions, but no unequivocal invasion is identified.

TERMINOLOGY

Definitions

- Noninvasive parathyroid neoplasm composed of chief cells with variable amounts of oxyphil and transitional cells
  - Shares features with parathyroid carcinoma, such as adherence to adjacent structures, mitotic activity, fibrosis, trabecular growth, and tumor cells within capsule, but lacks unequivocal capsular, vascular, or perineural invasion or invasion into adjacent structures
- Atypical parathyroid adenomas have been described as parathyroid tumors of uncertain malignant potential

ETIOLOGY/PATHOGENESIS

Sporadic

- Etiology not well understood
- Possible association with ionizing radiation

Inherited

- Hereditary hyperparathyroidism less common than sporadic
- CDC73 (HRPT2)-associated, less often MEN1 or MEN2A

Hyperparathyroidism-Jaw Tumor Syndrome

- Autosomal dominant
- Inactivating mutations in CDC73 (HRPT2) (1q21-q31) tumor suppressor gene that encodes parafibromin/CDC73
- Hyperparathyroidism, fibroosseous jaw tumors, kidney cysts, hamartomas, and Wilms tumors
- Parathyroid adenoma or carcinoma (increase risk of parathyroid carcinoma)
- Penetrance hyperparathyroidism 80%
- 15% develop parathyroid carcinoma

Familial Isolated Hyperparathyroidism

- Autosomal dominant, accounts for 1% hyperparathyroidism
- Cause unknown in most families, but CDC73 (HRPT2) (15%), MEN1, and area on chromosome 2 implicated

MEN1

- Autosomal dominant, high-penetrance germline mutation in MEN1 tumor suppressor gene (11q13) encoding menin protein
- Parathyroid adenoma, including atypical adenoma, and carcinomas occur in MEN1 but are less common than multiglandular parathyroid disease

CLINICAL ISSUES

Epidemiology

- Age
  - 5th decade (range: 3rd-7th decade)
- Sex
  - F > M

Presentation

- Often asymptomatic or vague symptoms of fatigue, weakness; gastrointestinal symptoms
- May be clinically indistinguishable from parathyroid carcinoma

  - However, atypical parathyroid adenoma generally lacks palpable neck mass seen in some carcinomas
  - Serum calcium elevated, but less than in carcinoma
    - Serum calcium levels may overlap, often intermediate calcium levels between typical adenomas and carcinomas
- Operative findings may not differentiate atypical parathyroid adenoma from carcinoma
  - Recent French study: Subset of patients with atypical adenoma had suspicious findings intraoperatively with adherence to adjacent tissues or thick capsule

Laboratory Tests

- Elevated serum calcium, < 13.5 mg/dL (rarely above 14 mg/dL), but lower mean calcium than in parathyroid carcinomas (however, overlap in calcium, often levels intermediate between typical parathyroid adenoma and carcinoma)

Natural History

- Usually cured by resection, but recurrences and persistent disease have been reported in some cases

Treatment

- Surgical resection of involved gland usually curative
- Intraoperative parathyroid hormone (PTH) monitoring helpful in ensuring removal of diseased gland(s)
- As intraoperative findings may be indistinguishable for atypical parathyroid adenoma and carcinoma, some are resected en bloc with ipsilateral lobe of thyroid
- Clinical follow-up to monitor for recurrent hypercalcemia

Prognosis

- Usually indolent behavior, but close clinical follow-up is recommended
- Loss of CDC73 (parafibromin) may be helpful predicting recurrence
- Parafibromin-positive atypical parathyroid adenomas usually do not recur
- Parafibromin-negative tumors have 10-20% risk of recurrence

MACROSCOPIC

General Features

- Single parathyroid gland involved
- May be adhered to adjacent thyroid tissue due to fibrosis and have thickened capsule
- Grossly and surgically may be difficult to differentiate atypical parathyroid adenoma from carcinoma

Size

- Variable: 2.2 cm, 6.5 g

MICROSCOPIC

Histologic Features

- Hypercellular parathyroid with some features of carcinoma (fibrosis, mitoses) but lack definitive invasive growth
- Intratumoral &/or peritumoral fibrosis
- May have entrapped tumor cells within capsule
- No extension of tumor beyond capsule (true invasion must be distinguished from entrapment of tumor cells)
- Hemosiderin deposition

- Cyst formation
- Mitoses may be present, but not atypical mitoses
- No necrosis
- No vascular invasion (caution as artifactual dislodgement of tumor cells must be differentiated from true vascular invasion)
- No perineural invasion
- No invasion into adjacent structures

ANCILLARY TESTS

Immunohistochemistry

- Parathyroid positive for neuroendocrine markers chromogranin and synaptophysin
- Parathyroid positive for parathyroid hormone
- Keratin positive, particularly CAM5.2 (most helpful keratin for neuroendocrine tumors)
- Negative for TTF-1, thyroglobulin, calcitonin (usually)
- Positive p27, Bcl-2, MDM2, and low Ki-67 in parathyroid adenomas and atypical adenomas (opposite to immunophenotype of carcinomas)
- Parafibromin (encoded by HRPT2)
  - Parafibromin (CDC73) often absent in parathyroid carcinoma and often present in parathyroid adenoma
  - Sporadic adenomas usually positive for parafibromin, while many carcinomas show loss of parafibromin
  - Parathyroid carcinomas in hemodialysis patients can show staining in primary and metastatic parathyroid carcinomas
  - CDC73 (HRPT2) encodes parafibromin/CDC73
  - Loss of nuclear parafibromin in CDC73 (HRPT2)-associated parathyroid carcinomas and adenomas
  - Complete loss of nuclear parafibromin expression in parathyroid carcinoma helpful as adenoma, including atypical adenoma, usually shows parafibromin expression
    - Parafibromin expression may be lost in parathyroid adenomas with germline CDC73/HRPT2 mutations
    - Parathyroid carcinomas in hemodialysis patients can show staining in primary and metastases
  - Parafibromin-positive atypical parathyroid adenomas usually do not recur
    - However, parafibromin-negative tumors may recur
      - These may be considered tumors of low malignant potential
  - Parafibromin helpful but requires rigorously controlled testing as variability among laboratories

Genetic Testing

- CDC73 (HRPT2) (tumor suppressor gene, 1q21-q31) encodes CDC73 (parafibromin) protein
  - CDC73 (HRPT2) mutation in familial and sporadic parathyroid carcinoma
  - CDC73 (HRPT2) mutation uncommon in sporadic adenomas, but identified in 20% of sporadic cystic adenomas (may be HPT-JT associated)

DIFFERENTIAL DIAGNOSIS

Parathyroid Carcinoma

- Parathyroid carcinomas and atypical parathyroid adenomas may both be large in size, have solid growth, intratumoral and peritumoral fibrosis, and mitoses
  - However, atypical parathyroid adenomas do not have invasion (capsular, vascular, perineural, or invasion into adjacent structures)
- May have palpable mass (unusual for parathyroid adenoma and atypical parathyroid adenoma)
- Larger than adenomas (including atypical adenomas), but overlap in size
- Serum calcium usually markedly elevated in parathyroid carcinoma (> 13 mg/dL), generally higher than in parathyroid adenoma and atypical parathyroid adenoma, but serum calcium levels may show overlap
- Often solid or trabecular growth; lacks well-defined follicular or acinar patterns often seen in adenomas
- Mitotic activity can be seen in atypical parathyroid adenomas and carcinomas, but atypical mitoses generally limited to parathyroid carcinomas
- Fibrosis and fibrous bands common in both parathyroid carcinoma and adenoma
- Tumor cells may be trapped in capsule of atypical parathyroid adenoma but lack definitive capsular invasion
- Vascular invasion (must distinguish true vascular invasion from tumor cells pushed into capsule)
- Complete loss of nuclear parafibromin expression in parathyroid carcinoma helpful as adenoma, including atypical adenoma, usually shows parafibromin expression
- Loss of expression of parafibromin, retinoblastoma protein, Bcl-2, p27, MDM2, and APC, and increased Ki-67 (MIB1) proliferative index > 5% and positivity for galectin (in single gland disease) favors parathyroid carcinoma

Thyroid Neoplasms

- Thyroid tumors usually show thyroglobulin (absent in parathyroid, but proteinaceous material in some parathyroid tumors can be difficult to differentiate on histology alone)
- Parathyroid neoplasms usually have well-defined cytoplasmic membranes (unlike thyroid)
- Thyroid often shows calcium oxalate crystals
- Thyroid follicular cell tumors positive for TTF-1 and thyroglobulin and negative for chromogranin, synaptophysin, and parathyroid hormone
- Medullary thyroid carcinomas and parathyroid tumors both lack colloid and have neuroendocrine chromatin
- Medullary thyroid carcinomas and parathyroid tumors both positive for chromogranin and synaptophysin
- Medullary thyroid carcinomas positive for TTF-1 and calcitonin (parathyroid tumors negative for TTF-1, but calcitonin can be variable)

DIAGNOSTIC CHECKLIST

Clinically Relevant Pathologic Features

- Elevated serum calcium; can overlap with that of parathyroid carcinoma
- Palpable neck mass generally absent in parathyroid adenoma, including atypical parathyroid adenoma

- Intraoperative findings can be indistinguishable as parathyroid adenomas can be adhered to adjacent structures and have thick capsule similar to carcinoma

Pathologic Interpretation Pearls

- Atypical parathyroid adenomas can show fibrosis, mitotic figures, and cells trapped in capsule
- Atypical parathyroid adenomas do not show definitive invasion (no capsular, vascular, or perineural invasion, or invasion into adjacent structures)

SELECTED REFERENCES

1. Clark CM et al: Atypical parathyroid adenoma with diffuse fibrosis. Ear Nose Throat J. 96(2):57-58, 2017
2. Dobrinja C et al: Effectiveness of intraoperative parathyroid monitoring (ioPTH) in predicting a multiglandular or malignant parathyroid disease. Int J Surg. 41 Suppl 1:S26-S33, 2017
3. Marchiori E et al: Specifying the molecular pattern of sporadic parathyroid tumorigenesis-The Y282D variant of the GCM2 gene. Biomed Pharmacother. 92:843-848, 2017
4. Pandya C et al: Genomic profiling reveals mutational landscape in parathyroid carcinomas. JCI Insight. 2(6):e92061, 2017
5. Agarwal A et al: Molecular characteristics of large parathyroid adenomas. World J Surg. 40(3):607-14, 2016
6. Cakir B et al: Evaluation of preoperative ultrasonographic and biochemical features of patients with aggressive parathyroid disease: is there a reliable predictive marker? Arch Endocrinol Metab. 60(6):537-544, 2016
7. Christakis I et al: Parathyroid carcinoma and atypical parathyroid neoplasms in MEN1 patients; a clinico-pathologic challenge. The MD Anderson case series and review of the literature. Int J Surg. 31:10-6, 2016
8. Christakis I et al: Differentiating Atypical Parathyroid Neoplasm from Parathyroid Cancer. Ann Surg Oncol. 23(9):2889-97, 2016
9. Hosny Mohammed K et al: Parafibromin, APC, and MIB-1 Are Useful Markers for Distinguishing Parathyroid Carcinomas From Adenomas. Appl Immunohistochem Mol Morphol. ePub, 2016
10. Hu Y et al: Diagnostic performance of parafibromin immunohistochemical staining for sporadic parathyroid carcinoma: a meta-analysis. Endocrine. 54(3):612-619, 2016
11. Kumari N et al: Role of Histological Criteria and Immunohistochemical Markers in Predicting Risk of Malignancy in Parathyroid Neoplasms. Endocr Pathol. 27(2):87-96, 2016
12. Mele M et al: Recurrence of Hyperparathyroid Hypercalcemia in a Patient With the HRPT-2 Mutation and a Previous Parathyroid Carcinoma in Hyperparathyroidism-Jaw Tumor Syndrome. Int J Endocrinol Metab. 14(2):e35424, 2016
13. Saeger W et al: [Grading of neuroendocrine tumors.] Pathologe. 37(4):304-13, 2016
14. Sanpaolo E et al: EZH2 and ZFX oncogenes in malignant behaviour of parathyroid neoplasms. Endocrine. 54(1):55-59, 2016
15. Diaconescu MR et al: Clinicopathological phenotype of parathyroid carcinoma: therapeutic and prognostic aftermaths. Chirurgia (Bucur). 110(1):66-71, 2015
16. Favere AM et al: Association between atypical parathyroid adenoma and neurofibromatosis. Arch Endocrinol Metab. 59(5):460-6, 2015
17. Karaarslan S et al: The Role of Parafibromin, Galectin-3, HBME-1, and Ki-67 in the Differential Diagnosis of Parathyroid Tumors. Oman Med J. 30(6):421-7, 2015
18. Quinn CE et al: Modern experience with aggressive parathyroid tumors in a high-volume New England referral center. J Am Coll Surg. 220(6):1054-62, 2015
19. Schneider R et al: Immunohistochemical expression of e-cadherin in atypical parathyroid adenoma. World J Surg. 39(10):2477-83, 2015
20. Gill AJ: Understanding the genetic basis of parathyroid carcinoma. Endocr Pathol. 25(1):30-4, 2014
21. Kawashima ST et al: Primary hyperparathyroidism due to atypical vertically long cystic adenoma. Endocrinol Diabetes Metab Case Rep. 2014:140086, 2014
22. Korpi-Hyövälti E et al: CDC73 intragenic deletion in familial primary hyperparathyroidism associated with parathyroid carcinoma. J Clin Endocrinol Metab. 99(9):3044-8, 2014
23. Kruijff S et al: Negative parafibromin staining predicts malignant behavior in atypical parathyroid adenomas. Ann Surg Oncol. 21(2):426-33, 2014
24. LiVolsi VA et al: Parathyroid: The pathology of hyperparathyroidism. Surg Pathol Clin. 7(4):515-31, 2014
25. Pazienza V et al: Identification and functional characterization of three NoLS (nucleolar localisation signals) mutations of the CDC73 gene. PLoS One. 8(12):e82292, 2013
26. Andreasson A et al: Molecular characterization of parathyroid tumors from two patients with hereditary colorectal cancer syndromes. Fam Cancer. 11(3):355-62, 2012
27. Erovic BM et al: Biomarkers of parathyroid carcinoma. Endocr Pathol. 23(4):221-31, 2012
28. Guarnieri V et al: CDC73 mutations and parafibromin immunohistochemistry in parathyroid tumors: clinical correlations in a single-centre patient cohort. Cell Oncol (Dordr). 35(6):411-22, 2012
29. Rodriguez C et al: Parathyroid carcinoma: a difficult histological diagnosis. Eur Ann Otorhinolaryngol Head Neck Dis. 129(3):157-9, 2012
30. Sulaiman L et al: Genome-wide and locus specific alterations in CDC73/HRPT2-mutated parathyroid tumors. PLoS One. 7(9):e46325, 2012
31. Cavaco BM et al: Identification of de novo germline mutations in the HRPT2 gene in two apparently sporadic cases with challenging parathyroid tumor diagnoses. Endocr Pathol. 22(1):44-52, 2011
32. DeLellis RA: Parathyroid tumors and related disorders. Mod Pathol. 24 Suppl 2:S78-93, 2011
33. Demiralay E et al: Morphological evaluation of parathyroid adenomas and immunohistochemical analysis of PCNA and Ki-67 proliferation markers. Turk Patoloji Derg. 27(3):215-20, 2011
34. Juhlin CC et al: Absence of nucleolar parafibromin immunoreactivity in subsets of parathyroid malignant tumours. Virchows Arch. 459(1):47-53, 2011
35. Niramitmahapanya S et al: Sensitivity of HRPT2 mutation screening to detect parathyroid carcinoma and atypical parathyroid adenoma of Thai patients. J Med Assoc Thai. 94 Suppl 2:S17-22, 2011
36. Witteveen JE et al: Downregulation of CASR expression and global loss of parafibromin staining are strong negative determinants of prognosis in parathyroid carcinoma. Mod Pathol. 24(5):688-97, 2011
37. Zhang Y et al: Endocrine tumors as part of inherited tumor syndromes. Adv Anat Pathol. 18(3):206-18, 2011
38. Juhlin CC et al: Parafibromin and APC as screening markers for malignant potential in atypical parathyroid adenomas. Endocr Pathol. 21(3):166-77, 2010
39. Fernandez-Ranvier GG et al: Defining a molecular phenotype for benign and malignant parathyroid tumors. Cancer. 115(2):334-44, 2009
40. Fraser WD: Hyperparathyroidism. Lancet. 374(9684):145-58, 2009
41. Osawa N et al: Diagnosis of parathyroid carcinoma using immunohistochemical staining against hTERT. Int J Mol Med. 24(6):733-41, 2009
42. Cetani F et al: Hyperparathyroidism 2 gene (HRPT2, CDC73) and parafibromin studies in two patients with primary hyperparathyroidism and uncertain pathological assessment. J Endocrinol Invest. 31(10):900-4, 2008
43. DeLellis RA et al: Primary hyperparathyroidism: a current perspective. Arch Pathol Lab Med. 132(8):1251-62, 2008
44. Delellis RA: Challenging lesions in the differential diagnosis of endocrine tumors: parathyroid carcinoma. Endocr Pathol. 19(4):221-5, 2008
45. DeLellis RA: Parathyroid carcinoma: an overview. Adv Anat Pathol. 12(2):53-61, 2005
46. DeLellis RA et al: Paraneoplastic endocrine syndromes: a review. Endocr Pathol. 14(4):303-17, 2003
47. Kameyama K et al: Parathyroid carcinomas: can clinical outcomes for parathyroid carcinomas be determined by histologic evaluation alone? Endocr Pathol. 13(2):135-9, 2002
48. DeLellis RA: The neuroendocrine system and its tumors: an overview. Am J Clin Pathol. 115 Suppl:S5-16, 2001
49. DeLellis RA. Tumors of the Parathyroid Gland. AFIP Atlas of Tumor Pathology Series 3, Fascicle 6. Washington DC: American Registry of Pathology, 1-102, 1991
50. Jackson MA et al: CDC73-Related Disorders 1993
51. Woolner LB et al: Tumors and hyperplasia of the parathyroid glands; a review of the pathological findings in 140 cases of primary hyperparathyroidism. Cancer. 5(6):1069-88, 1952
52. Black BK et al: Tumors of the parathyroid; a review of twenty-three cases. Cancer. 3(3):415-44, 1950
53. Bauer W et al: Carcinoma of parathyroid gland. N Engl J Med. 239(23):894-6, 1948
54. Black BM: Adenocarcinoma of parathyroid origin with hyperparathyroidism, local recurrence and metastases; report of case. Mayo Clin Proc. 22(1):8-14, 1947

Atypical Parathyroid Adenoma vs. Parathyroid Carcinoma

Feature	Atypical Parathyroid Adenoma	Parathyroid Carcinoma
Symptomatic	Unusual	Yes
Palpable mass	Unusual	Yes
Serum calcium	Elevated, often intermediate serum calcium levels between typical parathyroid adenoma and carcinoma	Markedly elevated (> 13 mg/dL)
Tumor size	Tumors can overlap in size	Larger
Vascular invasion	No	Yes
Perineural invasion	No	Yes
Invasion into adjacent structures	No (but cells can be trapped in capsule)	Yes
Metastases	Usually not; most atypical adenomas have indolent behavior	Yes
Growth pattern	Acinar, follicular, may be sheet-like	Monotonous, patternless
Cellular features	Usually chief cells, but can have mixed cell types, can show endocrine atypia	Monotonous, high nuclear:cytoplasmic ratio, prominent nucleoli
Mitoses	Can be present but fewer than carcinomas	Yes (often higher mitotic rate than adenomas)
Atypical mitoses	Usually not	Yes
Proliferation markers (Ki-67)	Low to moderate, may be intermediate between typical parathyroid adenoma and carcinoma	Moderate to high
Fibrous bands	Yes	Yes
Proliferation p27, Bcl-2, MDM2, Ki-67	Positive/high for p27, Bcl-2, MDM2; low/moderate Ki-67	Negative/low for p27, Bcl-2, MDM2; positive/high Ki-67
Parafibromin (CDC73)	Parafibromin-positive atypical adenomas usually do not recur, but parafibromin-negative tumors have 10-20% risk of recurrence and may be considered tumors of low malignant potential	Parafibromin often lost

Thick Fibrous Bands

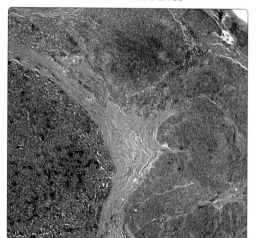

Irregular Growth Pattern

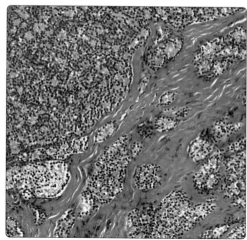

(Left) *Atypical parathyroid adenoma with prominent fibrous bands is shown. Although these tumors show atypical features, they lack unequivocal invasion. Atypical parathyroid adenomas are usually associated with indolent behavior.* **(Right)** *Atypical parathyroid adenoma with fibrous bands and irregular growth pattern is shown. True invasion must be differentiated from fibrous bands and tumor cells trapped within the capsule.*

Irregular and Solid Growth Pattern

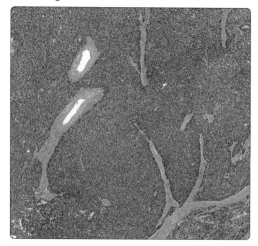

Chief Cells

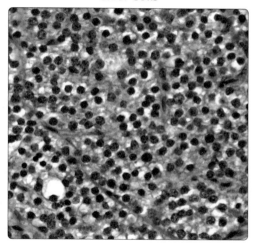

(Left) *The solid and irregular growth is concerning in this parathyroid tumor, but no unequivocal capsular invasion, vascular invasion, or invasion into adjacent structures was identified. Thus, a diagnosis of atypical parathyroid adenoma was made.* **(Right)** *Atypical parathyroid adenoma is composed predominantly of chief cells with sheet-like growth. This high-magnification picture shows uniform chief cells with well-defined cytoplasmic borders and round nuclei.*

Chief Cells Around Vessels

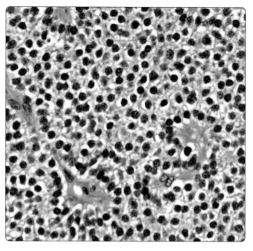

Mitosis and Cytological Atypia

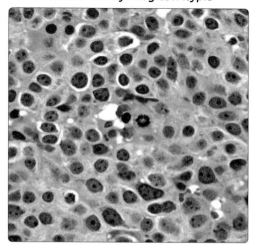

(Left) *This atypical parathyroid adenoma is composed of chief cells with round, hyperchromatic nuclei arranged around vascular spaces. These tumors may show some atypical features (fibrous bands, mitoses, etc.) but lack unequivocal invasion.* **(Right)** *This parathyroid carcinoma shows cytologic atypia and mitotic activity. Mitotic activity is not in itself diagnostic of malignancy as it can also be seen in atypical parathyroid adenoma and other parathyroid lesions. A diagnosis of parathyroid carcinoma requires invasion.*

Parathyroid Carcinoma

TERMINOLOGY

- Malignant parathyroid parenchymal neoplasm

ETIOLOGY/PATHOGENESIS

- Most parathyroid carcinomas are sporadic but increased incidence in patients with HPT-JT syndrome
- HPT-JT: Autosomal dominant disorder of hyperparathyroidism, fibroosseous jaw tumors, kidney cysts, hamartomas, and Wilms tumors
- FIH: Autosomal dominant; accounts for 1% of primary hyperparathyroidism: Adenoma or hyperplasia
- Multiple endocrine neoplasia 1 (MEN1): Autosomal dominant; only rare case of parathyroid carcinoma reported
- MEN2A: 20-30% have parathyroid hyperplasia or adenoma with only rare reports of carcinoma

CLINICAL ISSUES

- Markedly elevated serum calcium (> 13 mg/dL), PTH, alkaline phosphatase

- *CDC73* (HRPT2) mutations in familial and some sporadic, can be new germline mutation

MICROSCOPIC

- Require invasive growth with capsular, vascular, perineural, or invasion into adjacent structures
- Histologic features in sporadic and HPT-JT parathyroid lesions similar, but HPT-JT lesions may be cystic

ANCILLARY TESTS

- Positive for chromogranin, synaptophysin, CAM5.2, PTH; negative for TTF-1, thyroglobulin, calcitonin
- Loss of parafibromin nuclear staining in many
- *CDC73* (HRPT2) mutation (tumor suppressor gene, encodes parafibromin)
- *MEN1* mutation (tumor suppressor gene)
- *RET* mutation (protooncogene)
- Cyclin-D1/*CCND1*

Parathyroid Carcinoma Gross Appearance

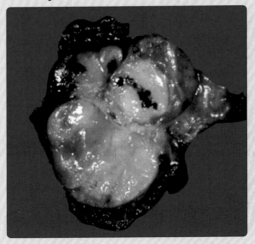

Nodular Growth Pattern

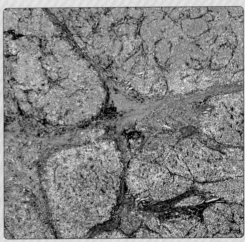

(Left) Cut section of a parathyroid carcinoma (PC) shows a firm, tan-yellow-gray, nodular cut surface with a bosselated appearance, invading into adjacent structures. (Right) The low-power view of this PC shows an irregular, nodular growth pattern. Nests of tumor cells are separated by fibrous bands.

Invasive Growth Pattern

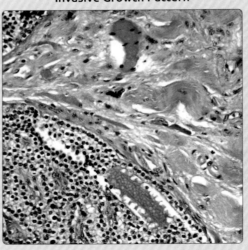

Invasion Into Thyroid

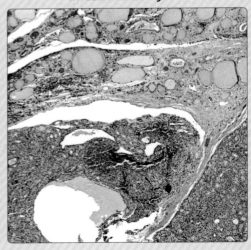

(Left) This routine hematoxylin and eosin-stained section of a PC show tumor cells invading into the sternocleidomastoid muscle. Invasive growth is diagnostic of malignancy in parathyroid. (Right) The thyroid parenchyma is compressed and invaded by this PC. Invasion into adjacent structures is diagnostic of malignancy in parathyroid lesions. Parathyroid with adherence to the thyroid can also occur in benign parathyroid diseases.

TERMINOLOGY

Abbreviations

- Parathyroid carcinoma (PC)

Definitions

- Malignant neoplasm of parathyroid parenchymal cells (chief cells, oxyphilic cells, transitional cells, water/clear cells, or mixtures of cell types)

ETIOLOGY/PATHOGENESIS

Sporadic

- Most parathyroid carcinomas are sporadic
- Unlike *CDC73* germline associated PCs, most sporadic PCs arise de novo
- Predisposing factors poorly understood
  - Possible association with prior ionizing radiation
- Reports of PC occurring in setting of secondary parathyroid hyperplasia and celiac disease
- Substantial minority (20%) of clinically sporadic PCs actually have germline *CDC73* mutation

Inherited

- Increased incidence PC in patients with *CDC73*-related disorders, such as hyperparathyroidism-jaw tumor (HPT-JT) syndrome

Hyperparathyroidism Jaw-Tumor Syndrome

- Autosomal dominant
- Inactivating mutation tumor suppressor gene *CDC73* (HRPT2) on 1q21-q31
  - 80% of mutations truncating (frameshift and nonsense), most involve exon 1
  - *CDC73* (HRPT2) encodes parafibromin (CDC73) protein
- Disorder of hyperparathyroidism, fibroosseous jaw tumors, kidney cysts, hamartomas, and Wilms tumors
- 80% present with hyperparathyroidism
  - Hyperparathyroidism usually develops by late adolescence
  - Penetrance of hyperparathyroidism is 80%
  - Parathyroid adenoma or carcinoma
  - 15% develop PC
- Germline *CDC73* (HRPT2) mutations identified in subset of patients with *CDC73* (HRPT2) mutation-positive carcinomas

Familial Isolated Hyperparathyroidism

- Autosomal dominant; accounts for 1% of primary hyperparathyroidism (parathyroid is only endocrine organ involved), adenoma, or hyperplasia
- Increased risk of PC has been reported but may be due to inclusion of HPT-JT cases
- Cause unknown in most families, but *CDC73* (HRPT2) gene (15%), *MEN1* gene, and area on chromosome 2 implicated

CDC73-Related Disorders

- Inactivating mutation tumor suppressor gene *CDC73* (HRPT2) on 1q21-q31
  - CDC73 transcript spans 2.7 kb
  - CDC73 protein binds RNA polymerase II as part of PAF1 transcriptional regulatory complex, mediates H3K9 methylation that silences expression of cyclin-D1

- *CDC73* mutation present in familial predisposition to PC (as with HPT-JT, familial isolated hyperparathyroidism)
- CDC73 protein regulates gene expression and inhibits cell proliferation
- Somatic inactivating *CDC73* mutations in some sporadic parathyroid carcinomas
  - Up to 75% *CDC73* inactivation but may be higher as mutations may be outside of coding region sequenced in clinical testing and some research studies
  - Germline CDC73 mutations present in substantial minority (20%) of clinically sporadic-appearing PC
- Additional genes may be involved for malignant behavior
  - *CCND1* overexpressed in many PCs

Multiple Endocrine Neoplasia 1

- Autosomal dominant, high penetrance, germline mutation in *MEN1* tumor suppressor gene (11q13); results in truncated menin protein
- 20% of patients with primary parathyroid hyperplasia have multiple endocrine neoplasia 1 (MEN1), but only rare case of PC reported in MEN1
- Loss of heterozygosity and somatic *MEN1* mutations identified in some PCs
- Somatic *MEN1* mutations occur in 15-20% of sporadic adenomas and occasionally in sporadic carcinomas
- 0.28% to 0.70% of MEN1 patients have PC

Multiple Endocrine Neoplasia 2A

- 20-30% with MEN2A have parathyroid hyperplasia or adenoma (only rare reports of carcinoma)

CLINICAL ISSUES

Epidemiology

- Incidence
  - 1-2% of primary hyperparathyroidism (parathyroid adenoma: 80-85%; parathyroid hyperplasia: 15%)
  - < 1 case per million population
  - Reports: Up to 5% of hyperparathyroidism due to carcinoma in Italy and Japan
  - Parathyroid carcinoma occurs in 10-15% of patients with HPT-JT syndrome
- Age
  - Middle-aged and older adults (mid 40s to mid 50s; mean: 56 years; range: 15-89 years)
  - 1 decade earlier than parathyroid adenomas
- Sex
  - M = F (unlike adenomas, which are more frequent in females)

Site

- Arises in site of parathyroid gland
  - Similar to parathyroid adenomas, carcinomas can also occur in ectopic sites

Presentation

- Most PCs are functional, and patients are symptomatic, but nonfunctional tumors occur
  - Fatigue, weakness, weight loss, nausea, polyuria, polydipsia, renal disease, bone disease
  - Bone disease (osteitis fibrosa cystica, diffuse osteopenia, subperiosteal bone resorption, skull involvement, fractures) common in PC

- o Renal disease (nephrolithiasis, nephrocalcinosis, decreased renal function) common in carcinoma
- o Prominent symptoms, particularly renal and bone involvement, concerning for malignancy
- o Parathyroid adenomas usually asymptomatic or vague, mild symptoms
- Palpable neck mass in 30-75% (unusual for adenoma)
- Recurrent laryngeal nerve paralysis very worrisome for carcinoma
- Local recurrence of parathyroid adenoma is worrisome for carcinoma but can be parathyromatosis

Laboratory Tests

- Extremely high serum calcium levels (> 13 mg/dL) more common in carcinoma
- Markedly elevated PTH levels (> 1,000 ng/L)
- High serum alkaline phosphatase activity (> 200 IU/L)

Natural History

- Usually recur 1st in neck then metastasize to cervical and mediastinal lymph nodes, lung, bone, and liver
- Frequent locoregional progression after surgery
- Average time between surgery and 1st recurrence is 3 years, but recurrences may be delayed for decades
- Metastatic sites: Lymph node (#1 metastatic site), lung (#1 distant metastatic site), bone, liver
- Death usually due to uncontrollable hypercalcemia

Treatment

- Surgical approaches
  - o 1st-line treatment en block resection of parathyroid tumor and surrounding structures, usually ipsilateral thyroid lobe at 1st surgery (better local control and disease-free survival)
  - o Risk progression associated with margin status
- Drugs
  - o Inoperable PC management may include calcimimetics to control hypercalcemia and bisphosphonates to control bone resorption
  - o Chemotherapy effectiveness unclear
  - o Few reports of immunomodulating therapeutic approaches with vaccines
- Radiation
  - o Patients treated with surgery and postoperative radiation may have lower risk of locoregional progression and improved cause-specific survival

Prognosis

- Recurrences associated with marked hypercalcemia
- 5-year survival up to 78-85%; 10-year survival 49-70%
- Best chance for cure is surgical resection en bloc with adjacent tissues, often ipsilateral thyroid lobe
- Tumors treated with extensive surgery associated with improved survival
- Significant risk of locoregional disease progression after surgery
  - o Tend to recur locally and spread to contiguous structures in neck
  - o Involve ipsilateral thyroid, strap muscles, recurrent laryngeal nerve, esophagus, and trachea
- Postoperative radiation may be associated with decreased risk progression and improved survival

- Metastases usually occur late and involve cervical lymph nodes, lung, and liver
- Negative prognostic factors include older age, larger tumor size, male sex, metastatic lymph nodes
- Main cause of death in patients with parathyroid carcinoma is parathyroid hormone-induced hypercalcemia

IMAGING

General Features

- Tc-99m sestamibi scintigraphy or sonography identifies location but does not separate adenoma from carcinoma
- Mass noted on CT and MR, often no specific features

MACROSCOPIC

General Features

- Large, firm tumors; may be variably encapsulated, poorly circumscribed
  - o Lobulated appearance due to thick, fibrous bands
  - o May be grossly encapsulated and resemble adenomas
- May be adherent to or invasive into adjacent structures
- Large parathyroid adenomas, especially with cystic change, can become fibrotic and adhere to adjacent structures

Size

- Large tumors (mean: 6.7 g; range: 1.5 to > 50.0 g)
  - o Generally larger than adenomas but overlap in size can occur

MICROSCOPIC

Histologic Features

- Diagnosis of malignancy requires documented metastasis or invasive growth involving adjacent structures: Thyroid and soft tissues, capsular &/or extracapsular blood vessels or perineural spaces
  - o Vascular invasion involves capsular vessels or vessels in surrounding soft tissues
  - o Tumor should be attached to vessel wall and fibrin should be present
  - o Endothelial lining may or may not be present
- Capsular invasion of tumor beyond thickened capsule identified in 60%
  - o Entrapment of cells in capsule can occur in adenomas, especially if cystic or fibrotic (must be distinguished from true capsular invasion)
- Fibrous bands common (up to 90%) but not specific
  - o Often subdivide tumors from peritumoral capsule
  - o Parathyroid adenomas can be fibrotic, especially if cystic or hemorrhagic degeneration
  - o Parathyroid hyperplasia, particularly secondary hyperplasia, can also show fibrous bands
- Invasion of vessels in thickened capsule or surrounding soft tissue (most specific feature for carcinoma, seen in 15% of cases)
  - o Artifactual dislodgement of tumor cells floating in vessels must be differentiated from true vascular invasion in which tumor cells at least partially attach to vessel wall and may or may not be surrounded by endothelial cells
- Perineural invasion

- Solid growth pattern with sheets of cells or closely packed nests or trabecular growth but can show follicular or other growth patterns, even rare carcinosarcomatous growth pattern
    - Prominent growth patterns (follicular and acinar) common in adenomas and uncommon in carcinomas
- Cellular monotony common, but occasional cases pleomorphic
    - High nuclear:cytoplasmic ratios
    - Prominent nucleoli (macronucleoli)
    - Foci of pleomorphic cells with hyperchromatic nuclei should not be mistaken for atypia of carcinoma, as "endocrine atypia" is often seen in benign parathyroid lesions
- Often composed of chief cells, intermediate in size, round to oval nuclei, dense chromatin, and may not have prominent nucleoli
    - Cytomorphology in some of these cases indistinguishable from adenomas
- Usually composed of chief cells but can have variable oncocytes, transitional oncocytes, clear cells and spindle cells
- Oncocytic PCs have identical criteria for malignancy as those composed predominantly of chief cells
- Mitotic figures identified in at least 80% of carcinomas but also in up to 70% of adenomas
    - Mitotic activity more prominent in carcinomas than adenomas
- Atypical mitoses strongly favor parathyroid carcinoma
- Suggested triad of macronucleoli, > 5 mitoses per 50 HPF, and necrosis associated with aggressive behavior in PC
- Histologic features in sporadic and HPT-JT parathyroid lesions similar, but HPT-JT lesions may be cystic (30%)
- PCs can be composed entirely of oxyphil (oxyphil PC) or clear cells (clear cell PC)
    - Same criteria used to diagnose these variants

ANCILLARY TESTS

Immunohistochemistry

- Positive for chromogranin and synaptophysin
- Positive for keratin (CAM5.2 most helpful keratin for neuroendocrine tumors)
- Positive for parathyroid hormone but may be less extensive than in adenomas
- Negative for TTF-1, thyroglobulin, calcitonin (usually)
- Ki-67 (MIB-1) elevated > 4% (higher than in adenomas)
- p27 (cyclin-dependent kinase inhibitor protein) decreased expression in PCs compared to adenomas
- Carcinomas often low/absent p27, MDM2, and higher Ki-67 labeling index
    - Adenomas often positive for p27, Bcl-2, and MDM2 and low Ki-67 labeling index
- Keratin 14 reported negative in oxyphil carcinomas and positive in oxyphil adenomas
- GCM2-positive (transcription factor) regulatory gene in parathyroid development
- GATA3 positive (transcription factor)
- Galectin-3 and PEP9.5 positive
- APC, CDKN1B, and Bcl-2 negative or weakly positive
- Parafibromin (CDC73)

- CDC73 (HRPT2) encodes parafibromin/CDC73
- Loss of nuclear parafibromin in CDC73 (HRPT2)-associated PCs and adenomas
- Complete loss of nuclear or nucleolar parafibromin expression in PC helpful for differentiating from parathyroid adenoma, which usually shows intact nuclear and nucleolar parafibromin expression
    - Parafibromin expression may be lost in parathyroid adenomas associated with germline CDC73/HPRT2 mutations
    - PCs in hemodialysis patients can show staining in primary and metastasis
- Parafibromin helpful but requires rigorously controlled testing as variability among laboratories
- Possible prognostic significance parafibromin in parathyroid carcinoma
    - Parafibromin-negative parathyroid carcinomas higher risk recurrence and decreased 5- and 10-year survivals (59% and 23%, respectively)

Genetic Testing

- CDC73 (HRPT2) mutation (tumor suppressor gene, 1q21-q31, encodes CDC73/parafibromin protein)
    - Strong association CDC73 (HRPT2) mutation in familial and sporadic parathyroid cancer
        - CDC73 (HRPT2) mutation uncommon in sporadic adenomas but identified in 20% of sporadic cystic adenomas
    - 15% with HPT-JT [caused by germline CDC73 (HRPT2) inactivating mutation] develop PC
    - Germline CDC73 (HRPT2) mutations identified in subset of patients with mutation-positive carcinomas
        - Consider genetic testing in patients with PC
        - Substantial minority of clinically sporadic PCs may have germline mutation
        - Up to 75% of PCs have CDC73 inactivation
        - Clinical testing may not identify all mutations inactivating CDC73 mutations, as may be located outside coding region evaluated
        - Patients with PC may be offered germline CDC73 mutation testing
- MEN1 mutation (tumor suppressor gene, 11q13, results in truncated menin protein)
    - Somatic MEN1 inactivation of loss of heterozygosity in 15-20% of sporadic adenomas but not frequent in PCs
    - Loss of heterozygosity and somatic MEN1 mutations in some PCs
    - Only rare cases of PC identified in MEN1
- RET mutation (protooncogene, 10q11.2)
    - Only rare case reports of parathyroid carcinomas in MEN2A
- Cyclin-D1/CCND1 (11q13)
    - Genetic alterations in cyclin-D1/CCND1 (parathyroid adenoma) gene, 11q13, in 5-8% of parathyroid neoplasms
    - Loss of chromosome 11 frequent in parathyroid adenomas, and frequent chromosomal gain in parathyroid carcinomas in FISH studies
    - Cyclin-D1/CCND1 encodes cyclin-D1 (regulator of cell cycle progression from G1 to S phase), and cyclin-D1 overexpression observed in neoplastic parathyroid

— Lack of definitive genotype-phenotype correlation limits utility

- Loss of 1p and 13q relatively common in parathyroid carcinomas whereas loss of 11q (*MEN1* gene location) most common abnormality in parathyroid adenoma
- Loss of chromosome 11 common in parathyroid adenoma; gain of chromosome 11 in carcinoma, particularly in those who die of disease
- Loss of heterozygosity on 13q [*RB1* (RB) and *BRCA2* gene location] in carcinomas, but specific abnormalities of *RB1* (RB) or *BRCA2* not identified by sequencing
- Candidate oncogenes: PRUNE2, PIK3CA, KMT2D, MTOR, ADCK1

DIFFERENTIAL DIAGNOSIS

Parathyroid Adenoma

- Benign neoplasm of thyroid chief, oxyphil, transitional, water-clear cells, or mixtures of cell types
- Serum calcium elevated but often not as high as carcinoma (often > 13)
- Usually asymptomatic or vague symptoms, often identified by screening serum calcium
- No palpable mass
- Fibrous bands and scattered mitoses but usually lack atypical mitoses
- No unequivocal invasive growth (no capsular, vascular, or perineural invasion or invasion into adjacent structures)
- Mixture of cellular patterns rather than monotonous or trabecular growth of carcinomas
- Cells may show foci of endocrine atypia

Atypical Parathyroid Adenoma

- Noninvasive parathyroid neoplasm composed of chief cells with variable oncocytes and transitional oncocytes, with some features of PC
  - Adherence to adjacent structures, mitotic activity, fibrous bands, trabecular growth, and tumor cells within capsule
    - However, no unequivocal capsular, vascular, or perineural invasion or invasion into adjacent structures

Thyroid Follicular Neoplasm

- Follicular growth, may have colloid, lack well-defined cytoplasmic membranes
- Oxyphilic parathyroid adenomas must be distinguished from Hürthle cell thyroid tumors
- Positive for TTF-1 and thyroglobulin; negative for PTH, chromogranin, and synaptophysin

Parathyromatosis

- Rare cause of hyperparathyroidism
- Caused by inadvertent autotransplantation of tissue from previous operations or hyperfunction of tissue left behind in development
- Multiple nests of hyperfunctioning parathyroid tissue scattered throughout fibrous or fibrofatty tissue or muscle of lower neck or superior mediastinum
- Features favoring parathyroid carcinoma over parathyromatosis: Markedly elevated serum calcium, palpable mass, vascular or perineural invasion, infiltrative growth, prominent mitotic activity

Medullary Thyroid Carcinoma

- Positive for calcitonin and CEA, negative for PTH
- Both medullary thyroid carcinoma and parathyroid lack colloid and are positive for neuroendocrine markers chromogranin and synaptophysin and keratin (particularly CAM5.2)

DIAGNOSTIC CHECKLIST

Clinically Relevant Pathologic Features

- Palpable neck mass (rare for adenoma)
- Symptomatic (fatigue, weakness, weight loss, nausea, polyuria, polydipsia, renal disease, bone disease)
  - Presence of bone and renal disease worrisome for malignancy
- Markedly elevated serum calcium (> 13 mg/dL), PTH, alkaline phosphatase
- *CDC73* (HRPT2) mutations in familial and some sporadic; can be new germline mutation (consider genetic testing in patients with parathyroid carcinoma)
- En bloc resection of tumor and surrounding structures best chance for cure
- Locoregional recurrences common, can have prolonged clinical course
- Death due to uncontrolled hypercalcemia

Pathologic Interpretation Pearls

- Requires invasive growth for diagnosis of PC (capsular, vascular, perineural, into adjacent structures)
- Mitoses, fibrosis, fibrous bands can be seen in PC and adenoma
- Atypical mitoses
- Sheet-like or trabecular growth
- Monotonous cellular morphology, high nuclear:cytoplasmic ratios, macronucleoli

TNM Staging of Tumors of Parathyroid Glands (WHO 2017)

- T: Primary tumor
  - TX: Primary tumor cannot be assessed
  - TX: No evidence of primary tumor
  - Tis: Atypical parathyroid neoplasm
  - T1: Localized to parathyroid gland with extension limited to soft tissue
  - T2: Direct invasion into thyroid gland
  - T3: Direct invasion into recurrent laryngeal nerve, esophagus, trachea, skeletal muscle, adjacent lymph nodes, or thymus
  - T4: Direct Invasion into major blood vessels or spine
- N: Regional lymph nodes
  - NX: Regional lymph nodes cannot be assessed
  - N0: No regional lymph nodes metastases
  - N1: Regional lymph nodes metastases
  - N1a: Metastases to level VI (pretracheal, paratracheal, prelaryngeal/Delphian lymph nodes, or upper/superior mediastinum lymph nodes
  - N1b: Metastases to unilateral, bilateral or contralateral cervical (levels I, II, II, IV, V) or retropharyngeal lymph nodes
- M: Distant metastases
  - M0: No distant metastases
  - M1: Distant metastases

Stage

- There is not enough data to propose formal staging system (WHO 2017)

REPORTING

Various Systems Proposed

- No generally accepted staging system for parathyroid carcinoma
  - System of low- and high-risk groups based on extent of invasion and nodal and distant metastases
  - System dividing minimally and widely invasive based on extent of capsular and vascular invasion

SELECTED REFERENCES

1. Angelousi A et al: Molecular targeted therapies in adrenal, pituitary and parathyroid malignancies. Endocr Relat Cancer. 24(6):R239-R259, 2017
2. Araujo Castro M et al: Giant parathyroid adenoma: differential aspects compared to parathyroid carcinoma. Endocrinol Diabetes Metab Case Rep. 2017, 2017
3. Barazeghi E et al: A role for TET2 in parathyroid carcinoma. Endocr Relat Cancer. 24(7):329-338, 2017
4. Christakis I et al: Postoperative local-regional radiation therapy in the treatment of parathyroid carcinoma: The MD Anderson experience of 35 years. Pract Radiat Oncol. ePub, 2017
5. Cinque L et al: Novel association of MEN1 gene mutations with parathyroid carcinoma. Oncol Lett. 14(1):23-30, 2017
6. DeLellis et al: Parathyroid carcinoma. From Lloyd RV et al: WHO Classification of Tumours of Endocrine Organs. 4th ed. Paris: IARC Press. 146-52, 2017
7. Dobrinja C et al: Effectiveness of intraoperative parathyroid monitoring (ioPTH) in predicting a multiglandular or malignant parathyroid disease. Int J Surg. 41 Suppl 1:S26-S33, 2017
8. Goldenberg M et al: Parathyroid carcinoma in a patient with three prior parathyroid adenomas. Ear Nose Throat J. 96(6):E48-E49, 2017
9. Guarnieri V et al: Large intragenic deletion of CDC73 (exons 4-10) in a three-generation hyperparathyroidism-jaw tumor (HPT-JT) syndrome family. BMC Med Genet. 18(1):83, 2017
10. Pandya C et al: Genomic profiling reveals mutational landscape in parathyroid carcinomas. JCI Insight. 2(6):e92061, 2017
11. Pappa A et al: Simultaneous incidental parathyroid carcinoma and intrathyroid parathyroid gland in suspected renal failure induced hyperparathyroidism. Surg J (N Y). 3(1):e23-e24, 2017
12. Ryhänen EM et al: A nationwide study on parathyroid carcinoma. Acta Oncol. 56(7):991-1003, 2017
13. Sadacharan D et al: Hypercalcaemic encephalopathy due to metastatic parathyroid carcinoma. BMJ Case Rep. 2017, 2017
14. Silva-Figueroa AM et al: Prognostic scoring system to risk stratify parathyroid carcinoma. J Am Coll Surg. ePub, 2017
15. Suganuma N et al: Non-functioning parathyroid carcinoma: a case report. Surg Case Rep. 3(1):81, 2017
16. Verdelli C et al: Epigenetic alterations in parathyroid cancers. Int J Mol Sci. 18(2), 2017
17. Arnold A: Major molecular genetic drivers in sporadic primary hyperparathyroidism. Trans Am Clin Climatol Assoc. 127:235-244, 2016
18. Christakis I et al: Parathyroid carcinoma and atypical parathyroid neoplasms in MEN1 patients; a clinico-pathologic challenge. The MD Anderson case series and review of the literature. Int J Surg. 31:10-6, 2016
19. Betea D et al: Parathyroid carcinoma: challenges in diagnosis and treatment. Ann Endocrinol (Paris). 76(2):169-77, 2015
20. Fountas A et al: The emerging role of denosumab in the long term management of parathyroid carcinoma-related refractory hypercalcemia. Endocr Pract. 1-18, 2015
21. Shifrin A et al: Primary and metastatic parathyroid malignancies: a rare or underdiagnosed condition? J Clin Endocrinol Metab. 100(3):E478-81, 2015
22. Yu W et al: Whole-exome sequencing studies of parathyroid carcinomas reveal novel PRUNE2 mutations, distinctive mutational spectra related to APOBEC-catalyzed DNA mutagenesis and mutational enrichment in kinases associated with cell migration and invasion. J Clin Endocrinol Metab. 100(2):E360-4, 2015
23. Gill AJ: Understanding the genetic basis of parathyroid carcinoma. Endocr Pathol. 25(1):30-4, 2014
24. Hsu KT et al: Is central lymph node dissection necessary for parathyroid carcinoma? Surgery. 156(6):1336-41; discussion 1341, 2014
25. Sadler C et al: Parathyroid carcinoma in more than 1,000 patients: a population-level analysis. Surgery. 156(6):1622-9; discussion 1629-30, 2014
26. Singh Ospina N et al: Prevalence of parathyroid carcinoma in 348 patients with multiple endocrine neoplasia type 1 - case report and review of the literature. Clin Endocrinol (Oxf). ePub, 2014
27. Cetani F et al: CDC73 mutational status and loss of parafibromin in the outcome of parathyroid cancer. Endocr Connect. 2(4):186-95, 2013
28. Costa-Guda J et al: Allelic imbalance in sporadic parathyroid carcinoma and evidence for its de novo origins. Endocrine. 44(2):489-95, 2013
29. DeLellis RA: Parathyroid tumors and related disorders. Mod Pathol. 24 Suppl 2:S78-93, 2011
30. Fang SH et al: Parathyroid cancer. Endocr Pract. 17 Suppl 1:36-43, 2011
31. Juhlin CC et al: Absence of nucleolar parafibromin immunoreactivity in subsets of parathyroid malignant tumours. Virchows Arch. 459(1):47-53, 2011
32. Witteveen JE et al: Downregulation of CASR expression and global loss of parafibromin staining are strong negative determinants of prognosis in parathyroid carcinoma. Mod Pathol. 24(5):688-97, 2011
33. Zhang Y et al: Endocrine tumors as part of inherited tumor syndromes. Adv Anat Pathol. 18(3):206-18, 2011
34. Okamoto T et al: Parathyroid carcinoma: etiology, diagnosis, and treatment. World J Surg. 33(11):2343-54, 2009
35. Delellis RA: Challenging lesions in the differential diagnosis of endocrine tumors: parathyroid carcinoma. Endocr Pathol. 19(4):221-5, 2008
36. Kelly TG et al: Surveillance for early detection of aggressive parathyroid disease: carcinoma and atypical adenoma in familial isolated hyperparathyroidism associated with a germline HRPT2 mutation. J Bone Miner Res. 21(10):1666-71, 2006
37. Krebs LJ et al: HRPT2 mutational analysis of typical sporadic parathyroid adenomas. J Clin Endocrinol Metab. 90(9):5015-7, 2005
38. Erickson LA et al: Oxyphil parathyroid carcinomas: a clinicopathologic and immunohistochemical study of 10 cases. Am J Surg Pathol. 26(3):344-9, 2002
39. Sandelin K et al: Prognostic factors in parathyroid cancer: a review of 95 cases. World J Surg. 16(4):724-31, 1992

Nested Growth Pattern

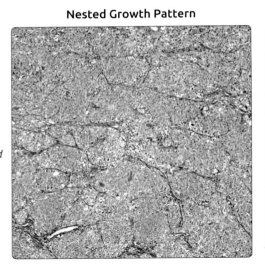

Cellular Monotony

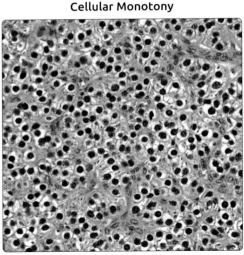

(Left) *This low-power microphotography reveals an unusual nested growth pattern in a case of PC. The nests of tumor cells are separated by a thin fibrovascular stroma.* (Right) *Monotonous cytomorphology in PC is shown. Tumor cells have increased nuclear:cytoplasmic ratios and little variation in nuclear size and shape. Note well-defined cytoplasmic membranes of parathyroid tissue.*

Increased Mitotic Activity

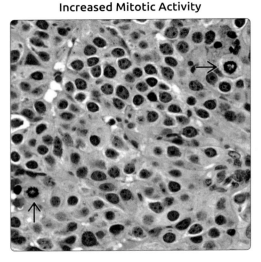

Capsular and Vascular Invasion

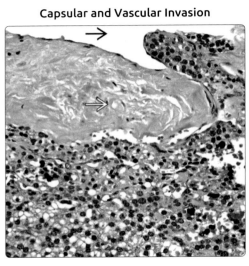

(Left) *PC may have some degree of nuclear atypia and may show prominent nucleoli. This illustration also shows mitotic figures ➡. Oxyphil carcinomas are usually functional and much larger than oxyphil adenomas. Similar to conventional PCs, invasion is required to diagnose malignancy.* (Right) *This picture illustrates tumor cells invading through the capsule ➡ into a vascular space ➡. Capsular invasion beyond thickened capsule is present in ~ 60% of cases and vascular invasion in ~ 15% of cases.*

Vascular Invasion

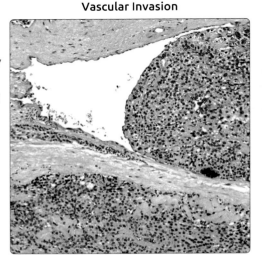

Invasion Into Thyroid

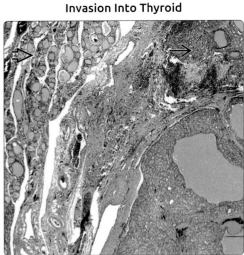

(Left) *Tumor thrombus is seen in a vessel within the thickened capsule of a PC. Vascular invasion is essentially diagnostic of malignancy in parathyroid. Dislodgement of tumor cells floating in a vessel should be differentiated from true vascular invasion.* (Right) *PC ➡ is shown invading into the perithyroidal tissue (thyroid parenchyma ➡). Invasive growth, including invasion into adjacent structures, is diagnostic of malignancy in PC.*

Trabecular Growth Pattern

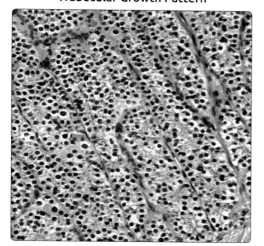

Parathyroid Carcinoma With Spindle Cells

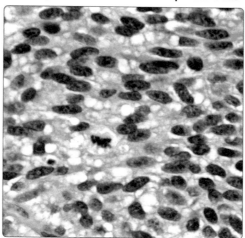

(Left) PC composed by chief cells with a trabecular growth pattern is shown. PCs usually have monotonous or trabecular growth. Other patterns of growth (follicular, acinar) are less common. (Right) PC with spindling cells with stippled neuroendocrine-type chromatin can be mistaken for other tumors such as medullary thyroid carcinoma. In difficult cases, immunoperoxidase studies can be helpful. A mitosis is seen.

Oxyphilic Parathyroid Carcinoma

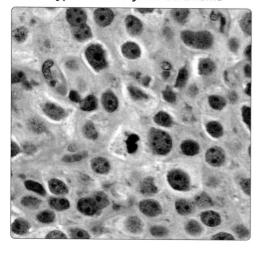

Infiltrative Growth Pattern

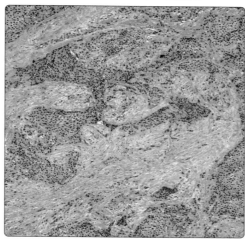

(Left) Oxyphilic parathyroid carcinoma shows multiple mitotic figures. Although mitotic figures can be seen in both parathyroid adenomas and carcinomas, they are more common in carcinomas. The triad of macronucleoli, > 5 mitosis/50 HPF and necrosis are associated with aggressive behavior in PC. (Right) This low-power view of a PC shows a highly infiltrative growth with islands of tumor cells infiltrating fibrous tissue.

Vascular Invasion

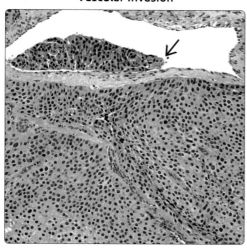

Metastatic Parathyroid Carcinoma

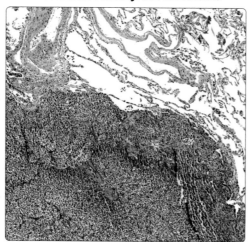

(Left) Vascular invasion ⊡ is one of the most definitive features of malignancy in PC, but it occurs in only ~ 15% of cases. The true vascular invasion is defined as in which the tumor cells are at least partially attached to the vessel wall and may or may not be surrounded by endothelial cells. (Right) The lung is one of the most common sites of distant metastasis of PC. The usual metastatic sites are lymph nodes, lung, bone, and liver.

Secondary Tumors, Parathyroid Gland

TERMINOLOGY

- Secondary involvement of parathyroid can occur from tumors metastasizing to or directly extending into parathyroid

ETIOLOGY/PATHOGENESIS

- Patients usually have history of malignancy
  - Breast, lung, malignant melanoma, hematolymphoid, thyroid, etc.
  - Parathyroid involvement may be underestimated as often not sampled

CLINICAL ISSUES

- Hyperparathyroidism and hypercalcemia may be presenting findings if metastasis is to parathyroid adenoma or hyperplasia
- Hypoparathyroidism from parathyroid destruction is unusual
- May present with neck mass

MACROSCOPIC

- Mass or microscopic involvement of parathyroid

MICROSCOPIC

- Microscopic features correlate with those of secondary tumor with surrounding parathyroid tissue

ANCILLARY TESTS

- Immunoperoxidase studies very helpful
- Parathyroid: Chromogranin, synaptophysin, parathyroid hormone, keratin (CAM5.2)
- Other tumors: TTF-1, thyroglobulin, GCDFP-15, keratins, CD45, melan-A, PSA

TOP DIFFERENTIAL DIAGNOSES

- Parathyroid carcinoma, metastasis to or direct extension of tumor to parathyroid

Metastatic Carcinoma

Metastatic Carcinoma to Parathyroid Adenoma

(Left) Metastatic carcinoma ⇒ (immunophenotypically compatible with breast primary carcinoma) to a parathyroid adenoma ⊟ is shown in this image. Metastases to the parathyroid are extraordinarily rare.
(Right) This metastatic carcinoma ⇒ forms an irregular mass in a parathyroid adenoma ⊟. Tumors secondarily involve the parathyroid via metastasis to the parathyroid or direct extension into the parathyroid.

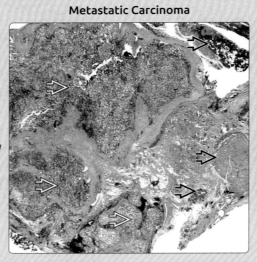

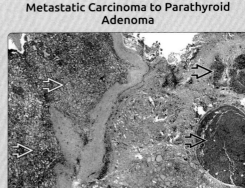

Atypical Cells in Metastatic Carcinoma

Parathyroid Adenoma

(Left) Metastatic carcinoma cells with marked cytologic atypia are shown. The immunophenotype of the metastatic carcinoma was compatible with breast primary and different from the immunophenotype of the surrounding parathyroid adenoma cells. (Right) The cells of parathyroid adenoma display monotonous cytomorphologic features and lack the significant atypia and mitotic activity that is observed in the tumor metastatic (not shown) to this parathyroid adenoma.

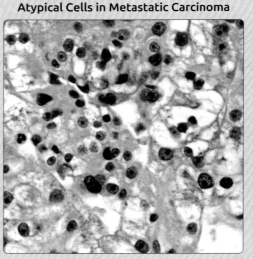

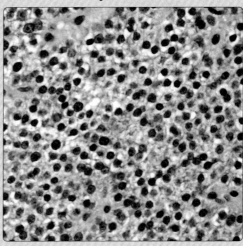

TERMINOLOGY

Definitions

- Secondary tumors can involve parathyroid gland by direct extension or by metastasis from another site

ETIOLOGY/PATHOGENESIS

Direct Extension

- Thyroid carcinoma most common (also laryngeal)
- Involvement of parathyroid by papillary thyroid carcinoma noted in 20 of 911 cases (most by direct invasion, but 2% were by metastases)

Metastasis From Another Site

- Breast, hematolymphoid, malignant melanoma, lung, prostate most common; others occur (kidney, stomach, salivary gland, tongue, seminoma, hepatocellular, etc.)
- May be predilection of spread to endocrine tumors usually seen in tumor to tumor spread due to rich blood supply of endocrine tissues and tumors

CLINICAL ISSUES

Epidemiology

- Incidence
  - Rarely identified during life
    - Parathyroid involvement may be underestimated as often not sampled
  - In thyroid carcinomas surgeries in which parathyroid glands were removed and evaluated, up to 4% had involvement by thyroid carcinoma
  - Autopsy studies show 0.2-11.9% of patients with known cancer have involvement of parathyroid
    - Occurred most often in patients with extensive metastases
- Age
  - Adults, age consistent with primary cancer type
- Sex
  - Dependent on type of carcinoma
    - Breast carcinoma (females), prostate (males), other tumors both males and females

Presentation

- Neck mass in patient with history of malignancy
- Hyperparathyroidism if tumor metastasizes to parathyroid adenoma or hyperplasia rather than normal parathyroid
- Hypoparathyroidism due to destruction of parathyroid tissue by metastatic tumor is rare
- Hypercalcemia reported in patients with metastatic cancer spread to parathyroid without histologic confirmation of hyperparathyroidism
  - Possibly alternative mechanism for malignant hypercalcemia

MACROSCOPIC

General Features

- Tumefactive mass involving parathyroid

MICROSCOPIC

Histologic Features

- Tumefactive mass with surrounding parathyroid tissue
- 2 different cell types (parathyroid and metastatic tumor cells)
- Histology of tumor secondarily involving parathyroid reflect known features of primary
- In tumor to tumor metastases, metastatic tumor's histologic features reflect features of primary whereas parathyroid tissue is hypercellular, such as in parathyroid adenoma
- Surrounding parathyroid tissue may be hypercellular if metastasis to parathyroid tumor or hyperplastic parathyroid gland

ANCILLARY TESTS

Immunohistochemistry

- Immunostains helpful to confirm diagnosis
- Parathyroid: Positive for chromogranin, synaptophysin, and PTH, and negative for TTF-1 and thyroglobulin
- Keratin confirms epithelial differentiation of tumor secondarily involving parathyroid
  - Parathyroid tissue also positive for keratin (CAM5.2)
- Other immunostains helpful (mammaglobin, GCDFP-15, estrogen receptor, melan-A/mart-1, TTF-1, HepPar, PSA, S100, etc.)

DIFFERENTIAL DIAGNOSIS

Parathyroid Carcinoma

- Marked hypercalcemia, elevated PTH
- Chromogranin, synaptophysin, PTH, CAM5.2

Metastatic or Direct Extension of Tumor to Parathyroid

- Usually history of cancer
- Tumefactive mass in background of parathyroid gland or parathyroid adenoma
- Immunostains helpful: Breast (CK7, GCDFP-15, mammaglobin, estrogen), lung (CK7, TTF-1), hematolymphoid (CD45), thyroid (keratin, TTF-1, thyroglobulin), hepatocellular (HepPar, albumin), prostate (PSA), melanoma (S100, Melan-A/MART-1), etc.

DIAGNOSTIC CHECKLIST

Clinically Relevant Pathologic Features

- Rare, usually history of malignancy
- Parathyroid involvement may be underestimated as parathyroid glands not often sampled

Pathologic Interpretation Pearls

- 2 distinct cell types: Parathyroid cells and secondary tumor cells
- Clinical situation and immunostains often used to confirm diagnosis

SELECTED REFERENCES

1. Torregrossa L et al: Metastasis of renal cell carcinoma to the parathyroid gland 16 years after radical nephrectomy: a case report. Oncol Lett. 12(5):3224-3228, 2016

Differential Diagnosis of Tumors Secondarily Involving Parathyroid

Tumor/Tissue	Chr	Syn	CK	TTF-1	Cal	Other
Parathyroid	Positive	Positive	Positive (CAM5.2)	Negative	Negative, but variable	Parathyroid hormone
Breast carcinoma	Negative	Negative	Variable	Negative	Negative	Mammaglobin, GCDFP-15, estrogen
Follicular/papillary thyroid	Negative	Positive	Positive	Positive	Negative	Thyroglobulin
Medullary thyroid	Positive	Positive	Positive (CAM5.2)	Positive	Positive	CEA
Hepatocellular carcinoma	Negative	Negative	Positive	Negative	Negative	HepPar, albumen
Prostatic adenocarcinoma	Negative	Negative	Positive	Negative	Negative	PSA, PAP
Malignant melanoma	Negative	Negative	Negative	Negative	Negative	S100, melan-A, HMB-45
Lung carcinoma	Negative	Negative	Positive	Positive	Negative	
Hematolymphoid	Negative	Negative	Negative	Negative	Negative	CD45 (LCA)

Chr = chromogranin; Syn = synaptophysin; CK = keratin; Cal = calcitonin.

2. Shifrin A et al: Primary and metastatic parathyroid malignancies: a rare or underdiagnosed condition? J Clin Endocrinol Metab. 100(3):E478-81, 2015
3. Ofo E et al: Renal cell carcinoma metastasis to the parathyroid gland: a very rare occurrence. Int J Surg Case Rep. 5(7):378-80, 2014
4. Lee SH et al: Concurrence of primary hyperparathyroidism and metastatic breast carcinoma affected a parathyroid gland. J Clin Endocrinol Metab. 98(8):3127-30, 2013
5. Chrisoulidou A et al: Parathyroid involvement in thyroid cancer: an unforeseen event. World J Surg Oncol. 10:121, 2012
6. Lee HE et al: Tumor-to-tumor metastasis: hepatocellular carcinoma metastatic to parathyroid adenoma. Pathol Int. 61(10):593-7, 2011
7. Ito Y et al: Clinical significance of extrathyroid extension to the parathyroid gland of papillary thyroid carcinoma. Endocr J. 56(2):251-5, 2009
8. Venkatraman L et al: Primary hyperparathyroidism and metastatic carcinoma within parathyroid gland. J Clin Pathol. 60(9):1058-60, 2007
9. Tang W et al: Parathyroid gland involvement by papillary carcinoma of the thyroid gland. Arch Pathol Lab Med. 126(12):1511-4, 2002
10. Gattuso P et al: Neoplasms metastatic to parathyroid glands. South Med J. 81(11):1467, 1988
11. Inoshita T et al: Tumor-to-tumor metastasis: malignant melanoma metastatic to parathyroid adenoma. Mil Med. 150(6):323-5, 1985
12. de la Monte SM et al: Endocrine organ metastases from breast carcinoma. Am J Pathol. 114(1):131-6, 1984
13. Horwitz CA et al: Secondary malignant tumors of the parathyroid glands. Report of two cases with associated hypoparathyroidism. Am J Med. 52(6):797-808, 1972

Metastatic Carcinoma to Parathyroid Adenoma

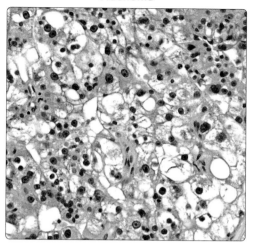

Parathyroid Adenoma

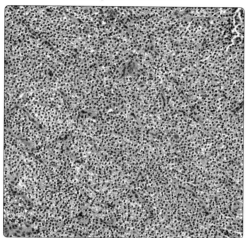

(Left) *Metastatic tumor with marked nuclear pleomorphism and atypia is identified in this field. This tumor was metastatic to a parathyroid adenoma.* **(Right)** *These parathyroid adenoma cells are positive for CAM5.2, chromogranin, synaptophysin, and parathyroid hormone, markers that were all negative in the metastatic carcinoma to the parathyroid adenoma. Thus, the 2 tumors were cytologically and immunophenotypically distinct.*

Metastatic Carcinoma

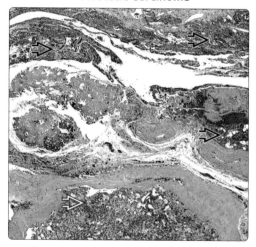

Metastatic Carcinoma to Parathyroid Adenoma

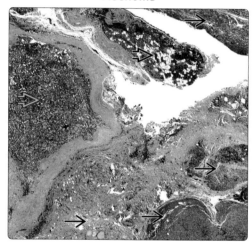

(Left) *Metastatic carcinoma ⮕, compatible with breast primary, involves a parathyroid adenoma ⮕. The tumors are histologically and immunophenotypically distinct.* **(Right)** *This image shows metastatic carcinoma ⮕ to parathyroid adenoma ⮕. Both tumors are cellular, but the parathyroid adenoma lacks the marked cytologic atypia of the metastatic carcinoma. A rim of normal parathyroid tissue is present ⮕.*

Metastatic Carcinoma in Vessel

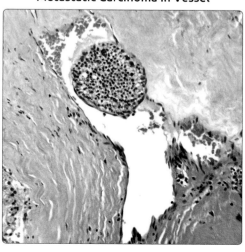

Rhabdomyoma

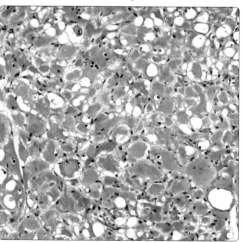

(Left) *High-power photomicrograph shows a focus of metastatic carcinoma in a vessel that was adjacent to a large focus of metastatic carcinoma involving a parathyroid adenoma.* **(Right)** *This is an unusual case of a rhabdomyoma involving a parathyroid gland, which appeared to be the result of direct extension of the tumor to involve the parathyroid.*

SECTION 3
Adrenal Glands

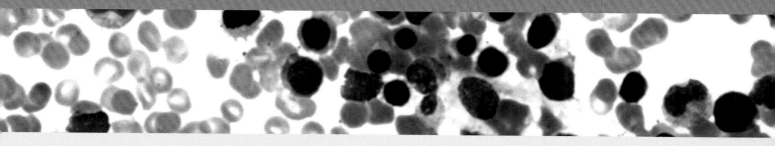

TERMINOLOGY

- Normal adrenal tissue in aberrant locations
- Synonyms: Ectopic adrenal, accessory adrenal, adrenal rests

ETIOLOGY/PATHOGENESIS

- Common sites consistent with remnants of adrenal ridge
  - Near adrenals, kidneys, ovaries, testis, spermatic cord
- Uncommon sites not readily explained
  - Gallbladder, lung, thyroid, anterior cranial fossa, choroid plexus, cranial nerve, spinal cord, placenta
- Medulla not usually present because developmental guidance cues are disrupted

CLINICAL ISSUES

- Incidental finding in > 30% of unselected autopsies; 1.6-2.5% of inguinoscrotal surgeries on pediatric patients
- Can mimic metastatic or primary carcinoma
  - Problematic in frozen sections of donor organs or during cancer staging

- Occasionally become hyperplastic or neoplastic

MICROSCOPIC

- Architecturally, cytologically, and immunohistochemically resemble normal adrenal cortex
- Usually no adrenal medulla
- Heterotopia in common sites usually involves fat and connective tissue; in rare sites, more likely intraparenchymal
- Capsule can be absent or incomplete when intraparenchymal in liver or other organs
- Anatomic zonation can be less developed in intraparenchymal sites

ANCILLARY TESTS

- Same as normal adrenal cortex
  - Inhibin (+)
  - Melan-A (+)
  - Synaptophysin (+)

Ectopic Adrenal Tissue in Periadrenal Fat

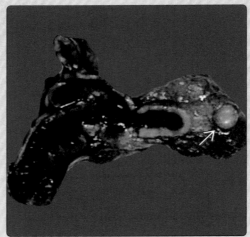

Ectopic Adrenal From Periadrenal Fat

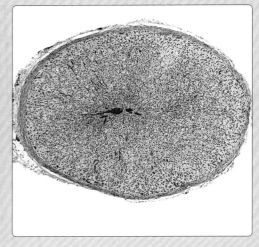

(Left) *Gross photograph shows a section of normal adrenal with a 2-mm ectopic adrenal in the adjacent fat ➡. The yellow color of the ectopic adrenal is the same as the normal cortex, a diagnostic clue.* (Right) *H&E shows a 2-mm ectopic adrenal with focal adherent fat. The ectopic gland consists of mature cortical tissue with zona glomerulosa, fasciculata, and reticularis. The medulla is absent.*

Adrenal Cortical Tissue in Donor Kidney

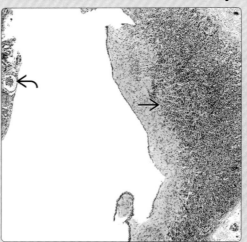

Adrenal Cortical Rest in Term Placenta

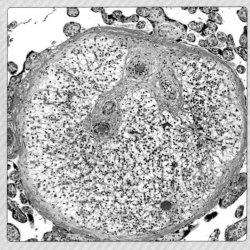

(Left) *H&E shows an unencapsulated ectopic adrenal cortex ➡ in the wall of a renal cyst from a donor kidney sampled to rule out malignancy prior to transplantation. A glomerulus ➡ is present at the opposite wall of the cyst.* (Right) *Ectopic adrenal in the placenta is a rare finding, possibly arising from stem cells in the placenta. Anatomic zones can be less developed than in retroperitoneal regions.*

TERMINOLOGY

Synonyms

- Ectopic adrenal, accessory adrenal, adrenal rests

Definitions

- Normal adrenal tissue in aberrant locations
  - Usually pertains to accessory adrenal tissue; sometimes applied to malformations in which complete adrenal is abnormally located

ETIOLOGY/PATHOGENESIS

Basis in Embryology

- Normal adrenal cortex forms from mesoderm-derived adrenal ridge in coelomic epithelium extending from T6-L1 near dorsal mesentery, medial to gonadal ridge
- Normal adrenal medulla forms from neuroectodermal progenitors that migrate from nearby developing sympathetic chains and secondarily colonize cortical primordium
- Medullary precursors do not usually colonize ectopic cortex because anatomical and chemical guidance cues are disrupted

Origins of Heterotopia

- Common sites are consistent with remnants of adrenal ridge that persist in original vicinity or migrate with gonads
- Rare sites are not readily explained; possibly abnormal migration or differentiation of adrenal progenitor or stem cells

CLINICAL ISSUES

Epidemiology

- Incidence
  - Incidental finding in > 30% of unselected autopsies; 1.6-2.5% of inguinoscrotal surgeries on pediatric patients
  - No apparent gender predilection

Site

- Common sites include periadrenal fat, celiac axis, broad ligament, mesovarium, testicular adnexa, spermatic cord, inguinal hernia sacs
- Less common to rare sites include upper pole of kidney, ovary, testis, liver, pancreas
- Very rare sites include colon, gallbladder, lung, thyroid, anterior cranial fossa, choroid plexus, cranial nerve, spinal cord, placenta
- Heterotopia in common sites usually involves fat and connective tissue; in rare sites, more likely intraparenchymal

Presentation

- Usually incidental finding during surgery or imaging
  - Can mimic metastatic or primary carcinoma
- Occasionally give rise to adrenal cortical carcinoma or adenoma, functional or nonfunctional
- Can become hyperplastic in patients with elevated ACTH
  - Congenital adrenal hyperplasia, Cushing syndrome

MACROSCOPIC

General Features

- Yellow-brown tissue resembling normal adrenal cortex
- Usually sharply circumscribed, encapsulated, round-to-oval nubbins
  - Typically < 5 mm; range: < 0.5 mm to ~ 2 cm reported
- Capsule can be absent or incomplete when intraparenchymal in liver or other organs

MICROSCOPIC

Histologic Features

- Architecturally normal adrenal cortical tissue
  - Variable proportions of fetal and adult cortex in fetuses and neonates
  - Mature cortex in adults
  - Medulla usually absent
    - Most likely to be present in ectopic adrenals close to celiac plexus (up to 50% reported); least likely in sites distant from abdomen
- Occasional associated findings include dystrophic calcification, ovarian thecal metaplasia

Cytologic Features

- Usually cytologically normal fetal or mature adult cortex
- Cytomegaly can be present in fetal rests

ANCILLARY TESTS

Immunohistochemistry

- Same as normal adrenal cortex
  - Inhibin (+), melan-A (+), synaptophysin (+); helpful in differential diagnosis

DIFFERENTIAL DIAGNOSIS

Leydig Cell Rests

- Contain Reinke crystalloid; often associated with nerve fibers

Extraadrenal Paraganglia

- Sometimes consist of clear cells resembling adrenal cortex
- Inhibin (-), chromogranin-A (+)

Renal Cell Carcinoma

- Histological and cytological features of malignancy
- Inhibin (-), CD10(+)

Adrenal Cortical Carcinoma

- Histological and cytological features of malignancy

Other Tumors

- Morphology and immunohistochemistry specific to tumor type

SELECTED REFERENCES

1. Liu Y et al: Ectopic adrenocortical adenoma in the renal hilum: a case report and literature review. Diagn Pathol. 11:40, 2016
2. Senescende L et al: Adrenal ectopy of adult groin region: a systematic review of an unexpected anatomopathologic diagnosis. Hernia. 20(6):879-885, 2016
3. Bonne L et al: Epididymal adrenal rest tissue in a patient with congenital adrenal hyperplasia. JBR-BTR. 97(3):193-4, 2014
4. Zhong H et al: Growth patterns of placental and paraovarian adrenocortical heterotopias are different. Case Rep Pathol. 2013:205692, 2013
5. Ye H et al: Intrarenal ectopic adrenal tissue and renal-adrenal fusion: a report of nine cases. Mod Pathol. 22(2):175-81, 2009
6. Drut R et al: Vascular malformation and choroid plexus adrenal heterotopia: new findings in Beckwith-Wiedemann syndrome? Fetal Pediatr Pathol. 25(4):191-7, 2006

TERMINOLOGY

- Grossly or microscopically abnormal anatomical configuration of complete adrenal gland
  - Include cortical extrusions, adhesion to other organs, complete or incomplete fusion with other organs, midline adrenal fusion, hypoplasia, agenesis

ETIOLOGY/PATHOGENESIS

- Etiologies of most adrenal malformations are unknown
- Midline adrenal fusion and other adrenal shape abnormalities often associated with asplenia syndromes, neural tube defects, and renal anomalies
- Adrenal hypoplasia can be caused by hereditary mutations of *NROB1, SF1, MC2R, MRAP, POMC*, and other genes

CLINICAL ISSUES

- Most common malformations are sporadic abnormalities of capsule

- Cortical extrusions can histologically mimic infiltrating cortical neoplasia
- Adrenal union or fusion can be radiologically misdiagnosed as mass lesions in kidney or liver
- Distinct hereditary adrenal hypoplasia syndromes associated with specific mutated genes
  - Can include severe glucocorticoid &/or mineralocorticoid insufficiency in infants, growth and pigmentation abnormalities in older patients
  - X-linked congenital adrenal hypoplasia is most common hereditary cause
    - Frequently accompanied by hypogonadotrophic hypogonadism

TOP DIFFERENTIAL DIAGNOSES

- Cortical extrusions vs. infiltrating cortical neoplasia
  - Differential diagnosis is based on familiarity with this anatomic variant and absent histological signs of malignancy

Adrenal Cortical Extrusion

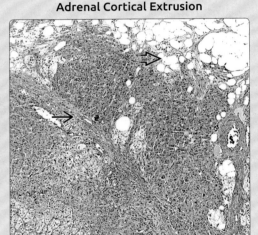

Adrenal Cortical Extrusion

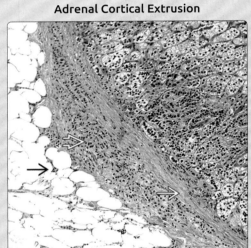

(Left) *Extrusion of benign adrenal cortical cells beyond the capsule ➡ of this hyperplastic adrenal extends into the periadrenal fat ➡.* (Right) *H&E shows an area with mild and focal extrusion of adrenal cortical cells ➡ through the capsule ➡ of this normal adrenal gland and into the periadrenal adipose tissue ➡.*

Adrenal-Renal Fusion (Incomplete Fusion)

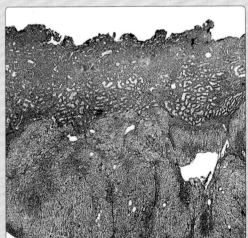

Midline Adrenal Fusion

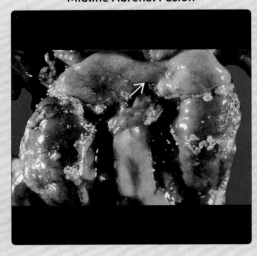

(Left) *Because it is fused to the kidney, this hyperplastic adrenal cortical tissue has an irregular border with the kidney, raising clinical suspicion of an invasive cortical tumor.* (Right) *This image shows a midline adrenal fusion ➡. (Courtesy E. Lack, MD.)*

TERMINOLOGY

Definitions

- Grossly or microscopically abnormal anatomical configuration of complete adrenal gland
  - Cortical extrusions (a.k.a. cortical protrusions)
    - Cortical cells extending beyond adrenal capsule
  - Adhesion
    - Adrenal tissue attached to different organ with intervening capsule
  - Incomplete union (a.k.a. incomplete fusion)
    - Adrenal partially merged with different organ with partially missing intervening capsule
  - Complete union
    - Entire adrenal incorporated into different organ
  - Midline adrenal fusion (a.k.a. horseshoe adrenal)
    - Single horseshoe- or butterfly-shaped adrenal in preaortic midline location
  - Hypoplasia
    - Small adrenals with defective cortical development
  - Agenesis
    - Complete absence of 1 or both adrenals

ETIOLOGY/PATHOGENESIS

Developmental Anomaly

- Malformations
  - Usually sporadic types
    - Cortical extrusions, adhesion to kidney or liver, incomplete or complete union with kidney or liver
  - Types variably associated with congenital disorders
    - Midline adrenal fusion: > 50% of cases associated with asplenia syndrome ("bilateral right-sidedness"), 37% with neural tube defects, 29% with renal anomalies or renal agenesis, 3% with Cornelia de Lange syndrome
    - Sporadic hypoplasia
      - □ Most common cause is anencephaly
      - □ Also seen with other CNS abnormalities affecting hypothalamic pituitary axis
    - Agenesis
      - □ Some cases possibly familial, gene unknown
      - □ Ipsilateral adrenal agenesis reported in ~ 10% of patients with unilateral renal agenesis
    - Accentuation of cortical extrusions, intermingling of cortex and medulla, sprouting of axon-like processes from medulla
      - □ Congenital adrenal hyperplasia
    - Cortical cytomegaly, cysts, medullary nodules
      - □ Beckwith-Wiedemann syndrome
- Hereditary hypoplasia [adrenal hypoplasia congenita (AHC)]
  - X-linked disease caused by mutation of *NROB1,* encoding DAX1 transcription factor
    - Most common hereditary type
      - □ Still very rare; estimated prevalence 1 per 70,000 to 1 per 600,000
      - □ DAX1 is required for development of definitive cortex but not fetal cortex
  - Autosomal dominant AHC
    - Caused by mutations of *NR5A1,* encoding SF1 transcription factor

- SF1 cooperates with DAX1 in normal adrenal development
  - IMAGe association (intrauterine growth restriction, metaphyseal dysplasia, AHC, and genital abnormalities)
    - Maternal overexpression of gain-of-function mutations in imprinted gene *CDKN1C* encoding cell cycle checkpoint protein p57kip2
    - Loss-of-function mutations in same gene found in 5-10% of sporadic Beckwith-Wiedemann syndrome cases and ~ 40% of familial cases
- Other genetic/hereditary causes of adrenal hypoplasia
  - ACTH receptor mutations; loss of receptor function
    - Familial glucocorticoid deficiency types 1 and 2; caused by autosomal recessive mutations of ACTH receptor [melanocortin-2 receptor (MC2R) or melanocortin-2 receptor accessory protein (MRAP)]
  - Mutations of proopiomelanocortin (*POMC*) gene
  - Defective development of pituitary corticotrophs
    - Isolated: *TBX19* mutation encoding TPIT transcription factor
    - Combined: *HESX, PROP1, LHX4* mutations

CLINICAL ISSUES

Presentation

- Cortical extrusions
  - Extremely common incidental finding/anatomical variant
  - Become more prominent in glands with cortical hyperplasia
  - Can be mistaken for capsular invasion in glands with cortical neoplasms
- Adrenal-hepatic and adrenal-renal adhesion or union
  - Incidental findings, hepatic most common; hepatic and adrenal occasionally concurrent
- Hypoplasia
  - Presentation depends on underlying etiology
    - Consider in differential diagnosis of adrenal insufficiency
  - Can include severe glucocorticoid &/or mineralocorticoid insufficiency in infants, growth and pigmentation abnormalities in older patients
    - Most common hereditary cause is X-linked AHC caused by *NROB1* mutations
    - Patients with defective DAX1 typically present with severe salt wasting in infancy, but some have onset during childhood or, rarely, present with adrenal failure as adults
    - Typically affects males; female carriers of *NROB1* mutations very rarely have symptoms
    - While *NROB1* mutations are associated with hypogonadotropic hypogonadism, *NR5A1* mutations cause gonadal dysgenesis, elevated gonadotropins and undervirilization
- Other malformations
  - Found as components of congenital/hereditary disorders or as rare incidental findings
  - Usually found at autopsy; sometimes found by sonography or radiology
- Agenesis
  - Usually found at autopsy

MICROSCOPIC

Histologic Features

- Cortical extrusions
  - Small groups of adrenal cortical cells extending into or beyond adrenal capsule
  - Unencapsulated or encapsulated
  - No underlying carcinoma
  - Sometimes traverse capsule at sites of small capsular blood vessels
  - Cytologically bland; lack features of malignancy
- Midline adrenal fusion
  - Histologically normal adrenals joined across midline
- Adrenal-hepatic or adrenal-renal union
  - Normal adrenal merged with hepatic or renal parenchyma
- Hypoplasia
  - Histology depends on underlying etiology
  - Infant adrenals with congenital adrenal hypoplasia can show cytomegaly and decreased fetal zone
    - Cytomegaly seen in X-linked AHC and in IMAGe association
    - Cytomegaly not reported in hypoplastic adrenals of autosomal recessive AHC
  - Adrenals in familial glucocorticoid deficiency show selective sparing of zona glomerulosa

DIFFERENTIAL DIAGNOSIS

Neoplasms

- Adrenal cortical extrusions and fusions must be differentiated from infiltrating cortical neoplasia
- Other primary or metastatic tumors
  - Renal cell carcinoma
    - Especially important in pretransplant frozen sections of donor kidney and liver
  - Other clear cell tumors

DIAGNOSTIC CHECKLIST

Pathologic Interpretation Pearls

- Consider adrenal-renal and adrenal-hepatic fusions before diagnosing malignancy
  - Differential diagnosis is based on familiarity with anatomic variants and absent histological signs of malignancy
    - Immunohistochemistry [(inhibin(+), melan-A(+), SF1(+)] can be helpful in diagnosis

SELECTED REFERENCES

1. Borges KS et al: Mutations in the PCNA-binding site of CDKN1C inhibit cell proliferation by impairing the entry into S phase. Cell Div. 10:2, 2015
2. Brett EM et al: Genetic forms of adrenal insufficiency. Endocr Pract. 21(4):395-9, 2015
3. Ali JM et al: Late onset X-linked adrenal hypoplasia congenita with hypogonadotropic hypgonadism due to a novel 4-bp deletion in exon 2 of NR0B1. J Pediatr Endocrinol Metab. 27(11-12):1189-92, 2014
4. Durković J et al: Low estriol levels in the maternal marker screen as a predictor of X-linked adrenal hypoplasia congenita: case report. Srp Arh Celok Lek. 142(11-12):728-31, 2014
5. Phillips K et al: IMAGe association: report of two cases in siblings with adrenal hypoplasia and review of the literature. Pediatr Dev Pathol. 17(3):204-8, 2014
6. Rojek A et al: A novel mutation in the NR0B1 (DAX1) gene in a large family with two boys affected by congenital adrenal hypoplasia. Hormones (Athens). 13(3):413-9, 2014
7. Xu XQ et al: Novel mutations in DAX1 of X-linked adrenal hypoplasia congenita over several generations in one family. Endocr Pract. 19(4):e105-11, 2013
8. Darcan S et al: Gonadotropin-dependent precocious puberty in a patient with X-linked adrenal hypoplasia congenita caused by a novel DAX-1 mutation. Horm Res Paediatr. 75(2):153-6, 2011
9. Folligan K et al: [Hypoplasia adrenal congenita of anencephalic type: two cases with pituitary abnormalities and review of literature.] Morphologie. 95(308):26-33, 2011
10. Sethuraman C et al: Bilateral absence of adrenal glands: a case series that expands the spectrum of associations and highlights the difficulties in prenatal diagnosis. Fetal Pediatr Pathol. 30(2):137-43, 2011
11. Chung TT et al: Phenotypic characteristics of familial glucocorticoid deficiency (FGD) type 1 and 2. Clin Endocrinol (Oxf). 72(5):589-94, 2010
12. Taide DV et al: Adrenal masses associated with Beckwith Wiedemann syndrome in the newborn. Afr J Paediatr Surg. 7(3):209-10, 2010
13. Ye H et al: Intrarenal ectopic adrenal tissue and renal-adrenal fusion: a report of nine cases. Mod Pathol. 22(2):175-81, 2009
14. Strouse PJ et al: Horseshoe adrenal gland in association with asplenia: presentation of six new cases and review of the literature. Pediatr Radiol. 32(11):778-82, 2002
15. Kyritsi EM et al: Familial or sporadic adrenal hypoplasia syndrome. MDText.com. 2000
16. Honma K: Adreno-hepatic fusion. An autopsy study. Zentralbl Pathol. 137(2):117-22, 1991

Perivascular Adrenal Cortical Extrusion

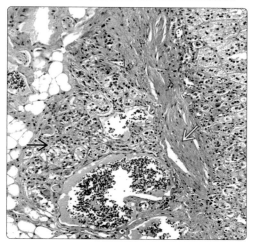

Adrenal-Renal Fusion

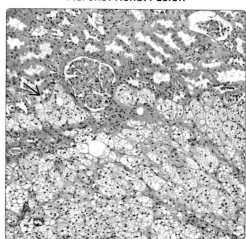

(Left) *Extrusion of normal cortical cells* ⊒ *into periadrenal fat is present in an area of the adrenal capsule* ⊒ *is penetrated by small blood vessels.* (Right) *This specimen shows incomplete adrenal-renal fusion with hyperplastic adrenal cortical tissue partly inside the renal capsule* ⊒.

Congenital Adrenal Hypoplasia

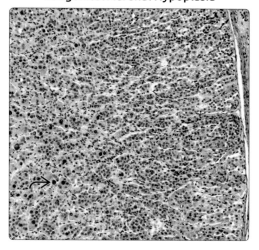

Cytomegaly in Adrenal Hypoplasia

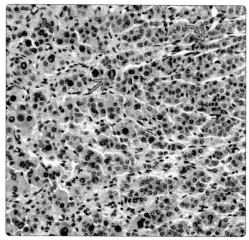

(Left) *H&E of a hypoplastic adrenal shows focal cytomegaly* ⊒ *in a 15-day-old male infant with hyponatremia and hyperkalemia. The combined adrenal weight was 3 grams.* (Courtesy H. Kozakewich, MD.) (Right) *In X-linked adrenal hypoplasia congenita, cytomegaly* ⊒ *occurs in the fetal cortex but not in the adult cortex* ⊒.

Novel Adrenal Cortical Malformation

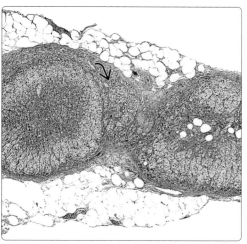

Novel Adrenal Malformation

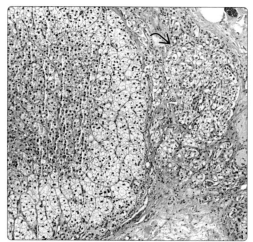

(Left) *The cortex of this unusual adult adrenal contained a series of discontinuous nodules devoid of medulla with intervening medullary tissue* ⊒. (Right) *Medullary tissue* ⊒ *is present external to cortical nodules, which are devoid of medulla in an unusual malformed adult adrenal.*

TERMINOLOGY

- Large adrenal cortical cells with abundant eosinophilic cytoplasm and atypical nuclei

ETIOLOGY/PATHOGENESIS

- Incidental finding in fetal or neonatal adrenal cortex or sporadically associated with intense or prolonged fetal stimulation or stress, erythroblastosis fetalis, prenatal infections, etc.
- Beckwith-Wiedemann syndrome
- Adrenal hypoplasia congenita (AHC), most often with X-linked *DAX1* mutation

CLINICAL ISSUES

- Most common in premature infants or newborns, occasional focal finding in adults
- Probably involutes in most cases with regression of fetal cortex

- Genetic testing needed for patients with AHC and family members

MACROSCOPIC

- Grossly normal, enlarged or hypoplastic adrenals, depending on etiology

MICROSCOPIC

- Large, polyhedral "cytomegalic" cells in fetal adrenal cortex
  - o Abundant eosinophilic cytoplasm
  - o Enlarged hyperchromatic nuclei with occasional nuclear pseudoinclusions
  - o Absent mitotic figures, low Ki67 labeling
  - o Multinucleation rare

TOP DIFFERENTIAL DIAGNOSES

- Cytomegalovirus infection: Associated with necrosis, inflammation, viral cytopathic effect

---

Cytomegaly in Regressing Fetal Cortex

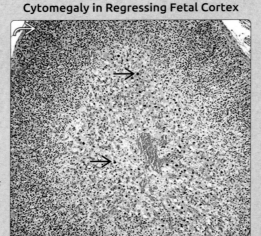

Cytologic Features of Adrenal Cytomegaly

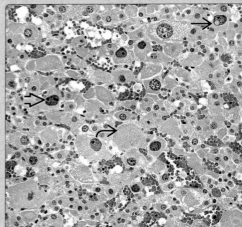

(Left) Cytomegaly is usually restricted to the fetal cortex, which regresses postnatally. This image shows scattered megalic cells ➡ in the involuting fetal cortex, which is being replaced by the definitive cortex ➡. (Right) Cytomegalic cells exhibit abundant eosinophilic cytoplasm ➡ and hyperchromatic nuclei ➡. Occasionally, intranuclear vacuoles and pseudoinclusions ➡ may be present.

Ki-67 Labeling in Megalic and Normal Cortical Cells

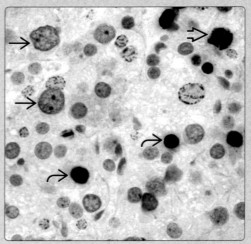

Congenital Adrenal Hypoplasia

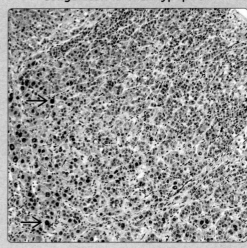

(Left) Megalic cells ➡ show little Ki-67 staining, unlike cortical tumors. In this slide of involuting fetal cortex, Ki-67 stains ingrowing definitive cortical cells ➡ and an apoptotic megalic cell ➡. (Right) Adrenal cortical cytomegaly ➡ occurs in congenital adrenal hypoplasia, especially with X-linked DAX-1 mutation and hypogonadotrophic hypogonadism.

TERMINOLOGY

Definitions

- Presence of markedly enlarged ("megalic"), variably sized cells with cytologic atypia within adrenal cortex

ETIOLOGY/PATHOGENESIS

Reported Sporadic Associations

- Incidental finding in neonatal adrenal cortex
- Intense or prolonged fetal stimulation or stress
- Erythroblastosis fetalis
- Prenatal viral infections
- Diaphragmatic hernia

Hereditary and Syndromic Disorders

- Beckwith-Wiedemann syndrome
- Adrenal hypoplasia congenita (AHC), most often with X-linked *DAX1* mutation
  - *DAX1* required for development of definitive cortex but not fetal cortex
  - Also feature of AHC in IMAGe association (intrauterine growth restriction, metaphyseal dysplasia, adrenal hypoplasia congenita, and genital abnormalities), associated with heterozygous mutation in *CDKN1C*
  - Not reported in hypoplastic adrenals of autosomal recessive AHC caused by mutations of *SF1*, which cooperates with *DAX1* in normal adrenal development

Molecular Basis

- DNA quantitation by image analysis suggests cytomegaly is reflection of polyploidy due to partial DNA replication &/or other modes of polyploidization
  - Up to 25x normal amount of DNA reported

CLINICAL ISSUES

Epidemiology

- Incidence
  - Present in 6.5% of premature stillborns, 3% of newborn autopsies, and 0.8% of pediatric autopsies
- Age
  - Common finding in infancy and early childhood; rare in normal adults
- Sex
  - No apparent gender predilection except in AHC; male predominance with *DAX1* mutation

Site

- Usually affects cells of fetal cortex
- Can be bilateral or unilateral, focal or diffuse

Natural History

- Probably involutes in most cases with regression of fetal cortex

Prognosis

- Depends on associated conditions; no prognostic implications in incidental cases
- Genetic testing needed for patients with AHC and family members

- Patients with *DAX1* mutation typically present with severe salt wasting in infancy, but some have onset during childhood or, rarely, present with adrenal failure as adults; female carriers of *DAX1* mutation very rarely have symptoms

MACROSCOPIC

General Features

- Adrenal cortex grossly normal, enlarged or hypoplastic depending on etiology

MICROSCOPIC

Histologic Features

- Enlarged polyhedral cells, usually confined to fetal adrenal cortex; distribution focal or diffuse

Cytologic Features

- Cells can measure > 150 μm
- Abundant eosinophilic cytoplasm
- Enlarged hyperchromatic nuclei; can be markedly pleomorphic
  - Occasional intranuclear pseudoinclusions
  - Multinucleation rare
  - Mitotic figures absent; Ki-67 labeling extremely rare

DIFFERENTIAL DIAGNOSIS

Adrenal Cytomegalovirus Infection

- Often seen in AIDS or other immunosuppressed states
- Cells have basophilic cytoplasm with large intranuclear inclusions surrounded by clear halo and cytoplasmic inclusions
- In situ hybridization and immunohistochemistry may be used to detect cytomegalovirus (CMV)
- Necrosis, fibrosis, and inflammation present with CMV

SELECTED REFERENCES

1. Brett EM et al: Genetic forms of adrenal insufficiency. Endocr Pract. 21(4):395-9, 2015
2. Phillips K et al: IMAGe association: report of two cases in siblings with adrenal hypoplasia and review of the literature. Pediatr Dev Pathol. 17(3):204-8, 2014
3. Lu DY et al: Automated in situ hybridization and immunohistochemistry for cytomegalovirus detection in paraffin-embedded tissue sections. Appl Immunohistochem Mol Morphol. 17(2):158-64, 2009
4. Trevisan M et al: Human cytomegalovirus productively infects adrenocortical cells and induces an early cortisol response. J Cell Physiol. 221(3):629-41, 2009
5. McCabe ER: DAX1: Increasing complexity in the roles of this novel nuclear receptor. Mol Cell Endocrinol. 265-266:179-82, 2007
6. Lehmann SG et al: Structure-function analysis reveals the molecular determinants of the impaired biological function of DAX-1 mutants in AHC patients. Hum Mol Genet. 12(9):1063-72, 2003
7. Noguchi S et al: Adrenal cytomegaly: two cases detected by prenatal diagnosis. Asian J Surg. 26(4):234-6, 2003
8. Li M et al: Molecular genetics of Wiedemann-Beckwith syndrome. Am J Med Genet. 79(4):253-9, 1998
9. Fasano M et al: Proliferative activity of adrenal glands with adrenocortical cytomegaly measured by MIB-1 labeling index. Pediatr Pathol Lab Med. 16(5):765-76, 1996
10. Ong BB et al: Adrenal cytomegaly associated with diaphragmatic hernia: report of a case. Malays J Pathol. 18(2):121-3, 1996
11. Favara BE et al: Adrenal cytomegaly: quantitative assessment by image analysis. Pediatr Pathol. 11(4):521-36, 1991
12. Gau GS et al: Fetal adrenal cytomegaly. J Clin Pathol. 32(3):305-6, 1979

CLASSIFICATION

- ACTH-dependent cortical hyperplasia
  - Congenital adrenal hyperplasia
- ACTH-independent micronodular adrenal cortical disease
- Primary macronodular cortical hyperplasia
  - "AIMAH" and related terms no longer appropriate
  - Independent of ACTH from extraadrenal sources but often not truly ACTH-independent
  - Ectopic expression of ACTH, other hormones and G-protein-coupled receptors (GPCRs) in adrenal cortical cells causes paracrine or autocrine stimulation

CLINICAL ISSUES

- "ACTH-independent" cortical hyperplasias increasingly recognized
- Autonomously functioning hyperplasias resemble adenomas in biochemical testing
- PPNAD and PMAH comprise ~ 10% of "ACTH-independent" Cushing syndrome and can mimic cortical neoplasms

- Many PMAH cases associated with *ARMC5* mutations and meningiomas

MICROSCOPIC

- Congenital and secondary ACTH-dependent hyperplasia
  - Bilateral diffuse and nodular expansion of zona fasciculata; varying populations of clear, lipid-containing cells and eosinophilic, lipid-depleted cells
- ACTH-independent micronodular hyperplasia
  - Multiple nodules, microscopic to ~ 1 cm; large, globular cells, usually with eosinophilic granular cytoplasm containing brown pigment define PPNAD
  - Intervening cortex usually atrophic
- Primary macronodular hyperplasia
  - Large nodules of clear and lipid-depleted cells, normal or atrophic intervening cortex; occasional unusual features including focal oncocytic or myxoid change; can be asynchronous or unilateral

Diffuse Adrenal Hyperplasia: Cut Surface

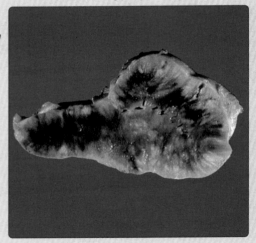

Lipid-Containing and Lipid-Depleted Cells

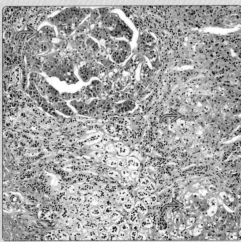

(Left) *ACTH-dependent hyperplasia usually shows diffusely thickened cortex with streaks and patches of yellow lipid-containing cells and brown lipid-depleted cells. (Courtesy R. DeLellis, MD.)* (Right) *Mild to moderate ACTH-dependent cortical hyperplasia shows enlarged lipid-containing cells ➡, compact lipid-depleted cells ➡, and lipid-containing cells resembling normal zona fasciculata ➡.*

Primary Pigmented Nodular Adrenal Disease

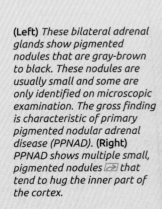

Multiple Pigmented Nodules

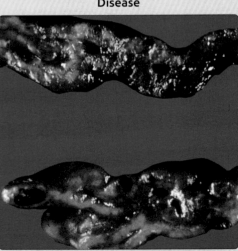

(Left) *These bilateral adrenal glands show pigmented nodules that are gray-brown to black. These nodules are usually small and some are only identified on microscopic examination. The gross finding is characteristic of primary pigmented nodular adrenal disease (PPNAD).* (Right) *PPNAD shows multiple small, pigmented nodules ➡ that tend to hug the inner part of the cortex.*

TERMINOLOGY

Definitions

- ACTH-dependent cortical hyperplasia
  - Synonym: Secondary adrenal cortical hyperplasia
  - Cortical cell proliferation driven by ACTH, which may be pituitary-derived or ectopic
- ACTH-independent cortical hyperplasia
  - Synonym: Primary adrenal cortical hyperplasia
  - Encompasses etiologically diverse group of diseases in which autonomous cortical cell proliferation is driven by varied genetic and signaling mechanisms

ETIOLOGY/PATHOGENESIS

ACTH-Dependent Cortical Hyperplasia

- Secondary hyperplasia in genetically normal patients
  - ACTH-dependent cortical hyperplasia caused by perturbations of hypothalamic-pituitary axis in patients with normal steroid synthesizing ability
    - Can be physiological response to chronic stress or pathological response to abnormally increased ACTH
    - Abnormally increased ACTH can be derived from pituitary adenoma or hyperplasia (Cushing disease) or can be ectopic from neuroendocrine tumor (most often small cell carcinoma)
      - ☐ Ectopic CRH drives ACTH production in rare cases
- Congenital adrenal hyperplasia (CAH)
  - ACTH-dependent cortical hyperplasia caused by mutations of genes encoding steroid synthesizing enzymes
    - Autosomal recessive inheritance; 1 in 16,000 individuals; 1 in 600 with nonclassic disease (one of most common recessive human genetic diseases)
    - Enzymes most commonly involved are 21-hydroxylase, 11b-hydroxylase, 3b-hydroxysteroid dehydrogenase, 17a-hydroxylase; glucocorticoid deficiency causes loss of feedback inhibition and increased ACTH secretion
    - Rare variant is lipoid adrenal hyperplasia, caused by mutations of StAR (steroidogenic acute regulatory protein), which transports cholesterol to mitochondria to begin steroid biosynthesis

ACTH-Independent Micronodular Adrenal Cortical Disease

- Proposed classification in 3 groups
  - Primary pigmented nodular adrenal cortical disease (PPNAD) as part of Carney complex, isolated PPNAD, isolated micronodular adrenocortical disease (i-MAD) without pigmentation
    - i-MAD has early onset, may be distinct entity or variant of PPNAD
- ~ 50% of cases familial, usually as component of Carney complex, others apparently sporadic
- Different germline mutations lead to increased cyclic AMP production, no strict correlation between pathology and genotype

- Germline inactivating mutations or deletions in regulatory R1A subunit of protein kinase A (*PRKAR1A*), which causes Carney complex, present in some patients with isolated PPNAD, inactivating mutations in phosphodiesterases 11A or 8B (*PDE11A*, *PDE8B*) in some cases of i-MAD, copy number gains of protein kinase A catalytic subunit alpa (*PRKACA*) in micronodular and occasional macronodular hyperplasias
  - Somatic *CTNNB1* mutations accompany germline mutations in some cases
- Can present as unilateral disease mimicking adenoma

Primary Macronodular Adrenal Hyperplasia

- Historically many synonyms, most recently ACTH-independent macronodular cortical hyperplasia (AIMAH)
- Other synonyms: ACTH-independent massive bilateral adrenal disease (AIMBAD), primary bilateral macronodular adrenal hyperplasia (PBMAH), bilateral macronodular adrenal hyperplasia (BMAH), autonomous macronodular adrenal hyperplasia (AMAH), massive macronodular adrenocortical disease (MMAD), macronodular hyperplasia with marked adrenal enlargement (MHMAE)
- Rare cause of Cushing syndrome (CS); < 2% of all endogenous CS cases; prevalence of subclinical cases unknown
- Can be hereditary or sporadic; apparently sporadic cases often harbor occult germline mutations
- Multiple causative genes, overlapping pathophysiology
- Inactivating germline mutations of *ARMC5* most common cause (> 50% of apparently sporadic and familial cases)
  - Different somatic mutations inactivate the 2nd allele in each nodule
- Other associations
  - Multiple endocrine neoplasia type 1; inactivating germline mutations of *MEN1* tumor suppressor gene, no loss of heterozygosity (LOH) in adrenal cortical tissue
    - Bilateral adrenal cortical enlargement in ~ 20% of MEN1 patients in some studies, macronodular hyperplasia in ~ 6%
  - Adenomatous polyposis coli; inactivating germline mutation of APC tumor suppressor gene that normally inhibits Wnt/β-catenin signaling, 2nd allele in adrenal tissue inactivated by mutation or LOH
  - Hereditary leiomyomatosis and renal cell carcinoma (HLRCC); inactivating germline mutation of Krebs cycle enzyme fumarate hydratase (FH), 2nd allele in adrenal tissue inactivated by mutation or LOH
    - Frequency of adrenal lesions in HLRCC estimated 7.8% in series of 255 patients
  - McCune-Albright syndrome; not hereditary, early post zygotic and somatic mutations in stimulatory (Gsα) G protein gene *GNAS* cause increased cyclic AMP production
    - Somatic mosaicism causes variable organ involvement, adrenal involvement rare
- Pathophysiology
  - Ectopic expression of peptide or amine hormones and G-protein-coupled receptors (GPCRs) in adrenal cortical cells, resulting in paracrine or autocrine stimulation
    - Associated with *ARMC5* mutations but possibly also factor in other hyperplastic conditions

- Ectopic ACTH expressed in adrenal cortex, not limited to cases with *ARMC5* mutation ("AIMAH" and related synonyms no longer appropriate)
  - □ Release of ectopic ACTH is triggered by aberrantly expressed receptors for various ligands (e.g., gastric inhibitory polypeptide (GIP), luteinizing hormone, vasopressin, serotonin; ectopic receptors for GIP may cause "food-dependent" cortisol release
  - □ Ectopic ligands including vasopressin and serotonin may provide further stimulation
  - Mechanisms underlying aberrant receptor expression still unclear
  - ○ Genetic abnormalities in melanocortin receptor or cyclic AMP signaling pathway components not common or consistent

CLINICAL ISSUES

Presentation

- **ACTH-dependent cortical hyperplasia in genetically normal patients**
  - ○ Manifestations range from asymptomatic to Cushing syndrome, depending on etiology and severity of hyperplasia
- **Congenital adrenal hyperplasia**
  - ○ 3 main groups of 21 hydroxylase deficiency
    - **Complete 21 hydroxylase deficiency (classic syndrome)**
      - □ Absent aldosterone leads to hyponatremia, hyperkalemia, acidosis, hypotension; absent cortisol causes increased ACTH and adrenal cortical hyperplasia with shunting of corticosteroid precursors to androgenic pathways, leading to virilization (adrenogenital syndrome)
      - □ Occasionally develop adrenal adenomas and myelolipomas
    - **Partial 21 hydroxylase deficiency (nonclassic syndrome)**
      - □ Some aldosterone, sufficient to prevent salt wasting; some cortisol, but still causes increased ACTH, cortical hyperplasia, increased androgens and virilization
    - **Cryptic syndrome**
      - □ Biochemical and genetic abnormality with subclinical presentation
  - ○ In congenital lipoid hyperplasia, all cortical steroids, including gonadal steroids, decrease
    - Classic disease usually fatal, surviving patients show hypogonadotropic hypogonadism, novel mutations cause milder disease
- **Micronodular adrenal cortical disease**
  - ○ Usually Cushing syndrome; sometimes cyclic or subclinical
  - ○ Bimodal age distribution: Early childhood and 2nd to 3rd decade, female predilection
- **Primary macronodular adrenal hyperplasia (PMAH)**
  - ○ Caused by aberrant receptors
    - Cushing syndrome, sometimes hyperaldosteronism, subclinical cases underdiagnosed
    - Strong association of *ARM5* mutation with meningiomas

- Cortical cells with *ARM5* mutation often hypofunctional; large adrenal size required before clinical evidence of function
  - □ Glands can be large enough to simulate neoplasm, especially if unilateral
  - ○ McCune-Albright syndrome: Cushing syndrome in infants and young children, may remit later in life
  - ○ MEN1: usually clinically silent

IMAGING

General Features

- **Micronodular adrenal cortical disease**
  - ○ Nodules in patients < 10 years old usually 0.5-3 mm
    - May not be detectable by CT or MR
  - ○ In older patients, usually < 5 mm, can be up to 1-2 cm
    - Detectable by CT or MR
  - ○ Nodules isodense or mildly hyperdense to rest of adrenal gland on CT
  - ○ With MR, nodules have lower T1- and T2-weighted signal intensity than adjacent cortical tissue
- **Primary macronodular adrenal hyperplasia**
  - ○ Glands massively enlarged, multiple macronodules up to 5 cm
  - ○ Large nodules isointense relative to muscle with T1-weighted sequences and hyperintense relative to liver with T2-weighted sequences

MACROSCOPIC

General Features

- **Congenital adrenal hyperplasia**
  - ○ Bilateral enlarged glands with cerebriform or convoluted external surface
  - ○ Diffuse or diffuse and nodular cortical enlargement depending on genetic basis, cortex may be mostly brown rather than yellow because of lipid depletion; Myelolipomas occasionally develop, especially in poorly controlled cases
  - ○ In congenital lipoid hyperplasia, cholesterol accumulation gives gland lucent yellow appearance
- **Other ACTH-dependent hyperplasia**
  - ○ Bilateral usually diffuse enlargement, sometimes small superimposed nodules, variable lipid depletion
- **ACTH-independent micronodular adrenal cortical disease**
  - ○ Usually bilateral, can be asynchronous and appear unilateral
  - ○ Adrenals usually ~ normal size with multiple pigmented or nonpigmented nodules usually < 1 cm; larger nodules/adenomas occasionally superimposed
- **Primary macronodular adrenal hyperplasia**
  - ○ Usually bilateral, can be asynchronous and appear unilateral
  - ○ Large adrenals (can be > 80 g) with large yellow nodules, variable lipid depletion, and normal or atrophic intervening cortex

MICROSCOPIC

Histologic Features

- **Congenital and other ACTH-dependent hyperplasia**

- Diffuse or diffuse and nodular expansion of zona fasciculata; varying populations of clear, lipid-containing cells and compact, lipid-depleted cells
- **PPNAD and isolated micronodular hyperplasia**
  - Multiple pigmented or nonpigmented nodules, microscopic to ~ 1 cm
    - Large, globular cells with eosinophilic granular cytoplasm containing brown pigment define PPNAD
    - Intervening cortex usually atrophic
  - Nodules tend to be deep in zona reticularis in classic micronodular hyperplasias
    - Expanding spectrum of nodule distribution recently found in cases with PRKACA amplification, including intracapsular and extracapsular nodules
  - Nodules and cortex show variable expression of immunohistochemical markers
    - Nodules with somatic *CTNNB1* mutation may show β-catenin translocation
- **Primary macronodular adrenal hyperplasia**
  - Large nodules of clear and lipid-depleted cells; normal or atrophic intervening cortex
  - Myelolipomatous foci may be prominent; occasional unusual features including oncocytic or myxoid change
  - Because of genetic mosaicism, adrenals in McCune-Albright syndrome can show segmental hyperplasia coexisting with secondary zona fasciculata atrophy (bimorphic adrenocortical disease)
  - Nodules and cortex show variable expression of immunohistochemical markers
    - Nodules associated with APC may show β-catenin translocation

ANCILLARY TESTS

Genetic Testing

- Congenital adrenal hyperplasia: Germline mutations in *CYP21A2* gene
- PMAH: Germline mutations in *ARMC5* gene (> 50% of sporadic and familial PMAH, association with meningiomas)
  - Other testing suggested by syndromic associations

DIAGNOSTIC CHECKLIST

Pathologic Interpretation Pearls

- Atrophy of cortex between nodules can be indicative of ACTH-independent nodular cortical hyperplasia
- Because of genetic mosaicism, adrenals in McCune-Albright syndrome can show coexisting diffuse and nodular hyperplasia, zona fasciculata atrophy, and zona glomerulosa hyperplasia (bimorphic adrenocortical disease)

SELECTED REFERENCES

1. Lowe KM et al: Cushing syndrome in Carney Complex: clinical, pathologic, and molecular genetic findings in the 17 affected Mayo Clinic patients. Am J Surg Pathol. 41(2):171-181, 2017
2. Yamazaki Y et al: Histopathological classification of cross-sectional image-negative hyperaldosteronism. J Clin Endocrinol Metab. 102(4):1182-1192, 2017
3. Gourgari E et al: Bilateral adrenal hyperplasia as a possible mechanism for hyperandrogenism in women with polycystic ovary syndrome. J Clin Endocrinol Metab. 101(9):3353-60, 2016
4. Kim H et al: Carney complex with multiple cardiac myxomas, pigmented nodular adrenocortical hyperplasia, epithelioid blue nevus, and multiple calcified lesions of the testis: A case report. J Pathol Transl Med. 50(4):312-4, 2016
5. Kirschner LS et al: 5th International ACC Symposium: The new genetics of benign adrenocortical neoplasia: hyperplasias, adenomas, and their implications for progression into cancer. Horm Cancer. 7(1):9-16, 2016
6. Stratakis CA: Carney complex: A familial lentiginosis predisposing to a variety of tumors. Rev Endocr Metab Disord. 17(3):367-371, 2016
7. Villares Fragoso MC et al: The role of gsp mutations on the development of adrenocortical tumors and adrenal hyperplasia. Front Endocrinol (Lausanne). 7:104, 2016
8. Angelousi A et al: McCune Albright syndrome and bilateral adrenal hyperplasia: the GNAS mutation may only be present in adrenal tissue. Hormones (Athens). 14(3):447-50, 2015
9. Drougat L et al: Genetics of primary bilateral macronodular adrenal hyperplasia: a model for early diagnosis of Cushing's syndrome? Eur J Endocrinol. 173(4):M121-31, 2015
10. El Ghorayeb N et al: Multiple aberrant hormone receptors in Cushing's syndrome. Eur J Endocrinol. 173(4):M45-60, 2015
11. Fragoso MC et al: Genetics of primary macronodular adrenal hyperplasia. J Endocrinol. 224(1):R31-R43, 2015
12. Zhang Y et al: Classification and surgical treatment for 180 cases of adrenocortical hyperplastic disease. Int J Clin Exp Med. 8(10):19311-7, 2015
13. Al-Bahri S et al: Giant bilateral adrenal myelolipoma with congenital adrenal hyperplasia. Case Rep Surg. 2014:728198, 2014
14. Carney JA et al: Primary pigmented nodular adrenocortical disease: the original 4 cases revisited after 30 years for follow-up, new investigations, and molecular genetic findings. Am J Surg Pathol. 38(9):1266-73, 2014
15. Carney JA et al: Germline PRKACA amplification leads to Cushing syndrome caused by 3 adrenocortical pathologic phenotypes. Hum Pathol. ePub, 2014
16. Duan K et al: Clinicopathological correlates of adrenal Cushing's syndrome. J Clin Pathol. ePub, 2014
17. Raff H et al: Physiological basis for the etiology, diagnosis, and treatment of adrenal disorders: Cushing's syndrome, adrenal insufficiency, and congenital adrenal hyperplasia. Compr Physiol. 4(2):739-69, 2014
18. Carney JA et al: Primary bimorphic adrenocortical disease: cause of hypercortisolism in McCune-Albright syndrome. Am J Surg Pathol. 35(9):1311-26, 2011
19. Flück CE et al: Characterization of novel StAR (steroidogenic acute regulatory protein) mutations causing non-classic lipoid adrenal hyperplasia. PLoS One. 6(5):e20178, 2011
20. Yoshida M et al: A case of ACTH-independent macronodular adrenal hyperplasia associated with multiple endocrine neoplasia type 1. Endocr J. 58(4):269-77, 2011
21. Zografos GN et al: Primary pigmented nodular adrenocortical disease presenting with a unilateral adrenocortical nodule treated with bilateral laparoscopic adrenalectomy: a case report. J Med Case Reports. 4:230, 2010
22. Paris F et al: Isolated Cushing's syndrome: an unusual presentation of McCune-Albright syndrome in the neonatal period. Horm Res. 72(5):315-9, 2009
23. Tadjine M et al: Detection of somatic beta-catenin mutations in primary pigmented nodular adrenocortical disease (PPNAD). Clin Endocrinol (Oxf). 69(3):367-73, 2008
24. Burgess JR et al: Adrenal lesions in a large kindred with multiple endocrine neoplasia type 1. Arch Surg. 131(7):699-702, 1996

(Left) *This case of severe diffuse adrenal cortical hyperplasia caused by ectopic ACTH from small cell lung cancer shows only a few streaks of residual, yellow, lipid-containing cells* ➔. *A small amount of gray entrapped medulla* ➔ *is also evident.* **(Right)** *Primary macronodular hyperplasia shows multiple cortical nodules > 1 cm* ➔. *The residual overlying and intervening cortex* ➔ *appears atrophic or normal.*

Adrenal Hyperplasia: Gross Cut Surface

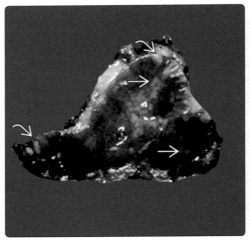

Multiple Macro Adrenal Nodules

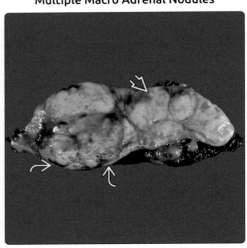

(Left) *H&E shows diffuse cortical hyperplasia and lipid depletion caused by ectopic ACTH from small cell lung cancer. A few lipid-containing cortical cells* ➔ *and entrapped medulla* ➔ *are also evident. The findings are those of severe diffuse hyperplasia in response to ectopic ACTH.* **(Right)** *Individual nodules in primary macronodular adrenal hyperplasia (PMAH) can have distinct characteristics, as shown by the varied degrees of lipid depletion in this case.*

Cortical Hyperplasia

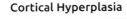
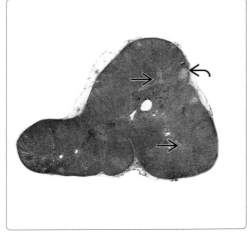

Primary Macronodular Adrenal Hyperplasia

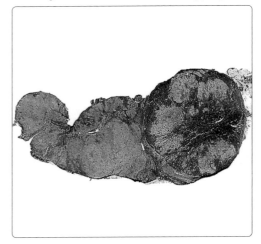

(Left) *This case of severe diffuse hyperplasia, caused by ectopic ACTH from small cell lung cancer, shows hypertrophied, globoid, lipid-depleted adrenocortical cells* ➔ *on the right and focal, residual, lipid-containing cells* ➔ *on the left.* **(Right)** *This case of primary macronodular cortical hyperplasia shows residual atrophic zona fasciculata* ➔ *compressed between lipid-containing* ➔ *and lipid-depleted* ➔ *cortical nodules.*

Lipid-Depleted Cortical Nodule

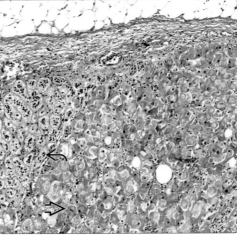

Adrenal Cortical Hyperplasia

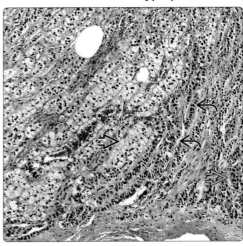

Lipid-Rich Predominant Cells

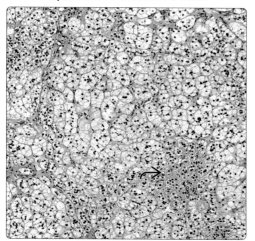

Lipomatous Metaplasia Within Hyperplasia

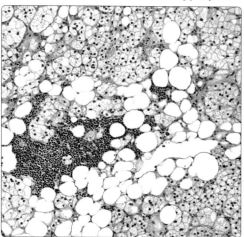

(Left) *Nodules in primary macronodular hyperplasia usually consist predominantly of lipid-containing cells with a minor component of lipid-depleted cells* ➱. (**Right**) *Common findings in macronodular hyperplasia are lymphocytic aggregates and multifocal lipomatous changes.*

Oncocytes and Lipid-Rich Cells

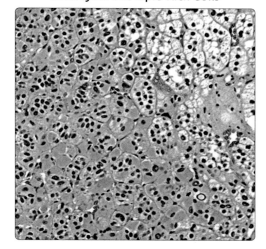

Distinct Nodules

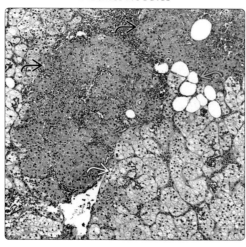

(Left) *Scattered oncocytes are occasionally found in primary macronodular hyperplasia. This field shows oncocytes distinguished from adjacent lipid-depleted and lipid-containing cells by their larger size and granular, eosinophilic cytoplasm.* (**Right**) *Oncocytic nodules* ➱ *were present in this case of primary macronodular hyperplasia adjacent to lipid-rich cells* ➱ *nodules and lipomatous metaplasia* ➱.

Pigmented Nodule

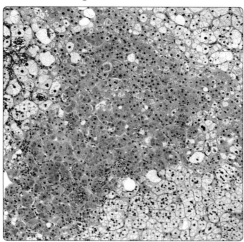

Primary Macronodular Hyperplasia

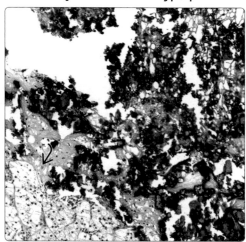

(Left) *Foci of pigmented cortical cells forming a nodule are an occasional finding in primary macronodular hyperplasia. These nodules are adjacent to lipid-rich nodules.* (**Right**) *Large nodules may show areas of infarction and dystrophic calcification adjacent to lipid-rich cells* ➱.

Adrenal Medullary Hyperplasia

TERMINOLOGY

- Increase in mass of adrenal medullary cells and expansion of these cells into areas of gland where they are not normally present

ETIOLOGY/PATHOGENESIS

- Adrenal medullary hyperplasia (AMH) is precursor of pheochromocytomas (PCCs) in MEN2 syndrome
- AMH common in MEN2A and MEN2B
  - Absent or very rare in other PCC/paraganglioma syndromes
- Bilateral diffuse AMH in patients with *SDHB* and *MAX* mutation

MACROSCOPIC

- Adrenal medulla normally confined to central region (body) of gland
  - Medullary hyperplasia often identifiable by gross extension of gray medullary tissue into alae and tail

- Patients with MEN2 syndromes usually have diffuse and nodular hyperplasia involving both glands
- Nodules are gray to tan and may compress adjacent cortex

MICROSCOPIC

- Nodules can occur with little or no diffuse hyperplasia
- Histology shows medullary hyperplasia composed of proliferation of cells containing normal cellular architecture
  - As opposed to nests of cytologically atypical polygonal cells that characterize pheochromocytoma

TOP DIFFERENTIAL DIAGNOSES

- Distinction between AMH and PCC can be challenging
- Cutoff of 1 cm to differentiate PCC from hyperplastic nodule is arbitrary
- Presence of unilateral vs. bilateral disease may be helpful in distinguishing AMH from PCC
- Unilateral AMH has been reported in isolated and familial AMH

Adrenal Medullary Expansion in MEN2

Hyaline Granules in MEN2

(Left) *Adrenal gland from a patient with multiple endocrine neoplasia type 2A (MEN2A) shows diffuse medullary expansion ➡, characteristic of adrenal medullary hyperplasia (AMH), and a well-defined nodule ➡.* (Right) *AMH in a patient with MEN2 syndrome shows medullary cells ➡ within the adrenal cortex ➡. The presence of hyaline granules ➡ is usually present in MEN2.*

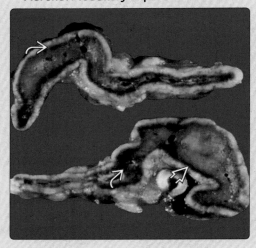

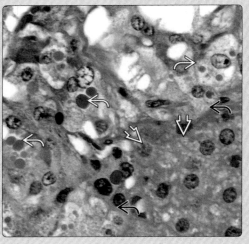

SDHB Preservation Within Medulla

SDHB Loss

(Left) *SDHB immonostin shows the presence of granules within the medullary cells, indicating the presence of the wild-type SDHB.* (Right) *Endothelial cells ➡ with granular immunopositivity for SDHB serve as intrinsic controls to indicate wild-type SDHB. Tumor cells ➡ with mutation of SDHB shows no immunoreactivity. Immunohistochemistry might also be useful screening for MAX mutations.*

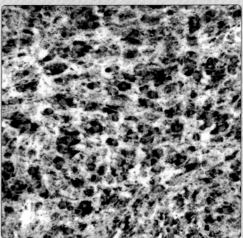

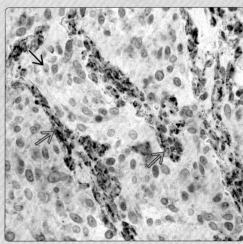

TERMINOLOGY

Abbreviations

- Adrenal medullary hyperplasia (AMH)

Definitions

- Increase in mass of adrenal medullary cells and expansion of these cells into areas of gland where they are not normally present
- Benign change in adrenal gland characterized by disproportionate enlargement of medulla compared with cortex
  - Considered adrenal cortex to medulla ratio of < 10:1
- Arbitrarily, lesions of < 1 cm in diameter are called AMH
  - Expected that majority of these are early lesions and, if left in situ, would grow to pheochromocytoma (PCC)
- Increased cell number in sympathoadrenal or parasympathetic paraganglia

ETIOLOGY/PATHOGENESIS

Familial Medullary Hyperplasia

- Known to be precursor lesion of MEN2 syndromes
- Other predisposing genetic syndromes not typically associated with AMH
  - Identification of adrenal medullary hyperplasia considered diagnostic of MEN2 syndrome
  - Bilateral diffuse adrenal medullary hyperplasia in patient with *SDHB* mutation
  - Familial pheochromocytoma with germline mutations in *MAX* (MYC associated factor X) gene
    - Both nodular and diffuse AMH belong to spectrum of *MAX*-related disease

Hyperplasia Associated With Genetic Disorders

- Bilateral adrenal medullary hyperplasia 1st described in 1966
  - Significance was not understood until identification of *RET* protooncogene
    - Now, association of AMH and MEN2 syndromes well established
- AMH is precursor of pheochromocytomas in MEN2 syndrome
  - Common in MEN2A and MEN2B
- AMH known to be absent or very rare in other PCC/paraganglioma syndromes
  - Report of bilateral diffuse adrenal medullary hyperplasia in patient with *SDHB* mutation
- AMH and hyperplasia of extraadrenal sympathetic paraganglia in Beckwith-Wiedemann syndrome (BWS) noted by Beckwith in 1969 description
  - Now seems less consistent than cortical abnormalities
- Mature chromaffin cell nodules (sometimes present in fetuses with BWS) suggest extraadrenal paraganglia developing within adrenals

As Precursor Lesion

- Because of link between *RET* mutations and adrenal medullary hyperplasia, it is hypothesized that medullary hyperplasia is precursor lesion that will eventually develop into PCC given enough time

- Similar pattern of progression from hyperplasia to malignancy seen in other endocrine tumors, such as medullary thyroid cancer and adrenal cortical tumors

Sporadic Adrenal Medullary Hyperplasia

- Sporadic AMH reported in different settings
  - In patients with cystic fibrosis
  - In infants dying of sudden infant death syndrome (SIDS)
  - Cushing syndrome
  - In sporadic forms of Beckwith-Wiedemann syndrome
  - Other rare causes

Compensatory Physiological Hyperplasia

- Extensively documented in parasympathetic paraganglia; mostly carotid body, sometimes vagal
  - Presumed association with hypoxia: Occurs in humans and animals living at high altitude; also reported in lung disease, cystic fibrosis, and cyanotic heart disease
  - Controversial association of hyperplastic paraganglia with SIDS

CLINICAL ISSUES

Presentation

- AMH may present with signs of catecholamine excess or be discovered incidentally after adrenalectomy for PCC
- Hyperplasia of extraadrenal paraganglia usually studied in autopsy series of patients dying from other causes

MACROSCOPIC

General Features

- Patients with MEN2 syndromes usually have diffuse and nodular hyperplasia involving both glands
  - Characteristically in these patients, medullary hyperplasia involves tail
- Nodules gray to tan and may compress adjacent cortex
- Adrenal medulla normally confined to central region (body) of gland
  - AMH often identifiable by gross extension of gray medullary tissue into alae and tail
  - Nodules often superimposed on diffuse hyperplasia
  - Mild diffuse hyperplasia may require morphometry for confirmation (usually not done in practice)
- On gross examination, as well as radiologic imaging, medullary hyperplasia has poorly defined nodules
  - Unlike PCC, which usually presents as enlarged adrenal nodule arising from medulla
- Hyperplasia of other paraganglia usually not identifiable macroscopically

Size

- Morphometrically calculated weight of 1 normal adrenal medulla: 0.3-0.5 g (~ 10% of total adrenal weight)
  - AMH often begins as diffuse ↑ in volume and weight
- Carotid body weight ↑ with age
  - Average normal combined weight in adults: < 15 mg (> 30 mg suggests hyperplasia)

MICROSCOPIC

Histologic Features

- Shows medullary hyperplasia composed by proliferation of cells containing normal cellular architecture
  - As opposed to nests of cytologically atypical polygonal cells that characterize PCC
  - In MEN2-associated medullary hyperplasia, hyaline globules may be present
  - Hyperplastic medullary cells may show various growth patterns: Alveolar, diffuse or solid, and trabecular
  - Sometimes, hyperplastic cells are arranged in small nests separated by thin fibrous tissue
- Presence of adrenal medullary tissue in tail indicates presence of adrenal medullary hyperplasia
- Classic AMH shows diffuse medullary expansion with increasing atypia and superimposed nodules
- Adrenal medullary nodules can occur with little or no diffuse hyperplasia
- Medulla does not represent > 1/3 of gland thickness, with cortex on each side comprising other 2/3
  - However, significant cortical atrophy, usually due to exogenous steroid administration, alters ratio and can mimic medullary hyperplasia
    - Careful evaluation of cortical anatomy and cytology required before diagnosis of AMH
- Normal carotid body divided by thick fibrous septa into variable number of lobes
  - Lobes further divided by thin septa into lobules
    - Lobules contain clusters (zellballen) of chief cells with peripheral sustentacular cells
  - Carotid body hyperplasia at high altitude
    - ↑ number of lobes and larger lobes with ↑ cellularity caused by chief cell hyperplasia
  - Studies variably report proportionate or disproportionate ↑ of sustentacular cells, especially in hyperplasia unrelated to high altitude

ANCILLARY TESTS

Immunohistochemistry

- Neuroendocrine markers highlight medullary cells
  - Chromogranin-A
  - Synaptophysin
  - NSE
  - CD56
  - S100 identifies sustentacular cells
- SDHA and SDHB immunostains help identify *SDHx*-associated inherited cases

DIFFERENTIAL DIAGNOSIS

Pheochromocytoma

- Distinction between AMH and PCC can be challenging
  - Cutoff of 1 cm to differentiate PCC from hyperplastic nodule is arbitrary
    - Some PCCs may be < 1 cm
    - Benign adrenal nodules in patients with MEN2B can be monoclonal
    - Both AMH and PCC often monoclonal
    - Best to consider nodular hyperplasia and small PCCs as part of continuum of same disease process

- Presence of unilateral vs. bilateral disease may be helpful in distinguishing AMH from PCC
  - Unilateral AMH has been reported in isolated and familial AMH
- Altered macroscopic appearance and histology probably more meaningful
- PCCs have characteristic alveolar pattern (zellballen) with variably sized nests of tumor cells surrounded by thin-walled vessels and thin bands of fibrous tissue
- Some PCCs lack organoid pattern and instead may show diffuse growth pattern
- Some PCCs show mosaic-like pattern of often large cells with granular basophilic cytoplasm admixed with cells that have amphophilic to slightly eosinophilic cytoplasm
- Some PCCs formed by small cells with ample eosinophilic cytoplasm with occasional bizarre cells

Metastatic Carcinoma

- Can be distinguished by characteristic morphological features
- Distinguished by immunohistochemical profile
  - Positivity for chromogranin, synaptophysin, NSE, and CD56 in AMH
  - Characteristic positivity for S100 in sustentacular cells, when present, helps identify AMH

DIAGNOSTIC CHECKLIST

Pathologic Interpretation Pearls

- Adrenals removed for PCC should be carefully examined for additional nodules as clue to presence of MEN2

SELECTED REFERENCES

1. Romanet P et al: Pathological and genetic characterization of bilateral adrenomedullary hyperplasia in a patient with germline MAX mutation. Endocr Pathol. ePub, 2016
2. Yang L et al: Diagnosis and treatment of adrenal medullary hyperplasia: experience from 12 cases. Int J Endocrinol. 2014:752410, 2014
3. Mete O et al: Precursor lesions of endocrine system neoplasms. Pathology. 45(3):316-30, 2013
4. Grogan RH et al: Bilateral adrenal medullary hyperplasia associated with an SDHB mutation. J Clin Oncol. 29(8):e200-2, 2011
5. Berthon A et al: Constitutive beta-catenin activation induces adrenal hyperplasia and promotes adrenal cancer development. Hum Mol Genet. 19(8):1561-76, 2010
6. Powers JF et al: Ret protein expression in adrenal medullary hyperplasia and pheochromocytoma. Endocr Pathol. 14(4):351-61, 2003
7. Diaz-Cano SJ et al: Clonal patterns in phaeochromocytomas and MEN-2A adrenal medullary hyperplasias: histological and kinetic correlates. J Pathol. 192(2):221-8, 2000
8. Carney JA et al: Adrenal medullary disease in multiple endocrine neoplasia, type 2: pheochromocytoma and its precursors. Am J Clin Pathol. 66(2):279-90, 1976
9. DeLellis RA et al: Adrenal medullary hyperplasia. A morphometric analysis in patients with familial medullary thyroid carcinoma. Am J Pathol. 83(1):177-96, 1976

Gross Cut Surface

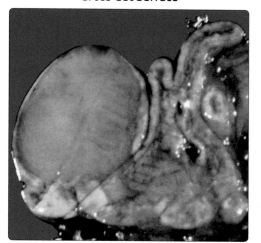

Alveolar Architecture

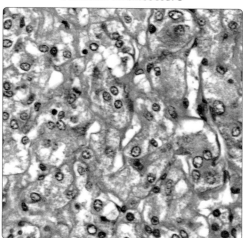

(Left) *Familial medullary hyperplasia is most commonly present in patients with MEN2A and MEN2B and associated with pheochromocytoma. The involvement is usually bilateral, diffuse, and nodular, and often extends to both alae and the tail of the adrenal gland.* **(Right)** *The hyperplastic medullary cells may show various growth patterns: Alveolar, solid, or trabecular. This example of AMH shows an alveolar growth pattern.*

Alveolar and Trabecular Architecture

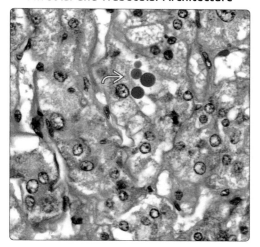

Distinct Cell Morphology

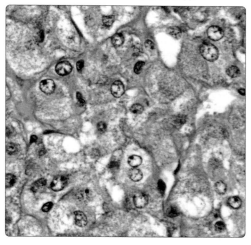

(Left) *Photomicrograph shows an area of AMH in a patient with MEN2 with a mixed alveolar-trabecular growth pattern. Note the presence of hyaline granules ➘, usually present in MEN2.* **(Right)** *In areas of AMH, the hyperplastic cells may be arranged in small nests of cells, or as single cells, separated by thin fibrous tissue.*

Intermixed Adrenal Cortical Cells

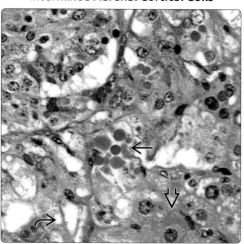

Scattered Hyaline Globules

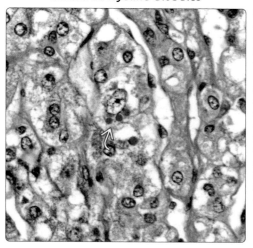

(Left) *Patients with MEN2 syndrome may have diffuse and nodular AMH. This picture shows medullary cells ➔ within the adrenal cortex ➔. The presence of hyaline granules ➔ is usually present in MEN2.* **(Right)** *H&E shows that diffuse AMH has cells arranged in cords and is composed of medullary cells with ample granular basophilic cytoplasm and small nuclei. There is mild nuclear pleomorphism. Rare hyaline ➘ globules are noted.*

ETIOLOGY/PATHOGENESIS

- *Mycobacterium tuberculosis* is most common bacterial cause worldwide
- *Histoplasma* is common fungal cause
- CMV is most common adrenotropic agent in HIV patients
- Adrenal cortical infection and necrosis may also contribute to electrolyte imbalance and circulatory collapse in emerging viral infections including Ebola hemorrhagic fever and Middle East respiratory syndrome

CLINICAL ISSUES

- Infectious adrenalitis with adrenal insufficiency are underdiagnosed causes of morbidity and death
- Fatal adrenal crisis can be 1st sign of adrenal insufficiency
- Variable recovery after resolution of infections

MICROSCOPIC

- Pathology varies with specific organism, immune status, and other host factors

- ○ **Tuberculosis**: Chronic inflammation, giant cells, and caseation; granulomas can be less developed than with TB in other sites; possibly due to high local steroid concentration
- ○ **Other bacteria**: Neutrophilic abscesses, organisms sometimes seen, sometimes with blood vessel invasion
- ○ **Viral infections**: Lesions vary from focal necrosis to diffuse destruction of gland
  - **CMV**: Large cells with amphophilic intranuclear inclusions and granular basophilic cytoplasmic inclusions, mixed inflammation, variable necrosis
  - **Herpes and Varicella-Zoster**: Eosinophilic intranuclear inclusions, variable necrosis, minimal inflammation

TOP DIFFERENTIAL DIAGNOSES

- **Autoimmune adrenalitis**: Lymphoplasmacytic infiltrate; no granulomas, no neutrophils
- **Lymphoma/leukemia**: Monomorphic, monotypic infiltrate, often cytologically distinctive

Tuberculosis Gross Cut Surface

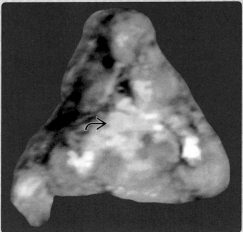

Granulomas in Tuberculosis

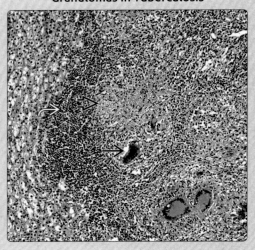

(Left) *Adrenal gland affected by tuberculosis shows extensive areas of caseous geographic necrosis ➡ involving both the cortex and the medulla.* (Right) *In adrenal tuberculosis, the granulomas are often less developed than in tuberculosis at other sites. Lymphocytes ➡, giant cells ➡, and foci of caseous material ➡ are present. Adrenocortical tissue is at left.*

Gross of Herpes Simplex Infection

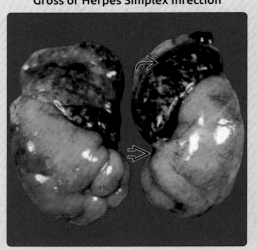

Herpes Simplex Inclusions

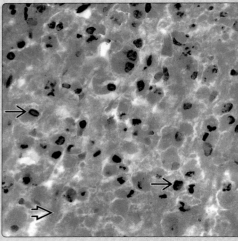

(Left) *Gross photo of transplacental herpes simplex infection shows multiple pinpoint areas of necrosis and calcification within the adrenal cortices ➡. The kidneys ➡ appear externally normal.* (Right) *In disseminated Herpes simplex, adrenal cortical cells show eosinophilic intranuclear inclusions ➡ and necrosis ➡.*

ETIOLOGY/PATHOGENESIS

Infectious Agents

- Many organisms infect adrenal glands, including bacteria, viruses, fungi, and parasites
- Infectious agent, histological manifestations, and severity of damage depend on tropism, immune status, and other host factors
  - Bacteria
    - *Mycobacterium tuberculosis* (TB) prevalent in developing countries
    - Others include *Pseudomonas*, *Treponema pallidum*, *Listeria*, *Neisseria meningitidis*, *Streptococcus pneumoniae*, *Staphylococcus aureus*, and *Haemophilus*
  - Fungi
    - *Histoplasma* is most common fungus infecting adrenal
    - Others include *Cryptococcus, Coccidioides, Paracoccidioides, Blastomyces, and Candida* spp.
  - Viruses
    - CMV is most common adrenotropic infectious agent in AIDS patients
    - Other viral infections: Herpesvirus group, Varicella-Zoster, HIV, coxsackie B, echovirus, Epstein-Barr virus, adenovirus
      - □ Adrenal cortical infection and necrosis may also contribute to electrolyte imbalance and circulatory collapse in Ebola hemorrhagic fever, Middle East respiratory syndrome, and other emerging viral infections
  - Parasites: Uncommon in developed countries, regional variations worldwide
    - Organisms include *Echinococcus* spp. (~ 7% of adrenal cysts), *Leishmania* spp., *Microspsora* spp., *Trypanosoma cruzi*
- Waterhouse-Friderichsen syndrome is secondary adrenal manifestation of systemic bacterial infection
  - Usually occurs in children < 2 years old, occasional occult cases in adults with septicemia
  - *Neisseria meningitidis* is most common causative organism
  - Others include *Streptococcus pneumoniae*, group B *Streptococcus*, *Haemophilus influenzae*, *Pseudomonas aeruginosa*
  - Mechanism(s) still unclear; may involve stress-induced increase in ACTH, increased adrenal blood flow, cytokine activation, bacterial toxins, adrenal vasospasm, disseminated intravascular coagulation

CLINICAL ISSUES

Presentation

- Adrenalitis usually secondary to systemic infection but can be isolated finding; usually bilateral
  - TB adrenalitis seen in up to 6% of patients with active TB, *Histoplasma* adrenalitis in 30-50% of patients with disseminated *H. capsulatum*
  - Adrenalitis in HIV/Aids: Direct adrenal infection by HIV plus multiple potential opportunistic agents
    - CMV adrenalitis in ~ 50% of AIDS patients, sometimes without apparent other organ involvement
  - HSV adrenalitis associated with congenital/neonatal disseminated HSV
    - Infection usually acquired during passage through birth canal, ~ 1/500-1/1500 births, ~ 20% of infections disseminated
    - Occasional cases with transplacental infection
- Iatrogenic or endogenous hypercortisolism increases susceptibility and masks adrenal insufficiency
  - Stimulation of hypothalamic-pituitary-adrenal axis by stress of systemic infection
  - "Pseudo-Cushing" caused by antiretroviral agents in some patients
  - Possible direct effects of CMV on steroidogenesis

Prognosis

- Uncontrolled or undetected infection can proceed to acute or chronic adrenal insufficiency, underdiagnosed causes of morbidity and death
  - Occur in 5-8% of patients with HIV infection, up to 47% with advanced AIDS
  - TB is most common infectious cause worldwide; histoplasmosis is most common fungal cause
  - Fatal adrenal crisis (acute adrenal insufficiency) can be 1st sign of adrenal insufficiency
- Variable recovery after resolution of infections
- Waterhouse-Friderichsen syndrome fatal in majority of cases

IMAGING

General Features

- In active TB infection: Enlarged glands with hypoattenuating necrotic areas ± calcifications in CT or x-ray; MRI may show marginal enhancement with persistent hypointensity of central areas
- Atrophy in advanced cases

MACROSCOPIC

General Features

- **Adrenal TB**: Glands up to 2-3x normal size; fibrocaseous tissue involving cortex and medulla is most prominent feature
- **Histoplasma**: Gland enlargement, caseation variably present
- **Systemic infections** with *Pseudomonas* spp. and *Listeria* spp.: Sharply punched-out necrotic areas
- **CMV, herpes, coxsackie B, and echovirus**: Punched-out or confluent areas of necrosis and hemorrhage
- **Waterhouse-Friderichsen syndrome**: Extensive hemorrhagic necrosis, usually bilateral

MICROSCOPIC

Histologic Features

- **Bacterial and fungal infections**
  - **Tuberculosis**: Chronic inflammation, giant cells, and caseation
    - Granulomas can be less developed than with TB in other sites; possibly due to high local steroid concentration
    - Subcapsular granulation tissue and calcifications in older lesions; medullary destruction
  - **Histoplasmosis and other fungi**: Epithelioid histiocytes, granulomas, and caseation variably present

- – Fungal emboli in small vessels with some fungi
- – Microscopic abscesses in disseminated candidiasis
  - o **Other bacteria**: Neutrophilic abscesses, organisms sometimes seen, sometimes with blood vessel invasion
  - o **Congenital syphilis**: Capsular and cortical fibrosis
- **Viral infections**: Lesions vary from focal necrosis to diffuse destruction of gland
  - o **CMV**
    - – Enlarged ("megalic") cells
    - – Amphophilic intranuclear inclusions with clear halo (Cowdry type A inclusions) plus granular basophilic cytoplasmic inclusions
    - – Variable necrosis, mixed inflammation
  - o **Herpesvirus and Varicella-Zoster**
    - – Smudged eosinophilic intranuclear inclusion without halo (Cowdry type B inclusions) in early or primary infections
    - – Large intranuclear inclusion with halo (Cowdry type A) may be found in older lesions
    - – Multinucleated giant cells, nuclear molding
    - – Variable necrosis, minimal inflammation
- **Waterhouse-Friderichsen syndrome**: Extensive hemorrhagic necrosis
  - o Hemorrhage begins in zona reticularis and extends toward capsule and medulla; zona glomerulosa may be partly spared
  - o Small fibrin thrombi suggesting diffuse intravascular coagulation variably present in sinusoids,
  - o Healing adrenals may show stippled calcification and fibrosis

ANCILLARY TESTS

Histochemistry

- Special stains for suspected microorganisms
- Immunohistochemistry or in situ hybridization for optimal detection of virus-infected cells

DIFFERENTIAL DIAGNOSIS

Inflammatory Conditions

- **Autoimmune adrenalitis**: Lymphoplasmacytic infiltrate; no granulomas and no neutrophils
- **Focal lymphocytic infiltration in adrenal cortex of elderly**: Possibly preclinical manifestation of autoimmune adrenalitis; variable focal or patchy lymphocytic infiltrate, little or no cortical destruction
- **Sarcoidosis:** Noncaseating granulomas, often fused but discrete, other stigmata of systemic involvement

Lymphoma/Leukemia

- Monomorphic, monotypic infiltrate, often cytologically distinctive

SELECTED REFERENCES

1. Rushworth RL et al: Adrenal crises: perspectives and research directions. Endocrine. 55(2):336-345, 2017
2. El Sayed SM et al: Updates in diagnosis and management of Ebola hemorrhagic fever. J Res Med Sci. 21:84, 2016
3. Chan JF et al: Middle East respiratory syndrome coronavirus: another zoonotic betacoronavirus causing SARS-like disease. Clin Microbiol Rev. 28(2):465-522, 2015
4. Chrousos GP et al: Hypothalamic-pituitary-adrenal axis in HIV infection and disease. Endocrinol Metab Clin North Am. 43(3):791-806, 2014
5. Rai B et al: Transient acute adrenal insufficiency associated with adenovirus serotype 40 infection. BMJ Case Rep. 2014, 2014
6. Upadhyay J et al: Tuberculosis of the adrenal gland: a case report and review of the literature of infections of the adrenal gland. Int J Endocrinol. 2014:876037, 2014
7. Tormos LM et al: The significance of adrenal hemorrhage: undiagnosed Waterhouse-Friderichsen syndrome, a case series. J Forensic Sci. 58(4):1071-4, 2013
8. Centers for Disease Control and Prevention (CDC): trends in tuberculosis–United States, 2010. MMWR Morb Mortal Wkly Rep. 60(11):333-7, 2011
9. Trevisan M et al: Human cytomegalovirus productively infects adrenocortical cells and induces an early cortisol response. J Cell Physiol. 221(3):629-41, 2009
10. Burrill J et al: Tuberculosis: a radiologic review. Radiographics. 27(5):1255-73, 2007
11. Guo YK et al: Addison's disease due to adrenal tuberculosis: contrast-enhanced CT features and clinical duration correlation. Eur J Radiol. 62(1):126-31, 2007
12. Ma ES et al: Tuberculous Addison's disease: morphological and quantitative evaluation with multidetector-row CT. Eur J Radiol. 62(3):352-8, 2007
13. Paolo WF Jr et al: Adrenal infections. Int J Infect Dis. 10(5):343-53, 2006
14. Wang YX et al: CT findings of adrenal glands in patients with tuberculous Addison's disease. J Belge Radiol. 81(5):226-8, 1998
15. Hayashi Y et al: Focal lymphocytic infiltration in the adrenal cortex of the elderly: immunohistological analysis of infiltrating lymphocytes. Clin Exp Immunol. 77(1):101-5, 1989

CMV Inclusions

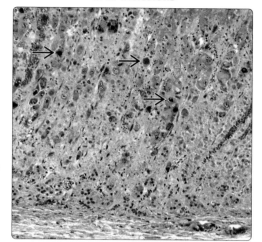

CMV Inclusion

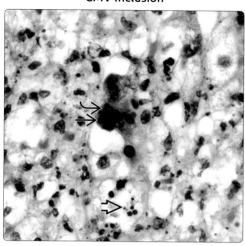

(Left) *Disseminated CMV infection in the adrenal gland of a child with congenital immunodeficiency is shown. This specimen was obtained at autopsy and shows necrosis and many large cells ⇥ that contain viral inclusions.* (Right) *In cytomegalovirus infection, the adrenal gland shows enlarged cells with amphophilic nuclear inclusions ⇥ with clear halo, cytoplasmic inclusions ⇗, and variable necrosis ⇥.*

Histoplasmosis

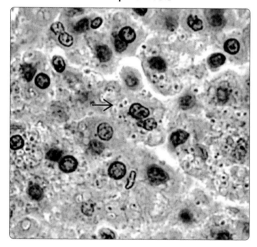

Waterhouse-Friderichsen Syndrome

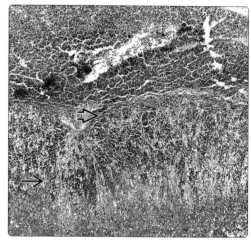

(Left) *Histoplasma capsulatum ⇥ is seen as tiny yeasts in the cytoplasm of macrophages admixed with cortical cells. Fixation artifact resembles an unstained capsule.* (Right) *An adrenal gland section in Waterhouse-Friderichsen syndrome shows cortical ⇥ and subcapsular hemorrhage dissecting into the surrounding fibroadipose tissue ⇥.*

Waterhouse-Friderichsen Syndrome

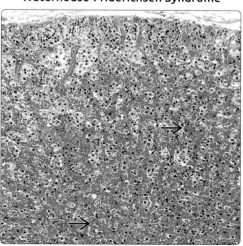

Posthemorrhagic Calcification

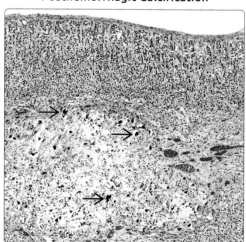

(Left) *Higher magnification of the adrenal cortical hemorrhage is shown with associated necrosis of the adrenal cortical cells ⇥.* (Right) *Posthemorrhagic calcification ⇥ is illustrated in this adrenal section. Note the stippled calcification. (From DP: Nonneoplastic Pediatrics.)*

KEY FACTS

TERMINOLOGY

- Adrenal cortical destruction by immunologically mediated mechanisms: Addison adrenalitis

CLINICAL ISSUES

- Progressive, predominantly T-cell mediated cortical destruction
  - Leads to adrenal insufficiency (Addison disease) in untreated cases
- Most of cortical tissue must be destroyed before Addison disease manifests
- Subclinical adrenal insufficiency can become clinically acute under stressful conditions
- Acute adrenal insufficiency (adrenal crisis) is life-threatening, often occurs in patients with chronic insufficiency subjected to stress
  - Critical finding is hypotension; others include nausea, vomiting, hypoglycemia, abdominal pain, confusion

- Patients with 1 autoimmune disorder at increased risk for others
  - ~ 50% of patients with autoimmune adrenalitis have other autoimmune endocrine disorders

MICROSCOPIC

- Lymphocytic and lymphoplasmacytic inflammatory infiltrate preferentially attacks adrenal cortex, leading to cortical cell necrosis
- Medulla relatively preserved and can extend to capsule
- Degenerating cortical cells coexist with hypertrophied, eosinophilic, lipid-depleted cells stimulated by increased ACTH
- Advanced disease: Cortex destroyed with fibrosis

ANCILLARY TESTS

- CD3 stain shows numerous T-lymphocytes interspersed between cells of adrenal cortex
- Other lymphoid markers demonstrate polyphenotypic inflammatory cell population

Adrenal Cortical Morphology

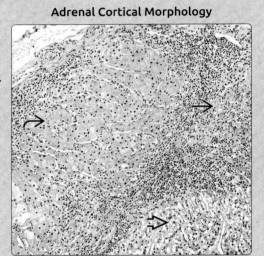

Chronic Autoimmune Adrenalitis

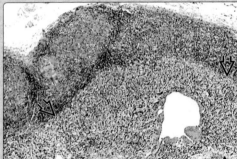

(Left) In autoimmune adrenalitis (AA), degenerating cortical cells ⮡ coexist with hypertrophied cells ➡ stimulated by increased ACTH. The medulla ⮕ is relatively preserved. (Courtesy F. van Nederveen, MD.) (Right) In advanced AA, cortex can be entirely destroyed and medulla ⮕ can extend to the capsule. (Courtesy F. van Nederveen, MD.)

Inflammatory Infiltrate

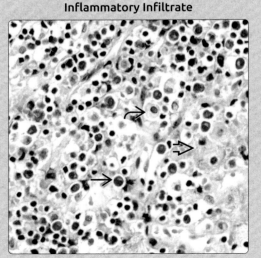

T-Lymphocytes

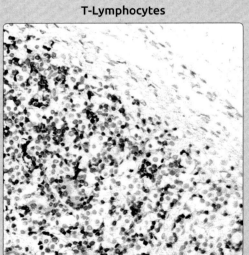

(Left) Inflammation in AA is mostly lymphocytic with variable numbers of plasma cells ⮕ and histiocytes ⮕ admixed with degenerating cortical cells ⮕. (Courtesy F. van Nederveen, MD.) (Right) This immunohistochemical stain for CD3 shows numerous T-lymphocytes interspersed between cells of the adrenal cortex in adrenilitis. (Courtesy F. van Nederveen, MD.)

TERMINOLOGY

Abbreviations

- Autoimmune adrenalitis (AA)

CLINICAL ISSUES

Presentation

- Can be isolated process or accompany other autoimmune disorders
  - Autoimmune polyglandular syndrome type 1 (APS-1) [a.k.a. autoimmune polyendocrinopathy-candidiasis ectodermal dystrophy (APECED)]
    - Defined by at least 2 of the following triad: Chronic mucocutaneous candidiasis, hypoparathyroidism, Addison disease (in ~ 60% of cases)
    - Other associations include: Type 1 diabetes, hypergonadotropic hypogonadism, autoimmune gastritis/pernicious anemia, malabsorption, hepatitis, asplenism, alopecia, keratitis, vitiligo, enamel dysplasia
    - Often sequential presentation: Candidiasis before age 5 years, then hypoparathyroidism followed by AA and other associations
    - Autosomal recessive inheritance, mutations of autoimmune regulator (AIRE) gene; onset in infancy, F ~ = M
  - Autoimmune polyglandular syndrome type 2 (APS-2)
    - Defined by Addison disease plus either type 1 diabetes or autoimmune thyroid disease
    - Other associations include vitiligo, hypergonadotropic hypogonadism, autoimmune gastritis/pernicious anemia, celiac disease, myasthenia gravis, and stiff man syndrome
    - Polygenic inheritance involving HLA genes encoding class 2 major histocompatibility complex (MHC) proteins; adolescent to early adult onset, F > M
    - Most prevalent APS syndrome: At least 1.5-4.5/100,000; many occult subclinical cases
  - Immunodeficiency, polyendocrinopathy, enteropathy, X-linked syndrome (IPEX)
    - Rare disease usually presenting very early in life, usual clinical triad of watery diarrhea, eczema, and polyendocrinopathy (most common type 1 diabetes)
    - X-linked inheritance, mutations of FOXP3 causing loss of regulatory T-cell function

Natural History

- Progressive, predominantly T-cell mediated cortical destruction leading to adrenal insufficiency (Addison disease) in untreated cases
  - Antibodies against cortical cell constituents variably present, probably secondary to cortical destruction
    - Antibodies can reflect disease progression, but often persist after treatment
- 80-90% adrenal cortical destruction necessary for signs and symptoms to become apparent
  - Chronic adrenal insufficiency: Clinical manifestations include hyperpigmentation, weakness, fatigue, orthostatic hypotension, sometimes salt craving
  - Acute adrenal insufficiency (adrenal crisis): Life-threatening, usually occurs in patients with chronic insufficiency subjected to physiological stress
    - Critical finding is hypotension; others include nausea, vomiting, hypoglycemia, abdominal pain, confusion

MACROSCOPIC

General Features

- Glands initially normal size (4-5 g)
- Bilateral, markedly shrunken glands in end stages (can weigh < 2 g)

MICROSCOPIC

Histologic Features

- Predominantly lymphocytic inflammatory infiltrate preferentially attacks adrenal cortex, leading to cortical cell necrosis
  - Lymphoid nodules with occasional germinal centers
  - Plasma cells and histiocytes variably present
- Degenerating cortical cells coexist with hypertrophied, eosinophilic, lipid-depleted cells stimulated by increased ACTH
- **Advanced disease**
  - Cortex almost completely destroyed; extensive fibrosis
  - Medulla relatively preserved and can extend to capsule

ANCILLARY TESTS

Immunohistochemistry

- CD3 stain shows numerous T-lymphocytes interspersed between cells of adrenal cortex
- Other lymphoid markers demonstrate polyphenotypic inflammatory cell population

DIFFERENTIAL DIAGNOSIS

Infections

- Tuberculosis: Caseous necrosis, Langerhans-type giant cells, granulomas
  - Destruction of both cortex and medulla
- Other infections: HIV, CMV, Cryptococcus, Histoplasma

Lymphoma/Leukemia

- Monomorphous, monotypic, cytologically atypical
- No cortical predilection

Myelolipomatous Change

- Fat cells, lymphocytes, and hematopoietic precursors in cortex
- No tissue destruction

Focal Lymphocytic Infiltrates

- Focal aggregates of lymphocytes in cortex
  - Small, focal, no tissue destruction
  - Sometimes seen in conjunction with lipomatous change

SELECTED REFERENCES

1. Rushworth RL et al: Adrenal crises: perspectives and research directions. Endocrine. 55(2):336-345, 2017
2. Akirav EM et al: The role of AIRE in human autoimmune disease. Nat Rev Endocrinol. 7(1):25-33, 2011
3. Husebye ES et al: Autoimmune polyendocrine syndromes: clues to type 1 diabetes pathogenesis. Immunity. 32(4):479-87, 2010
4. Betterle C et al: Autoimmune polyglandular syndrome Type 2: the tip of an iceberg? Clin Exp Immunol. 137(2):225-33, 2004

KEY FACTS

TERMINOLOGY

- Classification as "primary" or "secondary" amyloidosis is now replaced by classification according to specific amyloid protein

CLINICAL ISSUES

- Adrenal involvement can be localized or can be component of systemic disease
- Adrenal glands are commonly involved in amyloid A amyloidosis
- Subclinical abnormalities are relatively frequent
  - Occasional life-threatening addisonian crisis
  - Assessment of adrenal cortical function should be considered in patients with systemic or renal amyloidosis
- Any type of amyloid can be incidental finding

MACROSCOPIC

- Gland may be enlarged or normal size
- Gross involvement is firm, waxy, and pale yellow-gray

MICROSCOPIC

- Amyloid deposits 1st in zona fasciculata, then reticularis, and lastly glomerulosa

ANCILLARY TESTS

- Congo red stain with apple-green birefringence in polarized light is most commonly used generic amyloid stain
- Immunostaining can help to identify specific proteins in amyloid deposits but is often unreliable
- Mass spectrometry is current method of choice for definitive identification of major amyloid subtypes and their variants; can be performed with fresh or paraffin-embedded tissue

TOP DIFFERENTIAL DIAGNOSES

- Fibrosis or hyaline sclerosis can resemble amyloid but do not show green birefringence after Congo red stain

Advanced Amyloidosis

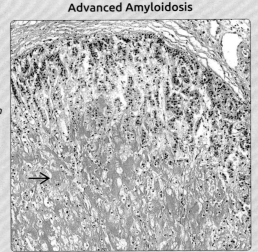

Patchy Predominantly Perivascular Distribution of Amyloid

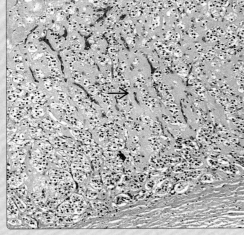

(Left) In advanced stage adrenal amyloidosis, there is diffuse, complete or nearly complete replacement of the zona fasciculata with pink homogeneous material ➡. (Right) Amyloid deposition ➡ may be patchy in patients with subclinical disease.

Adrenal Amyloidosis

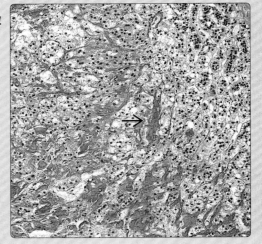

Characteristic Apple-Green Birefringence of Amyloid

(Left) Congo red stain gives amyloid a salmon red color ➡. (Right) Adrenal amyloidosis shows apple-green birefringence ➡ under polarized light after staining with Congo red.

TERMINOLOGY

Definitions

- Extracellular deposits of amyloid protein in adrenal parenchyma
- Traditional clinical classification as "primary" or "secondary" amyloidosis is replaced by classification according to specific protein
  - Primary amyloidosis usually light-chain amyloidosis (AL)
  - Secondary amyloidosis usually amyloid A (AA)
  - Currently ~ 30 amyloidogenic proteins known, with adrenal involvement documented only in a few

ETIOLOGY/PATHOGENESIS

Amyloidogenic Proteins

- Varies with different amyloid proteins
- Common denominator is abnormal protein folding that results in fibrillar protein deposits with shared morphological and staining characteristics
  - Abnormal proteins with increased amyloidogenic tendency compared to their normal counterparts
    - AL derived from IgG-light chains in multiple myeloma, plasma cell dyscrasias, or localized monoclonal B-cell dyscrasias
    - Transthyretin amyloidosis (ATTR) derived from mutant transthyretin in familial amyloidotic polyneuropathy
  - Secondary large elevations in concentrations of normal amyloidogenic proteins under altered physiological conditions
    - AA amyloidosis derived from serum amyloid A (SAA) protein produced in response to chronic inflammation or infection
    - β_2-microglobulin amyloidosis ($A\beta_2M$) in dialysis patients
  - Long-term exposure to normal, mildly amyloidogenic proteins at normal concentrations in susceptible individuals
    - Senile transthyretin amyloidosis (senile ATTR) caused by accumulation of normal transthyretin in elderly patients

Pathogenesis

- Amyloidogenic proteins have antiparallel, β-pleated sheet tertiary structure, accounting for Congo red staining and apple-green birefringence under polarized light
  - Resistance to metabolic processing leads to accumulation and interference with physiologic functioning
- Amyloid deposits composed of amyloidogenic protein and nonfibrillary glycoproteins serum-derived amyloid P [(SAP), apolipoprotein E, and glycosaminoglycans]
  - SAP is also known as amyloid P component

CLINICAL ISSUES

Epidemiology

- Incidence
  - ~ 40% of patients with systemic amyloidosis show adrenal involvement
    - Adrenal gland is 1 organ commonly involved in AA amyloidosis

- Involvement less frequent in AL and others
  - Adrenal amyloidosis mostly detected in autopsy studies and few small clinical studies
    - Age-related amyloid accumulation reported starting in 6th decade
    - Intracellular amyloid with no interstitial deposits reported in 68% of 108 autopsy cases of individuals 85 years and older studied for prevalence and characterization of local amyloid
    - Identities of reported intracellular amyloids mostly not established
- Age
  - AL and AA amyloidosis: Typically 50-70 years old
  - Familial forms: < 40 years old
- Sex
  - M:F = 2:1 overall

Site

- Usually bilateral involvement
- Affects adrenal cortex more often than medulla: Deposits 1st in zona fasciculata, followed by zona reticularis, and lastly zona glomerulosa

Presentation

- Can be localized to adrenal or be component of systemic disease
- Usually clinically asymptomatic
  - Subclinical adrenal cortical dysfunction commonly accompanies renal amyloidosis
  - Can cause acute adrenal insufficiency in occasional patients
  - May be localized incidental finding in elderly patients (senile amyloidosis)
- Any type of amyloid can be incidental finding

Laboratory Tests

- Basal and provocative cortical function tests

Treatment

- Options, risks, complications
  - Treat underlying disease
  - Different treatments directed against specific types of systemic amyloidosis
  - No specific approach to adrenal involvement other than possibility of hormone replacement

Prognosis

- Variable

IMAGING

Radiographic Findings

- Adrenal glands normal in size or mildly enlarged

MACROSCOPIC

General Features

- Cut surface pale yellow to gray, firm, and waxy

Size

- Normal or mildly enlarged; combined weight usually < 35 g

MICROSCOPIC

Histologic Features

- Involvement patchy or diffuse, occasionally multinodular
- Interstitial and perivascular pink homogeneous hyaline material 1st deposited in zona fasciculata, then reticularis and glomerulosa; involvement of medulla usually accompanied by advanced findings in cortex
- In advanced stage, complete to near complete replacement of zona fasciculata
- Adrenal amyloid often preceded or accompanied by deposits in periadrenal fat and blood vessels and around central vein; relative amounts of involvement of these tissues not predictable

Identification of Amyloid Protein

- Immunohistochemistry
- Immunofluorescence
- Electron microscopy
- Proteomics

ANCILLARY TESTS

Histochemistry

- Congo red
  - Reactivity: Positive
  - Congo red shows red-orange deposits under nonpolarized light; apple-green birefringence under polarized light required for specificity
    - Nonspecific red staining by Congo red can be seen with collagen, fibrin, or other protein deposits; collagen can be refractile but not usually green ± Congo red
    - In contrast to fibrillar collagen, amyloid fibrils are only birefringent after Congo red
  - Red without polarization (also called "congophilia")
    - Elastic fibers are congophilic but not birefringent
  - Small amyloid quantities may make it difficult to demonstrate apple-green birefringence
  - Metachromatic stains such as crystal violet or fluorescent stains such as thioflavin T or S are sometimes employed
    - Fluorescent stains less specific than Congo red

Immunohistochemistry

- Immunostaining by light, fluorescence, or electron microscopy used to identify specific proteins in amyloid deposits (AA, AL, ATTR, $A\beta_2M$)
  - Staining not always reliable because of chemical modifications, conformational changes, cross-linking, presence of serum proteins, glycosaminoglycans, light chain variability
    - Deglycosylation or other unmasking methods sometimes employed
    - Definitive amyloid protein identification may require mass spectrometry
- SAP nonfibrillar minor component of most amyloid deposits

Immunofluorescence

- Staining depends on type of amyloid
  - AL: Single light chain predominate
  - AA: Neither or both light chains stain

Electron Microscopy

- Fibrils
  - Nonbranching, nonperiodic
  - Interlacing arrays of 10-15 nm unbranched fibrils
    - Accurate measurement important
  - Cotton wool appearance of deposits at low magnification (~ 5,000x)
  - Electron-lucent core at ~ 100,000x

Mass Spectrometry

- Current method of choice for definitive identification of amyloid subtypes and their variants; can be performed with fresh or paraffin-embedded tissue

DIFFERENTIAL DIAGNOSIS

Fibrosis or Hyaline Sclerosis

- Congo red staining with apple-green birefringence favors amyloid

Immunoglobulin Deposition Diseases Without Amyloid

- Congo red is negative

DIAGNOSTIC CHECKLIST

Pathologic Interpretation Pearls

- Amorphous hyaline deposits
- Stain with Congo red ("congophilic") and subsequently show green birefringence with polarized light
- Immunostaining by light, fluorescence, or electron microscopy used to identify specific proteins in amyloid deposits (AA, AL, ATTR, $A\beta_2M$)
- Electron microscopy demonstrates interlacing arrays of 10-15 nm unbranched fibrils
  - Cotton wool appearance of deposits at low magnification (~ 5,000x)

SELECTED REFERENCES

1. Dogan A: Amyloidosis: Insights from proteomics. Annu Rev Pathol. 12:277-304, 2017
2. Ozdemir D et al: Endocrine involvement in systemic amyloidosis. Endocr Pract. 16(6):1056-63, 2010
3. Lloyd RV et al: Endocrine diseases. Atlas of Nontumor Pathology. Washington, DC: Armed Forces Institute of Pathology and American Registry of Pathology, 2002
4. Koike H et al: Distinct characteristics of amyloid deposits in early- and late-onset transthyretin Val30Met familial amyloid polyneuropathy. J Neurol Sci. 287(1-2):178-84, 2009
5. Gündüz Z et al: The hormonal and radiological evaluation of adrenal glands, and the determination of the usefulness of low dose ACTH test in patients with renal amyloidosis. Ren Fail. 23(2):239-49, 2001
6. Röcken C et al: Senile amyloidoses of the pituitary and adrenal glands. Morphological and statistical investigations. Virchows Arch. 429(4-5):293-9, 1996
7. Bohl J et al: Age-related accumulation of congophilic fibrillar inclusions in endocrine cells. Virchows Arch A Pathol Anat Histopathol. 419(1):51-8, 1991
8. Danby P et al: Adrenal dysfunction in patients with renal amyloid. Q J Med. 76(281):915-22, 1990
9. Eriksson L et al: Age-related accumulation of amyloid inclusions in adrenal cortical cells. Am J Pathol. 136(2):461-6, 1990
10. Guttman PH: Addison's disease: a statistical analysis of 566 cases and study of pathology. Arch Pathol. 10:742-895, 1930

Immunohistochemical Stain for Amyloid A

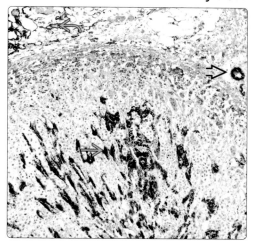

Subendothelial and Perivascular Amyloid

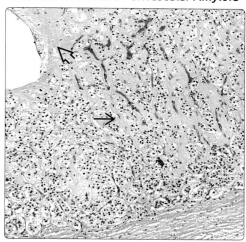

(Left) *Immunohistochemical stain for Amyloid A shows the presence of amyloid in the zona fasciculata ➡ of the adrenal, in periadrenal adipose tissue ➡, and in the wall of a small periadrenal artery ➡.* (Right) *This H&E photomicrograph shows an early subendothelial deposition of amyloid in the zona fasciculata ➡ with extensive deposition around the central vein ➡.*

Amyloid in Periadrenal Blood Vessels

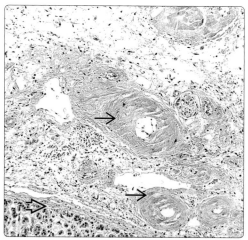

Selective Amyloid Deposition in Zona Fasciculata

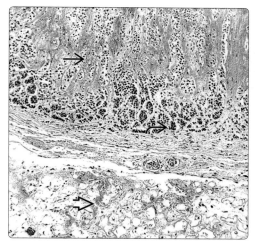

(Left) *Congo red shows marked deposition of amyloid in blood vessels ➡ adjacent to an adrenal ➡ that was itself minimally involved. The thickening of the vessel walls gives a homogeneous appearance.* (Right) *Congo red shows selective amyloid deposition in zona fasciculata ➡ with sparing of zona glomerulosa ➡ in an adrenal from a patient with AA amyloidosis with an intermediate stage of adrenal involvement. Extensive amyloid deposition is seen in the periadrenal fat ➡.*

Fibrillar Ultrastructure of Amyloid

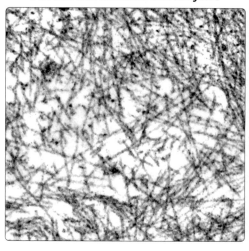

Fluorescent Staining of Amyloid With Thioflavin T

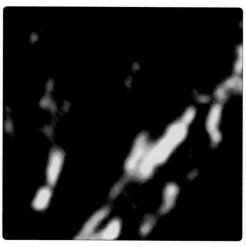

(Left) *Electron micrograph shows criss-crossed arrays of straight, nonbranching, 10-15 nm fibrils characteristic of all types of amyloid.* (Right) *Thioflavin T stain shows yellow fluorescent amyloid deposits. Fluorescent stains are very sensitive for detecting amyloid but less specific than Congo red with polarized light. Immunostaining by light, fluorescence, or electron microscopy is needed to identify specific proteins in amyloid deposits (AA, AL, ATTR, Aβ$_2$M).*

TERMINOLOGY

- Adrenal incidentaloma (AI): Adrenal mass, usually > 1 cm in diameter, discovered during radiologic examination performed for indications other than adrenal disease

CLINICAL ISSUES

- Goal of initial work-up to distinguish benign from malignant and nonfunctioning from functioning tumors
- In review of 34 studies, diagnoses were adenomas (41%), metastatic tumors (19%), adrenocortical carcinomas (10%), myelolipomas (8%), pheochromocytomas (4.5%), cysts (2%)
- Adrenal 4th most common site for extranodal metastasis after lung, liver, and bone; bilateral in 40-50% of cases
- All protocols require initial comprehensive clinical, radiologic, and hormonal evaluations to exclude primary or secondary malignancies or hypersecretion syndromes

ANCILLARY TESTS

- Fine-needle aspiration (FNA) biopsy with cytology and cell block for IHC sometimes helpful

  ○ Not recommended for initial work-up of AI
  ○ May rule out metastases or infection in cases with normal hormonal function and suspicious imaging characteristics; ~ 33-46% of adrenal FNA for metastatic malignancies
  ○ Panels of IHC markers required depend on specific diagnoses considered
    – Markers for normal or neoplastic adrenal cortex include SF1, inhibin, melan-A, synaptophysin, calretinin
      □ Sensitivity and specificity for individual markers differ for normal cortex, adenoma and carcinoma
  ○ Potentially challenging differential diagnoses
    – Metastatic clear cell renal cell carcinoma vs. adrenal cortical adenoma or carcinoma
      □ Renal cell carcinoma markers recently reported to be most sensitive and specific include carbonic anhydrase IX (CAIX), RCC, and pax-8; CD10, CAM5.2
    – High-grade metastatic adenocarcinoma vs. adrenal cortical carcinoma

Work-Up of Adrenal Incidentalomas

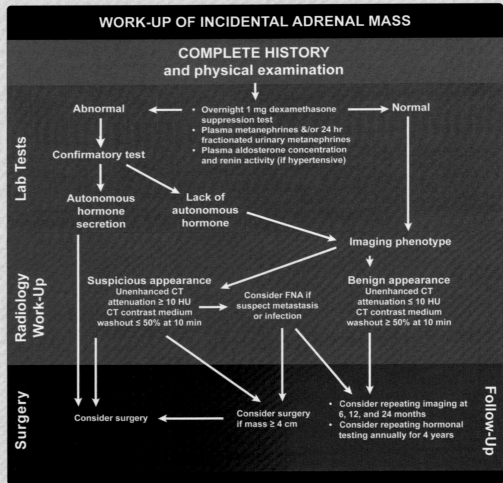

All protocols for evaluation of adrenal incidentalomas require initial comprehensive clinical, radiologic, and hormonal evaluations in order to distinguish benign from malignant and nonfunctioning from functioning tumors. (Modified from Young, 2007.)

TERMINOLOGY

Synonyms

- Adrenal incidentaloma (AI)

Definitions

- Adrenal mass, usually > 1 cm in diameter, discovered during radiologic examination performed for indications other than adrenal disease

CLINICAL ISSUES

Epidemiology

- Incidence
  - Increasingly detected with advances in imaging technology
    - Present in ~ 4% of CT scans in general population; 10-15% bilateral
  - Autopsy studies suggest overall prevalence ~ 2%
- Age
  - ~ 60% of cases between 6th and 8th decades (mean age: 56 ± 12.9 years)
  - Prevalence varies with age of patient and reason for diagnostic work-up
    - < 30 years (1%), middle aged (3%), elderly (10%)

Presentation

- In review of 34 studies (3,377 patients), diagnoses were cortical adenomas (41%), metastatic tumors (19%), cortical carcinomas (10%), myelolipomas (8%), pheochromocytomas (4.5%), and cysts (2%)
  - ~ 90% nonfunctioning in recent series
    - 5-20% show autonomous subclinical cortisol hypersecretion (subclinical Cushing syndrome)
  - Most common functioning AI: Cortisol-secreting adenomas (5-47%), pheochromocytomas (1.6-23%), aldosteronomas (1.6-3.8%)
  - Most primary tumors unilateral; bilaterality raises suspicion of metastases
- Tumors with predilection for adrenal metastasis: Lung (35-60%), breast, melanoma
  - Adrenal 4th most common site for extranodal metastasis after lung, liver, and bone
  - Adenocarcinomas most frequent tumor type
  - Metastases bilateral in 40-50% of cases
- Rare lesions encountered in some series
  - Tuberculosis or other infection
  - Congenital adrenal hyperplasia
  - Primary macronodular cortical hyperplasia
    - Cushing syndrome can be diagnosed in up to ~ 35% of bilateral cortical incidentalomas

Laboratory Tests

- Autonomous glucocorticoid production (Cushing syndrome or subclinical Cushing syndrome); overnight 1 mg dexamethasone suppression test, 73-100% sensitivity and 90% specificity
- Adrenocortical carcinoma: Sex hormone production; dehydroepiandrosterone, 17-hydroxyprogesterone, testosterone

- Hyperaldosteronism: Upright plasma aldosterone concentration to plasma renin ratio, sensitivity and specificity > 90%
- Pheochromocytoma: Plasma metanephrines &/or 24 hour fractionated urinary metanephrines; sensitivity and specificity > 90%

Diagnostic Evaluation

- Optimal work-up varies according to different protocols; all require initial comprehensive clinical, radiologic, and hormonal evaluations
- Endocrinological work-up precedes further imaging
- Goal of initial work-up to distinguish benign from malignant and nonfunctioning from functioning tumors; complete evaluation will help classify AI
  - **Lesions that can be followed clinically**: Benign, nonfunctional
  - **Lesions that will require surgical removal**: Adrenocortical carcinoma, pheochromocytoma, primary aldosteronism, Cushing syndrome
  - Current literature suggests size cut-off of 4 cm because most cortical carcinomas > 4 cm
  - Regardless of size, any adrenal mass with imaging phenotype suspicious for malignancy or pheochromocytoma should be considered for surgical removal
- Potential pitfalls
  - Cystic lesions may be functional or nonfunctional tumors
  - Subclinical Cushing syndrome
  - Possible rare progression of cortical adenoma to carcinoma

Follow-Up

- Surveillance recommended for nonfunctioning adenomas (typically < 4 cm) and nonresectable masses
- Any mass with clinically overt hormonal disturbance should be considered for removal
  - Management of subclinical Cushing controversial
  - Primary aldosteronism may be managed medically, especially if patients poor surgical candidates
- Most protocols recommend clinical and hormonal testing annually up to 4 years, typically with 1-3 radiologic assessments in 1st 2 years
  - Repeat imaging or hormonal evaluation after 2 years not proven to increase overall sensitivity for diagnosis of malignancy but might detect rare outlier cases
    - Extremely rare transition of apparently benign lesions to cortical carcinoma reported after > 5 years
  - Progression from nonfunctional to functional lesions rare but significant
    - Long-term study of clinically silent incidentalomas showed 1.79% new cases of subclinical Cushing, 0.7% overt Cushing, and 0.4% pheochromocytomas over mean follow-up of 44.2 months
      - ~ 3% of patients eventually underwent surgery

IMAGING

General Features

- CT most frequently employed imaging modality
  - Tumor size, density, and heterogeneity significantly associated with malignancy

○ Unenhanced and enhanced CT have been utilized
  – Density ≤ 10 Hounsfield units (HU) on unenhanced CT suggests benign lipid-rich cortical adenoma
  – Enhanced CT evaluated if density > 10 HU
  – Absolute percentage washout of ≥ 60% at 15 minutes or 50% at 10 minutes supports benignity
○ Recent guidelines from European Society of Endocrinology and European Network for the Study of Adrenal Tumors (ENSAT) aim to reduce cost and burden of repeated imaging
  – Strongest evidence base to confirm benign adrenal lesion is attenuation value of < 10 HU on NECT; if lesions homogeneous, < 4 cm, and not associated with adrenal cortical hyperfunction, no further imaging follow-up recommended
    □ Evidence base for 2nd- and 3rd-line imaging modalities to exclude malignancy considered weak
  – Long-term follow-up should be limited to lesions not unequivocally characterized as benign or < 4 cm and those with 20% increase in size over 12 months
  – Special circumstances
    □ Urgent assessment of adrenal masses recommended in children, adolescents, pregnant women, and adults younger than 40 years of age because of higher likelihood of malignancy
    □ MR rather than CT suggested for children, adolescents, pregnant women, and adults younger than 40 years of age
    □ Imaging and management of patients with frailty and poor general health should be proportional to potential clinical gain
• Hyperintense lightbulb sign not always present on T2-weighted MR for pheochromocytoma

MACROSCOPIC

General Features

• Most adrenal cortical lesions typically yellow, similar to normal cortex
• Pheochromocytomas gray to pink-tan, may show hemorrhage and cystic change
• Appearance of metastases varies according to tumor type
  ○ Adenocarcinoma may be mucinous and translucent; yellow renal cell carcinomas may resemble cortical tumors

ANCILLARY TESTS

Cytology

• Fine-needle aspiration (FNA) biopsy with cytology and cell block for IHC sometimes helpful
  ○ Not recommended for initial work-up of AI
  ○ May consider to rule out metastases or infection in cases with normal hormonal function and suspicious imaging characteristics; ~ 33-46% of adrenal FNA for metastatic malignancies
  ○ Panels of IHC markers required depend on specific diagnoses considered
    – Markers for normal or neoplastic adrenal cortex include SF1, inhibin, melan-A, synaptophysin, calretinin
      □ Sensitivity and specificity for individual markers differ for normal cortex, adenoma, and carcinoma

○ Potentially challenging differential diagnoses
  – Clear cell renal cell carcinoma vs. adrenal cortical adenoma or carcinoma
    □ Adrenal involvement in ~ 60% of radical nephrectomies and 90% of patients at autopsy
    □ Presence of renal mass clue but not always evident
    □ Renal cell carcinoma markers recently reported to be most sensitive and specific include carbonic anhydrase IX (CAIX), RCC, and pax-8; others include CD10, CAM5.2
  – High-grade metastatic adenocarcinoma vs. adrenal cortical carcinoma
    □ Metastatic adenocarcinomas often positive for mucin, cytokeratins (AE1/AE3), CEA

SELECTED REFERENCES

1. Belmihoub I et al: From benign adrenal incidentaloma to adrenocortical carcinoma: an exceptional random event. Eur J Endocrinol. 176(6):K15-K19, 2017
2. Foo E et al: Predicting malignancy in adrenal incidentaloma and evaluation of a novel risk stratification algorithm. ANZ J Surg. ePub, 2017
3. Huei TJ et al: Large adrenal leiomyoma presented as adrenal incidentaloma in an AIDS patient: A rare entity. Med J Malaysia. 72(1):65-67, 2017
4. Loh HH et al: The natural progression and outcomes of adrenal incidentaloma: a systematic review and meta-analysis. Minerva Endocrinol. 42(1):77-87, 2017
5. Sahdev A: Recommendations for the management of adrenal incidentalomas: what is pertinent for radiologists? Br J Radiol. 90(1072):20160627, 2017
6. Costantino C et al: Metastatic renal cell carcinoma without evidence of a renal primary. Int Urol Nephrol. 48(1):73-7, 2016
7. Fassnacht M et al: Management of adrenal incidentalomas: European Society of Endocrinology Clinical Practice Guideline in collaboration with the European Network for the Study of Adrenal Tumors. Eur J Endocrinol. 175(2):G1-G34, 2016
8. Drougat L et al: Genetics of primary bilateral macronodular adrenal hyperplasia: a model for early diagnosis of Cushing's syndrome? Eur J Endocrinol. 173(4):M121-31, 2015
9. Li H et al: Immunohistochemical distinction of metastases of renal cell carcinoma to the adrenal from primary adrenal nodules, including oncocytic tumor. Virchows Arch. 466(5):581-8, 2015
10. Patrova J et al: Clinical outcomes in adrenal incidentaloma: experience from one center. Endocr Pract. 21(8):870-7, 2015
11. Else T et al: Adrenocortical carcinoma. Endocr Rev. 35(2):282-326, 2014
12. Zografos GN et al: Subclinical Cushing's syndrome: current concepts and trends. Hormones (Athens). 13(3):323-37, 2014
13. Kapoor A et al: Guidelines for the management of the incidentally discovered adrenal mass. Can Urol Assoc J. 5(4):241-7, 2011
14. Muth A et al: Cohort study of patients with adrenal lesions discovered incidentally. Br J Surg. 98(10):1383-91, 2011
15. Song JH et al: Incidentally discovered adrenal mass. Radiol Clin North Am. 49(2):361-8, 2011
16. Comlekci A et al: Adrenal incidentaloma, clinical, metabolic, follow-up aspects: single centre experience. Endocrine. 37(1):40-6, 2010
17. Grogan RH et al: Adrenal incidentaloma: does an adequate workup rule out surprises? Surgery. 148(2):392-7, 2010
18. Nieman LK: Approach to the patient with an adrenal incidentaloma. J Clin Endocrinol Metab. 95(9):4106-13, 2010
19. Young WF Jr: Clinical practice. The incidentally discovered adrenal mass. N Engl J Med. 356(6):601-10, 2007

Metastatic Squamous Cell Carcinoma

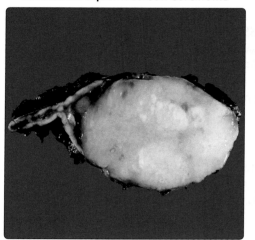

Adrenal Cortical Adenoma

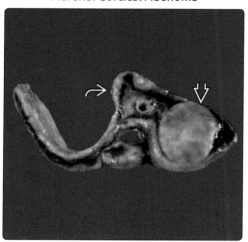

(Left) *This gross specimen shows an adrenal gland with metastatic squamous cell lung cancer.* (Right) *Adrenal cortical adenomas are the most common incidentalomas. This small adenoma ➡, identifiable as a cortical lesion by its yellow color, was most likely nonfunctional because the adjacent cortex is not atrophic ➡. Close follow-up would likely have been the recommended clinical course.*

Metastatic Adenocarcinoma

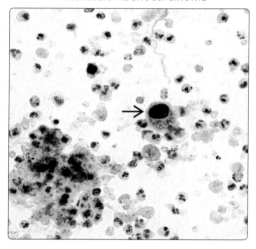

Pheochromocytoma

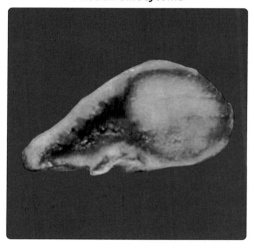

(Left) *Fine-needle aspiration (FNA) biopsy may be helpful for potential metastases or infection. Here, FNA shows adenocarcinoma of the lung ➡ metastatic to the adrenal gland.* (Right) *Even small pheochromocytomas, as in this gross specimen, are often functional.*

Metastatic Renal Cell Carcinoma

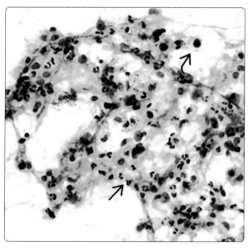

Cystic Pheochromocytoma

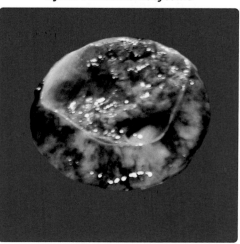

(Left) *This FNA Pap stain of a metastatic clear cell renal cell carcinoma shows classic intricate vessels with inflammatory cells ➡ and clinging tumor cells ➡. (Courtesy Yimin Ge.)* (Right) *This pheochromocytoma has been largely replaced by a cyst that contains degenerating blood and debris.*

CLASSIFICATION

- Usual classification based on type of lining (endothelial or epithelial cysts) or absence of lining (pseudocysts)
- Various classifications have been employed and do not necessarily reflect pathogenesis
- Some reports classify cystic neoplasms as epithelial cysts, while others limit definition to mesothelial-type inclusion cysts
- Some group endothelial cysts and pseudocysts as vascular cysts

ETIOLOGY/PATHOGENESIS

- Endothelial cysts thought to usually arise from preexisting vascular lesions, most often of lymphatic vessels
- Pseudocysts caused by intraadrenal hemorrhage
- Neoplasms with extensive cystic degeneration or recanalizing hemorrhage can mimic nonneoplastic endothelial cysts, epithelial cysts, or pseudocysts

- Excluding cystic neoplasms, most "epithelial" cysts probably mesothelial

CLINICAL ISSUES

- Nonneoplastic cysts can mimic neoplasms clinically and in imaging studies
- Neoplasms can masquerade as nonneoplastic cysts

MICROSCOPIC

- Endothelial cysts: Flat endothelial lining
- Pseudocysts: No endothelial or epithelial lining
- Epithelial cysts: Flat or columnar lining, sometimes ciliated

TOP DIFFERENTIAL DIAGNOSES

- Most important consideration is nonneoplastic cyst vs. pseudocyst arising in tumor; distinction made by thorough sampling of cyst wall and immunohistochemistry if needed

Lymphangiomatous Cyst

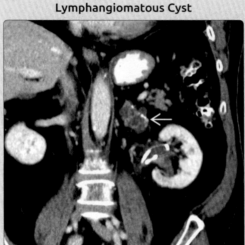

Lymphangiomatous Cyst: Cut Surface

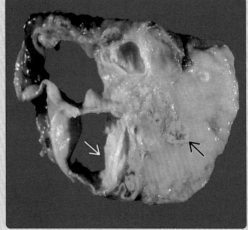

(Left) This multilocular adrenal cyst with calcification ➡ was incidentally discovered on CT imaging in a patient with renal cell carcinoma. (Right) Gross photo shows an incidentally discovered multilocular lymphangiomatous cyst with smooth lining ➡ and residual adrenal cortex ➡.

Nonneoplastic Adrenal Pseudocyst

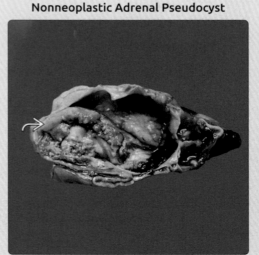

Adrenal Pseudocyst Wall

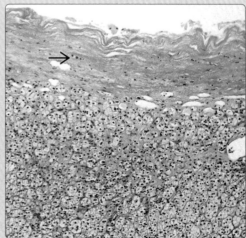

(Left) This large adrenal pseudocyst contains a smooth lining wall with adherent degenerating thrombus ➡. (Right) This adrenal pseudocyst is lined only by fibrous tissue, which contains occasional inflammatory cells ➡.

TERMINOLOGY

Definitions

- Endothelial cysts (vascular cysts) have endothelial lining, subcategorized by histology into lymphangiomatous and angiomatous types
- Epithelial cysts have epithelial lining; some reports limit definition to inclusion-type cysts, others include cystic neoplasms
- Pseudocysts (hemorrhagic cysts) have no lining; essentially hematomas or their residua
- Parasitic cysts caused by parasitic infestation

ETIOLOGY/PATHOGENESIS

Endothelial Cysts

- Probably derived from preexisting vascular malformation or ectasia
- Some may arise from recanalization of organizing hemorrhage

Epithelial Cysts

- Mostly mesothelial/peritoneal-type inclusion cysts if cystic neoplasms excluded
  ○ Embryonal cysts might be ciliated variants of inclusion cysts (tubal metaplasia) or other types of embryonal remnants
  ○ Retention cysts in early classifications were analogous to cysts in exocrine glands; either do not actually exist or are extraordinarily rare

Pseudocysts

- Hemorrhage into nonneoplastic adrenal tissue
  ○ Acute trauma, adrenal vein thrombosis, hemorrhagic diathesis, neonatal adrenal infarction
- Hemorrhage &/or cystic degeneration of adrenal cortical neoplasm or pheochromocytoma
  ○ Mural tumor nodules, including cortical carcinoma, identified in 6/32 lesions classified as pseudocysts in 2004 report

Parasitic Cysts

- Usually secondary to systemic disease; most echinococcal

CLINICAL ISSUES

Epidemiology

- Incidence
  ○ Endothelial cysts
    – 45% of cysts in autopsy studies and 2-24% of clinically symptomatic lesions
  ○ Epithelial cysts
    – 9% of cysts, rare if cystic neoplasms excluded
  ○ Pseudocysts
    – 39% of cysts in autopsy studies, most common clinically recognized subtype
    – 18.7-44% association with neoplasm: 30% pheochromocytomas, 23% adrenal cortical carcinomas, 23% adenomas; others include neuroblastomas, schwannomas, myelolipomas, primary adrenal lymphoma, metastases
      □ 7% associated with malignancy
  ○ Parasitic cysts
    – 7% of cysts in developing countries, mainly due to *Echinococcus* or *Leishmania*
- Age
  ○ Most common in 3rd-5th decades
- Sex
  ○ Female predominance (2-3:1)

Presentation

- Mostly unilateral with no side predominance, 8-15% bilateral
- Incidental findings on imaging studies, during surgery for other abdominal pathologies or at autopsy
- Widespread use of fetal ultrasound has led to increased detection of fetal/congenital adrenal cysts
- Usually asymptomatic
  ○ When large, may present with gastrointestinal symptoms, abdominal &/or flank pain, or palpable mass
  ○ Anaphylactic shock may be caused by rupture of hydatid cyst

Laboratory Tests

- Biochemical testing to exclude adrenal carcinomas or pheochromocytomas

Treatment

- Surgical approaches
  ○ Cysts > 5 cm or progression of cyst size
  ○ Unclear radiologic impression
  ○ Endocrine activity
- Conservative approach
  ○ Small and asymptomatic lesions

Unusual Associations of Adrenal Gland Cysts

- Beckwith-Wiedemann syndrome (BWS)
  ○ Single or multiple hemorrhagic macrocysts up to 8 cm
  ○ Occasionally develop in infants with BWS; can be congenital; male predominance (~ 5:1)
  ○ Probably arise from hemorrhage into microcysts during developmental involution of provisional cortex
  ○ Can be mistaken for neoplasms because of atypical cytomegalic cells in lining
- Heterotopic thyroid tissue
  ○ Very rare, adult adrenals; 1 cystic example reported
- Teratoma
  ○ 1 report of mature cystic teratoma (dermoid cyst) within adrenal; more often, retroperitoneal teratomas adjacent to adrenal mimic intraadrenal cysts

IMAGING

Endothelial Cysts

- Usually unilateral, variable size, with thin wall, smooth borders, and pure cystic internal structure; lymphangiomatous cysts often show septa and loculation
- CT attenuation usually < 20 HU with no enhancement after contrast injection; occasionally rim enhancement caused by compression of normally enhancing adjacent adrenal tissue
- MR imaging may show homogeneous lesion with low T1 and high T2 intensity with no soft tissue component or internal enhancement

Epithelial Cysts

- CT may show unilateral cysts with thin walls and smooth borders that do not enhance after contrast

Pseudocysts

- Interval change in size and appearance with evolution to homogeneous content
- Scintigraphic investigations are indicated in cysts with endocrine activity
- Metaiodobenzylguanidine (MIBG)-scintigraphy may be used for evaluation of tumors producing catecholamines and to exclude distant metastases

Parasitic Cysts

- Hydatid cysts show characteristic imaging appearance: Hydatid sand, floating membranes or daughter cysts, and septal or mural calcifications
  - Diagnostic sensitivity of ultrasound in abdominal echinococcosis 93-98%

MACROSCOPIC

General Features

- **Endothelial cysts**: Usually < 2 cm; lymphangiomatous type often multilocular, filled with clear or milky fluid; smooth lining
- **Epithelial cysts**: Uni- or multilocular, smooth lining
- **Pseudocysts**: Can be large (up to 50 cm); unilocular; thick, fibrous walls
- **Parasitic cysts**: Thick walls ± calcification, may contain parasites and ova

MICROSCOPIC

Histologic Features

- **Endothelial cysts**: Flat endothelial lining, no proliferating endothelium; lymphangiomatous type often shows multiple loculations up to ~ 1.5 cm, no smooth muscle in wall
- **Epithelial cysts**: Flat or columnar lining, sometimes ciliated, similar to mesothelial/peritoneal inclusion cysts in other organs; compressed cortical cells may be present in wall
- **Pseudocysts**: No endothelial or epithelial lining, thick fibrous wall, often with calcification, hemosiderophages and chronic inflammation

ANCILLARY TESTS

Immunohistochemistry

- All endothelial cysts positive for CD31, lymphangiomatous cysts stain for podoplanin (antibody D2-40), capillary endothelial cysts often stain focally for VWF
- Epithelial cysts stain for keratins: AE1/AE3, CAM5.2

Fine-Needle Biopsy

- FNA with aspiration of cyst fluid may be considered in bland cysts; inadvisable with suspected pheochromocytoma or *Echinococcus* infection

DIFFERENTIAL DIAGNOSIS

Nonneoplastic Cysts vs. Cystic Neoplasms

- Adrenal cortical adenoma or carcinoma or pheochromocytoma, primarily seen in adults

- Important differential in fetuses and infants is nonneoplastic pseudocyst vs. cystic neuroblastoma
  - Cysts in Beckwith-Wiedemann syndrome can be challenging because of cytomegaly and atypia
- Distinction by thorough sampling of cyst wall, immunohistochemistry if needed [inhibin for cortical tumor, chromogranin-A (CgA) for pheochromocytoma; synaptophysin more sensitive than CgA for neuroblastoma but also positive in normal and neoplastic cortex]
- Different types of nonneoplastic cysts distinguished by presence or absence of lining and by type of lining

DIAGNOSTIC CHECKLIST

Pathologic Interpretation Pearls

- If cyst lining present, differentiate endothelial cysts from epithelial cysts and pseudocysts
- Pseudocysts should be carefully examined for mural tumor nodules to rule out cystic neoplasm

SELECTED REFERENCES

1. Carsote M et al: Cystic adrenal lesions: focus on pediatric population (a review). Clujul Med. 90(1):5-12, 2017
2. Chakraborty PP et al: Pure cystic adrenal space-occupying lesion: always rule out cystic pheochromocytoma. BMJ Case Rep. 2016, 2016
3. Findeis-Hosey JJ et al: Von Hippel-Lindau disease. J Pediatr Genet. 5(2):116-23, 2016
4. White M et al: First report of congenital adrenal cysts and pheochromocytoma in a patient with mosaic genome-wide paternal uniparental disomy. Am J Med Genet A. 170(12):3352-3355, 2016
5. Saadai P et al: The pathological features of surgically managed adrenal cysts: a 15-year retrospective review. Am Surg. 79(11):1159-62, 2013
6. Sebastiano C et al: Cystic lesions of the adrenal gland: our experience over the last 20 years. Hum Pathol. 44(9):1797-803, 2013
7. Taide DV et al: Adrenal masses associated with Beckwith Wiedemann syndrome in the newborn. Afr J Paediatr Surg. 7(3):209-10, 2010
8. Wedmid A et al: Diagnosis and treatment of the adrenal cyst. Curr Urol Rep. 11(1):44-50, 2010
9. Suh J et al: True adrenal mesothelial cyst in a patient with flank pain and hematuria: a case report. Endocr Pathol. 19(3):203-5, 2008
10. Carvounis E et al: Vascular adrenal cysts: a brief review of the literature. Arch Pathol Lab Med. 130(11):1722-4, 2006
11. Hagiuda J et al: Ectopic thyroid in an adrenal mass: a case report. BMC Urol. 6:18, 2006
12. Akçay MN et al: Hydatid cysts of the adrenal gland: review of nine patients. World J Surg. 28(1):97-9, 2004
13. Erickson LA et al: Cystic adrenal neoplasms. Cancer. 101(7):1537-44, 2004
14. Bedri S et al: Mature cystic teratoma involving adrenal gland. Endocr Pathol. 13(1):59-64, 2002
15. Nadler EP et al: Adrenal masses in the newborn. Semin Pediatr Surg. 9(3):156-64, 2000
16. Torres C et al: Vascular adrenal cysts: a clinicopathologic and immunohistochemical study of six cases and a review of the literature. Mod Pathol. 10(6):530-6, 1997
17. Fukushima N et al: Mesothelial cyst of the adrenal gland. Pathol Int. 45(2):156-9, 1995
18. McCauley RG et al: Benign hemorrhagic adrenocortical macrocysts in Beckwith-Wiedemann syndrome. AJR Am J Roentgenol. 157(3):549-52, 1991
19. Gaffey MJ et al: Unusual variants of adrenal pseudocysts with intracystic fat, myelolipomatous metaplasia, and metastatic carcinoma. Am J Clin Pathol. 94(6):706-13, 1990

Lymphangiomatous Cyst: Cut Surface

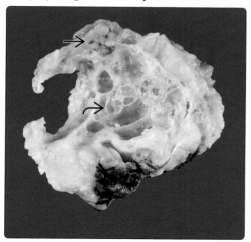

Pseudocyst Developing in Cortical Adenoma

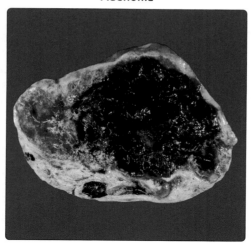

(Left) *Gross photo of lymphangiomatous cyst shows extensive septation and internal loculation* ➡. *There is minimal residual bright yellow adrenal cortex* ➡. **(Right)** *Gross photo of adrenal gland shows a pseudocyst developing within a hemorrhagic adrenal cortical adenoma.*

Lymphangiomatous Cyst

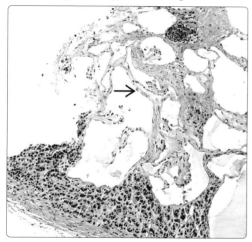

Hemorrhagic Adrenal Cortical Adenoma

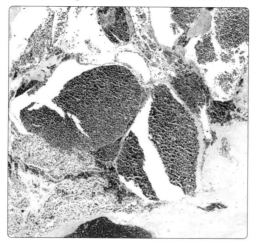

(Left) *Endothelial cysts are defined by smooth and flat endothelial lining* ➡ *and absence of proliferating endothelium. These lesions immunoexpress endothelial markers.* **(Right)** *This adrenal cortical adenoma with recent hemorrhage shows neovascularization by cystically dilated, endothelial-lined channels.*

Lymphangiomatous Cyst

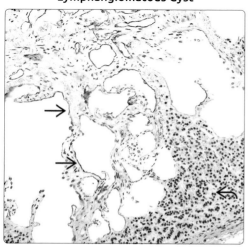

Cortical Adenoma With Endothelial-Lined Cysts

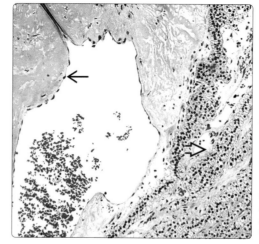

(Left) *Lining of a lymphangiomatous cyst stains for podoplanin, a lymphatic endothelial marker with antibody D2-40* ➡. *Normal adrenal cortex is present at the periphery of the lesion* ➡. **(Right)** *This dilated channel lined by capillary endothelium* ➡ *in a hemorrhagic cortical adenoma illustrates overlapping cyst categories; a hemorrhagic neoplasm might develop an endothelial lining (endothelial cyst), retain its own lining (epithelial cyst), or have no lining (pseudocyst). Residual adenoma is present at the periphery* ➡.

Adrenal Cysts

Adrenal Glands

Cystic Pheochromocytoma

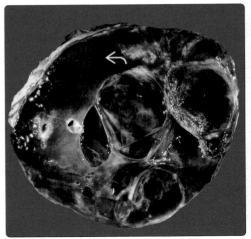

Rim Calcification

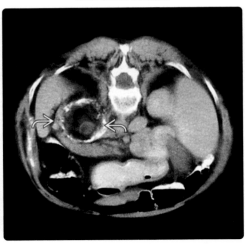

(Left) Gross photo shows a pheochromocytoma with hemorrhagic infarction and cyst formation. Older infarcted areas have undergone cystic change, while recently infarcted areas are diffusely hemorrhagic ➤. (Right) CT scan shows extensive rim calcification ➤ in a longstanding mature cystic teratoma (dermoid cyst) involving the adrenal gland.

Cystic Pheochromocytoma

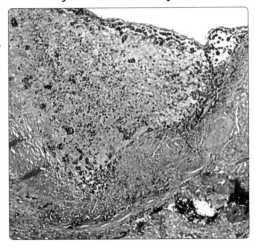

Mature Cystic Teratoma

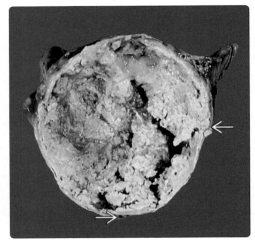

(Left) This pheochromocytoma contains an evolving pseudocyst with a thick fibrous wall, absent lining, and lumen containing degenerating blood and hemosiderophages. (Right) Gross photo shows an extremely rare example of a mature cystic teratoma (dermoid cyst) within an adrenal gland. Attenuated adrenal cortex is seen at the periphery ➤. More often, a teratoma adjacent to the adrenal mimics an adrenal cyst.

Cystic Pheochromocytoma With Calcification

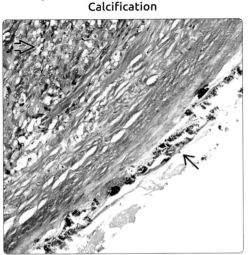

Adrenal Teratoma

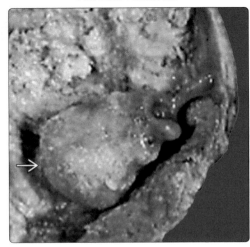

(Left) In longstanding cysts, calcification can be seen within the cyst walls. This is an example of calcification ➤ in the thick fibrous wall of a pseudocyst evolving in a pheochromocytoma. There is no lining epithelium, but residual pheochromocytoma ➤ is seen outside of the cyst. (Right) Gross examination of this mature cystic teratoma shows a single nubbin of mature teratomatous tissue ➤ attached to the cyst wall.

Hemorrhagic Macrocysts in Beckwith-Wiedemann Syndrome

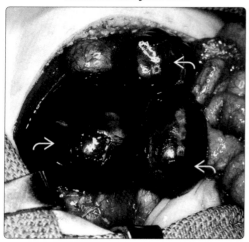

Congenital Cystic Neuroblastoma

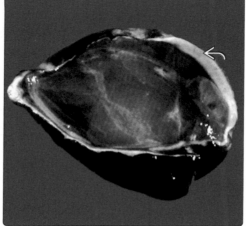

(Left) *Intraoperative photograph shows multiple large, congenital, hemorrhagic adrenal cysts* ⊅ *in an infant with Beckwith-Wiedemann syndrome (BWS).* (Right) *Gross photo shows a unilocular congenital adrenal cyst filled with fibrin and blood. A small amount of adrenal cortex is present at the periphery* ⊅*. Although the gross appearance suggests a nonneoplastic pseudocyst, extensive sampling showed nests of neuroblastoma in the cyst wall.*

Hemorrhagic Cyst With Cytomegaly in Beckwith-Wiedemann Syndrome

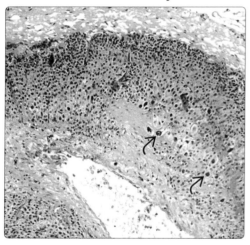

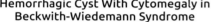

Congenital Cystic Neuroblastoma

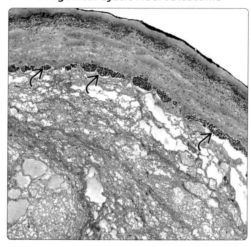

(Left) *The lining of this macrocyst from an infant with BWS contains scattered hyperchromatic, large cortical cells* ⊅ *that are typical of BWS but suggest neoplasia in the differential diagnosis.* (Right) *This congenital cystic neuroblastoma has a thick fibrous wall and fibrin-filled lumen. Extensive sampling shows only a few small nests of neuroblastoma* ⊅ *in the cyst lining.*

Beckwith-Wiedemann Syndrome

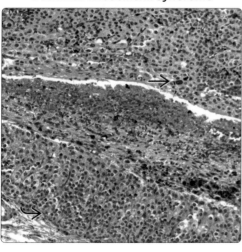

Congenital Cystic Neuroblastoma

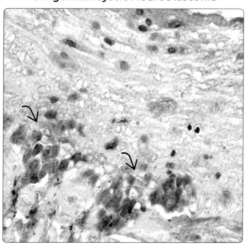

(Left) *Cytomegaly* ⊅ *in this hemorrhagic cyst is confined to the centrally located remnants of involuting fetal cortex and is absent from the mature cortex on the opposite cyst wall* ⊅*. The distribution suggests the cysts result from bleeding as the fetal cortex is replaced by adult cortex.* (Right) *Immunohistochemistry for synaptophysin shows small groups of tumor cells* ⊅ *focally positive for synaptophysin in cell bodies and short processes.*

KEY FACTS

TERMINOLOGY

- Adrenal incidentaloma
- Adrenal mass discovered incidentally by radiological imaging

CLINICAL ISSUES

- No clinical symptoms or signs at time of presentation
- With dedicated adrenal imaging to access lipid content
  - Lipid-rich tumors followed by observation
  - Tumors that are lipid poor, tumors with heterogeneity, and tumors with subclinical hormone excess should be considered for surgery

MICROSCOPIC

- Many different architectural patterns
  - Trabecular, alveolar, ribbon-like, and pseudoglandular
- Can have lipomatous, myelolipomatous, osseous metaplasia
- May have areas of oncocytic differentiation

- Medulla may show compressive features
- Sclerosis, cystic degeneration, and hemorrhage may be present

ANCILLARY TESTS

- Positive for adrenal cortical markers, such as SF1, synaptophysin, inhibin, and Melan-A
- *CTNNB1* mutations result in Wnt/β-catenin activation
  - Nuclear localization seen on immunohistochemistry
- Presence of activated mTOR pathway has been described

TOP DIFFERENTIAL DIAGNOSES

- Adrenal cortical carcinoma
- Functional adrenal cortical adenoma
- Pheochromocytoma
- Metastatic carcinoma (usually from kidney and lung)
  - Metastatic carcinomas are positive for cytokeratin and negative for inhibin

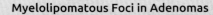

Myelolipomatous Foci in Adenomas

Myxoid Adrenal Adenoma

(Left) *Most adrenal cortical adenomas are well-circumscribed ➡, yellow-orange or tan masses. Some tumors may have foci of myelolipomatous metaplasia, giving to the tumor a variegated appearance. This picture shows the irregular red area of myelolipomatous metaplasia ➡.* (Right) *Photograph illustrates a large adrenal cortical adenoma, which has extensive myxoid changes, giving the microcystic gross cut surface appearance. Myxoid changes can be seen in all adenomas, and it is also seen in carcinoma.*

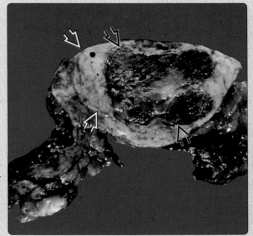

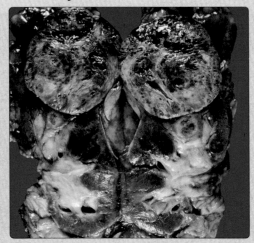

Lipomatous Metaplasia

Cellular Pleomorphism

(Left) *Lipomatous metaplasia ➡ is usually present in these neoplasms. Myelolipomatous metaplasia is also commonly identified within adrenal cortical adenomas.* (Right) *Photomicrograph of a nonfunctional adrenal cortical adenoma demonstrates cellular pleomorphism and large, binucleated atypical cells (so-called endocrine atypia). An intranuclear inclusion is present ➡.*

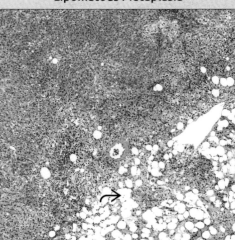

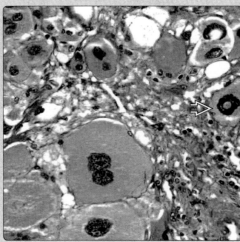

TERMINOLOGY

Abbreviations

- Adrenal cortical adenoma (ACA)

Synonyms

- Adrenal incidentaloma
- ACA with eucortisolism

Definitions

- Benign epithelial tumor of adrenal cortical cells in absence of clinical symptoms
- Adrenal mass discovered incidentally by radiologic examination
  - Hormone tests: Nonfunctional lesion

CLINICAL ISSUES

Epidemiology

- Incidence
  - Detected in 1.4-2.9% of autopsies
  - Found in 4.5% of all CT scans as incidental findings
  - More common in aging population
    - Present in 10% of those aged 70 years

Presentation

- No clinical symptoms or signs at time of presentation

Laboratory Tests

- Nonfunctional lesion

Prognosis

- With dedicated adrenal imaging to access lipid content
  - Lipid-rich tumors followed by observation only
  - Tumors that are lipid poor, tumors with heterogeneity, and tumors with subclinical hormone excess should be considered for surgery
- Optimal frequency and duration of follow-up for adrenal incidentaloma is uncertain
- Increased mortality both from cardiovascular disease and infections in patients with adrenal incidentaloma and low-grade excess cortisol

IMAGING

MR Findings

- Early dynamic serial gadolinium-enhanced MR aids in characterization of adrenal tumors

CT Findings

- Found on abdominal CT scans in ~ 5-10% of patients

MACROSCOPIC

General Features

- Nodules may be bilateral and multiple
- Nodules can be intracortical, sometimes even extruding from cortex into capsule showing mushroom appearance

MICROSCOPIC

Histologic Features

- Can have different architectural patterns
  - Trabecular
  - Alveolar
  - Ribbon-like
  - Pseudoglandular
- May have areas of oncocytic differentiation
- Cortical atrophy in remaining ipsilateral or contralateral cortex may be sign of hypercortisolism
- Can have lipomatous, myelolipomatous, and sometimes osseous metaplasia
- Medulla may show compressive features
- If large, then degenerative changes such as sclerosis, cystic degeneration, and hemorrhage may be present

ANCILLARY TESTS

Immunohistochemistry

- Positive for adrenal cortical markers: SF1, synaptophysin, inhibin-α, Melan-A
- Negative for chromogranin and cytokeratins

Genetic Testing

- *CTNNB1* mutations result in Wnt/β-catenin activation
  - Adenomas with this mutation tends to be larger and nonfunctioning
- Presence of activated mTOR pathway has been described

DIFFERENTIAL DIAGNOSIS

Adrenal Cortical Carcinoma

- Not well circumscribed; shows invasive pattern
- Frequently shows hemorrhage and necrosis
- Mitotic rate is usually > 5/50 HPF

Adrenal Cortical Adenoma (Functional)

- Based on hormonal secretory status

Pheochromocytoma

- Negative for inhibin and positive for chromogranin

Metastatic Carcinoma

- Immunohistochemistry will differentiate metastatic tumor from adrenal primaries

SELECTED REFERENCES

1. Papanastasiou L et al: Concomitant alterations of metabolic parameters, cardiovascular risk factors and altered cortisol secretion in patients with adrenal incidentalomas during prolonged follow-up. Clin Endocrinol (Oxf). 86(4):488-498, 2017
2. Fassnacht M et al: Management of adrenal incidentalomas: European Society of Endocrinology Clinical Practice Guideline in collaboration with the European Network for the Study of Adrenal Tumors. Eur J Endocrinol. 175(2):G1-G34, 2016
3. De Martino MC et al: Characterization of the mTOR pathway in human normal adrenal and adrenocortical tumors. Endocr Relat Cancer. 21(4):601-13, 2014
4. Kanthan R et al: Three uncommon adrenal incidentalomas: a 13-year surgical pathology review. World J Surg Oncol. 10:64, 2012
5. Suzuki T et al: Small adrenocortical tumors without apparent clinical endocrine abnormalities. Immunolocalization of steroidogenic enzymes. Pathol Res Pract. 188(7):883-9, 1992
6. Copeland PM: The incidentally discovered adrenal mass. Ann Intern Med. 98(6):940-5, 1983

Aldosterone-Producing Adenomas

TERMINOLOGY

- Conn syndrome
- Adrenal adenoma that secretes aldosterone, resulting in hypertension, hypokalemia/normokalemia, and suppressed plasma renin activity

MACROSCOPIC

- Single, unilateral, and well circumscribed
- Homogeneous, yellow-orange ("canary yellow")

MICROSCOPIC

- Pushing borders
- Pseudocapsule (sometimes may appear to be real capsule due to compression of adjacent structures by adenoma)
- Large, lipid-rich cells are most common, which give tumor its characteristic yellow color
- Spironolactone bodies: Small intracytoplasmic eosinophilic inclusions with laminated appearance

ANCILLARY TESTS

- Positive for adrenal cortical markers, such as SF1, calretinin, inhibin, and Melan-A
- Negative for cytokeratin and chromogranin
- CYP11B2 and CYP11B1 antibodies
  - Different expression between normal, hyperplastic, and neoplastic
- Somatic genetic alterations of genes that encode plasma membrane potassium or calcium channels
  - Somatic mutations of *KCNJ5* gene, which encodes GIRK4 potassium channels
    - Present in ~ 40% of aldosterone-producing adenomas
  - Aldosterone-producing adenomas that lack *KCNJ5* mutations may have *ATP1A1*, *ATP2B3*, and *CACNA1D* mutations

TOP DIFFERENTIAL DIAGNOSES

- Other adrenocortical adenomas and pheochromocytoma

(Left) *Cross section through an adrenal mass shows the classic "canary yellow" color of an aldosterone-secreting adenoma. Another characteristic of these tumors is the pushing borders ⊠.*
(Right) *High magnification of an aldosterone-secreting adenoma shows a nesting pattern (one of the characteristic patterns), as well as large lipid-rich cells, which are usually the predominant cell type.*

Yellow Cut Surface

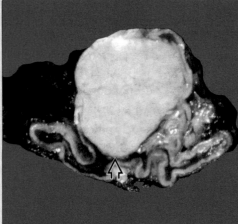

Large Lipid-Rich Cells

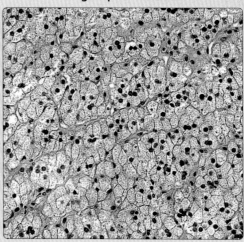

(Left) *Gross photo shows an adrenal cortical adenoma with central hemorrhage and infarction ⊠. The viable adenoma is bright yellow. Normal compressed adrenal can be identified focally ⊠.*
(Right) *The adenoma cells are arranged in a mixed pattern, with areas of solid sheets of cells and in areas with cord-like arrangement. The cells have a pale pink cytoplasm, and the round nuclei are centrally located with minute nucleoli.*

Adrenal Adenoma With Hemorrhage

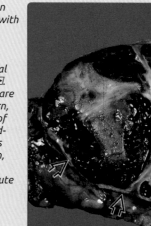

Solid Arrangement

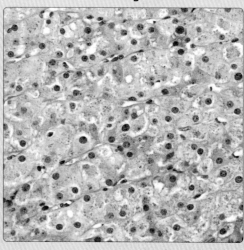

TERMINOLOGY

Abbreviations

- Aldosterone-producing adenoma (APA)

Synonyms

- Primary hyperaldosteronism
- Adrenal aldosterone-secreting adenoma
- Conn syndrome

Definitions

- Aldosterone production related to adrenal cortical lesion is called primary aldosteronism (or Conn syndrome)
- Adrenal adenoma which secretes aldosterone, resulting in hypertension, hypokalemia/normokalemia, higher rates of cardiovascular diseases and suppressed plasma renin activity

CLINICAL ISSUES

Epidemiology

- Incidence
  - Most common form of secondary hypertension
  - 5-10% in patients with hypertension
  - Around 20% in patients with resistant hypertension
  - Very few population-based studies on incidence of Conn syndrome exist
- Age
  - Peak incidence occurs in 3rd to 5th decades of life
- Sex
  - Predilection for female patients

Presentation

- Hypertension
  - Higher incidence of cardiovascular and cerebrovascular disease than those with essential hypertension
- Hypokalemia/normokalemia
- Metabolic alkalosis
- Mild hypernatremia (143-147 mEq/L)

Treatment

- Surgical approaches
  - Laparoscopic adrenalectomy
    - Based on results of adrenal venous sampling
    - Hypertension and hypokalemia should be corrected preoperatively with spironolactone

Prognosis

- As in most adrenal cortical adenomas, prognosis is determined by severity of endocrine manifestations

IMAGING

MR Findings

- Smooth contour and homogeneous
- Tumor may enhance mildly or even look darker than rest of gland
- Less intense than fat, greater than muscle, and similar to liver on both T1 and T2

CT Findings

- Well defined
- Homogeneous
- Attenuation values are usually less than normal adrenal
- Adrenal venous sampling
  - Differentiates unilateral disease from bilateral hyperaldosteronism

MACROSCOPIC

General Features

- Small (may vary 0.5-6.0 cm)
- Unilateral
- Solitary
- Round/ovoid
- Sharply demarcated by pseudocapsule
- Homogeneous, yellow-orange ("canary yellow")

MICROSCOPIC

Histologic Features

- Pushing borders
- Tumor cells arranged in nesting/alveolar pattern, short cords, anastomosing trabeculae, or mixture of patterns
- Pseudocapsule (sometimes may appear to be real capsule due to compression of adjacent structures by adenoma)
- Although uncommon, there can be areas of lipomatous and myelolipomatous metaplasia
- Can be hyperplasia of zona glomerulosa in nonneoplastic adrenal remnant

Cytologic Features

- Can be cells resembling those of zona glomerulosa, fasciculata, and reticularis and "hybrid" cells (capable of elaborating hormones from either zona glomerulosa or zona fasciculata)
- High N:C ratio; eosinophilic cells with few vacuoles (similar to those of zona glomerulosa) together with compact cells (resembling those of zona reticularis) tend to be distributed in periphery of adenoma
- Large lipid-rich cells are most common, which give tumor its characteristic yellow color
  - Distributed toward center of tumor
- Balloon cells may be present as well
- Spironolactone bodies: Small intracytoplasmic eosinophilic inclusions with laminated appearance usually surrounded by clear halo
  - Occur in patients treated with spironolactone and appear on cells of zona glomerulosa and in cells of aldosterone producing adenomas

ANCILLARY TESTS

Immunohistochemistry

- Used mainly to differentiate adrenal cortical adenomas from other adrenal tumors, as well as to recognize them when they spread to other sites of body
  - Used for differential diagnosis with pheochromocytomas and metastatic tumors
- Positive for adrenal cortical markers, such as SF-1, inhibin, and Melan-A
- Focally positive for synaptophysin; however, negative for chromogranin, which differentiates it from pheochromocytomas
- Negative for cytokeratin

- Antibodies against enzymes aldosterone synthase (CYP11B2) and 11β-hydroxylase (CYP11B1)
  - Different expression between normal/hyperplastic and neoplastic aldosterone-producing cells

In Situ Hybridization

- Gene *CYP11B2* can be used for postoperative differentiation of unilateral adenoma vs. bilateral adrenal hyperplasia

Genetic Testing

- Underlying mechanisms that result in excessive and autonomous aldosterone production was elucidated by next-generation sequencing studies
  - Somatic genetic alterations of genes that encode plasma membrane potassium or calcium channels
  - Somatic mutations of *KCNJ5* gene, which encodes GIRK4 potassium channels
    - Cause loss of ion selectivity increased intracellular calcium resulting in constitutive aldosterone production
    - Present in ~ 40% of APAs
    - *KCNJ5* mutations are associated with female sex, young patient age at diagnosis and more marked primary aldosteronism
    - APAs with *KCNJ5* mutations are larger and associated with zona fasciculata-like histological appearance
  - APAs that lack *KCNJ5* mutations may have mutations of *ATP1A1, ATP2B3,* and *CACNA1D*
- Adrenal miRNA
  - miR-24 seems to regulate CYP11B1 and CYP11B2 expression

Serologic Testing

- Testing guidelines per Endocrine Society (2008) for patients with otherwise unexplained hypertension and hypokalemia
  - Plasma renin activity (PRA) and plasma renin concentration (PRC): Very low, < 1 ng/mL per hour for PRA and undetectable for PRC
  - Plasma aldosterone concentration (PAC) to PRA ratio: > 30-50 (normal: 4-10)
  - 24-hour urine collection: Potassium > 30 mEq/day in patient with hypokalemia; aldosterone > 12 μg/day
- Confirmatory tests: Aldosterone suppression testing with oral sodium loading or saline infusion test

Electron Microscopy

- Cells with abundant intracytoplasmic lipid and others with barely any lipid vacuoles
- Prominent smooth endoplasmic reticulum
- Mitochondria have tubulovesicular cristae
- Spironolactone bodies consist of central core with amorphous electron-dense material surrounded by numerous concentric membranes continuous with endoplasmic reticulum

DIFFERENTIAL DIAGNOSIS

Other Adrenocortical Adenomas

- Hormonal secretion is key in differentiation
- Histologically they all look similar

Pheochromocytoma

- Negative for inhibin and positive for chromogranin

Metastatic Carcinoma

- Immunohistochemistry is key for differentiation
  - Metastatic carcinomas are negative for inhibin and positive for cytokeratin
- Primary sites of these tumors are usually lung and kidney

DIAGNOSTIC CHECKLIST

Pathologic Interpretation Pearls

- Clinical presentation triad: Hypertension, hypokalemia, and metabolic alkalosis
- Homogeneous and well-defined lesions both on CT and MR
- Small, solitary, and unilateral tumors
- Canary yellow color on gross examination
- Pushing borders with pseudocapsule
- Multiple cell types
- Most common cell is large, lipid-rich cell, which is mostly located at center of tumor
- Positive for inhibin and Melan-A
- Negative for cytokeratin

SELECTED REFERENCES

1. Chang CH et al: Arterial stiffness and blood pressure improvement in aldosterone-producing adenoma harboring KCNJ5 mutations after adrenalectomy. Oncotarget. 8(18):29984-29995, 2017
2. Fernandes-Rosa FL et al: Somatic and inherited mutations in primary aldosteronism. J Mol Endocrinol. 59(1):R47-R63, 2017
3. Maiolino G et al: Quantitative value of aldosterone-renin ratio for detection of aldosterone-producing adenoma: the aldosterone-renin ratio for primary aldosteronism (AQUARR) study. J Am Heart Assoc. 6(5), 2017
4. Omata K et al: Genetic and histopathologic intertumor heterogeneity in primary aldosteronism. J Clin Endocrinol Metab. 102(6):1792-1796, 2017
5. Scholl UI et al: Macrolides selectively inhibit mutant KCNJ5 potassium channels that cause aldosterone-producing adenoma. J Clin Invest. 127(7):2739-2750, 2017
6. Wu VC et al: The prevalence of CTNNB1 mutations in primary aldosteronism and consequences for clinical outcomes. Sci Rep. 7:39121, 2017
7. Nakamura Y et al: Expression of CYP11B2 in aldosterone-producing adrenocortical adenoma: regulatory mechanisms and clinical significance. Tohoku J Exp Med. 240(3):183-190, 2016
8. Nishimoto K et al: Case report: nodule development from subcapsular aldosterone-producing cell clusters causes hyperaldosteronism. J Clin Endocrinol Metab. 101(1):6-9, 2016
9. Åkerström T et al: Genetics of adrenocortical tumours. J Intern Med. 280(6):540-550, 2016
10. Monticone S et al: Understanding primary aldosteronism: impact of next generation sequencing and expression profiling. Mol Cell Endocrinol. 399C:311-320, 2015
11. Amar L et al: Progress in primary aldosteronism: mineralocorticoid antagonist treatment in aldosterone producing adenoma. Eur J Endocrinol. ePub, 2014
12. Fernandes-Rosa FL et al: Genetic spectrum and clinical correlates of somatic mutations in aldosterone-producing adenoma. Hypertension. 64(2):354-61, 2014
13. Funder JW: Genetics of primary aldosteronism. Front Horm Res. 43:70-8, 2014
14. Konosu-Fukaya S et al: 3β-hydroxysteroid dehydrogenase isoforms in human aldosterone-producing adenoma. Mol Cell Endocrinol. ePub, 2014
15. Nakamura Y et al: Dissecting the molecular pathways of primary aldosteronism. Pathol Int. 64(10):482-9, 2014
16. Nakamura Y et al: Adrenal CYP11B1/2 expression in primary aldosteronism: immunohistochemical analysis using novel monoclonal antibodies. Mol Cell Endocrinol. 392(1-2):73-9, 2014
17. Ono Y et al: Different expression of 11β-hydroxylase and aldosterone synthase between aldosterone-producing microadenomas and macroadenomas. Hypertension. 64(2):438-44, 2014
18. Volpe C et al: Primary aldosteronism; functional histopathology and long-term follow-up after unilateral adrenalectomy. Clin Endocrinol (Oxf). ePub, 2014

Immunohistochemistry

Antibody	Reactivity	Staining Pattern	Comment
	Positive	Not applicable	CYP11B2 immunohistochemistry helps in diagnosis of primary aldosteronism
SF1	Positive	Nuclear	
Inhibin	Positive	Cell membrane & cytoplasm	
Mart-1	Positive	Cytoplasmic	
melan-A103	Positive	Cytoplasmic	
calretinin	Positive	Cytoplasmic	
Chromogranin-A	Negative		Helps to discriminate from pheochromocytoma
CK7	Negative		Helps to discriminate from other epithelial tumors
CK20	Negative		Helps to discriminate from other epithelial tumors
AE1/AE3	Negative		Helps to discriminate from other epithelial tumors
EMA	Negative		Helps to discriminate from other epithelial tumors
CD10	Negative		Helps to discriminate from renal cell carcinoma
Hep-Par1	Negative		Helps to discriminate from hepatocellular carcinoma
HMFG	Negative		
RCC	Negative		Helps to discriminate from renal cell carcinoma
HMB-45	Negative		

Differential Diagnosis of Adrenal Cortical Adenoma

Neoplasm	Inhibin	Melan-A	Chrg	Syn	Hep-Par1	CD10	SF1
Adrenocortical adenoma	Positive	Positive	Negative	Positive (57%)	Negative	Negative	Positive
Pheochromocytoma	Negative	Negative	Positive	Positive	Negative	Negative	Negative
Hepatocellular carcinoma	Negative	Negative	Negative	Negative	Positive	Positive (61%)	Negative
Renal cell carcinoma	Negative	Negative	Negative	Negative	Negative	Positive	Negative

Chrg = chromogranin; Syn = synaptophysin.

19. Williams TA et al: Somatic ATP1A1, ATP2B3, and KCNJ5 mutations in aldosterone-producing adenomas. Hypertension. 63(1):188-95, 2014

20. Zennaro MC et al: An update on novel mechanisms of primary aldosteronism. J Endocrinol. ePub, 2014

21. Nanba K et al: Histopathological diagnosis of primary aldosteronism using CYP11B2 immunohistochemistry. J Clin Endocrinol Metab. 98(4):1567-74, 2013

22. Robertson S et al: MicroRNA-24 is a novel regulator of aldosterone and cortisol production in the human adrenal cortex. Hypertension. 62(3):572-8, 2013

23. Funder JW et al: Case detection, diagnosis, and treatment of patients with primary aldosteronism: an endocrine society clinical practice guideline. J Clin Endocrinol Metab. 93(9):3266-81, 2008

24. Schteingart DE: The 50th anniversary of the identification of primary aldosteronism: a retrospective of the work of Jerome W. Conn. J Lab Clin Med. 145(1):12-6, 2005

25. Enberg U et al: Postoperative differentiation between unilateral adrenal adenoma and bilateral adrenal hyperplasia in primary aldosteronism by mRNA expression of the gene CYP11B2. Eur J Endocrinol. 151(1):73-85, 2004

26. Stowasser M et al: Primary aldosteronism--careful investigation is essential and rewarding. Mol Cell Endocrinol. 217(1-2):33-9, 2004

27. Walz MK: Extent of adrenalectomy for adrenal neoplasm: cortical sparing (subtotal) versus total adrenalectomy. Surg Clin North Am. 84(3):743-53, 2004

28. Young WF Jr: Primary aldosteronism: management issues. Ann N Y Acad Sci. 970:61-76, 2002

29. Dunnick NR et al: CT in the diagnosis of primary aldosteronism: sensitivity in 29 patients. AJR Am J Roentgenol. 160(2):321-4, 1993

30. Melby JC: Diagnosis of hyperaldosteronism. Endocrinol Metab Clin North Am. 20(2):247-55, 1991

31. Young WF Jr et al: Primary aldosteronism: diagnosis and treatment. Mayo Clin Proc. 65(1):96-110, 1990

32. Aiba M et al: Spironolactone bodies in aldosteronomas and in the attached adrenals. Enzyme histochemical study of 19 cases of primary aldosteronism and a case of aldosteronism due to bilateral diffuse hyperplasia of the zona glomerulosa. Am J Pathol. 103(3):404-10, 1981

33. Eto T et al: Ultrastructural types of cell in adrenal cortical adenoma with primary aldosteronism. J Pathol. 128(1):1-6, 1979

34. Melby JC: Identifying the adrenal lesion in primary aldosteronism. Ann Intern Med. 76(6):1039-41, 1972

35. Conn JW: Plasma renin activity in primary aldosteronism. Importance in differential diagnosis and in research of essential hypertension. JAMA. 190:222-5, 1964

36. Janigan DT: Cytoplasmic bodies in the adrenal cortex of patients treated with spirolactone. Lancet. 1(7286):850-2, 1963

37. Conn JW: Primary aldosteronism. J Lab Clin Med. 45(4):661-4, 1955

(Left) Cross section shows several classic findings in aldosterone-producing tumors: A round, small, well-circumscribed mass ⊋ with pushing borders and a homogeneous, yellowish color; and hyperplasia of the zona glomerulosa ⊋ located at the remnant, nontumoral, adrenal gland, which is very frequently seen in aldosterone-secreting adenomas. (Right) Gross photo shows the typical golden yellow color in aldosterone-producing tumors with characteristic pushing borders ⊋.

Adrenal Adenoma and Hyperplasia

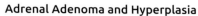
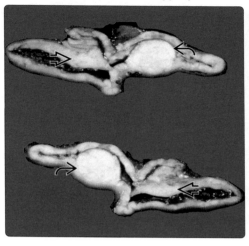

Pushing Borders

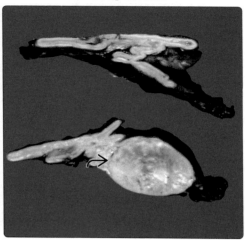

(Left) Low-power view of an aldosterone-producing adenoma highlights normal compressed adrenal ⊋, separated from the tumor by a thin fibrous pseudocapsule ⊋. (Right) High magnification of an aldosterone-producing adenoma has the characteristic spironolactone bodies ⊋, which are small intracytoplasmic eosinophilic inclusions with a laminated appearance usually surrounded by a clear halo, which appear in patients treated with spironolactone.

Interface of Adenoma and Normal Adrenal

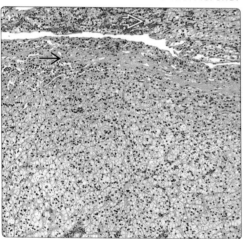

Spironolactone Bodies

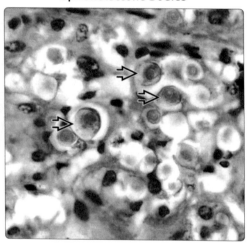

(Left) Low magnification of an aldosterone-secreting adenoma shows several characteristic features seen in these tumors. Lipomatous metaplasia ⊋ is intermixed with tumoral cells in a diffuse architecture or different morphological patterns and may coexist as nesting pattern and cords. (Right) High magnification of an aldosterone-producing tumor highlights the lipomatous metaplasia ⊋ present within the clear cells of the adenoma ⊋.

Lipomatous Metaplasia

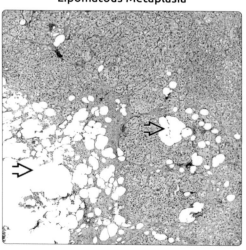

Adenoma With Lipomatous Changes

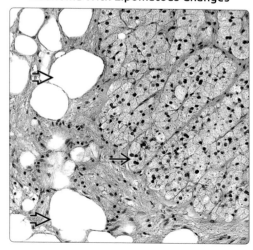

Aldosterone-Producing Adenomas

Well-Circumscribed Gross Cut Surface

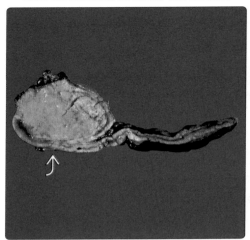

Bright Yellow Cut Surface

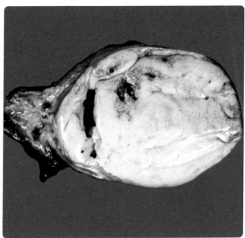

(Left) This gross photograph illustrates typical features of aldosterone-secreting adenomas, the golden yellow color and the sharp borders between the tumor and the remnant nontumoral adrenal parenchyma ➡. In this case, the remnant adrenal is normal. (Right) Aldosterone-producing adenomas have a bright yellow cut surface, related to the high steroid content. Areas of punctate hemorrhage or larger areas with hemorrhage may be present.

Lipid-Rich and Lipid-Poor Cells

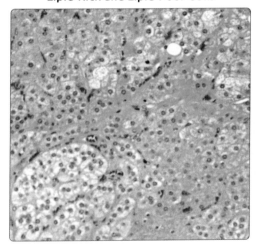

Nesting Pattern

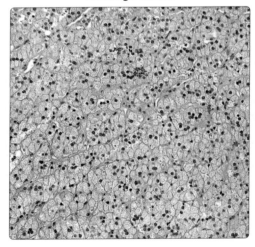

(Left) This photomicrograph shows an aldosterone-producing adenoma composed by cells with lipid-rich cytoplasm, intermixed with areas with cells with lipid-poor cytoplasm. (Right) A low-power view of an aldosterone-secreting adenoma shows the characteristic nesting pattern. The cells have a pale lipid-rich cytoplasm with small nuclei.

Aldosterone-Producing Adenoma

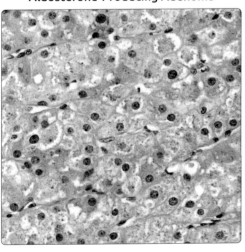

Lipid-Rich Cells

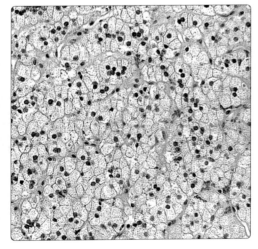

(Left) The adenoma cells are arranged in a mixed pattern, with areas of solid sheets of cells and in areas with cord-like arrangement. The cells have a pale-pink cytoplasm, and the round nuclei are centrally located with minute nucleoli. (Right) A high magnification of an aldosterone-secreting adenoma shows a nesting pattern (one of the characteristic patterns), as well as large lipid-rich cells, which are usually the predominant cell type.

Cortisol-Producing Adenomas

TERMINOLOGY

- Benign neoplasm arising from adrenal cortical cells with cortisol hypersecretion
- Cortisol-hypersecretion typically results in ACTH-independent Cushing syndrome

CLINICAL ISSUES

- Adrenal origin comprises ~ 20% of Cushing syndrome etiologies
- Weight gain, central obesity, facial rounding, hirsutism, hypertension, osteoporosis, skin striae

MICROSCOPIC

- Smooth "pushing" borders without well-defined fibrous capsule
- Cells are larger than in normal adrenal and have pleomorphic nuclei
- Nuclei are single, round/oval, with chromatin margination and single dot-like nucleolus
- Mixed composition of pale-staining lipid-rich cells and cells with lipid-poor compact cytoplasm

ANCILLARY TESTS

- Positive for adrenal cortical markers, such as SF-1, GATA6, inhibin, and Melan-A
- Positive for synaptophysin; negative for chromogranin
- Gain-of-function somatic mutations of *PRKACA* gene
  - Somatic *PRKACA* mutations result in unilateral cortisol-producing adrenal adenoma
  - Found in 35-65% in patients with cortisol-secreting adenoma and overt Cushing syndrome
  - *PRKACA* mutations are not observed in other forms of adrenal Cushing syndrome

TOP DIFFERENTIAL DIAGNOSES

- Other adrenocortical adenomas and adrenal cortical carcinoma
- Pheochromocytoma

Cortisol-Producing Adenoma Cut Surface

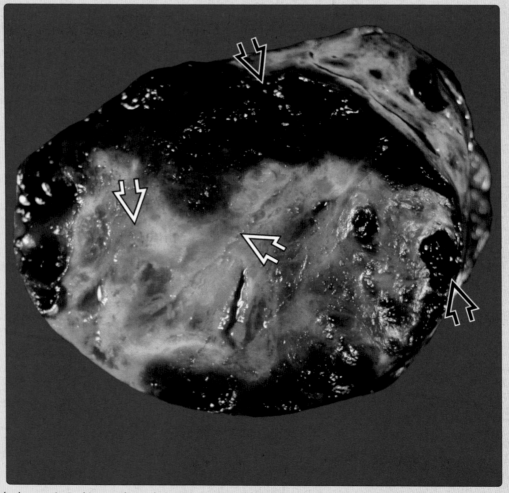

Adrenal cortical adenoma in Cushing syndrome has a tan-orange surface and mottled zones of darker pigmentation ⇨ due to accumulation of lipofuscin and lipid depletion of the neoplastic cells. Areas of hemorrhage ⇨ are also present in this tumor.

Cortisol-Producing Adenomas

TERMINOLOGY

Abbreviations
- Adrenal cortical adenoma (ACA)

Synonyms
- Cortisol-producing adrenocortical adenoma
- Cortisol-producing adrenal adenoma
- Cushing syndrome
- Functional adrenal adenoma

Definitions
- Benign neoplasm arising from adrenal cortical cells with cortisol hypersecretion
- Cortisol-hypersecretion typically results in ACTH-independent Cushing syndrome

CLINICAL ISSUES

Epidemiology
- Incidence
  - True incidence is unknown
  - Adrenal comprises 20% of Cushing syndrome etiologies
  - According to some literature, incidence of ACAs is low if "incidentalomas" are excluded
  - Typically unilateral, solitary, and benign
- Age
  - Can occur in any age group
- Sex
  - Any, but with female predilection

Presentation
- Weight gain
- Central obesity
- Supraclavicular and dorsocervical fat pads
- Facial rounding (moon face) and plethora
- Easy bruising
- Poor wound healing
- Purplish-red skin striae
- Proximal muscle weakness
- Hypertension
- Hyperglycemia
- Osteoporosis
- Hirsutism
- Infertility
- Susceptibility to opportunistic infections
- Cognitive/emotional changes

Treatment
- Surgical unilateral adrenalectomy

IMAGING

MR Findings
- Homogeneous
- Signal intensity less than fat but greater than muscle
- Similar intensity to liver on T1 and T2

CT Findings
- Well defined with smooth borders, homogeneous
- Attenuation values less than normal adrenal tissue
- May enhance after contrast administration

MACROSCOPIC

General Features
- Generally solitary, unilateral, and unicentric
- Rarely bilateral (contralateral adenoma is sometimes nonhyperfunctional)
- Cross section: Yellow or golden-yellow or tan-orange
- Geographic or mottled zones of dark pigmentation may be present
  - Due to lipid depletion of neoplastic cells as well as lipofuscin accumulation
- Necrosis, coarse lobulation, and cystic changes are rare (as compared to carcinomas)
- When diffusely dark brown or black: "Black adenoma"

Size
- Average diameter is 3.6 cm (1.5-6.0 cm)
- Usually < 50 g
- If > 100 g, considered carcinoma until proven otherwise

MICROSCOPIC

Histologic Features
- Smooth "pushing" borders without well-defined fibrous capsule
- Broad fields of pale-staining, lipid-rich cells with uniform nuclei
- Architectural patterns are cells in nesting or alveolar arrangement with delicate intersecting vasculature and areas of short cords
- Distinct cell borders mimicking cells of zona fasciculata
- Mixed pattern with oxyphilic and clear cells
  - Mixed composition of pale-staining, lipid-rich cells and cells with lipid-poor compact cytoplasm
- May have areas of lipomatous or myelolipomatous metaplasia
- Mitotic figures are very rare
- Some may have degenerative features: Fibrosis, organizing fibrin-rich thrombi within sinusoids, dystrophic calcification, or even metaplastic bone
- Myxoid changes are rare; however, when present they should prompt suspicion of borderline or malignant tumor

Cytologic Features
- Clear cytoplasm which, at higher magnification, is finely vacuolated due to intracytoplasmic lipid droplets
- Cells are larger than in normal adrenal and have pleomorphic nuclei
- Nuclei are single, round/oval, with chromatin margination and single dot-like nucleoli
  - Intranuclear inclusions may be present

ANCILLARY TESTS

Serologic Testing
- According to European Network for the Study of Adrenal Tumors (ENSAT), following tests should be performed when suspicious of functional adenoma
  - Fasting blood glucose
  - Potassium
  - Cortisol
  - ACTH

- 24-hour urinary free cortisol
- Fasting serum cortisol at 8 am following 1 mg dose of dexamethasone at bedtime
- Adrenal androgens (DHEAS, androstenedione, testosterone, 17-OH progesterone)
- Serum estradiol in men and postmenopausal women

Immunohistochemistry

- Used to confirm diagnosis, to differentiate from pheochromocytoma, or when tumors occur in unusual locations in abdomen or spinal canal
- Positive for adrenal cortical markers, such as SF-1, GATA6, inhibin, and Melan-A
- Can also be positive for synaptophysin and NSE (do not mistake for pheochromocytoma)
- Negative for chromogranin
- Negative for cytokeratin
- In cortisol-producing adenomas, steroidogenic enzymes are abundantly expressed in tumor cells, such as
  - 17α-hydroxylase/17
  - 20-lase (CYP17A1)
  - 3β-hydroxysteroid dehydrogenase (HSD3B)
  - 11β-hydroxylase (CYP11B1)
- Immunoreactivity of the following are detected in tumor cells
  - HSD3B2
    - HSD3B2 but not HSD3B1 was mainly involved in cortisol overproduction in cortisol-producing adenomas
  - CYP11B1
  - CYP17A1
  - Steroidogenic factor-1 (SF1[NR5A1]),
  - GATA6
  - Nerve growth factor induced-B (NGFIB[NR4A1])
    - NR5A1, GATA6, and NR4A1 were all considered to play important roles in cortisol overproduction through regulating *CYP11B1* gene transcription

Genetic Testing

- Mean number of comparative genomic hybridization changes in carcinomas is 7.6 (range: 1-15), while adenomas have mean of 1.1 changes (range: 0-4)
- Chromosomal loci implicated in adrenal cortical tumorigenesis include
  - Activation of oncogenes on chromosomes 5 and 12
  - Inactivation of tumor suppressor genes on chromosome arms 1p and 17p
- Gain-of-function somatic mutations of *PRKACA* gene
  - Location: 10p13.1
  - Protein: Protein kinase A catalytic subunit alpha (PKA C-alpha)
  - Somatic *PRKACA* mutations result in unilateral cortisol-producing adrenal adenoma
  - Found in 35-65% in patients with cortisol-secreting adenoma and overt Cushing syndrome
    - Also found in patients with subclinical Cushing syndrome of patients
  - *PRKACA* mutations are not observed in other forms of adrenal Cushing syndrome
    - Germline duplications of this gene results in bilateral adrenal hyperplasia

- Encodes catalytic subunit of cyclic AMP-dependent protein kinase mutation results in Leu206Arg substitution within evolutionary conserved region of P+1 loop
  - Region interacts with PKA regulatory subunit encoded by *PRKAR1A*
    - Leading to constitutive PKA activation
  - *PRKAR1A* mutations occur in Carney complex
  - Carney complex causes Cushing syndrome due to primary pigmented nodular adrenal cortical disease
    - Mutations in *PRKAR1A*
      - Located 17q24.2
      - Protein: cAMP-dependent protein kinase type 1-alpha regulatory subunit (PRKAR1A)
- Adrenal miRNA
  - miR-24 seems to modulate CYP11B1 and CYP11B2 expression

Electron Microscopy

- Abundant amount of intracytoplasmic lipid droplets
- Some may have little or no lipid
- Abundant smooth endoplasmic reticulum
- Mitochondria can be prominent with cristae that have tubular or vesicular profile (similar to normal cells of zona fasciculata)

DIFFERENTIAL DIAGNOSIS

Other Adrenocortical Adenomas

- Differentiation is based on hormonal secretory status
- Clinical symptoms specific for each hormone will help in differential
- Morphology will rarely help in differentiating these adenomas

Pheochromocytoma

- Negative for inhibin and positive for chromogranin

Metastatic Carcinoma

- Most metastatic carcinomas to adrenal are originally from lung or kidney
- Immunohistochemistry differentiates these tumors
  - Negative for inhibin and Melan-A and positive for cytokeratin

DIAGNOSTIC CHECKLIST

Pathologic Interpretation Pearls

- Unilateral
- Solitary
- Usually benign neoplasms
- Cross section: Yellow or golden yellow
- Geographic or mottled zones of dark pigmentation may be present
- Smooth pushing borders
- Broad fields of pale-staining, lipid-rich cells with uniform nuclei
- Clear cytoplasm that is finely vacuolated due to intracytoplasmic lipid droplets
- Mixed cell population with small compact eosinophilic cells and pale-staining lipid-rich cells
- Positive for inhibin, synaptophysin, and Melan-A
- Negative for cytokeratin and chromogranin

SELECTED REFERENCES

1. Wagner-Bartak NA et al: Cushing syndrome: diagnostic workup and imaging features, with clinical and pathologic correlation. AJR Am J Roentgenol. 209(1):19-32, 2017
2. de La Villéon B et al: Long-term outcome after adrenalectomy for incidentally diagnosed subclinical cortisol-secreting adenomas. Surgery. 160(2):397-404, 2016
3. Kubota-Nakayama F et al: Expression of steroidogenic enzymes and their transcription factors in cortisol-producing adrenocortical adenomas: immunohistochemical analysis and quantitative real-time polymerase chain reaction studies. Hum Pathol. 54:165-73, 2016
4. Nanba K et al: Double adrenocortical adenomas harboring independent KCNJ5 and PRKACA somatic mutations. Eur J Endocrinol. 175(2):K1-6, 2016
5. Ronchi CL et al: Genetic landscape of sporadic unilateral adrenocortical adenomas without PRKACA p.Leu206Arg Mutation. J Clin Endocrinol Metab. 101(9):3526-38, 2016
6. Saroka RM et al: No postoperative adrenal insufficiency in a patient with unilateral cortisol-secreting adenomas treated with mifepristone before surgery. Clin Med Insights Endocrinol Diabetes. 9:31-6, 2016
7. Tirosh A et al: Diurnal plasma cortisol measurements utility in differentiating various etiologies of endogenous Cushing syndrome. Horm Metab Res. 48(10):677-681, 2016
8. Zheng S et al: Comprehensive pan-genomic characterization of adrenocortical carcinoma. Cancer Cell. 30(2):363, 2016
9. Åkerström T et al: Genetics of adrenocortical tumours. J Intern Med. 280(6):540-550, 2016
10. Beuschlein F et al: Constitutive activation of PKA catalytic subunit in adrenal Cushing's syndrome. N Engl J Med. 370(11):1019-28, 2014
11. Di Dalmazi G et al: Novel somatic mutations in the catalytic subunit of the protein kinase A as a cause of adrenal Cushing's syndrome: a European multicentric study. J Clin Endocrinol Metab. 99(10):E2093-100, 2014
12. Duan K et al: Clinicopathological correlates of adrenal Cushing's syndrome. J Clin Pathol. ePub, 2014
13. Robertson S et al: MicroRNA-24 is a novel regulator of aldosterone and cortisol production in the human adrenal cortex. Hypertension. 62(3):572-8, 2013
14. Wilmot Roussel H et al: Identification of gene expression profiles associated with cortisol secretion in adrenocortical adenomas. J Clin Endocrinol Metab. 98(6):E1109-21, 2013
15. Lau SK et al: Mixed cortical adenoma and composite pheochromocytoma-ganglioneuroma: an unusual corticomedullary tumor of the adrenal gland. Ann Diagn Pathol. 15(3):185-9, 2011
16. Lloyd RV: Adrenal cortical tumors, pheochromocytomas and paragangliomas. Mod Pathol. 24 Suppl 2:S58-65, 2011
17. Papotti M et al: Adrenocortical tumors with myxoid features: a distinct morphologic and phenotypical variant exhibiting malignant behavior. Am J Surg Pathol. 34(7):973-83, 2010
18. Yaneva M et al: Genetics of Cushing's syndrome. Neuroendocrinology. 92 Suppl 1:6-10, 2010
19. Fassnacht M et al: Clinical management of adrenocortical carcinoma. Best Pract Res Clin Endocrinol Metab. 23(2):273-89, 2009
20. McNicol AM: A diagnostic approach to adrenal cortical lesions. Endocr Pathol. 19(4):241-51, 2008
21. Stratakis CA: Cushing syndrome caused by adrenocortical tumors and hyperplasias (corticotropin-independent Cushing syndrome). Endocr Dev. 13:117-32, 2008
22. Tissier F: [What's new in bilateral adrenal cortex pathology?.] Ann Pathol. 28 Spec No 1(1):S35-8, 2008
23. Giordano TJ: Molecular pathology of adrenal cortical tumors: separating adenomas from carcinomas. Endocr Pathol. 17(4):355-63, 2006
24. Cassarino DS et al: Spinal adrenal cortical adenoma with oncocytic features: report of the first intramedullary case and review of the literature. Int J Surg Pathol. 12(3):259-64, 2004
25. Tung SC et al: Bilateral adrenocortical adenomas causing ACTH-independent Cushing's syndrome at different periods: a case report and discussion of corticosteroid replacement therapy following bilateral adrenalectomy. J Endocrinol Invest. 27(4):375-9, 2004
26. Sugawara A et al: A case of aldosterone-producing adrenocortical adenoma associated with a probable post-operative adrenal crisis: histopathological analyses of the adrenal gland. Hypertens Res. 26(8):663-8, 2003
27. Zhang PJ et al: The role of calretinin, inhibin, melan-A, BCL-2, and C-kit in differentiating adrenal cortical and medullary tumors: an immunohistochemical study. Mod Pathol. 16(6):591-7, 2003
28. Loy TS et al: A103 immunostaining in the diagnosis of adrenal cortical tumors: an immunohistochemical study of 316 cases. Arch Pathol Lab Med. 126(2):170-2, 2002
29. Sidhu S et al: Comparative genomic hybridization analysis of adrenocortical tumors. J Clin Endocrinol Metab. 87(7):3467-74, 2002
30. Wieneke JA et al: Corticomedullary mixed tumor of the adrenal gland. Ann Diagn Pathol. 5(5):304-8, 2001
31. Brown FM et al: Myxoid neoplasms of the adrenal cortex: a rare histologic variant. Am J Surg Pathol. 24(3):396-401, 2000
32. Munro LM et al: The expression of inhibin/activin subunits in the human adrenal cortex and its tumours. J Endocrinol. 161(2):341-7, 1999
33. Pelkey TJ et al: The alpha subunit of inhibin in adrenal cortical neoplasia. Mod Pathol. 11(6):516-24, 1998
34. Kato S et al: Cushing's syndrome induced by hypersecretion of cortisol from only one of bilateral adrenocortical tumors. Metabolism. 41(3):260-3, 1992
35. Kepes JJ et al: Adrenal cortical adenoma in the spinal canal of an 8-year-old girl. Am J Surg Pathol. 14(5):481-4, 1990
36. Unger PD et al: Lipid degeneration in a pheochromocytoma histologically mimicking an adrenal cortical tumor. Arch Pathol Lab Med. 114(8):892-4, 1990
37. Neville AM et al: Histopathology of the human adrenal cortex. Clin Endocrinol Metab. 14(4):791-820, 1985
38. Bertagna C et al: Clinical and laboratory findings and results of therapy in 58 patients with adrenocortical tumors admitted to a single medical center (1951 to 1978). Am J Med. 71(5):855-75, 1981
39. Harrison JH et al: Proceedings: tumors of the adrenal cortex. Cancer. 32(5):1227-35, 1973

Immunohistochemistry

Antibody	Reactivity	Staining Pattern	Comment
SF1	Positive	Nuclear	
Inhibin	Positive	Cell membrane & cytoplasm	
Mart-1	Positive	Cytoplasmic	
Synaptophysin	Positive	Cell membrane and cytoplasm	
melan-A103	Positive	Cytoplasmic	
Chromogranin-A	Negative		Helps to discriminate from pheochromocytoma
CK7	Negative		Helps to discriminate from other epithelial tumors
CK20	Negative		Helps to discriminate from other epithelial tumors
AE1/AE3	Negative		Helps to discriminate from other epithelial tumors
EMA	Negative		Helps to discriminate from other epithelial tumors
CD10	Negative		Helps to discriminate from renal cell carcinoma
Hep-Par1	Negative		Helps to discriminate from hepatocellular carcinoma
HMFG	Negative		
RCC	Negative		Helps to discriminate from renal cell carcinoma
HMB-45	Negative		

Differential Diagnosis of Adrenal Cortical Adenoma

Neoplasm	Inhibin	Melan-A	Chrg	Syn	Hep-Par1	CD10
Adrenocortical adenoma	Positive	Positive	Negative	Positive (~60%)	Negative	Negative
Pheochromocytoma	Negative	Negative	Positive	Positive	Negative	N/A
Hepatocellular carcinoma	Negative	Negative	Negative	Negative	Positive	Positive (61%)
Renal cell carcinoma	Negative	Negative	Negative	Negative	Negative	Positive

Chrg = chromogranin; Syn = synaptophysin.

Criteria for Differentiation Between Adenoma and Carcinoma

Criteria	Adenoma	Carcinoma
Hormonal production	Often functional	Usually nonfunctional
Gross	Weight < 50 g	Weight > 100 g
Tumor gross color	Variable	Variable; does not differentiate
Circumscription	Well circumscribed	Invasive
Hemorrhage	Absent	Frequent
Necrosis	Absent	Frequent
Capsular invasion	Absent	Usually present
Invasion into adjacent tissues	Absent	Usually present
Intratumoral fibrosis	May be present	May be present
Myxomatous degeneration	May be present	May be present
Cytology	May have cytological atypia	Cytological atypia present
Histology	Atypia may be present	Atypia present
Necrosis	Necrosis absent	Present; confluent necrosis
Mitosis	Rare	> 5/50 HPF
Venous invasion	Absent	Present

Cortisol-Producing Adenoma

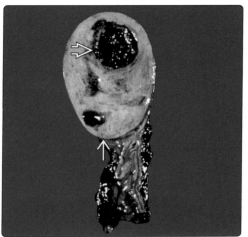

Degenerative Changes in Adenomas

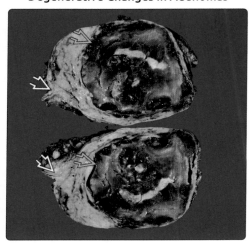

(Left) *Cross section from a cortisol-secreting adenoma shows the typical round, well-circumscribed ➡, yellow-orange appearance. This tumor has foci of dark discoloration ➡ that can be attributed to an old hemorrhage, area of lipid depletion of the tumor cells, or increased lipofuscin pigment.* (Right) *This well-circumscribed yellow-orange adrenal cortical adenoma shows a large central area of degenerative changes ➡. There is only a small rim of residual adrenal ➡.*

Adenoma Compressing Adjacent Adrenal

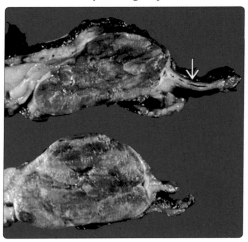

Adenoma With Myelolipomatous Area

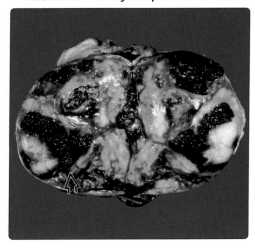

(Left) *This well-circumscribed adenoma has a mottled appearance with areas of dark discoloration due to compact eosinophilic cytoplasm of the tumor cells by lipid depletion and increased lipofuscin pigment. Note the marked atrophy of the attached adrenal cortex ➡.* (Right) *This large adrenal cortical adenoma has the characteristic bright yellow color with areas of myelolipomatous metaplasia ➡ and degenerative changes.*

Gross Cut Surface

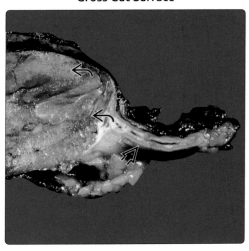

Adenoma-Adrenal Interface

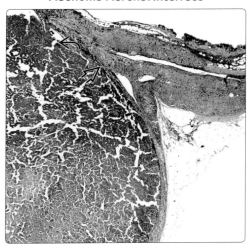

(Left) *This close-up view of adenoma highlights the mottled zones of dark pigmentation ➡. These areas are composed of lipid-depleted cells and cells with accumulation of lipofuscin pigment. Note the marked atrophy of the residual adrenal cortex ➡.* (Right) *This low-power view of a cortisol-producing adrenal cortical adenoma shows a sharp demarcation ➡ between the normal adrenal parenchyma, contrasting with the "pushing" borders of the adenoma ➡.*

(Left) *The tumor cells in cortisol-producing adrenal adenomas are arranged in a solid pattern with cytoplasmic lipofuscin pigment ⇨, a gradation in cell size, and a varying amount of lipid.* **(Right)** *The tumor cells are arranged in short cords or clusters. Individual tumor cells contain abundant lipid, which appears as numerous clear vacuoles ⇨. There is variation in nuclear size.*

Characteristic Histopathology

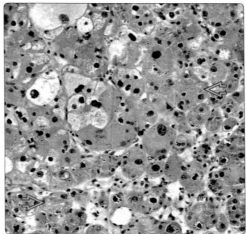

Abundant Lipid and Vacuolization

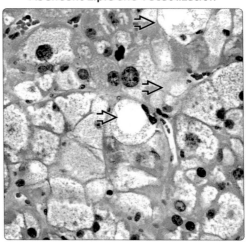

(Left) *Cortisol secreting adenomas are usually composed by cells with abundant granular eosinophilic cytoplasm. Some of the cells may present with clearing.* **(Right)** *The tumor cells in this cortisol-producing adrenal cortical adenoma are present within the central vein. There is an associated fibrin thrombus within the lumen ⇨, compressing the adjacent normal adrenal cortex ⇨.*

Eosinophilic Cytoplasm

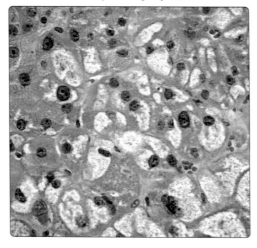

Adrenal Central Vein Thrombus

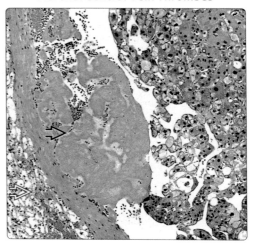

(Left) *Cortisol-secreting adrenal cortical adenoma composed of cells with eosinophilic cytoplasm that contains pigmented granular material ⇨ is shown. Note the presence of extracellular pigment within the stroma ⇨.* **(Right)** *Higher power view shows a cortisol-secreting adrenal cortical adenoma composed of cells with large cytoplasm, granular brown pigment, enlarged hyperchromatic nuclei, and some with prominent nucleoli. This illustrates the granular aspect of the pigment that represents lipofuscin ⇨.*

Intra- and Extracellular Lipofuscin Pigment

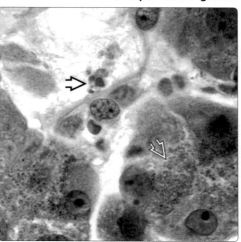

Lipofuscin Pigment

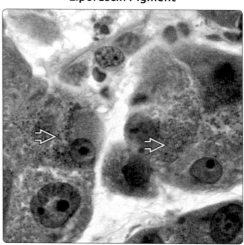

Cytology Features

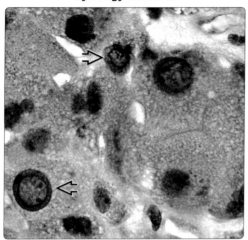

Intranuclear Pseudoinclusions

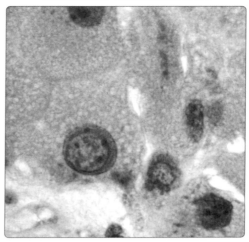

(Left) *This cortisol-producing adrenal cortical adenoma is composed of large cells with eosinophilic cytoplasm and enlarged hyperchromatic nuclei. Some cells show a prominent intranuclear pseudoinclusion ⊳.* (Right) *In adrenal cortical adenomas the nuclei tend to be small. However, in focal areas of a tumor, large bizarre nuclei may be present. Also, some tumors may contain large nuclei with intranuclear pseudoinclusions.*

Synaptophysin

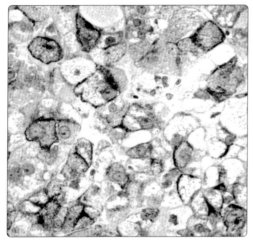

α-Inhibin Immunohistochemistry

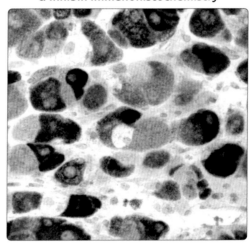

(Left) *Synaptophysin is present in adrenal cortical tumors in a moderately weak membranous and cytoplasmic pattern. This positivity is usually less intense than in pheochromocytoma.* (Right) *Immunoreactivity for a-inhibin as well as for Melan-A is sensitive but not specific for adrenal cortical tumors. The tumor cells have variably intense cytoplasmic granular immunopositivity. In contrast with other epithelial tumors, the tumor cells are negative for cytokeratin and EMA.*

Proliferative Index

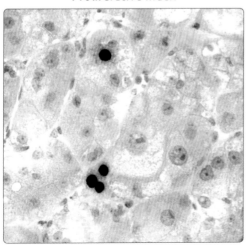

Immunonegative for Chromogranin

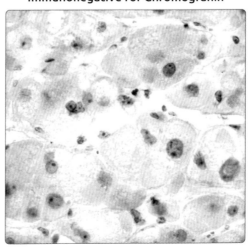

(Left) *Immunohistochemistry for Ki-67 reveals a low proliferative index in the benign cortisol-secreting adrenal cortical adenomas. These findings correlate with a very low mitotic index.* (Right) *Immunohistochemistry in adrenal cortical adenoma is characteristically negative for chromogranin. The tumor cells in these tumors are also negative for CK7, CK20, AE1/AE3, S100, and CD10, aiding in the differential diagnosis with other epithelial neoplasms.*

Sex Hormone-Producing Adenoma

KEY FACTS

CLINICAL ISSUES

- Secretion of sex hormones is more commonly observed in adrenal cortical carcinoma
- Rare sex hormone-producing adenomas
  - Only few cases reported
  - Usually tend to be in form of carcinoma more than adenoma
- Correlation with biochemical and endocrinologic data is essential for diagnosis
  - Androgen excess in females lead to hirsutism, amenorrhea, virilization
  - Estrogen excess in males results in gynecomastia and impotence
- Feminizing adrenal cortical neoplasms occur mostly between ages of 25-45
- Virilizing tumors, on other hand, are more prevalent in pediatric population

MACROSCOPIC

- Testosterone-producing neoplasms have average weight of 473 g
- Feminizing neoplasms have average weight of 1,000 g

MICROSCOPIC

- Cells resemble those of zona reticularis (responsible for sex steroids) and are compact with eosinophilic cytoplasm
- Attached adrenal remnant and contralateral adrenal cortex are not atrophic due to lack of glucocorticoid excretion

ANCILLARY TESTS

- Positive for SF1, synaptophysin, inhibin, and Melan-A
- Negative for chromogranin and cytokeratins

TOP DIFFERENTIAL DIAGNOSES

- Pheochromocytoma
- Adrenal cortical carcinoma and other adenomas
- Metastatic carcinoma

Gross Cut Surface

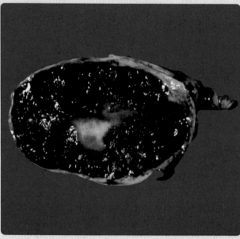

Oncocytic Neoplasm With Diffuse Growth

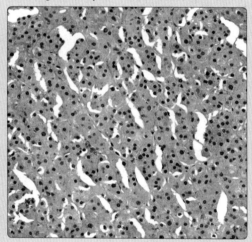

(Left) Gross photograph shows a cross section of an adrenal cortical neoplasm. This neoplasm is well circumscribed, encapsulated, and hemorrhagic with central degenerative changes. These are all frequent features of sex hormone-producing adenomas. (Right) High magnification shows an adrenal cortical adenoma that secretes sex steroids. This picture shows eosinophilic cells with abundant cytoplasm that resemble those cells in the zona reticularis.

Synaptophysin Reactivity

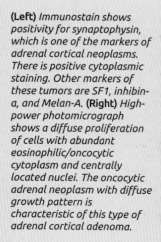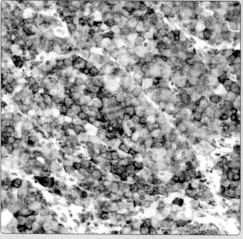

Cytological Features

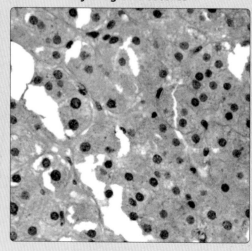

(Left) Immunostain shows positivity for synaptophysin, which is one of the markers of adrenal cortical neoplasms. There is positive cytoplasmic staining. Other markers of these tumors are SF1, inhibin-a, and Melan-A. (Right) High-power photomicrograph shows a diffuse proliferation of cells with abundant eosinophilic/oncocytic cytoplasm and centrally located nuclei. The oncocytic adrenal neoplasm with diffuse growth pattern is characteristic of this type of adrenal cortical adenoma.

TERMINOLOGY

Definitions

- Adrenal cortical adenoma with virilization &/or feminization

CLINICAL ISSUES

Epidemiology

- Incidence
  - Secretion of sex hormones is more commonly observed in adrenal cortical carcinoma
  - Only few cases of virilizing adrenal cortical adenomas
    - Only 10 virilizing adrenal tumors were described out of 190 cortical tumors collected over 3 years (5.3%)
- Age
  - Feminizing adrenal cortical neoplasms occur mostly between 25-45 years
  - Virilizing tumors, on other hand, are more prevalent in pediatric population

Presentation

- Virilization &/or feminization syndromes
  - Androgen excess in females leads to hirsutism, amenorrhea, virilization
  - Estrogen excess in males results in gynecomastia and impotence

Laboratory Tests

- Correlation with biochemical and endocrinologic data is essential for diagnosis

Natural History

- Rare tumors, usually tend to be in form of carcinomas more than adenomas (when present)

Treatment

- Surgical approaches
  - Adrenalectomy is treatment of choice

Prognosis

- Potential for malignancy
- Feminizing adrenal cortical neoplasms have tendency to be ominous

IMAGING

CT Findings

- Well circumscribed
- Smooth contour, round to oval in shape

MACROSCOPIC

General Features

- May be encapsulated and well circumscribed
- Those that are very large can have ominous characteristics like hemorrhage and necrosis

Size

- Testosterone-producing neoplasms have average weight of 473 g
- Feminizing neoplasms have average weight of 1,000 g; most measure > 12 cm in diameter

MICROSCOPIC

Histologic Features

- Cells resemble those of zona reticularis (responsible for sex steroids) and are compact with eosinophilic cytoplasm
- Attached adrenal remnant and contralateral adrenal cortex are not atrophic due to lack of glucocorticoid excretion

ANCILLARY TESTS

Immunohistochemistry

- Positive for SF1, synaptophysin, inhibin, and Melan-A
- Negative for chromogranin and cytokeratins

DIFFERENTIAL DIAGNOSIS

Pheochromocytoma

- Positive for chromogranin
- Negative for inhibin

Adrenal Cortical Carcinoma

- Hemorrhage and necrosis are frequently seen
- Invasive pattern, as opposed to well-circumscribed pattern of these lesions
- Mitotic rate is > 5/50 HPF

Other Adrenal Cortical Adenomas

- Based on hormonal secretory status and clinical symptoms

Metastatic Carcinoma

- Differential based on immunohistochemistry and morphology
  - Carcinomas are positive for cytokeratin
- Most frequent metastatic carcinomas are from kidney and lung origin

SELECTED REFERENCES

1. Ronchi CL et al: Genetic landscape of sporadic unilateral adrenocortical adenomas without PRKACA p.Leu206Arg mutation. J Clin Endocrinol Metab. 101(9):3526-38, 2016
2. Raymond VM et al: An oncocytic adrenal tumour in a patient with Birt-Hogg-Dubé syndrome. Clin Endocrinol (Oxf). 80(6):925-7, 2014
3. Assie G et al: Gene expression profiling in adrenocortical neoplasia. Mol Cell Endocrinol. 351(1):111-7, 2012
4. Akishima-Fukasawa Y et al: Malignant adrenal rest tumor of the retroperitoneum producing adrenocortical steroids. Endocr Pathol. 22(2):112-7, 2011
5. Lloyd RV: Adrenal cortical tumors, pheochromocytomas and paragangliomas. Mod Pathol. 24 Suppl 2:S58-65, 2011
6. Gruschwitz T et al: Improvement of histopathological classification of adrenal gland tumors by genetic differentiation. World J Urol. 28(3):329-34, 2010
7. Isaacs H Jr: Fetal and newborn adrenocortical tumors. Fetal Pediatr Pathol. 29(2):99-107, 2010
8. Lim YJ et al: Virilizing adrenocortical oncocytoma in a child: a case report. J Korean Med Sci. 25(7):1077-9, 2010
9. Danilowicz K et al: Androgen-secreting adrenal adenomas. Obstet Gynecol. 100(5 Pt 2):1099-102, 2002
10. Del Gaudio AD et al: Virilizing adrenocortical tumors in adult women. report of 10 patients, 2 of whom each had a tumor secreting only testosterone. Cancer. 72(6):1997-2003, 1993
11. Mattox JH et al: The evaluation of adult females with testosterone producing neoplasms of the adrenal cortex. Surg Gynecol Obstet. 164(2):98-101, 1987
12. Pollock WJ et al: Virilizing Leydig cell adenoma of adrenal gland. Am J Surg Pathol. 10(11):816-22, 1986
13. Coslovsky R et al: Female pseudohermaphroditism with adrenal cortical tumor in adulthood. J Endocrinol Invest. 8(1):63-5, 1985
14. Gabrilove JL et al: Feminizing adrenocortical tumors in the male. a review of 52 cases including a case report. Medicine (Baltimore). 44:37-79, 1965

Primary Pigmented Nodular Adrenocortical Disease

TERMINOLOGY

- Rare cause of ACTH-independent Cushing syndrome that may occur sporadically or in autosomal dominant familial form associated with Carney complex
- Characterized by bilateral adrenocortical hyperplasia

ETIOLOGY/PATHOGENESIS

- Familial as part of Carney complex
- Sporadic
- Autoimmune origin

CLINICAL ISSUES

- Corticotropin-independent Cushing syndrome
- Treatment: Bilateral adrenalectomy for Cushing syndrome

MACROSCOPIC

- Small- to normal-sized adrenal glands with multiple small, pigmented nodules

MICROSCOPIC

- Nodules are composed of cells with compact eosinophilic cytoplasm and abundant brown, granular pigment (lipofuscin)

ANCILLARY TESTS

- Most patients with Carney complex and PPNAD have inactivating mutations in *PRKAR1A*
  - Nonsense mutations, splice-site mutations, and loss of heterozygosity of *PRKAR1A* gene
- Mutations of *PDE11A* and *PDE8B* genes

TOP DIFFERENTIAL DIAGNOSES

- Cushing syndrome caused by primary cortisol-producing adrenocortical adenoma
- Corticotropin (ACTH)-independent bilateral macronodular adrenal hyperplasia
- Cushing disease
- Malignant melanoma

Numerous Pigmented Nodules

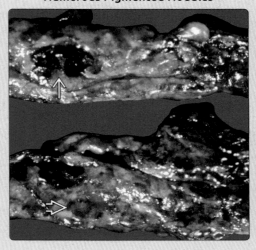

Multiple Nodules and Myelolipomatous Foci

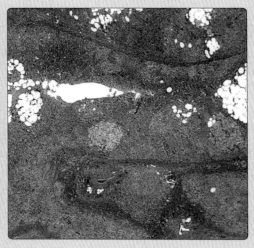

(Left) These bilateral adrenal glands show pigmented nodules that are jet black to gray-brown ➡. These nodules are usually small; however, some are macronodules resulting from a confluence of smaller nodules ➡. (Right) The microscopic evaluation of primary pigmented nodular adrenocortical disease (PPNAD) is less obvious than the gross examination. The pigmented nodules are small, round or oval, or may have irregular contours. The adjacent adrenal cortical tissue shows atrophy and lipomatous metaplasia.

PPNAD With Lipomatous Foci

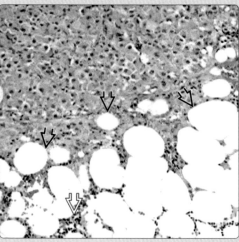

Pigment Deposits

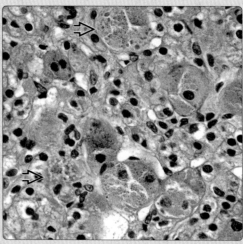

(Left) This nodule has focal compact cells with eosinophilic cytoplasm and prominent lipomatous metaplasia ➡ with a small component of lymphocytic infiltration ➡. (Right) The intranodular cells in PPNAD have lipid-depleted, compact, eosinophilic cytoplasm. Some have abundant, finely granular cytoplasmic lipofuscin pigment ➡ with focal accumulation of pigment.

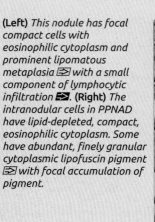

TERMINOLOGY

Abbreviations

- Primary pigmented nodular adrenocortical disease (PPNAD)

Synonyms

- Primary pigmented nodular adrenal disease
- Isolated or sporadic primary pigmented nodular adrenocortical disease (iPPNAD)
- PPNAD associated with Carney complex (CNC)
- Adrenocortical dysplasia
- Bilateral micronodular hyperplasia

Definitions

- Rare form of primary bilateral adrenal disease that is often associated with adrenocorticotropic hormone (ACTH)-independent Cushing syndrome (CS)
- Characterized by bilateral micronodular adrenocortical hyperplasia
- Can be inherited in autosomal dominant manner associated with CNC
- Nonfamilial, or isolated or sporadic (iPPNAD) forms also exist

ETIOLOGY/PATHOGENESIS

Etiology

- Unknown
- **Familial**
  - Can occur in familial form, inherited as autosomal dominant trait when associated with CNC
    - Known genetic heterogeneity in CNC
    - PPNAD is most frequent endocrine manifestation of CNC, occurring in ~ 1/4 of patients
- **Sporadic**
  - Can occur as nonfamilial isolated or sporadic form (iPPNAD)
- **Autoimmune origin**
  - May result from adrenal-stimulating antibodies, which stimulate corticotropin receptor sites in adrenal cortex

Genetic Abnormality

- Disorder has been mapped to genomic loci on chromosomes 2q15-16 and 17q22-24
- Inactivating mutations of *PRKAR1A* gene on 17q22-24 have been reported in most patients with CNC
- Inactivating mutations of phosphodiesterase 11A (*PDE11A*) located at 2q31-2q35 have been identified in sporadic PPNAD
- Despite known genetic heterogeneity in CNC, in most cases, PPNAD in its sporadic or isolated forms (iPPNAD) is caused by inactivating heterozygous mutations of *PRKAR1A* gene
  - Polypyrimidine tract mutation of *PRKAR1A* gene leading to probable mild alteration of PRKAR1A mRNA splicing
  - Compared with mutations described for *PRKAR1A* gene, exon 7 IVS del([-]7 → [-]2) has low penetrance and is almost exclusively associated with iPPNAD
- Strong genotype-phenotype correlation in CNC &/or PPNAD for *PRKAR1A* mutation

Pathogenesis

- All genetic events lead to constitutive activation of cAMP/PKA pathway, which results in hyperglucocortisolism and adrenocortical hyperplasia

CLINICAL ISSUES

Epidemiology

- Age
  - Patients with PPNAD in both sporadic and familial forms usually present in late childhood/early adulthood
- Sex
  - Slight female predominance

Presentation

- Most patients with PPNAD also have multiple neoplasia syndrome within CNC
- PPNAD in its sporadic or isolated forms is rare
- **Familial form as part of CNC: Autosomal dominant**
  - In addition to PPNAD, which is most common endocrine manifestation, CNC patients have
    - Myxomas
    - Spotty skin pigmentation
    - Cutaneous abnormalities
    - Schwannomas
    - Testicular tumors, including Leydig cell tumor and large cell calcifying Sertoli cell tumors
    - Mammary myxoid fibroadenoma
    - Pituitary macroadenoma
    - Psammomatous melanotic schwannoma
- **Sporadic or isolated Corticotropin-independent Cushing syndrome (iPPNAD)**
  - Establishing diagnosis of PPNAD can be challenging, particularly when PPNAD is only manifestation of disease; some signs are
    - Weight gain
    - Fatigue
    - Muscle weakness
    - Moon face
    - Facial flushing
    - Buffalo hump
    - Striae marks
    - Bruises
    - Depression, anxiety, and irritability
    - Irregular or absent menstrual periods in females

Laboratory Tests

- Plasma cortisol is usually moderately elevated without diurnal rhythm
- Plasma ACTH is low or undetectable
- Hypercortisolism is resistant to high-dose dexamethasone suppression test (HDDST), metyrapone stimulation, and corticotropin-releasing hormone stimulation

Treatment

- Surgical approaches
  - Bilateral adrenalectomy is treatment of choice for PPNAD in patients with Cushing syndrome

Prognosis

- Most tumors are slow growing without malignant potential

- Life span is decreased in patients with CNC due to increased incidence of sudden death caused by heart myxoma or its complications
- Genetic screening and long-term follow-up
- 90% of patients with CNC will develop other endocrine &/or nonendocrine tumors over time

IMAGING

CT Findings

- Bilateral irregular adrenal margins with nodules
- Size of adrenal can be normal

MACROSCOPIC

General Features

- Small to normal-sized adrenal glands
  - Rarely, slight increase in adrenal gland size
- Multiple small cortical nodules, 0.1-0.3 cm in diameter involving both glands
- Nodules may be pigmented, either brown or black
  - Some nodules may be pale to bright yellow

MICROSCOPIC

Histologic Features

- Nodules composed of cells with compact eosinophilic cytoplasm and abundant brown, granular pigment (lipofuscin)
- Cell nuclei are vesicular and may contain prominent eosinophilic nucleoli
- Intervening cortical tissue is atrophic

ANCILLARY TESTS

Serologic Testing

- Elevated basal cortisol
- Low ACTH
- High 24-hour urinary free cortisol
- Nonsuppressed cortisol after HDDST suggests ACTH-independent Cushing syndrome

Immunohistochemistry

- Increased expression of glucocorticoid receptor

Genetic Testing

- PPNAD in its sporadic or isolated forms (iPPNAD) is caused by inactivating heterozygous mutations of *PRKAR1A* gene, encoding regulatory subunit type I-α of cAMP-dependent protein kinase A (PKA)
  - Compared with other mutations described for *PRKAR1A* gene, exon 7 IVS del([-]7 → [-]2) has low penetrance and is almost exclusively associated with iPPNAD
- Most patients with CNC and PPNAD have inactivating mutations in *PRKAR1A*
  - Nonsense mutations, splice-site mutations, and loss of heterozygosity of *PRKAR1A* gene
  - Because disease-associated mutations result in complete loss of function, there is generally poor correlation between phenotype and genotype
- Mutations of *PDE11A* and *PDE8B* genes

DIFFERENTIAL DIAGNOSIS

Corticotropin (ACTH)-Independent Bilateral Macronodular Adrenal Hyperplasia

- Associated with tumefactive enlargement of both adrenal glands
- Also associated with bilateral adrenocortical nodules, but nodules are much larger
- On imaging, there is marked asymmetric nodularity throughout most of adrenal glands
- Associated with markedly enlarged adrenal glands
- Marked distortion of cortical architecture composed of lipid-rich cells with some lipid-depleted cells showing atrophy between nodules

Cushing Syndrome Caused by Primary Cortisol-Producing Adrenocortical Adenoma

- Patient presents with Cushing syndrome
- Lab: High cortisol, low ACTH
- Well-demarcated tumor lesion inside adrenal gland
- Gross: Single tumor nodule with expansile appearance, adjacent to grossly normal adrenal gland
- Tumor cells arranged in short cords or alveoli

Cushing Disease

- ACTH-dependent hypercortisolism caused by pituitary adenoma
- Lab: High cortisol, high ACTH
- MR shows mass in anterior pituitary gland
- Diffuse enlargement of adrenal cortex
- Grossly, diffuse adrenocortical hyperplasia
- Microscopically, diffuse adrenocortical hyperplasia without pigment deposition

Metastatic Malignant Melanoma

- Both diseases involve both adrenal glands
  - Immunohistochemistry for S100, HMB-45, Melan-A can readily separate both diseases

DIAGNOSTIC CHECKLIST

Pathologic Interpretation Pearls

- Adrenal glands usually normal in size
- Scattered small pigmented nodules ranging from light gray, gray-brown, dark brown, to jet black
- Histologically, pigmented nodules are round or oval; sporadic and familial forms have similar findings
- Unencapsulated nodules of mixed lipid-rich and lipid-depleted adrenocortical cells with expansile borders
- Intracytoplasmic pigment is lipofuscin

SELECTED REFERENCES

1. Kiefer FW et al: PRKAR1A mutation causing pituitary-dependent Cushing disease in a patient with Carney complex. Eur J Endocrinol. 177(2):K7-K12, 2017
2. Lowe KM et al: Cushing syndrome in Carney complex: clinical, pathologic, and molecular genetic findings in the 17 affected Mayo Clinic patients. Am J Surg Pathol. 41(2):171-181, 2017
3. Bram Z et al: PKA regulatory subunit 1A inactivating mutation induces serotonin signaling in primary pigmented nodular adrenal disease. JCI Insight. 1(15):e87958, 2016
4. Mineo R et al: A novel mutation in the type Iα regulatory subunit of protein kinase A (PRKAR1A) in a Cushing's syndrome patient with primary pigmented nodular adrenocortical disease. Intern Med. 55(17):2433-8, 2016

Immunohistochemistry in PPNAD

Immunostain	Cortical Nodules	Cortical Atrophy	Cortical Extrusions
Synaptophysin	Positive	Negative	Positive
Vimentin	Negative	Positive	Positive
Inhibin-A	Positive	Positive	Positive
Melan-A	Positive	Positive	Positive
CD56	Negative	Positive	Positive
β-catenin	Positive	Positive	Positive
Ki-67	Positive	Negative	Positive

Primary pigmented nodular adrenocortical disease = PPNAD.

Modified from Carney, et al, 2014.

5. Schernthaner-Reiter MH et al: MEN1, MEN4, and Carney complex: pathology and molecular genetics. Neuroendocrinology. 103(1):18-31, 2016

6. Stratakis CA: Carney complex: a familial lentiginosis predisposing to a variety of tumors. Rev Endocr Metab Disord. 17(3):367-371, 2016

7. Berthon AS et al: PRKACA: the catalytic subunit of protein kinase A and adrenocortical tumors. Front Cell Dev Biol. 3:26, 2015

8. Carney JA et al: Primary pigmented nodular adrenocortical disease: the original 4 cases revisited after 30 years for follow-up, new investigations, and molecular genetic findings. Am J Surg Pathol. 38(9):1266-73, 2014

9. Carney JA et al: Germline PRKACA amplification leads to Cushing syndrome caused by 3 adrenocortical pathologic phenotypes. Hum Pathol. 46(1):40-9, 2014

10. Guillaud Bataille M et al: Systematic screening for PRKAR1A gene rearrangement in Carney complex: identification and functional characterization of a new in-frame deletion. Eur J Endocrinol. 170(1):151-60, 2014

11. London E et al: Differences in adiposity in Cushing syndrome caused by PRKAR1A mutations: clues for the role of cyclic AMP signaling in obesity and diagnostic implications. J Clin Endocrinol Metab. 99(2):E303-10, 2014

12. Almeida MQ et al: Activation of cyclic AMP signaling leads to different pathway alterations in lesions of the adrenal cortex caused by germline PRKAR1A defects versus those due to somatic GNAS mutations. J Clin Endocrinol Metab. 97(4):E687-93, 2012

13. Anselmo J et al: A large family with Carney complex caused by the S147G PRKAR1A mutation shows a unique spectrum of disease including adrenocortical cancer. J Clin Endocrinol Metab. 97(2):351-9, 2012

14. Rauschecker M et al: Molecular genetics of adrenocortical tumor formation and potential pharmacologic targets. Minerva Endocrinol. 37(2):133-9, 2012

15. Azevedo MF et al: The transcriptome that mediates increased cAMP signaling in PRKAR1A defects and other settings. Endocr Pract. 17 Suppl 3:2-7, 2011

16. da Silva RM et al: Children with Cushing's syndrome: primary pigmented nodular adrenocortical disease should always be suspected. Pituitary. 14(1):61-7, 2011

17. Li Z et al: Corticotropin-independent Cushing's syndrome in patients with bilateral adrenal masses. Urology. 77(2):417-21, 2011

18. Libé R et al: Frequent phosphodiesterase 11A gene (PDE11A) defects in patients with Carney complex (CNC) caused by PRKAR1A mutations: PDE11A may contribute to adrenal and testicular tumors in CNC as a modifier of the phenotype. J Clin Endocrinol Metab. 96(1):E208-14, 2011

19. Zhang Y et al: Endocrine tumors as part of inherited tumor syndromes. Adv Anat Pathol. 18(3):206-18, 2011

20. Almeida MQ et al: Carney complex and other conditions associated with micronodular adrenal hyperplasias. Best Pract Res Clin Endocrinol Metab. 24(6):907-14, 2010

21. Carney JA et al: Familial micronodular adrenocortical disease, Cushing syndrome, and mutations of the gene encoding phosphodiesterase 11A4 (PDE11A). Am J Surg Pathol. 34(4):547-55, 2010

22. Courcoutsakis N et al: CT findings of primary pigmented nodular adrenocortical disease: rare cause of ACTH-independent Cushing syndrome. AJR Am J Roentgenol. 194(6):W541, 2010

23. Peck MC et al: A novel PRKAR1A mutation associated with primary pigmented nodular adrenocortical disease and the Carney complex. Endocr Pract. 16(2):198-204, 2010

24. Pereira AM et al: Association of the M1V PRKAR1A mutation with primary pigmented nodular adrenocortical disease in two large families. J Clin Endocrinol Metab. 95(1):338-42, 2010

25. Storr HL et al: Familial isolated primary pigmented nodular adrenocortical disease associated with a novel low penetrance PRKAR1A gene splice site mutation. Horm Res Paediatr. 73(2):115-9, 2010

26. Bertherat J et al: Mutations in regulatory subunit type 1A of cyclic adenosine 5'-monophosphate-dependent protein kinase (PRKAR1A): phenotype analysis in 353 patients and 80 different genotypes. J Clin Endocrinol Metab. 94(6):2085-91, 2009

27. Iliopoulos D et al: MicroRNA signature of primary pigmented nodular adrenocortical disease: clinical correlations and regulation of Wnt signaling. Cancer Res. 69(8):3278-82, 2009

28. Stratakis CA: New genes and/or molecular pathways associated with adrenal hyperplasias and related adrenocortical tumors. Mol Cell Endocrinol. 300(1-2):152-7, 2009

29. Tadjine M et al: Detection of somatic beta-catenin mutations in primary pigmented nodular adrenocortical disease (PPNAD). Clin Endocrinol (Oxf). 69(3):367-73, 2008

30. Horvath A et al: Primary pigmented nodular adrenocortical disease and Cushing's syndrome. Arq Bras Endocrinol Metabol. 51(8):1238-44, 2007

31. Stratakis CA: Adrenocortical tumors, primary pigmented adrenocortical disease (PPNAD)/Carney complex, and other bilateral hyperplasias: the NIH studies. Horm Metab Res. 39(6):467-73, 2007

32. Bertherat J: Carney complex (CNC). Orphanet J Rare Dis. 1:21, 2006

33. Cazabat L et al: PRKAR1A mutations in primary pigmented nodular adrenocortical disease. Pituitary. 9(3):211-9, 2006

34. Groussin L et al: A PRKAR1A mutation associated with primary pigmented nodular adrenocortical disease in 12 kindreds. J Clin Endocrinol Metab. 91(5):1943-9, 2006

35. Horvath A et al: Serial analysis of gene expression in adrenocortical hyperplasia caused by a germline PRKAR1A mutation. J Clin Endocrinol Metab. 91(2):584-96, 2006

36. Groussin L et al: Adrenal pathophysiology: lessons from the Carney complex. Horm Res. 64(3):132-9, 2005

37. Lacroix A et al: Bilateral adrenal Cushing's syndrome: macronodular adrenal hyperplasia and primary pigmented nodular adrenocortical disease. Endocrinol Metab Clin North Am. 34(2):441-58, x, 2005

38. Libé R et al: Molecular genetics of adrenocortical tumours, from familial to sporadic diseases. Eur J Endocrinol. 153(4):477-87, 2005

39. Sandrini F et al: Clinical and molecular genetics of Carney complex. Mol Genet Metab. 78(2):83-92, 2003

40. Groussin L et al: Mutations of the PRKAR1A gene in Cushing's syndrome due to sporadic primary pigmented nodular adrenocortical disease. J Clin Endocrinol Metab. 87(9):4324-9, 2002

41. Carney JA: Carney complex: the complex of myxomas, spotty pigmentation, endocrine overactivity, and schwannomas. Semin Dermatol. 14(2):90-8, 1995

42. Sasano H et al: Primary pigmented nodular adrenocortical disease (PPNAD): immunohistochemical and in situ hybridization analysis of steroidogenic enzymes in eight cases. Mod Pathol. 5(1):23-9, 1992

43. Doppman JL et al: Cushing syndrome due to primary pigmented nodular adrenocortical disease: findings at CT and MR imaging. Radiology. 172(2):415-20, 1989

44. Carney JA et al: The complex of myxomas, spotty pigmentation, and endocrine overactivity. Medicine (Baltimore). 64(4):270-83, 1985

45. Shenoy BV et al: Bilateral primary pigmented nodular adrenocortical disease. Rare cause of the Cushing syndrome. Am J Surg Pathol. 8(5):335-44, 1984

(Left) *In addition to PPNAD, which is the most common endocrine manifestation, Carney complex patients have the characteristic findings of spotty skin pigmentation in the mucocutaneous regions around eyes and lips. (Courtesy J.A. Carney, MD.)* **(Right)** *The normal adrenal gland architecture in PPNAD is replaced by multiple nodules, most of which are unencapsulated ⇗ but some with a thin fibrous capsule ⇉. The adjacent adrenal is atrophic.*

Characteristic Pigmentation

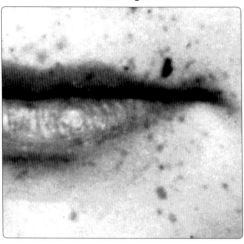

Low-Power View of PPNAD

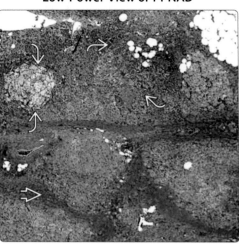

(Left) *Low power of an adrenal gland from a patient with PPNAD shows a nodule composed of cells with lipid-depleted cytoplasm ⇗ containing a small amount of finely granular lipofuscin pigment. Lipomatous metaplasia ⇗ is also present.* **(Right)** *Intranodular cells in PPNAD have lipid-depleted cytoplasm with finely granular to focally coarse cytoplasmic lipofuscin. The pigmented nodule cells may have pleomorphic nuclei and prominent nucleoli.*

Lipomatous Foci

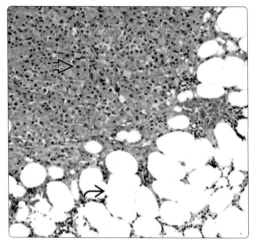

Lipid-Depleted Cells

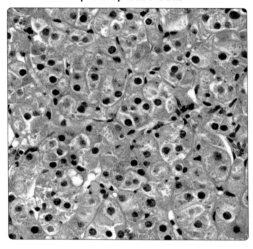

(Left) *The lipid-depleted, compact, and eosinophilic cells in PPNAD may have abundant, finely granular, cytoplasmic, orange-brown lipofuscin pigment with focal globular pigment formation ⇉. (Right) Cytologically, the cells are uniform, although occasional binucleated or cells with enlarged nuclei and prominent nucleoli can be seen. The lipid-poor eosinophilic cytoplasm may contain a finely granular, orange-brown lipofuscin pigment ⇗ with focal globular pigment.*

Pigment Deposition

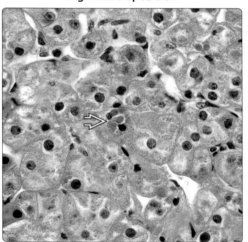

Lipofuscin Pigment

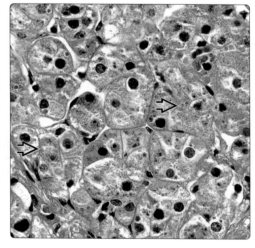

Small Cortical Nodules

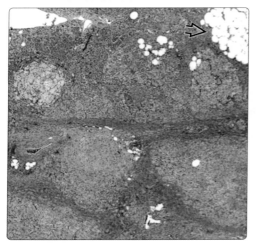

Extensive Pigment Deposition

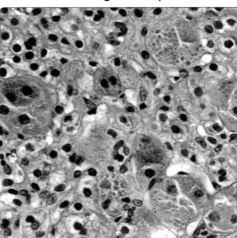

(Left) *Multiple nodules in PPNAD may be separated from each other by collagen bundles. The uninvolved adrenal cortex may show signs of atrophy and myelolipomatous metaplasia ➡. **(Right)** In some areas of the adrenal with PPNAD, there is extensive pigment deposition. The pigment often accumulates in the cytoplasm of the cells occupying the entire cytoplasm.*

Lipofuscin Accumulation

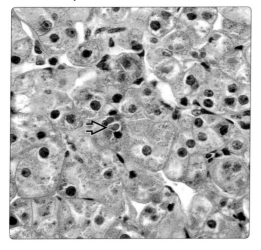

Clear Cytoplasm With Pigment

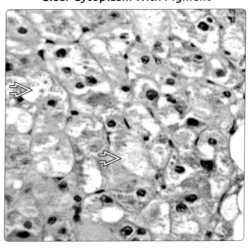

(Left) *The nodules are composed by enlarged globular cortical cells with granular eosinophilic cytoplasm with lipochrome pigment. The pigment often accumulates in the cytoplasm of the cells, forming a pigmented globule ➡. **(Right)** High-power view of a PPNAD nodule shows cells with abundant lipid-rich foamy and clear cytoplasm ➡ intermixed with cells that contain eosinophilic cytoplasm with finely granular orange-brown pigment (lipofuscin). Note slight nuclear pleomorphism.*

Malignant Melanoma

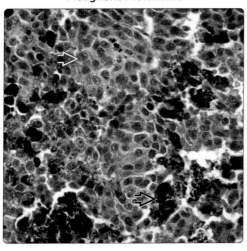

Cell Morphology in Melanoma

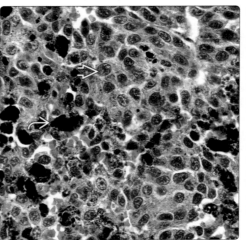

(Left) *Differential diagnosis of PPNAD: Primary adrenal melanoma shows pleomorphic cells and irregular nuclei ➡ with abundant brown granular pigment (melanin) ➡. The color of the pigment and immunohistochemistry will help in the diagnosis. **(Right)** Within the differential diagnosis of PPNAD is primary adrenal melanoma, which shows pleomorphic cells with irregular nuclei ➡ and abundant dark brown, coarsely granular melanin pigment ➡.*

Adrenal Cortical Oncocytoma

TERMINOLOGY

- Rare adrenal cortical epithelial neoplasm composed entirely of cells with large granular eosinophilic cytoplasms packed with mitochondria
- Oncocytic adrenocortical neoplasms

CLINICAL ISSUES

- Asymptomatic, often incidental finding

MACROSCOPIC

- Dark tan or mahogany brown, similar morphologic features as oncocytomas in other areas of the body
- Median size = 8.5 cm, median weight = 217.5 g

MICROSCOPIC

- Tumor is composed of polygonal cells with abundant, granular, intensely eosinophilic cytoplasm
- Most have diffuse, sheet-like pattern
- Prominent nuclear pleomorphism
- Eosinophilic nuclear pseudoinclusions

- Weiss system cannot be directly applied to oncocytic adrenal cortical neoplasms
  - Due to constant presence of diffuse growth pattern, eosinophilic cytoplasm, and high-grade nuclear features
- To diagnose tumor as adrenocortical oncocytoma, it must be considered benign according to Lin-Weiss-Bisceglia criteria
  - **Malignant**: Presence of any major criteria
  - **Borderline malignant potential**: Presence of any minor criteria
  - **Benign**: Absence of all criteria
- Lymphoid infiltrates can be seen

ANCILLARY TESTS

- Positive for SF1, synaptophysin, inhibin, and Melan-A
- Negative for HMB-45, S100, and EMA
- Most are negative for chromogranin and cytokeratin
- Positive for MES-13 (antimitochondrial antibody)

Adrenal Cortical Oncocytoma

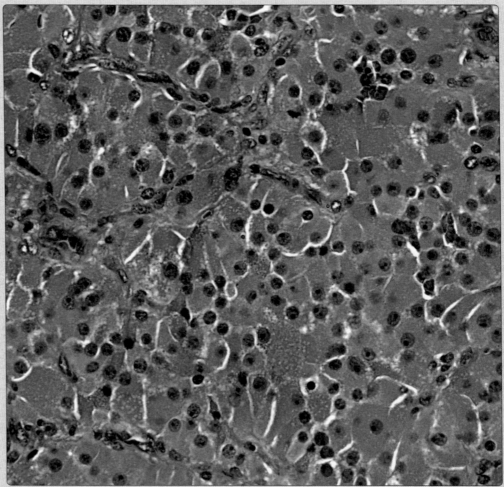

High-power view of a typical oncocytic adrenocortical neoplasm shows the large polygonal tumor cells with abundant, granular, eosinophilic cytoplasm in a diffuse architecture.

TERMINOLOGY

Synonyms
- Adrenal oncocytoma
- Oncocytic adrenal cortical adenoma
- Oncocytic adrenocortical neoplasms
- Incidentaloma

Definitions
- Rare adrenal cortical epithelial neoplasm composed entirely of large cells with granular eosinophilic cytoplasms packed with mitochondria

CLINICAL ISSUES

Epidemiology
- Incidence
  - Rare tumors that occur most frequently in salivary glands, kidneys, thyroid, parathyroids, and pituitary
  - Until recently, classification as separate entity in adrenal was debatable
- Age
  - Median: 46
- Sex
  - F:M (1.8:1)

Presentation
- Asymptomatic, often incidental finding
- Oncocytomas are usually nonfunctioning adenomas, but can be associated with androgen excess and virilization

Prognosis
- Usually considered benign in its biological behavior, however some carcinomas have been reported

MACROSCOPIC

General Features
- Dark tan or mahogany brown; similar morphologic features as oncocytomas in other areas
- Encapsulated mass with focal necrosis or hemorrhage

Size
- Median size: 8.5 cm
- Median weight: 217.5 g

MICROSCOPIC

Histologic Features
- Tumor is composed of polygonal cells with abundant, granular, intensely eosinophilic cytoplasm
- All or large percentage of tumor (> 90%) should be oncocytic to be called oncocytoma
- Most have diffuse, sheet-like pattern
- Isolated nuclear pleomorphism and prominent nucleoli
- Lymphoid infiltrates can be seen

Cytologic Features
- Prominent nuclear pleomorphism
- Eosinophilic nuclear pseudoinclusions
- Bizarre, multinucleated tumor giant cells can be seen; however, more common in malignant or borderline tumors

Criteria for Malignancy: Lin-Weiss-Bisceglia Criteria
- Major criteria
  - Mitotic rate > 5/50 HPF
  - Atypical mitotic figures
  - Venous invasion
- Minor criteria
  - Size > 10 cm &/or weight > 200 g
  - Necrosis (microscopic)
  - Capsular invasion
  - Sinusoidal invasion
- **Malignant**: Presence of any major criteria
- **Borderline malignant potential**: Presence of any minor criteria
- **Benign**: Absence of all criteria

ANCILLARY TESTS

Immunohistochemistry
- Positive for SF-1, synaptophysin, inhibin-α, and Melan-A
- Also positive for calretinin in most cases
- Negative for HMB-45, S100, and EMA
- Most negative for chromogranin and cytokeratin
- Positive for MES-13 (antimitochondrial antibody: Strong diffuse granular pattern)
- Reports of diffusely immunopositive for mitochondria and GLUT1

Serologic Testing
- Tumors considered nonfunctional, as they do not express enzymes involved in steroidogenesis

Electron Microscopy
- Numerous mitochondria and smooth endoplasmic reticulum in tumor cell cytoplasm

DIFFERENTIAL DIAGNOSIS

Adrenocortical Neoplasm
- ≥ 90% of cells in oncocytomas are oncocytes
- 50-90% oncocytes = mixed oncocytic/conventional
- < 50% oncocytes = conventional adrenocortical neoplasm with focal oncocytic differentiation
- Oncocytomas strongly positive for MES-13 (strong diffuse granular pattern), as opposed to weaker pattern in normal adrenocortical cells

Pheochromocytoma
- Negative for inhibin and positive for chromogranin

Renal Cell Carcinoma
- Negative for inhibin and synaptophysin
- Positive for CD10

Hepatocellular Carcinoma
- Negative for inhibin
- Positive for Hep-Par1

Metastatic Carcinoma
- Immunohistochemistry needed for differential diagnosis

Immunohistochemistry

Antibody	Reactivity	Staining Pattern	Comment
Inhibin	Positive	Cell membrane & cytoplasm	
SF1	Positive	Nuclear	
Melan-A103	Positive	Cytoplasmic	
Synaptophysin	Positive	Cytoplasmic	
mES-13	Positive	Cytoplasmic	
Calretinin	Positive	Nuclear & cytoplasmic	
Chromogranin-A	Negative		Helps to discriminate from pheochromocytoma
CK7	Negative		Helps to discriminate from other epithelial tumors
CK20	Negative		Helps to discriminate from other epithelial tumors
AE1/AE3	Negative		Helps to discriminate from other epithelial tumors
EMA	Negative		Helps to discriminate from other epithelial tumors
CD10	Negative		Helps to discriminate from renal cell carcinoma
S100	Negative		
RCC	Negative		Helps to discriminate from renal cell carcinoma
HMB-45	Negative		
Hep-Par1	Negative		Helps to discriminate from hepatocellular carcinoma

Differential Diagnosis of Oncocytoma

Features	Adrenal Cortical Adenoma	Adrenal Cortical Carcinoma	Oncocytoma
Size	Weight: < 50 g	Weight: > 100 g	Weight: 217 g
Gross characteristics	Well circumscribed, variable color	Invasive, variable color	Mahogany color
Cytology characteristics	May have atypia	Atypia present	Nuclear pleomorphism
Hormonal production	Often functional	Usually nonfunctional	Usually nonfunctional

Lin-Weiss-Bisceglia Criteria for Malignancy

Major Criteria	Minor Criteria
Mitotic rate > 5/50 HPF	Size > 10 cm &/or weight > 200 g
Atypical mitotic figures	Necrosis (microscopic)
Venous invasion	Capsular invasion
	Sinusoidal invasion

Malignant = presence of any major criteria; borderline malignant potential = presence of any minor criteria; benign = absence of all criteria.

DIAGNOSTIC CHECKLIST

Pathologic Interpretation Pearls

- Dark tan or mahogany brown grossly
- Tumor composed of polygonal cells with abundant, granular, intensely eosinophilic cytoplasm
- Do not apply Weiss criteria; instead use Lin-Weiss-Bisceglia criteria

SELECTED REFERENCES

1. Lam AK: Update on adrenal tumours in 2017 World Health Organization (WHO) of endocrine tumours. Endocr Pathol. ePub, 2017
2. Li H et al: Immunohistochemical distinction of metastases of renal cell carcinoma to the adrenal from primary adrenal nodules, including oncocytic tumor. Virchows Arch. 466(5):581-8, 2015
3. Yordanova G et al: Virilizing adrenal oncocytoma in a 9-year-old girl: rare neoplasm with an intriguing postoperative course. J Pediatr Endocrinol Metab. 28(5-6):685-90, 2015
4. Raymond VM et al: An oncocytic adrenal tumour in a patient with Birt-Hogg-Dubé syndrome. Clin Endocrinol (Oxf). 80(6):925-7, 2014
5. Sato N et al: Case report: adrenal oncocytoma associated with markedly increased FDG uptake and immunohistochemically positive for GLUT1. Endocr Pathol. 25(4):410-5, 2014
6. Mearini L et al: Adrenal oncocytic neoplasm: a systematic review. Urol Int. 91(2):125-33, 2013
7. Wong DD et al: Oncocytic adrenocortical neoplasms—a clinicopathologic study of 13 new cases emphasizing the importance of their recognition. Hum Pathol. 42(4):489-99, 2011
8. Sasano H et al: Recent advances in histopathology and immunohistochemistry of adrenocortical carcinoma. Endocr Pathol. 17(4):345-54, 2006
9. Bisceglia M et al: Adrenocortical oncocytic tumors: report of 10 cases and review of the literature. Int J Surg Pathol. 12(3):231-43, 2004
10. Sasano H et al: Adrenocortical oncocytoma. A true nonfunctioning adrenocortical tumor. Am J Surg Pathol. 15(10):949-56, 1991

Oncocytoma Gross Features

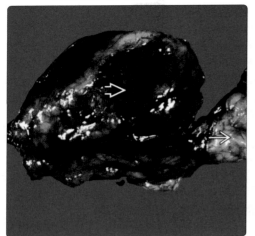

Well-Circumscribed Tumor

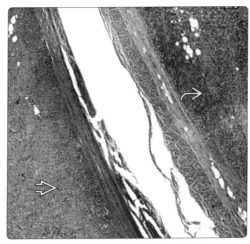

(Left) *Gross photo shows the external surface of an oncocytic neoplasm with the brown/mahogany tumor showing from behind the translucent capsule ⇒. Adjacent to the tumor, there is normal adrenal ⇒. The tumor is well circumscribed within the gland.* (Right) *Low-power photomicrograph shows a well-encapsulated neoplasm where the capsule separates the oncocytic neoplasm ⇒ from the normal adrenal ⇒.*

Oncocytic Cytoplasm

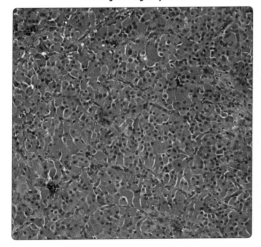

Solid Growth Pattern

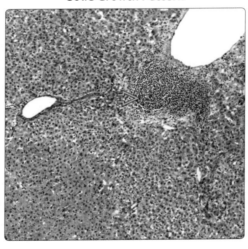

(Left) *High-power view shows the classic appearance of an oncocytic neoplasm. There is a diffuse pattern with sheets of polygonal, eosinophilic cells with an eosinophilic granular cytoplasm. There is nuclear pleomorphism as well, particularly at the top of this field.* (Right) *These oncocytic neoplasms may sometimes have lymphoid infiltrates, another characteristic of this type of tumor. The tumor is composed of large eosinophilic, polygonal cells, in sheets, with a focal lymphoid infiltrate ⇒.*

Large Cells With Ample Cytoplasm

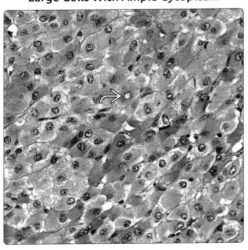

Synaptophysin Immunoreactivity

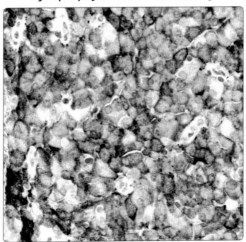

(Left) *H&E shows one of the cytologic characteristics of oncocytic neoplasms, which is the classic eosinophilic nuclear pseudoinclusion ⇒ typically seen in this tumor.* (Right) *Synaptophysin immunostaining shows both membranous and granular cytoplasmic positivity, a pattern seen in other adrenal neoplasms.*

TERMINOLOGY

- Catecholamine-secreting tumors from adrenal medulla or extraadrenal sympathetic paraganglia
  - Use of term pheochromocytoma (PCC) restricted to adrenal medulla
- Malignancy defined by documentation of metastases to sites where normal paraganglia not present
  - "Metastatic" preferred to "malignant" to avoid ambiguity

ETIOLOGY/PATHOGENESIS

- At least 30% of PCC hereditary; at least 20 susceptibility genes now known
- Most attributable to mutations in *RET*, *VHL*, *NF1*, *SDHB*, *SDHD*, *TMEM127*, and *MAX*
- *SDHx* mutations account for up to 80% of familial PCC/paraganglioma (PGL) aggregations, 30% of pediatric tumors, and > 40% of tumors that metastasize
- *SDHB* mutation associated with extraadrenal abdominal location, high probability of metastasis, and poor prognosis

CLINICAL ISSUES

- Identification of patients with hereditary PCC involves clinical assessment, biochemical testing, and pathology leading to genetic testing

MICROSCOPIC

- Classic pattern is small nests (zellballen) of neuroendocrine cells with interspersed small blood vessels

ANCILLARY TESTS

- Germline mutation testing vital for individual patient care and allows screening and early detection of disease in at-risk family members
- Immunohistochemistry for SDHB, SDHA, and MAX can serve as adjuncts genetic testing

TOP DIFFERENTIAL DIAGNOSES

- Adrenal cortical carcinoma
- Other neuroendocrine tumors

Pheochromocytoma

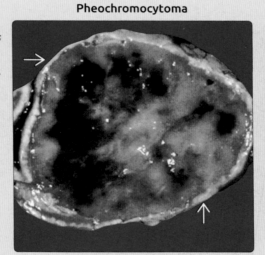

Carotid Body Paraganglioma

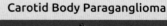

(Left) *The typical pheochromocytoma (PCC) has a gray-pink cut surface with areas of hemorrhage that distinguish it from the yellow-brown of adrenal cortex* ➡. (Right) *This gross photograph shows a carotid body paraganglioma encasing the carotid bifurcation (shown here in a transverse section* ➡) *and extensively invading the surrounding soft tissue.*

Pheochromocytoma

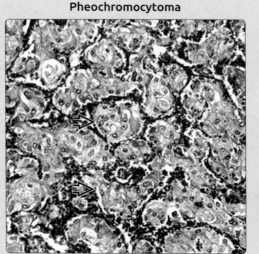

Carotid Body Paraganglioma

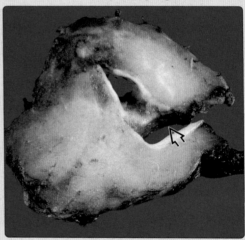

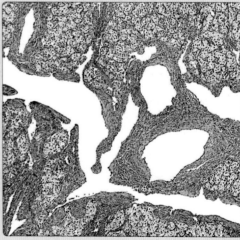

(Left) *The classic histologic pattern of pheochromocytoma is a small zellballen* ➡ *cellular arrangement with interspersed small blood vessels. The architecture is accentuated in this case by vascular congestion.* (Right) *Head and neck paragangliomas often show prominent zellballen, clear cells, and cavernous blood vessels mimicking vascular tumors or malformations.*

TERMINOLOGY

Abbreviations

- Pheochromocytoma (PCC)
- Paraganglioma (PGL)

Definitions

- Normal paraganglia consist of neural crest-derived neuroendocrine cells associated with sympathetic and parasympathetic nerves
  - Sympathetic (sympathoadrenal) paraganglia
    - Paraxial distribution in or near sympathetic ganglia and along branches of sympathetic nerves, predominantly those innervating pelvic and abdominal organs
    - Adrenal medulla in adults and organ of Zuckerkandl in fetuses are major sympathetic paraganglia; others microscopic
  - Parasympathetic (head and neck paraganglia)
    - Predominantly located along cranial and cervical branches of glossopharyngeal and vagus nerves
    - Carotid bodies are major parasympathetic paraganglia; others microscopic
- PCC and PGL are neuroendocrine tumors of neural crest origin that arise from adrenal medulla or extraadrenal paraganglia, respectively; PCC is intraadrenal sympathetic PGL
  - WHO definitions arbitrarily established terminology for tumors of paraganglia to eliminate previous inconsistent usage
    - By definition, PCC is neuroendocrine tumor arising from chromaffin cells of adrenal medulla; similar tumors in other locations are extraadrenal PGL, now abbreviated to just PGL
      - Sympathetic (sympathoadrenal) PGLs arise in vicinity of sympathetic chains and along sympathetic nerve branches in pelvic organs and retroperitoneum, sometimes mediastinum
      - Parasympathetic PGL arise mainly from branches of vagus and glossopharyngeal nerves in head and neck, sometimes mediastinum

ETIOLOGY/PATHOGENESIS

Hereditary Pheochromocytoma/Paraganglioma

- PCCs/PGLs have greatest degree of hereditary susceptibility of any human tumor
  - Up to 40% of PCCs/PGLs are hereditary
    - Occult germline mutations of hereditary susceptibility genes common in patients with apparently sporadic tumors
  - Striking genetic diversity; > 20 susceptibility genes now established
    - Up to ~ 32% of all individuals with PCC/PGL harbor germline mutation in one of 5 major susceptibility genes: VHL (~ 13%), SDHB (~ 8%), RET (~ 5%), SDHD (~ 5%), NF1 (~ 3%)
    - Less common: TMEM127 (~ 1-2%), MAX and SDHC (~ 1%), SDHA (< 1%)
    - Others very rare, some in single families or individuals

- Genotype-phenotype correlations affect tumor location, multiplicity, biochemical phenotype, risk of metastasis and syndromic associations
- Tumors with VHL or SDHx mutations have hypoxia-associated gene expression profile
- Tumors with RET and NF1 mutations characterized by expression of genes that mediate kinase signaling, translation initiation, protein synthesis, anabolic functions of activated RAS
  - Sporadic tumors or those with other mutations often segregate with one or other gene profile cluster; some may have intermediate profile

Sporadic Pheochromocytoma/Paraganglioma

- Majority of PCCs appear to arise sporadically
  - Germline mutations in known susceptibility genes may be seen in up to 16% of sporadic-appearing cases
- Somatic mutations of hereditary susceptibility genes relatively uncommon except for NF1
  - NF1 mutated in > 25% of sporadic tumors, VHL ~ 9%, RET ~ 5%
  - Changes in copy number of some hereditary susceptibility genes may be present
- Somatic mutations of common cancer driver genes occasionally present (HRAS, ATRX, VHL, EPAS1, TP53)
- New class of Wnt-altered PCCs/PGLs driven by MAML3 fusions and CSDE1 somatic mutations reported in 2017 Cancer Genome Atlas (TCGA) study
- Extremely low mutation burden in individual tumors; > 1 driver mutation rare

Environmental Influences

- High-altitude PGL in people and cattle living in mountainous areas of some countries
  - Possible modifier effect in genetically predisposed individuals
  - Mostly carotid PGL

CLINICAL ISSUES

Epidemiology

- Incidence
  - Precise incidence and prevalence not available because of varied reporting and occult cases; all current figures are estimates
  - Combined annual incidence of PCC and sympathetic PGL in all sites is ~ 0.4-9.5/million
    - < 3,000 cases each year in United States
  - Head and neck PGL (HNP) much rarer (~ 0.5-2/million)
- Age and sex
  - Most PCC and PGL present in 4th to 5th decades; ~ equal sex distribution
    - HNP shows female predominance
      - F:M ratio most pronounced in populations at high altitudes (up to 8:1)
  - Presentation in childhood strongly suggests hereditary susceptibility
  - Hereditary disease usually presents before age 40 but can present in elderly

Site

- Abdomen and pelvis: ~ 80-85% of all paragangliomas, ~ 98% of all sympathetic PGLs

- ~ 90% adrenal, 10% extraadrenal PGL
  - Extraadrenal abdominal & pelvic PGL ~ 1/10 as common as PCC in adults, up to 1/3 as common in children
- Head and neck: ~ 3% of all paragangliomas; ~ 100% of parasympathetic PGLs
  - Most are carotid (57%), followed by jugular (23%), vagal (~ 13%), and tympanic (~ 6%)
  - Head and neck sites account for ~ 0.6% of all tumors

Presentation

- Depends on tumor location
  - Sympathoadrenal PCCs/PGLs usually cause signs and symptoms of catecholamine excess
    - Tumors with *SDHB* gene mutation more likely than other sympathoadrenal PCCs/PGLs to be clinically silent
  - Parasympathetic PGLs usually clinically silent mass lesions
- Affected by genotype
  - Sporadic tumors solitary, usually in adults
  - Multiple tumors or tumors presenting in children suggest hereditary disease
  - Tumors with *RET* or *NF1* mutations almost always intraadrenal
  - Abdominal PGL or combination of sympathetic and parasympathetic PCC/PGL suggests *SDHx* mutation
- Confounded by complexity of tumor syndromes
  - Often highly varied penetrance and manifestation
  - Hereditary PCC/PGL syndromes may be found only after other stigmata point to hereditary basis (MEN2, VHL, NF1, SDH related)
    - New syndromic associations include gastrointestinal stromal tumors with *NF1* or *SDHx* mutations, renal cell CA with *VHL* or *SDHx*
    - Some patients develop only these tumors
  - Patients with occult germline mutations can present with apparently sporadic PCC/PGL
  - Mutations of some genes (e.g., *TMEM127*) cause hereditary but usually nonsyndromic PCC/PGL (no associated abnormalities)
  - *SDHD-* and *SDHAF2-* and *MAX*-related PGL show parent-of-origin dependent penetrance; tumor development only with paternal inheritance
  - Some PGL syndromic but not hereditary, e.g., Carney triad

Laboratory Tests

- Biochemical profile correlates with tumor genotype and location
- O-methylated metabolites more sensitive than corresponding catecholamines for tumor detection
  - PCC: Metanephrine &/or normetanephrine
  - Extraadrenal sympathetic PGL: Almost always normetanephrine &/or dopamine metabolite methoxytyramine
  - Head & neck PGL can lack ability for catecholamine biosynthesis or produce only methoxytyramine
  - Noradrenergic PCC raises suspicion of VHL disease
  - Dopamine/methoxytyramine: Sometimes produced by clinically nonfunctional tumors, especially with *SDHx* mutations, and tumors that metastasize

Treatment

- Complete surgical excision only cure
- Unresectable primary tumors and metastases can have long doubling time; active surveillance often viable option, especially to avoid complications in head and neck
- Potential new modalities target metabolic vulnerabilities caused by *SDHx* mutations

Prognosis

- Most patients with metastases eventually die from complications of excess catecholamines or destructive local growth

Malignancy

- WHO 2004 defined malignancy by presence of metastasis
  - Must be to sites where normal paraganglia not present to avoid confusion with new primary tumor
  - Term "metastatic" preferred to "malignant" to avoid ambiguity
- Currently, no generally accepted histological criteria to predict whether primary PCC or PGL will metastasize
  - Extensive local invasion alone poor predictor of metastasis
  - Limited predictive value of tumor size
- Risk of metastasis and prognosis vary with tumor location and genotype
  - ~ 10% metastasis for PCCs, > 20% for abdominal PGLs
  - Best predictor of metastasis is presence of *SDHB* mutation (> 30%)
    - After metastases occur, worst prognosis for tumors caused by *SDHB* mutation
- Staging system introduced in 8th edition of AJCC staging manual
  - Size > 5 cm **or** extraadrenal abdominal location automatically T2
  - Does not account for *SDHB* mutation
- Metastases can develop years or decades after resection of primary tumor
  - Currently recommended that no PCC/PGL be signed out as benign; all patients receive lifelong follow-up

IMAGING

General Features

- Anatomic imaging
  - MR: Very intense T2-weighted image (light bulb sign) classic but not always present
  - Contrast-enhanced CT
- Functional imaging
  - More specific because based on specific aspects of tumor phenotype
  - More sensitive for small tumors or metastases in bone
  - Efficacy of different functional imaging techniques varies according to tumor genotype and function
  - Somatostatin receptor imaging by PET/CT using recently developed DOTA; conjugated somatostatin analogs most sensitive modality

MACROSCOPIC

General Features

- Cut surface usually pink-gray to tan, distinguishes PCCs from yellow-gold of most adrenal cortical tumors
- Occasional tumors show patchy or diffuse brown pigmentation
- Hemorrhage and necrosis sometimes present
  - Extensive cystic change can result from resorbed hemorrhage
- Medullary hyperplasia, when present, may indicate hereditary form of disease

MICROSCOPIC

Histologic Features

- Classic pattern is small nests (zellballen) of neuroendocrine cells (chief cells) with interspersed small blood vessels
- Numerous variant and combined patterns exist, including diffuse growth, large zellballen, spindle cells, cell cords
- Sustentacular cells variably present, best seen with IHC
  - Possibly nonneoplastic cell type induced or attracted by tumor-derived factors
  - Rare or absent in metastases
- Cavernous blood vessels sometimes prominent, especially in HNP

Cytologic Features

- Tumor cells often smaller or larger than normal chromaffin cells, inconspicuous or large nucleoli
- Nuclear pseudoinclusions, embracing cells, extracellular hyaline globules variably present
- Basophilic, amphophilic, or clear cytoplasm
  - Clear cytoplasm particularly likely in parasympathetic PGL
- Extreme pleomorphism and hyperchromasia can be seen in benign tumors
- Mitoses usually rare

ANCILLARY TESTS

Immunohistochemistry

- Generic neuroendocrine markers chromogranin (CgA or CgB) and synaptophysin usually positive in chief cells; keratins usually negative
  - Can be expressed in patchy distribution and Golgi dot-like distribution in minimally functional or nonfunctional tumors
  - Parasympathetic PGL can be negative for CgA and positive for CgB
- Sustentacular cells stain for S100
- Tyrosine hydroxylase (TH) identifies ability to synthesize catecholamines
  - Helpful to discriminate PCC or PGL from other neuroendocrine tumors
  - Often negative in parasympathetic PGL
  - Elevated metanephrines or methoxytyramine after resection of TH(-) PGL suggests 2nd primary, not metastasis

- SDHB and SDHA important new markers for multiple purposes: Triage for genetic testing or surrogate test where testing not available; validate genetic sequence variants of unknown significance (VUS); assess whether any particular tumor part of syndrome or coincidental in patient with known or suspected SDHx mutation
  - SDHB protein lost in PCC/PGL with *SDHA*, *SDHB*, *SDHC*, or *SDHD* mutations; SDHA protein lost only when *SDHA* mutated
  - Endothelial cells serve as intrinsic positive controls
- MAX protein may similarly be lost in tumors with *MAX* mutations

Genetic Testing

- Germline mutation testing
  - Vital for individual patient care
  - Initiates screening and early detection of disease in at-risk family members
- Major genes causing hereditary PCCs/PGLs are *RET* (causes MEN2A and MEN2B), *VHL*, *NF1*, *SDHx*
- Caveat is that testing only detects abnormalities in genes added to testing panels, can fail to identify hereditary cases with mutations of uncommon susceptibility genes
  - New panels proposed to keep pace with newly discovered and rare genes

DIFFERENTIAL DIAGNOSIS

Adrenal Cortical Carcinoma

- Synaptophysin immunoreactivity present in both cortical and medullary tumors and should not be used in this differential diagnosis
- Chromogranin (-), TH(-), melan A(+), calretinin (+)

Other Neuroendocrine Tumors

- Neuroendocrine carcinomas and carcinoids, pancreatic endocrine tumors, medullary thyroid carcinoma
- Chromogranin and keratins positive
- TH usually negative but positive in some intestinal neuroendocrine tumors
- Tissue-specific hormones (e.g., calcitonin in medullary thyroid carcinoma, serotonin in intestinal neuroendocrine tumors) helpful, but some can be produced ectopically in PCC/PGL

Hepatocellular Carcinomas

- Absence of neuroendocrine markers, presence of keratins &/or tissue-specific markers

Renal Cell Carcinoma

- Absence of neuroendocrine markers, presence of keratins &/or CD10, RCC (renal cell carcinoma), and other tissue-specific markers

Alveolar Soft Part Sarcomas

- Absence of neuroendocrine markers, presence of soft tissue-specific marker: TFE3

Glomus Tumors and Glomangiomas

- Location: Outside distribution of paraganglia
- Presence of smooth muscle actin and muscle-specific actin

Tumor Distributions in Major Familial Paraganglioma Syndromes

Syndrome	Gene (Chromosome)	Adrenal	Other Sympathetic	Head & Neck	Other Tumors
MEN2A and MEN2B	*RET* (10q11)	(+++)	(+/-)	(+/-)	**Medullary thyroid carcinoma**, parathyroid adenoma (MEN2A only)
VHL	*VHL* (3p25-26)	(+++)	(++)	(+/-)	**RCC, clear cell type**, **hemangioblastoma**, endolymphatic sac tumor, pancreatic & intestinal NETs, epididymal papillary cystadenoma; cysts in liver, kidneys, and pancreas
NF1	*NF1* (17q11.2)	(+++)	(+/-)	(+/-)	**Neurofibroma**, MPNST, CNS gliomas, duodenal NET (typically somatostatinoma), GIST (typically small bowel, spindle cell type)
PGL 1-5	Familial paraganglioma syndromes, SDH related				**RCC, SDH-deficient type**, **GIST, SDH-deficient type** (typically gastric, epithelioid type), pituitary adenoma
No formal syndrome	*TMEM127* (2q11.2) (membrane protein involved in protein trafficking)	(+)	(+/-)	(+/-)	RCC (clear cell type)
No formal syndrome	*MAX* (14q23.3)	(+)			Renal oncocytoma

GIST = gastrointestinal stromal tumor; MPNST = malignant peripheral nerve sheath tumor; NET = neuroendocrine tumor; RCC = renal cell carcinoma.

Squamous Cell Carcinomas

- Absence of neuroendocrine markers, presence of keratins &/or p63

SELECTED REFERENCES

1. Currás-Freixes M et al: PheoSeq: A targeted next-generation sequencing assay for pheochromocytoma and paraganglioma diagnostics. J Mol Diagn. ePub, 2017
2. Fishbein L et al: Comprehensive molecular characterization of pheochromocytoma and paraganglioma. Cancer Cell. 31(2):181-193, 2017
3. Gasparotto D et al: Quadruple-negative GIST is a sentinel for unrecognized neurofibromatosis type 1 syndrome. Clin Cancer Res. 23(1):273-282, 2017
4. Schaefer IM et al: MAX inactivation is an early event in GIST development that regulates p16 and cell proliferation. Nat Commun. 8:14674, 2017
5. Korpershoek E et al: Complex MAX rearrangement in a family with malignant pheochromocytoma, renal oncocytoma, and erythrocytosis. J Clin Endocrinol Metab. 101(2):453-60, 2016
6. Brito JP et al: Testing for germline mutations in sporadic pheochromocytoma/paraganglioma: a systematic review. Clin Endocrinol (Oxf). 82(3):338-45, 2015
7. Dahia PL: Pheochromocytoma and paraganglioma pathogenesis: learning from genetic heterogeneity. Nat Rev Cancer. 14(2):108-19, 2014
8. Evenepoel L et al: Toward an improved definition of the genetic and tumor spectrum associated with SDH germ-line mutations. Genet Med. 17(8):610-20, 2015
9. Favier J et al: Paraganglioma and phaeochromocytoma: from genetics to personalized medicine. Nat Rev Endocrinol. 11(2):101-11, 2015
10. Hernandez KG et al: Familial pheochromocytoma and renal cell carcinoma syndrome: TMEM127 as a novel candidate gene for the association. Virchows Arch. 466(6):727-3, 2015
11. Bayley JP et al: Paraganglioma and pheochromocytoma upon maternal transmission of SDHD mutations. BMC Med Genet. 15:111, 2014
12. Korpershoek E et al: Adrenal medullary hyperplasia is a precursor lesion for pheochromocytoma in MEN2 syndrome. Neoplasia. 16(10):868-73, 2014
13. LeBlanc M et al: Synchronous adrenocortical neoplasms, paragangliomas, and pheochromocytomas: syndromic considerations regarding an unusual constellation of endocrine tumors. Hum Pathol. 45(12):2502-6, 2014
14. Lefebvre M et al: Pheochromocytoma and paraganglioma syndromes: genetics and management update. Curr Oncol. 21(1):e8-e17, 2014
15. Shuch B et al: The genetic basis of pheochromocytoma and paraganglioma: implications for management. Urology. 83(6):1225-32, 2014
16. Valencia E et al: Neurofibromatosis type 1 and GIST: is there a correlation? Anticancer Res. 34(10):5609-12, 2014
17. Dahia PL: Novel hereditary forms of pheochromocytomas and paragangliomas. Front Horm Res. 41:79-91, 2013
18. Dahia PL: The genetic landscape of pheochromocytomas and paragangliomas: somatic mutations take center stage. J Clin Endocrinol Metab. 98(7):2679-81, 2013
19. Rao JU et al: Genotype-specific abnormalities in mitochondrial function associate with distinct profiles of energy metabolism and catecholamine content in pheochromocytoma and paraganglioma. Clin Cancer Res. 19(14):3787-95, 2013
20. Rattenberry E et al: A comprehensive next generation sequencing-based genetic testing strategy to improve diagnosis of inherited pheochromocytoma and paraganglioma. J Clin Endocrinol Metab. 98(7):E1248-56, 2013
21. Toledo RA et al: In vivo and in vitro oncogenic effects of HIF2A mutations in pheochromocytomas and paragangliomas. Endocr Relat Cancer. 20(3):349-59, 2013
22. Burnichon N et al: MAX mutations cause hereditary and sporadic pheochromocytoma and paraganglioma. Clin Cancer Res. 18(10):2828-37, 2012
23. Janeway KA et al: Defects in succinate dehydrogenase in gastrointestinal stromal tumors lacking KIT and PDGFRA mutations. Proc Natl Acad Sci U S A. 108(1):314-8, 2011
24. Neumann HP et al: Germline mutations of the TMEM127 gene in patients with paraganglioma of head and neck and extraadrenal abdominal sites. J Clin Endocrinol Metab. 96(8):E1279-82, 2011
25. Stratakis CA et al: The triad of paragangliomas, gastric stromal tumours and pulmonary chondromas (Carney triad), and the dyad of paragangliomas and gastric stromal sarcomas (Carney-Stratakis syndrome): molecular genetics and clinical implications. J Intern Med. 266(1):43-52, 2009
26. van Nederveen FH et al: An immunohistochemical procedure to detect patients with paraganglioma and phaeochromocytoma with germline SDHB, SDHC, or SDHD gene mutations: a retrospective and prospective analysis. Lancet Oncol. 10(8):764-71, 2009
27. Wu D et al: Observer variation in the application of the pheochromocytoma of the adrenal gland scaled score. Am J Surg Pathol. 33(4):599-608, 2009

Pheochromocytoma With Mixed-Cell Population

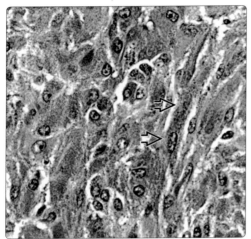

Pheochromocytoma With Spindle Cells

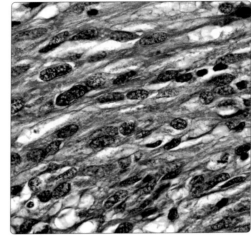

(Left) Spindle cells ⊞ can be a minor component of pheochromocytomas, as in this example. (Right) Some tumors are composed entirely of spindle cells, as in this example, and no classic pattern (zellballen) may be evident.

Pheochromocytoma With Mosaic-Like Pattern

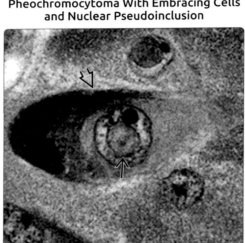

Pheochromocytoma With Embracing Cells and Nuclear Pseudoinclusion

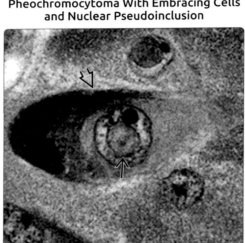

(Left) Some PCCs/PGLs, particularly if they are well fixed, show a mosaic-like pattern of often large cells with granular basophilic cytoplasm admixed with cells that have amphophilic to slightly eosinophilic cytoplasm. The basophilia is probably caused by abundant granin proteins, which are very acidic. (Right) This PCC shows a pair of "embracing" tumor cells ⊞ and a nuclear pseudoinclusion ➔. Nuclear pseudoinclusions are seen in both PCC/PGL and adrenal cortical tumors.

Pheochromocytoma With Extreme Atypia

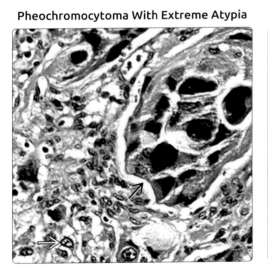

Pheochromocytoma With Small Cells and Diffuse Architecture

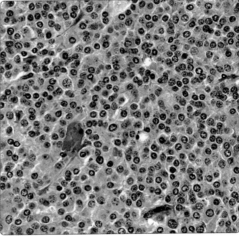

(Left) This photomicrograph of a pheochromocytoma shows large zellballen formed by large bizarre cells with ample cytoplasm and with extreme nuclear atypia ➔. The adjacent tumor tissue is composed of small tumor cells with no cellular pleomorphism ➔. (Right) Some PCCs/PGLs lack the typical pattern of small nests (zellballen) of neuroendocrine cells with interspersed small blood vessels and instead may show a diffuse growth pattern, as in this case.

Necrosis and Hemorrhage

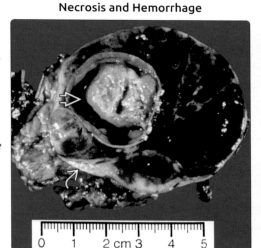

Necrosis

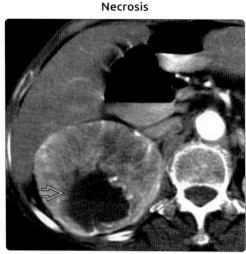

(Left) *Gross image shows the cut surface of a well-circumscribed adrenal PCC with a central area of necrosis ➡ and hemorrhage. Note small amount of residual adrenal cortex ➡. (Right) Axial CECT shows a large, well-circumscribed, moderately enhancing right adrenal PCC with a hypodense area of necrosis ➡.*

Large Cystic Pheochromocytoma

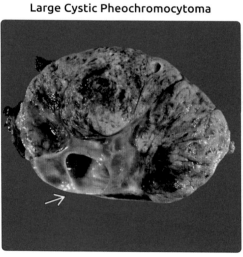

Gross Cut Surface

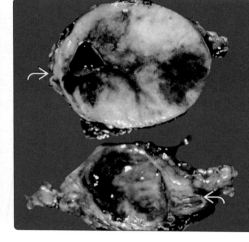

(Left) *This 14-cm pheochromocytoma contains a cyst formed by resorption of an old hemorrhagic infarct ➡. Recent areas of liquefactive degeneration and hemorrhage are also present. (Right) Gross image shows the cut surface of a well-circumscribed adrenal PCC with an area of hemorrhage. The gross appearance of PCCs is variable and may mimic other tumors. Small residual adrenal cortex is present ➡.*

Adrenal Medullary Hyperplasia and Pheochromocytoma

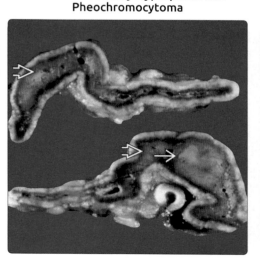

Gross Cut Surface

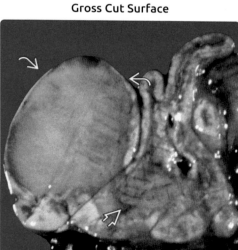

(Left) *This adrenal gland shows both MEN2-associated adrenal medullary hyperplasia ➡ and a microPCC ➡. Adrenal medullary hyperplasia is characteristic of MEN2. (Right) This adrenal gland shows both MEN2-associated PCC and adrenal medullary hyperplasia ➡, which is characteristic of MEN2. The cut surface is gray-pink, which distinguishes it from the yellow adrenal cortex ➡.*

Cytoplasmic Characteristics

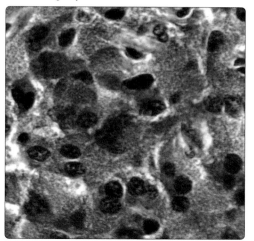

Mitosis and Eosinophilic Cytoplasm

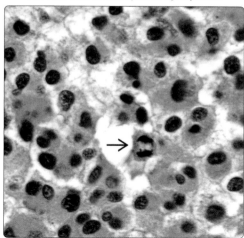

(Left) *PCC may contain cells with ample basophilic, amphophilic, or clear cytoplasm. This figure highlights the characteristic basophilic granular cytoplasm of some of these tumors.* (Right) *Although the classic histologic pattern of PCC is a zellballen pattern, numerous variants and combined patterns exist, including diffuse growth, large zellballen, spindle cells, and cell cords. Note the mitotic figure* ⇨.

Pleomorphic Cells

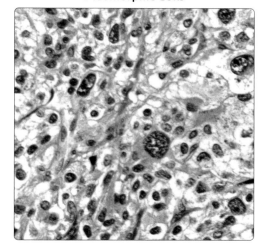

Hyaline Globules

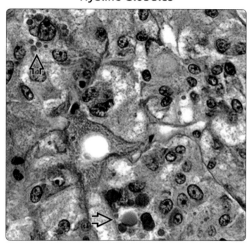

(Left) *The growth of this PCC is patternless with thin fibrous septa but lacking the zellballen cellular arrangement. There is marked variability in cell size with scattered pleomorphic cells surrounded by tumor cells with clear cytoplasm.* (Right) *The classic histologic pattern of PCC is a small zellballen cellular arrangement. Hyaline globules* ⇨ *are particularly conspicuous in PCCs of patients with MEN2.*

Unusual Architecture in Pheochromocytoma

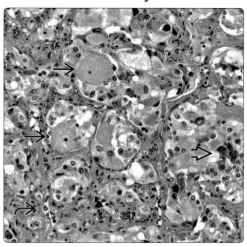

Unusual Architecture in Paraganglioma

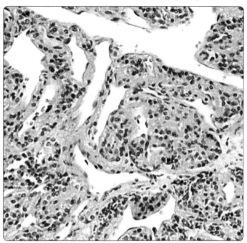

(Left) *This unusual PCC from a patient with MEN2A shows individual zellballen with degenerative changes* ⇨, *prominent thick-walled blood vessels* ⇨, *and scattered pigmented tumor cells* ⇨. (Right) *The tumor cells in this jugular PGL show an unusual pericyte-like distribution.*

(Left) *Immunohistochemistry for the proliferation marker Ki-67 ⇲ usually shows a low proliferative labeling index, often < 2-3%, in both primary and metastatic pheochromocytomas and paragangliomas, consistent with the usual slow doubling time of these tumors.* **(Right)** *A high Ki-67 labeling index is unusual in PCC/PGL and, when present, is sometimes associated with aggressive tumor behavior. This carotid PGL showed angioinvasion and extensive soft tissue infiltration.*

Paraganglioma

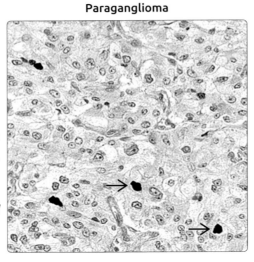

Carotid Body Paraganglioma

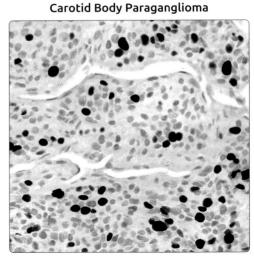

(Left) *Chromogranin-A immunostain shows granular immunoreactivity in the neuroendocrine cell nests between cavernous blood vessels in a carotid PGL. Note the negativity of the endothelial cells for this marker.* **(Right)** *S100 stain in a paraganglioma shows nuclear and cytoplasmic staining of sustentacular cells, which sometimes have conspicuous cytoplasmic processes ⇲. The chief cells are usually negative for this marker but sometimes show weak staining.*

Carotid Body Paraganglioma

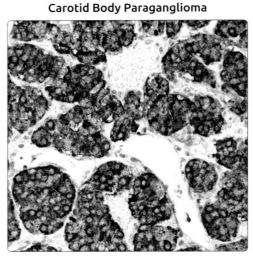

Paraganglioma

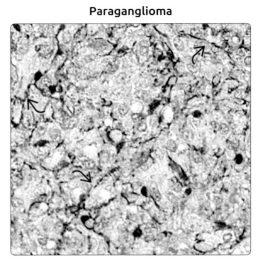

(Left) *Stain for tyrosine hydroxylase can be negative in parasympathetic PGL ⇲, which can be both clinically and biochemically nonfunctional. The adjacent nerve ⇲ is positive for tyrosine hydroxylase.* **(Right)** *Immunohistochemical stain for tyrosine hydroxylase is variably positive in pheochromocytomas, and most extraadrenal sympathetic PGL and TYH is necessary for synthesis of catecholamines.*

Carotid Body Paraganglioma

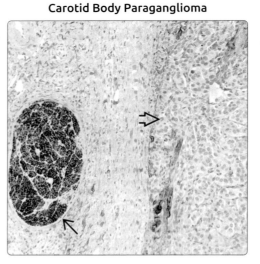

Pheochromocytoma

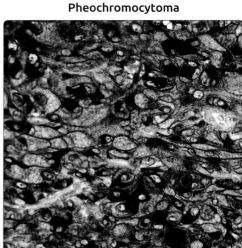

Endolymphatic Sac Tumor

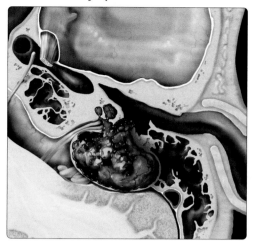

Endolymphatic Sac Tumor in VHL

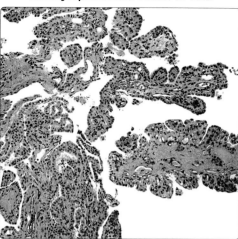

(Left) Axial graphic of temporal bone shows the typical appearance of endolymphatic sac tumor seen in patients with von Hippel-Lindau (VHL). The tumor is vascular, shows a tendency to fistulize the inner ear, and contains bone fragments within the tumor matrix. (Right) Endolymphatic sac tumors typically show a papillary architecture with fibrovascular cores and a single row of columnar epithelium with pale eosinophilic cytoplasm. These tumors are usually present in VHL syndrome.

VHL Syndrome

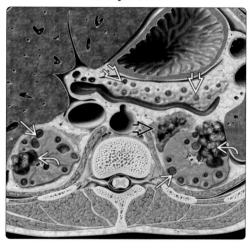

Pheochromocytoma in VHL

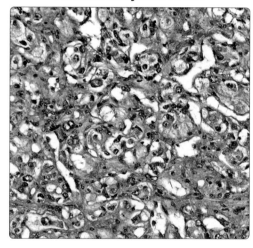

(Left) Graphic representation of abdominal lesions in VHL syndrome shows multiple bilateral renal cysts ➡, renal tumors ➡, pancreatic cysts ➡, and PCC ➡. PCC or PGL occurs in about 10-26% of VHL patients. (Right) This PCC from a patient with VHL shows a pattern of small cells with clear or slightly myxoid cytoplasm forming small zellballen with interspersed small blood vessels. This pattern is reported but inconsistently present in VHL disease.

Small Intestine GIST

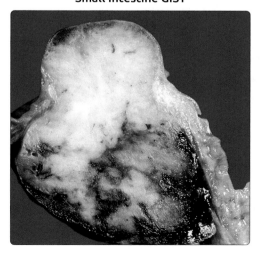

Gastric GIST

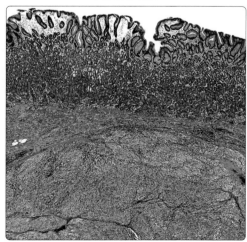

(Left) Gross photograph shows a small intestinal gastrointestinal stromal tumor (GIST). Small intestine is the typical location for GISTs in neurofibromatosis. (Right) Hematoxylin & eosin shows low magnification of a gastric GIST that involved the muscularis propria of the gastric body. The GIST associated with paragangliomas in SDHx syndromes are typically gastric, with predominantly epithelioid cytology and plexiform architecture.

TERMINOLOGY

- Composite pheochromocytoma (PCC) and composite paraganglioma (PGL) are tumors consisting of PCC or PGL combined with developmentally related neurogenic tumor
  - Ganglioneuroma (GN)
  - Ganglioneuroblastoma (GNB)
  - Neuroblastoma (NB)
  - Peripheral nerve sheath tumor

ETIOLOGY/PATHOGENESIS

- Mostly sporadic
- Some hereditary
  - Association with NF1
  - Germline *RET* or *VHL* mutations

CLINICAL ISSUES

- Usually indolent even when GNB or NB present; long-term follow-up required
- Histologic criteria unreliable in predicting biologic behavior

MICROSCOPIC

- Intimate mixture of architecturally complete tumor types
  - PCC/PGL almost always predominant component
  - 2nd component usually GN, followed by GNB, then NB, and rarely malignant peripheral nerve sheath tumor

ANCILLARY TESTS

- PCC/PGL chief cells show diffuse CgA and Syn staining while GN, GNB, and NB show weak focal staining mostly in processes
- Schwann cells and sustentacular cells stain for S100
- Neurofilament protein highlights axon-like processes

TOP DIFFERENTIAL DIAGNOSES

- Collision tumor
- Pure GN, GNB, or NB
- Tumor-to-tumor metastasis
- Mixed corticomedullary tumor

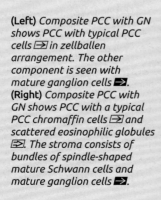

(Left) In composite pheochromocytoma (PCC) with ganglioneuroma (GN), the gross appearance is variable. The tumor is usually intraadrenal and is surrounded by a thin fibrous capsule, as shown in this gross photo. (Right) Gross photo of the cut surface of a composite PCC with GN shows a large, cystic tumor with a heterogeneous appearance.

Composite Pheochromocytoma Gross Surface

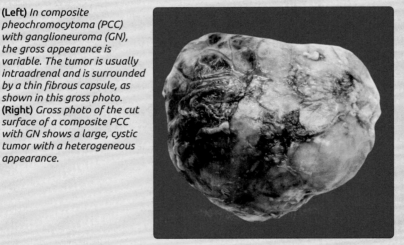

Composite Pheochromocytoma Cut Surface

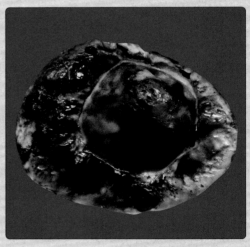

(Left) Composite PCC with GN shows PCC with typical PCC cells ⇨ in zellballen arrangement. The other component is seen with mature ganglion cells ➡. (Right) Composite PCC with GN shows PCC with a typical PCC chromaffin cells ⇨ and scattered eosinophilic globules ➡. The stroma consists of bundles of spindle-shaped mature Schwann cells and mature ganglion cells ➡.

Composite Pheochromocytoma Cells

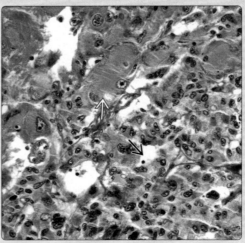

Composite Pheochromocytoma With Ganglioneuroma

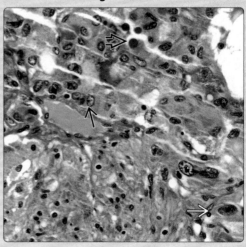

TERMINOLOGY

Abbreviations
- Pheochromocytoma (PCC)
- Paraganglioma (PGL)

Synonyms
- Composite or compound PCC
  - Compound adrenal medullary tumor
  - Mixed adrenal medullary tumor
  - Mixed neuroendocrine-neural tumor
- Composite PGL
  - Composite extraadrenal PCC
  - Compound PGL
  - Ganglioneuromatous PGL
  - Mixed neuroendocrine-neural tumor

Definitions
- Tumor consisting of PCC or PGL combined with developmentally related neurogenic tumor, such as ganglioneuroma (GN), ganglioneuroblastoma (GNB), neuroblastoma (NB), or malignant peripheral nerve sheath tumor (MPNST)
  - Pheochromocytoma or extraadrenal paraganglioma admixed with different, developmentally related type of tumor
    - 2nd component most frequently GN ~ 70-80%
    - GNB ~ 10-20%
    - Occasionally undifferentiated NB
    - Rarely MPNST
- Must be architecturally complete tumor patterns, not just scattered neurons
- No precise proportion of components specified in definition

ETIOLOGY/PATHOGENESIS

Genetic Basis
- Usually sporadic
- Occasionally associated with hereditary PCC/PGL syndromes
  - Disproportionate association with neurofibromatosis type 1 (NF1)
    - ~ 17% of PCC in NF1 show composite features
    - Composite PCC in NF1 sometimes bilateral, including cases with bilateral MPNST
  - Composite PCC reported in patients from several kindreds with germline RET mutations
    - Multiple endocrine neoplasia types 2A (MEN2A)
  - Isolated composite PCC reported with germline VHL mutation
  - Isolated composite PGL reported with germline SDHB deletion
- Hypothetical mechanisms for dual phenotype include transdifferentiation or pluripotent progenitor

CLINICAL ISSUES

Epidemiology
- Incidence
  - Composite PCC features seen in 3-9% of all PCCs
  - Composite PGLs extremely rare
    - 1/10 as frequent as composite PCC
- Age
  - Composite PCC usually occurs in adults
    - Average: 40-50 years (range 5-82 years)
    - Isolated cases in children or infants
  - Composite PGL have been reported from 15 months to 81 years
    - Early age at diagnosis and extraadrenal location reported in patient with germline SDHB deletion
- Sex
  - ~ equal distribution

Site
- PCC: Adrenal medulla
  - Usually identified as minor component during microscopic examination
  - Areas of GN or GNB reported in 3-9% of PCC
  - ~ 7% of cases bilateral
- Composite PGL
  - Most common extraadrenal site is urinary bladder and retroperitoneum
  - Also reported in filum terminale/cauda equina and posterior mediastinum
  - None reported in parasympathetic paraganglia of head and neck

Presentation
- Mass lesion similar to typical PCC or PGL
- Catecholamine excess and levels may vary
- A few cases with watery diarrhea, hypokalemia, achlorhydria (WDHA)
  - WDHA is caused by vasoactive intestinal peptide (VIP) produced mostly in neuronal component
    - VIP is potent vasodilator
    - Regulator of smooth muscle tone, epithelial cell secretion and blood flow in gastrointestinal tract
  - Syndrome is same as WDHA (Werner-Morrison) syndrome caused by ectopic VIP in pancreatic endocrine tumors
  - WDHA in children
    - Tumor arises from neural crest tissue of sympathetic ganglia or adrenal medulla

Laboratory Tests
- Levels of catecholamines may vary
- WDHA
  - Hypokalemia
  - Achlorhydria
  - Hypocalcemia
  - Hyperglycemia
  - Metabolic acidosis

Prognosis
- When 2nd component GN, prognosis same as for conventional PCC or PGL
  - Risk of metastases low
  - Can metastasize by lymphatic and hematogenous routes to lymph node, lung, bone, and liver
  - Most patients with metastasis eventually die from complications or destructive local growth
  - Metastases usually consist of PCC/PGL, rarely together with GN

- When metastases occur, they usually arise from tumors containing GNB, NB or MPNST
- When GNB or NB is 2nd component, behavior usually still indolent
  - Different from pediatric GNB or NB
  - Metastases most likely consist of GNB or NB, but sometimes contain 2 components
  - No recurrence with 5-year follow-up after complete surgical resection of tumors confined to adrenal
    - 5 years possibly too short
  - Metastases usually grow slowly, compatible with long clinical course
    - Life-long clinical and biochemical follow-up required
    - Some fatal cases reported
- Poor prognosis when MPNST present

IMAGING

General Features

- Usually similar to conventional PCC/PGL
- Heterogeneity in CT, US, or other modalities can suggest composite tumor if divergent differentiation extensive

MACROSCOPIC

General Features

- Composite pheochromocytoma and composite paraganglioma
  - Macroscopic features of both tumors similar
  - Usually well circumscribed
  - Size variable, up to 15 cm
  - Composite features often not grossly identifiable; depends on proportions of different components
  - Various components can have distinctive macroscopic features
    - PCC/PGL: Pink-gray to tan
    - GN: Pale gray and firm
    - GNB/NB: Soft, hemorrhagic, and may be necrotic

MICROSCOPIC

Histologic Features

- Mixture of tumor types with characteristic histology for each
- Transition may be abrupt or blended
- PCC/PGL almost always predominant component
  - Zellballen or variant patterns
- 2nd component usually GN (~ 60-80%) followed by GNB (20%), NB, and rarely MPNST
  - GN: Mature neurons (ganglion cells) in background of Schwann cells
  - GNB: Immature and maturing neurons, neuropil, Schwann cells
  - NB: Small round blue cells
  - MPNST: Malignant spindle cells, high mitotic count
    - Rhabdomyosarcomatous differentiation (triton tumor) reported

ANCILLARY TESTS

Immunohistochemistry

- Staining of PCC/PGL chief cells recapitulates normal chromaffin cells
  - Diffuse CgA and Syn staining corresponding to numerous cytoplasmic secretory granules
  - Decreased staining for CgA can help to identify areas of GN/GNB/NB
- Staining of GN, GNB, or NB recapitulates normal neurons
  - Weak focal CgA and Syn staining, often in linear or punctuate distribution
    - Neuronal secretory granules sparser than those in chromaffin cells
    - Distribution corresponds to axon-like processes where neuronal secretory granules accumulate
  - Increased staining for neurofilament protein (NFP), especially in axon-like processes
  - Sometimes increased staining for receptor tyrosine kinase RET and VIP
    - VIP most likely in mature or nearly mature neurons of GN and GNB
- Sustentacular cells in PCC/PGL and Schwann cells in GN/GNB stain for S100
- Both composite PCC and PGL have similar morphological features, except for the cauda equina PGLs, which can show extensive expression of keratins
- Ki-67 (MIB-1) staining highlights components with differences in cell proliferation
  - Highest in NB and MPNST, usually low in PCC/PGL, absent in ganglion cells
  - Can be robust in Schwann cells and endothelial cells

Genetic Testing

- *N-myc* not amplified in neuroblastic component
  - Different from pediatric GNB or NB
- Reduced expression of neurofibromin in Schwann cells and sustentacular cells of composite PCC
  - Seen in patients with and without evidence of neurofibromatosis
- Somatic loss-of-function mutation affecting *ATRX* identified

DIFFERENTIAL DIAGNOSIS

Collision Tumor

- Collision of developmentally unrelated tumors
  - e.g., PCC and adrenal cortical adenoma, carcinoma, or myelolipoma
- Collision of related but separate tumors originating adjacent to one another
  - e.g., PCC and GN
- Patterns of growth, intermixed cellular components, and immunohistochemistry usually allow distinction

Pure GN, GNB, or NB

- PCC/PGL component not present

Tumor-to-Tumor Metastasis

- Distinctive morphology and immunohistochemistry for each component
- Metastases from other neuroendocrine tumors potentially problematic

- o Metastatic medullary thyroid carcinoma in patients with MEN2 syndromes
  - – Stains for calcitonin, *TTF-1*
- PCC with melanoma or neuroendocrine carcinoma reported as variants of composite tumors
  - o Most likely to represent metastases from occult primary tumors
    - – Thorough clinical evaluation is critical

Mixed Corticomedullary Tumor

- Single mass composed of adrenal cortical tumor and PCC
  - o Might originate as collision tumor
  - o Cortical component positive for inhibin, negative for CgA
  - o PCC positive for CgA, negative for inhibin
  - o Syn should not be used for this differential diagnosis
    - – Immunoreactive Syn expressed in both cortex and medulla

DIAGNOSTIC CHECKLIST

Pathologic Interpretation Pearls

- Areas of decreased staining for CgA can help to identify composite features

SELECTED REFERENCES

1. Lam AK: Update on adrenal tumours in 2017 World Health Organization (WHO) of endocrine tumours. Endocr Pathol. ePub, 2017
2. Yamasaki M et al: Composite paraganglioma-ganglioneuroma concomitant with adrenal metastasis of medullary thyroid carcinoma in a patient with multiple endocrine neoplasia type 2B: a case report. Asian J Endosc Surg. 10(1):66-69, 2017
3. Comino-Méndez I et al: ATRX driver mutation in a composite malignant pheochromocytoma. Cancer Genet. 209(6):272-7, 2016
4. Namekawa T et al: Composite pheochromocytoma with a malignant peripheral nerve sheath tumor: case report and review of the literature. Asian J Surg. 39(3):187-90, 2016
5. Shida Y et al: Composite pheochromocytoma of the adrenal gland: a case series. BMC Res Notes. 8:257, 2015
6. Shawa H et al: Clinical and radiologic features of pheochromocytoma/ganglioneuroma composite tumors: a case series with comparative analysis. Endocr Pract. 20(9):864-9, 2014
7. Ende K et al: A 45-year-old female with hypokalemic rhabdomyolysis due to VIP-producing composite pheochromocytoma. Z Gastroenterol. 50(6):589-94, 2012
8. Kikuchi Y et al: Pheochromocytoma with histologic transformation to composite type, complicated by watery diarrhea, hypokalemia, and achlorhydria syndrome. Endocr Pract. 18(4):e91-6, 2012
9. Lau SK et al: Mixed cortical adenoma and composite pheochromocytoma-ganglioneuroma: an unusual corticomedullary tumor of the adrenal gland. Ann Diagn Pathol. 15(3):185-9, 2011
10. Fritzsche FR et al: Radiological and pathological findings of a metastatic composite paraganglioma with neuroblastoma in a man: a case report. J Med Case Reports. 4:374, 2010
11. George DJ et al: Composite adrenal phaeochromocytoma-ganglioneuroma causing watery diarrhoea, hypokalaemia and achlorhydria syndrome. Eur J Gastroenterol Hepatol. 22(5):632-4, 2010
12. Mahajan H et al: Composite phaeochromocytoma-ganglioneuroma, an uncommon entity: report of two cases. Pathology. 42(3):295-8, 2010
13. Alexandraki KI et al: Corticomedullary mixed adrenal tumor: case report and literature review. Endocr J. 56(6):817-24, 2009
14. Armstrong R et al: Succinate dehydrogenase subunit B (SDHB) gene deletion associated with a composite paraganglioma/neuroblastoma. J Med Genet. 46(3):215-6, 2009
15. Comstock JM et al: Composite pheochromocytoma: a clinicopathologic and molecular comparison with ordinary pheochromocytoma and neuroblastoma. Am J Clin Pathol. 132(1):69-73, 2009
16. Gupta R et al: Composite phaeochromocytoma with malignant peripheral nerve sheath tumour and rhabdomyosarcomatous differentiation in a patient without von Recklinghausen disease. J Clin Pathol. 62(7):659-61, 2009
17. Charfi S et al: [Composite pheochromocytoma associated with multiple endocrine neoplasia type 2B.] Ann Pathol. 28(3):225-8, 2008
18. Ercolino T et al: Uncommon clinical presentations of pheochromocytoma and paraganglioma in two different patients affected by two distinct novel VHL germline mutations. Clin Endocrinol (Oxf). 68(5):762-8, 2008
19. Ch'ng ES et al: Composite malignant pheochromocytoma with malignant peripheral nerve sheath tumour: a case with 28 years of tumour-bearing history. Histopathology. 51(3):420-2, 2007
20. Tatekawa Y et al: Composite pheochromocytoma associated with adrenal neuroblastoma in an infant: a case report. J Pediatr Surg. 41(2):443-5, 2006
21. Powers JF et al: Ret protein expression in adrenal medullary hyperplasia and pheochromocytoma. Endocr Pathol. 14(4):351-61, 2003
22. Wieneke JA et al: Corticomedullary mixed tumor of the adrenal gland. Ann Diagn Pathol. 5(5):304-8, 2001
23. Lam KY et al: Composite pheochromocytoma-ganglioneuroma of the adrenal gland: an uncommon entity with distinctive clinicopathologic features. Endocr Pathol. 10(4):343-352, 1999
24. Matias-Guiu X et al: Composite phaeochromocytoma-ganglioneuroblastoma in a patient with multiple endocrine neoplasia type IIA. Histopathology. 32(3):281-2, 1998
25. Brady S et al: Composite pheochromocytoma/ganglioneuroma of the adrenal gland associated with multiple endocrine neoplasia 2A: case report with immunohistochemical analysis. Am J Surg Pathol. 21(1):102-8, 1997
26. Franquemont DW et al: Immunohistochemical detection of neuroblastomatous foci in composite adrenal pheochromocytoma-neuroblastoma. Am J Clin Pathol. 102(2):163-70, 1994
27. Chetty R et al: Bilateral pheochromocytoma-ganglioneuroma of the adrenal in type 1 neurofibromatosis. Am J Surg Pathol. 17(8):837-41, 1993
28. Min KW et al: Malignant peripheral nerve sheath tumor and pheochromocytoma. A composite tumor of the adrenal. Arch Pathol Lab Med. 112(3):266-70, 1988
29. Tischler AS et al: The distribution of immunoreactive chromogranins, S-100 protein, and vasoactive intestinal peptide in compound tumors of the adrenal medulla. Hum Pathol. 18(9):909-17, 1987

Composite Tumor Cut Surface

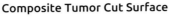

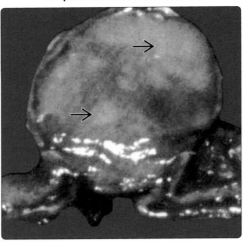

(Left) *In composite PCC with GN, the GN component can sometimes be identified grossly as firm, gray-white patches ⇨. (Right) Gross cut surface of a composite PCC with GN is shown. This component is difficult to identify but can be seen as firm, gray-white areas ⇨ within a background of grey or hemorrhagic color giving am heterogeneous appearance.*

Composite Tumor Cut Surface

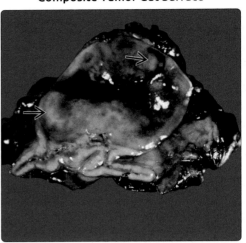

Composite Pheochromocytoma

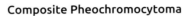

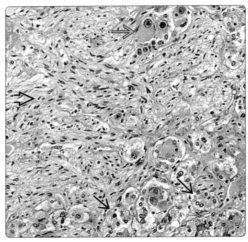

(Left) *Composite PCC with GN shows PCC with a typical zellballen pattern ⇨, stroma consisting of mature Schwann cells ⇨, and mature ganglion cells ⇨. (Right) Composite PCC with prominent neuromatous component shows PCC intermixed with the stromal component consisting of mature bundles of spindle-shaped Schwann cells and axon-like processes and ganglion cells.*

High-Power View Composite Tumor

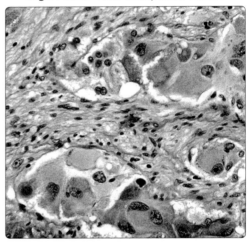

Pheochromocytoma and Schwann Stroma

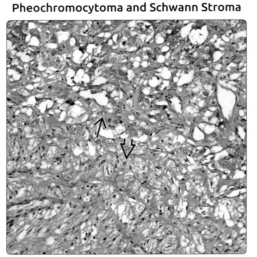

(Left) *Composite PCC with GN shows the PCC component with focally cystic zellballen pattern ⇨. The stroma is composed of mature Schwann cells ⇨. (Right) Composite PCC with GN shows PCC with a typical zellballen pattern and immunopositivity for S100 within sustentacular cells ⇨. The stroma of mature Schwann cells shows fibrillary positivity for S100 ⇨.*

Pheochromocytoma and Schwann Stroma

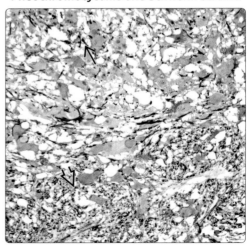

Composite Pheochromocytoma With Ganglioneuroma

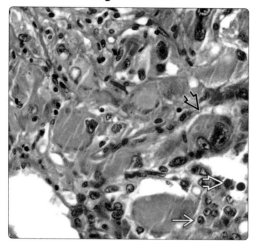

Composite Pheochromocytoma With Ganglioneuroma

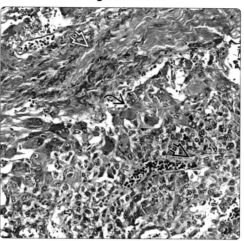

(Left) *Composite PCC with GN shows PCC ➡ containing eosinophilic globules ➡ with a stroma consisting of mature Schwann cells and mature ganglion cells ➡.* (Right) *This composite tumor consists of PCC ➡ with GN. The GN component shows stroma ➡ consisting of axons, Schwann cells, and mature ganglion cells ➡.*

Areas of Decreased Staining

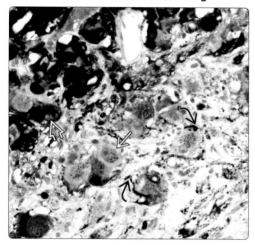

Composite Tumor RET Expression

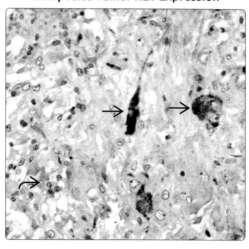

(Left) *CgA can reveal different components of composite tumors. This tumor shows intense cytoplasmic staining in PCC cells ➡, weak or absent staining in neuronal cell bodies ➡, and linear or punctate staining in neuronal processes ➡. Areas of decreased staining identify composite features.* (Right) *Receptor tyrosine kinase RET is strongly expressed by normal neurons but only minimally by adult chromaffin cells. This PCC with GN shows strong staining of scattered ganglion cells ➡ but not PCC cells ➡.*

Composite Tumor Axon-Like Processes

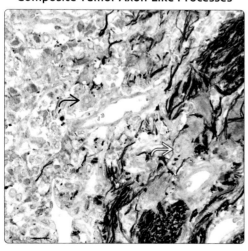

Composite Tumor Hormonal Production

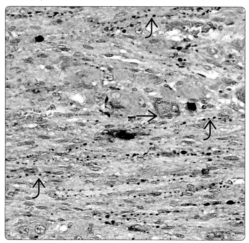

(Left) *Staining for neurofilament protein highlights axon-like processes, as shown in this tumor consisting of PCC with GN. Cell bodies of both PCC cells ➡ and neurons ➡ show weak or absent staining.* (Right) *Vasoactive intestinal peptide (VIP) is produced by normal neurons but not chromaffin cells. This PCC with GNB shows extensive VIP staining in a distribution ➡ corresponding to varicosities of neuronal processes where secretory vesicles accumulate. A few cell bodies show weak staining ➡.*

Myelolipoma, Adrenal Glands

TERMINOLOGY

- Tumor or tumor-like lesion composed of mature adipose tissue and hematopoietic elements

CLINICAL ISSUES

- Tumor discovered incidentally on radiographic examination for other reasons
- Benign process with no risk of recurrence
- ~ 3% of primary adrenal neoplasms

IMAGING

- Vast majority of tumors are unilateral and solitary
- T1-weighted MR images show high fat signal intensity

MACROSCOPIC

- Usually well-circumscribed, unencapsulated mass with variegated surface, soft and yellow to red, depending on proportion of components
- Cut surface is variegated
- Hemorrhage and infarction more common in large lesions

MICROSCOPIC

- Mixture of mature fat and trilineage maturation of mature and immature myeloid, erythroid, and megakaryocytic lines
- Rarely, osseous metaplasia, hemorrhage, and fibrosis
- **Caveat**: 1 reported case of ML colonized by lymphoma

TOP DIFFERENTIAL DIAGNOSES

- Pheochromocytoma
  - Rarely, myelolipomatous foci/metaplasia can be seen, but it is never dominant finding
- Adrenal cortical adenoma
  - Adenomas may have myelolipomatous foci
  - Adenoma must be dominant finding
- Adrenal lipoma
  - Adipocyte neoplasm without hematopoietic elements
- Adrenal cortical hyperplasia
  - Admixed lipomatous and myelolipomatous elements may be found

Small Adrenal Myelolipoma

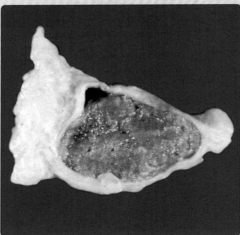

Large Adrenal Mass Cut Surface

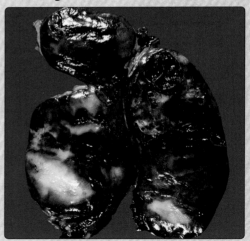

(Left) Grossly, this adrenal myelolipoma is a well-circumscribed, soft tan-yellow to focally red mass within and compressing the adrenal gland. (Right) Gross cut surface of the adrenal myelolipomas shows an area of soft yellow tissue intermixed with areas of red firmer tissue with focal cystic changes.

Fat and Hematopoiesis

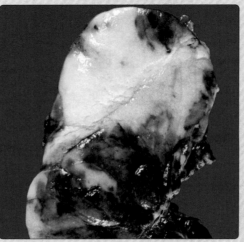

Residual Adrenal Tissue

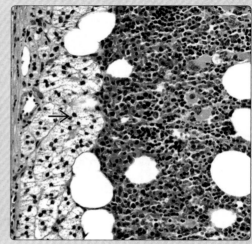

(Left) The cut surface of myelolipomas is usually variegated and shows a yellow and red to brown cut surface, which reflects the composition of both fat and hematopoietic elements. (Right) H&E shows the typical appearance of a myelolipoma with easily identifiable adrenal cells ➡ juxtaposed to bone marrow elements. Note the numerous megakaryocytes.

TERMINOLOGY

Abbreviations
- Myelolipoma (ML)

Synonyms
- ML of adrenal gland

Definitions
- Rare, benign tumor or tumor-like lesion composed of mature adipose tissue and variable amount of hematopoietic elements of various proportions

ETIOLOGY/PATHOGENESIS

Proposed Theories
- May result from metaplastic alterations of adrenal cortical or stromal cells
- Possibly related to bone marrow emboli
- Metaplasia of adrenal cortical cells
- Embryonic rests of bone marrow in adrenal gland
- May arise from uncommitted or pluripotential adrenal stromal cells
- Nonrandom X-chromosome inactivation has been reported, suggesting neoplastic process

CLINICAL ISSUES

Epidemiology
- Incidence
  - ~ 3% of primary adrenal neoplasms
  - Autopsy incidence of 0.01-0.20% depending on age group
- Age
  - Usually 5th-7th decades; rare before 30 years

Site
- Adrenal gland is most common location
  - Rarely, presacral region of retroperitoneum, mediastinum, liver, leptomeninges, lung, and gastrointestinal tract may be affected
- Most are unilateral
- Bilateral disease may be seen (< 7%)

Presentation
- Asymptomatic
  - Tumor discovered incidentally on radiographic examination for other reasons
- Symptomatic
  - Abdominal or flank pain, hematuria, palpable mass, hypertension, retroperitoneal hemorrhage
  - Rarely, endocrine dysfunction detected
    - Cushing syndrome, pituitary Cushing disease, Addison disease, virilism, and pseudohermaphroditism
- Not usually associated with disturbances of hematopoietic system

Treatment
- Options, risks, complications
  - Risk of rupture and hemorrhage in large tumors
    - Surgery recommended for these tumors
  - Small, clinically silent lesions can be watched (radiographic monitoring)
- Surgical approaches
  - Complete surgical excision prevents recurrence

Prognosis
- Benign process
- No recurrence risk

IMAGING

MR Findings
- Vast majority of tumors are unilateral and solitary
- T1-weighted MR images show high fat signal intensity

CT Findings
- Usually unilateral, solitary mass within adrenal gland, showing density identical to fat
- Inhomogeneous attenuation is common
- Rarely, calcifications may be seen

MACROSCOPIC

General Features
- Usually well-circumscribed, unencapsulated mass
  - Measuring up to 34 cm and 6,000 g
  - Contour can be smooth, wavy, or irregular
  - May blend with uninvolved adrenal cortex
- Soft and yellow to red, reflecting composition of fat and hematopoietic elements
- Cut surface is variegated
- Hemorrhage and infarction more common in large lesions

MICROSCOPIC

Histologic Features
- Mixture of mature adipose tissue and hematopoietic elements
- Full trilineage maturation of myeloid, erythroid, and megakaryocytic lines
- Rarely, osseous metaplasia, hemorrhage, and fibrosis
- **Caveat**: 1 reported case of ML colonized by lymphoma

DIFFERENTIAL DIAGNOSIS

Adrenal Cortical Adenoma and Hyperplasia
- Areas of adrenocortical cells present

Pheochromocytoma
- Positive for chromogranin-A

SELECTED REFERENCES

1. Lam A: Lipomatous tumours in adrenal gland: WHO updates and clinical implications. Endocr Relat Cancer. 24(3):R65-R79, 2017
2. Chakraborty PP et al: Bilateral adrenal myelolipoma in Cushing's disease: a relook into the role of corticotropin in adrenal tumourigenesis. BMJ Case Rep. 2016, 2016
3. Polamaung W et al: Asymptomatic bilateral giant adrenal myelolipomas: case report and review of literature. Endocr Pract. 13(6):667-71, 2007
4. Bishop E et al: Adrenal myelolipomas show nonrandom X-chromosome inactivation in hematopoietic elements and fat: support for a clonal origin of myelolipomas. Am J Surg Pathol. 30(7):838-43, 2006
5. Lam KY et al: Adrenal lipomatous tumours: a 30 year clinicopathological experience at a single institution. J Clin Pathol. 54(9):707-12, 2001
6. Saeger W: Pathology of adrenal neoplasms. Minerva Endocrinol. 20(1):1-8, 1995

Illustration of Myelolipoma

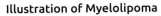
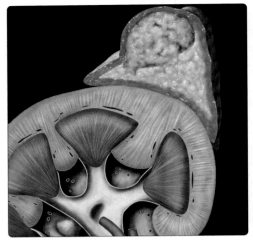

Large Adrenal Mass

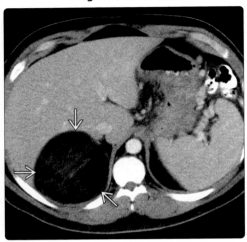

(Left) *Graphic demonstrates the fatty nature of a myelolipoma within the adrenal gland. It can raise the cortex and expand into the medullary region.* (Right) *There is a unilateral, single right adrenal mass ➡ with a density identical to fat. This is a characteristic appearance of adrenal myelolipoma. Rarely, areas of calcification may be present. Myelolipomas may be large, measuring up to 34 cm.*

Interface Between Adrenal and Tumor

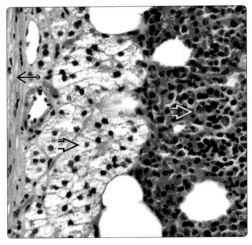

Bone Marrow With Megakaryocytes

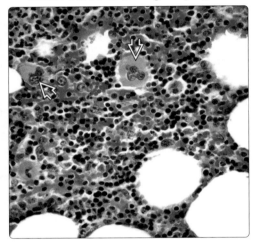

(Left) *Photomicrograph of a myelolipoma depicts the adrenal capsule ➡, the normal adrenal cells ➡, and the marrow elements ➡ that constitute a typical myelolipoma. The tumor is sharply separated from the adrenal tissue.* (Right) *High-power H&E shows the presence of marrow elements within a myelolipoma. The 3 cellular lineages of the bone marrow are usually present, and megakaryocytes ➡ are easily identifiable as large multinucleated cells with abundant cytoplasm.*

Relationship of Tumor and Cortical Cells

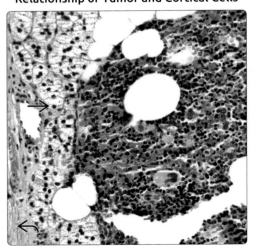

Scarce Hematopoietic Cells

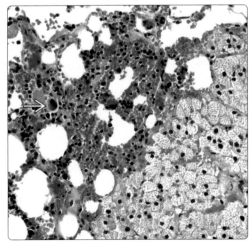

(Left) *In this myelolipoma, the adipose tissue and marrow components of the tumor compress the rim of normal adrenal tissue ➡ to a thin layer squeezed between the adrenal capsule ➡ and the tumor.* (Right) *The proportion of marrow elements in a myelolipoma can be variable. At low magnification, the appearance is that of hemorrhage within the adrenal gland. Closer inspection reveals a megakaryocyte ➡ that should prompt the search for the other marrow elements in this neoplasm.*

Residual Adrenal Cortical Cells

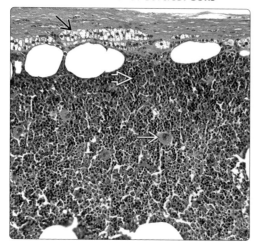

Demarcation of Tumor

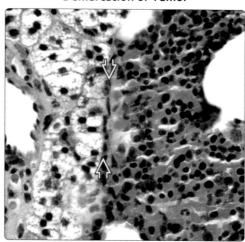

(Left) *There is a small rim of compressed adrenal cortical tissue ⇨ trapped between the adrenal capsule and the neoplasm ⇨. The tumor is composed of fat admixed with marrow elements; the megakaryocytes are usually easy to find ⇨.* (Right) *Myelolipomas are normally unencapsulated tumors. This micrograph shows a sharp demarcation ⇨ in the transitional area between the tumor and the adjacent uninvolved adrenal tissue with easily identifiable adrenal cells juxtaposed to bone marrow elements.*

Fibrous Capsule

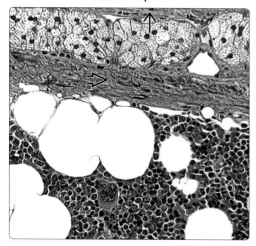

Lobulated Architecture

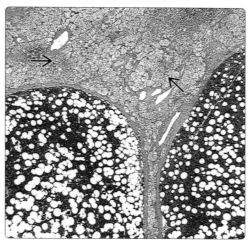

(Left) *Although most myelolipomas are devoid of a capsule, the neoplasm shown in this picture has a distinct tumor capsule ⇨ that separates it from the surrounding adrenal. Note that a portion of the adrenal capsule is also shown ⇨.* (Right) *Myelolipoma shows a lobulated architecture with trabeculae of adrenal cortex ⇨ surrounding the tumor nodules. The tumor nodule on the left shows extensive hemorrhage.*

Mixed Cell Population

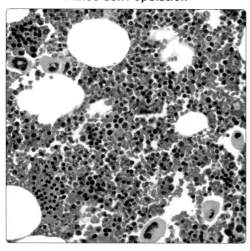

Cortical Cells and Myelolipoma

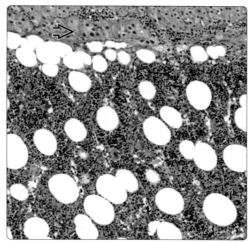

(Left) *The amount of adipose and bone marrow elements are variable. This tumor has trilineage hematopoiesis of mature and immature myeloid, erythroid, and megakaryocytic lines mixed with a small amount of mature fat.* (Right) *Adrenal cortical tissue is seen at the periphery of this lesion ⇨ and may sometimes be found within the tumor. Adipocytes are present throughout the proliferation. The proportion of fat and marrow components determine the overall gross appearance of the lesion.*

Benign Connective Tissue Tumor, Adrenal Glands

CLINICAL ISSUES

- Most found incidentally during autopsies

MICROSCOPIC

- **Hemangioma**
  - Large, cystically dilated vessels (cavernous type) with thin walls; intravascular thrombus and calcification may be present
- **Leiomyoma**
  - Features identical to benign smooth muscle tumors occurring in other sites
  - Cytologically bland-looking spindle cells in different planes of section with fibrillary cytoplasm, minimal or no atypia, no mitotic activity, and no necrosis
- **Lipoma**
  - Mature adipose tissue partially surrounded by thin, fibrous capsule

TOP DIFFERENTIAL DIAGNOSES

- Connective/mesenchymal tumors in general
  - Nonneoplastic cysts
  - Cystic lymphangioma
  - Cystic teratoma
- Hemangioma
  - Angiosarcoma
  - Lymphangioma
- Leiomyoma
  - Leiomyosarcoma
- Lipoma
  - Adrenal cortical adenoma with myelolipomatous metaplasia
  - Adrenal myelolipomas
  - Well-differentiated liposarcoma

Mature Adipocytes

Vascular Channels

(Left) Photomicrograph shows an adrenal lipoma. Mature adipose cells ⇨ are seen forming a well-circumscribed mass. Note the absence of hematopoietic elements and the absence of myelolipomatous metaplasia. (Right) Adrenal hemangioma is shown at medium power. This benign tumor is composed of cystically dilated vessels with thin walls ➡. Hemosiderin is present ➡. Normal adrenal tissue ⇨ is shown.

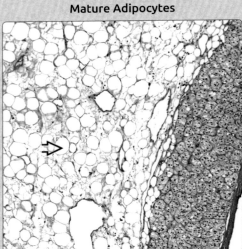
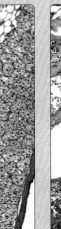
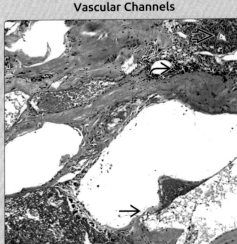

Caldesmon in Leiomyoma

Myelolipoma as Differential Diagnosis

(Left) Immunohistochemistry for caldesmon shows diffuse cytoplasmic staining in this adrenal leiomyoma. Other muscle markers can also be used for tumor characterization. (Right) The gross cut surface of this adrenal mass shows a focally homogeneous, yellow tissue admixed with bright red, homogeneous hemorrhagic area with focal cystic changes.

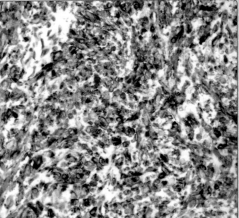
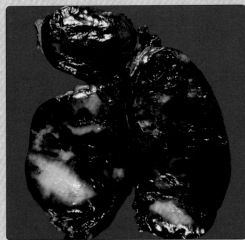

TERMINOLOGY

Synonyms

- Benign soft tissue tumors of adrenal glands, mesenchymal tumors, stromal tumors

Definitions

- Benign neoplasms arising from nonsteroid or noncatecholamine-producing cells

CLINICAL ISSUES

Presentation

- Usually small, asymptomatic tumors
- **Hemangioma**
  - Extremely rare; most found incidentally during autopsies
- **Leiomyoma**
  - Primary adrenal leiomyomas very rare
- **Lipoma**
  - Extremely rare, most incidentally found during autopsies
    - Few cases reported in literature

Treatment

- Local excision
  - Clinical follow-up may be treatment of choice

Prognosis

- Excellent; however, limited data available

IMAGING

Hemangioma

- Large, heterogeneous-enhancing mass with calcification (frequent), hemorrhage, necrosis, and phleboliths (not frequent but characteristic)

Leiomyoma

- Soft tissue attenuating mass on CT scan (nonspecific), usually associated with adrenal vein

Lipoma

- Low-density, well-circumscribed, ovoid mass with homogeneous imaging characteristics of fat and occasional calcifications

MACROSCOPIC

Hemangioma

- Red-brown mass with macrocystic, hemorrhagic surface

Leiomyoma

- Well-circumscribed, rubbery, gray-white tumors

Lipoma

- Well-circumscribed, yellow nodule with fat consistency and occasional calcifications

MICROSCOPIC

Histologic Features

- **Hemangioma**
  - Large, cystically dilated vessels with thin walls; intravascular thrombus or calcification may be present
  - Usually cavernous type
- **Leiomyoma**
  - Features identical to benign smooth muscle tumors occurring in other sites
    - Cytologically bland-looking spindle cells in different planes of section with fibrillary cytoplasm, minimal or no atypia, no mitotic activity, and no necrosis
- **Lipoma**
  - Mature adipose tissue partially surrounded by thin, fibrous capsule
    - In some areas, fat cells might be in contact with adrenal cortical cells

DIFFERENTIAL DIAGNOSIS

Connective/Mesenchymal Tumors in General

- Nonneoplastic cysts
- Cystic lymphangioma
- Cystic teratoma
- Rare lesions such as teratomas, schwannomas, ganglioneuromas, and neurofibromas

Hemangioma

- Angiosarcoma: Endothelioid features, necrosis, atypia, hobnail appearance
- Lymphangioma: Even more rare than hemangioma, and few cases reported would be best classified as adenomatoid tumor

Leiomyoma

- Leiomyosarcoma: Cellular atypia, tumor necrosis, mitosis, and other features of malignancy

Lipoma

- Adrenal cortical adenoma with myelolipomatous metaplasia
  - Composed of areas of cells resembling those seen in adrenal cortex intermixed with hematopoietic cells and adipose tissue
- Adrenal myelolipomas
  - Bone marrow elements should be present
- Well-differentiated liposarcoma
  - Characterized by lipoblasts, atypical cells, and plexiform vessels

DIAGNOSTIC CHECKLIST

Clinically Relevant Pathologic Features

- Very rare, usually small, asymptomatic tumors of adrenal

Pathologic Interpretation Pearls

- Differential diagnosis should be made with malignant counterpart of these neoplasms

SELECTED REFERENCES

1. Luo J et al: Lipoadenoma of the adrenal gland: report of a rare entity and review of literature. Int J Clin Exp Pathol. 8(8):9693-7, 2015
2. Kumar S et al: Large bilateral adrenal leiomyomas presenting as calcified adrenal masses: a rare case report. Korean J Urol. 55(5):363-6, 2014
3. Lack E: Tumors of the Adrenal Glands and Extraadrenal Paraganglia. AFIP Atlas of Tumor Pathology Series 4, Fascicle 8. Washington, DC: American Registry of Pathology, 2007
4. Milathianakis KN et al: Giant lipoma of the adrenal gland. J Urol. 167(4):1777, 2002
5. Büttner A: Lipoma of the adrenal gland. Pathol Int. 49(11):1007-9, 1999

TERMINOLOGY

- Malignant epithelial neoplasm of adrenal cortical cells

ETIOLOGY/PATHOGENESIS

- Adrenal cortical neoplasms are thought to arise through acquired genetic mutations in driver genes
- Li-Fraumeni syndrome
- Beckwith-Wiedemann syndrome
- Lynch syndrome
- Multiple endocrine neoplasia 1
- Familial adenomatous polyposis
- Carney complex
- Neurofibromatosis type 1

MICROSCOPIC

- Adrenal cortical carcinomas (ACCs) are subdivided on basis of mitotic frequency in
  - **Low grade**: ≤ 20 mitosis/50 HPF
  - **High grade**: > 20 mitosis/50 HPF

ANCILLARY TESTS

- Positive for synaptophysin, inhibin, Melan-A/Mart-1, and SF1 stains
- High prevalent role of *IGF2* overexpression
- *TP53* mutation and its dominant frequency in pediatric ACC and association with aggressive behavior
- Frequent and diversity of WNT pathway defects: *CTNNB1* point mutations and *ZNRF3* deletions
- Copy number alterations and whole genome doubling
- Important role of telomeres and telomerase reactivation
- Relative lack of targetable hotspot mutations
- Expression of *DLGAP5* (previously called *DLG7*) and *PINK1* identify carcinomas and tumors within borderline Weiss criteria

TOP DIFFERENTIAL DIAGNOSES

- Pheochromocytoma, renal cell carcinoma, metastatic tumors
- Adrenal cortical adenoma

Large Adrenal Mass

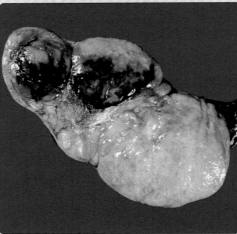

Adrenal Cortical Carcinoma

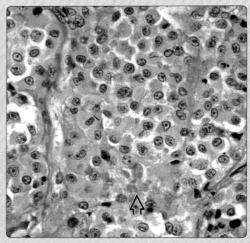

(Left) *Most adrenal carcinomas are large, solitary, and circumscribed tumors. The cut surface of this tumor shows a pale-yellow variegated appearance with areas of necrosis and hemorrhage.* (Right) *The growth pattern in adrenal cortical carcinomas (ACCs) are usually solid, broad trabecular, or large nested. This picture illustrates a tumor with broad trabecula composed of cells with ample eosinophilic cytoplasm and focal necrosis* ⭢.

Areas of Necrosis

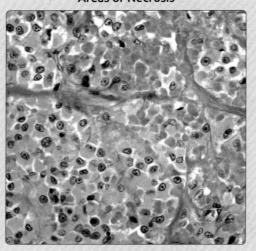

High Proliferative Index

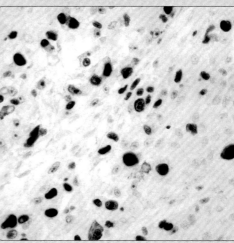

(Left) *This adrenal carcinoma in a patient with virilization is composed of large cells with eosinophilic cytoplasm and shows multifocal areas of necrosis. The cells have irregular nuclei with prominent nucleoli.* (Right) *The ACC in a patient with virilization syndrome shows a high proliferative index. The diagnostic evaluation of adrenal cortical tumors incorporate mitotic rate. ACC can be subdivided based on mitotic activity in low grade or high grade.*

TERMINOLOGY

Abbreviations

- Adrenal cortical carcinoma (ACC)

Synonyms

- Adrenocortical carcinoma

Definitions

- Malignant epithelial tumor of adrenal cortical cells

ETIOLOGY/PATHOGENESIS

Possible Multistep Process

- Adrenal cortical neoplasms are thought to arise through acquired genetic mutations in driver genes, with activation of key cellular signaling pathways
- Adrenal cortical hyperplasia and adenoma may represent precursor lesions
- Cumulative chromosomal alterations toward malignant transformation

Syndrome Association

- Li-Fraumeni syndrome (autosomal dominant)
- Beckwith-Wiedemann (autosomal dominant)
- Lynch syndrome
- Multiple endocrine neoplasia 1
- Familial adenomatous polyposis
- Carney complex
- Neurofibromatosis type 1
- Congenital adrenal hyperplasia

CLINICAL ISSUES

Epidemiology

- Incidence
  - 1 in every 4,000 adrenal tumors
  - 0.5-2.0 cases per million per year
  - Comprises ~ 3% of endocrine neoplasms
- Age
  - Bimodal distribution
    - 60-70 years
      - Peak in 5th decade
    - Early childhood
      - 0.21 per million per year
      - 0.3-0.4% of all neoplasms in this age
- Sex
  - Females affected more than males with ratio of 2.5:1.0
    - More often have functional tumors

Presentation

- 42-57% are hormonally functional
- Nonfunctional tumors are detected more often as radiographic techniques improve
- Most common presentation is associated with hormone oversecretions
  - Glucocorticoid
    - Cushing syndrome
    - Central obesity
    - Moon facies
    - Protein wasting, striae, and skin thinning
    - Muscle atrophy, osteoporosis
    - Diabetes, hypertension, gonadal dysfunction
    - Psychiatric disorders
  - Mineralocorticoid
    - Hypertension and hypokalemia
  - Androgens
    - Virilization in women
    - Excess testosterone in men
  - Estrogens
    - Very rare, yielding gynecomastia and testicular atrophy in men
    - Menstrual irregularities in women
- Mass
  - Flank pain due to compressive symptoms
- In children
  - Usually functional
  - May present: Virilization, precocious puberty, Cushing syndrome, or feminization

Laboratory Tests

- Serum or urinary hormone quantification
  - Hormones may not be bioactive
  - May require special methods for detection
  - Deoxycorticosterone, hydroxyprogesterone
  - Androstenedione, estrogens
  - Urine 17-ketogenic steroids or 17-ketosteroids may be elevated
  - Dehydroepiandrosterone sulfate (DHEAS)
- Dexamethasone suppression test

Treatment

- Options, risks, complications
  - Complications due to pituitary-hypothalamus-adrenal axis suppression
- Surgical approaches
  - Complete, radical surgical resection is treatment of choice
- Drugs
  - Mitotane
    - May help prolong recurrence-free survival after radical surgery
    - Can be used after incomplete resection or for metastatic disease
    - In patients not eligible for surgery
  - Chemotherapy regimens reported
    - Etoposide, doxorubicin, cisplatin, and mitotane
    - Streptozotocin and mitotane
    - Failure possibly due to high rate of multidrug resistance protein 1 (MDR1) gene expression
- Radiation
  - Radiotherapy can help control residual disease

Prognosis

- Aggressive disease with dismal prognosis
- Overall 5-year survival: 37-47%
- Key prognostic factors
  - Clinically relevant hypercortisolism
  - Resection margin status
  - Tumor stage correlates with survival
  - Tumor grade
  - Age > 50 years

- o Mitotic rate: Low grade (≤20/50 HPF) and high grade (> 20/50 HPF)
- o KI67 proliferative index: Significant prognostic and predictive power
- o High expression of *SF1* correlates with poorer outcome
- o Biomarkers *TOP2A*, *EZH2*, and *BARD1* might provide additional prognostic information
- o Expression of genes *BUB1B* and *PINK1* predicts prognosis
- o Carcinomas classified into 2 main molecular subgroups with distinct genomic alterations: C1A and C1B
- Nearly 40% have distant metastases at presentation
  - o Most common metastases to lymph nodes, lung, liver, and bone
  - o Rarely metastasizes to brain

IMAGING

Radiographic Findings
- Inhomogeneous masses with irregular borders and necrosis
- Usually show low tumor fat content
  - o Distinctly different from adenomas, which have high fat content

MR Findings
- Carcinoma tends to be large (> 5 cm)
- Irregular or invasive borders
- Decreased intracellular lipid and macroscopic fat
- Signal heterogeneity and necrosis
- Vena cava extension/invasion may be seen

CT Findings
- Heterogeneous, enhancing large mass
- Typically > 5 cm
- Frequently with displacement or invasion of adjacent organs
- Calcifications present in 30% of cases

PET Findings
- Helpful in determining distant metastases

MACROSCOPIC

General Features
- Bulky tumors with red-brown and fleshy, firm appearance
- Typically unilateral
  - o If bilateral, consider contralateral metastasis
- Large, solitary, circumscribed tumors
- Tan-yellow cut surface with areas of necrosis and hemorrhage

Sections to Be Submitted
- Sample foci of hemorrhage &/or necrosis
- Usually 1 section per cm, up to 15 sections

Size
- Often large: 10-14 cm
  - o Can range 1-25 cm

Weight
- Usually > 200 g
- Can be 10-5,000 g

MICROSCOPIC

Histologic Features
- Patternless sheets or nests of cells, solid arrangement
- Broad trabeculae and large nested
- Tumor encapsulation is rule: Thick fibrous capsule is associated with carcinoma
- May have
  - o High nuclear grade
  - o High mitotic counts
  - o Bizarre mitotic figures
  - o Venous invasion
- Necrosis may be abundant, specially in high-grade tumors
- Degenerative changes is usually focally identified
- Myxoid change may be present
- Capsular and lymphovascular invasion is usually identified
- Mitoses are strong predictors of ACC
  - o Diagnostic evaluation of adrenal cortical tumors incorporate mitotic rate
  - o ACC are subdivided on basis of mitotic frequency in
    - **Low grade:** ≤ 20 mitosis/50 HPF
    - **High grade:** > 20 mitosis/50 HPF
- In children, these features may not indicate malignancy
- Benign cortical tumors with oncocytic change can have some of these features

Cytologic Features
- Cells have clear to eosinophilic cytoplasm
- Nuclei range from bland to highly atypical
- Variable mitotic rate

ANCILLARY TESTS

Cytology
- Unable to separate benign from malignant adrenocortical lesions
- High nuclear pleomorphism, chromatin irregularities, and prominent nucleoli favor carcinoma
- FNA can be diagnostic for metastatic tumors

Immunohistochemistry
- Positive for
  - o Synaptophysin, Melan-A, Inhibin, SF1 stains

Genetic Testing
- Numerous studies have elucidated molecular pathogenesis of adrenal cortical tumors
  - o Leading to molecular classification
  - o Molecular evidence for adenoma to carcinoma progression
- **Gene expression profiling**
  - o Overexpression of *IGF2* is one of most highly expressed in carcinomas
  - o Expression of *DLGAP5* (previously called *DLG7*) and *PINK1* identify carcinomas and tumors within borderline Weiss criteria
  - o Somatic mutations of *TP53*, *CTNNB1*, or RB
- **MicroRNA expression profiling**
  - o MicroRNAs were shown to be deregulated in adrenocortical carcinoma
    - High miR-210 is associated with aggressiveness and poor prognosis

- **Integrated genomic characterization**
  - (1) High prevalent role of *IGF1* overexpression
  - (2) *TP53* mutation and its dominant frequency in pediatric ACC and association with aggressive behavior
  - (3) Frequent and diversity of WNT pathway defects: *CTNNB1* point mutations and *ZNRF3* deletions
    - Present in ~ 50% of ACC
  - (4) Copy number alterations and whole genome doubling
    - Complex pattern of chromosomal aberrations
      - Multiple regions of gains and losses
  - (5) Important role of telomeres and telomerase reactivation
  - (6) Relative lack of targetable hotspot mutations

Electron Microscopy

- Features of steroidogenesis
  - Abundant rough and smooth endoplasmic reticulum
  - Many mitochondria
  - Intracytoplasmic lipid droplets

DIFFERENTIAL DIAGNOSIS

Adrenal Cortical Adenoma

- Tends to be smaller and weigh less than carcinoma
- Often lacks mitotic figures, necrosis, and invasion
- Diagnosis of pediatric adrenal cortical tumors is difficult

Metastatic Tumors

- More likely to be bilateral
- Glandular, squamous, or small cell histology
- Often metastasizes to adrenal gland
  - Breast and lung carcinomas
  - Melanoma

Hepatocellular Carcinoma

- Confirm biopsy site
- Trabecular pattern, bile pigment, glandular arrangement
- Positive keratin, CEA, and Hep-Par1 stains

Renal Cell Carcinoma

- Pseudoalveolar pattern
- Extravasated erythrocytes
- Clear cytoplasm, prominent cell borders
- Positive for keratin, CD10, and EMA stains

Pheochromocytoma

- Different radiographic appearance, especially with scintigraphic studies
- Nested and zellballen pattern
- Basophilic cytoplasm, bizarre, isolated, atypical nuclei
- Positive for chromogranin, synaptophysin, and CD56 stains in paraganglia cells
- S100 protein positive sustentacular cells

DIAGNOSTIC CHECKLIST

Distinction Between Benign and Malignant Adrenal Cortical Neoplasms

- No single feature is diagnostic of carcinoma
- Multiple systems used for diagnosis (Weiss, Hough, van Slooten)

- Weiss criteria for malignancy in adrenal cortical tumors: Presence of ≥ 3 of these criteria correlates with malignant behavior
  - High-nuclear grade (Fuhrman grade IV)
  - Mitotic rate > 5 mitotic figures/50 HPF
  - Atypical mitotic figures
  - < 25% of tumor cells with clear/vacuolated cytoplasm
  - Diffuse architecture (> 1/3 of tumor)
  - Confluent tumor necrosis
  - Venous invasion (of smooth muscle walled vessels)
  - Sinusoidal invasion (no smooth muscle in vessel wall)
  - Capsular invasion

Assessment of Biological Aggression in ACC

- Mitotic grade
  - **Low-grade carcinoma:** ≤ 20 mitosis/50 HPF
  - **High-grade carcinoma:** > 20 mitosis/50 HPF

STAGING

European Network for Study of Adrenal Tumors (ENSAT)

- Stage I: Confined to gland, ≤ 5 cm
- Stage II: Confined to gland, > 5 cm
- Stage III: Extends beyond gland, into surrounding tissues but not into adjacent organs; positive regional lymph nodes or involvement of regional veins
- Stage IV: Distant metastases or adjacent organ involvement

SELECTED REFERENCES

1. Brown RE et al: Metformin and melatonin in adrenocortical carcinoma: morphoproteomics and biomedical analytics provide proof of concept in a case study. Ann Clin Lab Sci. 47(4):457-465, 2017
2. Else T et al: Adrenocortical carcinoma and succinate dehydrogenase gene mutations. Eur J Endocrinol. ePub, 2017
3. Jonker PKC et al: Epigenetic dysregulation in adrenocortical carcinoma, a systematic review of the literature. Mol Cell Endocrinol. ePub, 2017
4. Drelon C et al: EZH2 is overexpressed in adrenocortical carcinoma and is associated with disease progression. Hum Mol Genet. 25(13):2789-2800, 2016
5. Liu-Chittenden Y et al: Serum RARRES2 Is a prognostic marker in patients with adrenocortical carcinoma. J Clin Endocrinol Metab. 101(9):3345-52, 2016
6. Papathomas TG et al: An international Ki67 reproducibility study in adrenal cortical carcinoma. Am J Surg Pathol. 40(4):569-76, 2016
7. Zheng S et al: Comprehensive pan-genomic characterization of adrenocortical carcinoma. Cancer Cell. 29(5):723-36, 2016
8. Zheng S et al: Comprehensive pan-genomic characterization of adrenocortical carcinoma. Cancer Cell. 30(2):363, 2016
9. Asare EA et al: A novel staging system for adrenocortical carcinoma better predicts survival in patients with stage I/II disease. Surgery. 156(6):1378-86, 2014
10. Burotto M et al: Brain metastasis in patients with adrenocortical carcinoma: a clinical series. J Clin Endocrinol Metab. jc20142650, 2014
11. De Martino MC et al: Characterization of the mTOR pathway in human normal adrenal and adrenocortical tumors. Endocr Relat Cancer. 21(4):601-13, 2014
12. Erickson LA et al: Adrenocortical carcinoma: review and update. Adv Anat Pathol. 21(3):151-9, 2014
13. Hofland J et al: Inhibin alpha-subunit (INHA) expression in adrenocortical cancer is linked to genetic and epigenetic INHA promoter variation. PLoS One. 9(8):e104944, 2014
14. Lerario AM et al: Genetics and epigenetics of adrenocortical tumors. Mol Cell Endocrinol. 386(1-2):67-84, 2014
15. Mouat IC et al: Assessing biological aggression in adrenocortical neoplasia. Surg Pathol Clin. 7(4):533-41, 2014
16. Sasano H et al: Roles of the pathologist in evaluating surrogate markers for medical therapy in adrenocortical carcinoma. Endocr Pathol. 25(4):366-70, 2014

Immunohistochemistry

Antibody	Reactivity	Staining Pattern	Comment
Vimentin	Positive	Cytoplasmic	
Inhibin	Positive	Cytoplasmic	Nondiscriminating between adenoma and carcinoma
Melan-A103	Positive	Cytoplasmic	Nondiscriminating between adenoma and carcinoma
Calretinin	Positive	Nuclear & cytoplasmic	
SF1	Positive	Nuclear	
CK-PAN	Equivocal	Cytoplasmic	< 5% of tumor cells reactive
Synaptophysin	Positive	Cytoplasmic	Frequently expressed
CD56	Positive	Cytoplasmic	
CEA-M	Negative		Generally negative
Chromogranin-A	Negative		

Histologic Criteria for Distinguishing Benign From Malignant Adrenal Cortical Neoplasms

Weiss Criteria*	van Slooten System**
High nuclear grade; Fuhrman criteria used	Histologic criteria/**weight**
> 5 mitoses/50 HPF	Extensive regressive changes (necrosis, hemorrhage, fibrosis, calcification)/**5.7**
Atypical mitotic figures	Loss of normal structure/**1.6**
< 25% of tumor cells are clear cells	Nuclear atypia (moderate/marked)/**2.1**
Diffuse architecture (> 33% of tumor)	Nuclear hyperchromasia (moderate/marked)/**2.6**
Necrosis	Abnormal nucleoli/**4.1**
Venous invasion (smooth muscle in wall)	Mitotic activity (≥ 2/10 HPF)/**9.0**
Sinusoidal invasion (no smooth muscle in wall)	Vascular or capsular invasion/**3.3**
Capsular invasion	

Presence of 3 or more criteria highly correlates with malignant behavior. This system is the most used system for the diagnosis of adrenal cortical carcinoma.
**Histologic index > 8 correlates with malignant behavior.*

17. Raymond VM et al: Adrenocortical carcinoma is a Lynch syndrome-associated cancer. J Clin Oncol. 31(24):3012-8, 2013
18. de Krijger RR et al: Adrenocortical neoplasia: evolving concepts in tumorigenesis with an emphasis on adrenal cortical carcinoma variants. Virchows Arch. 460(1):9-18, 2012
19. Szabó PM et al: Underexpression of C-myc in adrenocortical cancer: a major pathogenic event? Horm Metab Res. 43(5):297-9, 2011
20. Giordano TJ: Adrenocortical tumors: an integrated clinical, pathologic, and molecular approach at the University of Michigan. Arch Pathol Lab Med. 134(10):1440-3, 2010
21. Giordano TJ et al: Molecular classification and prognostication of adrenocortical tumors by transcriptome profiling. Clin Cancer Res. 15(2):668-76, 2009
22. McNicol AM: A diagnostic approach to adrenal cortical lesions. Endocr Pathol. 19(4):241-51, 2008
23. McNicol AM: Lesions of the adrenal cortex. Arch Pathol Lab Med. 132(8):1263-71, 2008
24. Volante M et al: Pathological and molecular features of adrenocortical carcinoma: an update. J Clin Pathol. 61(7):787-93, 2008
25. Gross MD et al: PET in the diagnostic evaluation of adrenal tumors. Q J Nucl Med Mol Imaging. 51(3):272-83, 2007
26. van't Sant HP et al: The prognostic value of two different histopathological scoring systems for adrenocortical carcinomas. Histopathology. 51(2):239-45, 2007
27. Abiven G et al: Clinical and biological features in the prognosis of adrenocortical cancer: poor outcome of cortisol-secreting tumors in a series of 202 consecutive patients. J Clin Endocrinol Metab. 91(7):2650-5, 2006
28. Allolio B et al: Clinical review: Adrenocortical carcinoma: clinical update. J Clin Endocrinol Metab. 91(6):2027-37, 2006
29. Sasano H et al: Recent advances in histopathology and immunohistochemistry of adrenocortical carcinoma. Endocr Pathol. 17(4):345-54, 2006
30. Elsayes KM et al: Adrenal masses: MR imaging features with pathologic correlation. Radiographics. 24 Suppl 1:S73-86, 2004
31. Sidhu S et al: Clinical and molecular aspects of adrenocortical tumourigenesis. ANZ J Surg. 73(9):727-38, 2003
32. Wieneke JA et al: Adrenal cortical neoplasms in the pediatric population: a clinicopathologic and immunophenotypic analysis of 83 patients. Am J Surg Pathol. 27(7):867-81, 2003
33. Dackiw AP et al: Adrenal cortical carcinoma. World J Surg. 25(7):914-26, 2001
34. Stratakis CA: Genetics of adrenocortical tumors: Carney complex. Ann Endocrinol (Paris). 62(2):180-4, 2001
35. Weiss LM et al: Pathologic features of prognostic significance in adrenocortical carcinoma. Am J Surg Pathol. 13(3):202-6, 1989
36. Weiss LM: Comparative histologic study of 43 metastasizing and nonmetastasizing adrenocortical tumors. Am J Surg Pathol. 8(3):163-9, 1984
37. Hough AJ et al: Prognostic factors in adrenal cortical tumors. A mathematical analysis of clinical and morphologic data. Am J Clin Pathol. 72(3):390-9, 1979
38. Macfarlane DA: Cancer of the adrenal cortex; the natural history, prognosis and treatment in a study of fifty-five cases. Ann R Coll Surg Engl. 23(3):155-86, 1958

Radiologic Image

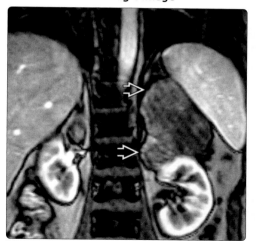

Large Adrenal Carcinoma

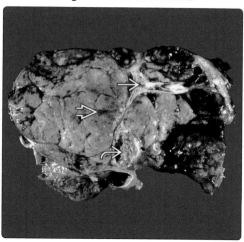

(Left) *Radiologic image shows a large left adrenal gland mass* ⇒ *pushing the kidney down and compressing the adjacent spleen. The interior is mottled and shows mixed intensity.* (Right) *This ACC presented as an irregularly shaped, bulky, unilateral mass and has a light brown variegated color. The cut surface shows extensive regressive changes, necrosis* ⇒*, hemorrhage* ⇒*, fibrosis and degeneration* ⇒*, and calcification.*

Gross Cut Surface With Extensive Necrosis

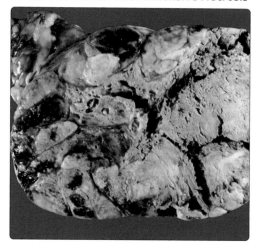

Cytological Features

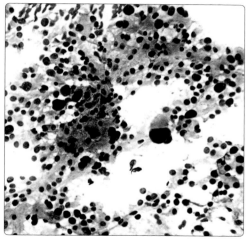

(Left) *This large ACC shows extensive necrosis and hemorrhage with only small areas of viable tumor. This gross appearance may mimic an adrenal pseudocyst.* (Right) *Cytologic diagnosis of ACC can be challenging. The degree of polymorphism and nuclear irregularity shown in this cytology favors carcinoma, confirmed on histological examination.*

Cellular Characteristics

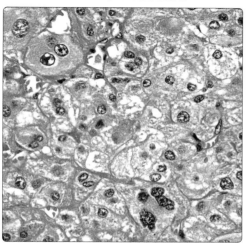

Degenerative Changes

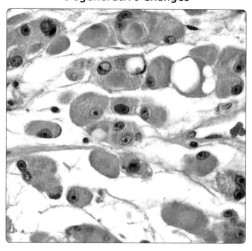

(Left) *High-magnification view of an ACC shows a tumor composed by slightly pleomorphic round cells with eosinophilic ample cytoplasm. There is mild nuclear pleomorphism and multinucleated tumor giant cells.* (Right) *H&E shows an ACC composed of large eosinophilic cytoplasm with pleomorphic nuclei and with prominent nucleoli. This area of the tumor shows dyscohesive cells with edematous stroma with degenerative changes.*

(Left) *This ACC, steroid-producing, present in a child, is composed by cells with ample eosinophilic cytoplasm. Occasional markedly enlarged multinucleated cells are identified.* **(Right)** *The finding of atypical mitosis is one of the Weiss criteria for malignancy. This tumor, present in a patient with Li-Fraumeni syndrome, shows numerous atypical mitosis.*

Pleomorphic Cell

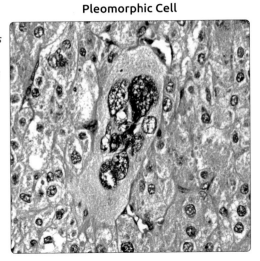

Atypical Mitosis

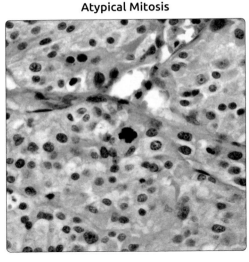

(Left) *This tumor, present in a patient with Li-Fraumeni syndrome, shows multifocal areas of tumor necrosis. Necrosis is one of the Weiss criteria for distinguishing benign from malignant cortical tumors. In the higher grade tumors, necrosis may be abundant.* **(Right)** *Myxoid changes may be present in adrenal cortical adenomas and in carcinomas, although these changes are more commonly seen in carcinomas.*

Foci of Necrosis in ACC

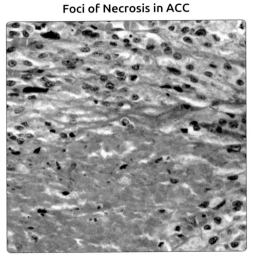

Myxoid Stromal Changes

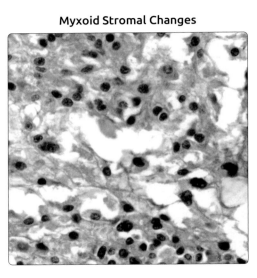

(Left) *The picture illustrates a strong synaptophysin immunoreactivity in the adrenal carcinoma in a patient with Li-Fraumeni syndrome. This stain is usually patchy. The tumors in these patients also stain positive for p53.* **(Right)** *ACC in a child with steroid-producing tumor shows patchy and variably focal staining for Melan A. These tumors are also positive for SF1, synaptophysin, and inhibin-alpha stains.*

Cytoplasmic Synaptophysin Reactivity

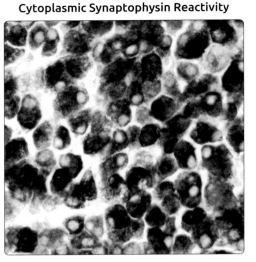

Melan A Immunoreactivity in ACC

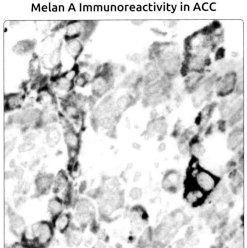

Lymphovascular Invasion

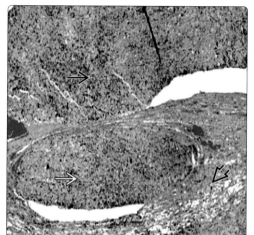

Vascular Invasion

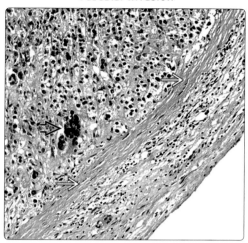

(Left) *Low-magnification view shows an area of juxtaposition between an ACC composed of small uniform cells ⇥ and the residual normal adrenal tissue ⇥. Tumor invasion of a large intraparenchymal vessel is shown ➡.* (Right) *This tumor invades a vessel wall ➡ and is composed of small, uniform cells with clear cytoplasm. Atypical cells with large irregular nuclei and a large bizarre multinucleated cell ⇥ are also shown.*

Necrosis

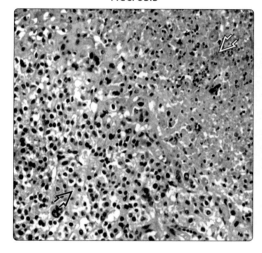

Distinct Cell Morphology

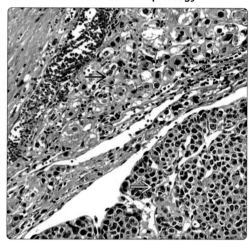

(Left) *Viable tumor ⇥ and necrosis ➡ are depicted. Tumor necrosis is an important histologic criterion in all schemes for differentiation between benign and malignant adrenal cortical neoplasms.* (Right) *H&E shows the interface between 2 distinct areas of an ACC. One area of tumor is made up of sheets of small, compact round cells with scant cytoplasm ➡. There is a sharp contrast in the cell size of this component compared to the other component ⇥.*

Metastases to Lung

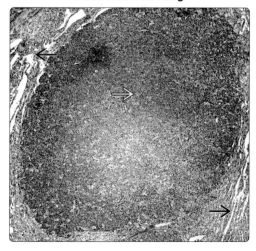

Lung With Metastatic Focus of ACC

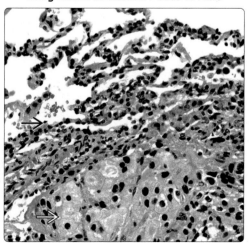

(Left) *H&E shows metastatic adrenal cortical carcinoma ➡ to lung parenchyma. The tumor mass is composed of small, compact eosinophilic cells and is surrounded by lung parenchyma ⇥.* (Right) *ACC metastatic to lung exhibits tumor cells ➡ with abundant, granular, oncocytic cytoplasm with round, uniform, hyperchromatic nuclei. Nuclear pleomorphism can be seen among tumor cells. The compressed adjacent lung parenchyma is seen ⇥.*

TERMINOLOGY

- Neuroblastic tumors of adrenal gland: Group of tumors arising from sympathoadrenal lineage of neural crest during development (WHO 2017)

MICROSCOPIC

- International Neuroblastoma Pathology Committee (INPC) classification
- **Neuroblastoma (schwannian stroma-poor)**
  - Cellular neuroblastic tumor without prominent schwannian stroma
    - **Undifferentiated**: No identifiable neuropil formation and supplementary diagnostic techniques required
    - **Poorly differentiated**: Diagnosis can be made by pure morphological criteria; differentiating neuroblasts < 5%; characteristic neuropil present
    - **Differentiating**: Usually abundant neuropil; differentiating neuroblasts > 5%

- **Ganglioneuroblastoma, intermixed (schwannian stroma-rich)**
  - Intermingled microscopic foci of neuroblastic elements in expanding schwannian stroma, constituting > 50% of tumor volume
- **Ganglioneuroblastoma, nodular (composite, schwannian stroma-rich/dominant and schwannian stroma-poor)**
  - Grossly identifiable neuroblastic nodular (stroma-poor) component coexisting with intermixed ganglioneuroblastoma (stroma-rich) or ganglioneuroma (stroma dominant) component
- **Ganglioneuroma (schwannian stroma-dominant)**
  - Predominantly composed of schwannian stroma without individually distributed neuronal elements
    - **Maturing ganglioneuroma**: Both maturing and mature ganglion cells
    - **Mature ganglioneuroma**: Exclusively mature ganglion cells in schwannian stroma

N-myc FISH Amplification

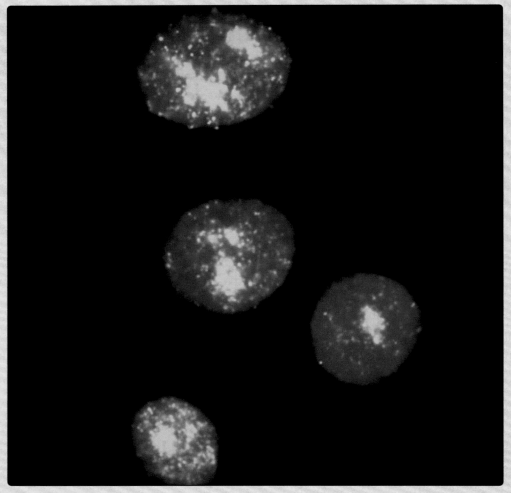

Fluorescence in situ hybridization (FISH) of neuroblastoma (NB) shows marked amplification of N-myc (multiple confluent green dots). The degree of N-myc amplification, higher or lower, is not correlated with a worse outcome.

TERMINOLOGY

Abbreviations

- Neuroblastoma (NB)
- Ganglioneuroblastoma (GNB)
- Ganglioneuroma (GN)

Synonyms

- Peripheral neuroblastic tumor

Definitions

- Neuroblastic tumors of adrenal gland: Group of tumors arising from sympathoadrenal lineage of neural crest during development (WHO 2017)
  - Included within broader classification of peripheral neuroblastic tumors
- International Neuroblastoma Pathology Classification (INPC) defines 4 categories of peripheral neuroblastic tumors
  - Neuroblastoma (schwannian stroma-poor)
  - Ganglioneuroblastoma, intermixed (schwannian stroma-rich)
  - Ganglioneuroblastoma, nodular (composite, schwannian-rich/dominant)
  - Ganglioneuroma (schwannian stroma-dominant)

ETIOLOGY/PATHOGENESIS

Developmental Anomaly

- Neuroblastic tumors arise from sympathoadrenal lineage of neural crest during development
  - Derived from primordial neural crest cells
    - These cells migrate from spinal cord to adrenal medulla and sympathetic ganglia
  - ~ 70% abdominal, and most located in adrenal glands
  - Other locations include abdominal ganglia, thoracic ganglia, pelvic ganglia, cervical sympathetic ganglia, and paratesticular region
- Caused by transformation of neural crest cells secondary to genetic or epigenetic events
- Events leading to tumorigenesis remain poorly understood
- May be preconception or gestational factors; some tumors congenital
- No definitive factors accepted to increase incidence

Ganglioneuroma

- Believed that all GN were once NB in early stage of tumor development
- Developmental anomaly
  - Postulated that tumor cells derived from neuroblasts in adrenal medulla
  - Most develop de novo
- Associated conditions
  - Polypoid GNs in GI tract associated with tumor syndromes
    - PTEN hamartoma tumor syndrome (Cowden disease), MEN2B, NF1, juvenile polyposis, and tuberous sclerosis
  - Most adrenal GNs sporadic
    - Some cases have been associated with Turner syndrome and MEN2

CLINICAL ISSUES

Epidemiology

- Incidence
  - Peripheral neuroblastic tumors 3rd most common childhood neoplasm
    - After leukemias and brain tumors
  - Most common neoplasms during 1st year of life
  - Most common extracranial solid tumors during 1st 2 years of life
  - Prevalence: 1/7,000 live births
- Age
  - 40% of patients diagnosed < 1 year of age
  - ~ 90% diagnosed < 5 years of age
  - ~ 20-30% congenital (some detected on US during pregnancy)
- Sex
  - M:F = 1.2:1
- Ethnicity
  - Less common in African Americans; very low incidence in "Burkitt lymphoma belt" in Africa
- GN
  - Age
    - 7 years or older
  - Sex
    - No predilection

Site

- Primary site reflects migration pattern of neural crest cells during fetal development and follows distribution of sympathetic ganglia
  - Abdomen (54%)
    - Adrenal (40%)
    - Abdominal ganglia (25%)
  - Thoracic ganglia (15%)
  - Cervical sympathetic ganglia (3-5%)
  - Pelvic ganglia (5%)
  - Rare tumors occur in paratesticular region
- GN
  - Most found in posterior mediastinum and retroperitoneum
  - 20-30% of all GNs occur in adrenal

Presentation

- Usually sporadic
  - Some autosomal dominant familial cases have been seen
- Depends on age of patient, location of tumor, and associated clinical syndromes
- Most have nonspecific symptoms
  - Fever, weight loss, diarrhea, anemia, hypertension
- Fetuses may have hydrops
- Palpable mass
- ~ 2/3 have metastasis on presentation
- "Blueberry muffin" baby
  - Blue-red cutaneous lesions in infants
- Opsoclonus/myoclonus syndrome ("dancing eyes, dancing feet")
- Complex and heterogeneous disease

- o Many factors, such as age at diagnosis and stage of disease, in addition to molecular, cellular, and genetic features of tumor, determine whether it will spontaneously regress or metastasize and become refractory to therapy
- GN
  - o Asymptomatic; incidental, painless mass
  - o Most tumors hormone silent
    - – Up to 37% can produce catecholamine, testosterone, and other hormones

Laboratory Tests

- Urine catecholamine metabolites and dopamine have been used for screening
- Lactate dehydrogenase
  - o > 1,500 IU/L associated with worse clinical outcome
- Ferritin
  - o > 142 ng/mL associated with worse clinical outcome
- NSE
  - o > 100 ng/mL associated with worse clinical outcome

Natural History

- Some cases undergo spontaneous regression, including stage IV-S
  - o Most in children under 1 year of age

Treatment

- Low risk
  - o Surgery or observation alone
- Intermediate risk
  - o Surgery and adjuvant chemotherapy
- High risk
  - o Induction chemotherapy
  - o Delayed tumor resection
  - o Radiation of primary site
  - o Myeloablative chemotherapy with stem cell recovery
- Metastases
  - o Bone
  - o Lymph nodes
  - o Liver
  - o Skin
- GN
  - o Definitive treatment surgical excision

Prognosis

- International Neuroblastoma Staging System (INSS) and International Neuroblastoma Risk Group (INRG) used to predict prognosis of patients with NB
- **INSS**
  - o Molecular facts
    - – *MYCN* status
      - □ *MYCN* amplification, detected by FISH or immunohistochemistry, present in ~ 25% NB
    - – DNA index: Ploidy
  - o Patient age
  - o INPC histology groups
    - – Favorable
    - – Unfavorable
      - □ Based on age of patient, histological type, and mitosis-karyorrhexis index (MKI) (defined as number of cells undergoing mitosis or karyorrhexis per 5,000 cells)

- o Clinical parameters
- **INGR**
  - o Patient age
  - o Histological category
  - o Grade of tumor differentiation
  - o Molecular factors
    - – MYCN status
    - – Ploidy
    - – Presence of unbalanced 11q aberration
      - □ High risk with aberration
- 5-year survival based on stage at time of diagnosis
  - o Stage I: > 90%
  - o Stage II: 70-80%
  - o Stage III: 40-70%
  - o Stage IV
    - – < 1 year old: > 60%
    - – 1-2 years old: 20%
    - – > 2 years old: 10%
  - o Stage IV-S: > 80%
- Patient age at diagnosis, stage of disease, and presence of *MYCN* amplification in NB cells are 3 strongest determinants of clinical outcome
- Adverse factors
  - o Older age at diagnosis
  - o Advanced stage of disease (except IV-S)
  - o High histologic grade of tumor
  - o Diploid DNA value
  - o *N-myc* (v-myc myelocytomatosis viral related oncogene, neuroblastoma derived) oncogene amplification and loss of chromosome 11q heterozygosity have been known to be indicative of poor prognosis
    - – MYCN expression profile still one of most robust and significant prognostic markers for NB outcome
  - o Cytogenetic abnormalities of chromosomes 1 and 17
  - o Pattern of urinary catecholamine excretion
  - o Increased levels of ferritin, NSE, LDH, creatine kinase BB, or chromogranin-A
  - o Abnormalities in ganglioside composition
  - o Lack of high affinity nerve growth factor receptors

Ganglioneuroma

- Excellent; a few cases reported of malignant transformation of GNs into malignant schwannoma and malignant peripheral nerve sheath tumor (MPNST)

IMAGING

General Features

- Extensive radiographic evaluation required to determine extent of disease and identify metastatic foci
- Calcifications often seen in central portion of tumor
- GN imaging
  - o MR
    - – Low nonenhanced T1-weighted signal, slightly high and heterogeneous T2-weighted signal, and late and gradual enhancement on dynamic MR
  - o CT
    - – Well-defined, sometimes encapsulated, solid mass inside adrenal gland
    - – Punctuate or discrete calcifications seen in almost 1/2 of GNs

Bone Scan

- Radiolabeled metaiodobenzylguanidine (MIBG) incorporates into catecholamine-secreting cells and can detect neuroblastoma

MACROSCOPIC

General Features

- Color and consistency depends on amount of stroma present (stroma-poor vs. stroma-rich tumors), hemorrhage and necrosis
- Usually solitary masses
- **NB (schwannian-stroma poor)**: Reach 10 cm and form soft, gray-pale mass with areas of hemorrhage
- **GNB, nodular type**: Soft, hemorrhagic nodules intermixed with tan-white tumor tissue
- **GNB, intermixed type**: Tan-white cut surface
- **NB (schwannian-stroma poor)**: Well-circumscribed, firm, multinodular mass with gray-white cut surface
- Cystic degeneration, hemorrhage, necrosis, and calcification can be seen

MICROSCOPIC

Histologic Features

- **Histopathological classification**: INPC defines 4 categories of neuroblastic tumors (NB, intermixed GNB, nodular GNB, and GN) and delineates distinction between them
- **Cytological features**
  - Neuroblasts
    - Small round blue cells with very scant cytoplasm
  - Homer Wright rosettes or pseudorosettes (uncommon)
    - Nuclei grouping in ring-like structures around central cores of tangled neuritic cell processes
  - Ganglionic differentiation
    - Cells enlarged
    - Increased eosinophilic or amphophilic cytoplasm
    - Nuclear chromatin pattern becomes vesicular
    - Must have synchronous differentiation of cytoplasm and nucleus
  - Neuropil
    - Fibrillar eosinophilic matrix
  - Mitotic-karyorrhectic index (MKI), applicable for stroma-poor tumors
    - Count of cells undergoing mitosis or karyorrhexis (per 5,000 cells)
      - Low: < 100 cells
      - Intermediate: 100-200 cells
      - High: > 200 cells
  - Schwann cells with spindled cytoplasm, wavy dark nuclei, and inconspicuous nucleoli admixed with ganglion cells
  - Ganglion cells exhibit abundant eosinophilic cytoplasm, large vesicular nuclei, and prominent nucleoli

INPC Classification

- **Neuroblastoma (Schwannian stroma-poor)**
  - Cellular neuroblastic tumor without prominent schwannian stroma
    - No ganglionic differentiation
    - No neuropil
    - No or minimal schwannian stroma

- Often requires immunohistochemistry for accurate diagnosis
  - 3 subtypes included
    - **Undifferentiated**
      - No identifiable neuropil formation and supplementary diagnostic techniques required
    - **Poorly differentiated**
      - Diagnosis can be made by pure morphological criteria
      - Characteristic neuropil present
      - Differentiating neuroblasts < 5%
    - **Differentiating**
      - Usually abundant neuropil
      - Differentiating neuroblasts > 5%
- **Ganglioneuroblastoma, intermixed (schwannian stroma-rich)**
  - Intermingled microscopic foci of neuroblastic elements in expanding schwannian stroma, constituting > 50% of tumor volume
    - Neuroblastic foci microscopic without grossly visible nodular formation
    - Neuroblastic foci composed of mixture of neuroblastic cells in various stages of differentiation
    - Neuropil background
- **Ganglioneuroblastoma, nodular (composite, schwannian stroma-rich/dominant and schwannian stroma-poor)**
  - Grossly identifiable neuroblastic nodular (stroma-poor) component coexisting with intermixed GNB (stroma-rich) or GN (stroma dominant) component
    - Proportion of component varies
    - Abrupt demarcation between stroma-poor NB and stroma-rich component
    - Fibrous pseudocapsule often seen surrounding NB component
    - > 50% schwannian stroma
- **Ganglioneuroma (schwannian stroma-dominant)**
  - Predominantly composed of schwannian stroma without individually distributed neuronal elements
  - Neuritic processes produced by ganglion cells enveloped by cytoplasm of Schwann cells
  - Characterized by the presence of ganglion cells individually distributed in schwannian stroma
  - 2 subtypes
    - **Maturing GN**: Both maturing and mature ganglion cells
    - **Mature GN**: Exclusively mature ganglion cells in schwannian stroma
      - Composed of mature ganglion cells, Schwann cell-like spindle cells, and nerve fibers
      - Variable size and number of intermixed ganglion cells in uniform spindle cell matrix
      - May show calcification, cystic change, and hemorrhage
      - Rare mixed composite NB and pheochromocytoma
- Do not classify posttreatment resections
  - "Neuroblastoma with treatment effect" is sufficient
- May classify metastatic disease if resection/biopsy pretreatment

ANCILLARY TESTS

Immunohistochemistry

- Tumor cells variably positive for neuronal markers
- Panel approach more appropriate, including synaptophysin, chromogranin, PGP9.5, CD56, NFP
- Tumor cells positive for neural crest markers, such as tyrosine hydroxylase and PHOX2B, and NB marker NB84
- NSE
  - Most sensitive but least specific
  - Found at least focally even in very undifferentiated NBs
- NB84(+) in almost all NBs
  - Not specific; occasionally positive in other small round cell tumors
- S100 protein
  - Mature Schwann cells S100 positive in intermixed GNB and in GN
  - Positive in schwannian stroma
- PHOX2B
  - Highly sensitive and specific IHC marker for peripheral neuroblastic tumors, including NB
  - Reliably distinguishes NB from histological mimics: Wilms tumor, Ewing sarcoma, and round cell sarcoma

Genetic Testing

- N-myc
  - Amplification associated with worse prognosis
  - Usually seen in advanced disease
  - MYCN is transcription factor that belongs to family of MYC oncoproteins, comprising c-MYC and MYCL genes
    - Can repress at least as many genes as it activates, thus proposing novel function of this protein in neuroblastoma biology
- DNA ploidy
  - Near-diploidy or tetraploidy associated with worse prognosis
  - Hyperdiploidy associated with better prognosis
- Loss of heterozygosity of 1p and 11q
  - Both associated with worse prognosis
- TrkA (high-affinity nerve growth factor receptor)
  - Increased expression associates with better prognosis

Electron Microscopy

- Wide range of cytologic differentiation
- Dense core of neurosecretory granules
  - Found in elongated cell processes
  - 100 nm in diameter
  - Dense core surrounded by clear halos and delicate outer membranes

Genetic Events

- By definition, this disease is caused by transformation of neural crest cells secondary to genetic and epigenetic events
- Tumorigenesis still poorly understood
- Young age of patients at onset of disease suggests role of preconceptional or gestational factors
- Neuroblastic tumors present as congenital tumors

Sporadic Neuroblastoma

- ~ 6-10% of sporadic NBs carry somatic ALK-activating mutations; additional 3-4% have high frequency of ALK gene amplification
  - These findings in familial and sporadic NB suggest that ALK is oncogenic driver in NB
    - Activating ALK mutations or amplifications, especially in presence of MYCN amplification, associated with lethal disease
    - ALK is promising target for molecular therapy in preclinical studies and clinical trials for NB
- Mutations in α-thalassemia/mental retardation syndrome X-linked (ATRX) among most common lesions in sporadic NB
  - ATRX encodes SWI/SNF chromatin-remodeling ATP-dependent helicase
    - ATRX mutations associated with X-linked mental retardation (XLMR) and α-thalassemia, suggesting that ATRX functions in various developmental processes
    - Important association between ATRX mutations and age at diagnosis of NB
      - Very young children (< 18 months of age) with stage 4 disease tend to have better prognosis than their older counterparts, and no ATRX mutations have been identified in this age group
      - ATRX mutations occur in 17% of children aged between 18 months and 12 years with stage 4 disease and in 44% of patients > 12 years who uniformly have very poor prognosis
      - Relationship between age at diagnosis and ATRX mutations significant

Genetic Susceptibility: Familial Neuroblastoma

- Familial NB is rare (1-2% of all NBs)
- Autosomal dominant inheritance pattern with incomplete penetration
- Usually diagnosed at earlier age than patients with sporadic cases (mean: 9 months vs. 17.3 months)
- ~ 20% have bilateral adrenal tumors and multifocal tumors
- Mutations in some signaling pathways important for development of sympathoadrenal lineage are associated with familial genetic syndromes
- Characterized by defects in development and predisposition to NB
- Germline mutations reported in familial NB located in PHOX2B and ALK
- 1st predisposition mutation identified in NB was in paired-like homeobox 2b (PHOX2B)
  - Encodes homeodomain transcription factor that promotes cell cycle exit and neuronal differentiation
    - Plays crucial part in development of neural crest-derived autonomic neurons
  - Perturbations in PHOX2B-regulated differentiation pathway in sympathoadrenal lineage of neural crest may contribute to NB tumorigenesis
- More common lesion associated with familial NB is in anaplastic lymphoma receptor tyrosine kinase (ALK) gene
  - Known natural ligands of ALK include pleiotrophin and midkine; ALK is expressed in developing sympathoadrenal lineage of the neural crest

- May regulate balance between proliferation and differentiation through multiple cellular pathways, including MAPK and RAS-related protein 1 (*RAP1*) signal transduction pathways
- *PHOX2B* can directly regulate *ALK* gene expression, providing connection between these 2 pathways that are mutated in familial NB

DIFFERENTIAL DIAGNOSIS

Ewing Sarcoma/Primitive Neuroectodermal Tumor

- Usually older patients
- Cells have finely stippled chromatin and glycogen-filled cytoplasm
- CD99 positivity
- Specific gene fusions, most commonly *EWSR1-FLI1*

Alveolar Rhabdomyosarcoma

- Cells with more pleomorphism and abundant cytoplasm
- Immunoreactivity for muscle markers (desmin, myogenin)
- t(1;13) or t(2;13) with *PAX-FOXO1* fusion

Lymphoma

- Lymphoid immunomarkers (CD45, CD3, CD20)

Ganglioneuroma

- Differs from intermixed GNB in having single cells instead of nests of cells within schwannian stroma
- Schwannoma
  - Strong S100 positivity; ganglion cells absent
- GNBs
  - Presence of neuroblasts

DIAGNOSTIC CHECKLIST

Clinically Relevant Pathologic Features

- Gross appearance
  - Cystic degeneration and calcification can be seen
- Microscopy
  - Small round blue cells with very scant cytoplasm
  - Homer Wright rosettes or pseudorosettes
  - Ganglionic differentiation
- MKI applicable for stroma-poor tumors
  - Count of cells undergoing mitosis or karyorrhexis (per 5,000 cells)

Pathologic Interpretation Pearls

- To assess classification based on degree of tumor differentiation
- High importance of cytogenetics
  - *N-myc* amplification associated with worse prognosis
  - Loss of heterozygosity of 1p and 11q associated with worse prognosis

SELECTED REFERENCES

1. He WG et al: Clinical and biological features of neuroblastic tumors: A comparison of neuroblastoma and ganglioneuroblastoma. Oncotarget. 8(23):37730-37739, 2017
2. Hung YP et al: PHOX2B reliably distinguishes neuroblastoma among small round blue cell tumors. Histopathology. ePub, 2017
3. Iacobone M et al: Adrenal ganglioneuroma: The Padua Endocrine Surgery Unit experience. Int J Surg. 41 Suppl 1:S103-S108, 2017
4. Lam AK: Update on adrenal tumours in 2017 World Health Organization (WHO) of endocrine tumours. Endocr Pathol. ePub, 2017
5. Shimada H et al: Neuroblastic tumors of the adrenal gland. In WHO classification of tumors of the endocrine organs. 196-203, 2017
6. Decarolis B et al: Treatment and outcome of ganglioneuroma and ganglioneuroblastoma intermixed. BMC Cancer. 16:542, 2016
7. Lee JH et al: Clinicopathological features of ganglioneuroma originating from the adrenal glands. World J Surg. 40(12):2970-2975, 2016
8. Newman EA et al: Recent biologic and genetic advances in neuroblastoma: Implications for diagnostic, risk stratification, and treatment strategies. Semin Pediatr Surg. 25(5):257-264, 2016
9. Abu-Arja R et al: Neuroblastoma in monozygotic twins with distinct presentation pathology and outcome: is it familial or in utero metastasis. Pediatr Blood Cancer. 61(6):1124-5, 2014
10. Barco S et al: Urinary homovanillic and vanillylmandelic acid in the diagnosis of neuroblastoma: report from the Italian Cooperative Group for Neuroblastoma. Clin Biochem. 47(9):848-52, 2014
11. Beltran H: The N-myc oncogene: maximizing its targets, regulation, and therapeutic potential. Mol Cancer Res. 12(6):815-22, 2014
12. Jrebi NY et al: Review of our experience with neuroblastoma and ganglioneuroblastoma in adults. World J Surg. 38(11):2871-4, 2014
13. Li L et al: Adrenal ganglioneuromas: experience from a retrospective study in a Chinese population. Urol J. 11(2):1485-90, 2014
14. Louis CU et al: Neuroblastoma: molecular pathogenesis and therapy. Annu Rev Med. ePub, 2014
15. Murga-Zamalloa C et al: ALK-driven tumors and targeted therapy: focus on crizotinib. Pharmgenomics Pers Med. 7:87-94, 2014
16. Murphy JM et al: Advances in the surgical treatment of neuroblastoma: a review. Eur J Pediatr Surg. 24(6):450-6, 2014
17. Shawa H et al: Adrenal ganglioneuroma: features and outcomes of 27 cases at a referral cancer centre. Clin Endocrinol (Oxf). 80(3):342-7, 2014
18. Shawa H et al: Clinical and radiologic features of pheochromocytoma/ganglioneuroma composite tumors: a case series with comparative analysis. Endocr Pract. 20(9):864-9, 2014
19. Waters AM et al: The interaction between FAK, MYCN, p53 and Mdm2 in neuroblastoma. Anticancer Agents Med Chem. 14(1):46-51, 2014
20. Williams P et al: Outcomes in multifocal neuroblastoma as part of the neurocristopathy syndrome. Pediatrics. 134(2):e611-6, 2014
21. Barone G et al: New strategies in neuroblastoma: therapeutic targeting of MYCN and ALK. Clin Cancer Res. 19(21):5814-21, 2013
22. Castel V et al: Emerging drugs for neuroblastoma. Expert Opin Emerg Drugs. 18(2):155-71, 2013
23. Cheung NK et al: Neuroblastoma: developmental biology, cancer genomics and immunotherapy. Nat Rev Cancer. 13(6):397-411, 2013
24. Gherardi S et al: MYCN-mediated transcriptional repression in neuroblastoma: the other side of the coin. Front Oncol. 3:42, 2013
25. Mei H et al: The mTOR signaling pathway in pediatric neuroblastoma. Pediatr Hematol Oncol. 30(7):605-15, 2013
26. Morgenstern DA et al: Current and future strategies for relapsed neuroblastoma: challenges on the road to precision therapy. J Pediatr Hematol Oncol. 35(5):337-47, 2013
27. Nonaka D et al: A study of gata3 and phox2b expression in tumors of the autonomic nervous system. Am J Surg Pathol. 37(8):1236-41, 2013
28. Schulte JH et al: Targeted therapy for neuroblastoma: ALK inhibitors. Klin Padiatr. 225(6):303-8, 2013
29. Sridhar S et al: New insights into the genetics of neuroblastoma. Mol Diagn Ther. 17(2):63-9, 2013
30. Navarro S et al: New prognostic markers in neuroblastoma. Expert Opin Med Diagn. 6(6):555-67, 2012
31. Capasso M et al: Genetics and genomics of neuroblastoma. Cancer Treat Res. 155:65-84, 2010
32. Maris JM: Recent advances in neuroblastoma. N Engl J Med. 362(23):2202-11, 2010
33. Matthay KK et al: Criteria for evaluation of disease extent by (123)I-metaiodobenzylguanidine scans in neuroblastoma: a report for the International Neuroblastoma Risk Group (INRG) Task Force. Br J Cancer. 102(9):1319-26, 2010
34. Rondeau G et al: Clinical and biochemical features of seven adult adrenal ganglioneuromas. J Clin Endocrinol Metab. 95(7):3118-25, 2010
35. Allende DS et al: Ganglioneuroma of the adrenal gland. J Urol. 182(2):714-5, 2009
36. Ambros PF et al: International consensus for neuroblastoma molecular diagnostics: report from the International Neuroblastoma Risk Group (INRG) Biology Committee. Br J Cancer. 100(9):1471-82, 2009
37. Cohn SL et al: The International Neuroblastoma Risk Group (INRG) classification system: an INRG Task Force report. J Clin Oncol. 27(2):289-97, 2009
38. Esiashvili N et al: Neuroblastoma. Curr Probl Cancer. 33(6):333-60, 2009
39. Okamatsu C et al: Clinicopathological characteristics of ganglioneuroma and ganglioneuroblastoma: a report from the CCG and COG. Pediatr Blood Cancer. 53(4):563-9, 2009

International Neuroblastoma Pathology Classification (INPC) With Favorable and Unfavorable Histological Groups in Neuroblastic Tumors

Age at Diagnosis	Favorable Histology Group	Unfavorable Histology Group
Any age	Ganglioneuroblastoma, intermixed (schwannian stroma-rich) Ganglioneuroma (schwannian stroma dominant) of either subtype (maturing or mature)	Neuroblastoma (schwannian stroma-poor) of undifferentiated subtype Neuroblastoma (schwannian stroma-poor) of any subtype with high MKI
< 18 months (< 548 days)	Neuroblastoma (schwannian stroma-poor) of poorly differentiated subtype with low or intermediate MKI Neuroblastoma (schwannian stroma-poor) of differentiating subtype with low to intermediate MKI	
16-60 months (548 days to 5 years)		Neuroblastoma (schwannian stroma-poor) of poorly differentiated subtype Neuroblastoma (schwannian stroma-poor) of differentiating subtype with intermediate MKI
> 60 months (> 5 years)		Neuroblastoma (schwannian stroma-poor) of any subtype

Modified from Shimada et al, Neuroblastic tumors of the adrenal, WHO 2017.

Neuroblastoma Staging System

Stage	Definition
I	Localized, confined tumor; complete gross excision; ipsilateral and contralateral nodes negative
IIA	Unilateral tumor; incomplete gross excision; identifiable ipsilateral and contralateral nodes negative
IIB	Unilateral tumor ± complete gross excision; identifiable ipsilateral nodes positive; identifiable ipsilateral and contralateral nodes negative
III	Tumor infiltrating across midline without positive nodes; or unilateral tumor with positive contralateral nodes
IV	Distant metastases to nodes, bone, bone marrow, liver, skin, &/or other organs not stage 4S
IV-S	Localized primary tumor (stage 1 or 2) with metastases limited to liver, skin, &/or bone marrow

40. De Bernardi B et al: Retrospective study of childhood ganglioneuroma. J Clin Oncol. 26(10):1710-6, 2008
41. Lack E: Tumors of the adrenal glands and extraadrenal paraganglia. In AFIP Atlas of Tumor Pathology Series 4, Fascicle 8. Washington, DC: American Registry of Pathology, 2007
42. Tornóczky T et al: Pathology of peripheral neuroblastic tumors: significance of prominent nucleoli in undifferentiated/poorly differentiated neuroblastoma. Pathol Oncol Res. 13(4):269-75, 2007
43. Sano H et al: International neuroblastoma pathology classification adds independent prognostic information beyond the prognostic contribution of age. Eur J Cancer. 42(8):1113-9, 2006
44. Peuchmaur M et al: Revision of the International Neuroblastoma Pathology Classification: confirmation of favorable and unfavorable prognostic subsets in ganglioneuroblastoma, nodular. Cancer. 98(10):2274-81, 2003
45. Shimada H: The International Neuroblastoma Pathology Classification. Pathologica. 95(5):240-1, 2003
46. Ambros IM et al: Morphologic features of neuroblastoma (Schwannian stroma-poor tumors) in clinically favorable and unfavorable groups. Cancer. 94(5):1574-83, 2002
47. Goto S et al: Histopathology (International Neuroblastoma Pathology Classification) and MYCN status in patients with peripheral neuroblastic tumors: a report from the Children's Cancer Group. Cancer. 92(10):2699-708, 2001
48. Shimada H et al: International neuroblastoma pathology classification for prognostic evaluation of patients with peripheral neuroblastic tumors: a report from the Children's Cancer Group. Cancer. 92(9):2451-61, 2001
49. Shimada H et al: Terminology and morphologic criteria of neuroblastic tumors: recommendations by the International Neuroblastoma Pathology Committee. Cancer. 86(2):349-63, 1999
50. Shimada H et al: The International Neuroblastoma Pathology Classification (the Shimada system). Cancer. 86(2):364-72, 1999
51. Brodeur GM et al: International criteria for diagnosis, staging, and response to treatment in patients with neuroblastoma. J Clin Oncol. 6(12):1874-81, 1988
52. Fletcher CD et al: Malignant nerve sheath tumour arising in a ganglioneuroma. Histopathology. 12(4):445-8, 1988

Sympathetic Chain

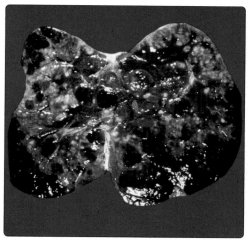

Clinical and Imaging Features

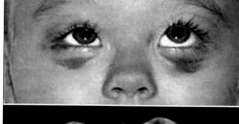

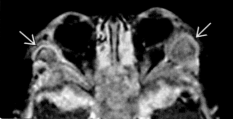

(Left) Graphic shows the anatomic extent of the sympathetic chain ➡ (including adrenal gland) from cervical region through mediastinum and abdomen to the inferior pelvis. NB can arise anywhere along the sympathetic chain. (Right) Child with bilateral orbital masses ➡ clinically presents with proptosis and ecchymosis.

Metastatic Neuroblastoma to Liver

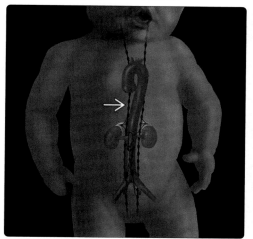

MR of Adrenal Tumor and Metastases to Liver

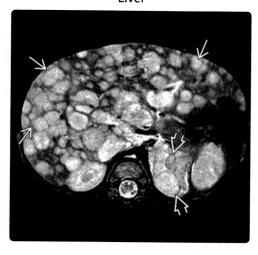

(Left) This specimen of liver shows diffuse involvement and extensive replacement by multiple deposits of metastatic NB. There are several foci of hemorrhage. (Right) Axial T2-weighted MR shows a left adrenal mass ➡, which proved to be NB. It was widely metastatic; the liver was filled with multiple high-signal nodular lesions ➡ with little normal remaining hepatic parenchyma.

MR of Mediastinal Tumor

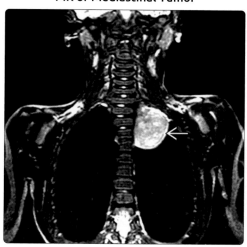

MR of Adrenal Neuroblastoma

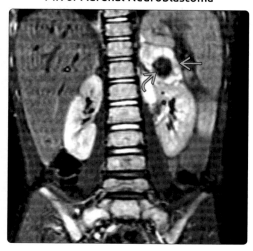

(Left) Coronal T2-weighted MR in a patient with ganglioneuroblastoma (GNB) shows a mildly hyperintense posterior mediastinal mass ➡ with no abnormality in the adjacent osseous marrow signal. (Right) Coronal T2-weighted MR shows NB ➡ of the left adrenal gland with an area of central necrosis ➡.

Characteristic Gross Appearance of GNB

Homogeneous Cut Surface of Ganglioneuroma

(Left) *This is a typical appearance of a nodular GNB. The hemorrhagic nodule ⮞ is stroma-poor NB, whereas the tan, fleshy rim ⮞ is either ganglioneuroma (GN) or intermixed GNB. The diagnosis of nodular GNB requires gross visible nodules.* (Right) *Gross photograph of the cut surface of GN shows a well-circumscribed mass with a yellow and whorled appearance. This appearance resembles a leiomyoma.*

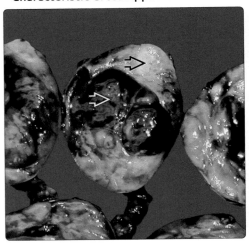

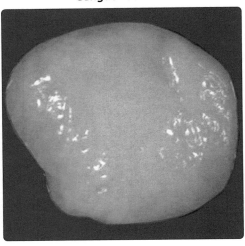

Cytomorphological Features

Characteristic Histopathological Findings

(Left) *In NB (schwannian stroma-poor), undifferentiated subtype, the cells have scant cytoplasm and rounded, deeply staining nuclei. On H&E, this could be mistaken for Ewing sarcoma, alveolar rhabdomyosarcoma, or lymphoma.* (Right) *H&E shows the typical low-power appearance of NB (schwannian stroma-poor), poorly differentiated. Small strips of schwannian stroma ⮞ separate the neuroblasts and neuropil, imparting a nested or multinodular appearance.*

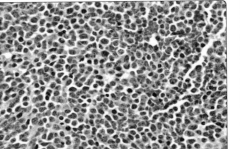

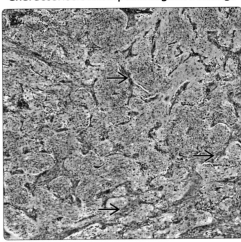

Round Cells and Neuropil

Areas of Necrosis

(Left) *NB (schwannian stroma-poor), poorly differentiated subtype shows sheets of small round cells ⮞ in aggregates within a background of neuropil ⮞.* (Right) *NBs are commonly hemorrhagic with areas of necrosis ⮞. These changes can also be seen after treatment. NBs that have undergone treatment should not be classified in the INPC system.*

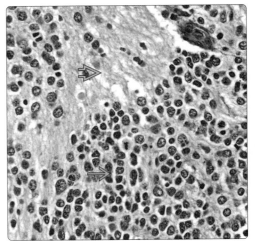

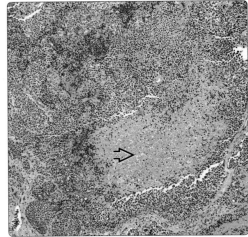

Nodular Areas

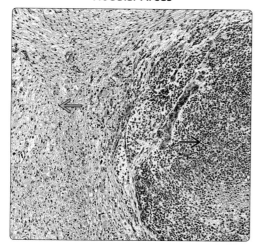

Schwannian Stroma

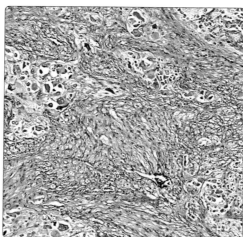

(Left) *This GNB, nodular (composite, NB schwannian stroma-rich/dominant and stroma poor) shows the pushing border between the stroma-poor NB component ⇨ and the intermixed GNB ⇨. A grossly visible nodule is required to diagnose nodular GNB.* **(Right)** *At least 50% of the tumor must be composed of schwannian stroma to make the diagnosis of GNB, intermixed (schwannian stroma-rich). This is characterized by spindled, wavy cells in bundles of varying cellularity.*

Prominent Stroma

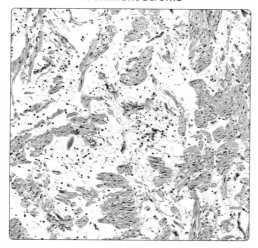

Neuroblasts and Ganglion Cells

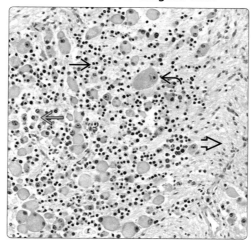

(Left) *This field of a GNB, intermixed, could be mistaken for neurofibroma (spindled wavy cells in a myxoid background). Adequate sampling, generally 1 section per centimeter of tumor, is required to make an accurate diagnosis.* **(Right)** *Higher magnification of GNB, intermixed (schwannian stroma-rich) shows details of neuroblasts ⇨, maturing neuroblasts ⇨, and ganglion cells ⇨ blending into the schwannian stroma ⇨.*

Mixed Cell Population With Neuropil and Schwannian Stroma

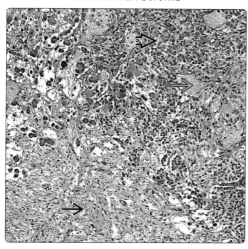

Clusters of Ganglion Cells

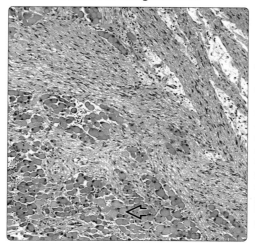

(Left) *Low magnification of GNB, intermixed (schwannian stroma-rich) shows clusters of maturing neuroblasts and ganglion cells ⇨, foci of neuropil ⇨, and areas of schwannian stroma ⇨.* **(Right)** *The neuroblastomatous component of this GNB, intermixed (schwannian stroma-rich) is predominantly made up of mature ganglion cells ⇨. The ganglion cells are present in clusters in this tumor, differing from the pattern in maturing GN in which they are present as single cells.*

Characteristics of Ganglion Cells

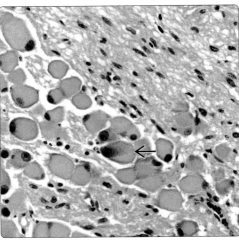

Neuroblastic Cells and Schwannian Stroma

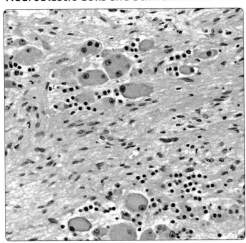

(Left) Mature ganglion cells ➡ are characterized by abundant eosinophilic to amphophilic cytoplasm, eccentric nuclei, and prominent nucleoli. Nissl substance may or may not be present. These cells are admixed with a schwannian stroma. (Right) This section of GNB, intermixed (schwannian stroma-rich) could be mistaken for a maturing GN. In maturing GN, the tumor is mainly composed of schwannian stroma, and individual neuroblastic cells merge into the schwannian stroma instead of forming distinct nests.

Neuropil Characteristics

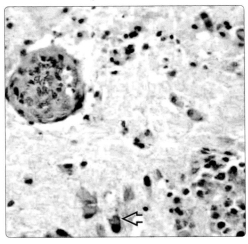

Site of Involvement

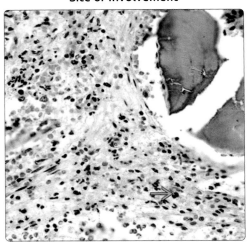

(Left) High-power view of GNB highlights the maturing ganglion cells ➡ in a background of neuropil. The neuropil is composed of a dense tangle of fibrillary, eosinophilic cytoplasmic processes. (Right) Bone marrow biopsy of metastatic NB shows small, hyperchromatic cells ➡ replacing hematopoietic precursors.

Diffuse Bone Marrow Involvement

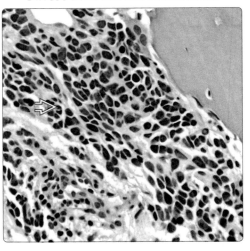

Focal Marrow Involvement

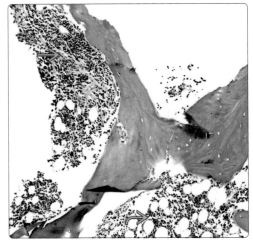

(Left) Core biopsy specimen of bone shows a focus of metastatic NB. The marrow has been extensively replaced by sheets of metastatic small round cell tumor ➡ and shows no areas with normal trilineage hematopoiesis. (Right) Core biopsy specimen of bone marrow shows normal marrow ➡ in the lower part of the field and a focus of metastatic neuroblastoma ➡ in the upper part. The normal bone marrow architecture is destroyed in the focus of metastatic tumor.

Ganglion Cells

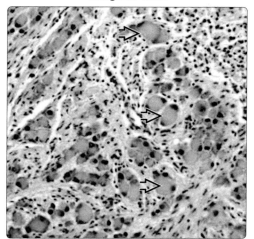

Interface of Adrenal Cortex and Ganglioneuroma

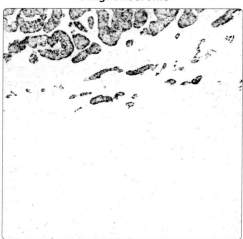

(Left) *GN (schwannian stroma-dominant) have a variable number of ganglion cells. This image shows numerous fully differentiated mature ganglion cells ⊇ in a paucicellular spindle Schwann cell-like stroma.* (Right) *Immunohistochemistry for melan-A highlights the normal adrenal cells, while the neoplastic cells are negative for this and other adrenal cortical markers, such as inhibin. Ganglioneuromas are usually positive for S100, NSE, NFP, synaptophysin, and chromogranin.*

Characteristic Immunoreactivity

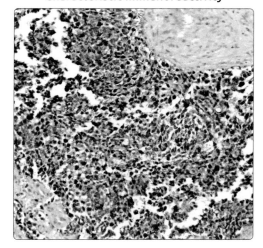

Marker of Neuroblastoma

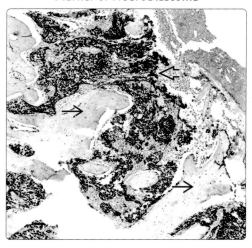

(Left) *NSE immunohistochemical staining of NB shows strong diffuse cytoplasmic positivity. NSE is a sensitive marker for NB, although nonspecific.* (Right) *In this bone marrow trephine specimen, there is diffuse immunoreactivity for NB antigen (NB84) in metastatic deposits of NB ⊇ that extend between bony trabeculae ⊇.*

Synaptophysin Stain

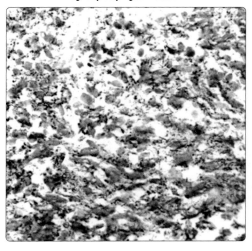

Pattern of ALK Staining

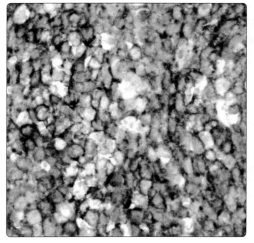

(Left) *Immunohistochemistry for synaptophysin shows membranous staining. Although not specific, this can be used for the differential diagnosis of other small round blue cell tumors, such as lymphoma, rhabdomyosarcoma, or Ewing sarcoma. These tumors are also positive for chromogranin and CD56.* (Right) *Immunohistochemistry for ALK1 in NB shows strong membranous staining. Activating mutations in ALK gene have been reported in NB and provide a potential therapeutic target.*

Malignant Melanoma, Adrenal Glands

TERMINOLOGY

- Primary malignant neoplasm of adrenal gland

CLINICAL ISSUES

- While adrenal gland metastases can be seen in context of metastatic malignant melanoma, primary adrenal melanoma (PAM) is extremely rare
  - ~ 25 cases reported
- Both adrenal melanomas and pheochromocytomas should be considered in differential diagnosis
  - When primary biochemical finding is increased urine dopamine excretion
- Adrenalectomy and nephrectomy
- PAM has high fatality rate

MICROSCOPIC

- Similar to melanoma arising in conventional sites
- May be amelanotic

ANCILLARY TESTS

- Positive immunostains: S100, Melan-A, HMB-45
- Negative immunostains: Synaptophysin, chromogranin
- Electron microscopy: Melanosomes and premelanosomes

TOP DIFFERENTIAL DIAGNOSES

- Metastatic malignant melanoma to adrenal
- Pigmented pheochromocytoma
- Pigmented adrenal lesions
- Primary pigmented nodular adrenal disease

DIAGNOSTIC CHECKLIST

- **Proposed diagnostic criteria include**
  - Presence of malignant melanoma in only 1 gland
  - No prior or current pigmented lesions in skin, mucosa, or eye
  - No history of removal of pigmented skin lesions
  - Failure to detect extraadrenal primary
    - Exclusion of adrenal metastasis

Pleomorphic Cells

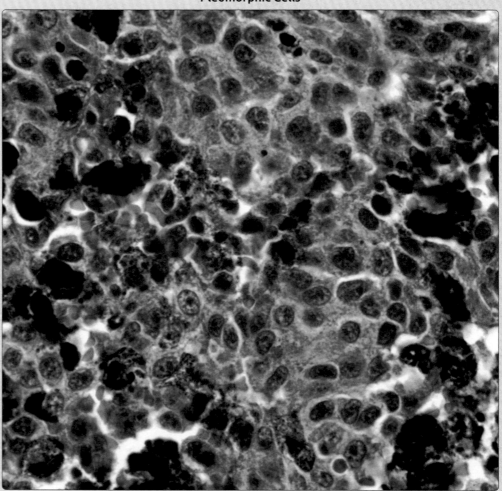

High-power view of an adrenal primary malignant melanoma shows cells with pleomorphic nuclei and prominent nucleoli with interspersed dark brown melanin pigment.

TERMINOLOGY

Abbreviations
- Primary adrenal melanoma (PAM)

Synonyms
- Primary malignant melanoma of adrenal gland

Definitions
- Adrenal neoplasm of melanocytes

ETIOLOGY/PATHOGENESIS

Origin
- Neural crest-derived cells in adrenal gland

CLINICAL ISSUES

Epidemiology
- Incidence
  - ~ 25 reported cases
- Age
  - Middle-aged adults

Presentation
- Painful flank mass, lymph node metastasis

Treatment
- Surgical approaches
  - Nephroadrenalectomy is procedure of choice

Prognosis
- Mortality near 100% within 2 years

IMAGING

CT Findings
- Primary melanoma of adrenal gland is usually voluminous, nonfunctional tumor
- Enlarged, well-encapsulated adrenal mass
- Heterogeneous contrast enhancement on computed tomographic (CT) scan

MACROSCOPIC

General Features
- Gray-brown-black with hemorrhage and necrosis

Size
- Reported cases ranged from 8-17 cm

MICROSCOPIC

Histologic Features
- Similar to melanoma arising in conventional sites
- Diagnosis is made on basis of histological and immunohistochemical studies
- Brown intracytoplasmic pigment present; may also be amelanotic

ANCILLARY TESTS

Immunohistochemistry
- Positive: S100, MART-1/Melan-A, and HMB-45
- Negative: Synaptophysin, chromogranin, and NSE

Electron Microscopy
- Presence of melanosomes and premelanosomes

DIFFERENTIAL DIAGNOSIS

Metastatic Malignant Melanoma to Adrenal
- Often bilateral
- Adrenal glands can be sites for metastatic dispersal of cutaneous or visceral melanomas in up to 50% of cases
  - Histological and immunohistochemical studies do not make it possible to differentiate metastatic tumors from primary melanomas
- Ainsworth criteria (1976)
  - Detailed clinical record indicating no prior existence of cutaneous melanomas or cutaneous lesions that may have reappeared
  - Careful cutaneous and ocular exploration to eliminate the presence of lesions
  - Exhaustive evaluation to eliminate any other visceral location
  - Pattern of recurrence concordant with the location site
  - From histological point of view, nontypical melanocytes are usually seen on periphery of lesions, which does not occur with secondary melanomas
- Use Carstens criteria to formally differentiate PAM from metastatic melanoma to adrenal
- Carstnes criteria (1984)
  - Neoplastic involvement of a single gland
  - Absence of melanoma in rest of organism
  - Absence of previous excisions of pigmented mucous, cutaneous or ocular lesions
  - Exclusion of any hidden pigmented lesion, preferably by autopsy

Pigmented Pheochromocytoma
- Clinical and laboratory findings related to catecholamine secretion
- Immunohistochemistry is useful
  - Positive: Chromogranin, synaptophysin, and NSE
  - Caution: HMB-45 is positive in up to 1/3 of pheochromocytomas
  - S100 highlights sustentacular cells but not tumor cells
  - Negative: S100 (tumor cells), MART-1/Melan-A

Pigmented Adrenal Lesions
- Pigmented adenomas
- Adrenal hematoma with hemosiderin-laden macrophages
- Tumors with neuromelanin (altered lipofuscin) may be confused with melanin

Primary Pigmented Nodular Adrenal Disease
- Adrenal gland may be of normal size
- Multiple small adrenal cortical nodules
- Cells composed of cell with compact eosinophilic cytoplasm, with abundant brown granular lipofuscin pigment
- Cell nuclei are usually small and round; may contain prominent nucleoli
- Intervening cortical tissue is atrophic

Immunohistochemistry Profile: PAM vs. Pigmented Pheochromocytoma

Immunostain	PAM	Pheochromocytoma
S100	Positive in tumoral cells	Negative in tumoral cells; highlights sustentacular cells
Melan-A/MART-1	Positive	Negative
HMB-45	Positive	Positive in up to 1/3 of cases
BRAF	Positive	
BAP1	Unknown	Not known in PAM
Chromogranin	Negative	Positive
Synaptophysin	Negative	Positive
NSE	Negative	Positive

PAM = primary adrenal melanoma.

DIAGNOSTIC CHECKLIST

Pathologic Interpretation Pearls

- Rule out adrenal metastasis
- Differentiate from pigmented pheochromocytomas

Carstens Criteria to Differentiate Primary vs. Metastatic Adrenal Melanoma

- Unilateral adrenal involvement
- No prior or current pigmented lesion of skin, mucosal surfaces, or eye
- Exclusion of hidden primary lesion by autopsy

SELECTED REFERENCES

1. Drouet C et al: Bilateral huge incidentalomas of isolated adrenal metastases from unknown primary melanoma revealed by 18F-FDG PET/CT. Clin Nucl Med. 42(1):e51-e53, 2017
2. Zage PE et al: CD114: A new member of the neural crest-derived cancer stem cell marker family. J Cell Biochem. 118(2):221-231, 2017
3. Barmpari ME et al: Adrenal malignant melanoma masquerading as a pheochromocytoma in a patient with a history of a multifocal papillary and medullary thyroid carcinoma. Hormones (Athens). 15(2):283-90, 2016
4. Kakkar A et al: Pigmented pheochromocytoma: an unusual variant of a common tumor. Endocr Pathol. 27(1):42-5, 2016
5. Maison N et al: Somatic RET mutation in a patient with pigmented adrenal pheochromocytoma. Endocrinol Diabetes Metab Case Rep. 2016:150117, 2016
6. Flaherty DC et al: Adrenalectomy for Metastatic Melanoma: Current Role in the Age of Nonsurgical Treatments. Am Surg. 81(10):1005-9, 2015
7. Blanco R et al: Massive bilateral adrenal metastatic melanoma of occult origin: a case report. Anal Quant Cytopathol Histpathol. 36(1):51-4, 2014
8. Ejaz S et al: Melanoma of unknown primary origin presenting as a rapidly enlarging adrenal mass. BMJ Case Rep. 2013, 2013
9. Avgerinos DV et al: Primary adrenal melanoma with inferior vena caval thrombus. Ann Thorac Surg. 94(6):2108-10, 2012
10. González-Sáez L et al: Primary melanoma of the adrenal gland: a case report and review of the literature. J Med Case Rep. 5:273, 2011
11. Bastide C et al: Primary malignant melanoma of the adrenal gland. Int J Urol. 13(5):608-10, 2006
12. Granero LE et al: Primary melanoma of the adrenal gland, a continuous dilemma: report of a case. Surg Today. 34(6):554-6, 2004
13. Zalatnai A et al: Primary malignant melanoma of adrenal gland in a 41-yr-old woman. Endocr Pathol. 14(1):101-5, 2003
14. Cuesta Alcalá JA et al: [Therapeutic approach in adrenal melanoma. review of the literature.] Arch Esp Urol. 54(7):685-90, 2001
15. Amérigo J et al: Primary malignant melanoma of the adrenal gland. Surgery. 127(1):107-11, 2000
16. Chetty R et al: Pigmented pheochromocytomas of the adrenal medulla. Hum Pathol. 24(4):420-3, 1993
17. Landas SK et al: Occurrence of melanin in pheochromocytoma. Mod Pathol. 6(2):175-8, 1993
18. Lallier TE: Cell lineage and cell migration in the neural crest. Ann N Y Acad Sci. 615:158-71, 1991
19. Dao AH et al: Primary malignant melanoma of the adrenal gland. a report of two cases and review of the literature. Am Surg. 56(4):199-203, 1990
20. Parker LA et al: Detection of adrenal melanoma with computed tomography. Urol Radiol. 8(4):209-10, 1986
21. Carstens PH et al: Primary malignant melanomas of the lung and adrenal. Hum Pathol. 15(10):910-4, 1984
22. Shnyrenkova OV: [Adrenal melanoblastoma with metastases.] Arkh Patol. 18(1):111-3, 1956
23. Poore JB et al: Adrenal-cortical carcinoma and melanocarcinoma in a 5-year-old Negro child. Cancer. 7(6):1235-41, 1954
24. Kniseley RM et al: Primary melanoma of the adrenal gland. Arch Pathol (Chic). 42:345-9, 1946

Intraadrenal Primary Melanoma

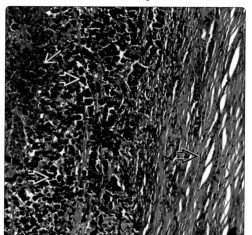

Compressed Adrenal Cortex

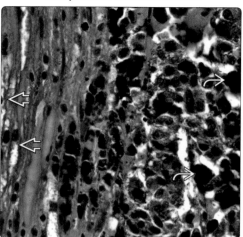

(Left) *H&E shows a primary adrenal melanoma with pigmented cells* ⮡ *surrounded by a fibrous capsule* ⮡. *The tumor is viable close to the capsule, and extensive area of necrosis is present* ⮡. (Right) *H&E shows polygonal melanoma cells with admixed melanin pigment deposition* ⮡. *Compressed adrenal cortical cells* ⮡ *are present within the fibrous bundles of the capsule.*

Pigmented Tumor

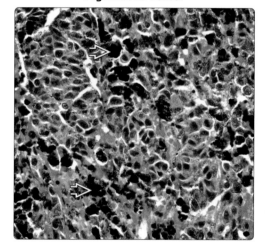

Tumor Necrosis

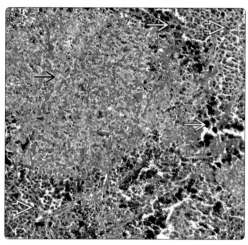

(Left) *Primary adrenal melanoma is a highly cellular neoplasm composed of polygonal cells with irregular nuclei and abundant brown granular pigment (melanin)* ⮡. *The tumor has a diffuse architecture, sometimes obstructed by the heavy melanin pigment.* (Right) *A focus of tumor necrosis* ⮡ *is surrounded by tumor cells* ⮡ *and with melanin pigment* ⮡. *Foci of necrosis are usually seen in larger tumors.*

Remnant Adrenal Cortex

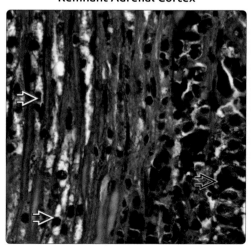

Differential Diagnosis

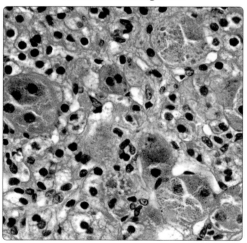

(Left) *H&E shows polygonal melanoma cells with admixed melanin pigment deposition* ⮡. *Compressed adrenal cortical cells* ⮡ *are present within the fibrous bundles of the capsule.* (Right) *Primary pigmented nodular adrenal disease represents a diagnostic pitfall as it also shows granular light brown pigment. However, note the pigmented cells to be adrenal cortical cells without nuclear pleomorphism. The pigment in these cases is lipofuscin.*

TERMINOLOGY

- Extremely rare malignancies with vascular differentiation

CLINICAL ISSUES

- Age: 41-85 years
- Adrenalectomy
- Biologically malignant neoplasms

MACROSCOPIC

- Grossly solid to cystic invasive mass

MICROSCOPIC

- Similar to angiosarcomas in other anatomical sites
- Irregularly anastomosing vessels
- Hobnailing endothelial cells
- Sheets or nests of large epithelioid cells
- Variable mitotic activity

ANCILLARY TESTS

- **Positive immunostaining**
  - Endothelial markers: FVIII, CD31, CD34, ERG, FLI-1
  - May have immunohistochemical stain for MYC (nuclear staining)
  - Epithelioid cells may stain for cytokeratin, EMA, vimentin, and TAG72
- **Negative staining**: S100, calretinin, HMB-45
- FISH: Copy number gain in chromosome 8

TOP DIFFERENTIAL DIAGNOSES

- Metastatic angiosarcoma
- Adrenal cortical adenoma
- Adrenal cortical carcinoma
- Metastatic carcinoma
- Malignant melanoma
- Epithelioid hemangioendothelioma
- Epithelioid hemangioma
- Papillary endothelial hyperplasia of adrenal gland

Interface of Tumor and Adrenal

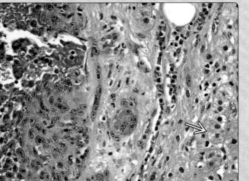

CD31 Membranous Staining

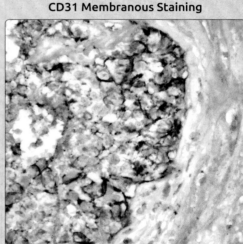

(Left) A small area with residual normal adrenal cortical tissue ➡ is compressed by a tumor consisting of large pleomorphic cells with prominent nucleoli and irregular vascular spaces. (Right) The adrenal is compressed by an expanding tumor mass. The tumor forms a solid and cystic mass, and the tumor cells have strong immunopositivity for endothelial markers. CD31 is the most sensitive marker. Many tumors also stain for CD34, ERG, and FLI-1.

Blood Lakes and Cellular Pleomorphism

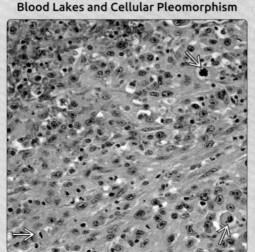

CD31 Immunoexpression

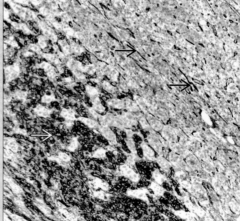

(Left) Numerous blood lakes within vascular channels are present, lined by cells with marked cellular pleomorphism and large nucleoli. Numerous mitosis ➡ are identified. (Right) CD31 immunostain supports the endothelial phenotype of the large epithelioid cells ➡. In this case, the tumor cells show strong cytoplasmic and membranous staining for CD31. The vasculature of the normal adrenal is also highlighted ➡.

TERMINOLOGY

Abbreviations

- Adrenal angiosarcoma (AAS)

Synonyms

- Primary adrenal angiosarcoma (PAA)
- Adrenal epithelioid angiosarcoma

Definitions

- Mesenchymal tumor of adrenal gland with endothelial differentiation

CLINICAL ISSUES

Epidemiology

- Incidence
  - Rare: About 39 cases reported
  - 1st case described in 1988
- Age
  - 41-85 years
- Sex
  - No significant gender preference

Presentation

- Asymptomatic (incidentaloma)
- Enlarging retroperitoneal mass ± pain
- Distant metastasis

Treatment

- Surgical approach
  - Adrenalectomy

Prognosis

- Biologically malignant neoplasms
- Variable prognosis
- Survival reported up to 13 years post adrenalectomy

IMAGING

General Features

- Suprarenal or retroperitoneal mass
- Usually large, unilateral, and solitary

CT and MR

- Useful in assessment of tumor extent, metastasis, nodal and venous spread

MACROSCOPIC

General Features

- Grossly well-circumscribed to ill-defined, invasive mass
- Solid to cystic with variegated cut surface

Size

- Reported 5-15 cm

MICROSCOPIC

Histologic Features

- PAA demonstrates epithelioid morphology with histologically malignant features
  - Tumor necrosis
  - High mitotic rates

- Associated with poor prognosis
- Cytologically malignant spindle and epithelioid cells that have capacity to form rudimentary blood vessels
- Similar to angiosarcoma (AS) in other anatomical sites
- Irregularly anastomosing vessels
- Hobnailing endothelial cells
- Sheets or nests of large epithelioid cells
- Areas of desmoplastic or fibromyxoid appearance
- Varying degrees of necrosis and hemorrhage

Cytologic Features

- AS shows range of cytomorphologic features
- Elongated to plump epithelioid cells
- Variable pleomorphism
- Intracytoplasmic vacuolization with occasional red blood cells
- Variable mitotic activity

ANCILLARY TESTS

Immunohistochemistry

- Immunopositivity for endothelial markers (CD31 and CD34), ERG, and FLI-1
- Epithelioid cells may stain with keratin and rarely with EMA
- MYC nuclear staining identified in 3 cases reported
  - De novo AS demonstrates variable MYC expression, with high-grade tumors showing significantly higher MYC expression than low-grade tumors
    - Suggests that MYC overexpression may play role in pathogenesis
    - MYC IHC may be prognostic &/or therapeutic biomarker in subset of these tumors
  - Radiation-associated AS associated with *MYC* gene amplification and protein overexpression
    - Whereas other radiation-associated vascular lesions (including atypical vascular lesions) are not associated with MYC overexpression

Genetic Testing

- Mutations in *PLCG1* and *KDR* genes and *MYC* amplification may be identified

Electron Microscopy

- Rod-shaped microtubulated bodies and intracytoplasmic lumen formation

FISH

- 2 of 3 cases with MYC immunopositivity showed polysomy of chromosome 8 without MYC amplification or rearrangement

DIFFERENTIAL DIAGNOSIS

Metastatic Angiosarcoma

- Extraadrenal primary site should be ruled out

Adrenal Cortical Adenoma and Carcinoma

- Especially in tumors with solid appearance and hemorrhage

Metastatic Carcinoma

- Epithelioid appearance and cytokeratin positivity

Malignant Melanoma

- HMB-45, Melan-A, and S100(+)

Immunohistochemistry

Antibody	Reactivity	Staining Pattern	Comment
CD31	Positive	Cell membrane & cytoplasm	Sensitive marker
CD34	Positive	Cell membrane & cytoplasm	40-100%
FVIIIRAg	Positive	Cell membrane	
AE1/AE3	Positive	Cell membrane & cytoplasm	35%
Ki-67	Positive	Nuclear	> 10% of cells in 72% cases
EMA	Positive	Cell membrane	Variable
FLI-1	Positive	Nuclear	
TAG72	Positive	Cell membrane & cytoplasm	
Vimentin	Positive	Cytoplasmic	
S100	Negative		Also negative for calretinin and HMB-45

Epithelioid Hemangioendothelioma

- Nests of plump endothelial cells
- No significant pleomorphism or mitotic activity

Adrenal Papillary Endothelial Hyperplasia

- Exceedingly rare process that radiologically mimics adrenal cortical carcinoma
- Pathologic differentiation from AS can be difficult

DIAGNOSTIC CHECKLIST

Pathologic Interpretation Pearls

- Endothelial cell immunomarkers

SELECTED REFERENCES

1. Harker D et al: MYC amplification in angiosarcomas arising in the setting of chronic lymphedema of morbid obesity. J Cutan Pathol. 44(1):15-19, 2017
2. Geller RL et al: Cytologic features of angiosarcoma: A review of 26 cases diagnosed on FNA. Cancer Cytopathol. 124(9):659-68, 2016
3. Udager AM et al: MYC immunohistochemistry in angiosarcoma and atypical vascular lesions: practical considerations based on a single institutional experience. Pathology. 48(7):697-704, 2016
4. Cornejo KM et al: MYC analysis by fluorescent in situ hybridization and immunohistochemistry in primary adrenal angiosarcoma (PAA): a series of four cases. Endocr Pathol. 26(4):334-41, 2015
5. Gusenbauer K et al: Angiosarcoma of the adrenal gland with concurrent contralateral advanced renal cell carcinoma: A diagnostic and management dilemma. Can Urol Assoc J. 9(5-6):E302-5, 2015
6. Hendry S et al: Epithelioid angiosarcoma arising in an adrenal cortical adenoma: A case report and review of the literature. Int J Surg Pathol. ePub, 2014
7. Fernandez AP et al: FISH for MYC amplification and anti-MYC immunohistochemistry: useful diagnostic tools in the assessment of secondary angiosarcoma and atypical vascular proliferations. J Cutan Pathol. 39(2):234-42, 2012
8. Schreiner AM et al: Primary adrenal epithelioid angiosarcoma showing rhabdoid morphology on air-dried smears. Diagn Cytopathol. 2011 Apr 6. doi: 10. 1002/dc. Epub ahead of print, 2169
9. Hart J et al: Epithelioid angiosarcoma: a brief diagnostic review and differential diagnosis. Arch Pathol Lab Med. 135(2):268-72, 2011
10. Nunes ML et al: 18F-FDG PET for the identification of adrenocortical carcinomas among indeterminate adrenal tumors at computed tomography scanning. World J Surg. 34(7):1506-10, 2010
11. Gambino G et al: Adrenal epithelioid angiosarcoma: a case report. Chir Ital. 60(3):463-7, 2008
12. Al-Meshan MK et al: An unusual angiosarcoma. A case report. Med Princ Pract. 13(5):295-7, 2004
13. Azurmendi Sastre V et al: [Adrenal spindle cell angiosarcoma. Report one case.] Arch Esp Urol. 57(2):156-60, 2004
14. Galmiche L et al: [Primary adrenal angiosarcoma.] Ann Pathol. 24(4):371-3, 2004
15. Sidoni A et al: [Primary adrenal angiosarcoma.] Pathologica. 95(1):60-3, 2003
16. Mayayo Artal E et al: [Epithelioid angiosarcoma of the adrenal gland. Report of a case.] Arch Esp Urol. 55(10):261-4, 2002
17. Pasqual E et al: Adrenal angiosarcoma: report of a case. Surg Today. 32(6):563-5, 2002
18. Tousi-Sadr HR et al: [Angiosarcoma of the adrenal gland.] Ugeskr Laeger. 164(7):911-2, 2002
19. Croitoru AG et al: Primary epithelioid angiosarcoma of the adrenal gland. Ann Diagn Pathol. 5(5):300-3, 2001
20. Invitti C et al: Unusual association of adrenal angiosarcoma and Cushing's disease. Horm Res. 56(3-4):124-9, 2001
21. Krüger S et al: Primary epithelioid angiosarcoma of the adrenal gland case report and review of the literature. Tumori. 87(4):262-5, 2001
22. Otal P et al: Imaging features of uncommon adrenal masses with histopathologic correlation. Radiographics. 19(3):569-81, 1999
23. Sasaki R et al: [A case of adrenal angiosarcoma.] Nippon Hinyokika Gakkai Zasshi. 86(5):1064-7, 1995
24. Jochum W et al: [Cytokeratin-positive angiosarcoma of the adrenal gland.] Pathologe. 15(3):181-6, 1994
25. Wenig BM et al: Epithelioid angiosarcoma of the adrenal glands. A clinicopathologic study of nine cases with a discussion of the implications of finding "epithelial-specific" markers. Am J Surg Pathol. 18(1):62-73, 1994
26. Ben-Izhak O et al: Epithelioid angiosarcoma of the adrenal gland with cytokeratin expression. Report of a case with accompanying mesenteric fibromatosis. Cancer. 69(7):1808-12, 1992
27. Fiordelise S et al: Angiosarcoma of the adrenal gland. Case report. Arch Ital Urol Nefrol Androl. 64(4):341-3, 1992
28. Bosco PJ et al: Primary angiosarcoma of adrenal gland presenting as paraneoplastic syndrome: case report. J Urol. 146(4):1101-3, 1991
29. Livaditou A et al: Epithelioid angiosarcoma of the adrenal gland associated with chronic arsenical intoxication? Pathol Res Pract. 187(2-3):284-9, 1991
30. Kareti LR et al: Angiosarcoma of the adrenal gland. Arch Pathol Lab Med. 112(11):1163-5, 1988
31. Kern WH et al: Angiosarcoma of lungs and adrenal gland: unusual clinical and pathologic manifestations. Minn Med. 50(9):1339-43, 1967
32. Rasore-Quartino A: [Congenital discordant adrenal tumor (angiosarcoma) in a monozygotic twin.] Pathologica. 59(873):153-8, 1967

Tumor Adrenal Interface

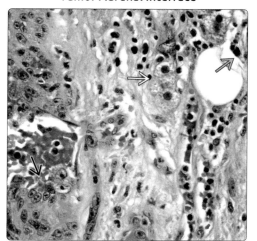

Angiosarcoma Interface With Adrenal

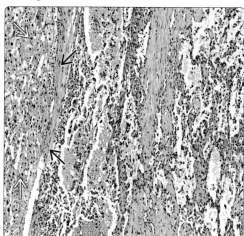

(Left) *Large epithelioid and pleomorphic cells line vascular spaces, invading and destroying adrenal cortical parenchyma, with only rare residual cells ⇒. Focally these cells form small tumor nodules ⇒. Fibrosis and hemosiderin deposition are present ⇒.* (Right) *A portion of residual normal adrenal parenchyma ⇒ is compressed by a tumor consisting of irregular vascular spaces and scattered red blood cells. A thin tumor capsule ⇒ is also present.*

Vascular Spaces

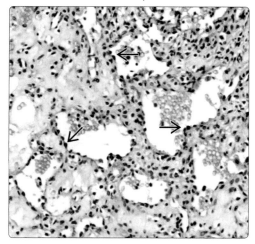

Vascular Spaces Highlighted By CD31

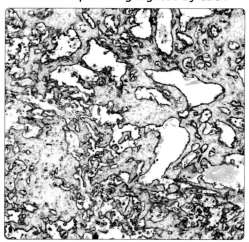

(Left) *High magnification reveals clusters of blood vessels with irregular sizes and shapes. Cells lining the vessels often have prominent nuclei that protrude into the lumen ⇒.* (Right) *Immunostain for CD31 reveals a complex network of irregular, immature, interconnecting blood vessels of various sizes. The epithelioid malignant endothelial cells also stain for the other endothelial markers such as CD34, ERG, and FLI-1.*

Large Epithelioid Cells

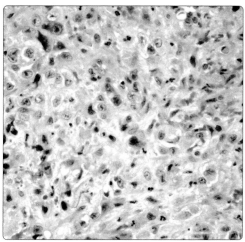

CD31 Immunopositivity

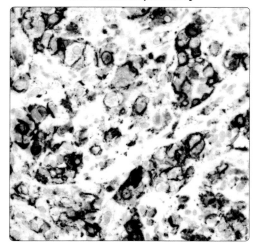

(Left) *Photomicrograph shows a metastatic adrenal angiosarcoma to the brain after many months post adrenalectomy for a primary adrenal angiosarcoma. Note the large epithelioid pleomorphic cells, some with red blood cells.* (Right) *This adrenal angiosarcoma has mestastasized to the brain. The large, bizarre epithelioid cells have membranous staining for CD31. In about 50% of cases, the tumor cells may also stain with epithelial markers, specially keratins and EMA.*

TERMINOLOGY

- Rare malignant smooth muscle tumor
- Likely arises from smooth muscle of adrenal vessels

ETIOLOGY/PATHOGENESIS

- Association with HIV and Epstein-Barr virus infection

CLINICAL ISSUES

- Enlarging abdominal mass
- Abdominal pain
- Generally poor prognosis
- Survival depends on feasibility of complete resection
- Metastasis most common to
  - Lung
  - Liver
  - Lymph nodes

MACROSCOPIC

- Soft to moderately firm, well-demarcated mass
- Hemorrhage, necrosis, and cystic degeneration
- Large tumors may invade adjacent organs
- Often completely replaces adrenal gland

MICROSCOPIC

- Spindle cell and pleomorphic types
- Fascicular arrangement of spindle cells
- Diffuse proliferation of pleomorphic large and polygonal cells
- Morphologic subtypes
  - Conventional spindled leiomyosarcoma
  - Pleomorphic type

ANCILLARY TESTS

- Positive stains
  - Actin, smooth muscle myosin, desmin, SMA, H-caldesmon, calponin

TOP DIFFERENTIAL DIAGNOSES

- Metastatic leiomyosarcoma

Leiomyosarcoma With Necrosis

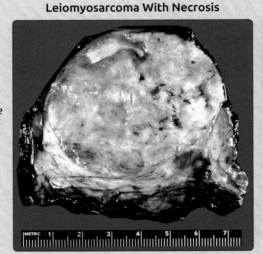

Gross Cut Surface Features

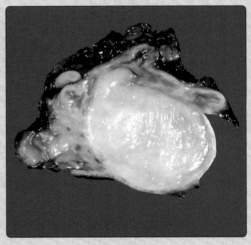

(Left) Cut surface of this primary leiomyosarcoma of the adrenal gland shows a firm, gray-white mass with necrosis, focal degenerative changes, with focal areas of hemorrhage and pigment deposition. (Right) Cut surface of this adrenal gland shows a well-demarcated, firm, gray-white mass compressing the adjacent adrenal gland. No hemorrhage or necrosis are identified. The gross differential diagnosis with leiomyoma is not possible.

Residual Cortex and Tumor Interface

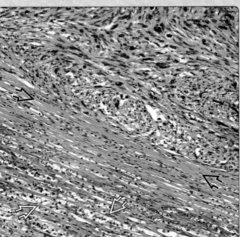

Marked Nuclear Pleomorphism

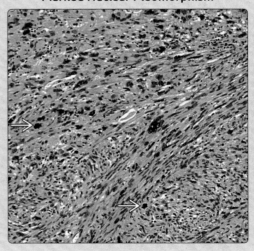

(Left) The residual adjacent adrenal cortical tissue ➡ is compressed by fascicles of pleomorphic spindle cells with numerous mitosis. A fibrous pseudocapsule is present ➡. (Right) High magnification shows fascicles of pleomorphic spindle cells with hyperchromatic, enlarged, and irregular nuclei. A multinucleated giant cell is shown. Multiple mitotic figures ➡ are also present.

TERMINOLOGY

Abbreviations
- Adrenal leiomyosarcoma (ALMS)

Synonyms
- Primary ALMS
- Pleomorphic ALMS (subtype)

Definitions
- Rare malignant smooth muscle tumor
  - Only ~ 30 cases reported in English literature
- Likely arises from smooth muscle of adrenal central vein

ETIOLOGY/PATHOGENESIS

Infectious Agents
- Association with HIV and Epstein-Barr virus infection has been suggested

CLINICAL ISSUES

Epidemiology
- Incidence
  - Few cases reported in literature
- Age
  - Range: 4th-7th decades of life
- Sex
  - No sex predilection

Presentation
- Enlarging abdominal mass ± pain

Treatment
- Surgical approaches
  - Radical resection may prolong survival
- Radiation
  - Used postoperatively for locally advanced disease
- Chemotherapy
  - Efficacy is poorly defined

Prognosis
- Biologically malignant neoplasms
- Generally poor prognosis
- Behavior correlated to histological grade
  - Mitosis, necrosis, atypia
- Survival depends on feasibility of complete resection
- Tumor-associated tissue eosinophilia may be associated with better prognosis

IMAGING

CT and MR
- Heterogeneous solid and cystic suprarenal mass
- Useful in assessment of tumor extent, metastasis, and venous spread

MACROSCOPIC

General Features
- Soft to moderately firm, well-demarcated mass
- Usually gray-white ± necrosis
- Hemorrhage, necrosis, and cystic degeneration

- Large tumors may invade adjacent organs
- Often completely replaces adrenal gland
- May invade vena cava and extend into heart
- Metastasis most common in lung and liver

MICROSCOPIC

Histologic Features
- General features
  - Tumor contains entrapped adrenal cortical cells
  - Variable mitotic activity
  - Neoplastic cells are spindle-shaped
  - Tumor cells demonstrate pleomorphism and hyperchromasia
  - Cytoplasm is fibrillar and eosinophilic
  - Nuclei are elongated with blunted ends
  - Degree of cytological atypia correlates with grade of tumor
  - Report of case of primary ALMS with marked tissue eosinophilia
    - Tumor-associated tissue eosinophilia may be associated with longer survival
- Morphologic subtypes
  - Conventional spindled leiomyosarcoma
    - Fascicular arrangement of spindle cells
    - Bundles intersect at wide angles
    - Cigar-shaped, blunt-ended nuclei
    - Variable nuclear atypia
  - Pleomorphic type
    - Diffuse proliferation of pleomorphic large and polygonal cells
    - Prominent nucleoli
    - Bizarre mitotic figures
    - Perivascular growth of tumor cells
    - Large, irregular zones of necrosis
    - Multinucleated giant cells

ANCILLARY TESTS

Immunohistochemistry
- Positive (smooth muscle markers)
  - Actin
  - Smooth muscle myosin
  - Desmin
  - H-caldesmon
  - Smooth muscle actin
  - Calponin
- Negative
  - S100
  - Myoglobin
  - CD34
  - CD117
  - HMB-45
  - DOG1
  - Cytokeratin

Electron Microscopy
- Pinocytotic membrane
- Thin filaments
  - With dense bodies
- Basal lamina

- Round-ended nuclei with indentations

DIFFERENTIAL DIAGNOSIS

Metastatic Leiomyosarcoma

- Rule out extraadrenal primary site

Leiomyoma

- Absence of atypia, mitosis, necrosis, and hemorrhage

Myofibroblastic Sarcoma

- Tumor cells have amphophilic cytoplasm
- Nuclei have tapered ends, instead of cigar-shaped, round ended
- Immunohistochemistry for smooth muscle markers patchy and weak
- EM shows myofibroblastic differentiation

Malignant Fibrous Histiocytoma

- Diagnosis of exclusion
- Highly pleomorphic and bizarre cells
- Lack of immunohistochemical line of differentiation

Synovial Sarcoma

- Positive for HMB-1 and CD99
- Cytogenetics (*SYT1-SSX1* and *SYT1-SSX2* fusion genes)

Fibrosarcoma

- Fascicles intersect at acute straight angles
- Herringbone pattern, hyperchromatic nuclei
- Negative or weakly positive for smooth muscle markers

Angiosarcoma

- Immature anastomosing vessels
- Positive for vascular endothelial markers (CD31, CD34, factor VIII)

DIAGNOSTIC CHECKLIST

Pathologic Interpretation Pearls

- Exclusion of metastatic leiomyosarcoma is needed before making diagnosis of primary ALMS

SELECTED REFERENCES

1. Tawbi HA et al: Pembrolizumab in advanced soft-tissue sarcoma and bone sarcoma (SARC028): a multicentre, two-cohort, single-arm, open-label, phase 2 trial. Lancet Oncol. ePub, 2017
2. Onishi T et al: Primary adrenal leiomyosarcoma with lymph node metastasis: a case report. World J Surg Oncol. 14(1):176, 2016
3. Khan IN et al: A retroperitoneal leiomyosarcoma presenting as an adrenal incidentaloma in a subject on warfarin. Case Rep Endocrinol. 2015:830814, 2015
4. Quildrian S et al: Primary adrenal leiomyosarcoma treated by laparoscopic adrenalectomy. Endocrinol Nutr. 62(9):472-3, 2015
5. Sonoda H et al: Complete Surgical Resection of a Leiomyosarcoma Arising from the Inferior Vena Cava. Case Rep Med. 2015:342148, 2015
6. Zhou Y et al: Primary adrenal leiomyosarcoma: a case report and review of literature. Int J Clin Exp Pathol. 8(4):4258-63, 2015
7. Bhalla A et al: Primary adrenal leiomyosarcoma: a case report and review of the literature. Conn Med. 78(7):403-7, 2014
8. Gulpinar MT et al: Primary leiomyosarcoma of the adrenal gland: a case report with immunohistochemical study and literature review. Case Rep Urol. 2014:489630, 2014
9. Lee S et al: Primary leiomyosarcoma of adrenal gland with tissue eosinophilic infiltration. Korean J Pathol. 48(6):423-5, 2014
10. Deshmukh SD et al: Primary adrenal leiomyosarcoma: a case report with immunohistochemical study and review of literature. J Cancer Res Ther. 9(1):114-6, 2013
11. Karaosmanoglu AD et al: Sonographic findings of an adrenal leiomyosarcoma. J Ultrasound Med. 29(9):1369-73, 2010
12. Hamada S et al: Bilateral adrenal leiomyosarcoma treated with multiple local therapies. Int J Clin Oncol. 14(4):356-60, 2009
13. Nanpo Y et al: Primary adrenal leiomyosarcoma: a case report. Nippon Hinyokika Gakkai Zasshi. 100(6):640-5, 2009
14. Van Laarhoven HW et al: The diagnostic hurdle of an elderly male with bone pain: how 18F-FDG-PET led to diagnosis of a leiomyosarcoma of the adrenal gland. Anticancer Res. 29(2):469-72, 2009
15. Goto J et al: A rare tumor in the adrenal region: neuron-specific enolase (NSE)-producing leiomyosarcoma in an elderly hypertensive patient. Endocr J. 55(1):175-81, 2008
16. Tomasich FD et al: Primary adrenal leiomyosarcoma. Arq Bras Endocrinol Metabol. 52(9):1510-4, 2008
17. Mohanty SK et al: Pleomorphic leiomyosarcoma of the adrenal gland: case report and review of the literature. Urology. 70(3):591, 2007
18. Wang TS et al: Leiomyosarcoma of the adrenal vein: a novel approach to surgical resection. World J Surg Oncol. 5:109, 2007
19. Lee CW et al: Primary adrenal leiomyosarcoma. Abdom Imaging. 31(1):123-4, 2006
20. Candanedo-González FA et al: Pleomorphic leiomyosarcoma of the adrenal gland with osteoclast-like giant cells. Endocr Pathol. 16(1):75-81, 2005
21. Wong C et al: Cold feet from adrenal leiomyosarcoma. J R Soc Med. 98(9):418-20, 2005
22. Kato T et al: Primary adrenal leiomyosarcoma with inferior vena cava thrombosis. Int J Clin Oncol. 9(3):189-92, 2004
23. Lujan MG et al: Pleomorphic leiomyosarcoma of the adrenal gland. Arch Pathol Lab Med. 127(1):e32-5, 2003
24. Thamboo TP et al: Adrenal leiomyosarcoma: a case report and literature review. Pathology. 35(1):47-9, 2003
25. Matsui Y et al: Adrenal leiomyosarcoma extending into the right atrium. Int J Urol. 9(1):54-6, 2002
26. Etten B et al: Primary leiomyosarcoma of the adrenal gland. Sarcoma. 5(2):95-9, 2001
27. Fernández JM et al: Primary leiomyosarcoma. a rare tumor of the adrenal gland. Arch Esp Urol. 51(10):1029-31, 1998
28. Gohji K et al: Bilateral adrenal tumours: a case report of an unusual manifestation of mesenteric leiomyosarcoma. Br J Urol. 79(3):479-80, 1997
29. Dugan MC: Primary adrenal leiomyosarcoma in acquired immunodeficiency syndrome. Arch Pathol Lab Med. 120(9):797-8, 1996
30. Zetler PJ et al: Primary adrenal leiomyosarcoma in a man with acquired immunodeficiency syndrome (AIDS). Further evidence for an increase in smooth muscle tumors related to Epstein-Barr infection in AIDS. Arch Pathol Lab Med. 119(12):1164-7, 1995
31. Lack EE et al: Primary leiomyosarcoma of adrenal gland. case report with immunohistochemical and ultrastructural study. Am J Surg Pathol. 15(9):899-905, 1991
32. Choi SH et al: Leiomyosarcoma of the adrenal gland and its angiographic features: a case report. J Surg Oncol. 16(2):145-8, 1981

Gross Necrotic Area

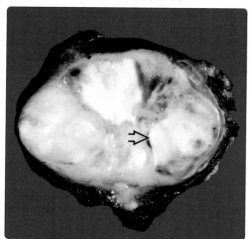

Interface of Adrenal and Leiomyosarcoma

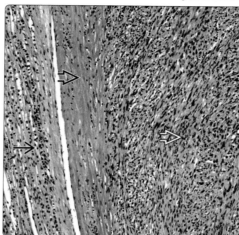

(Left) *Gross cut surface of this adrenal gland shows a well-demarcated, firm, gray-white mass with hemorrhage, necrosis ⮞, and degenerative changes.* **(Right)** *Low-power view shows an adrenal leiomyosarcoma ⮞ compressing the normal adrenal gland ⮞. A distinct fibrous capsule ⮞ is present and separates the spindle cell tumor from the surrounding normal gland.*

Spindle Cells

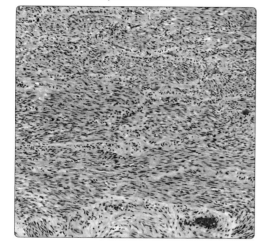

Storiform Pattern

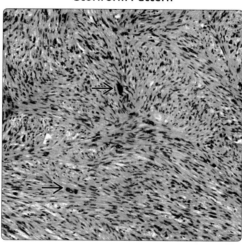

(Left) *Low power view of an adrenal low grade leiomyosarcoma shows the proliferation of spindle-shaped cells arranged in a fascicular pattern. The bundles of cells intersect at broad angles, and the eosinophilic cytoplasm is ill-defined. The nuclei of are small and mild nuclear pleomorphism seen.* **(Right)** *This image demonstrates the characteristic appearance of leiomyosarcoma composed of spindle cells in a storiform pattern. Few atypical cells with large, hyperchromatic nuclei are noted ⮞.*

Tumor Necrosis

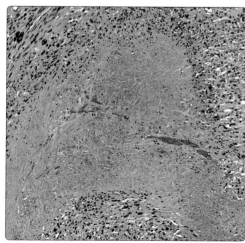

Necrosis

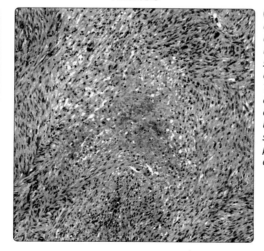

(Left) *This image shows an adrenal leiomyosarcoma with a focus of hemorrhage and tumor necrosis surrounded by spindle cells with marked cellular pleomorphism.* **(Right)** *This low-power view demonstrates the characteristic appearance of leiomyosarcoma composed of spindle cells in a storiform pattern with multifocal areas of necrosis.*

TERMINOLOGY

- Metastatic tumors involving adrenal glands
- Secondary tumors of adrenal cortex originate in extraadrenal locations and spread to adrenal gland by either metastasis or direct infiltration

CLINICAL ISSUES

- Adrenal gland 4th most common site of metastasis after lung, liver, and bones
- Adrenal metastasis reported in as many as 27% of cancer cases
- Bilateral metastases in ~ 50% of cases
- Secondary tumors more common than primary
- Common primary sources: Lungs, breast, stomach, esophagus, liver, kidney, ovaries, pancreas, bile duct, and colon

MICROSCOPIC

- Some tumors might histologically resemble primary site of origin
- Carcinoma, primarily adenocarcinoma, constitutes ~ 90% of metastatic tumors
- Some tumors challenging to diagnose, such as renal cell carcinoma, hepatocellular carcinoma, and melanoma

ANCILLARY TESTS

- Immunohistochemistry may provide valuable information in differential diagnosis
  - Should be based on patient history of primary malignancy
  - If adrenocortical carcinoma suspected instead, inhibin, SF1, melan-A, synaptophysin, calretinin, and vimentin can be used as confirmatory markers
  - Adrenal cortical tumors typically negative for cytokeratins

Granular Cut Surface

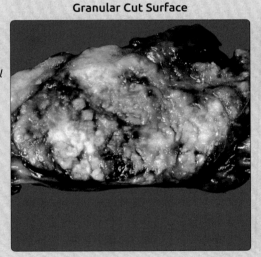

Cut Surface of Adrenal Tumor

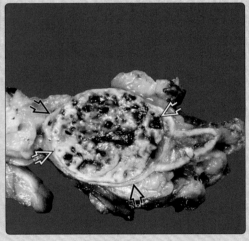

(Left) *Gross cut surface of an adrenal gland with a metastatic carcinoma shows a markedly granular tumor with areas of hemorrhage and focal necrosis. Primary adrenal tumors, benign or malignant, usually have a smooth cut surface.* (Right) *Gross cut surface of a metastatic renal cell carcinoma* ➟ *shows an irregular yellow tumor with focal hemorrhage. Residual cortex* ➥ *is present around the tumor. Kidney, lung, breast, and GI tract are the usual secondary adrenal tumors.*

Poorly Differentiated Carcinoma

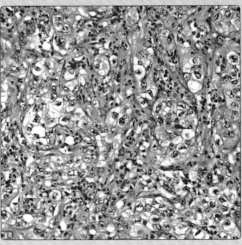

Immunohistochemistry

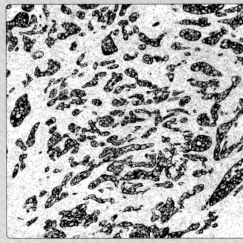

(Left) *H&E shows a metastatic poorly differentiated carcinoma to the adrenal. The patient had a primary lung neoplasm, and ancillary studies further confirmed a pulmonary origin for this tumor.* (Right) *Ancillary studies are very important on metastatic tumors to the adrenal to further characterize the origin of the tumor. This low-power view of an adrenal tumor shows strong CK7 positivity. CK7 highlights membranous staining in a secondary adrenal tumor.*

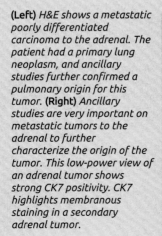

TERMINOLOGY

Synonyms

- Metastatic tumors involving adrenal glands

Definitions

- Secondary tumors of adrenal cortex originate in extraadrenal locations and spread to adrenal gland by either metastasis or direct infiltration

CLINICAL ISSUES

Presentation

- Adrenal metastasis reported in as many as 27% of cancer cases
- Adrenal gland 4th most common site of metastasis
  - After lungs, liver, and bones
    - High blood flow and sinusoidal vasculature are possible explanations for high incidence of metastases despite small size of organ
- Common primary sources: Lungs, breast, stomach, esophagus, liver, kidney, ovaries, pancreas, bile duct, and colon
  - Noncarcinoma primary sources: Lymphomas and sarcomas (angiosarcoma and Kaposi sarcoma in HIV-positive patients)
- Secondary tumors more common than primary
- ~ 80-90% of gland has to be involved to initiate symptoms of adrenal insufficiency
- Bilateral metastases present in ~ 50% of cases

Treatment

- Adrenalectomy for clinically isolated metastasis can prolong survival in selected patients

Prognosis

- Poor
  - Some studies show improved long-term survival after surgical resection

IMAGING

MR Findings

- Heterogeneous signal on T2 and sometimes T1, in which gland may appear iso- to hypointense to liver

CT Findings

- Smooth or lobulated contour
- May simulate adrenocortical adenoma
  - MR should be performed on any solitary adrenal mass on patients with known malignancy

MACROSCOPIC

General Features

- Depends on primary site of malignancy
- Lacks bright yellow of normal adrenal parenchyma

MICROSCOPIC

Histologic Features

- Depends on primary site
  - Some tumors might histologically resemble primary site of origin

- Carcinoma, primarily adenocarcinoma, constitutes ~ 90% of metastatic tumors
- Some tumors have similar morphological appearance as primary adrenal tumors
  - Immunohistochemistry may provide valuable information in diagnosis
- Some tumors can prove to be particularly challenging to diagnose
  - Renal cell carcinoma
  - Large cell neuroendocrine carcinoma of lung
  - Hepatocellular carcinoma
  - Melanoma

ANCILLARY TESTS

Immunohistochemistry

- Should be based on patient history of primary malignancy
  - If no previous history, immunostains may be used to rule in/out most common metastatic tumors (lungs, breast, kidney, stomach, esophagus, ovaries, pancreas, and colon) if morphology not helpful
- May provide valuable information in differential diagnosis
- When adrenocortical origin of tumor is within differential diagnosis, markers of adrenal cortical tumors should be performed
  - Inhibin
  - Calretinin
  - Melan-A
  - Synaptophysin
  - SF1
  - Vimentin
- Adrenal cortical tumors are typically negative for cytokeratin, CEA, and chromogranin
- Depending on tumor morphology and differential diagnosis, immunohistochemistry work-up for metastatic carcinoma could include
  - Cytokeratins
  - CEA
  - EMA
  - CDX-2
  - RCA
  - HEPAR
  - TTF-1
  - p40
  - p63
  - S100
  - HMB-45
  - Others

DIFFERENTIAL DIAGNOSIS

Adrenocortical Carcinoma

- As a rule, primary tumor has to be excluded 1st
- Usually broad trabecular growth pattern with anastomosing cords of 10-20 cells separated by delicate endothelial layer
- Cell borders usually well defined
- Presence of intracytoplasmatic eosinophilic globules
- Positive immunohistochemistry: Inhibin, calretinin, melan-A, synaptophysin, SF1, and vimentin

Immunohistochemistry Used in Primary Adrenal Cortical Neoplasms to Differentiate from Metastatic Neoplasms

Antibody	Reactivity	Staining Pattern
SF1	Positive	Cytoplasmic
Synaptophysin	Positive	Cytoplasmic
Inhibin-α	Positive	Cell membrane and cytoplasm
Melan-A	Positive	Cytoplasmic
calretinin	Positive	Cytoplasmic
CK-PAN	Negative	
EMA/MUC1	Negative	
CEA-M	Negative	
Chromogranin-A	Negative	

Metastatic Carcinoma

- If bilateral, should be strongly considered
- Clinical history of another primary malignancy
- Implants on adrenal surface
- Multiple tumor emboli in lymphatic spaces
- Immunohistochemistry should be performed to determine origin of primary site

Lymphoma

- Reported in 18-25% of patients at autopsy
- Patients with widespread disease
- Immunohistochemistry for B-cell and T-cell markers should be used for diagnosis

Sarcomas

- Rare
- Diagnosis of exclusion; HIV-positive patients

DIAGNOSTIC CHECKLIST

Clinically Relevant Pathologic Features

- Common primary sources: Lungs, breast, stomach, esophagus, liver, kidney, ovaries, pancreas, and colon

Pathologic Interpretation Pearls

- Consider metastatic tumors if very unusual histological pattern for adrenocortical carcinoma

SELECTED REFERENCES

1. Agarwal KK et al: FDG PET/CT in Carcinoma of the tongue with bilateral adrenal metastases. Clin Nucl Med. 42(2):123-124, 2017
2. Dagher J et al: Clear cell renal cell carcinoma: a comparative study of histological and chromosomal characteristics between primary tumors and their corresponding metastases. Virchows Arch. 471(1):107-115, 2017
3. Ganeshan D et al: Pattern and distribution of distant metastases in anaplastic prostate carcinoma: A single-institute experience with 101 patients. AJR Am J Roentgenol. 1-6, 2017
4. Imaoka Y et al: Adrenal failure due to bilateral adrenal metastasis of rectal cancer: A case report. Int J Surg Case Rep. 31:1-4, 2017
5. Kanaya N et al: A case of long-term survival after surgical resection for solitary adrenal recurrence of esophageal squamous carcinoma. Surg Case Rep. 3(1):61, 2017
6. Pardo Aranda F et al: Surgical treatment of lung cancer with synchronous adrenal metastases: Adrenalectomy first. Cir Esp. 95(2):97-101, 2017
7. Schieda N et al: Update on CT and MRI of adrenal nodules. AJR Am J Roentgenol. 1-12, 2017
8. Shaheen O et al: Esophageal cancer metastases to unexpected sites: A systematic review. Gastroenterol Res Pract. 2017:1657310, 2017
9. Ettaieb MH et al: Synchronous vs. metachronous metastases in adrenocortical carcinoma: An analysis of the Dutch Adrenal Network. Horm Cancer. 7(5-6):336-344, 2016
10. Fujimoto N et al: [Resection of hepatocellular carcinoma with synchronous bilateral adrenal metastasis.] Gan To Kagaku Ryoho. 43(12):1770-1772, 2016
11. Glenn JA et al: Management of suspected adrenal metastases at 2 academic medical centers. Am J Surg. 211(4):664-70, 2016
12. Jung J et al: Radiotherapy for adrenal metastasis from hepatocellular carcinoma: A multi-institutional retrospective study (KROG 13-05). PLoS One. 11(3):e0152642, 2016
13. Lomte N et al: Bilateral adrenal masses: a single-centre experience. Endocr Connect. 5(2):92-100, 2016
14. Mouka V et al: Solitary adrenal metastasis from early-stage dedifferentiated endometrial carcinoma: CT findings and review of the literature. J Obstet Gynaecol. 36(7):881-882, 2016
15. Singh Lubana S et al: Adrenal Metastasis from Uterine Papillary Serous Carcinoma. Am J Case Rep. 17:289-94, 2016
16. Taguchi T et al: Adrenal and thyroid metachronous metastases from renal cell carcinoma. Endocrine. 53(1):335-6, 2016
17. Tonyali S et al: Survival following laparoscopic adrenalectomy for solitary metastasis of lung cancer. Int Urol Nephrol. 48(11):1803-1809, 2016
18. Duregon E et al: Pitfalls in the diagnosis of adrenocortical tumors: a lesson from 300 consultation cases. Hum Pathol. 46(12):1799-807, 2015
19. Flaherty DC et al: Adrenalectomy for metastatic melanoma: Current role in the age of nonsurgical treatments. Am Surg. 81(10):1005-9, 2015
20. Lack EE: Tumors of the Adrenal Glands and Extraadrenal Paraganglia. In AFIP Atlas of Tumor Pathology Series 4, Fascicle 8. Washington, DC: American Registry of Pathology, 2007
21. Gufler H et al: Differentiation of adrenal adenomas from metastases with unenhanced computed tomography. J Comput Assist Tomogr. 28(6):818-22, 2004
22. Lam KY et al: Metastatic tumours of the adrenal glands: a 30-year experience in a teaching hospital. Clin Endocrinol (Oxf). 56(1):95-101, 2002
23. Kim SH et al: The role of surgery in the treatment of clinically isolated adrenal metastasis. Cancer. 82(2):389-94, 1998
24. Lack EE et al: Embryology, developmental anatomy, and selected aspects of non-neoplastic pathology. In Pathology of the Adrenal Glands. New York: Churchill Livingstone. 1-74, 1990
25. Twomey P et al: Successful treatment of adrenal metastases from large-cell carcinoma of the lung. JAMA. 248(5):581-3, 1982
26. Abrams HL et al: Metastases in carcinoma; analysis of 1000 autopsied cases. Cancer. 3(1):74-85, 1950

Small Tumor Foci Within Adrenal Cortex

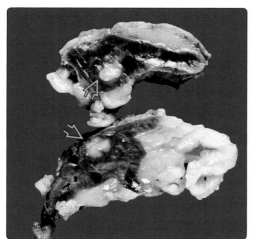

Renal Cell Carcinoma Metastatic to Adrenal

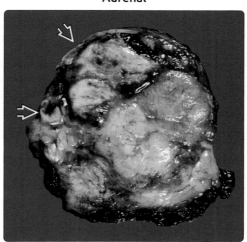

(Left) *Gross cut surface of an adrenal gland shows two small, white-gray tumor nodules ⇗ with irregular contours. The primary tumor was an insulin-producing neuroendocrine carcinoma of the pancreas.* (Right) *Gross cut surface of an adrenal gland shows a large, gray-pink and yellow tumor with multifocal areas of hemorrhage. The tumor occupies most of the gland with only a small rim of residual adrenal cortex ⇒ identified. The primary tumor was a renal cell carcinoma.*

Neuroendocrine Tumor in Adrenal

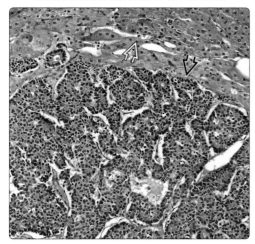

Hepatocellular Carcinoma

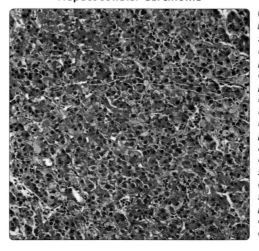

(Left) *This metastatic tumor ⇒ to the adrenal ⇒ gland shows a well-demarcated nodule with no capsule in a patient with known history of an insulin-producing pancreatic endocrine neoplasm. Immunohistochemistry for the hormone confirmed a pancreatic origin.* (Right) *Metastatic hepatocellular carcinoma to adrenal is shown. The sinusoidal pattern and morphology should raise suspicion for liver as the primary source. Hepatocellular antigen confirmed the diagnosis in this case.*

Metastatic Carcinoma to Adrenal

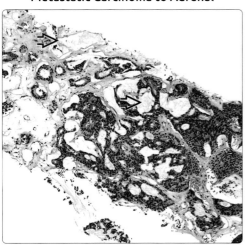

High-Grade Malignant Tumor

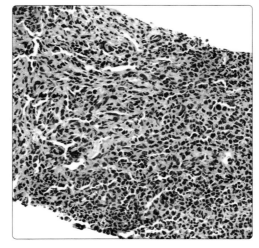

(Left) *Breast adenocarcinoma is a common cause of metastatic cancer to the adrenal. This tumor shows marked resemblance to the primary invasive ductal carcinoma. Mucin pools are present ⇒.* (Right) *Core biopsy shows a high-grade pleomorphic neoplasm with abundant mitotic figures. HMB-45, melan-A, and S100 were positive, supporting the diagnosis of a metastatic malignant melanoma.*

ETIOLOGY/PATHOGENESIS

- Li-Fraumeni syndrome
  - Accounts for most pediatric cases of adrenal cortical carcinoma (ACC)
    - ~ 50% of very early onset ACCs occur in children with germline *TP53* mutations
  - TP53 R337H mutation
- Beckwith-Wiedemann syndrome
  - Characterized by adrenal cytomegaly
  - Associated with adrenal cortical neoplasms
- Multiple endocrine neoplasia type 1
- Lynch syndrome
- Carney complex
- Familial adenomatous polyposis
- Neurofibromatosis type 1
- Hemihypertrophy
  - Adrenal cortical neoplasms have been associated with hemihypertrophy in children
- Congenital adrenal hyperplasia
  - Adrenal cortical adenoma and ACC have been associated with adrenogenital syndrome
- McCune-Albright syndrome

CLINICAL ISSUES

- Females have higher incidence until 5 years of age, after which sex difference disappears
- > 90% of children with adrenal cortical neoplasms present with symptoms of endocrine syndrome
  - Most common presentation is virilization
- Adrenal cortical tumors in children more frequently show adverse histologic features in clinically benign tumors as compared to adult tumors

MICROSCOPIC

- Different architectural patterns are seen
- Confluent necrosis is histologic feature; adverse prognostic finding if > 25%

Variegated Gross Cut Surface

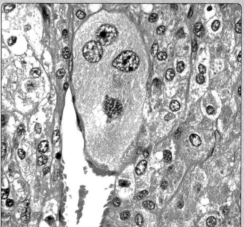

Large Eosinophilic Cells

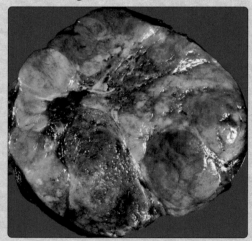

(Left) *Adrenal cortical carcinoma (ACC) cut surface shows a variegated appearance. This markedly enlarged adrenal gland is completely replaced by a irregularly shaped, bulky mass with a pale-brown cut surface. Multiple areas of yellow necrotic foci are identified.* (Right) *This picture illustrates the adrenal tumor in a child with sex-hormone-producing ACC. The cells are large with ample eosinophilic cytoplasm and with marked variation in nuclear size and shape.*

Large Multinucleated Cells

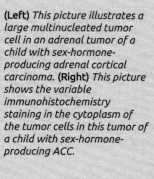

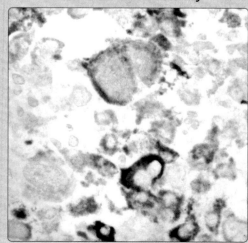

Melan-A Immunoreactivity

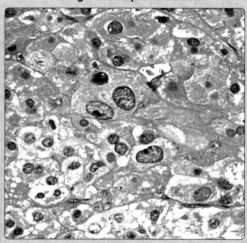

(Left) *This picture illustrates a large multinucleated tumor cell in an adrenal tumor of a child with sex-hormone-producing adrenal cortical carcinoma.* (Right) *This picture shows the variable immunohistochemistry staining in the cytoplasm of the tumor cells in this tumor of a child with sex-hormone-producing ACC.*

TERMINOLOGY

Abbreviations

- Adrenal cortical neoplasm (ACN)

Synonyms

- Adrenal cortical adenoma (ACA)
- Adrenal cortical carcinoma (ACC)
- Adrenal cortical tumor

Definitions

- Neoplasms arising from adrenal cortical cells
- Adrenal cortical carcinoma is malignant epithelial tumor of adrenal cortical cells
- ACA is benign epithelial tumor of adrenal cortical cells

ETIOLOGY/PATHOGENESIS

Sporadic

- Rare cases in children are nonsyndromic
- Wide variety of syndromes are associated with adrenal cortical tumors
  - ~ 50% of early onset ACCs occur in children with germline *TP53* mutations
  - Adult patients with ACC often harbor germline mutations causing hereditary syndromes, including Li-Fraumeni syndrome, Lynch syndrome, and multiple endocrine neoplasia type 1 (MEN1)

Li-Fraumeni Syndrome

- a.k.a. SBLA syndrome: **S**arcoma; **b**reast and **b**rain tumors; **l**eukemia, **l**aryngeal carcinoma, and **l**ung cancer; **a**drenal cortical carcinoma
- Li-Fraumeni syndrome accounts for most pediatric ACC cases
  - Roughly 50% of very early onset ACCs occur in children with germline *TP53* mutations
- Endometrial carcinoma
- Autosomal dominant mode of inheritance
- Alterations in *P53* tumor suppressor gene
- Most common associated neoplasms are soft tissue sarcomas, bone sarcomas, and breast carcinoma

Beckwith-Wiedemann Syndrome

- Involves chromosome 11p15.5 in ~ 80% of cases
  - *IGF2* and *KCNQ1OT1* are normally expressed from paternal allele
  - *H19*, *CDKN1C*, and *KCNQ1* are normally expressed from maternal allele
- Characterized by adrenal cytomegaly
- Associated with adrenal cortical neoplasms
- Characterized by embryonal tumor in childhood
  - Main tumors associated with Beckwith-Wiedemann syndrome are nephroblastoma, ACC, and hepatoblastoma
- Characteristic facies in early childhood (often normal by adulthood)
- Somatic overgrowth
- Classic triad
  - Exomphalos
  - Gigantism
  - Macroglossia

Congenital Adrenal Hyperplasia

- ACA and ACC have been associated with congenital adrenal hyperplasia (adrenogenital syndrome)
- Associated with testicular tumors of adrenal cortical type

Hemihypertrophy

- Adrenal cortical neoplasms have been associated with hemihypertrophy in children
- Adrenal neoplasms are not necessarily located ipsilateral to hemihypertrophy
- Other associated tumors are Wilms tumor, hepatoblastoma, and pheochromocytoma

Other Syndromes

- MEN1
- Carney complex
- McCune-Albright syndrome
- Neurofibromatosis type 1
- Familial adenomatous polyposis
- Lynch syndrome
- Hereditary nonpolyposis colorectal cancer

CLINICAL ISSUES

Epidemiology

- Incidence
  - ~ 20 new ACC cases per year
  - ~ 25 new cases of ACA per year in United States in patients < 20 years of age
  - Annual incidence is 3:1,000,000 patients < 20 years old
  - Females have higher incidence until 5 years of age, after which sex difference disappears
  - Adrenal cortical neoplasms constitute 0.2% of all malignancies observed in children
- Age
  - Average at presentation: 8 years old
    - Most cases occur in patients < 5 years old

Presentation

- > 90% of children with adrenal cortical neoplasms present with symptoms of endocrine syndrome
- Functionally active tumors account for > 80%
- Most common presentation is virilization
  - Expressed in females
    - Increased muscle mass, clitoromegaly, facial hair, pubic hair, deepening of voice
  - Expressed in males
    - Penile enlargement, pubic hair
- May present with Cushing syndrome
  - If so, syndrome is usually associated with virilization

Prognosis

- Adrenal cortical tumors in children more frequently show adverse histologic features in clinically benign tumors vs. adult tumors
- Adverse prognostic factors in pediatric tumors
  - Older age at diagnosis: > 5 years of age
  - Average tumor size: 12 cm
  - Tumor weight: > 400 g
  - Mitotic count: > 30 per 50 HPF
  - Average tumor necrosis: 60%
  - Vascular &/or capsular invasion

- ○ Tumor ploidy has been shown **not** to correlate with outcome
- Most frequent sites of metastases are lung and liver; other places are peritoneum, pleura/diaphragm, abdominal lymph nodes, and kidneys

Associated Neoplasms

- Beckwith-Wiedemann syndrome
  - ○ Wilms tumor
  - ○ Hepatoblastoma
  - ○ Rhabdomyosarcoma
  - ○ Neuroblastoma
- Li-Fraumeni syndrome (a.k.a. SBLA syndrome)
  - ○ Endometrial carcinoma

MACROSCOPIC

General Features

- Mostly unilateral; bilateral tumors are extremely rare

Size

- Wide range: 2.5-20 cm
- Tumors with better prognosis have average size of 6 cm, whereas those with worse prognosis have average size of 12 cm

MICROSCOPIC

Histologic Features

- Pediatric tumors differ from adult adrenal cortical neoplasms in that those features associated with malignancy in adults can sometimes be seen in clinically benign tumors in children
  - ○ Capsular invasion
  - ○ Confluent necrosis (adverse prognostic finding if > 25%)
  - ○ Vascular invasion
- Different architectural patterns are seen
  - ○ Alveolar pattern is most common pattern in ACA
  - ○ Trabecular (commonly seen in malignant neoplasms)
  - ○ Solid
- Mitotic grading of ACC divides tumors into 2 prognostically significant groups
  - ○ Low-grade carcinomas: < 20 mitosis per 50 HPF
  - ○ High-grade carcinomas: > 20 mitosis per 50 HPF

Cytologic Features

- Nuclear pleomorphism
- Some can have oncocytic features
- Nuclear hyperchromasia
- Mitosis: Few figures can be seen in clinically benign tumors; sign of malignancy if numerous (> 30 per 50 HPF)
- Intracytoplasmic hyaline globules

ANCILLARY TESTS

Immunohistochemistry

- Positive for adrenal cortical markers such as SF-1, inhibin, synaptophysin, chromogranin, and Melan-A
- Negative for cytokeratin and chromogranin
- May be positive for P53
- Ki-67 proliferative index has demonstrated significant prognostic and predictive marker

- SF-1: High expression correlates with poorer clinical outcome

DIFFERENTIAL DIAGNOSIS

Pheochromocytoma

- Positive for chromogranin
- Negative for inhibin and MART-1

Renal Cell Carcinoma

- Negative for chromogranin

Other Primary or Metastatic Neoplasms

- Neuroblastoma, Wilms tumor, hepatoblastoma

DIAGNOSTIC CHECKLIST

Genetic susceptibility

- Given wide variety of syndromes, it has been recommended that patients with ACC be screened for hereditary diseases associated with *TP53* mutation

SELECTED REFERENCES

1. Babińska A et al: Diagnostic and prognostic role of SF1, IGF2, Ki67, p53, adiponectin, and leptin receptors in human adrenal cortical tumors. J Surg Oncol. 116(3):427-433, 2017
2. Bulzico D et al: A novel TP53 mutation associated with TWIST1 and SIP1 expression in an aggressive adrenocortical carcinoma. Endocr Pathol. ePub, 2017
3. Lodish M: Genetics of adrenocortical development and tumors. Endocrinol Metab Clin North Am. 46(2):419-433, 2017
4. Macedo GS et al: p53 signaling pathway polymorphisms, cancer risk and tumor phenotype in TP53 R337H mutation carriers. Fam Cancer. ePub, 2017
5. Achatz MI et al: The inherited p53 mutation in the brazilian population. Cold Spring Harb Perspect Med. 6(12), 2016
6. Challis BG et al: Familial adrenocortical carcinoma in association with Lynch syndrome. J Clin Endocrinol Metab. 101(6):2269-72, 2016
7. Das S et al: Weineke criteria, Ki-67 index and p53 status to study pediatric adrenocortical tumors: Is there a correlation? J Pediatr Surg. 51(11):1795-1800, 2016
8. Else T et al: 5th International ACC Symposium: hereditary predisposition to childhood ACC and the associated molecular phenotype: 5th International ACC Symposium Session: Not Just for Kids! Horm Cancer. 7(1):36-9, 2016
9. Papathomas TG et al: Sarcomatoid adrenocortical carcinoma: a comprehensive pathological, immunohistochemical, and targeted next-generation sequencing analysis. Hum Pathol. 58:113-122, 2016
10. Zheng S et al: Comprehensive pan-genomic characterization of adrenocortical carcinoma. Cancer Cell. 29(5):723-36, 2016
11. Adachi H et al: Congenital hyperinsulinism in an infant with paternal uniparental disomy on chromosome 11p15: few clinical features suggestive of Beckwith-Wiedemann syndrome. Endocr J. 60(4):403-8, 2013
12. Choufani S et al: Molecular findings in Beckwith-Wiedemann syndrome. Am J Med Genet C Semin Med Genet. 163(2):131-40, 2013
13. Jacob K et al: Beckwith-Wiedemann and Silver-Russell syndromes: opposite developmental imbalances in imprinted regulators of placental function and embryonic growth. Clin Genet. Epub ahead of print, 2013
14. Kantaputra PN et al: A novel mutation in CDKN1C in sibs with Beckwith-Wiedemann syndrome and cleft palate, sensorineural hearing loss, and supernumerary flexion creases. Am J Med Genet A. 161A(1):192-7, 2013
15. Raymond VM et al: Adrenocortical carcinoma is a Lynch syndrome-associated cancer. J Clin Oncol. Epub ahead of print, 2013
16. Sidhu A et al: Infantile adrenocortical tumor with an activating GNAS1 mutation. J Clin Endocrinol Metab. 98(1):E115-8, 2013
17. Carney JA et al: Massive neonatal adrenal enlargement due to cytomegaly, persistence of the transient cortex, and hyperplasia of the permanent cortex: findings in Cushing syndrome associated with hemihypertrophy. Am J Surg Pathol. 36(10):1452-63, 2012
18. Netchine I et al: Imprinted anomalies in fetal and childhood growth disorders: the model of Russell-Silver and Beckwith-Wiedemann syndromes. Endocr Dev. 23:60-70, 2012
19. Malkin D: Li-fraumeni syndrome. Genes Cancer. 2(4):475-84, 2011
20. Michalkiewicz E et al: Clinical and outcome characteristics of children with adrenocortical tumors: a report from the International Pediatric Adrenocortical Tumor Registry. J Clin Oncol. 22(5):838-45, 2004

Adrenal Cortical Tumor as Part of Inherited Tumor Syndromes

Syndrome	Gene	Adrenal Pathology	Prevalence Among Patients With Adrenal Cortical Carcinoma
Li-Fraumeni syndrome	TP53	Adrenal cortical carcinoma	3-5% in adults 50-80% in children
HNPCC (Lynch syndrome)	MLH1, MSH2, MSH6, PMS2	Adrenal cortical carcinoma	~ 3% in adults
Multiple endocrine neoplasia 1	MEN1	Adrenal cortical adenoma and carcinoma	1-2% in adults
Beckwith-Wiedemann syndrome	CDKN1C, NSD1	Adrenal cortical carcinoma, adenoma, and hyperplasia	< 1%
Carney complex	PRKAR1A	Primary pigmented adrenal nodular disease (hyperplasia)	< 1%
Neurofibromatosis 1	NF1	Adrenal cortical carcinoma	< 1%
Familial adenomatous polyposis	APC	Adrenal cortical adenoma and carcinoma	< 1%
McCune-Albright syndrome	GNAS1	Adrenal nodular hyperplasia, adenoma and carcinoma	
Congenital adrenal hyperplasia	CYP21	Adrenal nodular hyperplasia; adrenal cortical adenoma and carcinoma	

21. Ribeiro RC et al: Childhood adrenocortical tumours. Eur J Cancer. 40(8):1117-26, 2004
22. Sarwar ZU et al: Congenital adrenocortical adenoma: case report and review of literature. Pediatr Radiol. 34(12):991-4, 2004
23. Hertel NT et al: Late relapse of adrenocortical carcinoma in Beckwith-Wiedemann syndrome. Clinical, endocrinological and genetic aspects. Acta Paediatr. 92(4):439-43, 2003
24. Wieneke JA et al: Adrenal cortical neoplasms in the pediatric population: a clinicopathologic and immunophenotypic analysis of 83 patients. Am J Surg Pathol. 27(7):867-81, 2003
25. Ribeiro RC et al: An inherited p53 mutation that contributes in a tissue-specific manner to pediatric adrenal cortical carcinoma. Proc Natl Acad Sci U S A. 98(16):9330-5, 2001
26. Liou LS et al: Adrenocortical carcinoma in children. Review and recent innovations. Urol Clin North Am. 27(3):403-21, 2000
27. Teinturier C et al: Clinical and prognostic aspects of adrenocortical neoplasms in childhood. Med Pediatr Oncol. 32(2):106-11, 1999
28. Bugg MF et al: Correlation of pathologic features with clinical outcome in pediatric adrenocortical neoplasia. A study of a Brazilian population. Brazilian Group for Treatment of Childhood Adrenocortical Tumors. Am J Clin Pathol. 101(5):625-9, 1994
29. Lack EE et al: Adrenal cortical neoplasms in the pediatric and adolescent age group. Clinicopathologic study of 30 cases with emphasis on epidemiological and prognostic factors. Pathol Annu. 27 Pt 1:1-53, 1992
30. Medeiros LJ et al: New developments in the pathologic diagnosis of adrenal cortical neoplasms. A review. Am J Clin Pathol. 97(1):73-83, 1992
31. Weiss LM et al: Pathologic features of prognostic significance in adrenocortical carcinoma. Am J Surg Pathol. 13(3):202-6, 1989
32. Li FP et al: A cancer family syndrome in twenty-four kindreds. Cancer Res. 48(18):5358-62, 1988
33. Neblett WW et al: Experience with adrenocortical neoplasms in childhood. Am Surg. 53(3):117-25, 1987
34. Cagle PT et al: Comparison of adrenal cortical tumors in children and adults. Cancer. 57(11):2235-7, 1986
35. Lynch HT et al: The sarcoma, breast cancer, lung cancer, and adrenocortical carcinoma syndrome revisited. Childhood cancer. Am J Dis Child. 139(2):134-6, 1985
36. Weiss LM: Comparative histologic study of 43 metastasizing and nonmetastasizing adrenocortical tumors. Am J Surg Pathol. 8(3):163-9, 1984
37. Hough AJ et al: Prognostic factors in adrenal cortical tumors. A mathematical analysis of clinical and morphologic data. Am J Clin Pathol. 72(3):390-9, 1979
38. Lynch HT et al: Genetic and pathologic findings in a kindred with hereditary sarcoma, breast cancer, brain tumors, leukemia, lung, laryngeal, and adrenal cortical carcinoma. Cancer. 41(5):2055-64, 1978
39. Schnakenburg KV et al: Congenital hemihypertrophy and malignant giant pheochromocytoma - a previously undescribed coincidence. Eur J Pediatr. 122(4):263-73, 1976
40. Li FP et al: Soft-tissue sarcomas, breast cancer, and other neoplasms. A familial syndrome? Ann Intern Med. 71(4):747-52, 1969
41. Fraumeni JF Jr et al: Primary carcinoma of the liver in childhood: an epidemiologic study. J Natl Cancer Inst. 40(5):1087-99, 1968
42. Fraumeni JF Jr et al: Adrenocortical neoplasms with hemihypertrophy, brain tumors, and other disorders. J Pediatr. 70(1):129-38, 1967
43. Fraumeni JF Jr et al: Wilms' tumor and congenital hemihypertrophy: report of five new cases and review of literature. Pediatrics. 40(5):886-99, 1967

Beckwith-Wiedemann syndrome

Extensive Necrosis

(Left) *This term infant with Beckwith-Wiedemann syndrome has a protuberant abdomen, secondary to enlarged liver and kidneys, and a large mouth with macroglossia. (Courtesy J. L. B. Byrne, MD.)* **(Right)** *ACCs tend to appear grossly as large solid masses in the suprarenal region, typically measuring > 5 cm. Focal areas of necrosis and hemorrhage are usually present.*

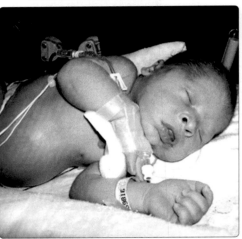

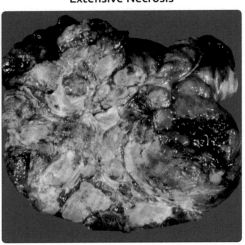

Adrenal Carcinoma With Liver Metastases

Adrenal Cortical Carcinoma

(Left) *Coronal graphic shows primary ACC with invasion into adjacent kidney. N1 and M1 disease is illustrated via an involved paraaortic lymph node ⊡ and multifocal hepatic metastases ⊡. (Right) Axial graphic demonstrates T4 right-sided ACC invading adjacent organs, including the right kidney, the liver, and the inferior vena cava.*

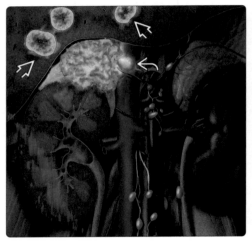

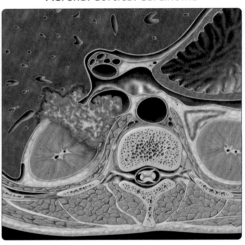

Adrenal Carcinoma Cut Surface

Metastases to Lung

(Left) *Gross photo shows a cross section of a large adrenal mass replacing the adrenal parenchyma in a young child. This ACC is yellow-tan, has irregular borders and necrosis, and weighs over 100 g.* **(Right)** *This photomicrography shows an H&E of the lung of a 6-month-old patient with ACC and metastases to the lung. The tumor cells have an ample and eosinophilic cytoplasm.*

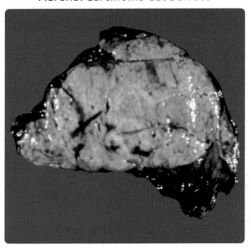

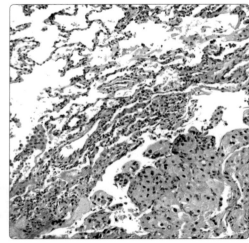

Adrenal Cortical Carcinoma

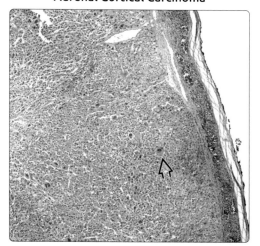

Encapsulated Adrenal Carcinoma

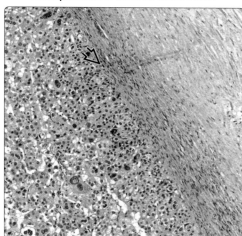

(Left) Photomicrograph shows a moderately well-circumscribed solid lesion with areas of necrosis and multiple enlarged cells with atypical nuclei ⊟ in a 20-day-old boy with an adrenal mass. (Right) Higher magnification of an ACC shows the interface ⊟ between the tumor and the fibrous capsule. The tumor has a predominantly trabecular and solid pattern and is composed of compact cells with nuclear atypia and focal nuclear pleomorphism.

Necrosis and Pleomorphism

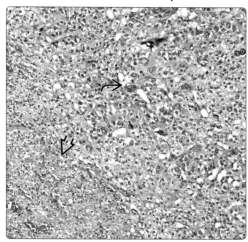

Tumor Cell Characteristics

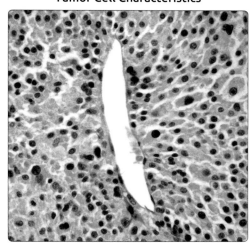

(Left) H&E shows an area of ACC with focal necrosis ⊟. The tumor cells have an eosinophilic cytoplasm with nuclear pleomorphism, atypia, and mitosis. Some of the cells are multinucleated ⊟. (Right) Higher magnification of an ACC shows a tumor has a predominantly solid pattern and is composed of compact eosinophilic cells with nuclear atypia and focal nuclear pleomorphism.

Lung Metastases

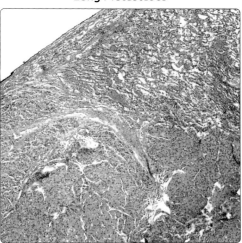

Oncocytic Carcinoma in Lung

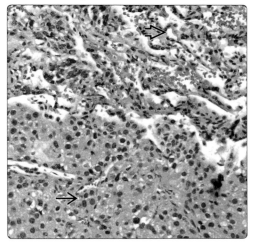

(Left) H&E shows lung metastasis from an ACC from a 6-year-old girl. The patient presented with multiple lesions in her lungs a few months after the diagnosis of ACC. Biopsy of those lesions showed metastatic carcinoma that was morphologically and immunophenotypically similar to the originally diagnosed ACC. (Right) Higher magnification shows a metastatic ACC ⊟ in the lung of a 6-year-old girl. Note the adjacent normal lung parenchyma ⊟.

Encapsulated Tumor

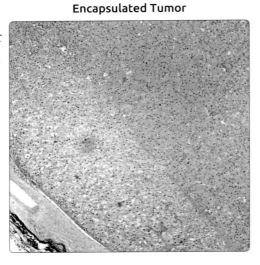

Focal Pleomorphism

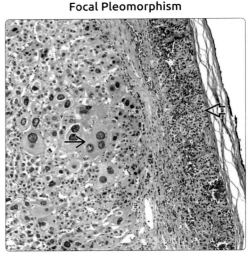

(Left) This tumor from a 6-year-old girl with virilizing ACC shows a well-circumscribed mass; however, the tumor also had multiple atypical mitosis and necrosis (not shown). All these features are suggestive of carcinoma (ACC). (Right) Higher magnification view of virilizing ACC shows the residual adrenal gland ⇨. There are numerous bizarre and multinucleated giant cells ⇨, some with intranuclear inclusions. This lesion has several features of malignancy.

Extensive Necrosis

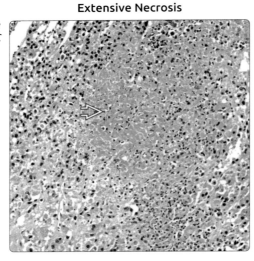

Myxoid Component

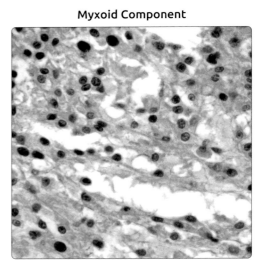

(Left) High-magnification view shows an area of virilizing ACC with necrosis ⇨ in the center of the field. Necrosis of > 50-60% is a feature seen in ACCs. (Right) Some adrenal cortical tumors may have focal areas with a myxoid stroma. ACCs more frequently have myxoid stroma than do the adrenal cortical adenomas.

Eosinophilic Granules

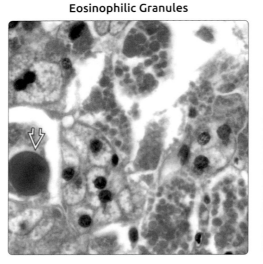

Necrosis

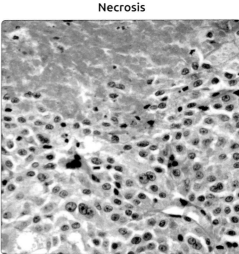

(Left) This picture of an unusual adrenal cortical neoplasm shows numerous giant eosinophilic granules and a large hyaline globule ⇨. (Right) The presence of necrosis is one of the Weiss criteria for malignancy in adrenal cortical tumors. This tumor from a patient with Li-Fraumeni syndrome and TP53 mutation shows multifocal areas of necrosis.

Newborn Adrenal

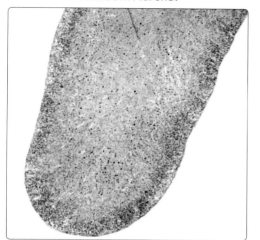

Adrenal Cytomegaly

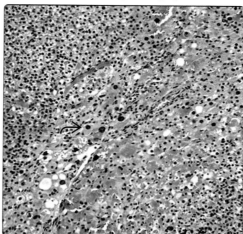

(Left) *This H&E section from an adrenal of a newborn with Beckwith-Wiedemann syndrome shows adrenal cortical cell cytomegaly. The large nuclei can be identified at this magnification.* (Right) *There are numerous enlarged and bizarre polyhedral cells ⊘ with eosinophilic granular cytoplasm and large hyperchromatic nuclei in adrenal cortex in patients with Beckwith-Wiedemann syndrome.*

ACC Pleomorphic Cells in Beckwith-Wiedemann Syndrome

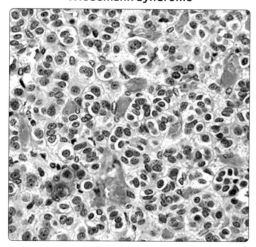

Synaptophysin

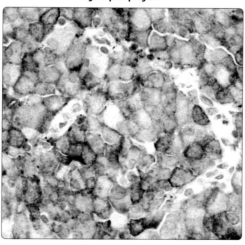

(Left) *High-power magnification shows an ACC in a patient with Beckwith-Wiedemann syndrome. In these patients, the adrenal neoplasms are usually associated with pleomorphism.* (Right) *ACCs usually have immunopositivity for synaptophysin, calretinin, Melan-A, SF-1, and inhibin a. Synaptophysin is present in these tumors in the cytoplasm and in cellular membranes and can be very weak in some tumors.*

Atypical Mitosis

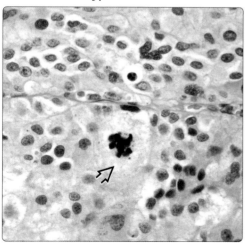

High Proliferative Index

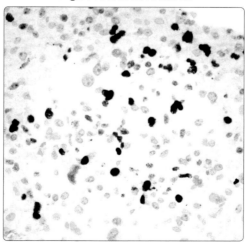

(Left) *This ACC has a diffuse growth pattern, and is composed by cells with eosinophilic cytoplasm and with the presence of atypical mitosis ⊘ and scattered pleomorphic cells.* (Right) *This picture illustrates a high Ki-67 proliferative index. ACCs are associated with a high proliferative rate and can be divided on the basis of mitotic activity in low grade or high grade.*

TERMINOLOGY FOR DEFINITIONS, STAGING, AND CANCER PROTOCOLS

- Adrenal cortical carcinoma is malignant epithelial tumor of adrenal cortical cells (WHO 2017)
- Adrenal cortical carcinomas are not usually graded on histological grounds
- Some features, such as high mitotic count, presence of atypical mitosis, high nuclear grade, vascular invasion, and tumor necrosis, are evaluated to confirm diagnosis of carcinoma
- Adrenal cortical carcinomas can be subdivided based on mitotic activity
  - Low grade: ≤ 20 mitoses per 50 HPF
  - High grade: > 20 mitoses per 50 HPF
- CAP cancer protocol applies only to adrenal cortical carcinoma and does not apply to any other adrenal tumor types

- Recent 2017 WHO Classification of Tumors of Endocrine Organs suggests use of European Network for Study of Adrenal Tumors (ENSAT) staging system
  - Stage I: Tumors confined to adrenal gland ≤ 5 cm
  - Stage II: Tumors confined to adrenal gland > 5 cm
  - Stage III: Tumors extend out of gland with or without involving adjacent organs
  - Stage IV: Tumors characterized by distant metastases
- TNM classification of tumors of adrenal cortex (8th edition, 2016)
  - T1: Tumors ≤ 5 cm, no extraadrenal invasion
  - T2: Tumors > 5 cm, no extraadrenal invasion
  - T3: Tumors of any size, with local invasion, but not invading adjacent organs
    - Kidney, diaphragm, renal vein, vena cava, pancreas, and liver
  - T4: Tumor of any size with invasion of adjacent organs

T4 Adrenal Cortical Carcinoma

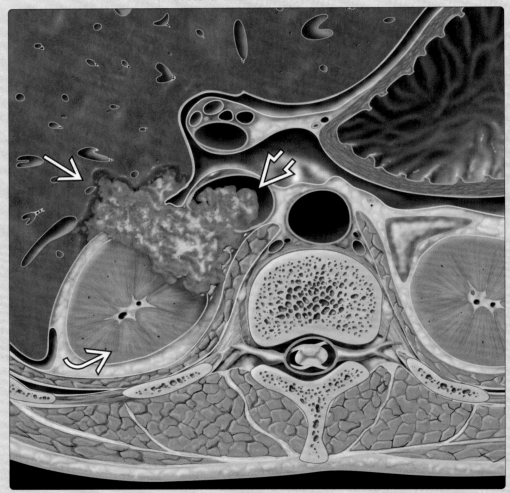

Axial graphic demonstrates T4 right-sided adrenal cortical carcinoma invading adjacent organs, including the right kidney ➡, the liver ➡, and the inferior vena cava ➡.

T1 Adrenal Cortical Carcinoma

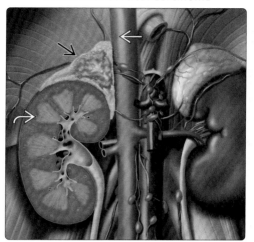

T2 Adrenal Cortical Carcinoma

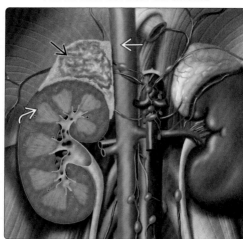

(Left) *Coronal graphic demonstrates T1 disease. The primary tumor ⊟ is ≤ 5 cm in its greatest dimension, limited to the adrenal gland without invasion of adjacent organs, including the kidney ⊟ or the inferior vena cava ⊟.* (Right) *Coronal graphic demonstrates T2 disease. The primary tumor ⊟ is > 5 cm in its greatest dimension, limited to the adrenal gland, and without invasion of adjacent organs, including the kidney ⊟ or inferior vena cava ⊟.*

T3 Adrenal Cortical Carcinoma

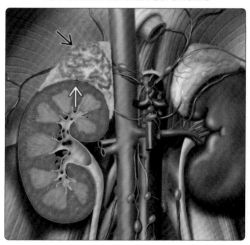

T4 Adrenal Cortical Carcinoma

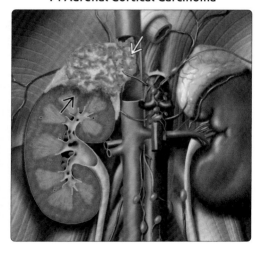

(Left) *Coronal graphic demonstrates T3 disease. The primary tumor may be any size with local invasion beyond the confines of the adrenal capsule, shown in the superolateral margin ⊟, but with no involvement of adjacent organs, such as the kidney ⊟.* (Right) *Coronal graphic demonstrates T4 disease. The primary tumor can be any size with local invasion beyond the confines of the adrenal capsule and into adjacent organs, including the kidney ⊟. Direct extension into the inferior vena cava is illustrated ⊟.*

T4 N1 M1 Adrenal Cortical Carcinoma

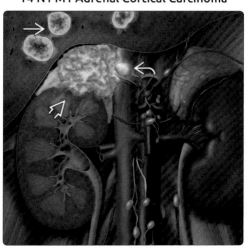

Tumor Grading by Mitotic Count

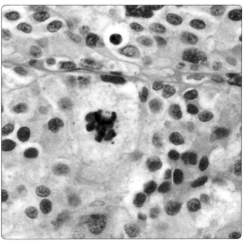

(Left) *Coronal graphic shows primary adrenal cortical carcinoma with invasion into the adjacent kidney, T4 ⊟. N1 and M1 disease is illustrated via an involved paraaortic lymph node ⊟ and multifocal hepatic metastases ⊟. This will be stage IV disease.* (Right) *Adrenal cortical carcinomas can be subdivided on the basis of mitotic frequency into low grade (≤ 20 mitoses per 50 HPF) and high grade (> 20 mitoses per 50 HPF).*

SECTION 4
Pituitary Gland

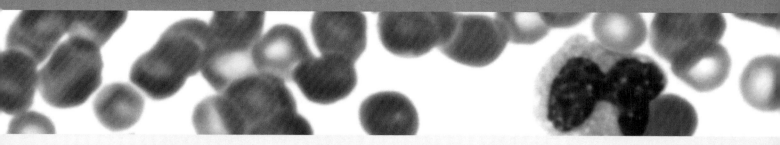

TERMINOLOGY

- Primary inflammatory hypophysitis is characterized by focal or diffuse inflammatory infiltration and ultimate destruction of pituitary gland
  - Histopathological categories: Lymphocytic, granulomatous, and xanthomatous hypophysitis
  - IgG4-related hypophysitis is rare form of primary hypophysitis
- Secondary hypophysitis is due to inflammation of nearby structure

ETIOLOGY/PATHOGENESIS

- Autoimmune cause has been suggested for lymphocytic hypophysitis

CLINICAL ISSUES

- Lymphocytic hypophysitis has strong female predilection (80% of cases) and is associated with puerperal period
- Association with other autoimmune disorders in ~ 25% of patients

MICROSCOPIC

- Lymphocytic hypophysitis displays lymphocytic infiltration predominantly of small, mature lymphocytes
- Granulomatous hypophysitis is composed of noncaseating granulomas associated with variable lymphocytic infiltrates
- IgG4-related hypophysitis displays dense plasmacytic infiltrates and minor component of lymphocytes and macrophages

TOP DIFFERENTIAL DIAGNOSES

- Hypophysitis secondary to craniopharyngioma or Rathke cleft cyst rupture
- Infectious diseases and sarcoidosis

Lymphocytic Hypophysitis

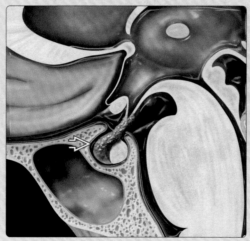

Neuroimaging of Infundibuloneurohypophysis

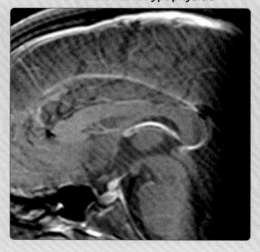

(Left) Sagittal graphic shows lymphocytic hypophysitis. Note the thickening of the infundibulum as well as infiltration into the anterior lobe of the pituitary gland ➡. (Right) Sagittal T1WI MR shows hyperintensity of pituitary gland and thickening of the infundibulum in a case of lymphocytic infundibuloneurohypophysitis.

Lymphocytic Hypophysitis

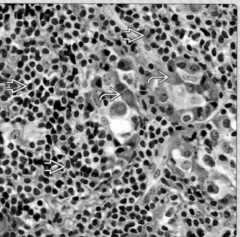

Granulomatous Hypophysitis

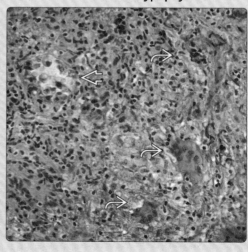

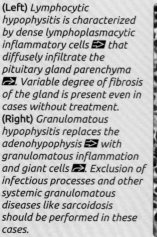

(Left) Lymphocytic hypophysitis is characterized by dense lymphoplasmacytic inflammatory cells ➡ that diffusely infiltrate the pituitary gland parenchyma ➡. Variable degree of fibrosis of the gland is present even in cases without treatment. (Right) Granulomatous hypophysitis replaces the adenohypophysis ➡ with granulomatous inflammation and giant cells ➡. Exclusion of infectious processes and other systemic granulomatous diseases like sarcoidosis should be performed in these cases.

TERMINOLOGY

Definitions

- **Primary hypophysitis**: Rare disorder characterized by focal or diffuse inflammatory infiltration and ultimate destruction of pituitary gland
  - Classified into 3 main histopathological categories
    - Lymphocytic hypophysitis
    - Granulomatous hypophysitis
    - Xanthomatous hypophysitis
  - IgG4-related hypophysitis has been regarded as a primary hypophysitis by some investigators
- **Secondary hypophysitis**: Inflammation of pituitary secondary to inflammation of nearby structure or systemic disease
  - Local causes include
    - Rupture of sellar cystic lesion (craniopharyngioma, Rathke cleft cyst, epidermoid cyst)
    - Meningitis
    - Osteomyelitis of sphenoid bone
  - Association with immunotherapy treatment targeting cytotoxic T-lymphocyte antigen 4 (CTLA-4)

ETIOLOGY/PATHOGENESIS

Autoimmune

- Suggested for lymphocytic hypophysitis
  - Circulating antipituitary antibodies detected in these patients
  - Candidate autoantibodies include α-enolase, growth hormone (GH), pituitary gland specific factors 1a and 2, and secretogranin-2
- Demonstration of antibodies directed against pituitary cells and association of other endocrine or immunologic diseases in number of patients has corroborated this hypothesis

IgG4-Related Hypophysitis

- Rare hypophysitis that may occur in isolation or in association with IgG4-related systemic diseases
- Proliferation of IgG4 antibodies has been associated with autoimmune and allergic disorders

Other Hypophysitis

- Etiology for granulomatous hypophysitis and xanthomatous hypophysitis unknown

CLINICAL ISSUES

Presentation

- All forms of primary hypophysitis present with signs of pituitary dysfunction and mass effect
  - Hyperprolactinemia is most frequent endocrine disturbance due to pituitary stalk effect &/or association with pregnancy
  - Hypopituitarism in particular may be seen in men
    - Isolated hormone deficiencies unusual; rare cases of isolated GH or ACTH deficiency have been reported
  - Headaches
  - Visual disturbances
  - Diabetes insipidus in cases of posterior pituitary involvement

- Lymphocytic hypophysitis can manifest as adenohypophysitis, infundibuloneurohypophysitis, or panhypophysitis
  - Peak incidence: 4th decade
    - Rarely involves children and elderly patients
  - Strong female predilection (80% of cases)
    - Strong association with pregnancy and puerperal period
  - Association with other autoimmune disorders in ~ 25% of patients
- Granulomatous hypophysitis
  - No gender predilection
  - No correlation with pregnancy
  - No correlation with other autoimmune disorders
- Xanthomatous hypophysitis is least common hypophysitis
  - No gender predilection
  - No correlation with pregnancy
  - No correlation with other autoimmune disorders
- IgG4-related hypophysitis may present isolated or in combination with other organs
  - Majority of reported cases have involvement of other organs

Treatment

- Corticosteroid therapy is main treatment for reduction of inflammatory response
  - Hormonal replacement therapy may be necessary depending upon pituitary dysfunction

Prognosis

- Partial or significant destruction of pituitary gland may occur due to either treatment or end-stage disease
  - Reduction of pituitary volume reported in almost 90% of patients
- Natural history is variable (some patients may improve spontaneously)
- Recurrence reported in ~ 18% of patients in one series

IMAGING

Radiographic Findings

- Neuroradiological studies show enlargement of pituitary gland in great majority of cases with frequent evidence of suprasellar extension
- Differentiation from pituitary adenoma may be challenging on neuroimaging

MACROSCOPIC

General Features

- Surgical specimen typically yellow and firm at gross examination, unlike soft pituitary adenomas

MICROSCOPIC

Histologic Features

- Lymphocytic hypophysitis
  - Infiltration of anterior pituitary by lymphocytes and plasma cells with occasional germinal centers
  - Parenchymal atrophy, variable degree of fibrosis, and residual lymphocytic infiltration at later stages of disease
  - Immunohistochemistry confirmatory of polytypic lymphoplasmacytic infiltrate

- Granulomatous hypophysitis
  - Well-formed, noncaseating granulomas associated with variable lymphocytic infiltrates
    - Special stains for microorganisms must be performed to rule out infectious causes
  - Variable parenchymal fibrosis
- Xanthomatous hypophysitis
  - Variable lymphoplasmacytic inflammatory infiltrates
  - Foamy macrophages with giant cell formation, necrosis, and hemosiderin deposition
- IgG4-related hypophysitis
  - Dense plasmacytic infiltrates and minor component of B lymphocytes and macrophages
  - Abundant IgG4(+) plasma cells [diagnostic criteria: > 10 IgG4(+) cells per HPF]
  - Dense fibrosis may be present

Cytologic Features

- Lymphocytic infiltration predominantly of small, mature lymphocytes without nuclear/cellular atypia

DIFFERENTIAL DIAGNOSIS

Hypophysitis Secondary to Craniopharyngioma or Rathke Cleft Cyst Rupture

- Dense lymphoplasmacytic inflammation with areas of xanthomatous changes at times
- Analysis of possible epithelium lining of cystic lesion may require several deeper levels on paraffin block

Infectious Processes

- Use histochemical stains for microorganisms or cultures when fresh tissues mandatory to rule out tuberculosis, fungal and bacterial causes

Sarcoidosis

- Clinical and laboratory data should be correlated with pathological analysis

Langerhans Cell Histiocytosis

- Immunohistochemical stains for CD1a and S100 diagnostic of LCH

Lymphoma

- Rare primary pituitary lymphoma and secondary involvement by systemic lymphoma
- Age at presentation differs with primary pituitary lymphoma involving older population

DIAGNOSTIC CHECKLIST

Clinically Relevant Pathologic Features

- Primary hypophysitis presents with signs of pituitary dysfunction and mass effect
- Pregnancy or postpartum period

Pathologic Interpretation Pearls

- Rich lymphoplasmacytic cell infiltration in absence of infectious or other more specific process, such as sarcoidosis

SELECTED REFERENCES

1. Bellastella G et al: Revisitation of autoimmune hypophysitis: knowledge and uncertainties on pathophysiological and clinical aspects. Pituitary. 19(6):625-642, 2016
2. Bernreuther C et al: IgG4-related hypophysitis is highly prevalent among cases of histologically confirmed hypophysitis. Brain Pathol. ePub, 2016
3. Faje A: Hypophysitis: evaluation and management. Clin Diabetes Endocrinol. 2:15, 2016
4. Shikuma J et al: Critical review of IgG4-related hypophysitis. Pituitary. ePub, 2016
5. Bando H et al: The prevalence of IgG4-related hypophysitis in 170 consecutive patients with hypopituitarism and/or central diabetes insipidus and review of the literature. Eur J Endocrinol. 170(2):161-72, 2014
6. Lammert A et al: Hypophysitis caused by ipilimumab in cancer patients: hormone replacement or immunosuppressive therapy. Exp Clin Endocrinol Diabetes. 121(10):581-7, 2013
7. Landek-Salgado MA et al: Growth hormone and proopiomelanocortin are targeted by autoantibodies in a patient with biopsy-proven IgG4-related hypophysitis. Pituitary. Epub ahead of print, 2011
8. Leporati P et al: IgG4-related hypophysitis: a new addition to the hypophysitis spectrum. J Clin Endocrinol Metab. 96(7):1971-80, 2011
9. Carpinteri R et al: Pituitary tumours: inflammatory and granulomatous expansive lesions of the pituitary. Best Pract Res Clin Endocrinol Metab. 23(5):639-50, 2009
10. Caturegli P et al: Pituitary autoimmunity: 30 years later. Autoimmun Rev. 7(8):631-7, 2008
11. Gutenberg A et al: Primary hypophysitis: clinical-pathological correlations. Eur J Endocrinol. 155(1):101-7, 2006
12. Bhansali A et al: Idiopathic granulomatous hypophysitis presenting as non-functioning pituitary adenoma: description of six cases and review of literature. Br J Neurosurg. 18(5):489-94, 2004
13. Leung GK et al: Primary hypophysitis: a single-center experience in 16 cases. J Neurosurg. 101(2):262-71, 2004

Lymphocytic Hypophysitis Involving Adenohypophysis

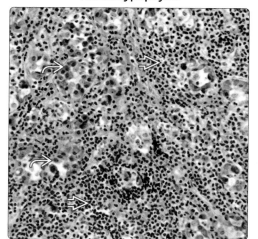

CD45 Immunohistochemistry in Lymphocytic Hypophysitis

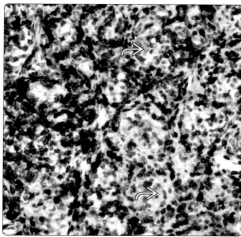

(Left) *Lymphocytic hypophysitis is characterized by infiltration of mature lymphocytes and plasma cells* ⮨ *in the anterior pituitary, destroying the adenohypophyseal cells* ⮨. (Right) *CD45 immunohistochemical stain highlights the dense lymphocytic inflammatory infiltrate in lymphocytic hypophysitis. T-lymphocytes composed most of the cells. There are scattered residual adenohypophyseal cells* ⮨ *(negative for the marker).*

End-Stage Lymphocytic Hypophysitis by H&E

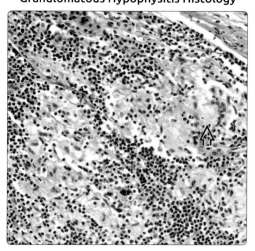

End-Stage Lymphocytic Hypophysitis by Reticulin

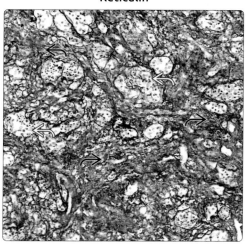

(Left) *H&E highlights end-stage lymphocytic hypophysitis showing extensive fibrosis* ⮨ *and lymphocytic infiltration* ⮨ *of anterior pituitary with scattered residual adenohypophyseal cells* ⮨. (Right) *Reticulin highlights end-stage lymphocytic hypophysitis displaying intense fibrosis* ⮨ *of the pituitary parenchyma with only scattered nests of residual cells* ⮨. *Destruction of the gland may occur independent of treatment.*

Granulomatous Hypophysitis Histology

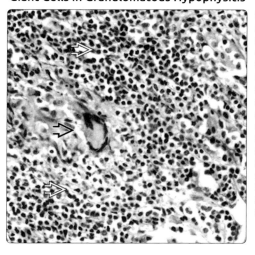

Giant Cells in Granulomatous Hypophysitis

(Left) *Granulomatous hypophysitis is characterized by noncaseous granulomatous inflammation* ⮨, *associated with variable lymphocytic infiltrate. Differential diagnosis includes infectious diseases and involvement by systemic granulomatous disorders.* (Right) *Granulomatous hypophysitis is characterized by severe lymphocytic infiltration* ⮨ *with scattered giant cells* ⮨ *within the adenohypophysis, destroying and replacing the adenohypophyseal cells.*

ETIOLOGY/PATHOGENESIS

- Physiological stimulation is best represented by lactotroph hyperplasia secondary to estrogen stimulation during pregnancy
- Thyrotroph hyperplasia may occur due to untreated primary hypothyroidism
- Ectopic secretion of hypothalamic-releasing hormones by neuroendocrine tumors is most common pathologic cause of pituitary hyperplasia
- Somatotroph hyperplasia may arise in setting of multiple endocrine neoplasia type 1, McCune-Albright, and X-linked acrogigantism syndromes
- Corticotroph hyperplasia may rarely be associated with Cushing disease

CLINICAL ISSUES

- Signs and symptoms of pituitary hormone hypersecretion mimicking secreting pituitary adenoma

- Identification of source of hypersecretion is crucial for treatment/management

IMAGING

- Diffuse enlargement of gland

MICROSCOPIC

- Anterior gland is composed of enlarged acini, which are mostly composed of single cell type with preserved reticulin network
- Focal or diffuse expansion of acini with preservation of reticulin pattern (reticulin stain)

ANCILLARY TESTS

- IHC for pituitary hormones identify hyperplastic cell population
- Other markers (S100, CD34) identify cellular components of pituitary gland intermixed between hyperplastic nodules

Pituitary Hyperplasia During Pregnancy

Lactotroph Hyperplasia During Pregnancy

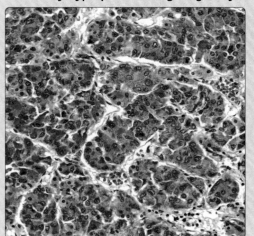
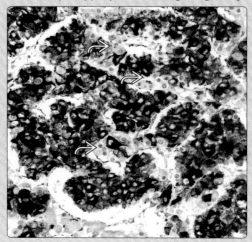

(Left) *Pituitary gland of an autopsy of a 27-year-old woman who died of DIC after delivery of a healthy baby. The pituitary was enlarged with diffuse expansion of the acini. The majority of the cells have acidophilic cytoplasm with large nuclei consistent with lactotroph cells.* (Right) *In the same patient, prolactin immunostain confirms lactotroph hyperplasia of pregnancy. Note that in addition to PRL(+) cells, several PRL(-) cells ➶ are present in the same acini, ruling out a lactotroph adenoma.*

Expansion of Acinar Structure in Pituitary Hyperplasia

Normal Acinar Structure in Pituitary Gland

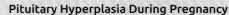
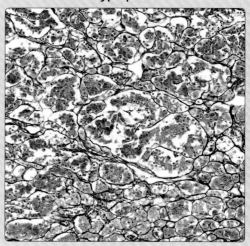
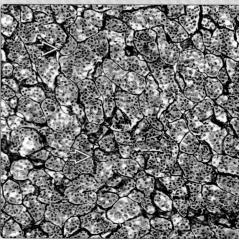

(Left) *Reticulin stain is crucial for diagnosis of hyperplasia, which shows expansion of the acini and preservation of the reticulin pattern, and its distinction from an adenoma. In comparison, reticulin stain of a normal adenohypophysis shows a relatively uniform distribution of acini.* (Right) *Reticulin stain of a normal adenohypophysis shows a relatively uniform distribution of acini surrounded by a reticulin network ➶.*

TERMINOLOGY

Definitions

- Cell proliferation driven by hormonal stimulus
- Rare and constitutes < 1% of sellar region surgical specimens

ETIOLOGY/PATHOGENESIS

Physiologic or Pathologic Mechanism

- Pituitary hyperplasia occurs secondary to hypersecretion of stimulating hormone by either physiologic or pathologic mechanism
- **Physiologic**
  - Stimulation due to estrogen secretion
    - Lactotroph hyperplasia during pregnancy
    - Hypertrophy of puberty mainly in females
- **Pathologic**
  - Ectopic secretion of hypothalamic-releasing hormones by neuroendocrine tumors is most common pathologic cause of pituitary hyperplasia
    - e.g., pancreatic and pulmonary growth hormone releasing hormone (GHRH)-secreting tumors producing somatotroph hyperplasia and pulmonary corticotropin releasing hormone (CRH)-secreting tumors producing corticotroph hyperplasia
  - Thyrotroph hyperplasia may occur due to untreated primary hypothyroidism
  - Corticotroph hyperplasia may rarely be associated with Cushing disease
- Genetic syndromes
  - Somatotroph hyperplasia may arise in setting of multiple endocrine neoplasia type 1, McCune-Albright, and X-linked acrogigantism syndromes

CLINICAL ISSUES

Presentation

- Signs and symptoms of pituitary hormone hypersecretion mimicking secreting pituitary adenoma
  - Acromegaly in cases of somatotroph or mammosomatotroph hyperplasia due to hypersecretion of GHRH
  - Cushing disease in cases of corticotroph hyperplasia due to hypersecretion of CRH
  - Primary hypothyroidism is main clinical presentation in cases of thyrotroph hyperplasia
  - Hyperprolactinemia in rare cases of idiopathic lactotroph hyperplasia

Treatment

- Identification of source of hypersecretion is crucial for treatment/management
  - Reversal of pituitary hyperplasia and hormonal imbalance should occur after treatment of primary disease

IMAGING

General Features

- Diffuse enlargement of gland

MACROSCOPIC

General Features

- Pituitary gland is enlarged and lacks well-defined lesion distinguishable from surrounding normal gland

MICROSCOPIC

Histologic Features

- Anterior gland is composed of enlarged acini, which are composed mostly of single cell type
- Focal or diffuse expansion of acini with preservation of reticulin pattern (reticulin stain)
- Hyperplasia may be diffuse within gland or focal with formation of nodules

ANCILLARY TESTS

Immunohistochemistry

- IHC for pituitary hormones identify hyperplastic cell population, and other markers (S100, CD34) identify cellular components of pituitary gland intermixed between hyperplastic nodules

DIFFERENTIAL DIAGNOSIS

Pituitary Adenoma, Including Corticotroph Cell Adenoma

- Reticulin stain helps in differentiating hyperplasia from adenoma
  - Differential diagnosis with adenoma is particularly significant in corticotroph cell hyperplasia

DIAGNOSTIC CHECKLIST

Pathologic Interpretation Pearls

- In pituitary hyperplasia, there is expansion of acini with preservation of reticulin pattern

SELECTED REFERENCES

1. Aquilina K et al: Nonneoplastic enlargement of the pituitary gland in children. J Neurosurg Pediatr. 7(5):510-5, 2011
2. Weiss DE et al: Ectopic acromegaly due to a pancreatic neuroendocrine tumor producing growth hormone-releasing hormone. Endocr Pract. 17(1):79-84, 2011
3. Nasr C et al: Acromegaly and somatotroph hyperplasia with adenomatous transformation due to pituitary metastasis of a growth hormone-releasing hormone-secreting pulmonary endocrine carcinoma. J Clin Endocrinol Metab. 91(12):4776-80, 2006
4. Ezzat S et al: Somatotroph hyperplasia without pituitary adenoma associated with a long standing growth hormone-releasing hormone-producing bronchial carcinoid. J Clin Endocrinol Metab. 78(3):555-60, 1994
5. Stefaneanu L et al: Pituitary lactotrophs and somatotrophs in pregnancy: a correlative in situ hybridization and immunocytochemical study. Virchows Arch B Cell Pathol Incl Mol Pathol. 62(5):291-6, 1992
6. Sano T et al: Growth hormone-releasing hormone-producing tumors: clinical, biochemical, and morphological manifestations. Endocr Rev. 9(3):357-73, 1988
7. Scheithauer BW et al: Pituitary gland in hypothyroidism. histologic and immunocytologic study. Arch Pathol Lab Med. 109(6):499-504, 1985
8. Thorner MO et al: Somatotroph hyperplasia. Successful treatment of acromegaly by removal of a pancreatic islet tumor secreting a growth hormone-releasing factor. J Clin Invest. 70(5):965-77, 1982

Sarcoidosis, Pituitary Gland

TERMINOLOGY

- Sarcoidosis is well-recognized systemic granulomatous process, which involves central nervous system in 5-15% of patients
  - Inflammatory multisystem disorder of unknown cause characterized by formation of noncaseating granulomas
- May involve hypothalamus and pituitary gland
  - Involvement of sellar region by sarcoidosis is overall infrequent occurrence, comprising < 1% of all intrasellar lesions

CLINICAL ISSUES

- Endocrine manifestations from neuro- &/or adenohypophysis failure
- Diabetes insipidus
- Most patients present with endocrine manifestations during course of systemic disease
- Hypogonadism is most frequently reported endocrine disorder in hypothalamic-pituitary sarcoidosis
- Hyperprolactinemia
- MR abnormalities disappear or improve under corticosteroid treatment, whereas most hormonal deficiencies are irreversible

MICROSCOPIC

- Well-formed, noncaseating granulomas with Langerhans or foreign body-like giant cells

TOP DIFFERENTIAL DIAGNOSES

- Primary granulomatous hypophysitis
- Infectious diseases
  - Tuberculosis, leprosy, Whipple disease, fungi
- Granulomatous systemic diseases
  - Wegener granulomatosis, Churg-Strauss syndrome, lymphomatoid granulomatosis
- Langerhans cell histiocytosis
- Germinoma with inflammatory cells

Sarcoid Granulomas

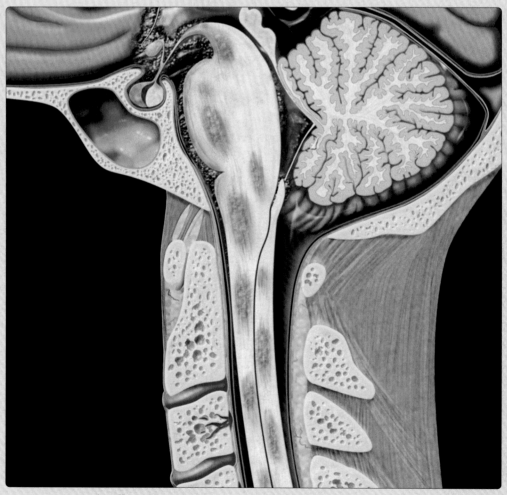

Any part of the nervous system can be affected by sarcoidosis, but the cranial nerves, hypothalamus, and pituitary gland are most commonly involved. Sagittal graphic depicts multiple intramedullary sarcoid granulomas in the brainstem and upper cervical cord. There is involvement of the pituitary stalk as well.

TERMINOLOGY

Definitions

- Inflammatory multisystem disorder of unknown cause characterized by formation of noncaseating granulomas
- May involve hypothalamus and pituitary gland

ETIOLOGY/PATHOGENESIS

Developmental Anomaly

- Genetic mechanisms may be implicated based on occasional familial clustering of cases
  ○ Association with certain HLA genotypes

Environmental Exposure

- Evidence that sarcoidosis results from genetically susceptible host's exposure to unidentified antigen with exacerbated Th1-immune response
  ○ Possible infectious factors
    – *Mycobacterium tuberculosis, Propionibacterium acnes, Rickettsia* species
  ○ Possible noninfectious factors
    – Pesticides, insecticides, pine pollen, silica, talc, metal dusts

CLINICAL ISSUES

Epidemiology

- Prevalence of clinical involvement of nervous system is estimated to be ~ 5-15%
- Disease is pathology of young adults between 20-40 years
- Prevalence is estimated between 8-10 per 100,000
- Pulmonary involvement is most frequent manifestation, but disease can affect every organ
- Any part of nervous system can be attacked by sarcoidosis, but cranial nerves, hypothalamus, and pituitary gland are most commonly involved
- Hypothalamic-pituitary (HP) manifestations are rare manifestations of sarcoidosis, occurring in < 1% of all intrasellar lesions
  ○ HP neurosarcoidosis accounts for 0.5% of cases of sarcoidosis and 1% of HP masses
- Sarcoid granulomas from HP region can also extend to and affect
  ○ Meninges
  ○ Parenchyma of brain
  ○ Brainstem subependymal layer of ventricular system
  ○ Choroid plexuses
  ○ Peripheral nerves
  ○ Blood vessels supplying nervous structures

Presentation

- Endocrine manifestations from neuro- &/or adenohypophysis failure
  ○ Diabetes insipidus
  ○ Hypopituitarism
    – Hypopituitarism is defined as 1 or more pituitary hormone deficits due to lesion in HP region
      □ Most common cause of hypopituitarism associated with sellar mass is pituitary adenoma
      □ Hypopituitarism should be considered within differential diagnosis in several other conditions, such as
      □ Other masses in sellar and parasellar region
      □ Brain damage caused by radiation and by traumatic brain injury
      □ Vascular lesions
      □ Infiltrative/immunological/inflammatory diseases (lymphocytic hypophysitis, sarcoidosis, and hemochromatosis)
      □ Infectious diseases and genetic disorders
  ○ Hyperprolactinemia with amenorrhea &/or galactorrhea due to "stalk effect"
- Most patients present with endocrine manifestations during course of systemic disease
- Recent series about HP involvement, including 9 patients, has suggested that gonadotropin deficiency was most frequent manifestation of disease
- In recent study of 24 patients with HP sarcoidosis, these are clinical symptoms found
  ○ Most patients reported clinical symptoms of pituitary deficiencies
  ○ Anterior pituitary deficiency was reported in 22 patients associated with posterior pituitary deficiency in 10 patients
  ○ Anterior pituitary deficiency was 1st symptom leading to diagnosis in 6 cases
  ○ Different manifestations were
    – Polyuria-polydipsia symptoms in 1/2 of cases
    – Asthenia: 8 cases
    – Decreased libido: 8 cases
    – Impotence: 3 cases
    – Decreased pilosity: 3 cases
    – Amenorrhea: 2 cases
    – Galactorrhea: 2 cases
    – Gynecomastia: 1 case

Treatment

- Depends on extent of systemic disease
- Corticosteroids, cytotoxic drugs, and immunomodulators
- Hormonal replacement
  ○ Testosterone
  ○ Estrogen and progesterone
  ○ Levothyroxine
  ○ Growth hormone
  ○ Hydrocortisone
- MR abnormalities improve under corticosteroid treatment, but most endocrine defects are irreversible

Prognosis

- Hormonal deficits may occur despite treatment of systemic disease

IMAGING

General Features

- Most cases show infundibulum involvement with thickness of pituitary stalk and involvement of anterior pituitary gland
- Association with brain parenchymal &/or meningeal lesions

Classification of Granulomatous Diseases Involving Pituitary Gland

Idiopathic	Infectious	Systemic Granulomatous Diseases	Neoplasias	Other Systemic Diseases
Granulomatous hypophysitis	Tuberculosis	Sarcoidosis	Langerhans cell histiocytosis	Crohn disease
	Leprosy	Wegener granulomatosis	Erdheim-Chester disease	Takayasu disease
	Whipple disease	Churg-Strauss syndrome	Germinoma	
	Fungal organisms	Lymphomatoid granulomatosis		

Radiographic Findings

- Absence of normal T1-weighted hyperintense signal of posterior pituitary
- Lesions are isointense to gray matter on T1-weighted and hyperintense on T2-weighted MR with homogeneous contrast enhancement

MICROSCOPIC

Histologic Features

- Involvement of neurohypophysis &/or adenohypophysis by well-formed, noncaseating granulomas
  - Aggregates of activated epithelioid histiocytes with Langerhans or foreign body-like giant cells
  - Moderate degree of lymphoplasmacytic infiltration
  - Variable degree of fibrosis of granulomas and parenchyma with chronicity of disease

DIFFERENTIAL DIAGNOSIS

Primary Granulomatous Hypophysitis

- Or granulomatous autoimmune hypophysitis
- Most common differential diagnosis
- Sometimes diagnosis of exclusion in absence of systemic sarcoidosis

Infectious Diseases

- Tuberculosis
- Leprosy
- Whipple disease
- Fungi
  - Histochemical stains for microorganisms &/or microbiological cultures should be performed to rule out infectious cause

Granulomatous Systemic Diseases

- Wegener granulomatosis
- Churg-Strauss syndrome
- Lymphomatoid granulomatosis
  - Detailed clinical and laboratory data are significant for differential diagnosis

Systemic Inflammatory Diseases

- Crohn disease
- Takayasu disease

Neoplasias

- Langerhans cell histiocytosis
- Germinoma with extensive inflammatory reaction
- Erdheim-Chester disease

SELECTED REFERENCES

1. Pekic S et al: Diagnosis of endocrine disease: expanding the cause of hypopituitarism. Eur J Endocrinol. 176(6):R269-R282, 2017
2. Al-Qudah ZA et al: Cranial nerve-VI palsy as the main clinical manifestation of neurosarcoidosis. Neurologist. 21(6):109-111, 2016
3. Anthony J et al: Hypothalamic-pituitary sarcoidosis with vision loss and hypopituitarism: case series and literature review. Pituitary. 19(1):19-29, 2016
4. Bongetta D et al: Systemic sarcoidosis unmasked by Cushing's disease surgical treatment. Case Rep Med. 2016:6405840, 2016
5. Diernaes JE et al: Unmasking sarcoidosis following surgery for Cushing disease. Dermatoendocrinol. 8(1):e983688, 2016
6. Prayson RA: Biopsy proven pituitary sarcoidosis presenting as a possible adenoma. J Clin Neurosci. 34:217-218, 2016
7. Badhey AK et al: Sarcoidosis of the head and neck. Head Neck Pathol. 9(2):260-8, 2015
8. Barberot-de Laubrière C et al: Hypophyseal neurosarcoidosis. Rev Prat. 62(8):1054, 2012
9. Langrand C et al: Hypothalamo-pituitary sarcoidosis: a multicenter study of 24 patients. QJM. 105(10):981-95, 2012
10. Marko NF et al: Sellar mass with vision loss and hypopituitarism. J Clin Neurosci. 19(9):1282; answer 1331, 2012
11. Kimball MM et al: Neurosarcoidosis presenting as an isolated intrasellar mass: case report and review of the literature. Clin Neuropathol. 29(3):156-62, 2010
12. Carpinteri R et al: Pituitary tumours: inflammatory and granulomatous expansive lesions of the pituitary. Best Pract Res Clin Endocrinol Metab. 23(5):639-50, 2009
13. Bihan H et al: Sarcoidosis: clinical, hormonal, and magnetic resonance imaging (MRI) manifestations of hypothalamic-pituitary disease in 9 patients and review of the literature. Medicine (Baltimore). 86(5):259-68, 2007
14. Hoitsma E et al: Neurosarcoidosis: a clinical dilemma. Lancet Neurol. 3(7):397-407, 2004

Pituitary and Infundibulum Sarcoidosis

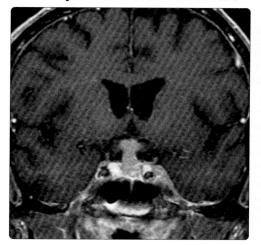

Pituitary Stalk Involvement

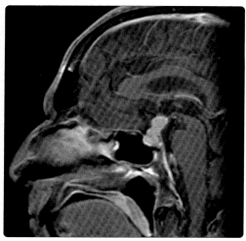

(Left) *Postcontrast T1WI MR shows a mass involving the infundibulum and anterior pituitary gland.* **(Right)** *Sagittal postcontrast T1WI MR shows an infiltrating lesion that enlarges the pituitary stalk and extends into the sellar region.*

Epithelioid and Giant Cells

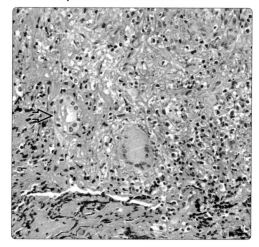

Giant Cell Granuloma

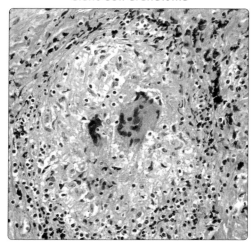

(Left) *Photomicrography shows residual acini of pituitary cells ⊟ seen intermixed with clustered epithelioid histiocytes and giant cells in a case of pituitary sarcoidosis.* **(Right)** *Biopsy of a pituitary gland shows the characteristic noncaseating granuloma with epithelioid histiocytes and multinucleated giant cells diffusely infiltrating the gland.*

Reticulin-Free Granulomas

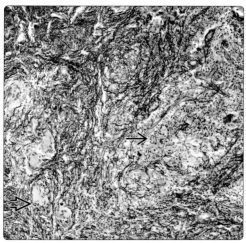

GH Immunohistochemistry

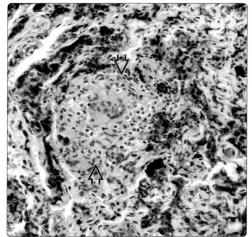

(Left) *Reticulin stain highlights the extensive fibrosis in a pituitary gland involved by sarcoidosis. Note the reticulin-free areas surrounding granulomas ⊟ and giant cells ⊟.* **(Right)** *Immunohistochemical stain for GH highlights GH-producing cells of the pituitary with negative staining in the sarcoid noncaseating granuloma ⊟ infiltrating the pituitary gland.*

KEY FACTS

TERMINOLOGY

- Pituitary apoplexy is defined by spontaneous infarction &/or hemorrhage of preexisting pituitary adenoma

CLINICAL ISSUES

- Apoplexy may have subclinical presentation with evidence of previous hemorrhage &/or necrosis
- Majority of cases present as acute event due to sudden increase in sellar contents with signs and symptoms of compression of sellar and surrounding structures
- Precipitating factors have been identified in almost 40% of cases of pituitary apoplexy
- Acute and emergent presentation with signs/symptoms of sellar and parasellar compression
- Apoplexy may also have subclinical presentation
- Treatment
  - Often, apoplexy constitutes medical and neurosurgical emergency
  - Supportive and clinical measures for stabilization of patients

MICROSCOPIC

- Combination of infarction and hemorrhage
- Extensive tumoral necrosis with ghost-like cells
- Breakdown of reticulin network helps to differentiate normal vs. tumoral pituitary
- Mostly nonfunctioning macroadenomas
  - Silent corticotroph adenomas are particularly prone to apoplexy
- Immunohistochemistry for pituitary hormones are important in distinguishing adenoma subtypes with aggressive behavior, such as silent corticotroph adenomas

TOP DIFFERENTIAL DIAGNOSES

- Subarachnoid hemorrhage
- Stroke
- Bacterial meningitis

Pituitary Adenoma Apoplexy Graphic

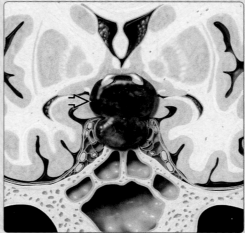

Pituitary Adenoma Apoplexy Histology

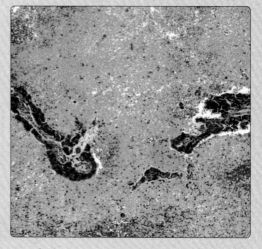

(Left) Coronal graphic shows a pituitary macroadenoma with suprasellar extension showing extensive acute hemorrhage ⊡ causing pituitary apoplexy. (Right) Apoplectic adenoma shows extensive areas of necrosis and focal hemorrhage. Remaining tumor cells are present surrounding blood vessels.

Apoplexy of Silent Corticotroph Adenoma

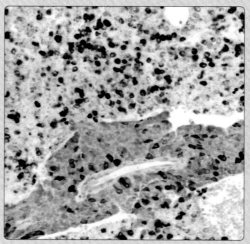

Pituitary Adenoma Apoplexy Organization

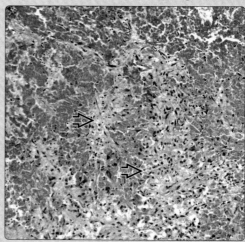

(Left) Silent corticotroph adenomas may commonly present with apoplexy. In this case, the patient did not present any clinical symptoms or laboratory data consistent with active Cushing disease. However, immunohistochemistry shows strong reactivity of viable and necrotic cells for adrenocorticotropic hormone. (Right) Focal organization of the necrotic adenoma shows incipient granulation tissue formation ⊡.

TERMINOLOGY

Synonyms

- Pituitary adenoma infarction
- Pituitary adenoma hemorrhage
- Pituitary apoplexy

Definitions

- Pituitary apoplexy is defined by spontaneous infarction &/or hemorrhage of preexisting pituitary adenoma

ETIOLOGY/PATHOGENESIS

Pituitary Adenoma

- Ischemia of adenoma results from outgrowing its blood supply

Compressive Features

- Compression (kinking) of superior hypophyseal artery against diaphragma sella

Vascular Disease

- Vasculopathy or abnormal blood vessels with tendency to hemorrhage

CLINICAL ISSUES

Presentation

- Majority of cases present as acute event due to sudden increase in sellar contents with signs and symptoms of compression of sellar and surrounding structures
  - Sudden and severe headaches
  - Hypopituitarism
  - Visual disturbances, cranial nerve palsies
  - Altered consciousness or coma
- Apoplexy may also have subclinical presentation with evidence of previous hemorrhage &/or necrosis seen by either neuroimaging or pathologic examination
- Age at presentation: 5th and 6th decades; slight male predominance (M:F = 1.6:1.0)
- Precipitating factors have been identified in almost 40% of cases of pituitary apoplexy
  - Systemic hypertension
  - Dynamic pituitary function test
  - Anticoagulant therapy; hormonal therapy (estrogens); initiation or withdrawal of dopaminergic agonist therapy
  - Head trauma
  - Pregnancy
  - Major surgery, particularly cardiovascular surgery

Treatment

- Often apoplexy constitutes medical and neurosurgical emergency
  - Acute endocrine deficits (including adrenal failure), present in ~ 70% of cases, should be corrected immediately
- Supportive and clinical measures for stabilization of patients
- Surgery has been advocated for improvement of visual field defects after clinical stabilization

IMAGING

General Features

- MR is radiologic test of choice and confirms diagnosis of pituitary apoplexy in great majority of patients
  - Both MR and MR angiogram are essential for distinguishing aneurysm from pituitary apoplexy

MR Findings

- Hemorrhagic tumors are hyperintense on T1- and hypointense on T2-weighted images in acute phases; blood products may be present in more chronic cases
- Infarcted tumors have low signal intensity on T1- and T2-weighted images with no contrast enhancement of tumor; rim enhancement may be present

MACROSCOPIC

General Features

- Surgical specimens are generally hemorrhagic and soft on inspection

MICROSCOPIC

Histologic Features

- Variable degree of acute hemorrhage ± evidence of previous hemorrhage (hemosiderin-laden macrophages)
- Extensive tumoral necrosis with ghost-like cells
  - Organization of hemorrhage may be present with infiltration of delicate fibroblastic network
  - Breakdown of reticulin network helps to differentiate normal vs. tumoral pituitary
  - Focal remaining viable adenoma cells may be present, particularly around blood vessels
- Majority of cases are nonfunctioning adenomas
  - Silent corticotroph adenomas are particularly prone to apoplexy
  - IHC for pituitary hormones are important in distinguishing adenoma subtypes with aggressive behavior, such as silent corticotroph adenomas

DIFFERENTIAL DIAGNOSIS

Critical Neurological Disorders

- Subarachnoid hemorrhage; stroke
- Bacterial meningitis

DIAGNOSTIC CHECKLIST

Pathologic Interpretation Pearls

- Variable degree of acute hemorrhage ± evidence of previous hemorrhage
- Extensive pituitary adenoma tumoral necrosis with ghost-like cells

SELECTED REFERENCES

1. Rajasekaran S et al: UK guidelines for the management of pituitary apoplexy. Clin Endocrinol (Oxf). 74(1):9-20, 2011
2. Semple PL et al: Pituitary apoplexy: correlation between magnetic resonance imaging and histopathological results. J Neurosurg. 108(5):909-15, 2008
3. Semple PL et al: Clinical relevance of precipitating factors in pituitary apoplexy. Neurosurgery. 61(5):956-61; discussion 961-2, 2007
4. Randeva HS et al: Classical pituitary apoplexy: clinical features, management and outcome. Clin Endocrinol (Oxf). 51(2):181-8, 1999

TERMINOLOGY

- Necrosis of pituitary associated with massive postpartum hemorrhage

ETIOLOGY/PATHOGENESIS

- Decreased blood flow to anterior pituitary gland in postpartum period
  - Usually caused by pituitary necrosis associated with massive hemorrhage during delivery
  - ~ 10% of Sheehan syndrome cases do not have documented or obvious postpartum bleeding
- Decreased blood flow to anterior pituitary due to nonobstetric causes
  - Trauma
  - Subarachnoid hemorrhage
  - Postsurgical procedures, in particular cardiovascular surgery
  - Anticoagulant therapy

- Pituitary apoplexy terminology is reserved for infarction of pituitary gland harboring pituitary adenoma, most often clinically nonfunctioning macroadenoma

CLINICAL ISSUES

- Partial or complete hypopituitarism

MICROSCOPIC

- In acute phase: Extensive necrosis of gland with ghost cell appearance of pituitary cells, hemorrhage, and minimal inflammatory response
- In subacute and chronic phases: Replacement of gland by various degrees of fibrosis

TOP DIFFERENTIAL DIAGNOSES

- Lymphocytic hypophysitis
- Pituitary apoplexy

Autopsy Specimen of Pituitary With Acute Infarction

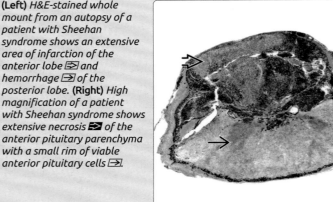

Anterior Pituitary Necrosis: Autopsy Specimen

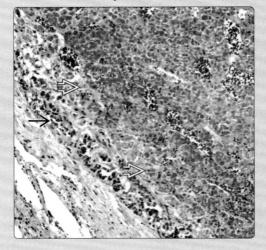

(Left) H&E-stained whole mount from an autopsy of a patient with Sheehan syndrome shows an extensive area of infarction of the anterior lobe ⊟ and hemorrhage ⊟ of the posterior lobe. (Right) High magnification of a patient with Sheehan syndrome shows extensive necrosis ⊟ of the anterior pituitary parenchyma with a small rim of viable anterior pituitary cells ⊟.

Anterior Pituitary Necrosis and "Ghost" Cells

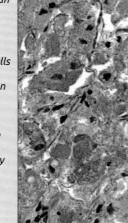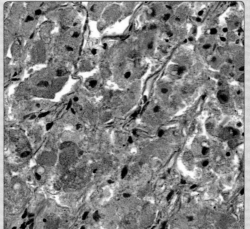

Anterior Pituitary Necrosis: GH Immunohistochemistry

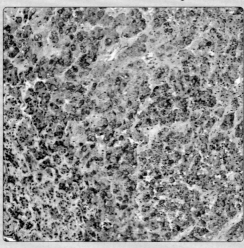

(Left) High magnification of an anterior pituitary gland in a patient with Sheehan syndrome emphasizing coagulative necrosis of the pituitary with "ghost"-like cells is shown. (Right) Extensive anterior pituitary necrosis can be appreciated in this GH immunostain. There is a lack of nuclei in the areas of necrosis, as seen in the acute phase of the process. This phase is also characterized by a ghost cell appearance of pituitary cells, hemorrhage, and minimal inflammatory response.

TERMINOLOGY

Synonyms

- Postpartum pituitary necrosis
- Postpartum pituitary infarction

Definitions

- Necrosis of pituitary associated with massive postpartum hemorrhage
  - First described in these terms by HL Sheehan in 1937

ETIOLOGY/PATHOGENESIS

Decrease of Blood Flow

- To anterior pituitary gland in postpartum period
  - Mechanisms of infarction still not completely understood
    - May be due to vasospasm or thrombosis caused by vascular compression
  - Conditions that increase risk of bleeding during childbirth and Sheehan syndrome include multiple pregnancies (twins or triplets) and placental problems
  - Compression of superior hypophyseal artery causing various degrees of ischemia
    - Pituitary lactotroph hyperplasia in late stages of pregnancy may result in compression of arterial supply
  - Sudden changes of arterial blood pressure during delivery
    - Mostly secondary to severe hypotension, shock, disseminated intravascular coagulopathy
    - Vasospasm due to fluctuation of blood pressure
  - ~ 10% of Sheehan syndrome cases do not have documented or obvious postpartum bleeding
- To anterior pituitary due to nonobstetric causes
  - Trauma
  - Subarachnoid hemorrhage
  - Postsurgical procedures, in particular cardiovascular surgery
  - Anticoagulant therapy

Pituitary Apoplexy

- Pituitary apoplexy terminology is reserved for infarction of pituitary gland harboring pituitary adenoma, most often clinically nonfunctioning macroadenoma

CLINICAL ISSUES

Presentation

- Partial or complete hypopituitarism
  - Hormonal deficiency may vary from single hormone to panhypopituitarism
    - Hypogonadism: 100% of cases
    - Prolactin and growth hormone deficiency: 100% of cases
    - Secondary hypothyroidism: 90% of cases
    - Hypocortisolism: 50% of cases
  - Latency between hemorrhage and symptom presentation varies from 2 months to 40 years (mean: 26.82 years)
- Most common clinical symptoms
  - Inadequate or failure of postpartum lactation
  - Amenorrhea or oligomenorrhea
  - Axillary and pubic hair loss
  - Adrenal insufficiency
  - Weakness and cold intolerance
  - Secondary infertility
  - Psychiatric disturbances
  - Fatigue
  - Low blood pressure

Treatment

- Hormone replacement therapy

Prognosis

- Frequency and severity in modern obstetrics is low
- Early diagnosis prevents severe complications, such as adrenal insufficiency and hypothyroidism crises; rare cases of spontaneous recovery have been reported

MACROSCOPIC

General Features

- Adenohypophysis may appear soft with grayish-red discoloration

MICROSCOPIC

Histologic Features

- Rarely is surgical pathology specimen
- In acute phase: Extensive necrosis of gland with ghost cell appearance of pituitary cells, hemorrhage, and minimal inflammatory response
- In subacute and chronic phases: Replacement of gland by various degrees of fibrosis

DIFFERENTIAL DIAGNOSIS

Lymphocytic Hypophysitis

- At initial and chronic phases due to similar clinical signs and symptoms of hypopituitarism
  - Lymphocytic hypophysitis lacks history of postpartum bleeding disorder

Pituitary Apoplexy

- May be 1st manifestation of previously undiagnosed pituitary macroadenoma
- Clinical manifestations are generally more acute and severe
  - Headaches, vomiting, visual changes, severe adrenal crisis

DIAGNOSTIC CHECKLIST

Pathologic Interpretation Pearls

- Variable extent of infarction, mostly accompanied by some degree of acute hemorrhage

SELECTED REFERENCES

1. Harbeck B et al: Life-threatening endocrine emergencies during pregnancy - management and therapeutic features. Gynecol Endocrinol. 1-5, 2017
2. Karaca Z et al: Sheehan syndrome. Nat Rev Dis Primers. 2:16092, 2016
3. Dökmetaş HS et al: Characteristic features of 20 patients with Sheehan's syndrome. Gynecol Endocrinol. 22(5):279-83, 2006
4. Feinberg EC et al: The incidence of Sheehan's syndrome after obstetric hemorrhage. Fertil Steril. 84(4):975-9, 2005
5. Kovacs K: Sheehan syndrome. Lancet. 361(9356):520-2, 2003
6. Sheehan HL: Post-partum necrosis of the anterior pituitary. J Path Bact. 45:189, 1937

TERMINOLOGY

- Rathke cleft cysts (RCCs) are benign cystic lesions of sella that occur due to accumulation of secretory material in Rathke cleft
- Epidermoid (EC) and dermoid cysts (DC) are benign cystic lesions that may develop in several areas of brain, including cerebellopontine angle, prepontine cisterns, and sellar region

CLINICAL ISSUES

- Clinical symptoms of these cystic lesions are mostly secondary due to compression of adjacent structures
  - Includes headaches, visual disturbances, hypopituitarism, and (only rarely) diabetes insipidus
- RCCs, ECs, and DCs account for ~ 1% of sellar lesions
- Surgical treatment is recommended for all symptomatic cystic lesions

IMAGING

- RCCs are well-defined cystic lesions with heterogeneous radiographic appearance depending upon cyst contents
- EC and DC show restricted diffusion on diffusion-weighted imaging may differentiate from other cystic lesions

MICROSCOPIC

- RCCs are lined by cuboidal ciliated cells with varied numbers of columnar and goblet cells
  - Squamous metaplasia and xanthogranulomatous reaction may be present in ~ 40% of RCCs
- ECs are lined by stratified squamous epithelium with "flaky" keratin formation, while DCs also contain adnexal structures such as hair follicles and glandular elements

TOP DIFFERENTIAL DIAGNOSES

- Papillary craniopharyngioma
  - In particular in RCC with squamous metaplasia and xanthomatous reaction

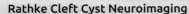

Rathke Cleft Cyst Neuroimaging

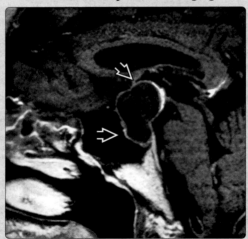

Rathke Cleft Cyst Graphic

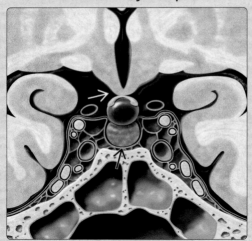

(Left) Sagittal T1-weighted MR of a patient with vision loss shows a Rathke cleft cyst (RCC) ➡ extending from the sella to the suprasellar area. (Right) Coronal graphic shows a typical suprasellar RCC interposed between the pituitary gland ➡ and the optic chiasm ➡.

Normal Rathke Cleft Epithelium

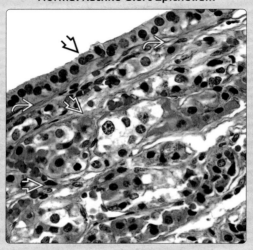

Rathke Cleft Epithelium With Goblet Cells

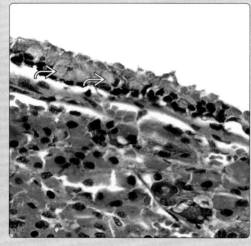

(Left) The Rathke cleft epithelium in a normal pituitary gland ➡ is composed of cuboidal to columnar cells with ciliated borders ➡. A delicate fibrous membrane or basal lamina ➡ is present between the epithelium and the gland. (Right) Goblet cells ➡ may also be present in the epithelium of the Rathke cleft. These cells may be present alone or intermixed with cuboidal to columnar cells. Goblet cells are commonly present in RCC lining.

TERMINOLOGY

Synonyms

- Pituitary cyst, colloid cyst of pituitary, intrasellar epithelial cyst

Definitions

- Rathke cleft cysts (RCCs) are benign cystic lesions of sella that occur due to accumulation of secretory material in Rathke cleft
- Epidermoid and dermoid cysts are benign cystic lesions that may develop in several areas of brain such as cerebellopontine angle, prepontine cisterns, and sellar region

ETIOLOGY/PATHOGENESIS

Developmental Anomaly

- RCCs are believed to develop from persistence and enlargement of Rathke cleft
- Epidermoid cysts (ECs) and dermoid cysts (DCs) are believed to develop from residual epithelial nests misplaced during closure of neural groove

CLINICAL ISSUES

Presentation

- RCCs account for < 1% of all primary intracranial masses; majority are incidental postmortem findings
  - Most symptomatic RCCs are ≥ 1 cm in size and represent ~ 5-9% of surgical lesions of sella
  - Clinical symptoms are due to compression of adjacent structures: Headaches, visual disturbances, hypopituitarism, and (only rarely) diabetes insipidus
  - Female predominance (2:1)
  - Mean age at presentation: 4th decade
- EC and DC are rare intracranial lesions; EC is more common than DC
  - Sellar and parasellar EC account for only 0.2-0.7% of sellar lesions
  - No gender predominance
  - Middle-aged patients
  - Clinical symptoms of mass effect similar to RCCs
    - Symptoms due to secondary hypophysitis and meningitis may occur in cases associated with cyst rupture

Treatment

- Surgical treatment is recommended for all symptomatic cystic lesions

Prognosis

- Recurrence of symptomatic RCC may occur in particular in cases with inflammatory reaction
- ECs may recur due to adherence of cyst walls to surrounding sellar structures

IMAGING

MR Findings

- RCCs are well-defined cystic lesions with heterogeneous radiographic appearance depending upon cyst contents

- EC and DC show restricted diffusion on diffusion-weighted imaging may differentiate from other cystic lesions

MACROSCOPIC

General Features

- RCCs are well-circumscribed lesions with smooth contours
  - Cyst contents are predominantly mucinous or gelatinous with yellow to pink hue
    - Greenish, viscous appearance (motor oil-like) in cases of previous hemorrhage or rupture
    - Purulent-like appearance in cases of rupture with secondary inflammation
- ECs are often adhesive lesions with encasing of surrounding nervous and vascular structures
  - Cyst contents have whitish mother-of-pearl appearance

MICROSCOPIC

Histologic Features

- RCCs are lined by cuboidal ciliated cells with varied numbers of columnar and goblet cells; occasional adenohypophyseal cells are also present
  - Squamous metaplasia may be present in ~ 40% of cases
  - Xanthogranulomatous changes may be present in 35-40% of cases
- ECs are lined by stratified squamous epithelium with "flaky" keratin formation, while DCs also contain adnexal structures such as hair follicles and glandular elements

DIFFERENTIAL DIAGNOSIS

Papillary Craniopharyngioma

- Particularly in RCC with squamous metaplasia and xanthomatous reaction
- Unlike EC and DC, papillary craniopharyngioma does not have formation of keratin

DIAGNOSTIC CHECKLIST

Clinically Relevant Pathologic Features

- RCC shows cuboidal epithelium with goblet cells
- EC and DC show stratified squamous epithelium with formation of "flaky" keratin

Pathologic Interpretation Pearls

- Inflammatory reaction with squamous metaplasia and xanthomatous changes may conceal diagnosis of craniopharyngioma

SELECTED REFERENCES

1. Uygur ER et al: Imaging of the sella and parasellar region. In Laws et al: Transsphenoidal Surgery. Philadelphia: Saunders Elsevier. 43-55, 2010
2. Park M et al: Differentiation between cystic pituitary adenomas and Rathke cleft cysts: a diagnostic model using MRI. AJNR Am J Neuroradiol. 36(10):1866-73, 2015
3. Zada G et al: Craniopharyngioma and other cystic epithelial lesions of the sellar region: a review of clinical, imaging, and histopathological relationships. Neurosurg Focus. 28(4):E4, 2010
4. Zada G et al: Surgical treatment of rathke cleft cysts in children. Neurosurgery. 64(6):1132-7; author reply 1037-8, 2009
5. Aho CJ et al: Surgical outcomes in 118 patients with Rathke cleft cysts. J Neurosurg. 102(2):189-93, 2005

Pituitary Gland

(Left) *Axial gross pathology shows a mucin-containing RCC ⇾ found incidentally at autopsy. (Courtesy E. Hedley-Whyte, MD.)* **(Right)** *RCCs are composed of cuboidal &/or columnar cells with a cilia border ⇾. The epithelial lining rests in a fibrous stroma that varies according to the pressure of the cyst and reactive changes. Proteinaceous materials compose the cyst contents ⇾.*

Rathke Cleft Cyst: Autopsy Specimen

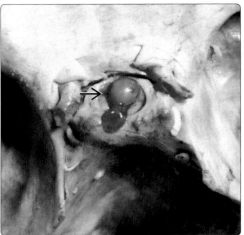

Rathke Cleft Cyst

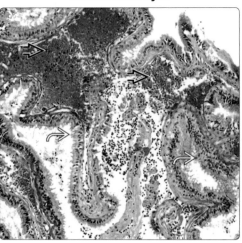

(Left) *Section of an RCC highlights the cystic contents, which are represented by proteinaceous colloid-like materials ⇾. In RCCs with squamous metaplasia, oil machinery-like contents, similar to craniopharyngiomas, may be present.* **(Right)** *An RCC shows incipient squamous metaplasia with pseudostratification of the epithelium. Note the presence of goblet cells ⇾ and ciliated cells ⇾ at the top of the cyst lining. Dense fibrosis ⇾ is present in the base of the cystic epithelial lining.*

Rathke Cleft Cyst Contents

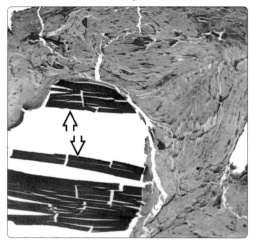

Squamous Metaplasia in Rathke Cleft Cyst

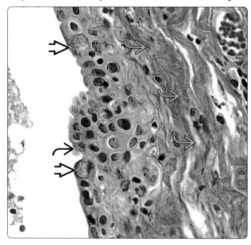

(Left) *A surgical specimen of an RCC with focal squamous metaplasia ⇾ and lymphoplasmacytic inflammation involving the adjacent anterior pituitary gland is shown. Secondary hypophysitis is a common complication of RCCs that have subclinical rupture.* **(Right)** *T1-weighted image MR of an epidermoid cyst is characterized by a large heterogeneous sellar and suprasellar mass with displacement of the optic chiasm.*

Rathke Cleft Cyst Histology

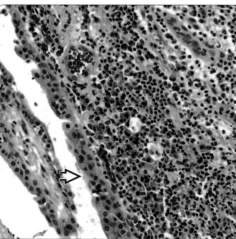

Neuroimaging of Epidermoid Cyst

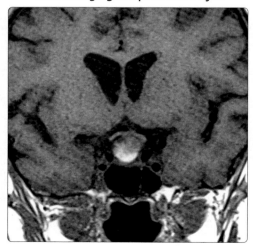

Epidermoid Cyst Histology

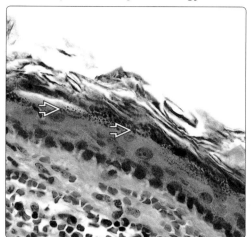

Keratin Formation in Epidermoid Cyst

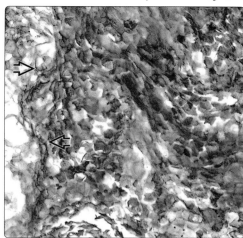

(Left) *High magnification of the epithelium lining of an epidermoid cyst displays stratified squamous epithelium with keratohyaline granular layer ➡ and dry ("flaky") keratin formation. The presence of true keratinization and "flaky" keratin differentiates epidermoid cysts from papillary craniopharyngiomas.* **(Right)** *Representative section of an epidermoid cyst contents composed solely of dry ("flaky") acellular keratin. Note the presence of eosinophilic and focally basophilic ➡ flakes.*

Epidermoid Cyst and Surrounding Stroma

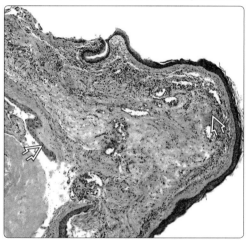

GFAP in Epidermoid Cyst With Invasion

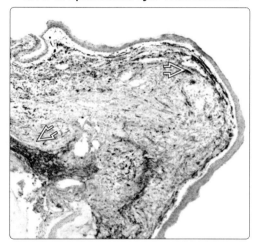

(Left) *Low-magnification view of an epidermoid cyst shows the stratified epithelium lining resting upon fibrous tissue and invading the brain ➡. Inflammation and reactive fibrosis are common features of the stroma.* **(Right)** *Invasion of the sellar region surrounding brain may be a severe complication of epidermoid cysts. GFAP immunohistochemistry demonstrates adhesion of the epidermoid cyst to the brain structures ➡.*

Xanthogranulomatous Inflammation in Epidermoid Cyst

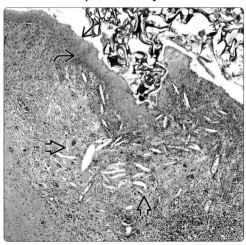

Papillary Craniopharyngioma

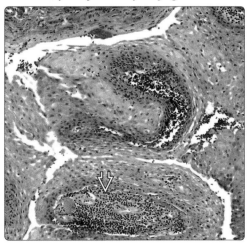

(Left) *Intense xanthogranulomatous reaction ➡ is present in this case of epidermoid cyst. Note the epithelium lining ➡ at the top of the photomicrograph.* **(Right)** *For comparison with epidermoid cyst, a section of a papillary craniopharyngioma shows papillary formations composed of pseudostratified epithelium, and a moderate degree of lymphocytic infiltrates in the fibrous vascular cores ➡.*

Empty Sella Syndrome

TERMINOLOGY

- Empty sella (ES) is characterized by herniation of subarachnoid space into sella turcica giving appearance of ES
- Incidence of ES reported in 5-23% of sella turcica examined by autopsy
- ES syndrome (ESS) may be primary or secondary

ETIOLOGY/PATHOGENESIS

- Primary ES is believed to be due to deficient diaphragma sella
- Secondary ES is attributed to partial destruction of pituitary gland within sella cavity

CLINICAL ISSUES

- In adults, ESS is more frequent in multiparous females and associated with systemic hypertension and obesity
  - F:M = 4:1
- Majority of cases are incidental findings

- Most common symptoms in adults include headaches, seizures, visual disturbances, and CSF rhinorrhea
- In children, ESS most often presents with endocrine symptoms
  - Growth hormone deficiency, hypogonadotrophic hypogonadism, delayed puberty
- Treatment is mostly centered in hormonal replacement

IMAGING

- Low-attenuation CSF-filled space compressing pituitary gland against floor and walls of sella ± enlargement

MICROSCOPIC

- Pituitary gland is flat and remodeled with no significant cellular abnormalities
- Mild degree of interstitial fibrosis may be present
- In secondary ES, specific pathology may be seen, including necrotic pituitary adenoma, chronic or remote evidence of infarction, variable degree of fibrosis

Empty Sella Graphic

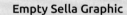

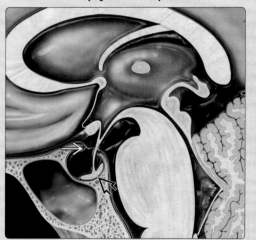

Empty Sella Autopsy Specimen

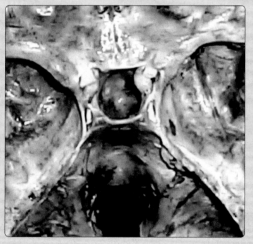

(Left) *Sagittal graphic shows an empty sella. The extension of arachnoid with cerebrospinal fluid through the diaphragma sellae ➡ flattens and displaces the pituitary gland ⇨ posteroinferiorly against the sellar floor.* (Right) *Superior view of the skull base shows an enlarged and empty sella turcica in a 78-year-old obese female patient who died of ischemic cardiomyopathy.*

Empty Sella Histology From Autopsy Specimen

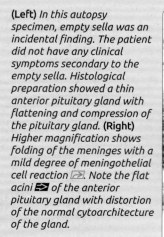

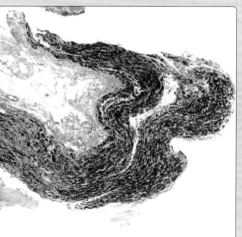

Empty Sella Histology

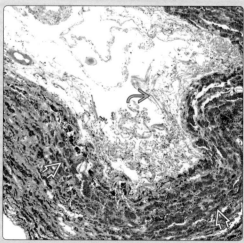

(Left) *In this autopsy specimen, empty sella was an incidental finding. The patient did not have any clinical symptoms secondary to the empty sella. Histological preparation showed a thin anterior pituitary gland with flattening and compression of the pituitary gland.* (Right) *Higher magnification shows folding of the meninges with a mild degree of meningothelial cell reaction ➡. Note the flat acini ⇨ of the anterior pituitary gland with distortion of the normal cytoarchitecture of the gland.*

TERMINOLOGY

Abbreviations

- Empty sella syndrome (ESS)

Definitions

- Empty sella is characterized by herniation of subarachnoid space into sella turcica giving appearance of ES
  - Cerebrospinal fluid (CSF) pressure inside sella turcica may build up leading to compression of pituitary gland
  - Associated remodeling of bony sella, stretching of stalk, and flattening of pituitary gland
- Combination of ES and pituitary dysfunction is termed ESS
- Incidence of ES reported in 5-23% of sella turcica examined by autopsy
- ESS may be primary or secondary

ETIOLOGY/PATHOGENESIS

Developmental Anomaly

- Primary ES is believed to be due to deficient diaphragma sella
  - Dynamic forces of pulsating CSF may cause remodeling of bony sella turcica and compression into pituitary gland

Environmental Exposure

- Secondary ES is attributed to partial destruction of pituitary gland within sella cavity
  - Common causes
    - Pituitary adenoma undergoing necrosis or hemorrhage
    - Pituitary atrophy due to hypophysitis
    - Traumatic damage
    - Surgery
    - Radiation therapy

CLINICAL ISSUES

Presentation

- In adults, more frequent in females (F:M = 4:1)
  - Associated with multiple pregnancies
  - Associated with systemic hypertension and obesity
- Most common symptoms in adults
  - Headaches, cranial nerve disorders, seizures, CSF rhinorrhea, and rarely dizziness
  - Visual field deficits, diplopia, blurred vision, optical neuritis, and mild papilledema
  - Hyperprolactinemia due to pituitary stalk effect is most common endocrine symptom
    - Partial or panhypopituitarism may also be present
- In children, no gender predilection
  - Symptoms are mostly endocrinologic: GH deficiency, hypogonadotrophic hypogonadism, delayed puberty
  - No association with obesity
  - May be associated to hypothalamic and pituitary developmental defects
  - May be associated with pituitary and hypothalamic tumors

Treatment

- Adjuvant therapy
  - Hormonal replacement
  - Dopamine agonist treatment in cases of hyperprolactinemia

Prognosis

- Most cases are incidental findings
  - Most symptomatic patients are children

IMAGING

Radiographic Findings

- Low-attenuation CSF-filled space compressing pituitary gland against floor and walls of sella
- Variable enlargement of sellar bony structure

MACROSCOPIC

General Features

- Various degrees of sellar turcica enlargement
- Thinning and opening of diaphragma sella
- Flattening of pituitary gland

MICROSCOPIC

Histologic Features

- Pituitary gland is flat and remodeled with no significant cellular abnormalities
- Mild degree of interstitial fibrosis may be present
- Invagination of meninges with various degrees of meningothelial cells reaction
- In secondary ES, specific pathology may be seen, including necrotic pituitary adenoma, chronic or remote evidence of infarction, variable degree of fibrosis

SELECTED REFERENCES

1. Melmed S et al: Disorders of the anterior pituitary and hypothalamus. In Longo DL et al: Harrison's Principles of Internal Medicine. 18th ed. New York: McGraw-Hill, 2011
2. Chiloiro S et al: Diagnosis of endocrine disease: primary empty sella: a comprehensive review. Eur J Endocrinol. ePub, 2017
3. Aijazi I et al: Primary empty sella syndrome presenting with severe hyponatremia and minimal salt wasting. J Ayub Med Coll Abbottabad. 28(3):605-608, 2016
4. Rahman SH et al: Delayed diagnosis of Cushing's disease in a pediatric patient due to apparent remission from spontaneous apoplexy. J Clin Transl Endocrinol Case Rep. 2:30-34, 2016
5. Dutta D et al: Multiple pituitary hormone deficiency, empty sella and ectopic neurohypophysis in Turner syndrome. Indian Pediatr. 52(9):803-4, 2015
6. Loh WJ et al: Symptomatic empty sella syndrome: an unusual manifestation of Erdheim-Chester disease. Endocrinol Diabetes Metab Case Rep. 2015:140122, 2015
7. Lubrano C et al: Severe growth hormone deficiency and empty sella in obesity: a cross-sectional study. Endocrine. 49(2):503-11, 2015
8. Paroder V et al: Absent sella turcica: a case report and a review of the literature. Fetal Pediatr Pathol. 32(5):375-83, 2013
9. Lenz AM et al: Empty sella syndrome. Pediatr Endocrinol Rev. 9(4):710-5, 2012
10. Giustina A et al: Primary empty sella: Why and when to investigate hypothalamic-pituitary function. J Endocrinol Invest. 33(5):343-6, 2010
11. Gallardo E et al: The empty sella: results of treatment in 76 successive cases and high frequency of endocrine and neurological disturbances. Clin Endocrinol (Oxf). 37(6):529-33, 1992
12. Buchfelder M et al: Results of dynamic endocrine testing of hypothalamic pituitary function in patients with a primary "empty" sella syndrome. Horm Metab Res. 21(10):573-6, 1989
13. Jaffer KA et al: "Empty" sella: review of 76 cases. South Med J. 72(3):294-6, 1979
14. Kaufman B et al: The ubiquitous "empty" sella turcica. Acta Radiol Diagn (Stockh). 13(1):413-25, 1972
15. Busch W: [Morphology of sella turcica and its relation to the pituitary gland.] Virchows Arch. 320(5):437-58, 1951

Pituitary Adenoma

TERMINOLOGY

- Pituitary adenoma (PA) is neoplastic proliferation of anterior pituitary hormone-producing cells (WHO 2017)
- Tumors are typically benign, but can be aggressive and invasive into adjacent structures

ETIOLOGY/PATHOGENESIS

- Majority of PAs are sporadic; some are part of inherited tumor syndrome
- PAs may be associated with the following familial syndromes
  - Multiple endocrine neoplasia type 1 and type 4
  - McCune-Albright syndrome
  - Carney complex
  - SDH-related familial paraganglioma and pheochromocytoma syndromes

CLINICAL ISSUES

- Constitute 15% of all intracranial neoplasms

- Hypersecretion of pituitary hormones including ACTH, PRL, GH, and TSH leading to endocrine syndromes
- Mass effects including hypopituitarism especially in clinically nonfunctioning adenomas
- Surgery is main modality of treatment for most PAs

MICROSCOPIC

- Chromophobic, acidophilic, or basophilic cells
- Architecture can predict cell type

ANCILLARY TESTS

- Immunohistochemistry for pituitary hormones, pituitary transcription factors, LMWK, and MIB-1
- Total breakdown of normal acinar architecture on reticulin stain is diagnostic of PA

(Left) *Gross image shows a pituitary macroadenoma that extends upward into the suprasellar cistern and laterally into the cavernous sinus.* **(Right)** *Cytoplasmic granularity gives 3 morphologically distinct cell types: Chromophobic, eosinophilic, and basophilic. This image shows a chromophobic pituitary adenoma with clear cells arranged in a diffuse, sheet-like pattern.*

Autopsy Image of Pituitary Macroadenoma

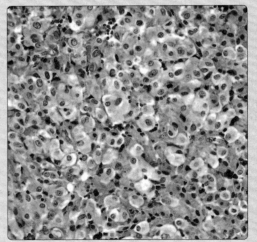

Pituitary Adenoma: Chromophobic Appearance

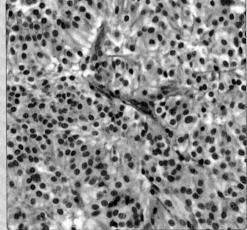

(Left) *This image is an example of an acidophilic pituitary adenoma composed of cells that exhibit bright cytoplasmic eosinophilia.* **(Right)** *Pituitary adenomas may display several histological arrangements. This adenoma shows papillary formations of chromophobic cells.*

Pituitary Adenoma: Acidophilic Appearance

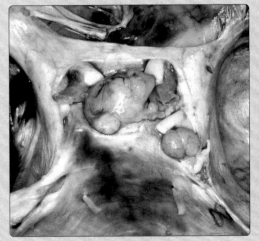

Pituitary Adenoma: Papillary Appearance

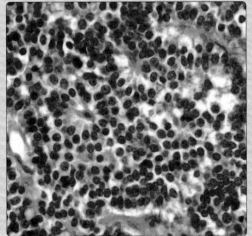

TERMINOLOGY

Abbreviations

- Pituitary adenoma (PA)

Definitions

- Pituitary adenoma is neoplastic proliferation of anterior pituitary hormone-producing cells (WHO 2017)
- Tumors are typically benign but can be aggressive and invasive into adjacent structures
- Usually arise in sella turcica but occasionally seen as ectopic lesion

ETIOLOGY/PATHOGENESIS

Etiology

- Genetic, epigenetic factors, hormonal stimulation, growth factors, and their receptors implicated in pituitary tumorigenesis

Pathogenesis

- Most adenomas are sporadic
- **Hormone regulatory pathways**
  - Hormonal stimulus or impaired feedback inhibition on hypothalamic-pituitary-target organ axes may underlie pathogenesis of PAs
    - Excess GHRH, CRH, TRH, or GnRH production
    - Target organ failure resulting in increased stimulation of hypothalamic-pituitary axes
- **Somatic genetics**
  - PAs are rarely affected by activating mutations of common oncogenes
  - Somatic mutations in *GNAS* gene have been identified in about 40% of sporadic somatotroph adenomas
  - Mutations in *USP8* (ubiquitin-specific protease 8) gene have been identified in about 36-62% of sporadic corticotroph adenomas
  - Epigenetically silenced tumor suppressors are found in sporadic PAs

Syndromic Diseases

- **Multiple endocrine neoplasia type 1**
  - Autosomal dominant disorder associated with germline mutation of *MEN1* tumor suppressor gene that encodes menin
  - Affected individuals usually develop growth hormone (GH) &/or prolactin (PRL)-secreting PAs
- **McCune-Albright syndrome**
  - Mosaic mutations of *GNAS* gene (Gαs protein; Gsp)
  - Affected patients develop somatotroph hyperplasia or somatotroph PAs
- **Carney complex**
  - Autosomal dominant disorder associated with germline mutations in *PRKAR1A* gene that encodes protein kinase-A regulatory subunit 1α
- **Multiple endocrine neoplasia type 4**
  - Autosomal dominant disorder associated with mutations of *CDKN1B* gene
  - Rare reported cases of somatotroph adenoma associated with hyperparathyroidism
- **SDH-related familial paraganglioma and pheochromocytoma syndromes**
  - Associated gene mutations include *SDHA*, *SDHB*, *SDHC*, *SDHD*, and *SDHAF2*

Isolated Pituitary Disease

- **Familial isolated pituitary adenoma (FIPA)**
  - Autosomal dominant disease with variable penetrance
    - 20% of patients affected by germline mutations in tumor suppressor aryl hydrocarbon receptor interacting protein (*AIP*)
    - No gene abnormality has been identified to date in majority of the FIPA families
  - *AIP* mutation-positive patients have characteristic clinical phenotype with usually young- or childhood-onset GH &/or PRL-secreting adenomas
- **Isolated familial somatotropinoma syndrome (IFS)**
  - About 50% of IFS kindreds exhibit mutations in *AIP* gene
- **X-linked acrogigantism syndrome**
  - Genetic defect is microduplication in chromosome Xq26.3 with upregulation of the *GPR101* gene
  - Majority of the patients < 5 years at diagnosis and present with hypersecretion of GH and PRL
  - Affected patients develop mixed somatotroph-lactotroph adenomas or pituitary hyperplasia

CLINICAL ISSUES

Epidemiology

- Incidence
  - Common, occurring in almost 20% of general population
  - Constitute 15% of all intracranial neoplasms
- Age
  - Majority of cases arise in the 5th to 7th decades
  - Uncommon in pediatric population
    - When present, may suggest familial syndrome
  - Incidence increases with age in autopsy studies

Presentation

- Clinically functioning adenomas with hypersecretion of pituitary hormones
  - Adrenocorticotrophic (ACTH) excess presents with Cushing disease or Nelson syndrome
  - GH excess causes acromegaly &/or gigantism
  - PRL excess presents with galactorrhea, amenorrhea, hypogonadism, and infertility
  - Thyrotropin (TSH) excess presents with hyperthyroidism and is sometimes associated with galactorrhea and hyperprolactinemia
  - Gonadotropin (FSH, LH) excess is extremely rare and may present with gonadal dysfunction
- Clinically nonfunctioning adenomas with mass effects symptoms
  - Symptoms include visual disturbances, headaches, hypopituitarism
- Hypopituitarism due to compression of nontumorous anterior pituitary parenchyma
- Mild hyperprolactinemia may be seeing due to compression of the pituitary stalk ("stalk effect")

Treatment

- Surgery is main modality of treatment for most PAs

- Pharmacotherapy is initial treatment for majority of prolactin-secreting adenomas and is used as adjuvant therapy when surgery cannot completely resect functioning adenoma
- Radiotherapy is used in treatment of patients with incompletely resected or recurrent aggressive neoplasms

Prognosis

- Best prognosticator is classification of PAs based on hormone content and cell structure
- Some PA subtypes are usually associated with invasive or aggressive behavior
  o Sparsely granulated somatotroph adenoma
  o Lactotroph adenoma in men
  o Acidophil stem cell adenoma
  o Crooke cell adenoma
  o Plurihormonal PIT-1-positive adenoma (previously called silent subtype 3 adenoma)

IMAGING

Radiographic Findings

- PAs are classified radiologically based on tumor size and degree of local invasion (Hardy classification)

MACROSCOPIC

General Features

- PAs are usually resected as multiple small pieces; majority of PAs exhibit soft tan gross appearance

MICROSCOPIC

Histologic Features

- Solid, diffuse, trabecular, sinusoidal, papillary growth patterns are common
- Adenoma reveals breakdown of normal acinar architecture on Gordon-Sweet silver stain
  o This distinguishes neoplasia from hyperplasia that retains acinar reticulin pattern
- Involvement of bone, posterior lobe, dura mater, or respiratory mucosa in invasive PAs
- Invasive PAs exhibiting increased mitotic activity &/or MIB-1/Ki-67 proliferative index > 3% should be considered high-risk tumor for recurrence and clinically aggressive behavior

ANCILLARY TESTS

Immunohistochemistry

- Most valuable tool in determination of cellular differentiation and classification of PAs
  o Hormones: GH, PRL, TSH-β, FSH-β, LH-β, ACTH, α-subunit
  o Transcription factors: PIT-1, SF1, and Tpit; other differentiating factors: ER-α, GATA2
- General neuroendocrine markers [chromogranin-A, synaptophysin, and neuron-specific enolase (NSE)]
- Other markers: LMWK (CAM5.2), MIB-1

DIFFERENTIAL DIAGNOSIS

Pituitary Hyperplasia

- Adenoma reveals total breakdown of normal acinar architecture on silver stain

Spindle Cell Oncocytoma/Pituicytoma

- Positive for TTF-1, vimentin, S100, EMA, and galactin-3; focally for GFAP
- Negative for chromogranin-A, synaptophysin, and keratin

Metastatic Neuroendocrine Carcinoma

- Negativity for pituitary hormones and transcription factors and positivity for other transcription factors (CDX-2, TTF-1, etc.) favors metastatic neuroendocrine carcinoma

SELECTED REFERENCES

1. Asa SL et al: From pituitary adenoma to pituitary neuroendocrine tumor (PitNET): an International Pituitary Pathology Club proposal. Endocr Relat Cancer. 24(4):C5-C8, 2017
2. Chandler CM et al: Cytomorphology of metastatic pituitary carcinoma to the bone. Diagn Cytopathol. 45(7):645-650, 2017
3. Glebauskiene B et al: Association of FGFR2 rs2981582, SIRT1 rs12778366, STAT3 rs744166 gene polymorphisms with pituitary adenoma. Oncol Lett. 13(5):3087-3099, 2017
4. Kiefer FW et al: PRKAR1A mutation causing pituitary-dependent Cushing disease in a patient with Carney complex. Eur J Endocrinol. 177(2):K7-K12, 2017
5. Marques NV et al: Frequency of familial pituitary adenoma syndromes among patients with functioning pituitary adenomas in a reference outpatient clinic. J Endocrinol Invest. ePub, 2017
6. Rostomyan L et al: AIP mutations and gigantism. Ann Endocrinol (Paris). 78(2):123-130, 2017
7. Rutkowski MJ et al: Atypical pituitary adenoma: a clinicopathologic case series. J Neurosurg. 1-8, 2017
8. Sahm F et al: WHO 2016 Classification: changes and advancements in the diagnosis of miscellaneous primary CNS tumours. Neuropathol Appl Neurobiol. ePub, 2017
9. Salvatori R et al: In-frame seven amino-acid duplication in AIP arose over the last 3000 years, disrupts protein interaction & stability and is associated with gigantism. Eur J Endocrinol. ePub, 2017
10. Schultz KAP et al: PTEN, DICER1, FH, and their associated tumor susceptibility syndromes: clinical features, genetics, and surveillance recommendations in childhood. Clin Cancer Res. 23(12):e76-e82, 2017
11. Shaid M et al: Genetics of pituitary adenomas. Neurol India. 65(3):577-587, 2017
12. Tufton N et al: Pituitary carcinoma in a patient with an SDHB Sutation. Endocr Pathol. ePub, 2017
13. Zhang Q et al: Germline mutations in CDH23, encoding cadherin-related 23, are associated with both familial and sporadic pituitary adenomas. Am J Hum Genet. 100(5):817-823, 2017
14. Beckers A et al: X-linked acrogigantism syndrome: clinical profile and therapeutic responses. Endocr Relat Cancer. 22(3):353-67, 2015
15. Hernández-Ramírez LC et al: Landscape of familial isolated and young-onset pituitary adenomas: prospective diagnosis in AIP mutation carriers. J Clin Endocrinol Metab. 100(9):E1242-54, 2015
16. Ma ZY et al: Recurrent gain-of-function USP8 mutations in Cushing's disease. Cell Res. 25(3):306-17, 2015
17. Perez-Rivas LG et al: The gene of the ubiquitin-specific protease 8 is frequently mutated in adenomas causing Cushing's disease. J Clin Endocrinol Metab. 100(7):E997-1004, 2015
18. Alband N et al: Familial pituitary tumors. Handb Clin Neurol. 124:339-60, 2014
19. Thakker RV: Multiple endocrine neoplasia type 1 (MEN1) and type 4 (MEN4). Mol Cell Endocrinol. Epub ahead of print, 2013
20. Xekouki P et al: Succinate dehydrogenase (SDHx) mutations in pituitary tumors: could this be a new role for mitochondrial complex II and/or Krebs cycle defects? Endocr Relat Cancer. 19(6):C33-40, 2012
21. DiGiovanni R et al: AIP mutations are not identified in patients with sporadic pituitary adenomas. Endocr Pathol. 18(2):76-8, 2007
22. Larkin S et al: Pathology and pathogenesis of pituitary adenomas and other sellar lesions. Endotext. 2017
23. Osamura R et al. Pituitary adenoma. In: WHO Classification of Tumours of the Endocrine Organs. 4th Ed. IARC: Lyon, pages 14-18

Immunohistochemical Classification of Pituitary Adenomas

Adenoma Type	Transcription Factor	Hormones	LMWK
GH-Producing Adenomas			
Densely granulated somatotroph adenoma	PIT-1	GH, α-SU	Perinuclear
Sparsely granulated somatotroph adenoma	PIT-1	GH	Fibrous bodies
Mammosomatotroph adenoma	PIT-1, ER-α	GH, PRL, α-SU	
Mixed somatotroph and lactotroph adenoma	PIT-1, ER-α	GH, PRL, α-SU	
Plurihormonal GH-producing adenoma	PIT-1, ER	GH, PRL, α-SU, TSH-β	
PRL-Producing Adenomas			
Sparsely granulated lactotroph adenoma	PIT-1, ER-α	PRL (Golgi pattern)	
Densely granulated lactotroph adenoma	PIT-1, ER-α	PRL (diffuse)	
Acidophilic stem cell adenoma		PRL (diffuse), GH (focal)	Fibrous bodies (few)
TSH-Producing Adenoma			
Thyrotroph adenoma	PIT-1, GATA2	TSH-β, α-SU	
ACTH-Producing Adenomas			
Densely granulated corticotroph adenoma	TPIT	ACTH	Diffuse pattern
Sparsely granulated corticotroph adenoma	TPIT	ACTH	Diffuse pattern
Crooke cell adenoma	TPIT	ACTH	Ring-like pattern
Gonadotropin-Producing Adenoma			
Gonadotroph adenoma	SF1, ER-α, GATA2	LH-β, FSH-β, α-SU	
Plurihormonal Adenomas			
Plurihormonal Pit-1-positive adenoma (previously called silent subtype 3 adenoma)	PIT-1 Other	GH, PRL, TSH-β, α-SU, ACTH (rarely)	
Unusual plurihormonal adenoma, NOS	Multiple: PIT-1 and TPIT	Multiple: usually PRL and ACTH	
Hormone-Negative Adenoma			
Null cell adenoma	Absent	Absent	

GH = growth hormone.

Genetic Predisposition to Pituitary Adenomas

Syndromic and Isolated Diseases	Associated Genes
Multiple endocrine neoplasia 1	*MEN1*
Multiple endocrine neoplasia 4	*CDKN1B*
SDH-related familial paraganglioma-pheochromocytoma syndromes	*SDHA, SDHB, SDHC, SDHD, SDHAF2*
DICER1 syndrome	*DICER1*
Carney complex	*PRKAR1A/CNC1*; rarely *PRKACA* and *PRKACB*
McCune-Albright syndrome	Mosaic *GNAS*
Neurofibromatosis	*NF1*
Familial isolated pituitary adenoma	*AIP*
X-linked acrogigantism syndrome	*GPR101*

Modified from WHO 2017.

(Left) *The pituitary is composed of neural tissue forming the posterior pituitary (PL) and pituitary stalk, epithelial neuroendocrine tissue forming the anterior lobe (AL), and the cystic remnants of the intermediate lobe (IL). The anterior pituitary is composed of cells with production of diverse hormones. Normal distribution of cells is shown (inset).* **(Right)** *Microadenomas are defined as tumor smaller than 1 cm in the largest dimension.*

Graphic of Normal Pituitary Gland

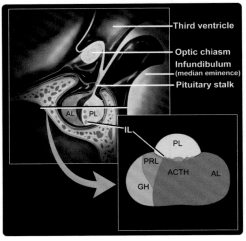

Pituitary Microadenoma

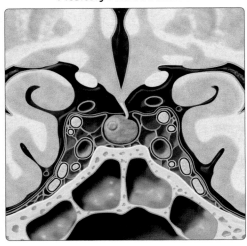

(Left) *MR shows a pituitary macroadenoma with suprasellar extension, sphenoid sinus, and cavernous sinus invasion.* **(Right)** *Coronal graphic illustrates a large pituitary macroadenoma extending superiorly to compress the body of the chiasm, thus compressing the bulk of the crossing nasal retinal fibers.*

Neuroimaging of Macroadenoma

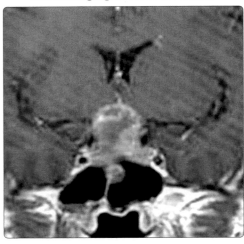

Macroadenoma With Suprasellar Extension

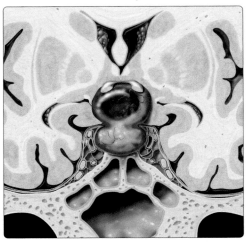

(Left) *Pituitary adenomas demonstrate a breakdown of normal acinar architecture. In this example, a microadenoma ⇒ shows definitive loss of the normal acinar pattern in comparison with the surrounding normal gland ⇒. (Right)* *Pituitary adenomas demonstrate a total breakdown of normal acinar architecture, as seen in this example, highlighting the loss of Wilder silver stain.*

Pituitary Microadenoma: Reticulin

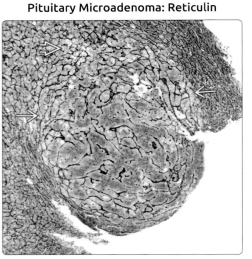

Pituitary Adenoma: Reticulin

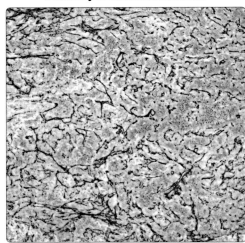

Pituitary Adenoma: Growth Hormone Immunohistochemistry

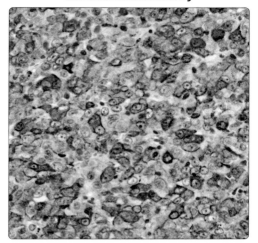

Pituitary Adenoma: ACTH Immunohistochemistry

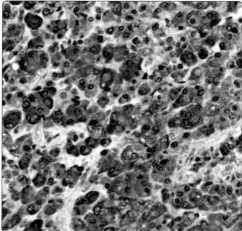

(Left) *Immunohistochemical stains for pituitary hormones are essential for the diagnosis of pituitary adenoma. In this example, strong and diffuse cytoplasmic reactivity is seen in a densely granulated somatotroph adenoma.* (Right) *Corticotroph adenomas most commonly are composed of densely granulated cells with diffuse cytoplasmic ACTH immunoreactivity.*

Pituitary Adenoma: PRL Immunohistochemistry

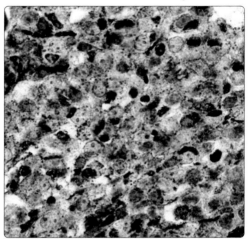

Pituitary Adenoma: LH-β Immunohistochemistry

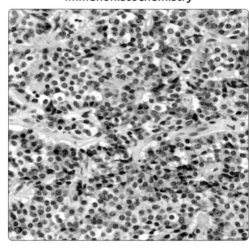

(Left) *In comparison to the densely granulated cells of corticotroph and somatotroph adenomas, lactotroph adenomas show sparse PRL reactivity with characteristic perinuclear Golgi-type of staining.* (Right) *Gonadotroph adenomas show only focal and sparse immunoreactivity for the gonadotropins, here exemplified by LH-β immunostaining.*

Pituitary Adenoma: Sinus Mucosa Invasion

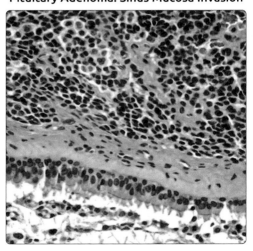

Pituitary Adenoma: Bone Invasion

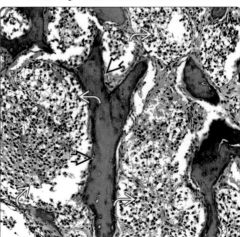

(Left) *Some pituitary adenomas may be associated with invasive or aggressive behavior and are called "invasive pituitary adenomas." Some PAs may grow inferiorly and invade the sphenoid sinus mucosa.* (Right) *This photomicrograph shows an invasive pituitary adenoma ➦ within bone marrow surrounded by bone trabeculae ➥.*

TERMINOLOGY

- Somatotroph adenoma (SA) is pituitary adenoma that mainly expresses growth hormone (GH) and arises from PIT-1 lineage

ETIOLOGY/PATHOGENESIS

- Most SAs are sporadic
- SAs may be component of multiple endocrine neoplasias type 1 (MEN1), Carney complex, McCune-Albright syndrome, familial isolated pituitary adenoma syndrome, succinate dehydrogenase-related hereditary pheochromocytoma/paraganglioma syndrome, and X-linked acrogigantism

CLINICAL ISSUES

- GH-producing adenomas constitute ~ 10-15% of resected adenomas
- Manifests as acromegaly &/or gigantism
  - Additional symptoms of mass effect in macroadenomas

- Surgery is primary treatment
- Best prognosticator is accurate histologic classification of SAs

MICROSCOPIC

- DGSA: Composed of acidophilic (eosinophilic) cells that exhibit diffuse, sinusoidal, and trabecular growth
- SGSA: Composed of chromophobic cells with fibrous bodies and arranged in diffuse growth
- Mammosomatotroph adenoma: Composed of acidophilic cells that exhibit diffuse or solid growth
- Mixed SA-lactotroph adenoma: Most commonly composed of DG somatotrophs (eosinophilic cells) and SG lactotrophs (chromophobic cells)

ANCILLARY TESTS

- Immunohistochemistry
  - DGSA: GH (strong and diffuse), α-subunit, PIT-1, LMWK (perinuclear)
  - SGSA: GH (weak and focal), PIT-1, LMWK (fibrous bodies)

Densely Granulated Somatotroph Adenoma

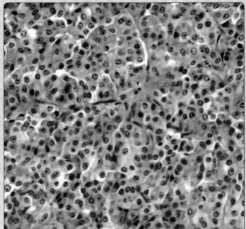

Densely Granulated Somatotroph Adenoma: GH Immunohistochemistry

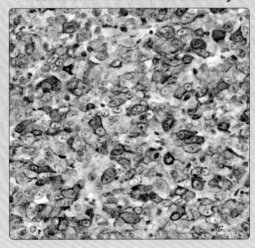

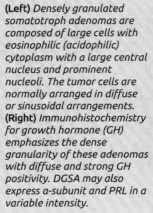

(Left) Densely granulated somatotroph adenomas are composed of large cells with eosinophilic (acidophilic) cytoplasm with a large central nucleus and prominent nucleoli. The tumor cells are normally arranged in diffuse or sinusoidal arrangements. **(Right)** *Immunohistochemistry for growth hormone (GH) emphasizes the dense granularity of these adenomas with diffuse and strong GH positivity. DGSA may also express a-subunit and PRL in a variable intensity.*

Sparsely Granulated Somatotroph Adenoma

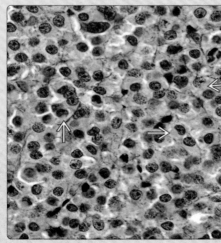

Sparsely Granulated Somatotroph Adenoma: GH Immunohistochemistry

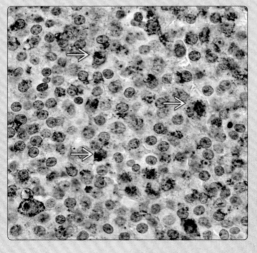

(Left) Sparsely granulated somatotroph adenomas are composed of chromophobic or slightly acidophilic cells with hyperchromatic nuclei. The nuclei may be displaced to the side due to the presence of fibrous bodies ➡, proteinaceous glassy cytoplasmic inclusions consistent with accumulation of keratin. **(Right)** *Immunopositivity for GH in sparsely granulated adenomas is sparse in the cells and focal in the tumor. A punctate ➡ almost Golgi pattern-like in lactotroph adenomas may be present.*

TERMINOLOGY

Abbreviations

- Somatotroph adenoma (SA)
- Growth hormone (GH)

Synonyms

- GH-secreting adenoma
- GH-producing adenoma
- Somatotropinoma
- GH cell adenoma

Definitions

- Pituitary adenoma that expresses mainly GH and arises from PIT-1 lineage
- Adenomas that cause GH excess are histologically classified into 5 clinically relevant subtypes
  - Densely granulated SA (DGSA)
  - Sparsely granulated SA (SGSA)
  - Mammosomatotroph adenoma
  - Mixed somatotroph and lactotroph adenoma
  - Plurihormonal GH-producing adenoma

ETIOLOGY/PATHOGENESIS

Somatic Genetics

- Most SAs are sporadic
- Activating somatic mutations in *GNAS* gene are associated in ~ 40% of somatic DGSA
- Somatic GH receptor mutations in somatotrophs have been reported in SGSA
- Truncated alternatively spliced form of GHRH receptor with limited signaling properties has also been described in SA

Familial Syndromes

- SAs may be component of
  - Multiple endocrine neoplasias types 1 (MEN1) and 4
  - Carney complex
  - McCune-Albright syndrome
  - Familial isolated pituitary adenoma syndrome
  - Succinate dehydrogenase-related hereditary pheochromocytoma/paraganglioma syndrome
  - X-linked acrogigantism
- Somatotroph hyperplasia may also be present in these familial syndromes, in particular MEN1, McCune-Albright syndrome, and Carney complex

CLINICAL ISSUES

Epidemiology

- Incidence
  - GH-producing adenomas constitute ~ 10-15% of resected adenomas
  - DGSA is more common than SGSA
  - Mammosomatotroph adenomas are most frequent in children and in young patients

Presentation

- Manifests as acromegaly &/or gigantism
  - Early signs of acromegaly appear in 3rd decade; however, features are subtle and, therefore, diagnosis is usually delayed for several years

- Hyperprolactinemia can be seen due to PRL production in bihormonal pituitary adenomas or due to pituitary stalk effect
- Signs and symptoms of mass effect, including headaches and visual disturbances, are commonly seen in macroadenomas
- Clinically nonfunctioning SAs, i.e., silent SAs, are rare

Treatment

- Surgery is primary treatment for most patients with acromegaly
- Somatostatin analogues (SSTs) are routinely used for patients who fail surgery or are not surgical candidates
  - SSTs do not usually cause clinically significant tumor shrinkage, but control symptoms and decrease soft tissue swelling to facilitate surgery
  - DGSAs are usually responsive to SSTs
  - SGSAs are less responsive to SSTs most likely related to small numbers of cytoplasmic SST receptors
- Pegvisomant
  - GH receptor antagonist
- Radiotherapy is selectively used

Prognosis

- Best prognosticator is accurate histologic classification of SAs
- SGSA is most aggressive subtype and needs to be distinguished from other subtypes
- Large and invasive tumors have poor long-term control

IMAGING

Radiologic Findings

- PAs are usually hypointense, distinguishing them from hyperplasia
- DGSAs are usually hypointense on T2 sequence of MR
- SGSAs are usually invasive macroadenomas

MACROSCOPIC

General Features

- SAs are soft and white to gray
- SGSAs are usually invasive macroadenomas

MICROSCOPIC

Densely Granulated Somatotroph Adenoma

- Composed of acidophilic (eosinophilic) cells that exhibit diffuse, sinusoidal, and trabecular growth
  - Cytoplasmic eosinophilic appearance correlates with dense secretory granules

Sparsely Granulated Somatotroph Adenoma

- Composed of chromophobic cells with diffuse growth
  - Chromophobic appearance correlates with sparse secretory granules
- Fibrous bodies may be seen on H&E sections
  - Nuclei exhibit pleomorphism and tend to be eccentric, pushed to cell periphery, and indented by fibrous bodies

Mammosomatotroph Adenoma

- Composed of acidophilic cells that exhibit diffuse or solid growth

Mixed Somatotroph and Lactotroph Adenoma

- Most commonly composed of densely granulated somatotrophs (eosinophilic cells) and sparsely granulated lactotrophs (chromophobic cells)

Plurihormonal GH-Producing Adenoma

- GH-producing dominant component usually exhibits densely granulated somatotroph or mammosomatotroph and thyrotroph differentiation
- Contain cells with thyrotroph differentiation

ANCILLARY TESTS

Histochemistry

- Breakdown of reticulin distinguishes adenoma from hyperplasia that retains reticulin network

Immunohistochemistry

- Plays critical role in classification of SAs
  - DGSAs
    - GH is diffusely positive
    - α-subunit is often expressed
    - PIT-1 is strongly expressed
    - LMWK (CAM5.2) reveals perinuclear pattern
  - SGSAs
    - GH is focally and weakly positive; α-subunit is usually negative
    - PIT-1 is strongly expressed
    - LMWK (CAM5.2) reveals globular juxtanuclear fibrous bodies
  - Mammosomatotroph adenomas
    - GH (diffuse), PRL (variably), and α-subunit are positive
    - PIT-1 and ER-α are diffusely expressed
    - LMWK (CAM5.2) reveals perinuclear pattern
  - Mixed somatotroph and lactotroph adenomas
    - GH (in somatotroph component), PRL (variably expressed with Golgi pattern), α-subunit (in somatotroph component) are positive
    - PIT-1 and ER-α are expressed
    - LMWK (CAM5.2) reveals perinuclear pattern
  - Plurihormonal GH-producing adenomas
    - GH, PRL, β-TSH, and α-subunit are variably expressed
    - PIT-1 and variable ER-α

Electron Microscopy

- DGSAs
  - Cytoplasm contains abundant large secretory granules measuring 400-600 nm
- SGSAs
  - Eccentric pleomorphic concave or multilobed nuclei
  - Secretory granules are sparse and range from 100-250 nm
  - Abundant fibrous bodies identified as juxtanuclear spherical accumulations of keratin filaments associated with variable amounts of endoplasmic reticulum and trapped secretory granules
- Mammosomatotroph adenomas
  - Monomorphic cells resembling densely granulated somatotrophs with exception of differences in secretory granule morphology and size
    - Pleomorphic and heterogeneous granules ranging from 150-1,000 nm

- Misplaced exocytosis similar to lactotroph cells
- Mixed somatotroph and lactotroph adenomas
  - Bicellular proliferation of distinct cell populations with ultrastructural features of DG somatotrophs and SG lactotrophs
- Plurihormonal GH-producing adenomas
  - Mixed ultrastructural features of PIT-1 lineage cells

DIFFERENTIAL DIAGNOSIS

Adenomas With Fibrous Body Formation

- SGSA is most common PA that exhibits abundant fibrous body formation; other entities may contain only occasional fibrous bodies
- Acidophil stem cell adenomas may contain occasional fibrous bodies
- Some DGSAs may reveal occasional fibrous bodies, and these are classified as "intermediate-type SA"
  - Since their biology does not differ from DGSA, they are classified in spectrum of DGSA

Somatotroph Hyperplasia

- Breakdown of acinar architecture on silver stain distinguishes adenoma from hyperplasia that has intact reticulin

Metastatic Neuroendocrine Carcinoma

- Demonstration of pituitary hormones and PIT-1 by immunohistochemistry rules out metastatic disease

Mixed or Plurihormonal Adenomas

- SAs may be diagnosed as plurihormonal adenomas due to use of less-specific antibodies against pituitary hormones
  - Antibodies against pituitary transcription factors are critical
- Trapped nontumorous cells can be mistaken as part of adenoma

SELECTED REFERENCES

1. Mete O et al: Somatotroph adenoma. In Lloyd RV et al: WHO Classification of Tumours of Endocrine Organs, 4th Ed. Lyon:IARC. 19-23, 2017
2. Gordon RJ et al: Childhood acromegaly due to X-linked acrogigantism: long term follow-up. Pituitary. 19(6):560-564, 2016
3. Hannah-Shmouni F et al: Genetics of gigantism and acromegaly. Growth Horm IGF Res. 30-31:37-41, 2016
4. Iacovazzo D et al: Germline or somatic GPR101 duplication leads to X-linked acrogigantism: a clinico-pathological and genetic study. Acta Neuropathol Commun. 4(1):56, 2016
5. Hernández-Ramírez LC et al: Landscape of familial isolated and young-onset pituitary adenomas: prospective diagnosis in AIP mutation carriers. J Clin Endocrinol Metab. 100(9):E1242-54, 2015
6. Lee CC et al: Stereotactic radiosurgery for acromegaly: outcomes by adenoma subtype. Pituitary. 18(3):326-34, 2015
7. Alband N et al: Familial pituitary tumors. Handb Clin Neurol. 124:339-60, 2014
8. Kato M et al: Differential expression of genes related to drug responsiveness between sparsely and densely granulated somatotroph adenomas. Endocr J. 59(3):221-8, 2012
9. Vortmeyer AO et al: Somatic GNAS mutation causes widespread and diffuse pituitary disease in acromegalic patients with McCune-Albright syndrome. J Clin Endocrinol Metab. 97(7):2404-13, 2012
10. Obari A et al: Clinicopathological features of growth hormone-producing pituitary adenomas: difference among various types defined by cytokeratin distribution pattern including a transitional form. Endocr Pathol. 19(2):82-91, 2008

Densely Granulated Somatotroph Adenoma: LMWK (CAM5.2)

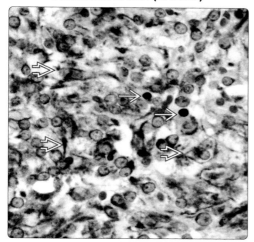

Sparsely Granulated Somatotroph Adenoma: LMWK (CAM5.2)

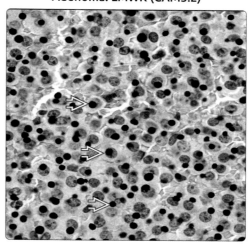

(Left) *In densely granulated somatotroph adenoma (DGSAs), keratin positivity is located in a perinuclear pattern ⇶. Occasional fibrous bodies ⇒ can be seen in "intermediate-type somatotroph adenomas," in which the tumor biology does not differ from densely granulated somatotroph adenomas.* (Right) *In sparsely granulated somatotroph adenomas, keratin immunohistochemistry reveals paranuclear keratin aggresomes, "fibrous bodies" ⇶. Note the displacement of the nucleus in several cells.*

Mammosomatotroph Adenoma

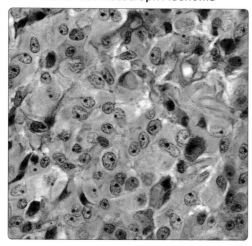

Mammosomatotroph Adenoma: GH

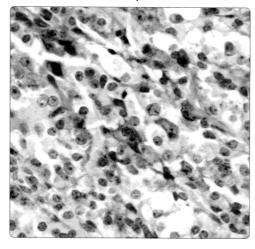

(Left) *Mammosomatotroph adenomas are quite similar to DGSA by H&E stain. The tumor cells are large, acidophilic, and with a large central nucleus with prominent nucleoli.* (Right) *Mammosomatotroph adenomas display immunoreactivity for GH and PRL in the same tumor cell in the same patient. In this picture, GH immunostain displays diffuse cytoplasmic positivity involving a moderate number of tumor cells.*

Mammosomatotroph Adenoma: PRL

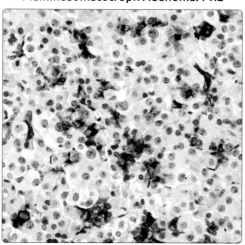

GH-Producing Adenomas: PIT-1

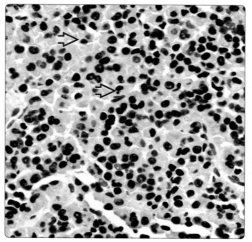

(Left) *In the same patient, PRL immunoreactivity was present in several tumor cells. Ultrastructure analysis confirmed a monocellular adenoma resembling densely granulated somatotrophs but with granular extrusion-like lactotroph cells.* (Right) *Regardless of the subtype, all GH-producing pituitary adenomas are strongly positive for PIT-1 ⇶. PIT-1 is also expressed in PRL- and TSH-producing pituitary adenomas.*

Lactotroph Adenoma

TERMINOLOGY

- Lactotroph adenomas (LA): Pituitary adenomas that express mainly PRL and arise from PIT-1 lineage adenohypophyseal cells
- Classified into 3 clinically relevant histological subtypes: SGLA, DGLA, and acidophilic stem cell adenoma

ETIOLOGY/PATHOGENESIS

- Majority of cases sporadic; familial cases associated most commonly with MEN1 and AIP-related FIPA

CLINICAL ISSUES

- LAs most common pituitary adenomas (30-50%)
- Most commonly occurs in adults, with peak around 3rd-4th decades; female predominance
- Women present mostly with galactorrhea &/or amenorrhea, and fertility problems
- Decreased libido and impotence can be seen in men

- Pharmacotherapy primary treatment modality for prolactinomas
- Lactotroph carcinomas most common malignant pituitary neuroendocrine tumor

MICROSCOPIC

- SGLA most common histological subtype of LA

ANCILLARY TESTS

- Immunohistochemistry
  - SGLA: PRL (Golgi pattern), PIT-1, ER-α
  - DGLA: PRL (diffuse pattern), PIT-1, ER-α
  - Acidophilic stem cell adenoma: PRL, GH (focal), LMWK (occasional fibrous bodies), PIT-1, ER-α

TOP DIFFERENTIAL DIAGNOSES

- Lactotroph hyperplasia
- Lymphocytic hypophysitis
- Lymphoma

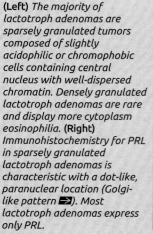

(Left) The majority of lactotroph adenomas are sparsely granulated tumors composed of slightly acidophilic or chromophobic cells containing central nucleus with well-dispersed chromatin. Densely granulated lactotroph adenomas are rare and display more cytoplasm eosinophilia. (Right) Immunohistochemistry for PRL in sparsely granulated lactotroph adenomas is characteristic with a dot-like, paranuclear location (Golgi-like pattern ➡). Most lactotroph adenomas express only PRL.

Lactotroph Adenoma

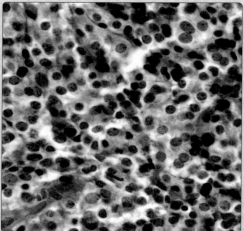

Sparsely Granulated Lactotroph Adenoma: PRL Immunohistochemistry

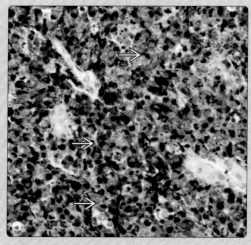

(Left) Unlike sparsely granulated adenomas, densely granulated lactotroph adenomas have diffuse cytoplasmic positivity for PRL ➡ and usually lack the characteristic Golgi pattern. (Right) Intense shrinkage of the tumor cells and extensive interstitial fibrosis is seen in adenomas from patients treated with dopamine agonists prior to surgical resection. The small tumor cells may be mistaken by lymphocytes. Immunostains for PRL and lymphoid markers are helpful for the correct diagnosis.

Densely Granulated Lactotroph Adenoma: PRL Immunohistochemistry

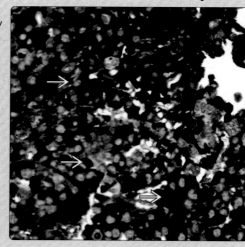

Lactotroph Adenoma: Post Dopamine Agonists Treatment

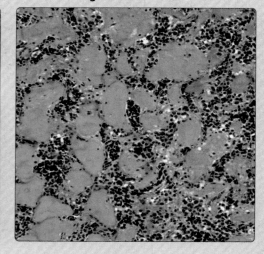

TERMINOLOGY

Abbreviations

- Lactotroph adenoma (LA)

Synonyms

- Lactotrope adenoma
- Prolactin (PRL)-secreting adenoma
- PRL-producing adenoma
- Prolactinoma

Definitions

- Pituitary adenomas that express mainly PRL and arise from PIT-1 lineage adenohypophyseal cells
- LAs classified into 3 clinically relevant histological subtypes
  - Sparsely granulated lactotroph adenoma (SGLA)
  - Densely granulated lactotroph adenoma (DGLA)
  - Acidophilic stem cell adenoma (ASCA)

ETIOLOGY/PATHOGENESIS

Pathogenesis

- Largely unknown
- Estrogen implicated in lactotroph proliferation during pregnancy, and some LAs grow faster during this time

Genetic Susceptibility

- Majority of cases sporadic
- Minority of pituitary adenomas associated with familial predisposition
- ~ 5% of all pituitary adenomas have genetic predisposition associated with
  - Multiple endocrine neoplasia type 1 (MEN1)
  - Multiple endocrine neoplasia type 4 (MEN4)
  - McCune-Albright syndrome
  - Familial isolated pituitary adenomas
  - SDH-related familial paraganglioma/pheochromocytoma syndromes
  - Carney complex
- Familial pituitary LAs mostly associated with MEN1

CLINICAL ISSUES

Epidemiology

- Incidence
  - LAs most common pituitary adenomas (30-50%)
  - Less common in surgical series due to successful pharmacotherapies
- Age
  - Most commonly occurs in adults, with peak around 3rd-4th decades
- Sex
  - Female predominance
  - In autopsy series, no gender predilection observed

Presentation

- Women present mostly with galactorrhea &/or amenorrhea, and fertility problems
- Decreased libido and impotence can be seen in men
- Women tend to have microadenomas
- Men tend to have invasive macroadenomas with visual field abnormalities and hypopituitarism
  - Giant adenomas (> 4 cm) usually seen in men
- Serum PRL levels correlate with adenoma size in majority of tumors
- Patients with acidophilic stem cell adenomas may have minor symptomatology of acromegaly or subtle biochemical evidence of GH excess

Treatment

- Pharmacotherapy is primary treatment modality for prolactinomas
  - SGLAs respond to dopamine agonists with rapid fall in serum PRL and tumor shrinkage
  - Response to pharmacotherapy usually low in non-SGLA, requiring require surgery
- Surgery most indicated in patients with resistance or intolerance to pharmacotherapy
  - Invasive macroadenomas may require surgery
- Radiotherapy indicated for cases that have failed surgery &/or medical treatment

Prognosis

- Histological classification plays important role in prognosis
  - SGLAs have better respond to dopamine agonists and usually have good prognosis
  - Acidophilic stem cell adenomas and DGLAs are more aggressive
- Lactotroph carcinomas are most common malignant pituitary neuroendocrine tumor

IMAGING

Radiologic Features

- Microadenomas are common in women with subtle radiological abnormalities
- Macroadenomas are common in males with evidence of suprasellar extension and as well downward invasion into sinuses or adjacent structures
- Downward invasion without upward extension is distinct finding of acidophilic stem cell adenoma

MACROSCOPIC

General Features

- Varies from soft, red, friable lesions to firm, white or gray tumors with fibrotic changes and calcifications

MICROSCOPIC

Sparsely Granulated Lactotroph Adenoma

- Most common histological subtype of LAs
  - Composed of chromophobic cells that exhibit solid, trabecular, or papillary growth
- May contain calcifications that may take form of psammoma bodies or extensive calcifications
- Endocrine amyloid deposition can also be seen

Densely Granulated Lactotroph Adenoma

- Composed of acidophilic cells that exhibit wide variation in architecture

Acidophilic Stem Cell Adenoma

- Composed of chromophobic or slightly eosinophilic cells that exhibit solid growth

- o Cytoplasmic eosinophilia is due to accumulation of mitochondria (oncocytic change)
- o Clear cytoplasmic vacuoles correspond to megamitochondria

Morphological Changes Due to Drugs

- Dopamine agonist "bromocriptine effects"
- o Significant shrinkage of tumor cell size, mainly affecting cell cytoplasm
- o Nuclei become irregular and hyperchromatic
- o Number of secretory granules is decreased and staining for PRL can be focal or even negative
- o Interstitial and perivascular fibrosis

ANCILLARY TESTS

Immunohistochemistry

- SGLA
- o PRL is intense and reveals juxtanuclear globular reactivity (Golgi pattern)
- o α-subunit (α-SU) usually negative
- o PIT-1 and ER-α strongly expressed
- DGLA
- o PRL is intense and reveals diffuse cytoplasmic reactivity
- o α-SU usually negative
- o PIT-1 and ER-α strongly expressed
- Acidophilic stem cell adenoma
- o PRL variable in intensity and distribution
  - – Rarely, Golgi-type staining can be seen
- o Focal GH positivity seen in majority of cases
- o Fibrous bodies can be present
  - – Even in absence of GH production by prolactinoma, oncocytic change with few fibrous bodies should suggest this neoplasm
- o PIT-1 and ER-α strongly expressed

Electron Microscopy

- SGLA
- o Polygonal cells with elongated cell processes and cytoplasm entirely filled with rough endoplasmic reticulum (RER)
- o Secretory granules sparse and spherical (150-300 nm)
- o Misplaced exocytosis or granular extrusion
  - – Characterized by extrusion of secretory granules along lateral cell surfaces
- DGLA
- o Less abundant RER, misplaced exocytoses
- o Numerous secretory granules (up to 700 nm)
- Acidophil stem cell adenoma
- o Numerous enlarged mitochondria, forming giant mitochondria with loss of cristae and harboring electron-dense tubular structures

DIFFERENTIAL DIAGNOSIS

Pituitary Hyperplasia

- Lactotroph hyperplasia are often mistaken for prolactinoma
- Disruption in reticulin network and immunostains for pituitary hormones critical for diagnosis

Lymphocytic Hypophysitis and Lymphoma

- LAs treated with dopamine agonists composed of small cells with hyperchromatic nuclei may mimic lymphocytic infiltrates similar to hypophysitis or even small cell lymphomas
- Use of lymphoid cell markers and PRL should be used to exclude this diagnosis

Adenomas With Fibrous Body Formation

- Lactotroph adenomas that exhibit occasional fibrous bodies should be classified as acidophil stem cell adenoma

SELECTED REFERENCES

1. Nose V et al. Lactotroph adenoma. In: WHO Classification of Tumours of Endocrine Organs, 4th Edition. Ed: Lloyd RV et al. IARC, Lyon. 24-27, 2017
2. Donegan D et al: Surgical outcomes of prolactinomas in recent era: Results of a heterogeneous group. Endocr Pract. 23(1):37-45, 2017
3. Lonser RR et al: Surgical management of Carney complex-associated pituitary pathology. Neurosurgery. 80(5):780-786, 2017
4. Marques P et al: Genetic aspects of pituitary adenomas. Endocrinol Metab Clin North Am. 46(2):335-374, 2017
5. McDonald WC et al: Steroidogenic factor 1, pit-1, and adrenocorticotropic hormone: A rational starting place for the immunohistochemical characterization of pituitary adenoma. Arch Pathol Lab Med. 141(1):104-112, 2017
6. Yeh T et al: Turner syndrome and pituitary adenomas: a case report and review of literature. J Pediatr Endocrinol Metab. 30(2):231-235, 2017
7. Livshits A et al: Pituitary tumors in MEN1: do not be misled by borderline elevated prolactin levels. Pituitary. 19(6):601-604, 2016
8. Seltzer J et al: Prolactin-secreting pituitary carcinoma with dural metastasis: Diagnosis, treatment, and future directions. World Neurosurg. 91:676.e23-8, 2016
9. Shimon I et al: Giant prolactinomas larger than 60 mm in size: a cohort of massive and aggressive prolactin-secreting pituitary adenomas. Pituitary. 19(4):429-36, 2016
10. Tirosh A et al: Current approach to treatments for prolactinomas. Minerva Endocrinol. 41(3):316-23, 2016
11. Delgrange E et al: Expression of estrogen receptor alpha is associated with prolactin pituitary tumor prognosis and supports the sex-related difference in tumor growth. Eur J Endocrinol. 172(6):791-801, 2015
12. Raverot G et al: Prognostic factors in prolactin pituitary tumors: clinical, histological, and molecular data from a series of 94 patients with a long postoperative follow-up. J Clin Endocrinol Metab. 95(4):1708-16, 2010
13. Kovacs K et al: Effects of medical therapy on pituitary tumors. Ultrastruct Pathol. 29(3-4):163-7, 2005
14. Stefaneanu L et al: Dopamine D2 receptor gene expression in human adenohypophysial adenomas. Endocrine. 14(3):329-36, 2001

Acidophilic Stem Cell Adenoma

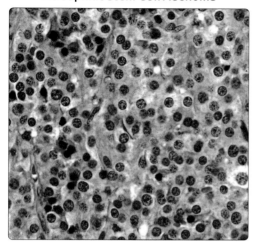

Acidophilic Stem Cell Adenoma: PRL Immunohistochemistry

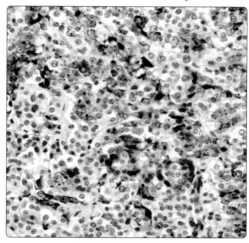

(Left) *Acidophilic stem cell adenomas are characterized by cells with acidophilic cytoplasm with focal oncocytic changes. These tumors tend to be macroadenomas and have a more aggressive behavior than the regular lactotroph adenoma. Patients may present with low levels of serum PRL comparable with the size of the tumor.* (Right) *Immunostaining for PRL is variable in acidophilic stem cell adenomas with cells displaying Golgi pattern and others with more diffuse reactivity. GH expression may occasionally be present.*

Acidophilic Stem Cell Adenoma: LMWK Immunohistochemistry

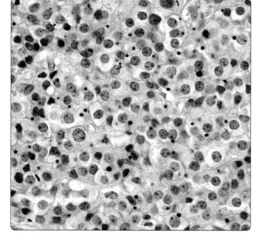

Acidophil Stem Cell Adenomas

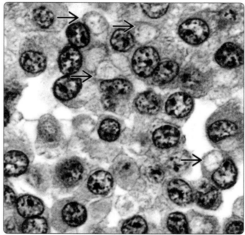

(Left) *Unlike lactotroph adenomas, acidophilic stem cell adenomas display fibrous bodies, highlighted here by keratin immunostaining. The fibrous bodies are similar to those seen in sparsely granulated somatotroph adenomas, but they are much less numerous.* (Right) *Acidophil stem cell adenomas may exhibit cytoplasmic vacuolization ➡ corresponding to giant mitochondria at the ultrastructural analysis.*

Acidophil Stem Cell Adenoma

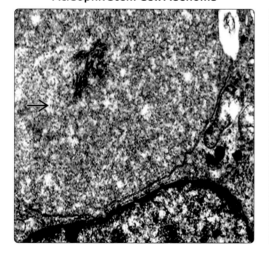

PRL-Producing Adenomas: PIT-1 Immunohistochemistry

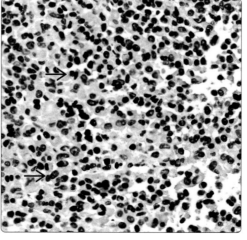

(Left) *A characteristic feature of acidophilic stem cell adenomas is juxtanuclear dilated giant mitochondria ➡. These dilated mitochondria may be seen by H&E.* (Right) *Regardless of the subtype, all PRL-producing adenomas are positive for PIT-1 ➡. PIT-1 is also expressed in the other acidophilic lineage adenomas, including somatotroph and thyrotroph adenomas.*

Thyrotroph Adenoma

TERMINOLOGY

- Pituitary adenomas that express mainly TSH and arise from PIT-1 lineage adenohypophyseal cells
- Thyrotroph adenoma (TA)
- Additional terminology: TSHoma, TSH-secreting adenoma, thyrotropinoma, TSH-producing adenoma

ETIOLOGY/PATHOGENESIS

- Most cases are sporadic adenomas with unknown etiology
- Patients with MEN1 may develop TAs

CLINICAL ISSUES

- Rare, constituting < 2% of all pituitary adenomas
- Most common in adults; predominantly in women
- Majority of TAs are clinically functioning adenomas associated with hyperthyroidism
- Clinically nonfunctioning (silent) TAs present with signs and symptoms of tumor mass
- Surgery is 1st line of treatment

IMAGING

- TAs are usually macroadenomas with extrasellar expansion

MICROSCOPIC

- Chromophobic polygonal, angulated, or spindle-shaped tumor cells that exhibit indistinct cell borders
- Stromal fibrosis is commonly observed

ANCILLARY TESTS

- β-TSH and α-SU: Usually positive
- PIT-1 and GATA2: Strongly expressed
- Membranous SSTR2A and SSTR5: In majority of TAs

TOP DIFFERENTIAL DIAGNOSES

- Plurihormonal PIT-1-positive adenomas
- Thyrotroph hyperplasia
- Paraganglioma
- Metastatic neuroendocrine carcinoma

Thyrotroph Adenoma Characteristics

Cellular Characteristics

(Left) *Thyrotroph adenomas are composed of chromophobic to slightly acidophilic cells with large central nuclei, most commonly arranged in diffuse pattern.* *(Right)* *Thyrotroph adenomas may be composed of chromophobic, angulated cells with a pleomorphic nucleus with prominent nucleoli that exhibit indistinct cell borders.*

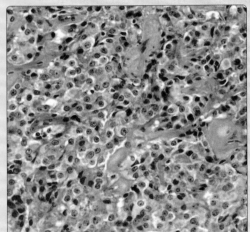
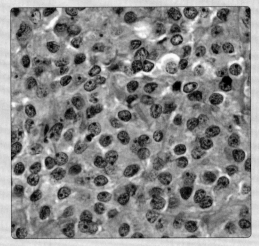

β-TSH Immunohistochemistry

Immunohistochemistry for β-TSH

(Left) *Immunostaining for β-TSH is variable in thyrotroph adenomas, including intense and diffuse positivity like this case. The immunopositivity may decorate the entire cytoplasm of the tumor cells.* *(Right)* *In other thyrotroph adenomas, only focal staining of the tumor cells is present, and the pattern of staining varies from one cell to the other.*

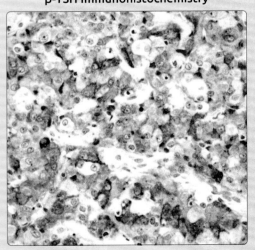
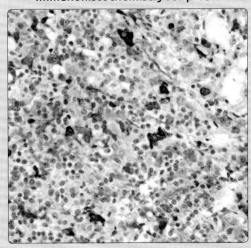

TERMINOLOGY

Abbreviations

- Thyrotroph adenoma (TA)

Synonyms

- TSH-producing adenoma
- TSHoma
- TSH-secreting adenoma
- Thyrotropinoma

Definitions

- Pituitary adenomas that mainly express TSH and arise from PIT-1 lineage adenohypophyseal cells

ETIOLOGY/PATHOGENESIS

Unknown

- Most cases are sporadic adenomas with unknown etiology

Hyperplasia-to-Neoplasia Transition

- Very few reported cases of TAs have developed in patients with longstanding primary hypothyroidism

Genetic Susceptibility

- Patients with MEN1 may develop TAs

CLINICAL ISSUES

Epidemiology

- Incidence
  - Rare, constituting < 2% of all pituitary adenomas
- Age
  - Most common in adults
  - In surgical series, age ranges from 21-74 years old
- Sex
  - Predominantly in women, especially clinically nonfunctioning TAs

Presentation

- Majority of TAs are clinically functioning adenomas associated with hyperthyroidism
  - Clinically, patients present with signs and symptoms of thyrotoxicosis in presence of normal or high serum TSH
  - In some patients, TSH excess is associated with galactorrhea and hyperprolactinemia due to lactotroph hyperplasia
  - Elevation of α-subunit is frequently found in patients with TAs
    - Molar ratio of α-subunit:TSH is elevated, distinguishing TAs from other nontumorous conditions with inappropriate TSH secretion
- Clinically nonfunctioning (silent) TAs are unassociated with hyperthyroidism
  - Present with symptoms related to mass effects and mild hyperprolactinemia due to stalk compression

Treatment

- Surgery is 1st line of treatment with endocrine remission in near 90% of cases
  - Poor surgical outcome is mostly related to invasive tumors
- Somatostatin analogues are effective in reducing TSH levels in most patients

- Radiation therapy has been recommended in cases with surgery and pharmacotherapy failure

Prognosis

- Ki-67 proliferative index has been reported as related to invasiveness and tumor size
- Invasive behavior commonly observed in these adenomas may preclude cure

IMAGING

Radiological Features

- TAs are usually macroadenomas with extrasellar expansion
  - Often exhibit invasion of cavernous sinuses
- Rare microadenomas can be present in mucoid wedge

MACROSCOPIC

General Features

- Usually large and invasive tumors
- May have firmer consistency than regular pituitary adenoma
- May sometimes exhibit calcifications

MICROSCOPIC

Histologic Features

- Chromophobic polygonal, angulated, or spindle-shaped tumor cells that exhibit indistinct cell borders
- Diffuse and solid growth pattern is common
- Cells may contain pleomorphic nuclei
- Stromal fibrosis is commonly observed
- Occasional calcifications forming psammoma bodies can be seen

ANCILLARY TESTS

Immunohistochemistry

- β-TSH and α-SU (usually) are positive
  - Immunoreactivity for β-TSH is variable
  - Tumor cells are frequently positive for both β-TSH and α-SU
    - Suggesting production and secretion of intact TSH from tumor cells
- TAs coexpress GH and PRL in ~ 84% of cases
- PIT-1 and GATA2 are strongly expressed
- TAs are strongly immunopositive for somatostatin receptor (SSTR) 2A and SSTR5
  - Membranous SSTR2A and SSTR5 immunoreactivity has been found in majority of TAs

Electron Microscopy

- Elongated cells resembling nontumorous thyrotrophs
- Cells exhibit distinct polarity with oval to spherical nuclei at 1 pole of cell
- Secretory granules are small (150-250 nm) and exhibit variable electron density
  - Occasionally, densely granulated tumors with larger secretory granules measuring up to 350 nm can be seen

DIFFERENTIAL DIAGNOSIS

Plurihormonal PIT-1-Positive Adenomas

- Prototypic of monomorphous PIT-1 lineage plurihormonal adenomas
  - Focal immunoreactivity for 1 or more PIT-1 lineage adenohypophyseal cell hormones (GH, PRL, β-TSH) is usually seen
  - Positivity for GH &/or PRL favors plurihormonal PIT-1-positive adenoma in sparsely granulated adenoma that reveals positivity for PIT-1 and β-TSH
- Both TAs and plurihormonal PIT-1-positive adenoma exhibit areas of stromal fibrosis
- Demonstration of nuclear inclusions "spheridia" is diagnostic

Plurihormonal Adenomas

- Use of polyclonal and concentrated antibodies against hormones can cause nonspecific cross reactivities; therefore, monoclonal antibodies against hormones and transcription factor antibodies are recommended
- Trapped nontumorous adenohypophyseal cells can be interpreted as component of adenoma

Thyrotroph Hyperplasia

- Patients with longstanding primary hypothyroidism may develop thyrotroph hyperplasia and even TA arising in background of hyperplasia
  - Only rarely these cases will be surgical pathology specimen
  - Serial sections are recommended when dealing with large pituitary lesions that exhibit expanded intact acinar architecture in order to exclude TA arising in background of thyrotroph hyperplasia
- Expanded intact acinar architecture on reticulin stain is characteristic of pituitary hyperplasia

Paraganglioma

- TAs can sometimes be difficult to distinguish from paragangliomas
- Positivity for PIT-1 and negativity for tyrosine hydroxylase favor TA

Metastatic Neuroendocrine Carcinoma

- Positivity for PIT-1 and β-TSH is diagnostic of TA

SELECTED REFERENCES

1. Gupta RK et al: T cell lymphoblastic lymphoma/leukemia within an adrenocorticotropic hormone and thyroid stimulating hormone positive pituitary adenoma: a cytohistological correlation emphasizing importance of intra-operative squash smear. Neuropathology. 37(4):358-364, 2017
2. Osamura RY et al: Thyrotroph adenoma. In Lloyd RV et al: WHO Classification of Tumours of Endocrine Organs. 4th ed. Lyon: IARC. 28-9, 2017
3. Sapkota S et al: Whole-exome sequencing study of thyrotropin-secreting pituitary adenomas. J Clin Endocrinol Metab. 102(2):566-575, 2017
4. Tjörnstrand A et al: Diagnosis of endocrine disease: diagnostic approach to TSH-producing pituitary adenoma. Eur J Endocrinol. ePub, 2017
5. Vargas G et al: An FSH and TSH pituitary adenoma, presenting with precocious puberty and central hyperthyroidism. Endocrinol Diabetes Metab Case Rep. 2017, 2017
6. Yu B et al: Clinical importance of somatostatin receptor 2 (SSTR2) and somatostatin receptor 5 (SSTR5) expression in thyrotropin-producing pituitary adenoma (TSHoma). Med Sci Monit. 23:1947-1955, 2017
7. Amlashi FG et al: Thyrotropin-secreting pituitary adenomas: epidemiology, diagnosis, and management. Endocrine. 52(3):427-40, 2016
8. Azzalin A et al: Comprehensive evaluation of thyrotropinomas: single-center 20-year experience. Pituitary. 19(2):183-93, 2016
9. Mouslech Z et al: TSH-secreting pituitary adenomas treated by gamma knife radiosurgery: our case experience and a review of the literature. Hormones (Athens). 15(1):122-8, 2016
10. Wang Q et al: Ectopic suprasellar thyrotropin-secreting pituitary adenoma: case report and literature review. World Neurosurg. 95:617.e13-617.e18, 2016
11. Johnston PC et al: Thyrotoxicosis with absence of clinical features of acromegaly in a TSH- and GH-secreting, invasive pituitary macroadenoma. Endocrinol Diabetes Metab Case Rep. 2015:140070, 2015
12. Rimareix F et al: Primary medical treatment of thyrotropin-secreting pituitary adenomas by first-generation somatostatin analogs: a case study of seven patients. Thyroid. 25(8):877-82, 2015
13. Yasuda A et al: A case of a TSH-secreting pituitary adenoma associated with evans' syndrome. Tokai J Exp Clin Med. 40(2):44-50, 2015
14. Chinezu L et al: Expression of somatostatin receptors, SSTR2A and SSTR5, in 108 endocrine pituitary tumors using immunohistochemical detection with new specific monoclonal antibodies. Hum Pathol. 45(1):71-7, 2014
15. Fujio S et al: Thyroid storm induced by TSH-secreting pituitary adenoma: a case report. Endocr J. 61(11):1131-6, 2014
16. Kamoun M et al: Coexistence of thyroid-stimulating hormone-secreting pituitary adenoma and graves' hyperthyroidism. Eur Thyroid J. 3(1):60-4, 2014
17. Beck-Peccoz P et al: 2013 European thyroid association guidelines for the diagnosis and treatment of thyrotropin-secreting pituitary tumors. Eur Thyroid J. 2(2):76-82, 2013
18. Scheithauer BW et al: Multiple endocrine neoplasia type 1-associated thyrotropin-producing pituitary carcinoma: report of a probable de novo example. Hum Pathol. 40(2):270-8, 2009
19. Simşek E et al: Pituitary hyperplasia mimicking pituitary macroadenoma in two adolescent patients with long-standing primary hypothyroidism: case reports and review of literature. Turk J Pediatr. 51(6):624-30, 2009
20. Wang EL et al: Clinicopathological characterization of TSH-producing adenomas: special reference to TSH-immunoreactive but clinically non-functioning adenomas. Endocr Pathol. 20(4):209-20, 2009
21. Foppiani L et al: TSH-secreting adenomas: rare pituitary tumors with multifaceted clinical and biological features. J Endocrinol Invest. 30(7):603-9, 2007
22. Umeoka K et al: Expression of GATA-2 in human pituitary adenomas. Mod Pathol. 15(1):11-7, 2002
23. Young M et al: Pituitary hyperplasia resulting from primary hypothyroidism mimicking macroadenomas. Br J Neurosurg. 13(2):138-42, 1999
24. Beck-Peccoz P et al: Thyrotropin-secreting pituitary tumors in hyper- and hypothyroidism. Acta Med Austriaca. 23(1-2):41-6, 1996

α-Subunit Immunohistochemistry

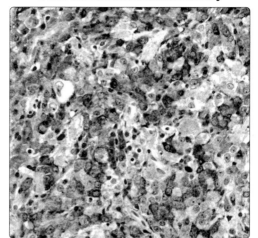

PIT-1 Immunopositivity

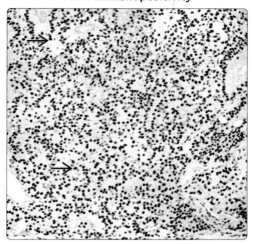

(Left) *In the majority of thyrotroph adenomas, α-subunit of the glycoproteins is immunopositive in addition to β-TSH.* (Right) *Thyrotroph adenomas are strongly and diffusely positive for PIT-1 ⊡. Other acidophilic lineage adenomas also express PIT-1, including somatotroph adenomas, lactotroph adenomas, and plurihormonal PIT-1-positive adenomas.*

Stromal Fibrosis

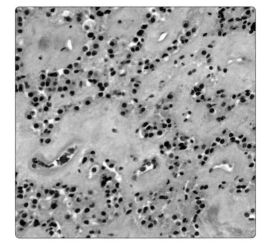

Reticulin Stain

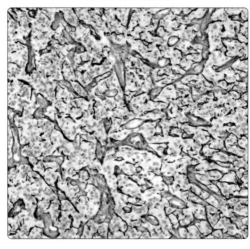

(Left) *Thyrotroph adenomas may exhibit a variable degree of stromal fibrosis. Calcifications may also be present. The stromal fibrosis gives a firm consistency to the adenomas that can be noted by the neurosurgeon during the surgical procedure.* (Right) *The stromal fibrosis can be better highlighted by special stains such as Wilder reticulin.*

Neuroimaging

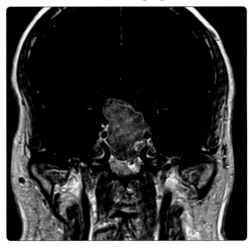

Invasive Pattern

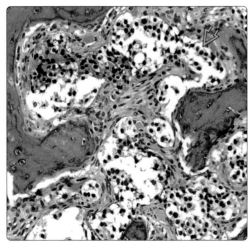

(Left) *Thyrotroph adenomas are most often macroadenomas with supra- and parasellar extension showing invasion of the cavernous sinus (T1-weighted MR post contrast).* (Right) *Thyrotroph adenomas are usually large and invasive adenomas. In this case, bone infiltration is evident with large groups of adenomatous cells ⊡ permeating the bone trabeculae.*

Corticotroph Adenoma

TERMINOLOGY

- Pituitary adenomas that express ACTH and other proopiomelanocortin (POMC) derived peptides and arises from TPIT-lineage adenohypophyseal cells
- Corticotroph adenomas (CAs) are classified into DGCA, SGCA, and Crooke cell adenoma

ETIOLOGY/PATHOGENESIS

- Majority of CAs sporadic
- Rare cases associated with MEN1, MEN4, Carney complex, and familial isolated pituitary adenoma
- Somatic mutations in *USP8* have been identified in ~ 36-62% of sporadic CA

CLINICAL ISSUES

- Cushing disease and CAs constitute 10-15% of all pituitary adenomas
- In adults, peak incidence is 30-40 years with female predominance (F:M = 8:1)
- Rare in pediatric population, where male predominance present
- Some CAs clinically silent

MICROSCOPIC

- Densely granulated (basophilic) to sparsely granulated (chromophobic) cells

ANCILLARY TESTS

- Immunohistochemistry
  - DGCA: ACTH (diffuse), LMWK, TPIT
  - SGCA: ACTH (weak), LMWK, TPIT
  - Crooke cell adenoma: ACTH (weak at cell periphery and perinuclear), LMWK (ring pattern), TPIT

TOP DIFFERENTIAL DIAGNOSES

- Corticotroph hyperplasia
- Metastatic carcinoma
- Gangliocytoma

Corticotroph Microadenoma

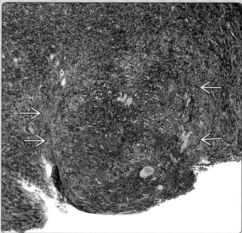

Corticotroph Microadenoma: ACTH

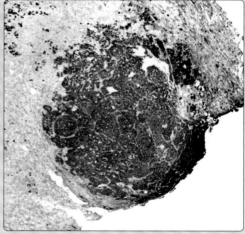

(Left) The majority of Cushing patients present with a corticotroph microadenoma ➡ as demonstrated in this 25-year-old woman. The adenomas are mostly basophilic and, as in this example, tend to have sharp tumor-gland interface. However, invasive tumor within the gland may also occur. (Right) Strong and diffuse immunoreactivity for ACTH is shown in this densely granulated corticotroph microadenoma.

Corticotroph Adenoma, Densely Granulated

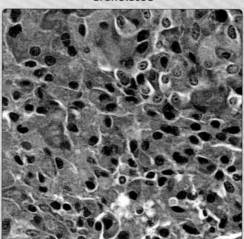

Corticotroph Adenoma, Densely Granulated: ACTH

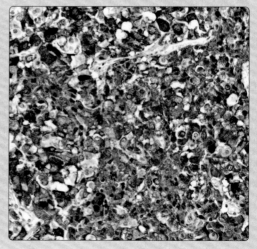

(Left) Densely granulated corticotroph adenoma (CA) is the most common subtype of CA. The adenoma cells typically have a basophilic, granular cytoplasm and a large, hyperchromatic nucleus with prominent nucleoli. (Right) In densely granulated CA, strong and diffuse immunostaining for ACTH is present. In the majority of CA, ACTH is the only pituitary hormone expressed by immunohistochemistry.

TERMINOLOGY

Abbreviations

- Corticotroph adenoma (CA)

Synonyms

- ACTH-producing adenoma
- ACTH-secreting adenoma
- Corticotropinoma
- Basophil adenoma
- ACTH cell adenoma
- ACTHoma

Definitions

- Pituitary adenomas that express ACTH and other proopiomelanocortin (POMC) derived peptides and arises from TPIT-lineage adenohypophyseal cells
- Adenomas causing ACTH excess classified into 3 clinically relevant histological subtypes
  - Densely granulated corticotroph adenoma (DGCA)
  - Sparsely granulated corticotroph adenoma (SGCA)
  - Crooke cell adenoma
- Although highly controversial, corticotroph hyperplasia has been reported as cause of Cushing disease
  - Cortical hyperplasia may rarely occur in setting of ectopic CRH-secreting neuroendocrine neoplasms

ETIOLOGY/PATHOGENESIS

Genetic Susceptibility

- Majority of CAs sporadic
- Rare cases have been reported in
  - Multiple endocrine neoplasia type 1 (MEN1)
  - Multiple endocrine neoplasia type 4 (MEN4)
  - Carney complex
  - Familial isolated pituitary adenoma (FIPA)
  - Tuberous sclerosis
    - Rare: Multiple endocrine neoplasia type 2 (MEN2) has only 1 case reported
- Germline mutations of *DICER1* described in pituitary blastoma, a rare infantile tumor associated with Cushing disease

Somatic Mutations

- Somatic mutations in *USP8*, leading to upregulated EGFR pathway, have been identified in ~ 36-62% of sporadic CA
- Rare CAs have somatic mutation in *GNAS1* and *PRKAR1A*

Epigenetic Silencing of Tumor Suppressors

- Reduced levels of expression, relative to normal pituitary gland, of CDKN1B/p27, CDKN2A/p16, and miR-493
  - Mutations have not been described
- Mice with RB, p27 or p18 gene deletions develop pituitary intermediate lobe tumors

CLINICAL ISSUES

Epidemiology

- Incidence
  - CAs constitute ~ 10-15% of all pituitary adenomas
  - Incidence of Cushing disease is ~ 1-10 cases per million per year
- Age
  - Peak incidence: 30-40 years
  - Rare in pediatric population
- Sex
  - In adults, female predominance (F:M = 8:1)
  - In children, male predominance

Presentation

- Signs and symptoms related to hypercortisolism
  - Centripetal obesity, hypertension, hyperglycemia, plethoric moon-shaped face, hirsutism, acne, menstrual irregularities, bruising, myopathy, osteoporosis, hypokalemia, hypernatremia, infections, and psychosis
- Severe pituitary-dependent ACTH excess may result in hyperpigmentation due to overproduction of POMC-derived MSH
- Nelson syndrome
  - Defined as rapid enlargement of CA following bilateral adrenalectomy
  - Characterized by muscle weakness and hyperpigmentation due to excess MSH
  - Rarely seen nowadays
- Sometimes CAs can be clinically silent

Treatment

- Main objective is to reduce ACTH levels to within normal range and normalize cortisol secretion
- Surgical resection main treatment
- Radiotherapy considered when surgery unsuccessful
- Medical therapy not widely used
- Temozolomide has proven valuable in small number of aggressive CAs

Prognosis

- Best prognosticator postoperative reduction in cortisol
- Silent CAs have more aggressive clinical behavior than other clinically nonfunctioning adenomas

IMAGING

Radiologic Features

- Microadenomas common (60-80%)
  - MR findings can sometimes be subtle, and microadenomas may not be identified or localized
  - Selective petrosal sinus sampling with CRH stimulation is useful to identify and localize lesions
    - MR with bilateral inferior petrosal sinus sampling
      - Failure to localize lesion common
      - ~ 10% of Cushing disease cases associated with no visible pituitary mass on MR
- Macroadenomas seen in patients with SGCAs, Crooke cell adenomas, and silent CAs
  - 5-10% macroadenomas
  - Silent corticotroph adenoma tend to present as macroadenomas invading cavernous sinuses

MACROSCOPIC

General Features

- Most CAs small (< 6 mm), soft, and red lesions

MICROSCOPIC

Densely Granulated Corticotroph Adenoma

- Basophilic cells exhibiting sinusoidal growth

Sparsely Granulated Corticotroph Adenoma

- Chromophobic cells exhibiting diffuse growth

Crooke Cell Adenoma

- Large chromophobic or slightly acidophilic tumor cells with nuclear pleomorphism
  - Crooke hyaline change in majority of tumor cells

Silent Corticotroph Adenomas

- Type 1 silent CA similar to DGCAs but unassociated with clinical evidence of excess ACTH
- Type 2 silent CA similar to SGCAs but unassociated with clinical evidence of excess ACTH

Crooke Hyaline Change

- In patients with glucocorticoid excess, normal corticotrophs develop accumulations of intermediate filament keratin that have glassy appearance on histology
  - This phenomenon, known as Crooke hyaline change, results in relocation of secretory granules to cell periphery and juxtanuclear location
- Intermediate lobe (basophil invasion zone) corticotrophs not sensitive to suppression of hypercortisolemia and unlikely to exhibit Crooke hyaline change
- Presence of this change in nontumorous adenohypophysis not diagnostic of CA in vicinity; it is diagnostic of hypercortisolism regardless of pathogenesis

ANCILLARY TESTS

Histochemistry

- PAS highlights basophilic granules of corticotrophs

Immunohistochemistry

- Densely granulated CA
  - Variably positive for ACTH (usually strong and diffuse); TPIT nuclear positivity
    - As of now, no commercial antibody for TPIT available
  - LMWK strongly expressed
- Sparsely granulated CA
  - Faintly positive for ACTH; TPIT nuclear positivity
  - LMWK less strong expressed than DGCA
- Crooke cell adenoma
  - Granular ACTH reactivity at cell periphery and adjacent to nucleus; TPIT nuclear positivity
  - Typical "ring-like" abundant LMWK

Electron Microscopy

- Densely granulated CA
  - Well-developed RER and Golgi complex
  - Dense secretory granules (150-450 nm)
    - Marked variability in electron density and shape (indented, teardrop, or heart shaped)
  - Intermediate filaments located predominantly around nucleus
- Sparsely granulated CA
  - Less well-developed organelles
  - Small, variably shaped granules (200-250 nm)
  - Keratin filaments fewer than DGCAs
- Crooke cell adenoma
  - Cytoplasm filled with intermediate filaments
  - Secretory granules limited to cell periphery and immediately adjacent to nucleus

DIFFERENTIAL DIAGNOSIS

Corticotroph Hyperplasia

- Breakdown of acinar architecture on silver stain is diagnostic of pituitary adenoma; hyperplasia characterized by expended but still intact acinar architecture

Metastatic Carcinoma

- Atypical large cells of Crooke cell adenoma may mimic metastatic carcinoma

Gangliocytoma

- Crooke cell adenoma may mimic gangliocytomas

SELECTED REFERENCES

1. Lonser RR et al: Cushing's disease: pathobiology, diagnosis, and management. J Neurosurg. 126(2):404-417, 2017
2. Mete O et al: Corticotroph adenoma. In: WHO Classification of Tumours of Endocrine Organs, 4th Edition. IARC: Lyon. 30-33, 2017
3. Fountas A et al: Cushing's syndrome due to CRH and ACTH co-secreting pancreatic tumor–presentation of a new case focusing on diagnostic pitfalls. Endocr Pathol. 26(3):239-42, 2015
4. Oldfield EH et al: Crooke's changes In Cushing's syndrome depends on degree of hypercortisolism and individual susceptibility. J Clin Endocrinol Metab. 100(8):3165-71, 2015
5. Perez-Rivas LG et al: The gene of the ubiquitin-specific protease 8 is frequently mutated in adenomas causing Cushing's disease. J Clin Endocrinol Metab. 100(7):E997-1004, 2015
6. Reincke M et al: Mutations in the deubiquitinase gene USP8 cause Cushing's disease. Nat Genet. 47(1):31-8, 2015
7. Seltzer J et al: Gene and protein expression in pituitary corticotroph adenomas: a systematic review of the literature. Neurosurg Focus. 38(2):E17, 2015
8. de Kock L et al: Pituitary blastoma: a pathognomonic feature of germ-line DICER1 mutations. Acta Neuropathol. 128(1):111-22, 2014
9. Xu Z et al: Silent corticotroph adenomas after stereotactic radiosurgery: a case-control study. Int J Radiat Oncol Biol Phys. 90(4):903-10, 2014
10. Raverot G et al: Clinical, hormonal and molecular characterization of pituitary ACTH adenomas without (silent corticotroph adenomas) and with Cushing's disease. Eur J Endocrinol. 163(1):35-43, 2010
11. Al Brahim NY et al: Complex endocrinopathies in MEN-1: diagnostic dilemmas in endocrine oncology. Endocr Pathol. 18(1):37-41, 2007
12. Scheithauer BW et al: Clinically silent corticotroph tumors of the pituitary gland. Neurosurgery. 47(3):723-9; discussion 729-30, 2000

Corticotroph Adenoma, Sparsely Granulated

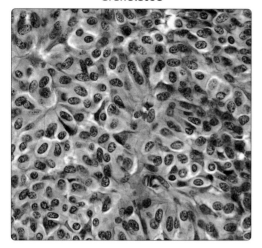

Corticotroph Adenoma, Sparsely Granulated: ACTH

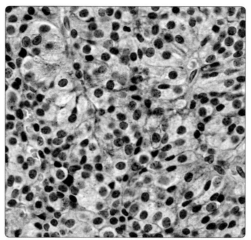

(Left) *Sparsely granulated CAs are composed of lightly basophilic or chromophobic cells. The cells contain more regular nucleus than the densely granulated adenomas. In this case, a hint of papillary formation is present.* (Right) *Unlike the densely granulated adenomas, ACTH immunoexpression in sparsely granulated CA is variable with faint and focal immunopositivity. Immunostaining for TPIT is confirmatory of the corticotroph differentiation.*

Crooke Cell Adenoma

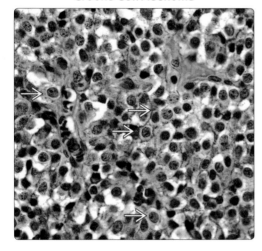

Crooke Cell Adenoma: ACTH

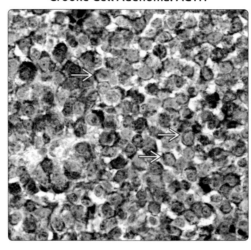

(Left) *Crooke cell adenomas are composed of > 60% of cells displaying Crooke changes, consistent with a target-like appearance of the tumor cells. In these cells, the secretory granules are displaced to the periphery of the cytoplasm* ➡. (Right) *Immunostain for ACTH highlights the displacement of the secretory granules to the periphery of the tumor cell cytoplasm* ➡, *a typical feature of Crooke cells.*

Crooke Cell Adenoma: LMWK

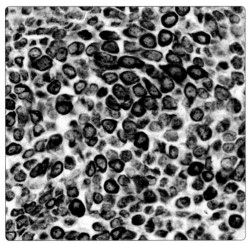

Corticotroph Adenoma: TPIT

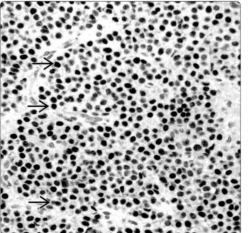

(Left) *Immunostain for keratin (CAM5.2) shows the typical accumulation of this intermediate filament in a ring-like positivity.* (Right) *Regardless of the histological subtype, all CAs are diffusely positive for TPIT* ➡. *Other pituitary adenomas are negative for TPIT. Of note, no commercial antibodies to TPIT are available at the moment.*

TERMINOLOGY

- Pituitary adenomas that express gonadotropin hormones, FSH and LH, and arise from SF1 (steroidogenic factor 1) lineage adenohypophyseal cells

ETIOLOGY/PATHOGENESIS

- GAs have been described in setting of MEN1 syndrome

CLINICAL ISSUES

- GAs common in middle-aged or older patients and have slight male predominance
- GAs represent most clinically nonfunctioning pituitary adenomas with symptoms of mass effect and hypogonadism
- Most common clinically nonfunctioning adenoma
- ~ 30% of surgically resected pituitary adenomas

IMAGING

- Usually presents as large macroadenoma with significant suprasellar or parasellar extension

MICROSCOPIC

- Composed of chromophobic cells with prominent sinusoidal, trabecular, or papillary architecture; prominent pseudorosette formations around blood vessels

ANCILLARY TESTS

- Immunohistochemistry
  - Variable immunopositivity for β-FSH, β-LH &/or α-subunit of glycoproteins
  - Immunoexpression of SF1, ER-α, and GATA
- Hormone immunonegative adenomas may be strongly positive for SF1 confirming gonadotroph differentiation

TOP DIFFERENTIAL DIAGNOSES

- Null cell adenoma
- Plurihormonal adenoma
- Acidophil stem cell adenoma
- Paraganglioma
- Metastatic neuroendocrine carcinoma

Gonadotroph Macroadenoma

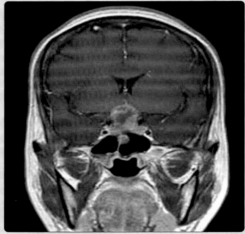

Gonadotroph Adenoma: Trabecular Pattern

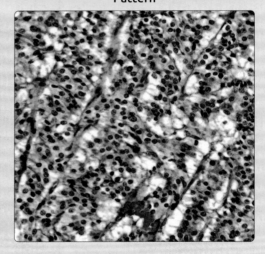

(Left) Gonadotroph adenomas (GAs) are the most common nonfunctioning pituitary adenomas. They usually lack a characteristic clinical syndrome and present when they have become large macroadenomas, as seen here. (Right) GAs are mostly composed of chromophobic cells with several histological patterns including nests, prominent trabecular and sinusoidal arrangements along blood vessels, as illustrated here.

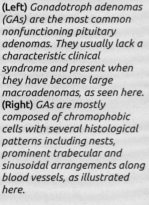

Gonadotroph Adenoma: Pseudorosette Pattern

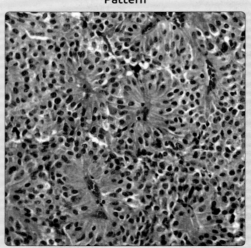

Gonadotroph Adenoma: Perivascular Arrangements

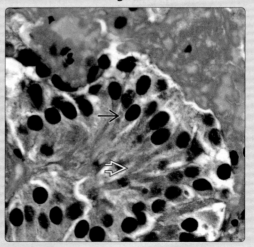

(Left) Differentiated GA shows typical growth of pseudopapillary and pseudorosette formations around blood vessels, as highlighted here. The tumor cells are elongated, showing marked cellular polarity. (Right) Marked polarity of cells with elongated cell processes ⇉ and eccentric nuclei ⇨ are characteristic of these perivascular arrangements. These tumors tend to exhibit variable positivity for gonadotropins.

TERMINOLOGY

Abbreviations
- Gonadotroph adenoma (GA)

Synonyms
- FSHoma
- LHoma
- FSH/LH cell adenoma

Definitions
- Pituitary adenomas that express gonadotropin hormones, FSH and LH, and arise from SF1 (steroidogenic factor 1) lineage adenohypophyseal cells

ETIOLOGY/PATHOGENESIS

Unknown
- Majority of cases sporadic
  - GAs have been described in setting of MEN1 syndrome

GnRH/Gonadal Steroid Imbalance
- Gonadotropin-releasing hormone (GnRH) and gonadal steroids regulate secretion of gonadotropins
- Patients with untreated, longstanding primary hypogonadism can develop GAs

CLINICAL ISSUES

Epidemiology
- Incidence
  - Most common clinically nonfunctioning adenoma
  - ~ 30% of surgically resected pituitary adenomas
- Age
  - Generally present in middle-aged or older patients but also occur in younger people
- Sex
  - Male predominance

Presentation
- GAs represent most clinically nonfunctioning pituitary adenomas
  - More often detected due to mass effects, including hypopituitarism and visual disturbances
  - Rarely symptoms or signs of gonadal dysfunction can be seen
- In premenopausal females and younger patients, these tumors are very rare
  - This population of patients may present with ovarian hyperstimulation syndrome symptoms, including
    - Menstrual disturbances
    - Abdominal distension
    - Abdominal or pelvic pain
- GAs more difficult to diagnose clinically in women
  - Perimenopausal and postmenopausal woman have physiologically increased serum gonadotropin levels
    - Thus making diagnosis of gonadotropin-producing adenoma difficult
- Hormonally active tumors most seen in men

Treatment
- Major aim in treatment of GA is to eliminate mass effect and correct hypopituitarism
- Surgery primary treatment for GAs
- Octreotide may reduce elevated gonadotropin levels in some patients
- Radiotherapy reserved for aggressive, recurrent, and invasive GAs

Prognosis
- Tumor recurrence at 10 years post surgery as high as 50%; depends on ability to completely resect tumor tissue

IMAGING

Radiologic Features
- Usually presents as large macroadenoma with significant suprasellar or parasellar extension
- Majority not invasive tumors; MR useful for determination of extent of invasion

MACROSCOPIC

General Features
- Usually large adenomas with soft consistency
- May exhibit areas of hemorrhage

MICROSCOPIC

Histologic Features
- Composed of chromophobic cells with prominent sinusoidal, trabecular, or papillary architecture; prominent pseudorosette formations around blood vessels
  - Differentiated tumors exhibit marked polarization of cells with elongated cell processes and eccentric nuclei
- Variable oncocytic change can be seen

ANCILLARY TESTS

Immunohistochemistry
- β-FSH, β-LH &/or α-subunit expressed in variable pattern of intensity and extension
  - Positivity usually focal
  - Most common combination β-FSH or β-LH and α-subunit
- SF1, ER-α, and GATA2 expressed
  - ER-α also expressed in mammosomatotrophs and lactotrophs
  - GATA2 also expressed in thyrotrophs
- Hormone immunonegative adenomas may be strongly positive for SF1, confirming gonadotroph differentiation

Electron Microscopy
- Heterogeneous ultrastructural features
  - Distinctive polar elongated cells with prominent cell processes in differentiated GAs
  - Round/polygonal cells in poorly differentiated GAs
  - Large and globular Golgi complexes
  - Variably small secretory granules (< 250 nm)
    - In differentiated cells, secretory granules tend to be localized at opposite pole from nucleus
  - When oncocytic change occurs, numerous mitochondria seen

DIFFERENTIAL DIAGNOSIS

Null Cell Adenoma

- Use of appropriate pituitary transcription SF1 immunostaining prevents these adenomas from being mistakenly diagnosed as null cell adenoma
  - Poorly differentiated GAs usually contain few secretory granules that cannot be detected immunohistochemically
    - Therefore, GAs can sometimes be negative for β-LH and β-FSH
- Similar to GAs, null cell adenomas can exhibit oncocytic change

Gonadotroph Hyperplasia

- Extremely rare condition that hardly ever would originate surgical pathology specimen
- Expanded acinar microarchitecture seen on silver stain diagnostic of hyperplasia

Plurihormonal Adenoma

- Use of polyclonal or suboptimally diluted antibodies against pituitary hormones can cause nonspecific false-positives in adenomas
- Trapped nontumorous gonadotrophs can be mistaken as component of another adenoma
  - And thus may be considered as plurihormonal adenoma

Acidophil Stem Cell Adenoma

- Variable oncocytic change seen in GAs mimic morphological features of acidophil stem cell adenoma
- Positivity for SF1 favors gonadotroph differentiation since acidophil stem cell adenomas are of PIT1-lineage

Paraganglioma and Metastatic Neuroendocrine Carcinoma

- Can be difficult to distinguish morphologically from GAs
  - GAs and metastatic neuroendocrine carcinomas can sometimes be negative for keratins
- While paragangliomas positive for tyrosine hydroxylase
  - Metastatic neuroendocrine carcinomas and GAs negative for tyrosine hydroxylase
- Negativity for pituitary transcription factors (PIT1, SF1, TPIT) and positivity for other transcription factors (CDX-2, TTF-1, etc.) favors metastatic neuroendocrine carcinoma in setting of appropriate clinical history

SELECTED REFERENCES

1. Caretto A et al: Ovarian hyperstimulation syndrome due to follicle-stimulating hormone-secreting pituitary adenomas. Pituitary. ePub, 2017
2. McDonald WC et al: Steroidogenic factor 1, pit-1, and adrenocorticotropic hormone: A rational starting place for the immunohistochemical characterization of pituitary adenoma. Arch Pathol Lab Med. 141(1):104-112, 2017
3. Yamada S et al. Gonadotroph adenoma. In: WHO Classification of Tumours of Endocrine Organs, 4th Edition. IARC: Lyon. 34-36, 2017
4. Cote DJ et al: Functional gonadotroph adenomas: Case series and report of literature. Neurosurgery. 79(6):823-831, 2016
5. Kontogeorgos G et al: The gonadotroph origin of null cell adenomas. Hormones (Athens). 15(2):243-7, 2016
6. Halupczok J et al: Ovarian hyperstimulation caused by gonadotroph pituitary adenoma–Review. Adv Clin Exp Med. 24(4):695-703, 2015
7. Lee M et al: SSTR3 is a putative target for the medical treatment of gonadotroph adenomas of the pituitary. Endocr Relat Cancer. 22(1):111-9, 2015
8. Nishioka H et al: The complementary role of transcription factors in the accurate diagnosis of clinically nonfunctioning pituitary adenomas. Endocr Pathol. ePub, 2015
9. Alband N et al: Familial pituitary tumors. Handb Clin Neurol. 124:339-60, 2014
10. Ntali G et al: Clinical review: Functioning gonadotroph adenomas. J Clin Endocrinol Metab. 99(12):4423-33, 2014
11. Kawaguchi T et al: Follicle-stimulating hormone-secreting pituitary adenoma manifesting as recurrent ovarian cysts in a young woman–latent risk of unidentified ovarian hyperstimulation: a case report. BMC Res Notes. 6:408, 2013
12. Fernández-Balsells MM et al: Natural history of nonfunctioning pituitary adenomas and incidentalomas: a systematic review and metaanalysis. J Clin Endocrinol Metab. 96(4):905-12, 2011
13. Fernandez A et al: Prevalence of pituitary adenomas: a community-based, cross-sectional study in Banbury (Oxfordshire, UK). Clin Endocrinol (Oxf). 72(3):377-82, 2010
14. Greenman Y et al: Non-functioning pituitary adenomas. Best Pract Res Clin Endocrinol Metab. 23(5):625-38, 2009
15. Benito M et al: Gonadotroph tumor associated with multiple endocrine neoplasia type 1. J Clin Endocrinol Metab. 90(1):570-4, 2005
16. Sano T et al: "Honeycomb Golgi" in pituitary adenomas: not a marker of gonadotroph adenomas. Endocr Pathol. 14(4):363-8, 2003
17. Asa SL et al: The transcription activator steroidogenic factor-1 is preferentially expressed in the human pituitary gonadotroph. J Clin Endocrinol Metab. 81(6):2165-70, 1996
18. Horvath E et al: Ultrastructural diagnosis of human pituitary adenomas. Microsc Res Tech. 20(2):107-35, 1992
19. Nicolis G et al: Gonadotropin-producing pituitary adenoma in a man with long-standing primary hypogonadism. J Clin Endocrinol Metab. 66(1):237-41, 1988
20. Kovacs K et al: Gonadotroph cell adenoma of the pituitary in a women with long-standing hypogonadism. Arch Gynecol. 229(1):57-65, 1980

Gonadotroph Adenoma: Oncocytic Changes

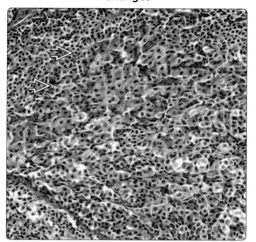

Gonadotroph Adenoma: Oncocytic Changes

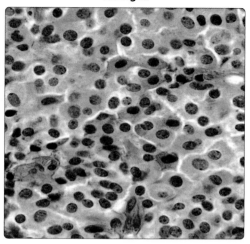

(Left) *Focal oncocytic changes* ⇒ *may be seen in GAs, characterized by granular eosinophilic cytoplasm due to accumulation of mitochondria. Note the focus of oncocytic cells surrounded by other more chromophobic cells.* (Right) *High magnification of the same case highlights the eosinophilic, granular cytoplasm of cells displaying oncocytic changes. Oncocytic changes may also occur in null cell adenomas.*

Gonadotroph Adenoma: BFSH

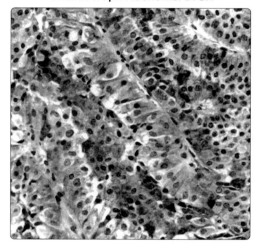

Gonadotroph Adenoma: BFSH

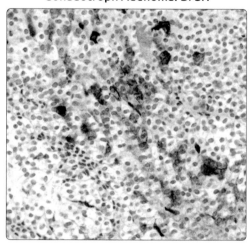

(Left) *Variable immunostaining for glycoprotein hormones may be detected in GA. In this example, strong and diffuse staining for β-FSH is present within the elongated cells surrounding blood vessels.* (Right) *In comparison with the previous adenoma, this case showed only faint and focal positivity, and immunoreactivity for β-FSH was present.*

Gonadotroph Adenoma: Transcription Factor

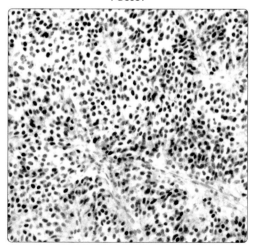

Gonadotroph Adenoma: ER-α

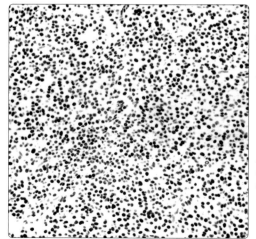

(Left) *GAs display strong nuclear expression of the steroidogenic factor 1 (SF1) that drives gonadotroph differentiation. In some GAs, glycoprotein hormonal expression may be minimal or absent. SF1 immunoexpression differentiates them from null cell adenomas.* (Right) *ER-α is variably expressed in GA tumor cells. ER-α can sometimes be weak or even negative due to poor tissue fixation.*

Null Cell Adenoma

KEY FACTS

TERMINOLOGY

- Null cell adenoma (NA)
- Adenomas composed of adenohypophyseal cells that do not exhibit any evidence of cell-type-specific differentiation using pituitary hormones, pituitary transcription factors, and ultrastructural features

ETIOLOGY/PATHOGENESIS

- No evidence of increased development of NAs in patients with syndromes associated with pituitary adenomas

CLINICAL ISSUES

- Incidence decreased significantly due to more strict pathologic criteria allowing accurate classification of hormone immunonegative adenomas
- Usually in elderly individuals (6th and 7th decades); slight male preponderance
- Clinically nonfunctioning neoplasms with mass effects, including hypopituitarism

- Surgical decompression and debulking remains main treatment of choice

IMAGING

- NAs are usually macroadenomas with parasellar and suprasellar extension

MICROSCOPIC

- Composed of chromophobic cells with solid and diffuse growth

ANCILLARY TESTS

- Negative for pituitary hormones and pituitary transcription factors

TOP DIFFERENTIAL DIAGNOSES

- Hormone-negative gonadotroph adenoma
- Metastatic neuroendocrine carcinoma
- Paraganglioma

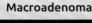

Macroadenoma

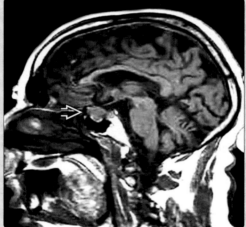

Sinusoidal Arrangement

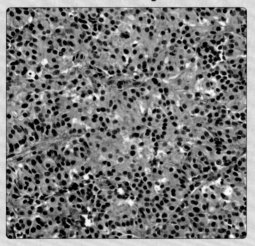

(Left) Null cell pituitary adenomas are clinically nonfunctioning neoplasms that present on imaging as invasive macroadenomas ➡, frequently with extrasellar extension. (Right) Null cell adenomas are composed of chromophobic or slightly eosinophilic cells arranged in a sinusoidal pattern with cells surrounding blood vessels. With the new and more strict classification criteria of null cell adenomas, the incidence of these adenomas has decreased significantly.

Cytologic Features

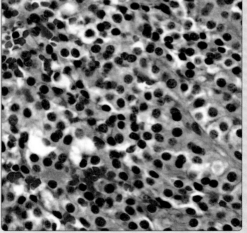

Negative Immunohistochemistry

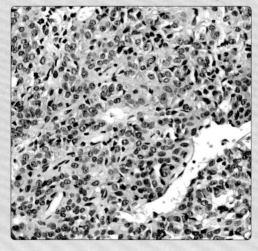

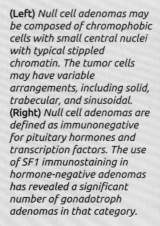

(Left) Null cell adenomas may be composed of chromophobic cells with small central nuclei with typical stippled chromatin. The tumor cells may have variable arrangements, including solid, trabecular, and sinusoidal. (Right) Null cell adenomas are defined as immunonegative for pituitary hormones and transcription factors. The use of SF1 immunostaining in hormone-negative adenomas has revealed a significant number of gonadotroph adenomas in that category.

TERMINOLOGY

Abbreviations

- Null cell adenoma (NA)

Definitions

- Adenomas composed of adenohypophyseal cells that do not exhibit any evidence of cell-type-specific differentiation using pituitary hormones and pituitary transcription factors by immunohistochemistry (WHO 2017)

ETIOLOGY/PATHOGENESIS

Genetic Susceptibility

- No evidence of increased development of NAs in syndromes associated with pituitary adenomas, including Carney complex or multiple endocrine neoplasia type 1

Somatic Genetics

- Cytogenetic alterations described in NAs overlap with findings seen in gonadotroph adenomas
  - No studies have been reported since new and more strict classification of NA

CLINICAL ISSUES

Epidemiology

- Incidence
  - Decreased significantly due to more strict histopathologic criteria
    - Accurate classification of hormone immunonegative adenomas has changed incidence of NAs
  - In old series, poorly differentiated gonadotroph adenomas negative for FSH-β or LH-β were considered NAs
    - However, use of SF-1, ER-α, and GATA2 confirm these tumors as gonadotroph adenomas
- Sex
  - Slight male preponderance is observed

Presentation

- Clinically nonfunctioning neoplasms with mass effects, including hypopituitarism

Treatment

- Surgical decompression and debulking remains main treatment of choice
- No effective pharmacotherapeutical option
- Radiotherapy is considered selectively for recurrent aggressive NAs

Prognosis

- Invasive macroadenomas usually recur when complete resection is not possible

IMAGING

Radiological Features

- NAs are usually macroadenomas with parasellar and suprasellar extension

MACROSCOPIC

General Features

- NAs are usually soft, yellow-tan lesions that may exhibit hemorrhagic and cystic changes

MICROSCOPIC

Histologic Features

- Composed of chromophobic cells with solid and diffuse growth
- Oncocytic change is commonly seen

ANCILLARY TESTS

Immunohistochemistry

- Negative for pituitary hormones (GH, PRL, β-TSH, β-FSH, β-LH, ACTH, and α-subunit)
- Negative for pituitary transcription factors (PIT-1, SF1 and TPIT) and other cofactors (GATA2 and ER-α)
- Variably positive for LMWK (CAM5.2), synaptophysin, and chromogranin

DIFFERENTIAL DIAGNOSIS

Hormone-Negative Gonadotroph Adenoma

- Use of pituitary cell-specific transcription factors is essential to classify accurately hormone-negative adenomas
- Positivity for SF1 &/or ER-α and GATA2 in hormone-negative adenoma is diagnostic of gonadotroph adenoma

Metastatic Neuroendocrine Carcinoma

- Past medical history of neuroendocrine carcinoma &/or positivity for other transcription factors favors possibility of metastatic neuroendocrine carcinoma

Paraganglioma

- Sellar paragangliomas are negative for keratins and positive for tyrosine hydroxylase
- NAs are negative for tyrosine hydroxylase and can be variably positive for keratins

Adenomas With Oncocytic Change

- Acidophilic stem cell adenomas, some gonadotroph adenomas, and NAs may exhibit oncocytic change
- Use of pituitary hormone and transcription factor antibodies is essential to classify adenomas with oncocytic change

SELECTED REFERENCES

1. Nishioka H et al: Null cell adenoma. In Lloyd RV et al.: WHO Classification of Tumours of Endocrine Organs. 4th Edition. Lyon:IARC. 37-38, 2017.
2. Kontogeorgos G et al: The gonadotroph origin of null cell adenomas. Hormones (Athens). 15(2):243-7, 2016
3. Balogun JA et al: Null cell adenomas of the pituitary gland: an institutional review of their clinical imaging and behavioral characteristics. Endocr Pathol. 26(1):63-70, 2015
4. Nishioka H et al: The complementary role of transcription factors in the accurate diagnosis of clinically nonfunctioning pituitary adenomas. Endocr Pathol. 26(4):349-55, 2015
5. Mayson SE et al: Silent (clinically nonfunctioning) pituitary adenomas. J Neurooncol. 117(3):429-36, 2014

TERMINOLOGY

- Plurihormonal adenoma (PHA): Pituitary adenomas producing > 1 pituitary hormone that cannot be accounted for by current concepts of adenohypophyseal cytodifferentiation
- WHO classification recommends following tumors included
  - Plurihormonal PIT-1-positive adenomas (previously called silent subtype III adenomas)
  - Clinically functioning adenomas, including GH-PRL-TSH secreting adenomas with acromegaly and thyroid dysfunction
  - Adenomas with unusual combinations of pituitary hormones that do not fit cytodifferentiation pattern

CLINICAL ISSUES

- All rare adenomas (< 1% of all adenomas)
- Most PHAs clinically nonfunctioning adenomas
  - Plurihormonal PIT-1-positive adenomas may present hyperprolactinemia, acromegaly, or hyperthyroidism

MICROSCOPIC

- Plurihormonal PIT-1-positive adenomas display chromophobic to slightly acidophilic cells with diffuse growth

ANCILLARY TESTS

- Plurihormonal PIT-1-positive adenomas show strong PIT-1 positivity
  - Focal GH, PRL, β-TSH, and α-subunit
  - Nuclear inclusions called "spheridia" characteristic by EM
- Other PHAs show unusual pituitary hormones immunopositivity; ACTH is rare

TOP DIFFERENTIAL DIAGNOSES

- Adenomas with trapped nontumorous adenohypophyseal cells
- Acidophilic stem cell adenoma
- Thyrotroph adenoma

Plurihormonal PIT-1-Positive Adenoma

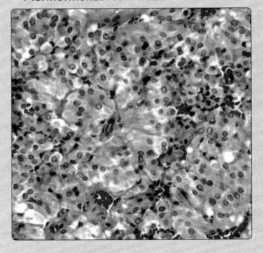

Plurihormonal PIT-1-Positive Adenoma

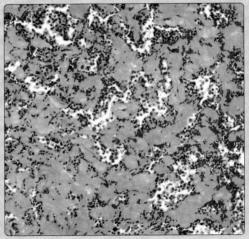

(Left) *Plurihormonal PIT-1-positive adenomas tend to be composed of large, chromophobic cells with large nuclei and prominent nucleoli. These adenomas used to be called silent subtype III adenoma.* **(Right)** *Plurihormonal PIT-1-positive adenomas may show variable degree of fibrosis. They may be clinically silent, but others may be clinically active, presenting with symptoms of mild hyperprolactinemia, acromegaly, and thyroid disturbances.*

Plurihormonal PIT-1-Positive Adenoma: Reticulin

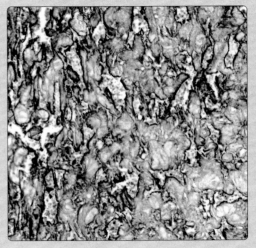

Plurihormonal PIT-1-Positive Adenoma: Cellular Atypia

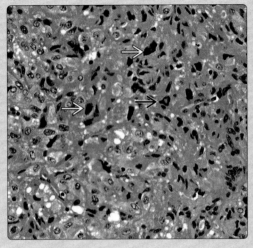

(Left) *Plurihormonal PIT-1-positive adenoma shows extensive stromal desmoplasia as demonstrated in a Wilder reticulin stain. The differential diagnosis of these adenomas includes thyrotroph adenomas that can also exhibit extensive desmoplasia.* **(Right)** *Plurihormonal PIT-1-positive adenomas may exhibit nuclear pleomorphism ➡ and nuclear inclusions ➡. Regardless of the presence of cellular atypia, these adenomas tend to have a more aggressive clinical behavior.*

TERMINOLOGY

Abbreviations

- Plurihormonal adenoma (PHA)

Synonyms

- Multihormonal adenoma
- Polyhormonal adenoma
- Multiple adenomas

Definitions

- PHA: Pituitary adenomas producing > 1 pituitary hormone that cannot be accounted for by current concepts of adenohypophyseal cytodifferentiation
- Can be divided into 2 types
  - Monomorphous PHA
    - Composed of 1 cell type that is capable of producing 2 (or rarely several) hormones
  - Plurimorphous PHA
    - Composed of at least 2 (or rarely more) cell different populations of cells
- WHO classification recommends following tumors included in this category
  - Plurihormonal PIT-1-positive adenomas (previously called silent subtype III adenomas)
  - Clinically functioning adenomas including GH-PRL-TSH secreting adenomas with acromegaly and thyroid dysfunction
  - Adenomas with unusual combinations of pituitary hormones by immunostaining that do not fit cytodifferentiation pattern
  - Adenomas with combinations of same cytodifferentiation (such as somatotroph adenomas with GH/PRL immunopositivity or gonadotroph adenomas with FSH/LH immunopositivity) are not considered PHA

ETIOLOGY/PATHOGENESIS

Largely Unknown

- Hypothesized as incidental occurrence of 2 separate monoclonal neoplastic components
- Alternatively, they might be derived from clonal expansions of primitive or uncommitted stem cells

Genetic Susceptibility

- A few cases of PIT-1-positive adenomas are associated with
  - Multiple endocrine neoplasia type 1 (MEN1)
  - Familial pituitary adenoma

CLINICAL ISSUES

Epidemiology

- Incidence
  - Plurihormonal PIT-1-positive adenoma described to account for < 1% of all adenomas
  - Other PHAs extremely rare
    - Reported incidence rates of double adenomas
      - 0.4-1.3% in surgical series
      - 0.9-1.85% in autopsies
    - Triple adenomas are rare in surgical series
- Age
  - Plurihormonal PIT-1-positive adenomas prevalent in younger patients (mean: 44.3 years)
    - No data regarding other rarer PHAs
- Sex
  - Plurihormonal PIT-1-positive adenomas have slight female predominance
    - No data regarding other rarer PHAs

Presentation

- Most PHAs clinically nonfunctioning adenomas
- Plurihormonal PIT-1-positive adenomas
  - Majority silent, although some may be associated with hyperprolactinemia, acromegaly, or hyperthyroidism
- Large PHAs with extensive suprasellar extension may cause mild hyperprolactinemia due to stalk compression
  - Other symptoms of mass compression include hypopituitarism and visual disturbances
- Clinical diagnosis is difficult distinguishing functioning plurihormonal adenomas and double adenomas
  - Due to combined hormone secretion

Treatment

- Surgery is main treatment; radiotherapy selectively considered in aggressive tumors

Prognosis

- Plurihormonal PIT-1-positive adenomas are aggressive tumors
  - Cavernous sinus invasion occurs in 67% of cases
  - Rate of persistent tumor is 59%
  - Recurrence rate of ~ 30%
- Plurihormonal PIT1-positive carcinomas have been reported

IMAGING

General Features

- PHAs usually macroadenomas with extrasellar extension

MACROSCOPIC

General Features

- Variable gross appearances

MICROSCOPIC

Monomorphous PHA

- Plurihormonal PIT-1-positive adenoma is prototype of monomorphous PHA
  - Chromophobe
    - Chromophobic to slightly acidophilic cells that exhibit solid and diffuse growth
  - Negative PAS reaction
- May exhibit stromal fibrosis

Polymorphous PHA

- Variable morphology

ANCILLARY TESTS

Immunohistochemistry

- Plurihormonal PIT-1-positive adenoma
  - PIT-1 is often diffusely and strongly expressed
  - Focal immunoreactivity for one or more PIT-1 lineage adenohypophyseal cell hormones
    - PRL, GH, β-TSH, and α-subunit

- ○ ER-α variably expressed
- ○ Plurihormonal PIT-1-positive adenomas may express somatostatin receptors
  - − Respond to long-acting somatostatin analogues
- Other unusual plurihormonal adenomas
  - ○ Multiple combinations of pituitary hormones
  - ○ PHAs rarely positive for ACTH

Electron Microscopy

- Plurihormonal PIT-1-positive adenoma
  - ○ Nuclear inclusions (so-called "spheridia") typical and helpful for confirmation of diagnosis
  - ○ Secretory granules usually sparse (100-200 nm) and located in cell processes

DIFFERENTIAL DIAGNOSIS

Adenomas With Trapped Nontumorous Adenohypophyseal Cells

- Trapped nontumorous cells can be mistaken for adenoma cells, and adenoma may be misclassified as PHA
  - ○ Careful analysis by H&E, reticulin stains, and serial sectioning with pituitary hormones helpful for discrimination of entrapped normal pituitary cells
  - ○ Presence of a few scattered cells positive for other hormones not unequivocal evidence of true plurihormonal adenoma
- Lineage-specific pituitary transcription factors highlight polymorphous phenotype and also confirm hormone reactivities

Acidophilic Stem Cell Adenoma

- Sometimes plurihormonal PIT-1-positive adenomas may present with hyperprolactinemia similar to patients with acidophilic stem cell adenomas
  - ○ Both are invasive macroadenomas
- Negativity for β-TSH and presence of oncocytic change and fibrous bodies should suggest acidophilic stem cell adenoma

Thyrotroph Adenoma

- Positivity for β-TSH observed in plurihormonal PIT-1-positive adenomas may mimic thyrotroph adenomas
- Positivity for GH or PRL should suggest possibility of plurihormonal PIT-1-positive adenoma
- Demonstration of spheridia will confirm this diagnosis

Metastatic Neuroendocrine Carcinoma

- Negativity for PIT-1 and positivity for other transcription factors (CDX-2, TTF-1, etc.) favors this diagnosis in setting of appropriate clinical history

SELECTED REFERENCES

1. Kontogeorgos G et al. Plurihormonal and double adenomas. In: WHO Classification of Tumours of Endocrine Organs, 4th Edition. Ed: Lloyd RV et al. IARC: Lyon. 39-40, 2017
2. Mete O et al: Overview of the 2017 WHO Classification of Pituitary Tumors. Endocr Pathol. ePub, 2017
3. Uraki S et al: Hypersecretion of ACTH and PRL from pituitary adenoma in MEN1, adequately managed by medical therapy. Endocrinol Diabetes Metab Case Rep. 2017, 2017
4. Mete O et al: Silent subtype 3 pituitary adenomas are not always silent and represent poorly differentiated monomorphous plurihormonal Pit-1 lineage adenomas. Mod Pathol. 29(2):131-42, 2016
5. Pereira BD et al: Monomorphous plurihormonal pituitary adenoma of Pit-1 lineage in a giant adolescent with central hyperthyroidism. Endocr Pathol. 27(1):25-33, 2016
6. Chin SO et al: Acromegaly due to a macroinvasive plurihormonal pituitary adenoma and a rectal carcinoid tumor. Endocrinol Metab (Seoul). 30(3):389-94, 2015
7. Cho HJ et al: Clinicopathologic analysis of pituitary adenoma: a single institute experience. J Korean Med Sci. 29(3):405-10, 2014
8. Rasul FT et al: Plurihormonal pituitary adenoma with concomitant adrenocorticotropic hormone (ACTH) and growth hormone (GH) secretion: a report of two cases and review of the literature. Acta Neurochir (Wien). 156(1):141-6, 2014
9. Villa A et al: A rare case of ACTH-LH plurihormonal pituitary adenoma: letter to the editor. Acta Neurochir (Wien). 156(7):1389-91, 2014
10. Jiang Z et al: Analysis of differential gene expression in plurihormonal pituitary adenomas using bead-based fiber-optic arrays. J Neurooncol. 108(3):341-8, 2012
11. Kannan S et al: A rare corticotroph-secreting tumor with coexisting prolactin and growth hormone staining cells. Case Rep Endocrinol. 2012:529730, 2012
12. Luk CT et al: Plurihormonal pituitary adenoma immunoreactive for thyroid-stimulating hormone, growth hormone, follicle-stimulating hormone, and prolactin. Endocr Pract. 18(5):e121-6, 2012
13. Maisnam I et al: Plurihormone secreting pituitary macroadenoma masquerading as thyrotoxicosis: Clinical presentation and diagnostic challenges. Indian J Endocrinol Metab. 16(Suppl 2):S315-7, 2012
14. Pawlikowski M: Immunohistochemical detection of dopamine D2 receptors in human pituitary adenomas. Folia Histochem Cytobiol. 48(3):394-7, 2010
15. Pawlikowski M et al: Plurihormonality of pituitary adenomas in light of immunohistochemical studies. Endokrynol Pol. 61(1):63-6, 2010
16. Al-Shraim M et al: Plurihormonal gonadotroph cell pituitary adenoma: report of a unique case. Clin Neuropathol. 2009 May-Jun;28(3):182-7. Erratum in: Clin Neuropathol. 30(3):157, 2011
17. Elhadd TA et al: A patient with thyrotropinoma cosecreting growth hormone and follicle-stimulating hormone with low alpha-glycoprotein: a new subentity? Thyroid. 19(8):899-903, 2009
18. Erickson D et al: Silent subtype 3 pituitary adenoma: a clinicopathologic analysis of the Mayo Clinic experience. Clin Endocrinol (Oxf). 71(1):92-9, 2009
19. Asa SL: Practical pituitary pathology: what does the pathologist need to know? Arch Pathol Lab Med. 132(8):1231-40, 2008
20. Trouillas J et al: Pituitary tumors and hyperplasia in multiple endocrine neoplasia type 1 syndrome (MEN1): a case-control study in a series of 77 patients versus 2509 non-MEN1 patients. Am J Surg Pathol. 32(4):534-43, 2008
21. Saeger W et al: Pathohistological classification of pituitary tumors: 10 years of experience with the German Pituitary Tumor Registry. Eur J Endocrinol. 156(2):203-16, 2007
22. Salehi F et al: Plurihormonality in pituitary adenomas associated with acromegaly. Endocr Pathol. 17(3):291-6, 2006
23. Horvath E et al: Silent adenoma subtype 3 of the pituitary–immunohistochemical and ultrastructural classification: a review of 29 cases. Ultrastruct Pathol. 29(6):511-24, 2005

Plurihormonal PIT-1-Positive Adenoma: PIT-1

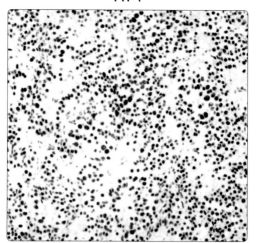

Plurihormonal PIT-1-Positive Adenoma: α-Subunit

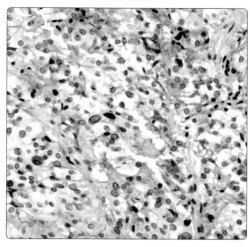

(Left) *Plurihormonal PIT-1-positive adenomas are by definition strongly and diffusely immunoreactive for the transcription factor PIT-1 that drives differentiation of the acidophilic lineage.* (Right) *In addition to PIT-1, plurihormonal PIT-1-positive adenoma may exhibit variable expression of PIT-1 lineage pituitary hormones including PRL, GH, TSH, and a-subunit. In this case, a-subunit and other pituitary hormones (TSH and PRL) were shown.*

Plurihormonal PIT-1-Positive Adenoma: β-TSH

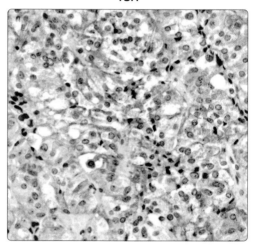

Plurihormonal PIT-1-Positive Adenoma: PRL

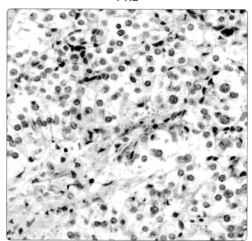

(Left) *β-TSH immunohistochemistry in the same case shows focal and weak immunoexpression.* (Right) *Prolactin is illustrated in the same case that showed a-subunit and β-TSH.*

Plurihormonal PIT-1-Positive Adenoma: ER-α

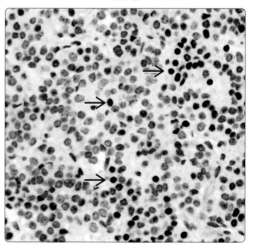

Plurihormonal PIT-1-Positive Adenoma

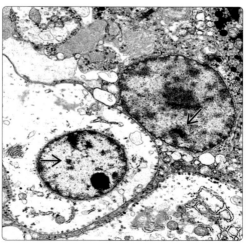

(Left) *ER-a ⮕ is variably expressed in plurihormonal PIT-1-positive adenomas but can also be negative. ER-a is also expressed in gonadotrophs, mammosomatotrophs, and lactotrophs.* (Right) *Large polar adenoma cells with sparse secretory granules and nuclear inclusions (so-called "spheridia") ⮕ are typical of plurihormonal PIT-1-positive adenoma*

TERMINOLOGY

- Low-grade epithelial neoplasm of sellar region related to Rathke pouch; 2 subtypes have been recognized
  - Adamantinomatous craniopharyngioma (ACP); papillary craniopharyngioma
  - Both variants are classified as WHO grade I tumors

CLINICAL ISSUES

- ACP common in children but arise at any age; PCP rare in children
- Growth delay may be presenting manifestation in children
- Surgical resection is primary treatment

IMAGING

- Suprasellar cystic mass with calcification

MACROSCOPIC

- ACP are cystic and contain thick, oil-like fluid described as "machinery oil"
- PCP are mostly solid, rubbery tumors

MICROSCOPIC

- Adamantinomatous CP
  - Palisading, stromal fibrosis, wet keratinization, calcification
- Papillary CP
  - Nonkeratinizing, pseudostratified epithelium arranged in large papillae; lacks wet keratin and calcification

ANCILLARY TESTS

- Adamantinomatous CP reveals aberrant nuclear β-catenin expression
- Papillary CP shows cytoplasmic BRAF V600E mutant protein expression

TOP DIFFERENTIAL DIAGNOSES

- Epidermoid cyst
- Rathke cleft cyst with extensive squamous metaplasia
- Pilocytic astrocytoma

(Left) *Adamantinomatous craniopharyngioma (CP) is composed of cords or islands of epithelial cells in a loose fibrous stroma with intervening cysts resembling adamantinoma. The outer layer of epithelium shows palisading* ➡. (Right) *Papillary CP is composed of mature squamous epithelium* ➡ *and lacks palisading, fibrosis, wet keratinization, and calcification; features that characterize adamantinomatous CP.*

Adamantinomatous Craniopharyngioma

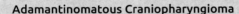
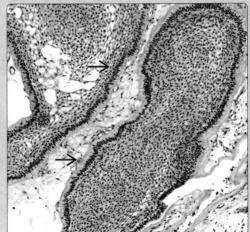

Papillary Craniopharyngioma

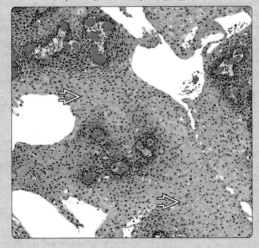

(Left) *Aberrant nuclear expression of β-catenin in a adamantinomatous craniopharyngioma. Note that the nuclear expression is not homogeneous within the epithelium and is most commonly seen in the cellular clusters or nodular whorls* ➡. (Right) *In papillary CP, the squamous epithelium shows strong cytoplasmic immunoexpression of V600E-mutant BRAF protein.*

β-Catenin Expression in ACP

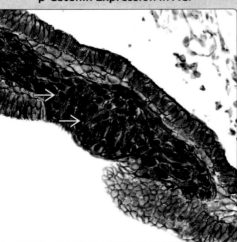

BRAF Expression in PCP

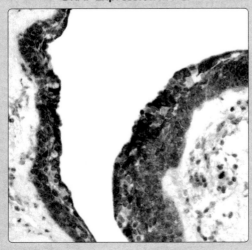

TERMINOLOGY

Abbreviations

- Craniopharyngioma (CP)

Definitions

- Low-grade epithelial neoplasm of sellar region related to Rathke pouch; 2 subtypes have been recognized
  - Adamantinomatous craniopharyngioma (ACP)
  - Papillary craniopharyngioma (PCP)

ETIOLOGY/PATHOGENESIS

CTNNB1 Mutations

- Have been documented in about 95% of ACP
- Aberrant nuclear immunopositivity of β-catenin correlates with mutation

BRAF V600E Mutations

- Have been documented in about 90% of PCP
- Cytoplasmic immunopositivity for V600E-mutant BRAF

CLINICAL ISSUES

Epidemiology

- Incidence
  - Represents ~ 3% of all intracranial tumors; 10% of tumors of all sellar region and is most frequent sellar tumor of childhood
- Age
  - ACPs common in all age groups; PCPs rare in children

Presentation

- Most common presenting symptoms are due to effects of sellar mass
- Growth delay may be presenting manifestation in children
- Diabetes insipidus seen in 25% of patients

Treatment

- Surgical resection is primary treatment
- Postoperative radiation to reduce risk of recurrence
- No medical therapy currently available

Prognosis

- Both variants are classified as WHO grade I tumors
- Significant morbidity and recurrence rates, up to 20% in cases of subtotal surgical resection, particularly in ACP
  - PCP appears less prone to postoperative recurrence due to higher success surgical resection

IMAGING

Radiologic Features

- Enlarged or eroded sella with suprasellar calcification in ~ 50% of patients
- Usually suprasellar cystic lesions, but may be cystic and solid on imaging

MACROSCOPIC

General Features

- ACP are cystic and contain thick, oil-like fluid described as "machinery oil"
- PCP are mostly solid, rubbery tumors

MICROSCOPIC

Adamantinomatous Craniopharyngioma

- Composed of cords or islands of epithelial cells in loose fibrous stroma with intervening cysts
- Outer layer of epithelium is palisaded
- "Wet keratin" associated with nuclear dropout to form ghost keratinocytes
- Cholesterol clefts, desquamated keratin, calcification
- Occasional inflammatory component and gliosis

Papillary Craniopharyngioma

- Composed of nonkeratinizing, pseudostratified squamous epithelium arranged in large papillae
- Lacks palisading, fibrosis, wet keratinization, and calcification features that characterize ACP

ANCILLARY TESTS

Immunohistochemistry

- Adamantinomatous CP reveals aberrant nuclear β-catenin expression
  - Nuclear staining can be focal and found in areas where morular structures are seen
- Papillary CP shows cytoplasmic BRAF V600E mutant protein expression

DIFFERENTIAL DIAGNOSIS

Epithelial Cysts of Sellar Region

- Hypocellular cystic CPs can be mistaken for epidermoid or Rathke cleft cyst (RCC)
- Epidermoid cysts are unilocular cysts lined by orderly stratified squamous epithelium; CPs have nodular and irregular appearance
- RCC with extensive squamous change can mimic PCP; use of BRAF V600E immunohistochemistry is helpful for differentiation

Pilocytic Astrocytoma

- Reactive gliosis in adjacent brain parenchyma can be mistaken for pilocytic astrocytoma

Xanthogranulomas of Sellar Region

- Considered reactive lesion most often related to rupture of RCC

SELECTED REFERENCES

1. Hölsken A et al: Adamantinomatous and papillary craniopharyngiomas are characterized by distinct epigenomic as well as mutational and transcriptomic profiles. Acta Neuropathol Commun. 4:20, 2016
2. Brastianos PK et al: Exome sequencing identifies BRAF mutations in papillary craniopharyngiomas. Nat Genet. 46(2):161-5, 2014
3. Buslei R et al: Common mutations of beta-catenin in adamantinomatous craniopharyngiomas but not in other tumours originating from the sellar region. Acta Neuropathol. 109(6):589-97, 2005
4. Buslei R, Rushing EJ, Giangaspero F, et al. Craniopharyngioma. In: Louis DN, Ohgaki H, Weistler OD, Cavenee C (Eds). WHO Classification of Tumours of the Central Nervous System. Revised 4th Edition. IARC: Lyon, pp 324-8, 2016

Pituitary Carcinoma

TERMINOLOGY

- Pituitary carcinoma (PC): Tumor of adenohypophysis exhibiting cerebrospinal &/or systemic metastases
- Conventional criteria of malignancy (nuclear atypia, cellular pleomorphism, mitotic activity, invasion, and necrosis) insufficient criteria for diagnosis

ETIOLOGY/PATHOGENESIS

- Most cases arise from progression of pituitary adenoma rather than de novo tumor

CLINICAL ISSUES

- Very rare (~ 0.1 cases per 100,000 population in Europe)
  - 6% of invasive adenomas in surveillance, epidemiology, and end result (SEER) database
- Majority (75%) endocrinologically functional tumors
  - Prolactin and ACTH are most frequent followed by clinically nonfunctioning tumors and GH- and TSH-producing tumors

- Treatment includes multimodality therapies (surgery, radiotherapy/radiosurgery, adjuvant chemotherapy)
- Poor prognosis (80% of patients die of disease-related causes)

MICROSCOPIC

- No histologic criteria to define PC
- Diagnosis of PC defined by confirmation of primary adenohypophyseal tumor and presence of metastases

ANCILLARY TESTS

- Neuroendocrine markers positivity similar to pituitary adenomas
- Pituitary hormones positivity similar to primary adenohypophyseal tumor
- Ki-67 labeling index is higher in PCs than in adenomas
- p53 expression present in PCs; expression in metastases higher than in primary tumor

MR of Invasive Pituitary Adenoma

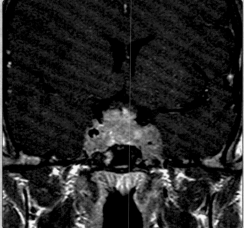

MR of Brain Metastases of Silent Corticotroph Adenoma

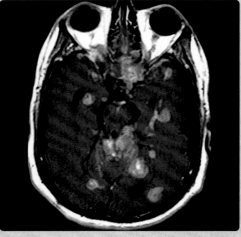

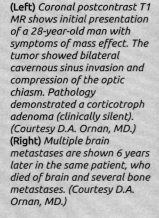

(Left) Coronal postcontrast T1 MR shows initial presentation of a 28-year-old man with symptoms of mass effect. The tumor showed bilateral cavernous sinus invasion and compression of the optic chiasm. Pathology demonstrated a corticotroph adenoma (clinically silent). (Courtesy D.A. Ornan, MD.) (Right) Multiple brain metastases are shown 6 years later in the same patient, who died of brain and several bone metastases. (Courtesy D.A. Ornan, MD.)

Pituitary Carcinoma Metastatic to Liver

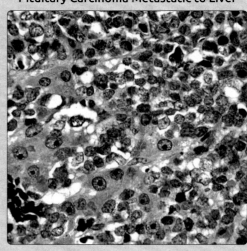

Pituitary Carcinoma Deposits

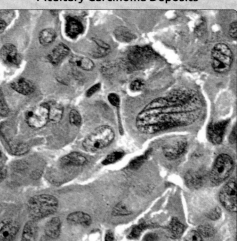

(Left) Partial hepatectomy specimen from a patient with history of pituitary tumor shows infiltration of liver parenchyma by a neuroendocrine neoplasm with immunoreactivity similar to the pituitary tumor. (Right) Pituitary carcinoma deposits may show solid arrangement of pleomorphic cells with an eosinophilic cytoplasm, nuclear pleomorphism, irregular nuclear membranes, and prominent nucleoli.

TERMINOLOGY

Abbreviations

- Pituitary carcinoma (PC)

Synonyms

- Pituitary adenocarcinoma

Definitions

- PC is strictly defined as tumor of adenohypophyseal cells that metastasizes cerebrospinally &/or is associated with systemic metastases (WHO 2017)
  - Conventional criteria of malignancy, such as nuclear atypia, pleomorphism, mitotic activity, necrosis, hemorrhage, &/or invasion, are insufficient criteria for diagnosis
- Definition is independent of histologic appearance
  - Local extension into adjacent structures is not criterion for malignancy
  - Brain invasion may be indicative of malignancy

ETIOLOGY/PATHOGENESIS

Genetics

- **Inherited**
  - Few cases of PC have been reported in multiple endocrine neoplasia type 1 and succinate dehydrogenase-related familial syndromes
    - However, no data supporting direct association of familial syndromes and PC

Pathophysiology

- Most cases arise from progression of pituitary adenoma rather than de novo tumor
  - Majority of cases arise in setting of invasive adenomas with multiple recurrences
- Systemic metastases most likely hematogenous
- Lymph node metastases most likely secondary to skull base and soft tissue involvement

Genetic Profile

- No conclusive data on genetic profile of PCs
- Several molecular and genetic alterations have been reported in isolated cases of both primary adenoma and carcinoma cases
  - *HRAS* point mutations; *RB1* gene alterations
  - Gains of chromosomes: 5, 7p, 13q22, 14q; LOH: 1p, 3p, 10q26, 11q13, 22q12
  - Overexpression of *ERBB2* (Her2/neu) in gonadotrophe carcinoma
  - 5 genes suggested to drive aggressive behavior
    - *CD44, TSG101, DGKZ, HTATIP2, GTF2H1*
  - *TP53* mutations are rare
  - MicroRNAs alterations: miR-122, miR-20a, miR-106B, miR-175p

CLINICAL ISSUES

Epidemiology

- Incidence
  - Very rare; ~ 0.1 cases per 100,000 population in Europe
    - 0.12% of adenohypophysial tumors in Germany
  - 6% of invasive adenomas in surveillance, epidemiology, and end result (SEER) database
- Age
  - Adults; median patient age at diagnosis is in 6th decade
  - Rarely in adolescents and children
- Sex
  - Slight female predilection
- Type of tumor
  - > 70% of reported PCs are either lactotroph or corticotroph carcinomas

Site

- Primary sellar
- Rarely ectopic: Only 2 cases reported
- Metastatic sites
  - Metastases frequently occur within craniospinal axis as result of dissemination in subarachnoid space
  - Craniospinal leptomeninges
  - Deep deposits in brain cortex and cerebellum
  - Systemic metastases
    - Are more commonly seen in liver, bone, lymph node, and lungs
    - Unusual sites include heart, pancreas, ovary and myometrium, middle ear, and orbit
  - Hematogenous metastases can occur via petrosal sinus

Presentation

- Premetastatic lesions and metastases can be hormonally active or clinically nonfunctioning, as conventional pituitary adenomas
- Majority (75%) endocrinologically functional
  - Prolactin and ACTH are most frequent followed by clinically nonfunctioning tumors and GH- and TSH-producing tumors
  - Presentations: Hyperprolactinemia, Cushing disease, acromegaly, hyperthyroidism, Nelson syndrome
- Diagnosis based on metastasis, often from multiple recurring, invasive adenoma
- De novo malignancy in adenoma extremely rare
- Interval to metastasis: 4 months to 30 years (mean: 10 years)
- Pituitary hormone levels do not permit distinction of adenoma from carcinoma
- Clinical signs specific to site of metastasis

Treatment

- Multimodality therapies (surgery, external beam radiotherapy, radiosurgery, adjuvant pharmacologic, and chemotherapy)
- Temozolomide therapy seems efficacious in several reported cases
  - Low MGMT immunoreactivity (< 10% of cells) correlates with higher response to temozolomide therapy
- Dopamine agonist response temporary in prolactin cell carcinomas

Prognosis

- Poor; mortality 6% at 1 year and 80% within 8 years
- Overall mean survival: 1 year: 57.1%; 10 years: 28.6%
- Survival shorter in systemic vs. craniospinal metastases

IMAGING

CT and MR Findings

- No features unique to PC when still restricted to sellar location
  - Most cases progressed from invasive pituitary adenoma often extending into parasellar structures
- Multifocal craniospinal deposits involving meninges and nerve roots, often in cauda equina
- Brain parenchyma infrequently involved by primary tumor

MACROSCOPIC

General Features

- Primary tumor of macroadenoma size (> 1 cm); all invasive
- Metastatic deposits may be single or multiple, nodular or diffuse
- Metastasis of PC indistinguishable from metastases of carcinomas of other organs

MICROSCOPIC

Histologic Features

- No histologic criteria define to PC
  - Diagnosis of PC defined by confirmation of primary adenohypophyseal tumor and presence of metastases
- Histologic features of cellular atypia, cellular pleomorphism, mitotic figures, and necrosis not sufficient for diagnosis
- Mitotic activity increased in carcinomas (up to 67%) but considerable overlap with adenomas
- In metastatic deposits, cellular atypia, pleomorphism, mitotic activity, and necrosis commonly present

ANCILLARY TESTS

Immunohistochemistry

- Neuroendocrine markers positivity similar to pituitary adenomas
  - Chromogranin-A, synaptophysin
- Pituitary hormones positivity similar to primary pituitary tumor
  - Most common PC lactotroph, followed by corticotroph and nonfunctioning tumors
- Ki-67 labeling index varies widely but is higher than in pituitary adenomas
  - Often higher in metastases
  - In primary lesions, values > 10% are associated with aggressive behavior
- p53 expression present in PCs; expression in metastases higher than in primary tumor
- β-catenin and p27 (cell cycle inhibitor widely expressed in normal pituitary), decreased in carcinomas
- Higher expression of several proteins in carcinomas:
  - Bcl-2, topoisomerase 2-α, cyclooxygenase-2, galectin-3, and VEGF
- Expression of enzyme MGMT (part of DNA repair system) in PCs is < 10% MGMT-positive cells

Electron Microscopy

- Does not distinguish adenoma from carcinoma

DIFFERENTIAL DIAGNOSIS

Metastatic Carcinoma From Other Organs

- Anaplasia more prominent in carcinoma from other organs
- Negative for pituitary hormones
- Synaptophysin positive only in neuroendocrine carcinomas
- Organ-specific markers positivity

Invasive Pituitary Adenoma

- Locally invasive tumor
- No metastases present
- Histologic features, immunohistochemical profile, electron microscopy, and proliferation markers cannot distinguish benign from malignant tumors

DIAGNOSTIC CHECKLIST

Clinically Relevant Pathologic Features

- History of pituitary adenoma mandatory for diagnosis

Pathologic Interpretation Pearls

- Disseminating lesions present in carcinoma
- Local infiltration not, in itself, indicator of carcinoma
- Useful to compare histologic appearance and immunohistochemical profile of metastatic focus with primary pituitary tumor
- No histologic, immunohistochemical, or ultrastructural finding conclusively separates pituitary adenomas from carcinomas

GRADING

Grading System

- No suitable grading system exists

SELECTED REFERENCES

1. Roncaroli F et al: Pituitary carcinoma. In Lloyd RV et al: WHO Classification of Tumours of Endocrine Organs. 4th ed. Ed. Lyon:IARC. 41-44, 2017
2. Wei Z et al: MicroRNA involvement in a metastatic non-functioning pituitary carcinoma. Pituitary. 18(5):710-21, 2015
3. Matsuno A et al: Molecular status of pituitary carcinoma and atypical adenoma that contributes the effectiveness of temozolomide. Med Mol Morphol. 47(1):1-7, 2013
4. Thakker RV: Multiple endocrine neoplasia type 1 (MEN1) and type 4 (MEN4). Mol Cell Endocrinol. 386(1-2):2-15, 2013
5. Zhou Y et al: Genetic and epigenetic mutations of tumor suppressive genes in sporadic pituitary adenoma. Mol Cell Endocrinol. 386(1-2):16-33, 2013
6. Moshkin O et al: Aggressive silent corticotroph adenoma progressing to pituitary carcinoma. the role of temozolomide therapy. Hormones (Athens). 10(2):162-7, 2011
7. Zhang Y et al: Endocrine tumors as part of inherited tumor syndromes. Adv Anat Pathol. 18(3):206-18, 2011
8. Lau Q et al: MGMT immunoexpression in aggressive pituitary adenoma and carcinoma. Pituitary. 13(4):367-79, 2010
9. Stilling G et al: MicroRNA expression in ACTH-producing pituitary tumors: up-regulation of microRNA-122 and -493 in pituitary carcinomas. Endocrine. 38(1):67-75, 2010
10. Scheithauer BW et al: Multiple endocrine neoplasia type 1-associated thyrotropin-producing pituitary carcinoma: report of a probable de novo example. Hum Pathol. 40(2):270-8, 2009
11. Gordon MV et al: Metastatic prolactinoma presenting as a cervical spinal cord tumour in multiple endocrine neoplasia type one (MEN-1). Clin Endocrinol (Oxf). 66(1):150-2, 2007
12. Tanizaki Y et al: P53 gene mutations in pituitary carcinomas. Endocr Pathol. 18(4):217-22, 2007

Metastatic Pituitary Carcinoma to Liver: Cytology

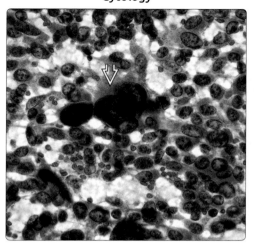

Metastatic Pituitary Carcinoma to Liver Appearance

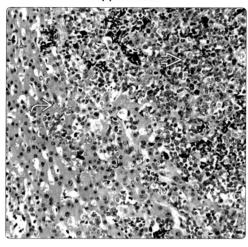

(Left) *Smear from a liver nodule shows a highly cellular neoplasm composed of rare giant cells ➡ present in the background of a monotonous population of cells with scant cytoplasm and nuclei with a homogeneous appearance.* (Right) *Low-power view shows metastatic pituitary carcinoma to the liver. The tumor infiltrates the hepatic sinusoids ➡ and forms solid sheets of tumor cells ➡ with regular nuclei lacking pleomorphism.*

Cellular Characteristics of Metastatic Pituitary Carcinoma to Liver

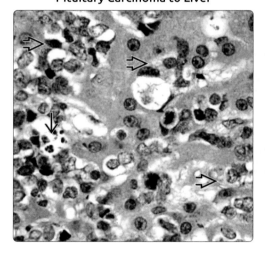

Pleomorphism and Mitosis in Metastatic Pituitary Carcinoma to Liver

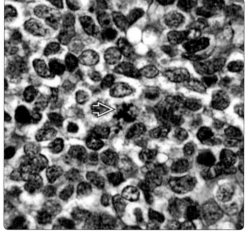

(Left) *H&E from a liver with metastatic pituitary carcinoma shows diffuse infiltration of the hepatic sinusoids ➡ by tumor cells. There are apoptotic bodies ➡ present within the tumor.* (Right) *Pituitary carcinoma metastatic to the liver shows a solid arrangement of cells with mild atypia, cellular pleomorphism, apoptosis, and the presence of an atypical mitosis ➡.*

Metastatic Pituitary Carcinoma to Liver: ACTH Immunopositivity

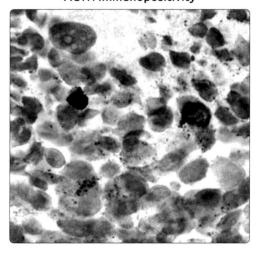

Metastatic Pituitary Carcinoma to Liver: Ki-67 Proliferative Index

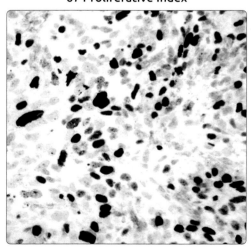

(Left) *ACTH immunostain of a smear from a liver tumor nodule shows positivity in the cytoplasm of scattered tumor cells. This immunopositivity was also present in the pituitary tumor of this patient.* (Right) *Immunohistochemistry for Ki-67 in a pituitary carcinoma metastatic to the liver shows a high proliferative index. p53 immunoexpression is often high and usually higher in metastatic sites than in the primary tumor.*

KEY FACTS

TERMINOLOGY

- Tumors composed of neoplastic ganglion cells
- Most tumors are associated with pituitary adenoma

ETIOLOGY/PATHOGENESIS

- No data regarding pathogenesis of isolated gangliocytoma
- Combined gangliocytoma-pituitary adenoma theories
  - Stimulation of hypothalamic trophic hormones
  - Transdifferentiation of pituitary adenomatous cells
  - Common precursor/stem cell origin

CLINICAL ISSUES

- Gangliocytomas are extremely rare
  - About 85% of cases have coexisting pituitary adenoma
- Slight female predominance
- No preferential age
- Endocrinopathies due to associated hormonally active adenoma
- Surgical resection is main treatment

MICROSCOPIC

- Large ganglion cells with abundant cytoplasm containing Nissl substance, embedded in rich neuropil-like matrix
- When intermingled with pituitary adenoma, ganglionic cells may be inconspicuous
- In acromegaly, sparsely granulated somatotroph adenoma is most common adenoma

ANCILLARY TESTS

- Ganglionic cells positive for neuronal markers
- Adenomatous cells positive for pituitary hormones according to specific adenoma subtype
- PIT-1 has been demonstrated in both adenomatous and ganglionic cells in mixed GC-somatotroph adenomas

TOP DIFFERENTIAL DIAGNOSES

- Normal hypothalamus
- Crooke cell adenoma
- Pituitary adenoma

Gangliocytoma

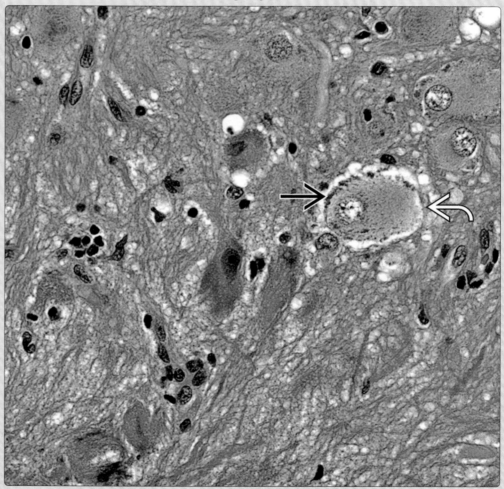

Sellar gangliocytomas are rare tumors and composed of large, mature ganglion cells ➡ with abundant cytoplasm that contain Nissl substance ➡ aggregated at the periphery of the cell body. Only the minority of these tumors are composed solely of ganglion cells.

TERMINOLOGY

Synonyms

- Pituitary adenoma-neuronal choristoma
- Adenohypophyseal choristoma
- Mixed gangliocytoma-adenoma
- Pituitary adenoma with gangliocytic component
- Ganglioneuroma

Definitions

- Tumor composed of neoplastic ganglion cells resembling hypothalamic neurons
  - Most tumors are associated with pituitary adenoma
- Gangliocytoma and mixed gangliocytoma-adenoma is a pituitary (intrasellar) tumor that contains ganglion (neuronal) cells, which are frequently mixed with pituitary adenoma or hyperplasia (WHO 2017)

ETIOLOGY/PATHOGENESIS

Unknown

- There is no significant data regarding pathogenesis of isolated sellar gangliocytoma
- 3 main hypotheses have been postulated for pathogenesis of combined gangliocytoma-pituitary adenoma
  - Stimulation of hypothalamic trophic hormones
    - Primary sellar gangliocytoma will induce adenoma by paracrine secretion of hypothalamic stimulating hormones
  - Transdifferentiation of pituitary adenomatous cells
    - Transitional cells with features of both adenomatous and ganglionic cells have been described by ultrastructural analysis
  - Common progenitor &/or stem cell
    - Combined tumors would derived from common progenitor/stem cell capable of differentiation in 2 cellular components
  - Recent description of pituitary transcription factor PIT-1 in both ganglionic and adenomatous cells raises possibility of either common origin or cellular transdifferentiation

CLINICAL ISSUES

Epidemiology

- Incidence
  - Gangliocytomas are extremely rare and ~ 85% of cases have coexisting pituitary adenoma
    - Gangliocytoma and mixed gangliocytoma associated with pituitary adenomas accounts for 0.25-1.26% of all sellar tumors (WHO 2017)
  - Female predominance is seen
  - No preferential age is reported

Presentation

- Tumor mass effect symptoms including hyperprolactinemia and visual disturbances
- Endocrinopathies due to associated hormonally active adenoma
  - Acromegaly (most common), amenorrhea-galactorrhea, and Cushing disease

Treatment

- Usually cured when complete surgical resection can be achieved
- Medical therapy targeted specifically to control hormone hypersecretion
- Radiation therapy in selected recurrent or aggressive tumors

Prognosis

- Prognosis is most related to associated pituitary adenoma subtype
- Extremely low proliferation potential
- Overall prognosis is good when complete resection is achieved
  - Of 23 cases reported in one series, only one case of intrasellar gangliocytomas associated with pituitary adenomas recurred 5 years after tumor resection

IMAGING

Radiological Features

- Cannot be differentiated from usual adenomas by imaging
- Sellar only or sellar and suprasellar, circumscribed, solid mass (hypointense in T1- and hyperintense in T2-weighted MR sequences)

MACROSCOPIC

General Features

- GC cannot be differentiated from usual adenomas by gross appearance and by imaging
- Heterogeneous gross features
  - Nodular, solid, or cystic

MICROSCOPIC

Gangliocytoma

- Composed of large ganglion cells with abundant cytoplasm containing Nissl substance and embedded in rich neuropil-like matrix
- Large nuclei and very prominent nucleoli; binucleated and multinucleated cells can be seen
- When combined with pituitary adenoma, ganglionic component may be inconspicuous

Pituitary Morphology Associated With Gangliocytomas

- In patients with acromegaly, sparsely granulated somatotroph adenoma is most common adenoma
- In patients with galactorrhea-amenorrhea, lactotroph adenomas and mixed somatotroph-lactotroph adenomas are reported
- In patients with Cushing disease, corticotroph adenomas have been reported

ANCILLARY TESTS

Immunohistochemistry

- Ganglionic elements are positive for neuronal markers including synaptophysin, NF, MAP2, and NeuN
- Adenomatous elements are positive for pituitary hormones according to specific adenoma subtype

- Sparsely granulated somatotroph adenoma is most commonly seen adenoma with sparse GH immunoreactivity and keratin-positive fibrous bodies
- Transcription factor PIT-1 has been demonstrated in both adenomatous and ganglionic elements in mixed gangliocytoma and somatotroph adenomas
- Peptide hormones can be detected in cytoplasm of ganglionic cells
  - GHRH, CRH, GnRH and other peptides including VIP and enkephalin have been demonstrated in
    - Tumors associated with Cushing disease contain CRH
      - But may also contain ACTH, β-lipotropin, and somatostatin
    - Tumors associated with precocious puberty contain GnRH
      - But may also contain CRH, oxytocin, and β-endorphin

Electron Microscopy

- Mature ganglionic cells with large nuclei and prominent nucleoli and neuronal process with neurotubules
- Transitional cells between ganglion cells and adenomatous cells have been described

DIFFERENTIAL DIAGNOSIS

Normal Hypothalamus

- Gangliocytomas are of low cellularity and can sometimes be difficult to distinguish from normal parenchyma

Crooke Cell Adenoma

- Large cells of Crooke cell adenoma may be mistaken for gangliocytoma
  - Positivity for neuronal markers and lack of ACTH and Tpit favors gangliocytoma

Pituitary Adenoma

- In combined gangliocytoma-pituitary adenoma, ganglionic component may be inconspicuous

SELECTED REFERENCES

1. Osamura RY et al: Gangliocytoma and mixed gangliocytoma-adenoma. In Lloyd RV et al: WHO Classification of Tumours of Endocrine Organs. 4th ed. IARC: Lyon. 48-9, 2017
2. Lopes MB et al: Mixed gangliocytoma-pituitary adenoma: insights on the pathogenesis of a rare sellar tumor. Am J Surg Pathol. 41(5):586-595, 2017
3. Sergeant C et al: Transdifferentiation of neuroendocrine cells: gangliocytoma associated with two pituitary adenomas of different lineage in MEN1. Am J Surg Pathol. 41(6):849-853, 2017
4. Cossu G et al: Gangliocytomas of the sellar region: a challenging diagnosis. Clin Neurol Neurosurg. 149:122-35, 2016
5. Serri O et al: An unusual association of a sellar gangliocytoma with a prolactinoma. Pituitary. 11(1):85-7, 2008
6. Kontogeorgos G et al: Ganglion cell containing pituitary adenomas: signs of neuronal differentiation in adenoma cells. Acta Neuropathol. 112(1):21-8, 2006
7. Kurosaki M et al: Intrasellar gangliocytomas associated with acromegaly. Brain Tumor Pathol. 19(2):63-7, 2002
8. Horvath E et al: Pituitary adenoma with neuronal choristoma (PANCH): composite lesion or lineage infidelity? Ultrastruct Pathol. 18(6):565-74, 1994
9. Asa SL et al: A case for hypothalamic acromegaly: a clinicopathological study of six patients with hypothalamic gangliocytomas producing growth hormone-releasing factor. J Clin Endocrinol Metab. 58(5):796-803, 1984

Mixed Gangliocytoma-Somatotroph Adenoma

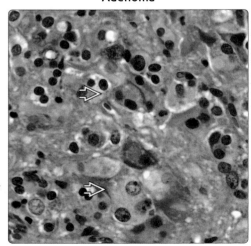

Mixed Gangliocytoma-Somatotroph Adenoma

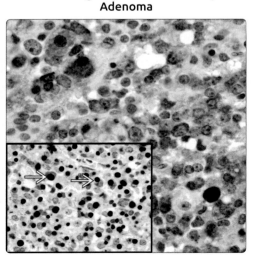

(Left) *The great majority of sellar gangliocytomas arise as combined tumors with a pituitary adenoma. Note in this figure, a ganglionic-rich area of a mixed tumor with several ganglionic cells, some of them bi- or multinucleated* ⇒. (Right) *In the same case, the adenomatous component is composed of a sparsely granulated somatotroph adenoma with uneven GH immunoreactivity within the tumor cells. The typical fibrous bodies are highlighted by keratin positivity* ⇒.

Mixed Gangliocytoma-Somatotroph Adenoma

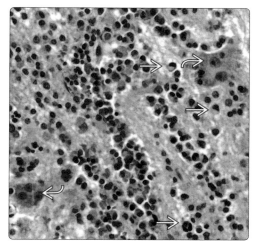

Composite Pituitary Tumor

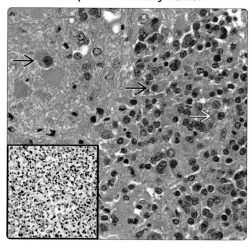

(Left) *In the same case, the tumor shows areas of adenomatous cells with a few ganglionic cells ⮌. The adenoma is composed of small acidophilic cells with fibrous bodies ➡ consistent with a sparsely granulated somatotroph adenoma.* (Right) *Composite gangliocytoma ➡ and sparsely granulated somatotroph adenoma with fibrous bodies ➡ are illustrated. The insert (lower left) highlights LMWK (CAM5.2) that reveals fibrous bodies.*

Mixed Gangliocytoma-Somatotroph Adenoma

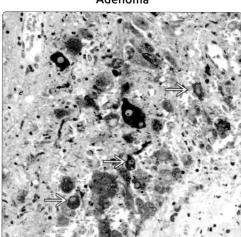

Mixed Gangliocytoma-Somatotroph Adenoma

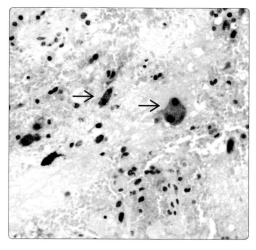

(Left) *In mixed gangliocytoma-pituitary adenoma, the ganglionic component is immunoreactive for neuronal markers including MAP2, like in this case. Note smaller cells ➡ that may represent transitional cells between adenomatous and ganglion cells also displaying positivity for MAP2.* (Right) *In the same case, the ganglionic component of mixed gangliocytoma-pituitary adenoma also shows strong nuclear reactivity for the neuronal marker NeuN ➡.*

CRH in Gangliocytoma

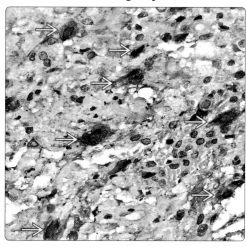

Gangliocytoma Neurofilament Stain

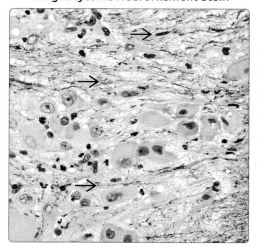

(Left) *Peptide hormones can be detected in the cytoplasm of neurons in gangliocytomas. Positivity for CRH ➡ is illustrated.* (Right) *In gangliocytomas, the large ganglionic cells are embedded in a rich neuropil-like stroma. Neurofilament immunohistochemistry ➡ highlights the neuronal processes in a sellar gangliocytoma.*

KEY FACTS

TERMINOLOGY

- Neuronal tumors of sellar region include paraganglioma, neuroblastoma, and neurocytoma

CLINICAL ISSUES

- Extremely rare in sella; involve adults
- Tumors mimic nonfunctioning pituitary adenomas with signs and symptoms of mass effect
- Surgical resection is treatment of choice
- Most paragangliomas are benign; diagnosis of malignancy requires evidence of metastatic spread
- Neurocytomas and neuroblastomas may show craniospinal dissemination; long-term follow-up is recommended

MICROSCOPIC

- Paragangliomas display sinusoidal growth pattern with solid nests or zellballen and anastomosing cords within delicate fibrovascular septa

- Neuroblastomas are composed of uniform small cells with hyperchromatic nuclei embedded in neuropil-like matrix
  - Pseudorosettes and Homer Wright rosettes are rare
- Neurocytomas have uniform, medium-sized cells with nuclei with neuroendocrine-like chromatin embedded in neuropil-like matrix
  - Small ganglion-like cells may be present

ANCILLARY TESTS

- Paragangliomas are positive for chromogranin-A, synaptophysin, and tyrosine hydroxylase
- Neuroblastomas and neurocytomas are positive for neuronal markers and negative for glial markers

TOP DIFFERENTIAL DIAGNOSES

- Null cell adenoma
- Metastatic carcinoma
- Olfactory neuroblastoma

Pituitary Paraganglioma Features

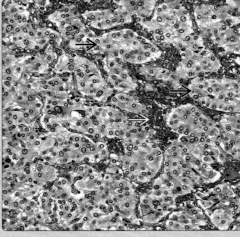

Paraganglioma: Chromogranin

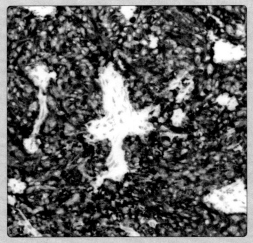

(Left) Paragangliomas have a sinusoidal growth pattern with solid nests or zellballen ➔ within delicate fibrovascular septa, which is typical. A congested appearance ➔ is present due to abundant vascularization. (Right) Sellar paragangliomas are strongly immunoreactive for neuroendocrine markers; such as chromogranin-A and synaptophysin. The differential diagnosis with null cell adenomas may be challenging and other peptide markers, including tyrosine hydroxylase, are quite helpful.

Paraganglioma: GFAP Reactivity

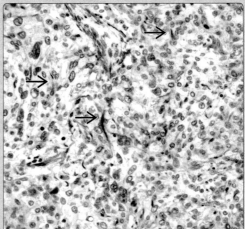

Patchy Tyrosine Hydroxylase Stain

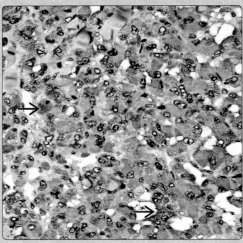

(Left) Sustentacular cells of paragangliomas are immunoreactive for S100 protein and GFAP ➔, as demonstrated in this case. (Right) Paragangliomas are positive for chromogranin-A, synaptophysin, and tyrosine hydroxylase, while they are negative for keratins. Positivity for tyrosine hydroxylase ➔ is illustrated in this example.

TERMINOLOGY

Definitions

- Neuronal tumors of sellar region include gangliocytoma, paraganglioma, neuroblastoma, and neurocytoma

ETIOLOGY/PATHOGENESIS

Genetic Susceptibility

- Paragangliomas known to be associated with germline mutations of *VHL* or SDH-related genes

CLINICAL ISSUES

Epidemiology

- Incidence
  - All of these tumors are extremely rare in sellar location
  - Usually occur in adults

Presentation

- Tumors can mimic nonfunctioning pituitary adenomas with signs and symptoms of mass effect
  - Headache, visual field changes, and sometimes hypopituitarism
  - Mild hyperprolactinemia

Treatment

- Surgical resection usually 1st treatment of choice, sometimes followed by radiotherapy

Prognosis

- Most paragangliomas are benign, and diagnosis of malignancy requires evidence of metastatic spread
- Neurocytomas and neuroblastomas may show craniospinal dissemination; long-term follow-up is recommended

IMAGING

Radiological Findings

- These tumors are indistinguishable from macroadenomas

MACROSCOPIC

General Features

- Paragangliomas have congested appearance due to abundant vascularization

MICROSCOPIC

Paraganglioma

- Sinusoidal growth pattern with solid nests or zellballen and anastomosing cords within delicate fibrovascular septa
- Composed of irregular polyhedral or elongated cells
- Nuclei exhibit neuroendocrine features

Neuroblastoma

- Uniform small cells with round to vesicular nuclei exhibiting fine chromatin and scant cytoplasm embedded in neuropil-like matrix
- Pseudorosettes and Homer Wright rosettes are rare
- Mitotic index is low

Neurocytoma

- Uniform, medium-sized cells with oval nuclei with stippled, neuroendocrine-like chromatin and small cytoplasm embedded in neuropil-like matrix
- Small, ganglion-like cells may be present
- Mitotic index is low

ANCILLARY TESTS

Paraganglioma

- Immunohistochemistry
  - Paragangliomas are positive for chromogranin-A, synaptophysin, and tyrosine hydroxylase and negative for keratins
  - S100 protein and GFAP highlight sustentacular cells
  - Loss of SDHB suggests possibility of familial paraganglioma syndrome due to SDH-related mutation

Neuroblastoma

- Immunohistochemistry
  - Tumor cells are variably positive for synaptophysin, NF, and MAP2; only focally and weakly positive for keratins
  - MIB-1 LI index is variable (10-50%) but has not shown correlation with tumor behavior

Neurocytoma

- Immunohistochemistry
  - Tumor cells are strongly positive for synaptophysin, NF, NeuN, and MAP-2; negative for glial markers (GFAP, OLIG2, S100)

DIFFERENTIAL DIAGNOSIS

Null Cell Adenoma vs. Paraganglioma

- Positivity for tyrosine hydroxylase confirms diagnosis of paraganglioma

Metastatic Carcinoma vs. Paraganglioma

- Immunohistochemical stains are essential for differentiation

Olfactory Neuroblastoma vs. Sellar Neuroblastoma

- Neuroimaging is important for precise primary location of lesion

SELECTED REFERENCES

1. Dwight T et al: Analysis of SDHAF3 in familial and sporadic pheochromocytoma and paraganglioma. BMC Cancer. 17(1):497, 2017
2. Gupta S et al: Composite pheochromocytoma/paraganglioma-ganglioneuroma: a clinicopathologic study of eight cases with analysis of succinate dehydrogenase. Endocr Pathol. ePub, 2017
3. Lopes MBS et al: Neuroblastoma. In Lloyd RV et al: WHO Classification of Tumours of Endocrine Organs. 4th ed. Lyon:IARC. 51, 2017
4. Mete et al: Neurocytoma. In Lloyd RV et al: WHO Classification of Tumours of Endocrine Organs. 4th ed. Lyon:IARC. 49-50, 2017
5. Osamura RY et al: Paraganglioma. In Lloyd RV et al: WHO Classification of Tumours of Endocrine Organs. 4th ed. Lyon:IARC. 50, 2017
6. Papathomas TG et al: SDHB/SDHA immunohistochemistry in pheochromocytomas and paragangliomas: a multicenter interobserver variation analysis using virtual microscopy: a Multinational Study of the European Network for the Study of Adrenal Tumors (ENS@T). Mod Pathol. 28(6):807-21, 2015

TERMINOLOGY

- Posterior pituitary tumors include pituicytoma, granular cell tumor of neurohypophysis, spindle cell oncocytoma, and sellar ependymoma

ETIOLOGY/PATHOGENESIS

- All 3 entities are believed to derive from pituicyte, specialized glial cell of neurohypophysis and infundibulum
- TTF-1 positivity seen in pituicytomas, spindle cell oncocytomas, and granular cell tumors supports their association with ventral neuroectoderm

CLINICAL ISSUES

- Posterior pituitary tumors are rare
- Most tumors occur in 5th and 6th decades of life
- Can mimic nonfunctioning pituitary adenomas
- Most of tumors have benign clinical course

MICROSCOPIC

- Spindle cell oncocytomas are composed of interlacing fascicles of spindle or epithelioid cells with eosinophilic cytoplasm
- Pituicytomas display elongated spindle-shaped cells with eosinophilic cytoplasm arranged in interlacing fascicles
- Granular cell tumors are composed of polygonal cells with abundant granular eosinophilic, PAS-positive cytoplasm

ANCILLARY TESTS

- Positive for TTF-1, S100 protein, vimentin, EMA, GFAP, and galectin-3
- Negative for neuroendocrine markers and pituitary hormones

TOP DIFFERENTIAL DIAGNOSES

- Pituitary adenoma
- Meningioma and schwannoma
- Normal neurohypophysis

Granular Cell Tumor of Neurohypophysis

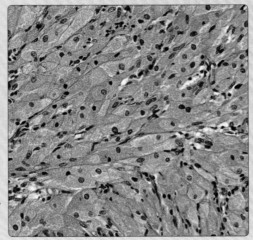

Pituicytoma

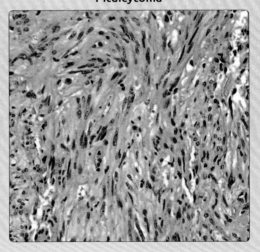

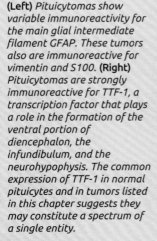

(Left) *Granular cell tumors of the neurohypophysis are composed of polygonal cells with granular cytoplasm and central nuclei. Unlike granular cell tumors of the peripheral nervous system, that are believed to be derived from Schwann cells, the pituitary tumors seem to be derived from pituicytes, the modified glia of the neurohypophysis and infundibulum.* (Right) *Pituicytomas are the prototype of tumors derived from the pituicytes. The tumors are formed by fibrillary cells with elongated nuclei and arranged in fascicles.*

Pituicytoma: GFAP Immunoreactivity

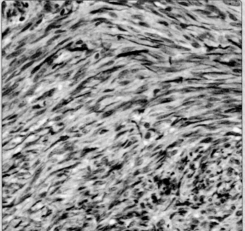

Pituicytoma: TTF-1 Immunoreactivity

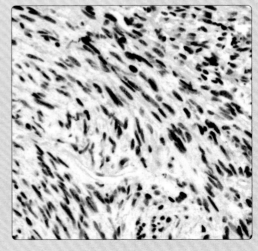

(Left) *Pituicytomas show variable immunoreactivity for the main glial intermediate filament GFAP. These tumors also are immunoreactive for vimentin and S100.* (Right) *Pituicytomas are strongly immunoreactive for TTF-1, a transcription factor that plays a role in the formation of the ventral portion of diencephalon, the infundibulum, and the neurohypophysis. The common expression of TTF-1 in normal pituicytes and in tumors listed in this chapter suggests they may constitute a spectrum of a single entity.*

TERMINOLOGY

Synonyms

- Term "pituicytoma" has been applied to variety of neoplasms
  - With advances understanding of this distinct group of neoplasms, these are now considered morphological spectrum of single nosological entity

Definitions

- Tumors of posterior pituitary are distinct group of low-grade neoplasms of sellar region, most likely constituting morphological spectrum of single nosological entity (WHO 2017)
- Posterior pituitary tumors include
  - Pituicytoma
  - Granular cell tumor of neurohypophysis
  - Spindle cell oncocytoma
  - Sellar ependymoma
- These tumors are believed to derive from pituicytes

ETIOLOGY/PATHOGENESIS

Cell of Origin

- All these 3 entities are believed to derive from pituicyte, specialized glial cell of neurohypophysis and infundibulum
- TTF-1 positivity seen in pituicytomas, spindle cell oncocytomas, and granular cell tumors supports their association with ventral neuroectoderm

CLINICAL ISSUES

Epidemiology

- Incidence
  - Posterior pituitary tumors are rare and represent < 1% of sellar lesions
    - Majority of tumors occur in adults and present in 5th and 6th decades of life
    - Granular cell tumors show M:F = 1:2
    - Pituicytomas are more prevalent in males (1.5:1 ratio)
    - Spindle cell oncocytomas have equal distribution between gender

Presentation

- These tumors can mimic nonfunctioning pituitary adenomas
  - Headache, visual field changes, and sometimes hypopituitarism
  - Mild hyperprolactinemia
    - Tissue destruction can result in hypothalamic hypopituitarism and decreased dopaminergic inhibition of prolactin
  - Sometimes hypopituitarism

Treatment

- Surgical resection usually 1st treatment of choice; radiotherapy may be used in recurrent tumors

Prognosis

- Most of tumors have benign clinical course
  - Local adhesion to adjacent structures may preclude total surgical resection with potential recurrences
  - Spindle cell oncocytomas can recur (1/3 of reported cases)
    - Recurrent tumors exhibit high proliferation rate or marked cellular atypia

IMAGING

Radiological Findings

- Spindle cell oncocytomas and pituicytomas are sharply demarcated, solid, contrast-enhancing masses indistinguishable from pituitary adenomas
- Granular cell tumors are well-demarcated dense lesions on CT and isointense on MR

MACROSCOPIC

General Features

- Spindle cell oncocytomas and pituicytomas are firm, solid lesions
  - Spindle cell oncocytomas may show areas of hemorrhage
- Granular cell tumors are firm, tan to gray, well-demarcated, unencapsulated, rubbery lesions

MICROSCOPIC

Spindle Cell Oncocytoma

- Composed of interlacing fascicles of spindle or epithelioid cells with eosinophilic cytoplasm
- Rare examples of spindle cell oncocytomas with atypical features exhibiting increased mitotic activity and nuclear atypia have been described

Pituicytoma

- Low-grade spindle cell tumor composed of glial cells originating in neurohypophysis or infundibulum
- Elongated spindle-shaped cells with eosinophilic cytoplasm arranged in interlacing fascicles or storiform pattern

Granular Cell Tumor of Neurohypophysis

- Composed of polygonal cells with abundant granular eosinophilic, PAS-positive cytoplasm

ANCILLARY TESTS

Spindle Cell Oncocytoma, Pituicytoma, and Granular Cell Tumor of Neurohypophysis

- Immunohistochemistry
  - Spindle cell oncocytomas, pituicytomas, and granular cell tumors share same immunoprofile
    - Positive for TTF-1, S100 protein, vimentin, EMA (variable), GFAP (variable), and galectin-3 (variable)
    - Spindle cell oncocytomas are diffusely positive for antimitochondrial markers
    - Granular cell tumors are diffusely positive for CD68 and other lysosomal markers
    - Negative for neuroendocrine markers (chromogranin, synaptophysin), pituitary hormones, pituitary transcription factors
- Ultrastructural features
  - Pituicytomas have well-formed intercellular junctions and desmosomes but no secretory granules
  - Spindle cell oncocytomas are rich in mitochondria

o Granular cell tumors are rich in lysosomes

DIFFERENTIAL DIAGNOSIS

Pituitary Adenoma

- Sometimes pituitary adenomas exhibit spindling that can mimic spindle cell oncocytoma/pituicytoma
  - o Positivity for TTF-1, S100 protein, and vimentin in addition to negativity for neuroendocrine markers, pituitary hormones, and pituitary transcription factors distinguishes them from pituitary adenoma

Meningioma and Schwannoma

- Spindle cell nature of cells may mimic pituicytomas and spindle cell oncocytomas
- Positivity for TTF-1 is essential since several markers (including vimentin, EMA, and S100) are shared by these entities

Normal Neurohypophysis

- Distinction of pituicytoma from normal neurohypophysis can be difficult
- Histochemical stains for axons (Bodian and Bielschowsky stains) and immunohistochemistry for neurofilaments demonstrate rich axonal complement of neurohypophysis not seen in pituicytoma

SELECTED REFERENCES

1. Billeci D et al: Spindle cell oncocytoma: report of two cases with massive bleeding and review of the literature. J Clin Neurosci. 39:39-44, 2017
2. Hagel C et al: Immunoprofiling of glial tumours of the neurohypophysis suggests a common pituicytic origin of neoplastic cells. Pituitary. 20(2):211-217, 2017
3. Sahm F et al: WHO 2016 classification: changes and advancements in the diagnosis of miscellaneous primary CNS tumours. Neuropathol Appl Neurobiol. ePub, 2017
4. Sali A et al: Spindle cell oncocytoma of adenohypophysis: review of literature and report of another recurrent case. Neuropathology. ePub, 2017
5. Brat DJ et al: Pituicytoma. In Louis DN et al: WHO Classification of Tumours of the Central Nervous System. 4th ed. Lyon: IARC. 332-33, 2016
6. Fuller GN et al: Granular cell tumour of the sellar region. In Louis DN et al: WHO Classification of Tumours of the Central Nervous System. 4th ed. Lyon: IARC. 329-31, 2016
7. Lopes MBS et al: Spindle cell oncocytoma. In Louis DN et al: WHO Classification of Tumours of the Central Nervous System. 4th ed. Lyon: IARC. 334-36, 2016
8. Neidert MC et al: Synchronous pituitary adenoma and pituicytoma. Hum Pathol. 47(1):138-43, 2016
9. Neidert MC et al: Coexisting pituicytoma and pituitary adenoma; a second coincidence?-reply. Hum Pathol. 55:205-6, 2016
10. Richer M et al: Coexisting pituicytoma and pituitary adenoma: a second coincidence? Hum Pathol. 55:204-5, 2016
11. Vuong HG et al: Spindle cell oncocytoma of adenohypophysis: report of a case and immunohistochemical review of literature. Pathol Res Pract. 212(3):222-5, 2016
12. Wang J et al: The clinicopathological features of pituicytoma and the differential diagnosis of sellar glioma. Neuropathology. 36(5):432-440, 2016
13. Hewer E et al: Suprasellar chordoid neoplasm with expression of thyroid transcription factor 1: evidence that chordoid glioma of the third ventricle and pituicytoma may form part of a spectrum of lineage-related tumors of the basal forebrain. Hum Pathol. ePub, 2015
14. Yoshimoto T et al: TTF-1-positive oncocytic sellar tumor with follicle formation/ependymal differentiation: non-adenomatous tumor capable of two different interpretations as a pituicytoma or a spindle cell oncocytoma. Brain Tumor Pathol. 32(3):221-7, 2015
15. Feng M et al: Surgical management of pituicytomas: case series and comprehensive literature review. Pituitary. 17(5):399-413, 2014
16. Saeed Kamil Z et al: TTF-1 expressing sellar neoplasm with ependymal rosettes and oncocytic change: mixed ependymal and oncocytic variant pituicytoma. Endocr Pathol. 25(4):436-8, 2014
17. Teti C et al: Pituitary image: pituicytoma. Pituitary. 18(5):592-7, 2014
18. Kleinschmidt-DeMasters BK et al: Update on hypophysitis and TTF-1 expressing sellar region masses. Brain Pathol. 23(5):495-514, 2013
19. Mete O et al: Spindle cell oncocytomas and granular cell tumors of the pituitary are variants of pituicytoma. Am J Surg Pathol. 37(11):1694-9, 2013
20. Karamchandani J et al: Pituicytoma of the neurohypophysis: analysis of cell proliferation biomarkers. Can J Neurol Sci. 39(6):835-7, 2012
21. Covington MF et al: Pituicytoma, spindle cell oncocytoma, and granular cell tumor: clarification and meta-analysis of the world literature since 1893. AJNR Am J Neuroradiol. 32(11):2067-72, 2011
22. Vajtai I et al: Spindle cell oncocytoma of the pituitary gland with follicle-like component: organotypic differentiation to support its origin from folliculo-stellate cells. Acta Neuropathol. 122(2):253-8, 2011
23. Coiré CI et al: Rapidly recurring folliculostellate cell tumor of the adenohypophysis with the morphology of a spindle cell oncocytoma: case report with electron microscopic studies. Clin Neuropathol. 28(4):303-8, 2009
24. Lee EB et al: Thyroid transcription factor 1 expression in sellar tumors: a histogenetic marker? J Neuropathol Exp Neurol. 68(5):482-8, 2009
25. Roncaroli F et al: 'Spindle cell oncocytoma' of the adenohypophysis: a tumor of folliculostellate cells? Am J Surg Pathol. 26(8):1048-55, 2002

Spindle Cell Oncocytoma

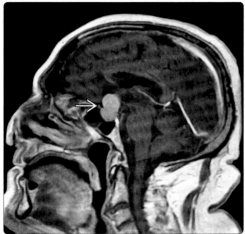

Spindle Cell Oncocytoma

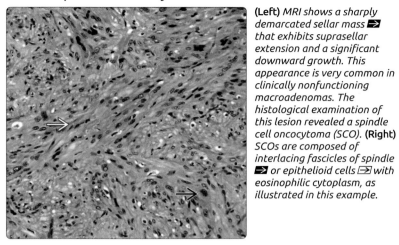

(Left) *MRI shows a sharply demarcated sellar mass ➡ that exhibits suprasellar extension and a significant downward growth. This appearance is very common in clinically nonfunctioning macroadenomas. The histological examination of this lesion revealed a spindle cell oncocytoma (SCO).* (Right) *SCOs are composed of interlacing fascicles of spindle ➡ or epithelioid cells ➡ with eosinophilic cytoplasm, as illustrated in this example.*

Spindle Cell Oncocytoma: S100 Immunoreactivity

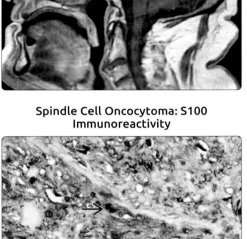

Spindle Cell Oncocytoma: TTF-1 Immunoreactivity

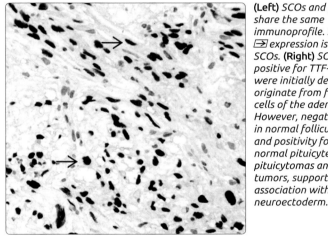

(Left) *SCOs and pituicytomas share the same immunoprofile. S100 protein ➡ expression is present in SCOs.* (Right) *SCOs are positive for TTF-1 ➡. SCOs were initially described to originate from folliculostellate cells of the adenohypophysis. However, negativity for TTF-1 in normal folliculostellate cells and positivity for TTF-1 seen in normal pituicytes, as well in pituicytomas and granular cell tumors, support their association with ventral neuroectoderm.*

Pituicytoma: Ultrastructure

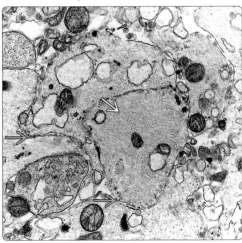

Spindle Cell Oncocytoma: Ultrastructure

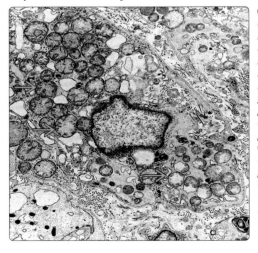

(Left) *SCOs and pituicytomas exhibit well-formed intercellular junctions ➡ and desmosomes. Their cytoplasm is variably filled with intermediate filaments ➡ but no cytoplasmic secretory granules. In this photomicrograph, the common features of pituicytoma are illustrated.* (Right) *There is little to distinguish SCOs from pituicytomas except the oncocytic change characterized by increased numbers of mitochondria ➡ in the cytoplasm of SCOs.*

TERMINOLOGY

- Secondary tumors are metastases to pituitary

ETIOLOGY/PATHOGENESIS

- Hematogenous spread or direct invasion
- Involvement of posterior lobe is more common

CLINICAL ISSUES

- Most common primary sites are breast, lung, and GI tract
- ~ 3-27% of patients with disseminated malignancy develop pituitary metastasis
- Diabetes insipidus is most common endocrinopathy
- Panhypopituitarism is very rare
- Because these tumors occur most frequently in terminal phase of malignancies, prognosis is usually poor
- Invasion of cavernous sinuses and associated structures causes ophthalmoplegia, visual field defects, ptosis, and headache

IMAGING

- Secondary tumors may mimic pituitary adenoma but are more common in neurohypophysis

MICROSCOPIC

- Correct diagnosis of these neoplasms requires detailed histological and immunohistochemical examination
- Most secondary tumors exhibit characteristic histology, suggesting type of differentiation

ANCILLARY TESTS

- Keratins, neuroendocrine markers, pituitary transcription factors, and cell differentiation immunomarkers
- Electron microscopy may be useful when neuroendocrine differentiation is equivocal

TOP DIFFERENTIAL DIAGNOSES

- Null cell adenoma
- Crooke cell adenoma
- Melanoma

Metastatic Neuroendocrine Carcinoma in Anterior Pituitary

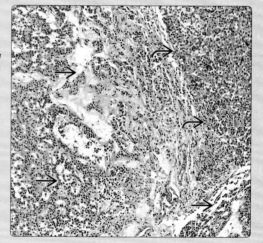

Metastasis to Neurohypophysis

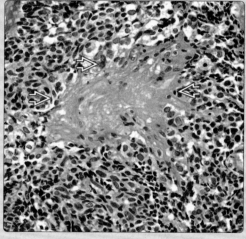

(Left) Solid and acinar architecture of metastatic tumors may mimic pituitary adenomas. Metastatic neuroendocrine carcinoma ➡ is illustrated. The right side of this image shows a normal anterior pituitary gland ➡. (Right) The posterior pituitary gland is most commonly involved by metastatic deposits. Here is an example of a metastatic small cell carcinoma of the lung to the posterior pituitary. Note a neuropil-like area with glial cells ➡ in the center of the figure.

Metastatic Lung Carcinoma to Anterior Pituitary

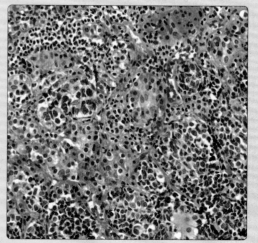

Metastatic Lung Carcinoma to Anterior Pituitary: TTF-1

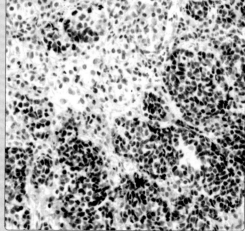

(Left) Metastatic small cell carcinoma of the lung into the anterior pituitary gland is shown. Nests of the malignant tumor cells infiltrate the gland, also inciting an inflammatory response. (Right) Immunohistochemical markers are essential for the differentiation of metastatic lesions from primary pituitary adenomas. In this small cell carcinoma in the same patient, immunoreactivity of the tumor cells for the transcription factor TTF-1 confirmed the lung origin of the metastasis.

TERMINOLOGY

Synonyms

- Metastatic tumors, pituitary tumor deposits

Definitions

- Secondary tumors of pituitary gland are neoplasms originated in extrahypophyseal cells that spread to pituitary

ETIOLOGY/PATHOGENESIS

Pathogenesis

- Secondary tumors of pituitary gland result from either hematogenous spread or direct invasion by bone metastases
- Hematogenous metastases result from abundant vascularity of this gland
- Involvement of posterior lobe is more common

CLINICAL ISSUES

Epidemiology

- Incidence
  - ~ 3-27% of patients with disseminated malignancy develop pituitary metastasis
    - Most common primary sites are breast, lung, and GI tract

Presentation

- Diabetes insipidus is most common endocrinopathy
  - Diabetes insipidus is exceptionally rare in pituitary adenoma and may raise possibility of metastasis in right clinical setting
- Invasion of cavernous sinuses and associated structures causes ophthalmoplegia, visual field defects, ptosis, and headache
- Panhypopituitarism is very rare
- Rare examples of metastatic carcinoma within pituitary adenoma have been reported

Treatment

- Palliative surgical decompression ± radiotherapy may be considered

Prognosis

- Because these tumors occur most frequently in terminal phase of malignancies, prognosis is usually poor

IMAGING

Radiological Features

- Secondary tumors may mimic pituitary adenoma but are more common in neurohypophysis
- Aggressive extrasellar invasion and involvement of cranial nerves is not common feature in pituitary adenomas
  - While pituitary macroadenomas tend to smoothly expand and remodel bone, metastatic tumors destroy bone

MACROSCOPIC

General Features

- Gross findings are variable

MICROSCOPIC

Histological Features

- Correct diagnosis of these neoplasms requires detailed histological and immunohistochemical examination
- Most secondary tumors exhibit characteristic histology, suggesting type of differentiation
- Solid and acinar architecture of metastatic tumors may mimic pituitary adenomas

ANCILLARY TESTS

Immunohistochemistry

- Keratins, neuroendocrine differentiation markers, and transcription factors are helpful

DIFFERENTIAL DIAGNOSIS

Pituitary Adenoma vs. Metastatic Neuroendocrine Carcinoma

- Metastatic neuroendocrine carcinoma (NEC) can mimic pituitary adenoma
  - Pituitary adenomas do not usually express peptides of thyroid, GI, and pancreas
  - Metastatic NEC can express ACTH, CRH, and GHRH but not GH, PRL, β-TSH, FSH, LH, and α-SU
  - In absence of pituitary hormones and pituitary transcription factors, these can be mistaken for null cell adenomas
    - TTF-1 can be expressed in poorly differentiated NEC, regardless of site of origin
    - SF1 can be positive in other steroid hormone-producing tumors, but chromogranin-A is usually negative in extrapituitary SF1 tumors
    - In absence of keratin, hormones, and transcription factors, positivity for tyrosine hydroxylase suggests paraganglioma
    - MIB-1 is usually high in metastatic carcinoma and low in pituitary adenoma

Crooke Cell Adenoma

- Large, atypical keratin (+) cells of Crooke cell adenoma may mimic metastatic carcinoma
- Demonstration of ACTH (along with Tpit) is valuable; however, metastatic NEC may produce ectopic ACTH

Melanoma

- Melanoma in sella is usually metastasis
- Markers of melanocytic differentiation are SOX10, S100 protein, melan-A, HMB-45, and tyrosinase

SELECTED REFERENCES

1. Osamura R et al. Secondary tumours. In: WHO Classification of Tumours of the Endocrine Organs. 4th Edition. IARC: Lyon; pages 63-64, 2017
2. Fassett DR et al: Metastases to the pituitary gland. Neurosurg Focus. 16(4):E8, 2004
3. Komninos J et al: Tumors metastatic to the pituitary gland: case report and literature review. J Clin Endocrinol Metab. 89(2):574-80, 2004
4. Morita A et al: Symptomatic pituitary metastases. J Neurosurg. 89(1):69-73, 1998

Mesenchymal and Hematopoietic Tumors, Pituitary Gland

KEY FACTS

TERMINOLOGY

- Mesenchymal tumors of sella are chordomas, meningiomas, vascular tumors, and tumors of fibroadipose tissue, bone, and cartilage
- Hematopoietic tumors encompass lymphoma, plasmacytoma, leukemia, and histiocytoses

ETIOLOGY/PATHOGENESIS

- Ionizing radiation (sellar sarcomas)

CLINICAL ISSUES

- Patients with mesenchymal tumors present with compressing mass symptoms, including visual disturbances and headaches
- Patients with Langerhans cell histiocytosis most commonly display symptoms of diabetes insipidus and rarely anterior pituitary deficiencies

MICROSCOPIC

- Chordomas composed of large polyhedral cells with vacuoles and areas of myxoid stroma
- Meningiomas composed of meningothelial cells with uniform nuclei and forming meningothelial whorls and fascicles
- Histiocytoses composed of epithelioid and histiocyte-like cells admixed with eosinophils, lymphocytes, and macrophages

ANCILLARY TESTS

- Chordomas usually positive for brachyury, S100 protein, EMA, and keratins
- Langerhans cell histiocytoses positive for S100 protein, CD1a, and langerin
  - *BRAF* V600E mutations common genetic change in Langerhans cell histiocytoses
- Lymphoid cell markers important to distinguish lymphoma from reactive lymphoproliferative disorders

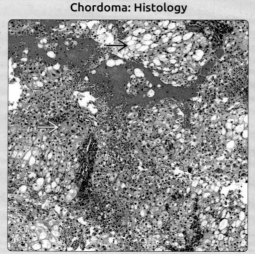

Chordoma: Histology

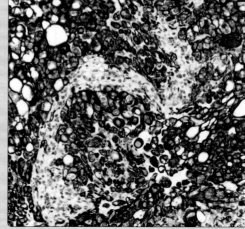

Chordoma: Keratin Immunoreactivity

(Left) *Chordomas are low-grade malignant neoplasms of notochord origin that exhibit a lobular pattern at low magnification. They are composed of cells with pale eosinophilic ➡ to somewhat clear and foamy cytoplasm (physaliphorous cells) ➡ with central round and bland nuclei.* (Right) *Chordomas are positive for S100 protein, EMA, keratins (specifically CK8, CK18, and CK19), HBME-1, and brachyury. Positivity for CK8 is illustrated in this example.*

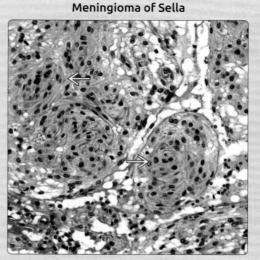

Meningioma of Sella

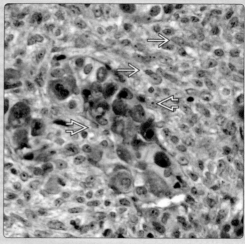

Pituitary Fibrosarcoma

(Left) *Meningiomas of the pituitary region commonly arise from the diaphragma sella or tuberculum sellae. Meningiomas exhibit a variety of morphological variants. In this example, syncytial arrangements and meningothelial whorls ➡ are easily seen.* (Right) *Malignant mesenchymal tumors rarely arise in the pituitary. Postradiation fibrosarcomas are the most common of these malignant tumors, like the case exemplified here. Note pituitary acini ➡ admixed the malignant spindle cells ➡.*

TERMINOLOGY

Definitions

- Variety of mesenchymal and hematopoietic tumors that may develop in sella
  o Mesenchymal tumors can be categorized as
    - Chordomas
    - Tumors of meninges
    - Vascular tumors
    - Tumors of fibroadipose tissue, bone, and cartilage
  o Hematopoietic tumors can be categorized as
    - Lymphomas and leukemias
    - Plasmacytoma
    - Histiocytoses

ETIOLOGY/PATHOGENESIS

Ionizing Irradiation

- Development of sellar sarcomas may be result of ionizing irradiation for pituitary adenoma

Dysfunction of Immune Responses

- Immune dysfunction may play role in pathogenesis of Langerhans cell histiocytoses

Genetic Predisposition

- Patients with neurofibromatosis type 2 (NF2) may develop sellar meningiomas

CLINICAL ISSUES

Epidemiology

- Incidence
  o Mesenchymal tumors of sella rare
    - Chordomas and chondrosarcomas account for 6% of all primary skull base tumors
    - Meningiomas constitute about 1% of tumors of sellar region
  o Lymphoma, leukemia, and histiocytoses usually systemic disorders

Presentation

- Chordomas are slow-growing, locally aggressive neoplasms occurring in patients over age 30
  o Pain, oculomotor disturbances, and cerebellopontine angle syndrome reported in patients with chordomas of clivus
- Meningiomas and other meningeal-related tumors manifest with compressing mass symptoms, including visual problems and headache
  o Incidentally found meningiomas may account for ~ 10%
- Majority of sarcomas secondary to radiation for pituitary lesions; very rare cases primary sarcomas
- Patients with Langerhans cell histiocytosis most commonly display symptoms of diabetes insipidus and rarely anterior pituitary deficiencies
- Sellar mass ± hypopituitarism can rarely be manifestation of lymphoma or leukemia

Treatment

- Surgery preferred initial approach for mesenchymal tumors; radiotherapy considered for incompletely resected lesions

- Postradiation sarcomas usually aggressive tumors
- Pituitary involvement with lymphoma/leukemia usually result of systemic disease
- Langerhans cell histiocytosis commonly treated with combined radiation therapy and chemotherapy

IMAGING

Radiological Features

- Chordomas thought to derive from remnants of notochord and occur in midline
  o Most often involve clivus and extend into sella with erosion of both areas
  o Usually calcified, lobulated, and osteolytic
  o Chordomas usually hyperintense on T2-weighted MR sequences
- Meningiomas mostly suprasellar lesions with hyperintensity on T2-weighted MR sequences
- Lymphomas of sella and hypothalamus hyperintense on T2-weighted MR sequences
  o Contrast enhancement usually uniform
- Histiocytoses usually ill-defined lesions mostly involving pituitary stalk
  o MR can detect small, multifocal lesions
  o Contrast-enhancing, hypodense masses on CT scan

MACROSCOPIC

General Features

- Chordomas have gelatinous and lobulated appearance with areas of calcification
- Meningiomas soft to fibrous lesions with multinodular gross appearance
- Vascular tumors soft lesions that contain areas of hemorrhage

MICROSCOPIC

Chordomas

- Cords and lobules of large, polyhedral cells with characteristic bubbly appearance
  o Term "physaliphorous" used to describe mucin and glycogen-containing vacuoles
- Cells separated by fibrous septa with extensive myxoid stroma that contains scattered stellate cells
- Some tumors may have more chondroid matrix and are denominated chondroid chordoma
  o Chondroid chordoma have similar biological behavior than regular chordoma
  o Dedifferentiated chordoma highly malignant biphasic neoplasm composed of typical chordoma and areas resembling fibrosarcoma, osteosarcoma, or pleomorphic undifferentiated high-grade sarcoma
    - Very rare variant in intracranial chordomas

Tumors of Meninges

- Meningiomas and solitary fibrous tumor/hemangiopericytoma may involve sella
- Meningiomas composed of meningothelial cells with uniform nuclei and forming meningothelial whorls and fascicles
  o At least 14 variants of meningiomas described by WHO, some with significant prognostic value

- Solitary fibrous tumor/hemangiopericytoma have spectrum of histological features ranging from spindle, fibrous cells arranged in fascicles to plump cells intermixed with branching, staghorn-like vessels

Vascular Tumors

- Benign cavernous hemangioma has been described in sella
- Glomangioma of sella thought to arise from gomitoli of pituitary stalk
- Sellar hemangioblastomas also reported in patients with von Hippel-Lindau disease

Tumors of Fibrous Tissue, Fat, Bone, & Cartilage

- Benign: Lipoma, myxoma, fibroma, giant cell tumor, chondromyxoid fibroma, chondroma, osteochondroma, enchondroma
- Malignant: Chondrosarcoma, osteosarcoma, rhabdomyosarcoma, leiomyosarcoma, alveolar soft part sarcoma, fibrosarcoma
- All these tumors extremely rare in sellar region

Histiocytoses

- **Langerhans cell histiocytosis**
  - Composed of epithelioid and histiocyte-like cells
  - Kidney-shaped, irregular nuclei and abundant cytoplasm
  - Usually admixed with eosinophils, chronic inflammatory cells, and foamy macrophages
- **Non-Langerhans cell histiocytoses**
  - Erdheim-Chester disease prototypic of rare systemic non-Langerhans cell histiocytoses
    - Accumulation of lipid-laden foamy histiocytes forming xanthomatous or xanthogranulomatous infiltrate
    - Variable stromal fibrosis
    - Occasional eosinophils, lymphocytic infiltrate with multinucleated giant cells

Lymphoma and Leukemia

- Lymphomas of sella or hypothalamus resemble systemic lymphomas
- Majority B-cell tumors with diffuse growth rather than follicular pattern
- Plasmacytomas may involve pituitary secondarily by involvement of sellar bone

ANCILLARY TESTS

Immunohistochemistry

- **Chordomas**
  - Positive for keratins, EMA, and S100 protein
  - Positive for brachyury (nuclear transcription factor regulating notochord development) and HBME-1
- **Meningiomas**
  - Positive for vimentin, EMA, SSR2
- Solitary fibrous tumor/hemangiopericytoma
  - Most significant positive for STAT6, diagnostic feature of these tumors
  - Positive for vimentin, CD34, CD99, Bcl-2
- **Histiocytoses**
  - Langerhans cells positive for S100 protein, CD1a, and langerin (CD207), and negative for CD45 and CD15
  - Immunostaining for BRAF mutated protein may be positive

  - Non-Langerhans cell histiocytosis positive for S100 protein, lysozyme, CD68, CD11c, and MAC387 but not langerin and CD1a

Genetic Testing

- *BRAF* V600E mutations common genetic change in Langerhans cell histiocytoses

DIFFERENTIAL DIAGNOSIS

Metastatic Renal Cell Carcinoma or Signet Cell Carcinoma vs. Chordoma

- Negativity for brachyury and lack of lobular architecture favor metastatic carcinoma
- Renal cell carcinomas exhibit prominent stromal vascularity when compared to chordomas

Chondrosarcoma vs. Chordoma

- Positivity for both EMA and keratins favors chordoma

Chordoid Meningioma vs. Chordoma

- Chordoid meningioma is an uncommon variant of meningioma with propensity for aggressive behavior and increased likelihood of recurrence
- EMA is usually positive in chordomas and chordoid meningiomas; keratins can be sometimes negative in chordoid meningiomas
- Nuclear transcription factor "brachyury" is only positive in chordomas

Lymphocytic Hypophysitis vs. Lymphoma

- Lymphocytes monophenotypical analysis by immunohistochemistry and monoclonality by molecular assays is mandatory

SELECTED REFERENCES

1. Huo Z et al: Clinicopathological features and BRAFV600E mutations in patients with isolated hypothalamic-pituitary Langerhans cell histiocytosis. Diagn Pathol. 11(1):100, 2016
2. Perry A et al. Meningioma. In: WHO classification of tumours of the central nervous system. Revised 4th Edition. IARC: Lyon. 232-245, 2016
3. Kwancharoen R et al: Clinical features of sellar and suprasellar meningiomas. Pituitary. 17(4):342-8, 2014
4. Schweizer L et al: Meningeal hemangiopericytoma and solitary fibrous tumors carry the NAB2-STAT6 fusion and can be diagnosed by nuclear expression of STAT6 protein. Acta Neuropathol. 125(5):651-8, 2013
5. Cho HY et al: Immunohistochemical comparison of chordoma with chondrosarcoma, myxopapillary ependymoma, and chordoid meningioma. Appl Immunohistochem Mol Morphol. 17(2):131-8, 2009
6. Oakley GJ et al: Brachyury, SOX-9, and podoplanin, new markers in the skull base chordoma vs chondrosarcoma differential: a tissue microarray-based comparative analysis. Mod Pathol. 21(12):1461-9, 2008
7. Almefty K et al: Chordoma and chondrosarcoma: similar, but quite different, skull base tumors. Cancer. 110(11):2457-67, 2007
8. Vujovic S et al: Brachyury, a crucial regulator of notochordal development, is a novel biomarker for chordomas. J Pathol. 209(2):157-65, 2006

Solitary Fibrous Tumor of Sella

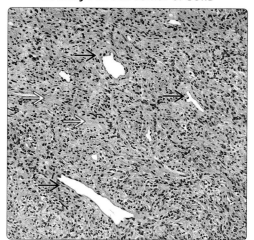

Solitary Fibrous Tumor: CD34

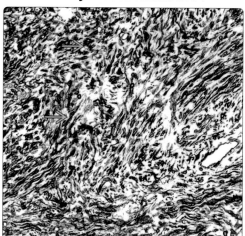

(Left) *Sellar solitary fibrous tumors are composed of a spindle cell proliferation that exhibits large, gaping sinusoidal spaces ("staghorn" configuration ➡). They often exhibit variable amounts of fibrosis, hyalinization ➡, or myxoid change.* (Right) *Diffuse positivity for CD34 ➡ is illustrated in a solitary fibrous tumor. Solitary fibrous tumors are positive for CD34, Bcl-2, and CD99. Nuclear STAT6 expression is diagnostic of these tumors.*

Glomangioma of Sella

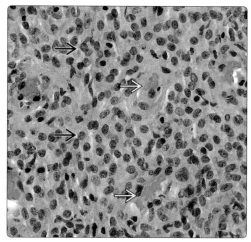

Glomangioma: SMA

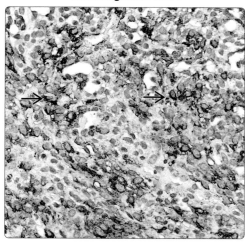

(Left) *Glomangiomas are rare sellar tumors composed of epithelioid cells ➡ surrounding prominent small, vascular channels ➡. The tumor cells have indistinct cell borders and monotonous nuclei.* (Right) *Glomangiomas are positive for vimentin and smooth muscle actin and are negative for CD34. Positivity for smooth muscle actin ➡ is illustrated in this sellar glomangioma.*

Plasmacytoma of Sella

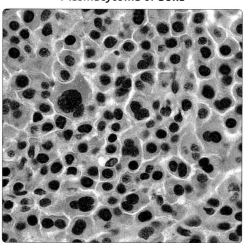

Histiocytosis of Sella

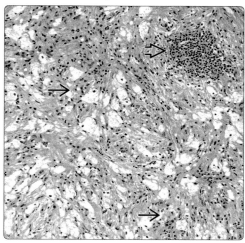

(Left) *Sellar plasmacytoma can mimic pituitary adenoma and metastatic neuroendocrine carcinoma. In this example, a sellar plasmacytoma is illustrated.* (Right) *Erdheim-Chester disease is prototypic of rare systemic non-Langerhans cell histiocytoses. It is characterized by accumulation of lipid-laden foamy macrophages ➡ forming xanthomatous or xanthogranulomatous infiltrate with occasional inflammation ➡ and stromal fibrosis.*

Pituitary

Pathology Case Summary (Checklist)

Procedure (select all that apply)

____	Transsphenoidal resection
____	Transcranial resection
____	Other (specify): _____
____	Not specified

Clinical Features

____	Functional
	Hormone excess (specify): _____
____	Clinically nonfunctioning

Tumor Size (from imaging)

____	Microadenoma (< 1 cm)
____	Macroadenoma (≥ 1 cm)
	Greatest dimension: _____ cm
	*Additional dimensions: _____ x _____ cm
____	Cannot be determined

*Received

*____	Fresh
*____	In formalin
____	Other

*Specimen Integrity

*____	Intact
*____	Fragmented

*Specimen Size

	_____ x _____ x _____ cm

*Specimen Weight

	*_____ g

Histologic Features

	Reticulin
	____ Intact
	____ Expanded
	____ Disrupted
	Infiltrating tumor
	____ Positive (specify tissue): _____
	____ Negative
	____ Cannot be determined

Immunohistochemistry

____	Adrenocorticotrophin (ACTH)
____	Growth hormone (GH)
____	Prolactin (PRL)
____	β-thyrotropin (TSH)
____	β-follicle-stimulating hormone (FSH)
____	β-luteinizing hormone (LH)
____	α-subunit
____	PIT-1
____	SF1
____	Tpit
____	Estrogen receptor (ER)

Pituitary (Continued)

Pathology Case Summary (Checklist)

____ Keratin (CAM5.2)

    ____ Diffuse

    ____ Fibrous bodies

    ____ Perinuclear

    ____ Membranous

____ MIB-1/Ki-67 proliferative index: _____ %

____ *Synaptophysin

____ *Chromogranin

____ Others (specify): _____

Additional Ancillary Studies

Specify: _____

Tumor Type: WHO Classification

Pituitary adenoma

  Subtype

    ____ Densely granulated corticotroph adenoma

    ____ Sparsely granulated corticotroph adenoma

    ____ Crooke cell adenoma

    ____ Densely granulated somatotroph adenoma

    ____ Sparsely granulated somatotroph adenoma

    ____ Mammosomatotroph adenoma

    ____ Mixed somatotroph-lactotroph adenoma

    ____ Sparsely granulated lactotroph adenoma

    ____ Densely granulated lactotroph adenoma

    ____ Acidophil stem cell adenoma

    ____ Thyrotroph adenoma

____ Plurihormonal Pit-1(+) adenoma

    ____ Unusual plurihormonal adenoma

    ____ Gonadotroph adenoma

    ____ Null cell adenoma

    ____ Other (specify): _____

Hyperplasia

    ____ Cell type (specify): _____

Pituitary carcinoma

    ____ Cell type (specify): _____

  Location of metastases: _____

Craniopharyngioma

    ____ Papillary

    ____ Adamantinomatous

Other

    ____ Gangliocytoma

    ____ Paraganglioma

    ____ Spindle cell oncocytoma

    ____ Pituicytoma

    ____ Granular cell tumor of sella

    ____ Other (specify): _____

Additional Pathologic Findings

Nontumorous adenohypophysis

Pituitary (Continued)

Pathology Case Summary (Checklist)

____ Present	
*____ Crooke hyaline change	
____ Not identified	
Neurohypophysis	
____ Present	
____ Not identified	

*Protocol applies to all adenomas and craniopharyngiomas of the pituitary gland. Primary neuronal tumors, lymphomas, sarcomas, and metastases are not included. *Data elements with asterisks are not required. These elements may be clinically important but are not yet validated or regularly used in patient management. Modified from Nosé V et al:Protocol for the examination of specimens from patients with primary pituitarytumors. Arch Pathol Lab Med. May;135(5):640-6, 2011.*

Pituitary Gland

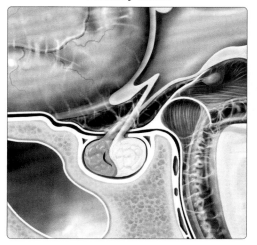

Pituitary Anterior and Posterior Lobes

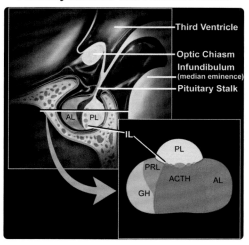

Third Ventricle · Optic Chiasm · Infundibulum (median eminence) · Pituitary Stalk · AL · PL · IL · PL · PRL · ACTH · AL · GH

(Left) *The adenohypophysis is comprised of the pars tuberalis, pars intermedia, and pars distalis. The neurohypophysis is comprised of the median eminence of hypothalamus, infundibulum, and pars nervosa.* (Right) *The pituitary is composed of neural tissue [the pituitary stalk and posterior lobe (PL)], epithelial tissue [the anterior lobe (AL)], and the cystic remnants of the intermediate lobe (IL). Normal distribution of ACTH, GH, and PRL cells is shown (inset).*

Pituitary Anatomic Relationships

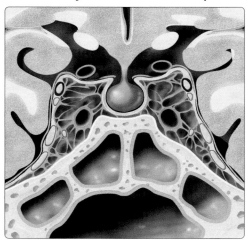

Pituitary Uniform Enlargement

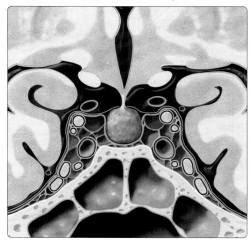

(Left) *The cranial nerves (oculomotor, trochlear, and 1st and 2nd divisions of trigeminal nerves) traverse the cavernous sinus within the lateral wall of the cavernous sinus. The only cranial nerve within the sinusoids of the cavernous sinus is the abducens nerve.* (Right) *Coronal graphic shows physiologic pituitary hyperplasia. The gland is uniformly enlarged and has a mildly convex superior margin.*

Pituitary Microadenoma

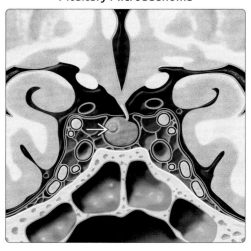

Pituitary Macroadenoma

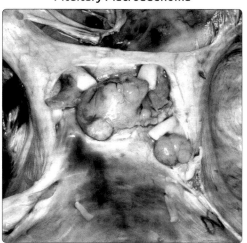

(Left) *Coronal graphic shows a small microadenoma ➜ that slightly enlarges the right side of the pituitary gland and deviates the infundibulum toward the left.* (Right) *Gross pathology shows a pituitary macroadenoma that extends upward through the diaphragma sellae into the suprasellar cistern and laterally into the cavernous sinus, which is partially unroofed.*

SECTION 5
Endocrine Pancreas

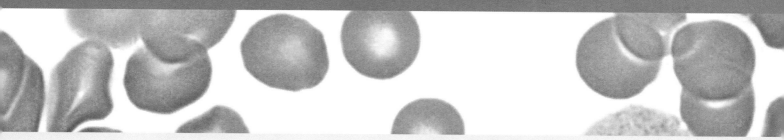

TERMINOLOGY

- WHO 2017 classifies PETs into 3 broad categories
  - **Well-differentiated neuroendocrine tumors (PanNETs)**
    - **PanNET G1**: < 2 mitoses/50 HPF, < 3% Ki-67 proliferative index
    - **PanNET G2**: 2-20 mitoses/50 HPF, 3-20% Ki-67 proliferative index
    - **PanNET G3**: > 20 mitoses/50 HPF, > 20% Ki-67 proliferative index
  - **Poorly differentiated pancreatic neuroendocrine carcinoma (PanNECs)**
    - **PanNEC (G3)**: > 20 mitoses/50 HPF, > 20% Ki-67 proliferative index
      - □ Small cell type
      - □ Large cell type
  - **Mixed neuroendocrine-nonneuroendocrine (ductal or acinar) neoplasms**

- In 10-20% of cases, well-differentiated PanNENs associated with hereditary syndromes
  - **Multiple endocrine neoplasia type 1**: ~ 80% have PETs (50% gastrinoma)
  - **von Hippel-Lindau syndrome**: Benign cysts and adenomas, which occur in 35-70% of VHL patients
    - Up to 60% of tumors contain clear cells or multivacuolated lipid-rich cells
  - **NF1**: Pancreatic somatostatinomas more rare than those of duodenal origin
  - **Tuberous sclerosis**: Rare
  - **Glucagon cell hyperplasia and neoplasia**: Unrelated to MEN1 and VHL
- Mutation in *MEN1* in ~ 45%, and *DAXX* or *ATRX* in ~ 45% of sporadic PanNETs
- ~ 15% sporadic PanNETs have alterations in *TSC2*, *PTEN*, *PIK3CA*
- Somatic mutations in *TP53*, *RB1*, *CDKN2A* in sporadic PanNECs

Pancreatic Tumor With Liver Metastases

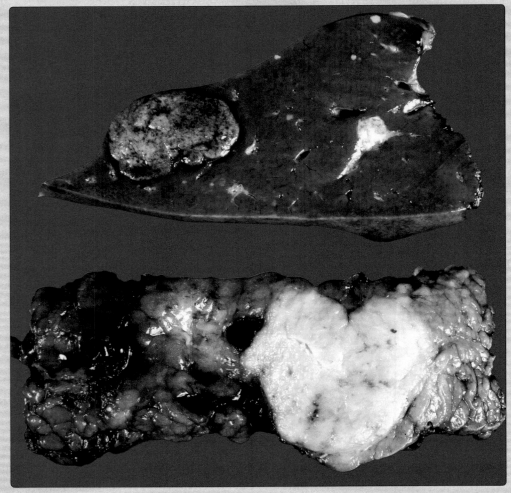

Pancreatic neuroendocrine tumor in a patient with Cushing syndrome shows a 3.8 cm, firm, tan-yellow cut surface. This ACTH-producing tumor metastasized to the liver.

TERMINOLOGY

Abbreviations

- Pancreatic neuroendocrine neoplasms (PanNENs)
- Pancreatic neuroendocrine tumor (PanNET)
- Pancreatic neuroendocrine carcinoma (PanNEC)

Synonyms

- Gastroenteropancreatic neuroendocrine tumors
- Pancreatic endocrine tumor
- Islet cell tumor
- Well-differentiated PET
- Poorly differentiated neuroendocrine carcinoma

Definitions

- PanNENs have significant neuroendocrine differentiation, with expression of synaptophysin and chromogranin (WHO 2017), including
  o Malignant well-differentiated neuroendocrine neoplasms, which are called PanNETs
  o Poorly differentiated neuroendocrine neoplasms, which are called PanNECs
- **PanNET**
  o Well-differentiated neuroendocrine neoplasms of low, intermediate, and high grade, composed of cells showing minimal to moderate atypia, displaying organoid patterns, and lacking necrosis
    - Expressing general markers or neuroendocrine differentiation: Diffuse and intense synaptophysin and usually also chromogranin staining
    - Expressing hormones: Usually intense, but not diffuse, either orthotopic or ectopic to pancreas
- **PanNEC**
  o Poorly differentiated high-grade neuroendocrine neoplasms composed of highly atypical small cells or intermediate to large cells
    - Expressing general markers or neuroendocrine differentiation: Diffuse or faint synaptophysin and focal to faint chromogranin-A staining
    - Rarely hormones; lacking expression of trypsin or chymotrypsin, markers of exocrine pancreas
- **Neuroendocrine-nonneuroendocrine neoplasm (MiNEN)**
  o Mixed neoplasm with neuroendocrine component combined with a nonneuroendocrine component: Typically ductal adenocarcinoma or acinar cell carcinoma
    - Both components high grade (G3)
      □ Occasionally, one component may be G2 or G1
    - Each component should account for > 30% of cell population
  o Diagnosis should give indication of cell component
    - Mixed acinar-neuroendocrine carcinoma
    - Mixed ductal-neuroendocrine carcinoma

Classification

- WHO 2017 classifies PETs into 3 broad categories
  o **PanNET**
    - **PanNET G1**: < 2 mitoses/50 HPF, < 3% Ki-67 proliferative index
    - **PanNET G2**: 2-20 mitoses/50 HPF, 3-20% Ki-67 proliferative index
    - **PanNET G3**: > 20 mitoses/50 HPF, > 20% Ki-67 proliferative index
  o **PanNECs**
    - **PanNEC (G3)**: > 20 mitosis/50 HPF, > 20% Ki-67 proliferative index
      □ Small cell type
      □ Large cell type
  o **MiNEN**
    - Tumors with both exocrine and endocrine features in morphologically uniform population, proven by double-labeled immunohistochemistry or EM
  o **Other tumors**
    - **Pancreatic neuroendocrine tumor with ductules**
    - Neuroendocrine microadenoma: < 0.5 cm
      □ Nonfunctional, discovered incidentally (surgery, radiographic, autopsy)
      □ Pancreatic head affected most commonly
      □ Often coexpress > 1 peptide
      □ Multiple microadenomas present in multiple endocrine neoplasia type 1 (MEN1) syndrome
- PanNETs can be classified as sporadic or inherited
  o In 10-20% of cases, well-differentiated PanNENs are associated with hereditary syndromes
    - MEN1
    - von Hippel-Lindau (VHL) syndrome
    - Neurofibromatosis
    - Tuberous sclerosis
    - Glucagon cell hyperplasia and neoplasia
- PanNETs divided in functional or nonfunctional
  o Functional: Associated with clinical syndromes caused by abnormal secretion of hormones
    - Insulinomas
    - Gastrinomas
    - Glucagonomas
    - VIPomas
  o Nonfunctional (~ 60% of all PanNENs)
    - Not associated with clinical hormone hypersecretion
    - May secrete pancreatic polypeptide and chromogranin; secreted at levels insufficient to cause symptoms

ETIOLOGY/PATHOGENESIS

Sporadic PanNET

- Majority of cases nonsyndromic (sporadic)
- No defined precursor lesions
  o Somatic mutations of *MEN1* gene identified in ~ 45%
  o Mutation in either *DAXX* or *ATRX* in ~ 45%
  o ~ 15% have alterations in *TSC2, PTEN, PIK3CA*
- Genetic alterations in PanNECs are different
  o Somatic mutations in *TP53, RB1, CDKN2A* (P16)

Syndromic PanNET

- Associated with MEN1, VHL, tuberous sclerosis (TS), NF1, and glucagon cell hyperplasia and neoplasia syndromes
- PETs associated with syndromes are associated with characteristic genetic abnormalities
- **MEN1**
  o *MEN1* gene
  o ~ 80% of cases have PETs
    - PETs diagnosed clinically in ~ 80% of patients with MEN1
    - This number approaches 100% in autopsy studies

o Patients with MEN1 have unique profile of hormonal function: 50% are gastrin-producing tumors, and 20% are insulin-producing tumors
  - In MEN1, duodenal gastrin-producing NETs are more common than those arising in pancreas
o MEN1 involvement of pancreas initially involves development of multiple small PETs, often microadenomas, associated with foci of nesidioblastosis or ductuloinsular complexes
o Presence of peliosis in islets and adenomas is curious feature
o Islet dysplasia: Normal-sized or slightly enlarged islets containing cells with mild cytologic atypia
  - Readily confirmed by immunohistochemistry that shows loss of normal spatial and quantitative arrangement of 4 main cell types
o Once islet dysplasia attains size of 0.5 mm, it is classified as microadenoma; islet dysplasia most frequently associated with MEN1
o MEN1 diagnosed in ~ 25% of patients who have gastrinoma and in ~ 5% of those who have insulin-producing PET
o In contrast to sporadic PETs, those associated with MEN1 tend to present at earlier age (30-50 years), have higher rate of postoperative recurrence, and are common cause of death in these patients
o MEN1-associated PETs display wide variety of molecular abnormalities, including chromosomal loss, chromosomal loss with duplication, mitotic recombination, or point mutation of wild-type MEN1 allele
o Similar to sporadic counterparts, exhibit inter- and intratumoral genetic heterogeneity, indicating chromosomal instability

- **VHL**
  o *VHL* gene
  o Pancreatic pathology in VHL usually takes form of benign cysts and microcystic or serous adenomas
    - Occur in 35-70% of VHL patients
    - Occur in young patients, are multiple and located anywhere in pancreas
    - Tumors said to be functionally inactive, although immunohistochemistry shows focal positivity for pancreatic polypeptide (PP), somatostatin, glucagon, &/or insulin in 30-40% of cases
    - Initially reported not to be associated with either microadenomas (endocrine cell foci, 0.5 cm in diameter) or nesidioblastosis; however, there is association of these findings with VHL
  o VHL-associated PETs tend to be arranged in trabeculae, glandular configurations, and solid foci
  o Characteristically, up to 60% of tumors contain clear cells or multivacuolated, lipid-rich cells in varying proportions
  o No data on VHL genotypic predisposition to PETs
  o Pancreatic tumors in patients with this disorder have been documented to exhibit loss of heterozygosity of normal *VHL* allele

- **TS**
  o *TSC1* and *TSC2* genes
  o Rare PETs have been reported in patients with TS
    - Not clear if causal association
  o Malignant PETs described in children

o Functional PETs reported to produce both insulin and gastrin
o TSC1 (hamartin) highly expressed in normal islet cells; loss of this tumor suppressor speculated to have etiologic role in these lesions

- **NF1**
  o *NF1* gene
  o Somatostatinomas of pancreas rarer than those of duodenal origin
    - 16x less common than duodenal somatostatinomas
  o Duodenal somatostatinomas occur in NF1 patients
    - NF1 accounted for 48% of duodenal somatostatinomas reported in literature
  o Occasional NF1 patients may have pancreatic gastrinoma, insulinoma, and nonfunctioning PET

- **Glucagon cell hyperplasia and neoplasia syndrome**
  o Germline *GCGR* mutation
  o Development of islet glucagon cell hyperplasia and glucagon cell microtumors and macrotumors
  o Only ~ 10 cases reported to date

CLINICAL ISSUES

Epidemiology

- Incidence
  o 2-5% of clinically detected pancreatic neoplasms
    - 1 per 100,000 people per year (USA)
    - 2-4 per million people per year for insulinoma
    - Asymptomatic type found in up to 1.5% of autopsies
  o ~ 20% of PET are MEN1 associated
  o Relative increase due to more sensitive diagnostic approaches
- Age
  o Peak: 30-60 years (mean: 50 years)
  o Syndrome-associated tumors (MEN1) tend to occur earlier (10-30 years)
- Sex
  o Equal distribution
    - Exception for somatostatinoma: F > M (2:1)
    - Exception for gastrinoma: M > F (1.2:1)

Site

- Entire pancreas may be affected; most common sites are body and tail
  o Somatostatinomas: More common in head
  o Gastrinoma: Head, duodenum, gastric antrum, and peripancreatic soft tissues
  o Glucagonoma: Tail most common
  o Vasoactive intestinal peptide (VIP)-oma: Most common in tail

Presentation

- **Functional PanNET**: Clinical syndromes related to excessive or inappropriate hormone or biogenic amine production
  o ~ 60%
  o Ectopic hormone: Gastrin, VIP, PP, ACTH, serotonin, and neurotensin
  o Pancreatic hormone: Insulin, glucagon, somatostatin, VIP
  o **Insulinoma syndrome** (~ 20%)

- Insulinoma is functioning, well-differentiated pancreatic neuroendocrine neoplasm composed of insulin-producing and pro-insulin-producing cells with uncontrolled insulin secretion causing hypoglycemic syndrome (WHO 2017)
- Whipple triad includes
  - □ Symptoms of hypoglycemia
  - □ Plasma glucose levels < 3.0 mmol/L
  - □ Relief of symptoms with administration of glucose
○ **Glucagonoma syndrome**
  - Glucagonoma is functioning, well-differentiated pancreatic neuroendocrine neoplasm composed of glucagon-producing and pre-proglucagon-derived peptide-producing cells with uncontrolled glucagon secretion causing glucagonoma syndrome (WHO 2017)
  - Skin rash (necrolytic migratory erythema) in 70% of patients
  - Rash usually starts in groin/perineum and migrates to distal extremities
  - Associated with angular stomatitis, cheilitis, atrophic glossitis, alopecia, onycholysis, vulvovaginitis, and urethritis
  - Marked weight loss (65%), mild diabetes mellitus (glucose intolerance) (50%), anemia (33%), diarrhea, depression (20%), deep vein thrombosis (12%)
○ **Somatostatinoma syndrome**
  - Somastotatinoma is functioning, well-differentiated pancreatic neuroendocrine neoplasm composed of somatostatin-producing neoplasm with uncontrolled somatostatin secretion causing somatostatinoma syndrome (WHO 2017)
  - Nonspecific findings, although diabetes mellitus, hypochlorhydria, gallbladder disease (cholelithiasis), diarrhea, steatorrhea, anemia, and weight loss may be present
  - Markedly elevated somatostatin serum/tumor levels define syndrome
○ **Gastrinoma syndrome** (~ 15%)
  - Gastrinoma is functioning, well-differentiated pancreatic neuroendocrine neoplasm composed of gastrin-producing G-cells with uncontrolled gastrin secretion causing Zollinger-Ellison syndrome (WHO 2017)
  - Increased gastrin results in gastric or duodenal ulcers, resulting in abdominal pain, diarrhea, vomiting, and weight loss
  - 25% of patients found to have MEN1 syndrome
○ **VIPoma syndrome**
  - VIPoma is functioning, well-differentiated pancreatic neuroendocrine neoplasm composed of VIP-producing and other hormone-like substance-producing cells with uncontrolled VIP secretion causing WDHA syndrome (WHO 2017)
  - a.k.a. Verner-Morrison syndrome
  - VIP excess produces voluminous watery diarrhea, hypokalemia, achlorhydria, and metabolic acidosis
  - Accounts for 80% of diarrheogenic tumors
○ **Serotonin-producing tumors**

- Functioning, well-differentiated pancreatic neuroendocrine neoplasm composed of serotonin-producing cells; rarely, release of serotonin can produce carcinoid syndrome (WHO 2017)
○ **ACTH-producing tumor with Cushing syndrome**
  - ACTH-producing tumor is functioning, well-differentiated pancreatic neuroendocrine neoplasm composed of ACTH-producing and ACTH-secreting cells causing Cushing syndrome (WHO 2017)
- **Nonfunctional PanNET**
  ○ Nonfunctioning, well-differentiated pancreatic neuroendocrine neoplasm occurring in patients with no paraneoplastic symptoms attributable to abnormal secretion of hormones or bioamines by tumor cells (WHO 2017)
  ○ Also called "inactive," "nonsyndromic," or "incidentally discovered"
  ○ Increased frequency more recently due to enhanced diagnostic imaging
    - Now, relative frequency ~70-80% of PanNETs
  ○ May have elevated hormone levels but not distinct syndrome
  ○ Large abdominal mass, abdominal or back pain, obstructive symptoms, pancreatitis
  ○ Jaundice may develop in large tumors located in head of pancreas
  ○ Large tumors usually nonfunctional

Laboratory Tests

- **Insulinoma**
  ○ Elevated plasma insulin and proinsulin concentrations by radioimmunoassay
    - Combined measures of insulin, proinsulin, C-peptide, and blood glucose help exclude factitious hyperinsulinemia
- **Glucagonoma**
  ○ Elevated fasting plasma glucagon concentration (usually 10-20x)
  ○ Tolbutamide or arginine stimulation tests may be used
  ○ ~ 20% will also have increased plasma gastrin levels
- **Somatostatinoma**
  ○ Elevated plasma somatostatin levels
- **Gastrinoma**
  ○ Secretin stimulation test (measures evoked gastrin levels)
  ○ 3 separate elevated fasting gastrin levels
  ○ Gastric acid secretion and pH

Treatment

- Options, risks, complications
  ○ Multidisciplinary approach mandatory
  ○ Before surgery, important to separate MEN1-associated tumors from solitary, nonsyndrome-associated, and malignant tumors
  ○ Pre- and intraoperative localization critical for management
  ○ Management of hormone production critical
  ○ Hormone replacement therapy if pancreatectomy performed
- Surgical approaches
  ○ Complete surgical resection

- – Enucleation or pancreas-preserving techniques, dependent on number of tumors, size, location, and duct association
  - o Debulking required for advanced disease
    - – May include adjacent organs (adrenal, stomach, spleen, and colon)
  - o Removal of hepatic metastases yields better outcome
    - – Surgery, hepatic artery embolization, &/or radiofrequency ablation
- Adjuvant therapy
  - o Usually employed for high-stage, malignant, &/or metastatic tumors
    - – Streptozocin, dacarbazine, doxorubicin, and 5-fluorouracil
  - o Includes chemoembolization for liver metastases
- Drugs
  - o Medical management frequently employed for metastatic disease
  - o Combined targeted therapies help to avoid molecular escape pathways
  - o Radionuclide peptide receptor targeted therapy (radioimmunotherapy)
    - – Somatostatin analogues radiolabeled with yttrium-90 or lutetium-177
  - o Long-acting somatostatin analogues palliate hormone syndromes
    - – Octreotide (Sandostatin), lanreotide, pasireotide
  - o Antiangiogenic (angiogenesis inhibitors) agents
    - – Bevacizumab, imatinib, EGFR inhibitors
  - o Biotherapy using interferon, mTOR inhibitors, and novel cytotoxic agents

Prognosis

- PanNETs generally slow-growing, with overall 5-year survival of 33%, 10-year survival of 17%, and 20-year survival of 10%
- Patients with PanNECs rarely survive 1 year
- Routine morphologic examination does not always predict behavior
  - o Metastatic disease (lymph nodes, liver) clinches malignant diagnosis
  - o Locally infiltrative disease, perineural and vascular invasion seen more often in malignant tumors
- Up to 30% of patients already have metastatic disease at diagnosis
  - o ~ 65% will develop metastatic disease at some point during disease course
- Survival depends on tumor size, functional status, and extent of local invasion
  - o Nonfunctional: 65% 5-year survival; 45% 10-year survival
  - o Functional: 45% 5-year survival (except insulinoma)
- Tumor behavior associated with functional status and specific hormone produced
  - o Nonfunctional tumors nearly all malignant (90%)
  - o **Insulinoma**: Has best prognosis
    - – Vast majority benign (~ 8% malignant)
    - – Early detection as result of symptoms while still small
  - o **Glucagonoma**
    - – ~ 60-70% have metastases at time of diagnosis
    - – Tumor size does not seem to correlate with behavior (most large)

- – Patients survive for many years due to slow tumor growth
  - o **Somatostatinoma**
    - – Generally large at time of diagnosis
    - – ~ 70% have metastases at time of diagnosis
    - – 75% 5-year survival (worse if metastases present)
- Long-term clinical follow-up required
  - o Metastases develop late
  - o Even when metastases identified, long-term survival common
- Adverse prognostic factors
  - o Metastasis to regional lymph nodes &/or liver
  - o Gross invasion into adjacent organs
  - o Angiolymphatic invasion and perineural invasion
  - o Rule of 2: > 2 cm, > 2 mitoses/10 HPF, > 2% proliferation index (Ki-67)
  - o Necrosis
  - o Functioning tumor (except insulinoma)
- Surgical margin, WHO 2010 grading, and TNM staging systems may all be meaningful prognostic factors impacting long-term survival of patients with p-NETs

IMAGING

Ultrasonographic Findings

- Endoscopic US: 20-65% sensitivity

MR Findings

- MR imaging: 25-60% sensitivity

Somatostatin Receptor Scintigraphy &/or Positron Emission Tomography

- Somatostatin analogues attach with high-affinity binding to receptors overexpressed by tumors
- Allows for detection of very small tumors
- Gastrinoma, somatostatinoma, glucagonoma, and VIPoma usually detected
- Insulinoma usually not detected

MACROSCOPIC

General Features

- Vast majority well demarcated, discrete/circumscribed, and solitary
  - o Multifocal tumors more common in MEN1
  - o White-gray-yellow, pink-red, or tan-brown
- Tend to be softer than adjacent pancreas

Size

- Overall range: < 0.5 up to 35 cm
- Microinsulinomas in MEN1 usually functionally silent, especially when multiple lesions
- Size as it relates to functional status and hormone produced
  - o Functional: Usually < 2 cm
    - – **Insulinomas**: < 2 cm
    - – **Somatostatinomas**: Mean: 5-6 cm
    - – **Glucagonomas**: Mean: 7 cm
  - o Nonfunctional: > 2 cm
  - o Microadenoma: < 0.5 cm but nearly always nonfunctioning
- Severity of symptoms does not correlate with size

- Larger tumors tend to be malignant: > 3 cm usually malignant

MICROSCOPIC

Histologic Features

- Variable patterns both between and within tumors
- Wide architectural and cytomorphologic appearance
  o Ribbon-like, trabecular, festooned, or gyriform
  o Solid, trabecular, glandular, tubuloacinar, or pseudorosette
- Cells are relatively uniform
  o Round, polygonal, plasmacytoid, spindled, elongated
  o Finely granular eosinophilic cytoplasm
  o Centrally located, round to oval, elongated nucleus
- Lipid-rich, clear cell (in VHL), oncocytic, and rhabdoid subtypes rare
- Nuclei show salt and pepper chromatin distribution
  o Clumped dense heterochromatin
- Stroma and fibrosis variably present
  o Amyloid seen in insulinoma
  o Psammoma bodies seen in somatostatinoma
  o Usually very richly vascularized stroma
- Invasion can be seen
  o Into peripancreatic soft tissue
  o Into adjacent organs (adrenal, kidney, stomach, bowel)
  o Lymph-vascular invasion
  o Perineural invasion
- Mitotic figures usually sparse (< 2/10 HPF)
  o Ki-67 required to document proliferation index
- Small cell carcinoma (poorly differentiated endocrine carcinoma) looks identical to pulmonary primaries and is rare

Well-Differentiated Pancreatic Neuroendocrine Neoplasm, G1/G2/G3

- Functioning
  o **Insulinoma** (most common type): β-cell derived
    – Nonfunctioning and microtumors not encapsulated
    – Predominantly solid, ribbon-like, trabecular, gland-like (tubular or acinar) growth
    – Amyloid unique to this tumor type (islet amyloid polypeptide or amylin)
  o **Gastrinoma** (2nd most common)
    – Many times, no primary tumor identified in spite of having lymph node metastases
    – High risk of malignant behavior, irrespective of size
  o **Glucagonoma** (3rd most common): α-cell derived
    – Glucagonomas commonly occur in tail of pancreas or attached to surface of pancreas
    – Few cells react with glucagon immunohistochemically
    – Nesidioblastosis may be present
  o **VIPoma** (4th most common)
    – Often react with other markers (growth hormone release hormone, α-human chorionic gonadotropin, PP)
  o **Somatostatinoma** (least common): δ-cell derived
    – Tend to have glands and psammoma bodies
    – Synaptophysin usually reactive; chromogranin weak

Poorly Differentiated Neuroendocrine Carcinoma, G3

- Functional or nonfunctional
- Metastases to liver
- **Small cell variant**: Diffuse, sheet-like arrangements of cells, geographic necrosis, mitotic figures > 10/10 HPF
  o Resembles small cell carcinoma of lung
- **Large cell neuroendocrine**
  o Resembles large cell neuroendocrine carcinoma of lung

ANCILLARY TESTS

Cytology

- Smears uniformly hypercellular
- Background tends to be "clean" without blood or debris
- Relatively monotonous small cells arranged individually, in loose clusters, or in pseudorosettes
  o May have flat sheets of several hundred cells
  o Perivascular attachment or distribution may be present
- Plasmacytoid appearance frequently seen
- Binucleation is common
- Cytoplasm varies from slight to abundant, amphophilic to eosinophilic to granular
- Nuclei round to oval, uniform with smooth contours, often eccentrically located
  o Stripped or naked nuclei may be seen
- Characteristically delicate to slightly granular, salt and pepper chromatin distribution
- Isolated atypical single cells occasionally seen

Immunohistochemistry

- Variety of neuroendocrine markers positive
  o Synaptophysin, chromogranin, NSE, CD56, CD57
    – Synaptophysin generally diffuse and strong
    – Chromogranin apical, may be less intense and focal
- Specific hormone products/prohormones can be found
  o Insulin, glucagon, somatostatin, gastrin, VIP, PP, serotonin
    – Some tumors may express SSTR2
  o Staining intensity and distribution pattern unrelated to symptom severity
  o Diffuse, basal, capillary pole, or focal staining seen
  o Hormones may be genetically impaired or altered and therefore undetected
  o Frequently, multiple hormones/peptides detected in same tumor
- In addition to usual pancreatic peptides, others can also be seen
  o Adrenocorticotrophic hormone, parathyroid-like hormone, calcitonin, growth hormone releasing hormone, serotonin

Flow Cytometry

- Nuclear ploidy does not separate benign and malignant tumors
  o If malignant tumors aneuploid, they have worse behavior

Genetic Testing

- Molecular genetics in PanNETs
  o *MEN1* gene somatically inactivated in ~ 45% of cases

- o In ~ 45% of PanNENs, mutations in one or both *DAXX* and *ATRX*
- o ~ 15% of PanNETs have alterations in mTOR pathway genes, as *TSC2*, *PTEN*, *PIK3CA*
- o HIF1A and VHL alterations also present in PanNETs
- Molecular genetics in PanNECs
  - o Mutations in distinct genes from PanNETs: *TP53*, *CDKN2A*, and *RB1*
- *MEN1* mutations present in ~ 20% of spontaneous neoplasms (most have losses of 11q13)
- *KRAS* and *SMAD4* not mutated
- Recurrent mutation in *YY1* gene in 30% of sporadic insulinomas
- Novel PHLDA3-mediated pathway of tumor suppression is important in development of PETs
  - o Genomic region of *PHLDA3* gene undergoes loss of heterozygosity at high frequency in human PETs
    - – This genetic change correlates with disease progression and poor prognosis

Electron Microscopy

- Shows secretory granules but can be quite variable depending on hormone produced

DIFFERENTIAL DIAGNOSIS

Solid Pseudopapillary Neoplasm

- Lacks clinical hormone syndrome; usually affects young women
- Usually large tumor; most often in body and tail but with mostly benign biologic outcome
- Degenerative papillary appearance with foamy histiocytes
- Oval nuclei with grooves, folds, or clefts
- Blood, necrosis, and cholesterol clefts
- Broad, hyalinized to myxoid septa
- PAS(+) hyaline globules
- Positive for CD56, NSE, and synaptophysin, which can cause misdiagnosis for PEN; negative for chromogranin

Ductal Adenocarcinoma

- Tends to show more significant pleomorphism
- Glandular architecture is prominent but also has single cell infiltration
- Mitotic figures usually easily identified, along with perineural invasion
- Nuclear chromatin irregular, heavy with prominent nucleoli
- Positive for CEA and MUC1, while lacking neuroendocrine markers

Acinar Cell Carcinoma

- Loose, acinar to clustered arrangement
- Significant granular, eosinophilic cytoplasm surrounding round nuclei with prominent, brightly eosinophilic nucleoli
- Positive for trypsin or chymotrypsin

Pancreatoblastoma

- Tumor of pediatric patients
- Small cell pattern but acinar in structure with eosinophilic, granular cytoplasm, along with squamous morules
- Hypercellular stroma may be prominent

Lymphoma/Plasmacytoma

- Dyscohesive cells with high nuclear:cytoplasmic ratio

- Plasmacytoma cells have eccentric nuclei, perinuclear hof zone, and clock face-type chromatin distribution
- Positive reactions with CD138, CD79a, kappa, or lambda light chain restriction

Localized Hyperplasia

- Islet cell hyperplasia or nesidioblastosis can give islet-glandular complexes
- Islet size may be difficult to ascertain, especially in chronic pancreatitis
- Normal islets show several hormones in appropriate distribution, while tumors typically show preponderance of one

Epithelioid Gastrointestinal Stromal Tumor

- Slightly spindled population but also monotonous
- Strongly positive for CD117 (C-kit) but negative for neuroendocrine markers

Metastatic Tumors to Pancreas

- Metastatic melanoma, renal cell carcinoma, colon adenocarcinoma
- Immunohistochemistry usually valuable in differentiating from PEN
  - o HMB-45, Melan-A/MART-1, S100, RCC, CD10, CK7, CK20, CDX-2

DIAGNOSTIC CHECKLIST

Clinically Relevant Pathologic Features

- Insulinoma: Hypoglycemia
- Glucagonoma: Skin rash (necrolytic migratory erythema)
- Gastrinoma: Zollinger-Ellison syndrome
- VIPoma: Verner-Morrison syndrome

Pathologic Interpretation Pearls

- Variable patterns between and within tumors and architectural appearance
  - o Ribbon-like, trabecular, festooned, or gyriform
  - o Solid, trabecular, glandular, tubuloacinar, or pseudorosette
- Nuclei show neuroendocrine salt and pepper chromatin
- Required to do Ki-67 to document proliferation index
- Amyloid seen in insulinoma
- Psammoma bodies seen in somatostatinoma

REPORTING

Key Elements to Report

- Tumor size
- Tumor invasion: Soft tissue, nerve, vessel
- Mitotic index
- Ki-67 proliferative index
- Staging

SELECTED REFERENCES

1. Carrera S et al: Hereditary pancreatic cancer: related syndromes and clinical perspective. Hered Cancer Clin Pract. 15:9, 2017
2. Chen L et al: Clinicopathological features and prognostic validity of WHO grading classification of SI-NENs. BMC Cancer. 17(1):521, 2017
3. Chiloiro S et al: Pancreatic neuroendocrine tumors in MEN1 disease: a mono-centric longitudinal and prognostic study. Endocrine. ePub, 2017
4. Conemans EB et al: Prognostic value of WHO grade in pancreatic neuro-endocrine tumors in Multiple Endocrine Neoplasia type 1: Results from the DutchMEN1 Study Group. Pancreatology. ePub, 2017

5. Federica G et al: KI-67 heterogeneity in well differentiated gastro-entero-pancreatic neuroendocrine tumors: when is biopsy reliable for grade assessment? Endocrine. ePub, 2017

6. Genç CG et al: A new scoring system to predict recurrent disease in grade 1 and 2 nonfunctional pancreatic neuroendocrine tumors. Ann Surg. ePub, 2017

7. Kolin DL et al: Expanding the spectrum of colonic manifestations in tuberous sclerosis: L-cell neuroendocrine tumor arising in the background of rectal PEComa. Endocr Pathol. ePub, 2017

8. Konukiewitz B et al: Somatostatin receptor expression related to TP53 and RB1 alterations in pancreatic and extrapancreatic neuroendocrine neoplasms with a Ki67-index above 20. Mod Pathol. 30(4):587-598, 2017

9. Love JE et al: CD200 Expression in neuroendocrine neoplasms. Am J Clin Pathol. 148(3):236-242, 2017

10. Murtha TD et al: A systematic review of proinsulin-secreting pancreatic neuroendocrine tumors. J Gastrointest Surg. 21(8):1335-1341, 2017

11. Oba A et al: A simple morphological classification to estimate the malignant potential of pancreatic neuroendocrine tumors. J Gastroenterol. ePub, 2017

12. O'Toole SM et al: Response to somatostatin analog therapy in a patient with von Hippel-Lindau disease and multiple pancreatic neuroendocrine tumors. Pancreas. 46(7):e57, 2017

13. Park JK et al: DAXX/ATRX and MEN1 genes are strong prognostic markers in pancreatic neuroendocrine tumors. Oncotarget. 8(30):49796-49806, 2017

14. Ricci C et al: Sporadic small (≤ 20 mm) nonfunctioning pancreatic neuroendocrine neoplasm: Is the risk of malignancy negligible when adopting a more conservative strategy? A systematic review and meta-analysis. Ann Surg Oncol. 24(9):2603-2610, 2017

15. Sharma A et al: Clinical profile of pancreatic cystic lesions in von Hippel-Lindau disease: A series of 48 patients seen at a tertiary institution. Pancreas. 46(7):948-952, 2017

16. Strosberg JR et al: The North American Neuroendocrine Tumor Society Consensus Guidelines for Surveillance and Medical Management of Midgut Neuroendocrine Tumors. Pancreas. 46(6):707-714, 2017

17. Tracht J et al: Grading and prognostication of neuroendocrine tumors of the pancreas: A comparison study of Ki67 and PHH3. J Histochem Cytochem. 65(7):399-405, 2017

18. Yang Z et al: Immunohistochemical characterization of the origins of metastatic well-differentiated neuroendocrine tumors to the liver. Am J Surg Pathol. 41(7):915-922, 2017

19. Yano M et al: Assessment of disease aggression in cystic pancreatic neuroendocrine tumors: A CT and pathology correlation study. Pancreatology. 17(4):605-610, 2017

20. Yonemori K et al: Impact of snail and E-cadherin expression in pancreatic neuroendocrine tumors. Oncol Lett. 14(2):1697-1702, 2017

21. Falconi M et al: ENETS Consensus Guidelines Update for the Management of Patients with Functional Pancreatic Neuroendocrine Tumors and Non-Functional Pancreatic Neuroendocrine Tumors. Neuroendocrinology. 103(2):153-71, 2016

22. Fielitz K et al: Characterization of pancreatic glucagon-producing tumors and pituitary gland tumors in transgenic mice overexpressing MYCN in hGFAP-positive cells. Oncotarget. 7(46):74415-74426, 2016

23. Hackeng WM et al: Aberrant Menin expression is an early event in pancreatic neuroendocrine tumorigenesis. Hum Pathol. 56:93-100, 2016

24. Jakobsen M et al: Mixed acinar-neuroendocrine carcinoma of the pancreas: a case report and a review. Histol Histopathol. 31(12):1381-8, 2016

25. Alkatout I et al: Novel prognostic markers revealed by a proteomic approach separating benign from malignant insulinomas. Mod Pathol. 28(1):69-79, 2015

26. Esposito I et al: Pathology, genetics and precursors of human and experimental pancreatic neoplasms: An update. Pancreatology. 15(6):598-610, 2015

27. Franchi G et al: Cytological Ki-67 in pancreatic endocrine tumors: a new "must"? Gland Surg. 3(4):219-21, 2014

28. Kamp K et al: Parathyroid hormone-related peptide (PTHrP) secretion by gastroenteropancreatic neuroendocrine tumors (GEP-NETs): clinical features, diagnosis, management, and follow-up. J Clin Endocrinol Metab. 99(9):3060-9, 2014

29. Massironi S et al: Gastrinoma and neurofibromatosis type 2: the first case report and review of the literature. BMC Gastroenterol. 14:110, 2014

30. Ohki R et al: PHLDA3 is a novel tumor suppressor of pancreatic neuroendocrine tumors. Proc Natl Acad Sci U S A. 111(23):E2404-13, 2014

31. Partelli S et al: GEP-NETS update: a review on surgery of gastro-entero-pancreatic neuroendocrine tumors. Eur J Endocrinol. 171(4):R153-62, 2014

32. Ricci C et al: WHO 2010 classification of pancreatic endocrine tumors. Is the new always better than the old? Pancreatology. 14(6):539-41, 2014

33. Yang M et al: Evaluation of the World Health Organization 2010 grading system in surgical outcome and prognosis of pancreatic neuroendocrine tumors. Pancreas. 43(7):1003-8, 2014

34. Chou A et al: von Hippel-Lindau syndrome. Front Horm Res. 41:30-49, 2013

35. Hatipoglu E et al: Von Hippel Lindau disease with metastatic pancreatic neuroendocrine tumor causing ectopic Cushing's syndrome. Neuro Endocrinol Lett. 34(1):9-13, 2013

36. Liu TC et al: Comparison of WHO Classifications (2004, 2010), the Hochwald grading system, and AJCC and ENETS staging systems in predicting prognosis in locoregional well-differentiated pancreatic neuroendocrine tumors. Am J Surg Pathol. 37(6):853-9, 2013

37. Thakker RV: Multiple endocrine neoplasia type 1 (MEN1) and type 4 (MEN4). Mol Cell Endocrinol. Epub ahead of print, 2013

38. McCall CM et al: Serotonin expression in pancreatic neuroendocrine tumors correlates with a trabecular histologic pattern and large duct involvement. Hum Pathol. 43(8):1169-76, 2012

39. Amato E et al: Chromosome 3p alterations in pancreatic endocrine neoplasia. Virchows Arch. 458(1):39-45, 2011

40. Batcher E et al: Pancreatic neuroendocrine tumors. Endocr Res. 36(1):35-43, 2011

41. Klöppel G: Classification and pathology of gastroenteropancreatic neuroendocrine neoplasms. Endocr Relat Cancer. 18 Suppl 1:S1-S16, 2011

42. Rindi G et al: Gastroenteropancreatic (neuro)endocrine neoplasms: the histology report. Dig Liver Dis. 43 Suppl 4:S356-60, 2011

43. Zhang L et al: Proposed histopathologic grading system derived from a study of KIT and CK19 expression in pancreatic endocrine neoplasm. Hum Pathol. 42(3):324-31, 2011

44. Zhang Y et al: Endocrine tumors as part of inherited tumor syndromes. Adv Anat Pathol. 18(3):206-18, 2011

45. Klöppel G et al: [The ENETS and UICC TNM classification of neuroendocrine tumors of the gastrointestinal tract and the pancreas: comment.] Pathologe. 31(5):353-4, 2010

46. Henopp T et al: Glucagon cell adenomatosis: a newly recognized disease of the endocrine pancreas. J Clin Endocrinol Metab. 94(1):213-7, 2009

47. Klöppel G et al: ENETS Consensus Guidelines for the Standards of Care in Neuroendocrine Tumors: towards a standardized approach to the diagnosis of gastroenteropancreatic neuroendocrine tumors and their prognostic stratification. Neuroendocrinology. 2009;90(2):162-6. Epub 2009 Aug 28. Erratum in: Neuroendocrinology. 2009;90(4):432. Neuroendocrinology. 2010;92(4):251. Neuroendocrinology. 92(3):197, 2010

48. Klöppel G et al: The ENETS and AJCC/UICC TNM classifications of the neuroendocrine tumors of the gastrointestinal tract and the pancreas: a statement. Virchows Arch. 456(6):595-7, 2010

49. Lewis RB et al: Pancreatic endocrine tumors: radiologic-clinicopathologic correlation. Radiographics. 30(6):1445-64, 2010

50. Niederle MB et al: Gastroenteropancreatic neuroendocrine tumours: the current incidence and staging based on the WHO and European Neuroendocrine Tumour Society classification: an analysis based on prospectively collected parameters. Endocr Relat Cancer. 17(4):909-18, 2010

51. Rindi G: The ENETS guidelines: the new TNM classification system. Tumori. 96(5):806-9, 2010

52. Arnold R et al: ENETS Consensus Guidelines for the Standards of Care in Neuroendocrine Tumors: follow-up and documentation. Neuroendocrinology. 90(2):227-33, 2009

53. Capelli P et al: Endocrine neoplasms of the pancreas: pathologic and genetic features. Arch Pathol Lab Med. 133(3):350-64, 2009

54. Eriksson B et al: ENETS Consensus Guidelines for the Standards of Care in Neuroendocrine Tumors: chemotherapy in patients with neuroendocrine tumors. Neuroendocrinology. 90(2):214-9, 2009

55. Hofer MD et al: Immunohistochemical and clinicopathological correlation of the metastasis-associated gene 1 (MTA1) expression in benign and malignant pancreatic endocrine tumors. Mod Pathol. 22(7):933-9, 2009

56. Garbrecht N et al: Somatostatin-producing neuroendocrine tumors of the duodenum and pancreas: incidence, types, biological behavior, association with inherited syndromes, and functional activity. Endocr Relat Cancer. 15(1):229-41, 2008

57. Schmitt AM et al: Islet 1 (Isl1) expression is a reliable marker for pancreatic endocrine tumors and their metastases. Am J Surg Pathol. 32(3):420-5, 2008

58. Chang MC et al: Clinicopathologic and immunohistochemical correlation in sporadic pancreatic endocrine tumors: possible roles of utrophin and cyclin D1 in malignant progression. Hum Pathol. 38(5):732-40, 2007

59. Lubensky IA et al: Molecular genetic events in gastrointestinal and pancreatic neuroendocrine tumors. Endocr Pathol. 18(3):156-62, 2007

60. Rindi G et al: TNM staging of foregut (neuro)endocrine tumors: a consensus proposal including a grading system. Virchows Arch. 449(4):395-401, 2006

61. Oberg K et al: Endocrine tumours of the pancreas. Best Pract Res Clin Gastroenterol. 19(5):753-81, 2005

62. Virgolini I et al: Nuclear medicine in the detection and management of pancreatic islet-cell tumours. Best Pract Res Clin Endocrinol Metab. 19(2):213-27, 2005

63. Soga J: Carcinoids and their variant endocrinomas. An analysis of 11842 reported cases. J Exp Clin Cancer Res. 22(4):517-30, 2003

Comparison of WHO Classifications of Pancreatic Neuroendocrine Neoplasms Over the Years

WHO 2000/2004	WHO 2010	WHO 2017
Well-differentiated endocrine tumor/carcinoma (WDET/WDEC)	Neuroendocrine tumor (NET) G1/G2	NET G1/G2/G3; well-differentiated neuroendocrine neoplasm (NEN)
Poorly differentiated endocrine carcinoma (PDEC)	Neuroendocrine carcinoma (NEC), large cell or small cell	NEC G3, large cell or small cell; poorly differentiated NEN

Grading and Clinicopathological Classification of Tumors of Endocrine Pancreas

2017 WHO Tumor Classification	Grading
Well-differentiated endocrine tumor, grade 1: (PanNET G1)	< 2 mitoses/50 HPF; < 3% Ki-67 proliferative index
Well-differentiated endocrine tumor, grade 2: (PanNET G2)	2-20 mitoses/50 HPF; 3-20% Ki-67 proliferative index
Well-differentiated neoplasm, grade 3: (PanNET G3)	> 20 mitoses/50 HPF or Ki-67 proliferative index > 20%

Immunohistochemistry

Antibody	Reactivity	Staining Pattern	Comment
Synaptophysin	Positive	Cell membrane and cytoplasm	Nearly every tumor cell positive; both solid pseudopapillary tumor (SPT) and acinar cell carcinoma (ACC) may be focally positive
PGP9.5	Positive	Cytoplasmic	Nearly every tumor cell positive
NSE	Positive	Cytoplasmic	Very low specificity
CD56	Positive	Cell membrane and cytoplasm	Usually accentuated on cell membrane
Chromogranin-A	Positive	Cytoplasmic	Granular reactivity, reflection of neurosecretory granules; less staining in less granulated tumors; SPT negative; ACC may be focally positive
E-cadherin	Positive	Cell membrane	SPT negative; ACC positive
CK-PAN	Positive	Cytoplasmic	Nearly all tumors
CK8/18/CAM5.2	Positive	Cytoplasmic	Most tumor cells
CK19	Positive	Cytoplasmic	Expression correlated with outcome
ISL1	Positive	Nuclear	Support pancreatic origin of metastases
CD117	Positive	Cell membrane	Abnormal expression linked to prognosis
PRP	Positive	Nuclear	If progesterone receptor positivity lost, associated with worse prognosis
NFP	Positive	Cytoplasmic	Present in few tumor cells
Trypsin	Negative		ACC positive; SPT negative
β-catenin	Negative		SPT positive; ACC negative

Pancreatic Tumor

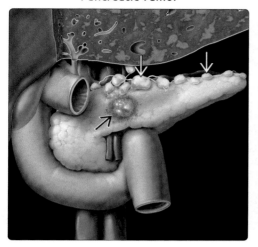

Well-Circumscribed Pancreatic Mass

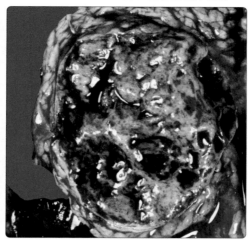

(Left) *Graphic demonstrates the anatomic relationship of the pancreas to the surrounding organs and vessels. A tumor ➡ is shown in relationship to the lymph nodes (seen along the upper border of the pancreas) ➡.* **(Right)** *This 3.5-cm mass in the head of the pancreas of a 26-year-old woman with MEN1 syndrome is well-circumscribed and shows a pale-pink cut surface with areas of cystic changes and hemorrhage.*

PanNET in Pancreatic Head

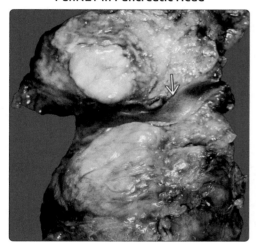

Cut Surface Appearance

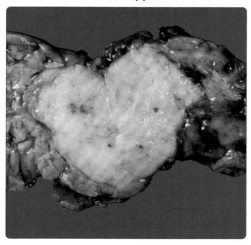

(Left) *Pancreas reveals a 3-cm, gray-white, firm and ill-defined mass underlying the main pancreatic duct. However, the main pancreatic duct ➡ appears to be not involved by the tumor.* **(Right)** *Pancreatic neuroendocrine tumor in a patient with Cushing syndrome shows a firm, tan-yellow cut surface that obliterates the pancreatic duct. Histologically, this was a well-differentiated PanPEN, intermediate grade. This 3.8-cm, ACTH-producing tumor metastasized to the liver.*

PanNET With Ductules

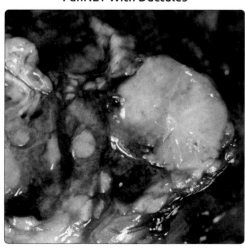

Mixed Ductal and Endocrine Carcinoma

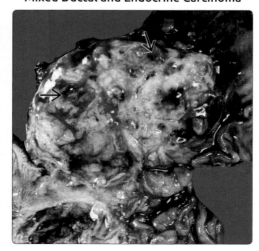

(Left) *Insulin-producing pancreatic neuroendocrine tumor with ductules is considered a variant of the pancreatic endocrine neoplasms. These tumors are known to have smaller size than typical PETs.* **(Right)** *This 6-cm, gray-white, friable, lobulated mass in the pancreatic head shows areas of small cystic formations ➡. Microscopically, this tumor had mixed ductal carcinoma and pancreatic neuroendocrine carcinoma.*

(Left) *CT image demonstrates a hypervascular mass ➡ in the body of the pancreas, a well-circumscribed lesion. Note that the pancreas shows marked fatty change, a finding more commonly identified in chronic pancreatitis.* **(Right)** *There is a complex mass ➡ (gastrinoma) in the tail of the pancreas expanding out into the surrounding tissues with increased vascularity. Note the metastatic foci ➡ in the liver, confirming pancreatic endocrine carcinoma.*

CT of Pancreatic Endocrine Tumor

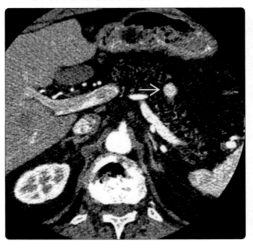

Pancreatic Endocrine Tumor

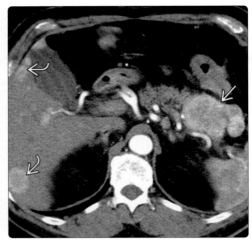

(Left) *Somatostatin receptor scintigraphy helps detect somatostatin receptor-positive lesions, like gastrinomas. They can be targeted by In-111-labeled octreotide. There is a large tumor in the head ➡, another in the body ➡, and a metastasis in the liver ➡.* **(Right)** *The duodenum in this patient with a 3-cm pancreatic head gastrinoma shows numerous submucosal nodules ➡. These nodules have the same immunophenotype as the pancreatic tumor.*

Pancreatic Endocrine Tumor

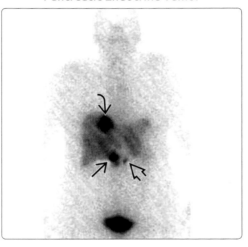

Gastrinoma With Duodenal Nodules

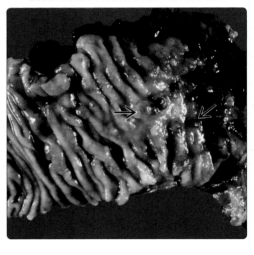

(Left) *The entire length of the small intestine shows multiple submucosal nodules associated with and contiguous to areas of serosal puckering. The primary tumor is a pancreatic neuroendocrine tumor, low grade.* **(Right)** *The small intestine of this patient with pancreatic neuroendocrine tumor had multiple submucosal nodules ranging 0.2-1.7 cm, spanning the length of the intestine. The largest nodule ➡ displays central cavitation.*

Metastatic PanPEN to Small Bowel

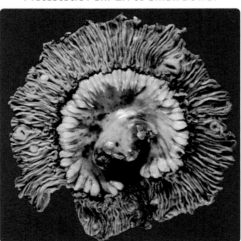

Metastatic Neuroendocrine Tumor

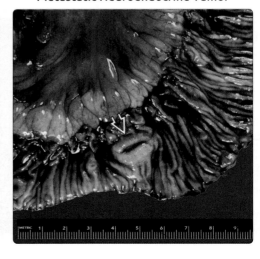

Cytology of Pancreatic Endocrine Neoplasm

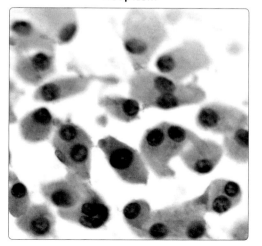

Pancreatic Neuroendocrine Tumor Cytology

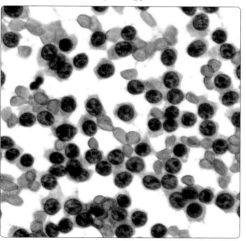

(Left) *H&E-stained smear of PanNET shows a uniformly monotonous population of epithelioid-plasmacytoid cells with ample pink cytoplasm. The nuclei are round to oval, uniform, and eccentrically located.* (Right) *PET smear demonstrates the characteristic loosely clustered epithelioid cells. The cells have pale-pink and small amount of cytoplasm with central nuclear placement. The nuclei have delicate salt and pepper nuclear chromatin.*

Well-Differentiated PanNET

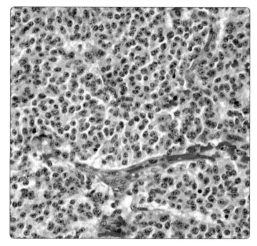

Intermediate-Grade PanNET

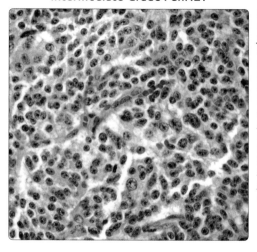

(Left) *A 3.5-cm tumor in the head of the pancreas in a 26-year-old woman with a family history of MEN1 shows a well-differentiated neuroendocrine tumor. This tumor, based on the mitotic count and on the Ki-67 proliferative index, is classified as intermediate grade.* (Right) *High-power view of this well-differentiated neuroendocrine tumor, intermediate grade, shows uniform cells with pale-pink cytoplasm and round nuclei with nucleoli.*

Large Cell Characteristics in PanNEC

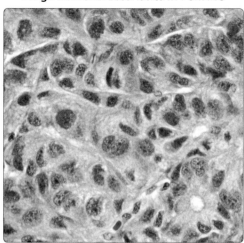

Large Cell Type PanNEC

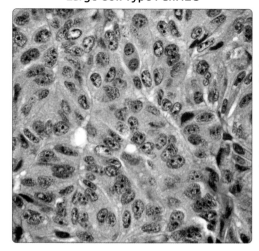

(Left) *Grade 3 pancreatic neuroendocrine carcinoma (poorly differentiated neuroendocrine neoplasm) shows a diffuse growth pattern with cells organized in a nested/organoid pattern with cytological atypia.* (Right) *Pancreatic neuroendocrine carcinoma (poorly differentiated neuroendocrine neoplasm) has a diffuse growth pattern and is composed by large cells with ample pink cytoplasm and large nuclei with prominent nucleoli.*

Trabecular Pattern of PanNEN

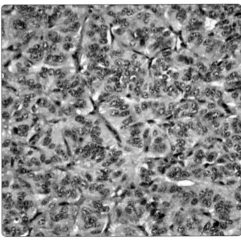

Ribbon-Like Pattern of PanNEN

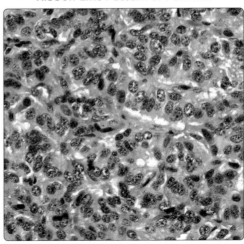

(Left) *Pancreatic endocrine neoplasm shows a trabecular architecture, which is characteristic of a PanNEN. The cytoplasm is pale, and the eccentrically located nuclei show salt and pepper chromatin.* **(Right)** *Ribbon-like to festooned architecture is characteristic for endocrine tumors of the pancreas. This tumor shows slightly more nuclear atypia. Generally, > 2 mitoses/50 HPF need to be found to suggest a more biologically aggressive behavior.*

Enlarged Islet

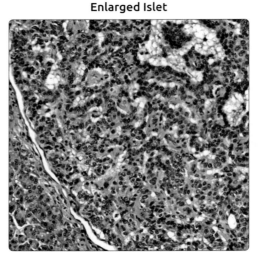

Chromogranin in Enlarged Islet

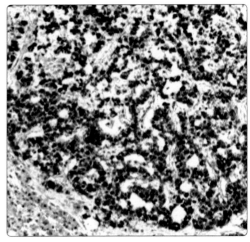

(Left) *Islet hyperplasia refers to slightly enlarged islets that contain neuroendocrine cells arranged in trabeculae and show loss of the normal spatial distribution and numbers of the normal main cell types. This is usually present in patients with MEN1, VHL, and glucagon hyperplasia and neoplasia.* **(Right)** *Immunohistochemistry for chromogranin-A in the pancreas of a patient with MEN1 shows a markedly enlarged islet. The pancreas also had multiple microadenomas, adenomas, and hyperplasia/dysplasia.*

Prominent Nucleoli in PanNET

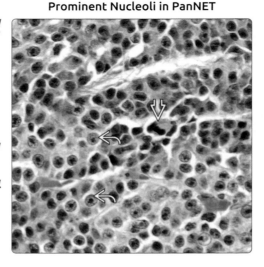

Microadenoma

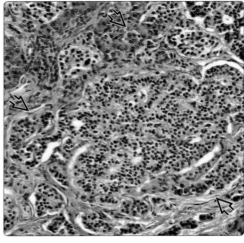

(Left) *PanNET in a 17-year-old boy with MEN1 was large and associated with islet cell hyperplasia. Note the prominent nucleoli ⇥ and mitoses ⬈. **(Right)** In the pancreas of patients with MEN1, there are typically multiple small (< 5 mm) neuroendocrine tumors, a finding that has been referred to as microadenomatosis. Note the irregular borders of the endocrine components ⇥.*

Psammoma Bodies in Insulinoma

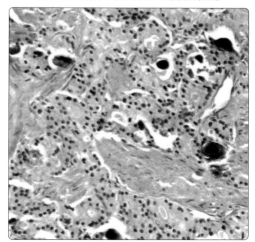

Paraganglioma-Like Pattern

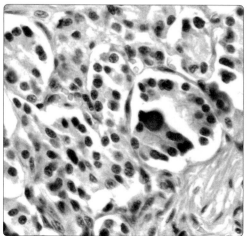

(Left) High-power view shows the characteristic medium-sized cells with ample eosinophilic cytoplasm and eccentrically located nuclei. There are areas of fibrosis and numerous psammoma bodies. (Right) Somatostatinoma have no distinctive histological features with other PanNETs, except that they may have a paraganglioma-like pattern. Rarely they may show a psammoma body, unlike the duodenal somatostatinoma, which have numerous psammoma bodies.

Organoid Arrangement

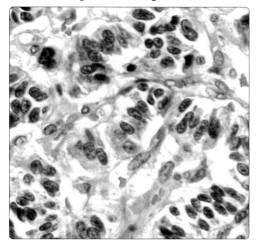

Focal Chromogranin Staining

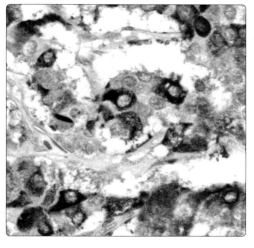

(Left) The pancreatic microadenomas seen in patients with MEN1, VHL, and NF are often accompanied by one or more macrotumors (diameter > 5 mm), some of which may become insulinomas or other hormone-producing tumors. (Right) Pancreatic neuroendocrine tumors usually have strong and diffuse staining for synaptophysin and only focal and apical staining for chromogranin A. In PanNETs with fewer secretory granules, chromogranin immunostaining is focal.

Pancreatic Endocrine Cell Proliferations

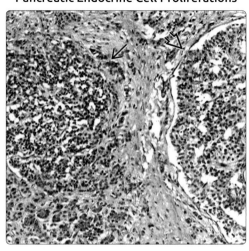

Pancreatic Endocrine Tumor/Hyperplasia

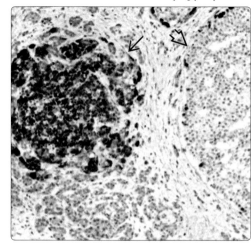

(Left) Two distinct pancreatic endocrine cell proliferations are shown in a case of MEN1. The lesion on the left ⇒ has irregular borders, and the lesion on the right ⇒ is well demarcated and larger. (Right) The smaller pancreatic endocrine lesion ⇒ is uniformly positive for glucagon (microadenoma), whereas the larger lesion ⇒ shows a pattern of distribution of glucagon similar to a normal islet, indicating hyperplasia.

(Left) *While the architectural pattern of the tumor is quite characteristic of a PanNET, it is important to note this tumor has invaded into the adjacent adrenal gland ➡. This is a finding associated with malignant or aggressive biologic behavior.* **(Right)** *H&E of liver in a 17-year-old boy with MEN1 shows metastases from the PET ➡ compressing the adjacent liver parenchyma ➡. Metastases were present at diagnosis.*

PanNET Invading Adrenal Gland

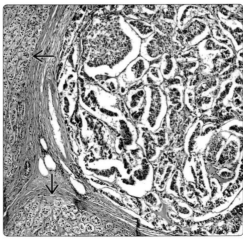

Metastases of PanNET to Liver

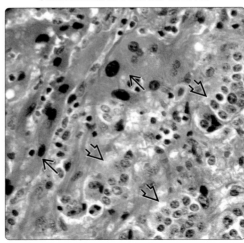

(Left) *H&E shows a mixed neuroendocrine-non-neuroendocrine (ductal) carcinoma. A solid neuroendocrine component ➡ positive for chromogranin is mixed with a poorly differentiated ductal component ➡ positive for trypsin.* **(Right)** *Mixed neuroendocrine-ductal carcinomas have a solid neuroendocrine component ➡ positive for chromogranin. The poorly differentiated ductal component ➡ is positive for trypsin (not shown) and negative for chromogranin.*

Mixed Pancreatic Tumor

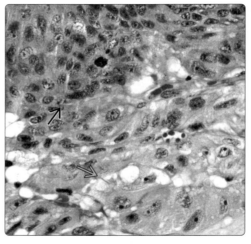

Chromogranin Staining in Mixed Tumors

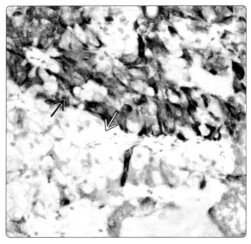

(Left) *Insulin-producing pancreatic neuroendocrine tumor with ductules is composed by an intimate association of the endocrine component with bland-appearing ductules. It is characterized by the presence of ductuloinsular units or complexes where endocrine cells could be seen budding off ducts singly or forming clusters within the wall of the ductules.* **(Right)** *Pancreatic neuroendocrine tumor with ductules is characterized by the strong association with insulin production by the endocrine cells.*

PanNET With Ductules

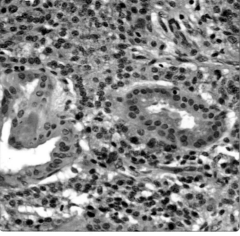

Insulin-Producing PanNET With Ductules

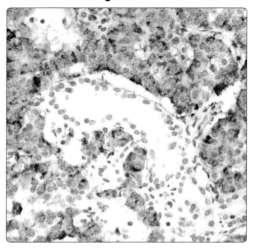

ACTH Immunopositivity in PanNET

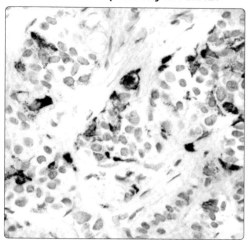

Membranous CD117 Expression

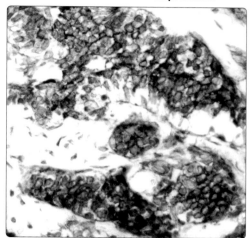

(Left) *This pancreatic neuroendocrine tumor in a patient with Cushing syndrome shows a well-differentiated PET, intermediate grade. This 3.8-cm tumor was an ACTH-producing tumor.* (Right) *Well-differentiated PanNET, intermediate grade, shows membranous staining for CD117. The immunopositivity for CD117 is related to prognosis.*

Strong Granular Cytoplasmic Staining

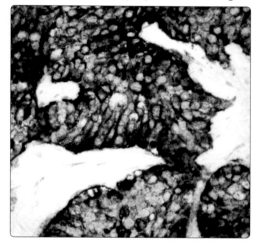

Insulin-Producing Tumor

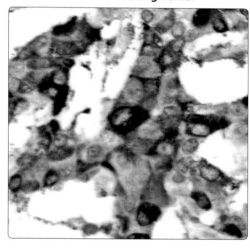

(Left) *This pancreatic neuroendocrine tumor has a large ribbon arrangement highlighted by the chromogranin A staining. There is strong and diffuse granular cytoplasmic staining.* (Right) *Multiple pancreatic microadenomas (< 5 mm) seen in patients with MEN1 and neurofibromatosis are often accompanied by 1 or more macroadenomas (diameter > 5 mm), some of which may become insulinomas, as seen here.*

Ki-67 Immunolabeling Index

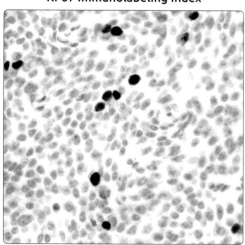

Ki-67 in PanNEC, Grade 3

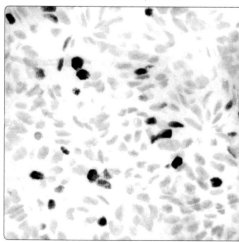

(Left) *This well-differentiated pancreatic neuroendocrine tumor is classified as intermediate grade by the WHO 2017, based on the mitotic count and Ki-67 proliferative index. The mitotic count was 2 mitosis per 10 HPF, and the Ki-67 proliferative index was 3.4%.* (Right) *This poorly differentiated pancreatic neuroendocrine neoplasm, classified as large cell neuroendocrine carcinoma, grade 3 has high mitotic index (> 20 mitoses per 10 HPF) and Ki-67 proliferative index > 20%.*

TERMINOLOGY FOR DEFINITIONS, STAGING, AND CANCER PROTOCOLS

- Pancreatic neuroendocrine neoplasms (PanNENs) have significant neuroendocrine differentiation with expression of synaptophysin and chromogranin (WHO 2017)
- 2017 WHO classification and grading of pancreatic neuroendocrine neoplasms divides these tumors into 3 categories
  o Well-differentiated PanNENs: Pancreatic neuroendocrine tumors (PanNETs)
    − PanNET G1 (< 3% Ki67 index and < 2 mitotic index)
    − PanNET G2 (3-20% Ki67 index and 2-20 mitotic index)
    − PanNET G3 (> 20% Ki67 index and > 20 mitotic index)
  o Poorly differentiated PanNENs: Pancreatic neuroendocrine carcinomas (PanNECs)
    − PanNEC G3 (> 20% Ki67 index and > 20 mitotic index)
      □ Small cell type
      □ Large cell type
  o Mixed neuroendocrine-nonneuroendocrine neoplasm

- Neuroendocrine tumors of pancreas have distinct cancer protocol from carcinoma of exocrine pancreas and from PanNECs
- Use of cancer protocol for incidentally identified pancreatic neuroendocrine tumors ≤ 0.5 cm, also defined as neuroendocrine microadenomas, is not required
- For resection specimens, TNM stage, based on macroscopic assessment of site, size, and metastases, should be reported
  o T1: Tumor limited to pancreas, < 2.0 cm in greatest dimension
  o T2: Tumor limited to pancreas, > 2.0 cm but not > 4 cm in greatest dimension
  o T3: Tumor limited to pancreas, > 4 cm in greatest dimension, or tumor invading duodenum or bile duct
  o T4: Tumor perforates visceral peritoneum or other organs or adjacent structures

T1 PanNET (G1 and G2)

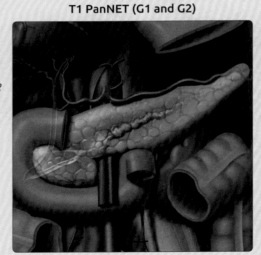

T2 PanNET (G1 and G2)

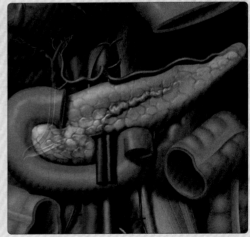

(Left) *Similar to exocrine pancreatic carcinoma, T1 disease is defined as a tumor confined to the pancreas and measuring ≤ 2 cm in the greatest dimension.* (Right) *T2 disease is defined as a tumor confined to the pancreas, ≥ 2 cm but < 4 cm in the greatest dimension.*

T3 PanNET (G1 and G2)

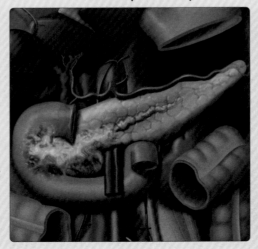

T4 PanNET (G1 and G2)

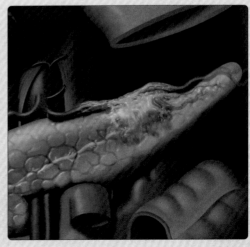

(Left) *In T3 disease, the tumor is limited to the pancreas, ≥ 4 cm in the greatest dimension, or tumor invading duodenum or bile duct. This graphic illustrates a tumor involving the duodenum but without involvement of the celiac axis or superior mesenteric artery.* (Right) *Involvement of the splenic artery is classified as T4 disease. In T4, the tumor perforates the visceral peritoneum or other organs or adjacent structures.*

T4 PanNET (G1 and G2)

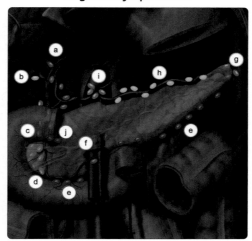

Regional Lymph Nodes

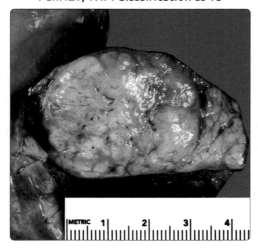

(Left) *This tumor involves the superior mesenteric artery* ⮕*. Tumors that involve the celiac axis or superior mesenteric artery are classified as T4.* **(Right)** *Important regional peripancreatic lymph node groups include (a) hepatic, (b) cystic duct, (c) posterior pancreaticoduodenal, (d) anterior pancreaticoduodenal, (e) inferior, (f) superior mesenteric, (g) splenic hilar, (h) superior, (i) celiac, and (j) pyloric. A minimum of 12 nodes are needed for adequate staging.*

PanNET, TNM Classification as T2

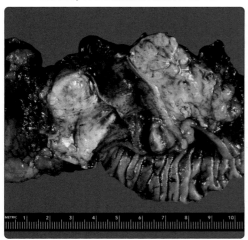

PanNET, TNM Classification as T3

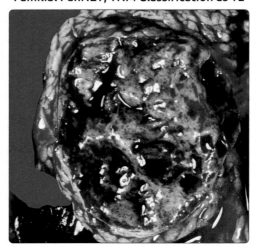

(Left) *The pancreatic head is noticeable for a 3.5-cm well-circumscribed mass, with a tan-yellow soft-cut surface. The mass does not involve the duodenum, the common bile duct, or the main pancreatic duct.* **(Right)** *This well-circumscribed, tan-yellow, firm pancreatic neuroendocrine tumor was located in the distal pancreas and measured 4.2 cm.*

Cystic PanNET, TNM Classification as T4

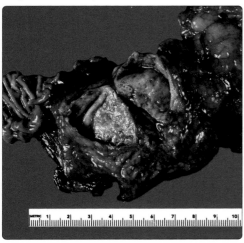

Familial PanNET, TNM Classification as T2

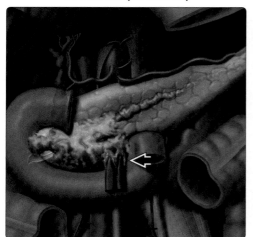

(Left) *This PanNET had extensive cystic changes with formation of a central cyst. The tumor measured 7.2 cm and invaded into adjacent structures, classified by TNM as T4.* **(Right)** *This 3.5-cm mass in the head of the pancreas of a patient with multiple endocrine neoplasia type 1 syndrome is well circumscribed and shows a pale pink cut surface with areas of cystic changes. The tumor does not invade surrounding structures.*

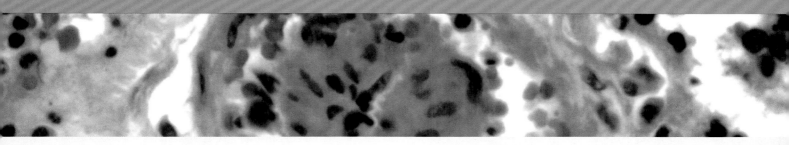

SECTION 6
Endocrine Skin

Merkel Cell Carcinoma

TERMINOLOGY

- High-grade neuroendocrine carcinoma of skin

ETIOLOGY/PATHOGENESIS

- Merkel cell polyomavirus
- Association with immunosuppression and ultraviolet light
- MCPV-negative tumors have high mutation burden associated with ultraviolet-induced DNA damage signature
  - Mutations in *RB1*, *TP53*, *NOTCH1*, *FAT1*

CLINICAL ISSUES

- Aggressive tumor occurring in sun-damaged skin of elderly

MICROSCOPIC

- High-grade tumor based in dermis with stippled (neuroendocrine-type) chromatin, diffuse or trabecular growth, and prominent mitotic activity
- May occur admixed with squamous cell or basal cell carcinoma

ANCILLARY TESTS

- Immunopositivity for CK20 (dot-like), chromogranin, synaptophysin, and (+/-) CK7; negative for TTF-1, CDX-2
- MCPV positive in up to 80% cases from United States and Europe, but less in Australia

TOP DIFFERENTIAL DIAGNOSES

- Small cell carcinoma of lung: Positive for CK7 and TTF-1; negative for CK20
- High-grade (small cell) carcinoma of salivary gland: Immunophenotype identical to Merkel cell carcinoma
- Other neuroendocrine metastases to skin
- High-grade squamous cell carcinoma of skin: Associated epidermal squamous dysplasia
- Basal cell carcinoma of skin: Basaloid, peripheral palisading, cleft artifact, CK20 negative

Merkel Cell Carcinoma

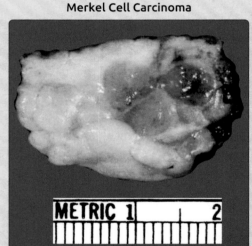

Merkel Cell Carcinoma With Mitotic Figures

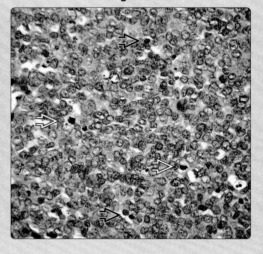

(Left) Gross photograph shows Merkel cell carcinoma forming a fleshy hemorrhagic mass based in the dermis, extending into the underlying subcutaneous tissue. (Right) Merkel cell carcinoma shows diffuse growth of cells with vesicular nuclei, prominent mitotic activity ⇾, and apoptotic cells ⇨.

Stippled Neuroendocrine Chromatin

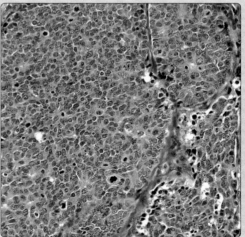

Neuroendocrine Chromatin and Mitotic Figures

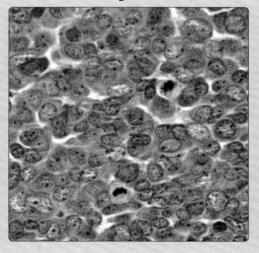

(Left) Merkel cell carcinoma shows prominent mitotic activity, apoptotic cells, and stippled neuroendocrine nuclei. (Right) High-power view shows stippled neuroendocrine chromatin in this Merkel cell carcinoma. The tumor is associated with prominent mitotic activity.

TERMINOLOGY

Abbreviations

- Merkel cell carcinoma (MCC)

Synonyms

- Trabecular carcinoma of skin

Definitions

- Neuroendocrine carcinoma of skin

ETIOLOGY/PATHOGENESIS

Merkel Cell Polyomavirus

- Recent studies have demonstrated clonal integration of polyomavirus in human MCC
  - Previously unknown polyomavirus was named Merkel cell polyomavirus (MCPV)
    - Small, circular, nonenveloped, double-stranded DNA virus
  - MCPV sequences found in majority of MCCs and corresponding metastases
  - MCPV DNA has been shown to be monoclonally integrated in tumor genome, indicating MCPV infection and integration preceded clonal expansion of tumor cells
  - Suggests MCPV may contribute to pathogenesis of MCC
- Monoclonal antibody (clone CM2B4) developed using recombinant peptide fragment unique to MCPV large T (LT)
  - 77-83% sensitivity compared with PCR; negative in MCPV-negative MCC & adjacent tissues
  - Some report that antibody is not specific for MCPV LT
    - Stains MCPV negative cases of MCC and nonneoplastic tissues (e.g., lymphocytes, sweat glands, etc.) that are negative for MCPV by PCR
    - 95% sensitivity and 83% specificity
- MCPV identified in 70-80% of MCC in United States and Europe
  - Australia much lower association with MCPV (25%)
    - Postulated relatively low sun exposure of North America and Europe may be associated with more virus-driven oncogenesis compared to highly sun-exposed, predominantly fair-skinned Australian population
  - Viral load in MCC determined by quantitative PCR
    - Viral copy numbers vary substantially
    - If viral genome integrated into host genome of carcinoma cells, viral load usually about 1 copy per cell or more
    - FISH study: Single viral signal in 90% of nuclei of MCC
  - Other tumors studied generally negative for MCPV: Prostate, colorectal, CNS, mesotheliomas, neuroendocrine tumors from various sites
    - Few CLLs (chronic lymphocytic leukemia/lymphoma) positive for MCPV, but unclear if virus integrated into genome
    - Rare small cell-undifferentiated carcinoma reported positive (1.3%)
- Seroprevalence MCPV in general population 46-88% (higher levels serum anti-MCPV IgG in patients with MCC positive for MCPV)
- High frequency of MCPV exposure and rarity of MCC suggest other events or molecular hits contribute to tumor development
- MCPV identified in normal tissues from immunocompetent and immunocompromised individuals (especially skin)
  - Quantitative PCR: MCPV widespread in human body, but very low levels (60x < MCC)

Merkel Cell Polyomavirus-Negative MCC

- Ultraviolet associated mutations
- More prevalent in some geographic regions with high sun exposure
- High mutation burden associated with ultraviolet-induced DNA damage signature
  - Mutations in RB1, TP53, NOTCH1, FAT1
    - Mutations or amplifications of possible clinical importance: PI3K pathway (PIK3CA, AKT1, PIK3CG) and MAP kinase pathway (HRAS, NF1)
  - MCPV-positive tumors have low mutation rates
- More often from most sun-exposed sites (head and neck) compared to other sites
- May be more aggressive
- MCC with mixed squamous differentiation usually negative for MCPV
- Reports of increased nuclear polymorphism, more abundant cytoplasm, and higher Ki-67 proliferative index

Risk Factors

- Immunocompromised states, particularly renal and cardiac transplant, lymphoma/leukemia, other cancers, HIV infection, immunosuppressant drugs, arsenic exposure
  - Immunocompromised 5-50x increased risk MCC
  - Younger age and worse prognosis for MCC in immunocompromised
- Natural and artificial sunlight
- Risk for developing MCC as 2nd malignancy in patients with multiple myeloma, chronic lymphocytic leukemia, lymphoma, malignant melanoma
- Patients with MCC at increased risk of developing subsequent cancer (salivary gland, biliary, and non-Hodgkin lymphoma) particularly during 1st year after diagnosis
- MCC can occur synchronous or metachronous with squamous cell and basal cell carcinomas
  - MCC also described admixed with squamous cell carcinoma and basal cell carcinoma

CLINICAL ISSUES

Epidemiology

- Incidence
  - 1,600 new cases each year in United States
  - Incidence increasing in past 20 years (aging population, increased prevalence immunosuppression, more accurate diagnoses)
- Age
  - Elderly (i.e., 7th decade) but wide age range
- Sex
  - M = F
- Ethnicity
  - Caucasians most commonly affected

Presentation

- Uncommon, aggressive tumor, occurring most often in sun-damaged skin of older patients
- Head and neck, particularly periorbital region, extremities, and other sites (trunk and oral/nasal mucosa and anogenital region)
- Painless, fast-growing, solitary erythematous nodule
- Paraneoplastic syndromes: cerebellar degeneration, Lambert-Eaton myasthenic syndrome, malignancy associated hyponatremia, and possibly increased incidence severe hyponatremia

Treatment

- Surgical excision (aggressive surgical management correlated with better prognosis)
- Sentinel lymph node biopsy (predictive of high short-term risk of recurrence or metastases)
- Therapeutic lymph node dissection (may prevent short-term regional lymph node recurrence)
- Radiation therapy following resection primary site and lymph node basin and head and neck (may improve locoregional control)
- Neoadjuvant chemotherapy: Little data available
- Chemotherapy: Often used in locally advanced or metastatic disease, but response often short-lived, and impact on overall survival uncertain
- Newer treatments such PD-1/PD-L1 inhibition show some promise and may be helpful in cases not amenable to surgery &/or radiation
  - Molecular characteristics are leading to potential therapeutic targets in MCC and clinical trials are ongoing

Prognosis

- Aggressive tumors
- 10-45% involve regional lymph nodes at presentation
- Lymph node involvement eventually identified in majority of patients
- Distant metastases (lymph node, liver, lung, brain, bone)
- 9,387 MCC in National Cancer Data Base Participant User File
  - 65% presented with local disease, 26% with nodal disease, 8% with distant disease
  - 5-year overall survival 51% for local, 35% for nodal, and 14% for distant disease
  - 5-year overall survival 40% with clinically occult and 27% for clinically detected regional nodal basin involvement
  - 336 cases with clinically detected nodal disease and unknown primary tumor better prognosis compared to cases presenting with concurrent primary tumor (42% vs. 27% survival)
- 4-5% of MCC are of unknown primary, but this subset represents 28-40% of MCC with clinically detected nodal disease
  - MCC of unknown primary has better prognosis than those with metastatic nodal MCC and concurrent primary tumor
- Frequent recurrence
- Poor prognostic factors: Large size (5 cm), invasion into subcutis, diffuse growth, male sex, recurrence, metastatic disease
  - Reports MCPV-negative tumors may be more aggressive, but controversial and not seen in all studies

MACROSCOPIC

General Features

- Fleshy tumor based in dermis; up to 4-5% occur as unknown primary

MICROSCOPIC

Histologic Features

- High-grade tumor usually based in dermis and generally without emanation from overlying epidermis
- Various histologic patterns such as solid, trabecular, and diffuse can be seen
  - Not of specific significance
  - Mixed patterns often identified
- High-grade neuroendocrine cells with vesicular nuclei with stippled chromatin and numerous mitoses
  - Reports of higher nuclear polymorphism and more abundant cytoplasm in MCPV-negative cases
- Can have intraepidermal component, and rare cases can be completely intraepidermal
- Can occur synchronous or metachronous with squamous cell carcinomas and basal cell carcinomas
  - MCC can be admixed with squamous cell carcinoma or basal cell carcinoma
    - Electron microscopy shows each component preserved, and transitional cell types not identified
    - MCC combined with squamous cell carcinoma generally MCPV-negative
  - MCC can have glandular, melanocytic, striated muscle, lymphoepithelioma-like features
- Cases of MCC primary to lymph node reported (up to 4-5% unknown primary)
  - Possible explanation spontaneous regression of cutaneous primary
    - But some have have better survival than expected for metastatic MCC to lymph node
  - Not possible to be certain which explanation most appropriate for these cases
    - Consider MCC in differential diagnosis of high-grade neuroendocrine carcinoma in lymph node, even in patients without history of MCC
- Neuroendocrine granules have been identified in a variety of common nonmelanocytic skin tumors, such as basal cell, sweat gland tumors, trichoblastoma, and trichofolliculoma
  - Rather nonspecific finding that correlates with plethora of reports of skin tumors showing focal staining for neuroendocrine markers

ANCILLARY TESTS

Immunohistochemistry

- Positive for CK20 (characteristic dot-like staining pattern; also seen in other low molecular weight keratins, e.g., CAM5.2)
- CK7 often negative, but ~ 14% of MCC positive for both CK20 and CK7
  - Rare cases reportedly CK7 positive and CK20 negative (would need to carefully rule out metastasis to skin)
  - CK20-negative cases usually MCPV negative and have ultraviolet signature mutations and recurrent *TP53* and *RB1* inactivation

- Positive for neuroendocrine markers chromogranin and synaptophysin
- Neurofilament protein, CD99, FLI-1, CD117, and pax-5 have been noted in some cases, but nonspecific
- Generally negative for TTF-1 and CDX-2
- CM2B4 (Merkel cell polyomavirus antibody, nuclear stain) positive in majority of cases
  - MCPV immunohistochemistry highly specific in all populations
  - Low incidence of MCPV-positive MCC in highly sun-exposed populations limits diagnostic utility in this setting

Cytogenetics and Molecular Genetics

- Comparative genomic hybridization studies have shown extensive genetic aberrations (gains > losses, frequent gains of whole chromosomes or arms)
- Common gains chromosomes 1, 5, 6, 18q, 20; rearrangements of 1p, 3q; gain of 5p; trisomy of 6; deletion of 1p (possible tumor suppressor gene), loss of 13 (increased survival in some)
- Mutations in *TP53* and *HRAS* gene
- *TP53* missense and nonsense mutations in subset
- MCPV-negative tumors associated with ultraviolet-associated mutations
  - High mutation burden associated with ultraviolet-induced DNA damage signature
  - Mutations in *RB1, TP53, NOTCH1, FAT1*
- Succinate-ubiquinone oxidoreductase subunit D (*SDHD*) tumor-suppressor gene alterations
- Allelic loss of 10q23
- KIT immunohistochemical expression common, but lack *KIT* activating mutations

DIFFERENTIAL DIAGNOSIS

High-Grade Neuroendocrine Carcinoma of Salivary Gland

- Immunophenotype identical to MCC (positive for chromogranin, synaptophysin, CK20)
- Must differentiate tumor metastatic to salivary gland lymph node vs. tumor primary to salivary gland

Small Cell Carcinoma of Lung

- Both MCC and small cell carcinoma of lung positive for chromogranin, synaptophysin, and CAM5.2
  - But small cell lung cancer usually positive for CK7 and TTF-1 and negative for CK20

Other Neuroendocrine Carcinomas

- Medullary thyroid carcinoma: Positive for chromogranin, synaptophysin, CAM5.2, CK7, TTF-1, and calcitonin; negative for CK20
- Atypical laryngeal carcinoid: Positive for chromogranin, synaptophysin, CAM5.2, CK7, and calcitonin; negative for CK20 and TTF-1
- Gastrointestinal carcinoid: Positive for chromogranin, synaptophysin, CAM5.2, CK20, and CDX-2 (foregut carcinoids); negative for CK7
- Pulmonary carcinoid: Positive for chromogranin, synaptophysin, CAM5.2, CK7, and TTF-1; negative for CDX-2 and CK20

Squamous Cell Carcinoma of Skin

- Usually involvement of overlying or adjacent epidermis (dysplasia or carcinoma in situ), may have squamous pearls or focal keratinization
- Positive for CK5/6, p63, and usually negative for CK20, synaptophysin, and chromogranin

Basal Cell Carcinoma of Skin

- Peripheral palisading, tumor cleft artifactual separation from associated dermis, lower grade cytologic features than MCC
- Positive for CK5/6 and p63, but usually negative for CK20, synaptophysin, and chromogranin

Lymphoma/Leukemia

- Similar diffuse growth pattern in dermis with high-grade cells
- Immunohistochemical markers helpful in differentiating these from MCC

DIAGNOSTIC CHECKLIST

Clinically Relevant Pathologic Features

- Aggressive tumors in sun-damaged skin of elderly
- May have lymph node metastases at diagnosis, and majority develop lymph node metastasis over time
- Associated with immunodeficiency and malignancies, and patients with Merkel cell may develop other malignancies

Pathologic Interpretation Pearls

- High-grade carcinoma based in dermis with stippled neuroendocrine chromatin, prominent mitoses, diffuse or trabecular growth
- Can occur with basal cell or squamous cell carcinoma
- Subset (4-5%) cases "primary" to lymph nodes or "unknown primary"
- Positive for CK20 (and +/- CK7), chromogranin, synaptophysin, and CAM5.2, and negative for TTF-1
  - Immunophenotype similar to high-grade neuroendocrine tumors of salivary gland
- MCPV positive in majority of cases from United States and Europe, but less common in Australia

STAGING

AJCC (8th Edition) Pathologic Stage Groups (pTNM)

- Based on 9,387 cases & literature
  - Stage 0: Tis, N0, M0 (in situ primary tumor, no LN or distant metastasis)
  - Stage I: T1, N0, M0 (primary tumor ≤ 2 cm, no LN or distant metastases)
  - Stage IIA: T2/T3, N0, M0 (T2 primary tumor > 2 cm but ≤ 5 cm, T3 primary tumor > 5 cm, no LN or distant metastases)
  - Stage IIB: T4, N0, M0 (primary tumor invades fascia, muscle cartilage, or bone, no LN or distant metastases)
  - Stage IIIA: T1-4, N1a(sn) or N1a, M0; **or** T0, N1b, M0
    - N1a: Clinically occult regional LN metastasis following LN dissection
    - N1a(sn): Clinically occult nodal metastasis identified only by sentinel lymph node biopsy
    - N1b: Clinically or radiologically detected regional LN metastasis, pathologically confirmed

- Stage IIIB: Any T1-4, N1b-3, M0 (no distant metastases)
  - N1b: Clinically or radiologically detected regional LN metastasis, pathologically confirmed
  - N2: In transit metastasis without LN metastasis
  - N3: In transit metastasis with LN metastasis
- Stage IV: Any T, any N, M1 (distant metastasis)
  - M1a: Metastasis to distant skin, distant subcutaneous tissue, or distant LN
  - M1b: Lung
  - M1c: All other distant sites

SELECTED REFERENCES

1. Garrett GL et al: Incidence of and risk factors for skin cancer in organ transplant recipients in the United States. JAMA Dermatol. 153(3):296-303, 2017
2. Moshiri AS et al: Polyomavirus-negative Merkel cell carcinoma: A more aggressive subtype based on analysis of 282 cases using multimodal tumor virus detection. J Invest Dermatol. 137(4):819-827, 2017
3. Strom T et al: Improved local and regional control with radiotherapy for Merkel cell carcinoma of the head and neck. Head Neck. 39(1):48-55, 2017
4. Cassler NM et al: Merkel cell carcinoma therapeutic Update. Curr Treat Options Oncol. 17(7):36, 2016
5. Gunaratne DA et al: Sentinel lymph node biopsy in Merkel cell carcinoma: a 15-year institutional experience and statistical analysis of 721 reported cases. Br J Dermatol. 174(2):273-81, 2016
6. Harms KL et al: Analysis of prognostic factors from 9387 Merkel cell carcinoma cases forms the basis for the new 8th Edition AJCC Staging System. Ann Surg Oncol. 23(11):3564-71, 2016
7. Harms PW et al: Next generation sequencing of cytokeratin 20-negative Merkel cell carcinoma reveals ultraviolet-signature mutations and recurrent TP53 and RB1 inactivation. Mod Pathol. 29(3):240-8, 2016
8. Iyer JG et al: Paraneoplastic syndromes (PNS) associated with Merkel cell carcinoma (MCC): A case series of 8 patients highlighting different clinical manifestations. J Am Acad Dermatol. 75(3):541-7, 2016
9. Liu W et al: Merkel cell polyomavirus infection and Merkel cell carcinoma. Curr Opin Virol. 20:20-27, 2016
10. Mauzo SH et al: Molecular characteristics and potential therapeutic targets in Merkel cell carcinoma. J Clin Pathol. ePub, 2016
11. Samimi M et al: Prognostic value of antibodies to Merkel cell polyomavirus T antigens and VP1 protein in patients with Merkel cell carcinoma. Br J Dermatol. 174(4):813-22, 2016
12. Walsh NM: Complete spontaneous regression of Merkel cell carcinoma (1986-2016): a 30 year perspective. J Cutan Pathol. 43(12):1150-1154, 2016
13. Grundhoff A et al: Merkel cell polyomavirus, a highly prevalent virus with tumorigenic potential. Curr Opin Virol. 14:129-37, 2015
14. Lai JH et al: Pure versus combined Merkel cell carcinomas: immunohistochemical evaluation of cellular proteins (p53, Bcl-2, and c-kit) reveals significant overexpression of p53 in combined tumors. Hum Pathol. 46(9):1290-6, 2015
15. Pulitzer MP et al: Cutaneous squamous and neuroendocrine carcinoma: genetically and immunohistochemically different from Merkel cell carcinoma. Mod Pathol. 28(8):1023-32, 2015
16. Wong SQ et al: UV-associated mutations underlie the etiology of MCV-negative merkel cell carcinomas. Cancer Res. 75(24):5228-34, 2015
17. Iwasaki T et al: Usefulness of significant morphologic characteristics in distinguishing between Merkel cell polyomavirus-positive and Merkel cell polyomavirus-negative Merkel cell carcinomas. Hum Pathol. 44(9):1912-7, 2013
18. Kuwamoto S et al: Association of Merkel cell polyomavirus infection with morphologic differences in Merkel cell carcinoma. Hum Pathol. 42(5):632-40, 2011
19. Kuwamoto S: Recent advances in the biology of Merkel cell carcinoma. Hum Pathol. 42(8):1063-77, 2011
20. Ly TY et al: The spectrum of Merkel cell polyomavirus expression in Merkel cell carcinoma, in a variety of cutaneous neoplasms, and in neuroendocrine carcinomas from different anatomical sites. Hum Pathol. Epub ahead of print, 2011
21. Paik JY et al: Immunohistochemistry for Merkel cell polyomavirus is highly specific but not sensitive for the diagnosis of Merkel cell carcinoma in the Australian population. Hum Pathol. 42(10):1385-90, 2011
22. Loyo M et al: Quantitative detection of Merkel cell virus in human tissues and possible mode of transmission. Int J Cancer. 126(12):2991-6, 2010
23. Duncavage EJ et al: Merkel cell polyomavirus: a specific marker for Merkel cell carcinoma in histologically similar tumors. Am J Surg Pathol. 33(12):1771-7, 2009
24. Sastre-Garau X et al: Merkel cell carcinoma of the skin: pathological and molecular evidence for a causative role of MCV in oncogenesis. J Pathol. 218(1):48-56, 2009
25. Shuda M et al: Human Merkel cell polyomavirus infection I. MCV T antigen expression in Merkel cell carcinoma, lymphoid tissues and lymphoid tumors. Int J Cancer. 125(6):1243-9, 2009
26. Feng H et al: Clonal integration of a polyomavirus in human Merkel cell carcinoma. Science. 319(5866):1096-100, 2008
27. Kassem A et al: Frequent detection of Merkel cell polyomavirus in human Merkel cell carcinomas and identification of a unique deletion in the VP1 gene. Cancer Res. 68(13):5009-13, 2008
28. Maza S et al: Impact of sentinel lymph node biopsy in patients with Merkel cell carcinoma: results of a prospective study and review of the literature. Eur J Nucl Med Mol Imaging. 33(4):433-40, 2006
29. Erickson LA et al: Cdx2 as a marker for neuroendocrine tumors of unknown primary sites. Endocr Pathol. 15(3):247-52, 2004
30. Erickson LA et al: Merkel cell carcinomas: expression of S-phase kinase-associated protein 2 (Skp2), p27, and proliferation markers. Endocr Pathol. 14(3):221-29, 2003
31. Cai YC et al: Cytokeratin 7 and 20 and thyroid transcription factor 1 can help distinguish pulmonary from gastrointestinal carcinoid and pancreatic endocrine tumors. Hum Pathol. 32(10):1087-93, 2001
32. Agoff SN et al: Thyroid transcription factor-1 is expressed in extrapulmonary small cell carcinomas but not in other extrapulmonary neuroendocrine tumors. Mod Pathol. 13(3):238-42, 2000
33. Inoue T et al: Spontaneous regression of merkel cell carcinoma: a comparative study of TUNEL index and tumor-infiltrating lymphocytes between spontaneous regression and non-regression group. J Dermatol Sci. 24(3):203-11, 2000
34. Chan JK et al: Cytokeratin 20 immunoreactivity distinguishes Merkel cell (primary cutaneous neuroendocrine) carcinomas and salivary gland small cell carcinomas from small cell carcinomas of various sites. Am J Surg Pathol. 21(2):226-34, 1997
35. Eusebi V et al: Neuroendocrine carcinoma within lymph nodes in the absence of a primary tumor, with special reference to Merkel cell carcinoma. Am J Surg Pathol. 16(7):658-66, 1992

Immunohistochemical Differential Diagnosis of Neuroendocrine Tumors

Tumor	CAM5.2	CK7	CK20	TTF-1	CDX-2
Lung carcinoid	Positive	21-80%	0%	69-95%	Few
Gastric carcinoid	Positive	13%	0%	0-2% focal weak	0-17%
Midgut carcinoid	Positive	0%	24%	0%	> 90%
Colon carcinoid	Positive	24% focal	35% focal	0%	Few
Pancreatic islet cell tumor	Positive	0-50% focal weak	0-14%	0%	30%
Lung small cell	Positive	11%	0-2%	90%	0%
Merkel cell	Positive	17%	95%	0%	0%

(Left) *Merkel cell carcinoma shows a diffuse growth pattern in the dermis and extending into the underlying subcutaneous tissue.* **(Right)** *Merkel cell carcinoma shows prominent mitotic activity and nuclei with stippled neuroendocrine chromatin. These tumors must be differentiated from visceral metastases to the skin, such as those from lung cancer or from lymphoproliferative disorders. In difficult cases, immunoperoxidase studies can be very helpful.*

Merkel Cell Carcinoma

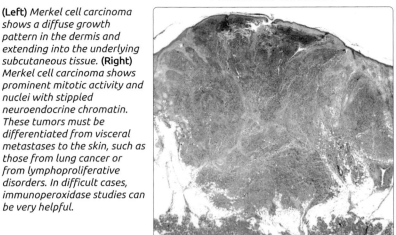

Merkel Cell Carcinoma With Mitotic Activity

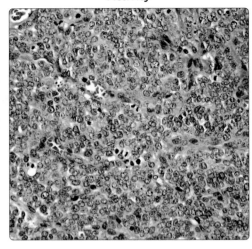

(Left) *CK20 shows characteristic immunopositivity in a Merkel cell carcinoma. Often, CK20 shows a dot-like staining pattern in these tumors. These tumors are usually positive for other low molecular weight keratins, such as CAM5.2.* **(Right)** *CK7 is usually negative in Merkel cell carcinoma. Merkel cell carcinomas can be positive for both CK20 and CK7, although most Merkel cell carcinomas are positive for CK20 and negative for CK7.*

CK20

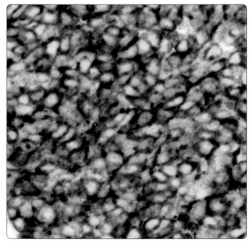

CK7

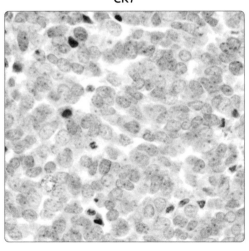

(Left) *Chromogranin-A staining in a Merkel cell carcinoma is shown. Merkel cell carcinomas are positive for neuroendocrine markers such as chromogranin and synaptophysin.* **(Right)** *Synaptophysin staining in a Merkel cell carcinoma is shown. Both Merkel cell carcinoma and small cell lung carcinoma will be positive for synaptophysin, chromogranin, and CAM5.2, but small cell lung carcinoma will usually also be positive for CK7 and TTF-1 and negative for CK20.*

Chromogranin-A

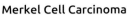

Synaptophysin

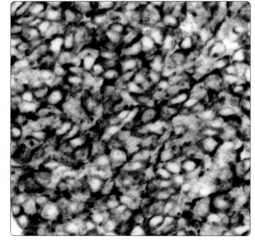

Merkel Cell Carcinoma Solid and Nested Growth

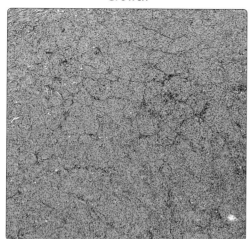

Nests and Nodules of Merkel Cell Carcinoma in Dermis

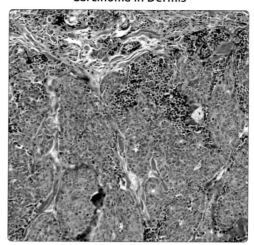

(Left) *Merkel cell carcinoma in the dermis shows a solid and nested growth pattern.* (Right) *Merkel cell carcinoma shows a nodular growth pattern in the dermis. The cells have characteristic stippled nuclei and prominent mitotic activity.*

Neuroendocrine Chromatin Stippling

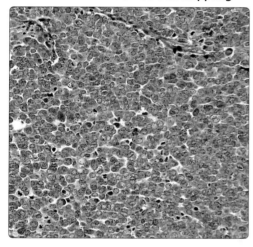

Merkel Cell Carcinoma Mitotic Figures

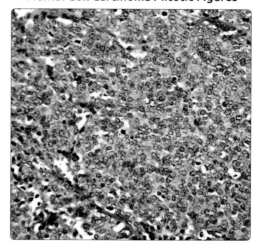

(Left) *Medium-power view of Merkel cell carcinoma is shown. This neuroendocrine tumor histologically can resemble high-grade small cell neuroendocrine carcinomas, such as from the lung. Immunoperoxidase studies can differentiate these tumors.* (Right) *Merkel cell carcinoma shows cells with vesicular nuclei with scant cytoplasm and prominent mitotic activity. Mitotic figures are usually identified in every field, reflecting the proliferative activity of these aggressive tumors.*

Sheet-Like Growth in Merkel Cell Carcinoma

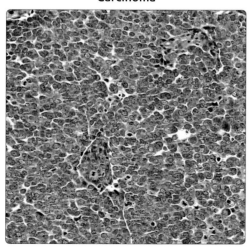

Merkel Cell Carcinoma

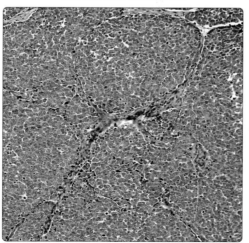

(Left) *Merkel cell carcinoma shows a sheet-like growth pattern, prominent mitotic activity, and nuclei with stippled neuroendocrine chromatin.* (Right) *Merkel cell carcinoma shows multiple nodules of tumor cells. These tumors must be differentiated from visceral metastases to the skin, such as those from lung cancer or lymphoproliferative disorders. Immunohistochemical studies are helpful in this distinction.*

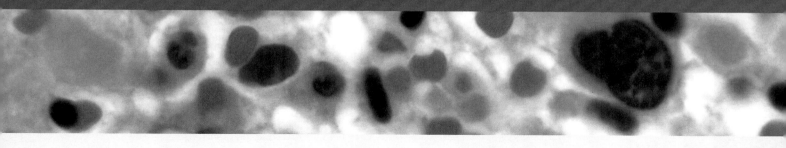

SECTION 7
Inherited Tumor Syndromes

KEY FACTS

TERMINOLOGY

- Multiple endocrine neoplasia type 1 (MEN1): Rare autosomal dominant disease resulting in proliferative lesions of multiple endocrine organs involving mainly parathyroid, endocrine pancreas/duodenum, and pituitary glands

ETIOLOGY/PATHOGENESIS

- MEN1 encodes menin, protein with multitude of functions and interactions and known tumor suppressor

CLINICAL ISSUES

- Hyperparathyroidism
- Pituitary tumors
- Endocrine pancreas/duodenal tumors
- Others including adrenal cortical lesions, cutaneous lesions, thymic carcinoids, and gastric ECLomas

MICROSCOPIC

- **Parathyroid hyperplasia**
  - All 4 glands are hypercellular with relative paucity of intraparenchymal fat
  - Predominant cell type is chief cell
- **Pituitary adenoma**
  - Composed of uniform, polygonal cells arrayed in sheets or cords with absence of reticulin network
  - Cytoplasm can be acidophilic, basophilic, or chromophobic depending on type and amount of secretory product
- **Duodenal &/or pancreatic endocrine tumors**
- Pancreatic endocrine tumors
  - Numerous nonfunctioning microadenomas (< 0.5 cm) spread throughout pancreas
- Duodenal endocrine tumors
  - Well-circumscribed nodule in mucosa or submucosa
- **Thymic and bronchial neuroendocrine tumors**
- **Adrenal cortical hyperplasia and tumors**
- **Skin: Collagenoma, angiofibroma, pigmented lesions**

Parathyroid Hyperplasia

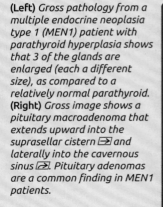 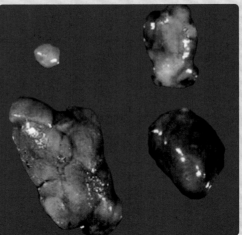

Pituitary Macroadenoma

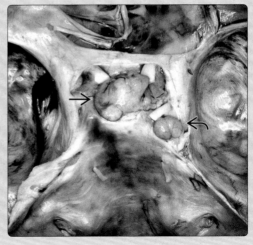

(Left) *Gross pathology from a multiple endocrine neoplasia type 1 (MEN1) patient with parathyroid hyperplasia shows that 3 of the glands are enlarged (each a different size), as compared to a relatively normal parathyroid.* (Right) *Gross image shows a pituitary macroadenoma that extends upward into the suprasellar cistern* ➡ *and laterally into the cavernous sinus* ➡. *Pituitary adenomas are a common finding in MEN1 patients.*

Pancreatic Microadenoma

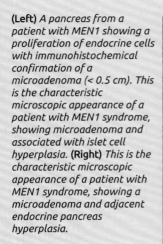 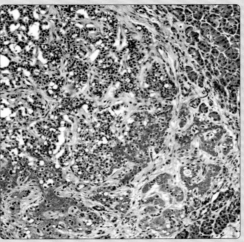

Glucagon Microadenoma

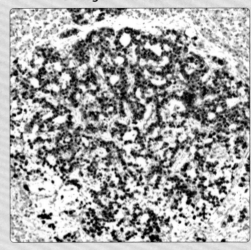

(Left) *A pancreas from a patient with MEN1 showing a proliferation of endocrine cells with immunohistochemical confirmation of a microadenoma (< 0.5 cm). This is the characteristic microscopic appearance of a patient with MEN1 syndrome, showing microadenoma and associated with islet cell hyperplasia.* (Right) *This is the characteristic microscopic appearance of a patient with MEN1 syndrome, showing a microadenoma and adjacent endocrine pancreas hyperplasia.*

TERMINOLOGY

Abbreviations

- Multiple endocrine neoplasia type 1 (MEN1)

Synonyms

- Wermer syndrome
- Multiple endocrine adenomatosis type 1
- Familial Zollinger-Ellison syndrome (ZES)

Definitions

- MEN1 is autosomal dominant disease caused by germline *MEN1* mutations leading to development of multifocal neoplastic endocrine lesions
  - Parathyroid glands, endocrine pancreas, duodenum, and anterior pituitary
  - Less commonly involving stomach, adrenal cortex, thymus, and lung
  - Various nonendocrine lesions occur in skin, soft tissue, and central nervous system

ETIOLOGY/PATHOGENESIS

Etiology

- Caused by mutations in *MEN1* gene at 11q13

Pathogenesis

- *MEN1* gene encodes 610-amino acid protein menin
  - Protein with multitude of functions and interactions and known tumor suppressor

CLINICAL ISSUES

Epidemiology

- Incidence
  - 1:20,000-40,000
- Age
  - Penetrance increases with age
- Sex
  - 1:1 sex distribution

Presentation

- **Hyperparathyroidism**
  - 1st clinical manifestation in most patients
  - Percentage of patients who develop biochemical evidence of hyperparathyroidism increases with age
    - 43% and 94% at age 20 and 50 years, respectively
  - Incidence of MEN1 among individuals aged < 40 years with primary hyperparathyroidism: 5-13%
  - Most are asymptomatic, severe cases with "moans, groans, bones, and stones" as hallmarks of hypercalcemia
  - Multiglandular disorder
  - High recurrence rate
- **Pituitary tumors**
  - 1st clinical manifestation of MEN1 in 17% (range: 10–25%) of patients
  - Prevalence in MEN1 of ~ 30-40% (range: 10-50%)
  - Suggested penetrance in MEN1 (aged > 16 years) of 38%
  - Patients with MEN1 with pituitary adenomas tend to be younger than patients with sporadic tumors
    - MEN1 adenomas: Mean patient age ± standard deviation = 35.1 ± 14.8 years

- Sporadic tumors: Mean patient age of 40 years
  - Prolactinomas (60%), nonsecreting adenomas (15%), growth hormone secreting adenoma (9-10%), adrenocorticotrophin secreting and thyrotroph adenomas (4-5%)
  - 10% of MEN1 pituitary adenomas show cosecretion by immunohistochemical methods
  - Women with PRL adenoma: Major clinical signs are amenorrhea, infertility, galactorrhea
  - Men with PRL adenoma: Hypogonadism
    - Men tend to have more macroadenomas, especially at young ages
  - GH adenoma: Acromegaly
  - ACTH-secreting adenoma: Cushing disease
- **Endocrine pancreatic/duodenal tumors**
  - Incidence of MEN1-associated duodenal and pancreatic NETs peaks at 40–60 years
  - Clinical manifestations in ~ 40% of patients with MEN1
  - Severe obstructive pancreatitis due to duct stenosis by macrotumors may occur
  - In as many as 80% of cases, tumors give rise to large periduodenal &/or peripancreatic lymph node metastases, which were formerly interpreted as gastrinoma primaries
    - ZES
      - Most frequent clinical manifestation related to duodenal &/or pancreatic gastrinoma observed in MEN1 patients
      - MEN1-associated ZES accounts for 20-30% of all ZES cases
      - Initial symptoms such as abdominal pain or gastroesophageal reflux disease caused by gastric acid hypersecretion
      - Severe complications include bleeding, perforation, and esophageal strictures
      - Source of gastrin excess is multicentric NETs typically in mucosa and submucosa of upper duodenum and sometimes at margin of ulcer
      - In 90% of MEN1 patients with ZES, lesions are often multiple, small, and located in duodenum
    - Insulinomas
      - 2nd most frequent pancreatic tumor in setting of MEN1
      - Hypoglycemia
    - Glucagonoma, VIPoma, and other pancreatic endocrine tumors
      - Occur in < 5% of MEN1 patients
      - > 70% of glucagonomas and 40% of VIPomas are malignant
      - Glucagonomas induce necrolytic migratory erythema associated with diabetes mellitus, which is secondary to abnormal glucagon secretion
      - VIPomas induce classic Verner-Morrison syndrome associated with watery diarrhea, hypokalemia, and achlorhydria
      - GHRH tumor causing acromegaly
    - Nonfunctioning pancreatic endocrine tumors
      - 20-40% of MEN1 patients
      - When misdiagnosed, often discovered after local compression &/or hepatic metastases
- **Others**

- o Adrenal cortical lesions
  - – Observed in 20-45% of MEN1 patients
  - – Often hyperplastic, ≤ 3 cm, bilateral, and nonfunctional
  - – Adrenal cortical carcinomas may be found bilaterally
  - – MEN1 cases more often associated with hyperaldosteronism
- o Cutaneous proliferations
  - – Present in 40-80% of MEN1 patients
  - – Variable histological forms
    - □ Collagenomas
    - □ Angiofibromas are multiple and often on face
    - □ Nodular lipomas are multicentric and show no recurrence after surgery
    - □ Café au lait macules
    - □ Confetti-like hypopigmented macules
    - □ Multiple gingival papules
- o Thymic and bronchial neuroendocrine tumor
  - – Observed in 5-10% of MEN1 patients
  - – Thymic carcinoids are predominantly in males
  - – Poor prognosis with local invasion, recurrence, and distant metastasis
  - – Account for ~ 25% of all thymic carcinoids
  - – Bronchial carcinoids (typical and atypical) are usually nonfunctioning
- o Gastric ECLomas
  - – Thought to originate from proliferation of enterochromaffin-like (ECL) cells in fundic mucosa
  - – Often small and multiple
  - – Can be treated with endoscopic polypectomy if lesion is < 1 cm
  - – Good prognosis
- o Central nervous system tumors
  - – Spinal ependymomas, meningioma, and astrocytoma have been described in MEN1 cases
- o Soft tissue tumors
  - – Esophageal leiomyoma
  - – Renal angiomyolipoma
  - – Malignant gastrointestinal stromal tumors
  - – Large visceral and intrathoracic lipomas
  - – Aggressive malignant peripheral nerve sheath tumor arising from adrenal ganglioneuroma
- o Breast Cancer
  - – Has been found in 6% of females with MEN1

Treatment

- **Hyperparathyroidism**
  - o Total parathyroidectomy with autotransplantation or subtotal resection of 3 1/2 parathyroid glands
    - – Multiglandular parathyroid involvement can be asymmetrical and asynchronous
  - o Prophylactic partial thymectomy is also considered: Mediastinal recurrence due to ectopic or supernumerary parathyroid glands in as many as 12% of cases
- **Pituitary adenoma**
  - o Conflicting data on treatment response
    - – Pharmacotherapy &/or surgery: Suboptimal response of functioning pituitary adenomas (earlier reports)
    - – Dopamine agonist therapy: Good response of lactotroph adenomas in adult patients with MEN1 (Netherlands cohort)

- **Endocrine pancreatic/duodenal tumors**
  - o Surgery

Prognosis

- Same prognosis for pituitary adenoma in MEN1 as in sporadic counterparts
- Malignancy of duodenal and pancreatic endocrine tumors
  - o Gastrinomas > 40%, glucagonoma > 80%, VIPoma > 40%, nonfunctioning tumor > 70%
- Increased risk of premature death, usually related to disease and its complications
  - o Main causes of death are thymic tumors, PanNETs, along with rare cases of aggressive adrenal tumors
  - o Female sex, family history of MEN1 and recent diagnosis are associated with lower risk of death
  - o Patients with small duodenal NETs have 15-year survival rate of nearly 100%

Diagnostic Criteria

- Criteria related to inherited cancers
  - o Age < 50 years,
  - o Positive family history
  - o Multifocal or recurrent neoplasia
  - o Presence of ≥ 2 of following
    - – Primary hyperparathyroidism with multiglandular hyperplasia &/or adenoma or recurrent primary hyperparathyroidism
    - – Duodenal &/or pancreatic endocrine tumors, gastric enterochromaffin-like tumors
      - □ Both functioning and nonfunctioning or multisecreting tumor
    - – Anterior pituitary adenoma
      - □ Functioning (GH-secreting tumor or acromegaly, prolactinoma)
      - □ Nonfunctioning or multisecreting
    - – Adrenocortical tumor
      - □ Both functioning and nonfunctioning
    - – Thymic &/or bronchial tube endocrine tumors (foregut carcinoids)
    - – 1st-degree relative with MEN1 according to above criteria

MACROSCOPIC

Hyperparathyroidism

- All 4 glands are generally grossly enlarged (> 6-8 mm), increased in weight (> 40-60 mg) and lobulated
- MEN1-associated multiglandular parathyroid lesions are composed of multiple monoclonal cell proliferations consisting of multiglandular adenomas

Pituitary Adenoma

- Soft, well-circumscribed lesion
  - o May be confined to sella turcica
  - o Larger lesions extend into suprasellar region and often compress optic chiasm
- MEN1-associated adenomas vs. nonassociated are more often to be
  - o Multiple (i.e., in 4-5% of cases vs. 0.1%)
  - o Multihormonal (i.e., in 10-39% of cases), with prolactin and growth hormone being most frequently detected

Duodenal &/or Pancreatic Endocrine Tumors

- Multiple well-circumscribed nodules in mucosa and submucosa of duodenum and within pancreatic parenchyma
- Diffuse microadenomatosis associated with 1 or several macrotumors (> 0.5 cm) is distinctive feature of pancreas in MEN1

MICROSCOPIC

Histologic Features

- **Parathyroid hyperplasia**
  - Multiglandular parathyroid lesions are suggested to be composed of multiple monoclonal proliferations, constituting multiple multiglandular microadenomas
  - All 4 glands are hypercellular with relative paucity of intraparenchymal fat
  - Architecturally, pattern in hyperplasia consists of cords or nests, or cells in glandular pattern as well as foci of solid sheets (nodular hyperplasia)
  - Predominant cell type is chief cell
    - Faintly eosinophilic cytoplasm and centrally placed, round, relatively monotonous nucleus without conspicuous nucleoli
    - Followed by oncocytic &/or clear cells
  - Mostly lack characteristic atrophic rim of nonlesional parathyroid tissue
- **Pituitary adenoma**
  - Composed of uniform, polygonal cells arranged in sheets or cords with absence of reticulin network
  - Cytoplasm can be acidophilic, basophilic, or chromophobic depending on type and amount of secretory product
  - Nuclei of neoplastic cells may be uniform or pleomorphic
  - Macroadenomas (76-85%) vs. sporadic cases
    - Significantly larger
    - Often more invasive
    - Higher Ki-67 proliferation index
    - More S100(+) folliculostellate cells
- **Pancreatic &/or duodenal endocrine tumors**
  - Pancreatic endocrine tumors
    - Diffuse microadenomatosis associated with 1 or several macrotumors (> 0.5 cm) is characteristic of pancreas in MEN1 syndrome
      - Numerous nonfunctioning microadenomas (< 0.5 cm) distributed throughout pancreas
    - Distinct trabecular/pseudoglandular pattern with conspicuous connective tissue stroma
    - Insulinomas with amyloid deposition
    - Tiny monohormonal glucagon cell proliferations that appear to originate from islets with hyperplastic glucagon cell component are composed of monoclonal cells
      - Characterized by loss of heterozygosity of 11q13, which is obviously required to transform hyperplastic cells into neoplastic proliferations
    - Islet hyperplasia and endocrine cell budding from ducts are not features
  - Duodenal endocrine tumors
    - Well-circumscribed mucosal or submucosal nodules
    - Well differentiated (grade 1)
    - Trabecular to pseudoglandular pattern
    - Cells have fine chromatin and inconspicuous nucleoli
    - Stain mainly for gastrin
    - Associated with focal hyperplastic changes of gastrin and somatostatin cells in duodenal crypts and Brunner glands
- **Others**
  - Adrenal nodular hyperplasia
  - Adrenal cortical carcinoma
  - Thymic and bronchial neuroendocrine tumors
  - Gastric ECLomas: Proliferation of enterochromaffin-like cells
  - TSH-producing pituitary carcinoma

ANCILLARY TESTS

Immunohistochemistry

- Pituitary adenoma can express 1 or several hormones
  - Prolactin, GH, ACTH, LH, FSH, and TSH
- Pancreatic endocrine tumor can express 1 or several hormones
  - Glucagon, insulin, pancreatic polypeptide, somatostatin, gastrin, vasointestinal polypeptide, serotonin, and calcitonin

Genetic Testing

- *MEN1* gene
  - Inherited as autosomal dominant trait or occurs de novo
  - Located on chromosome 11q13
  - Consists of 10 exons
  - Encodes menin
    - Protein with multitude of functions and interactions and known tumor suppressor
      - Multiple domains and interacting partners, ranging from transcription factors to histone deacetylase complexes
    - Scaffold protein with crystal structure that may associate with cell membrane and organelles and may be active in nucleus (regulates gene transcription)
- Mutation spectrum
  - > 400 different mutations described
  - Spread over entire coding and intronic sequence
    - 40% frameshift changes, 25% missense, 20% nonsense mutations
    - No significant genotype-phenotype correlations, with few exceptions
  - All somatic cells have inactivating mutation in 1 MEN1 allele, predisposing patient to development of tumors associated with condition
    - But neoplasms do not develop until loss of heterozygosity of normal *MEN1* allele occurs at tissue level
    - Therefore, loss of heterozygosity is essential for tumorigenicity, although other factors are also at play
  - Tissue-specific factors determine expression of *MEN1* mutations in specific organs
    - Range from menin expression levels and interacting proteins, such as mixed-lineage leukemia protein, to presence (or absence) of other genes that regulate cell growth and proliferation, such as *CDKN1B*
- Testing
  - Sequencing

– Genetic counseling useful for individuals and families with nonclassic MEN1 presentations

Serologic Testing

- Serum Ca, PTH: Hyperparathyroidism
- PRL, GH, ACTH, others: Pituitary adenoma
- Gastrin, insulin, glucagon, pancreatic polypeptide, and serum chromogranin-A: GI NET

DIFFERENTIAL DIAGNOSIS

Multiple Endocrine Neoplasia Type 4

- Autosomal dominant disease, caused by germline mutations of *CDKN1B*
- Resulting in phenotype similar to that of MEN1 characterized by neuroendocrine neoplasms, particularly in parathyroid glands, pituitary, and pancreas
- Patients presenting with MEN1-like changes but lacking germline MEN1 mutation should therefore be tested for *CDKN1B* mutation

Hyperparathyroidism-Jaw Tumor Syndrome

- Autosomal dominant disorder caused by mutation in *CDC73* (previously known as HRPT2*)* gene
- Often is caused by parathyroid adenoma or carcinoma and follows much more aggressive behavior

Multiple Endocrine Neoplasia Type 2

- Autosomal dominant tumor syndrome pattern caused by mutations of *RET* gene
- Characterized by various endocrine tumors involving thyroid, adrenals, and parathyroid
- Additional abnormalities affecting nonendocrine tissues may be present
- Subdivided into 3 groups
  o Familial medullary thyroid carcinoma, MEN2A, and MEN2B

Carney Complex

- Autosomal dominant syndrome caused by *PRKAR1A* mutations
- Multiple neoplasia syndrome featuring cardiac, endocrine, cutaneous, and neural tumors, as well as mucocutaneous pigmented lesions
- May involve several endocrine glands (adrenal cortex, pituitary, and thyroid)

Familial Isolated Pituitary Adenoma

- Defined as occurrence of pituitary adenomas of any type among ≥ 2 related family members in absence of MEN1 or Carney complex
- Autosomal dominant disease with low penetrance
- 20% of affected families harbor mutation in *AIP* gene

SELECTED REFERENCES

1. Chiloiro S et al: Pancreatic neuroendocrine tumors in MEN1 disease: a mono-centric longitudinal and prognostic study. Endocrine. ePub, 2017
2. Hyde SM et al: Genetics of multiple endocrine neoplasia type 1/multiple endocrine neoplasia type 2 syndromes. Endocrinol Metab Clin North Am. 46(2):491-502, 2017
3. Bartsch DK et al: Bronchopulmonary neuroendocrine neoplasms and their precursor lesions in multiple endocrine neoplasia type 1. Neuroendocrinology. 103(3-4):240-7, 2016
4. Concolino P et al: Multiple endocrine neoplasia type 1 (MEN1): an update of 208 new germline variants reported in the last nine years. Cancer Genet. 209(1-2):36-41, 2016
5. Ito T et al: Imaging in multiple endocrine neoplasia type 1: recent studies show enhanced sensitivities but increased controversies. Int J Endocr Oncol. 3(1):53-66, 2016
6. Pacheco MC: Multiple endocrine neoplasia: a genetically diverse group of familial tumor syndromes. J Pediatr Genet. 5(2):89-97, 2016
7. Thakker RV: Genetics of parathyroid tumours. J Intern Med. 280(6):574-583, 2016
8. Goudet P et al: MEN1 disease occurring before 21 years old: a 160-patient cohort study from the Groupe d'étude des Tumeurs Endocrines. J Clin Endocrinol Metab. 100(4):1568-77, 2015
9. Norton JA et al: Better survival but changing causes of death in patients with multiple endocrine neoplasia type 1. Ann Surg. 261(6):e147-8, 2015
10. Wells SA Jr et al: Revised American Thyroid Association guidelines for the management of medullary thyroid carcinoma. Thyroid. 25(6):567-610, 2015
11. Reid MD et al: Neuroendocrine tumors of the pancreas: current concepts and controversies. Endocr Pathol. 25(1):65-79, 2014
12. Thakker RV: Multiple endocrine neoplasia type 1 (MEN1) and type 4 (MEN4). Mol Cell Endocrinol. 386(1-2):2-15, 2013
13. Ito T et al: Zollinger-Ellison syndrome: recent advances and controversies. Curr Opin Gastroenterol. 29(6):650-61, 2013
14. Ito T et al: Causes of death and prognostic factors in multiple endocrine neoplasia type 1: a prospective study: comparison of 106 MEN1/Zollinger-Ellison syndrome patients with 1613 literature MEN1 patients with or without pancreatic endocrine tumors. Medicine (Baltimore). 92(3):135-81, 2013
15. Thakker RV et al: Clinical practice guidelines for multiple endocrine neoplasia type 1 (MEN1). J Clin Endocrinol Metab. 97(9):2990-3011, 2012
16. Daví MV et al: Presentation and outcome of pancreaticoduodenal endocrine tumors in multiple endocrine neoplasia type 1 syndrome. Neuroendocrinology. 94(1):58-65, 2011
17. Goudet P et al: Gender-related differences in MEN1 lesion occurrence and diagnosis: a cohort study of 734 cases from the Groupe d'etude des Tumeurs Endocrines. Eur J Endocrinol. 165(1):97-105, 2011
18. Hou R et al: A novel missense mutation in the MEN1 gene in a patient with multiple endocrine neoplasia type 1. Endocr Pract. 17(3):e63-7, 2011
19. Marsh DJ et al: Multiple endocrine neoplasia: types 1 and 2. Adv Otorhinolaryngol. 70:84-90, 2011
20. Mohrmann I et al: A de novo 0.57 Mb microdeletion in chromosome 11q13.1 in a patient with speech problems, autistic traits, dysmorphic features and multiple endocrine neoplasia type 1. Eur J Med Genet. 54(4):e461-4, 2011
21. Newey PJ et al: Role of multiple endocrine neoplasia type 1 mutational analysis in clinical practice. Endocr Pract. 17 Suppl 3:8-17, 2011
22. Nosé V et al: Protocol for the examination of specimens from patients with primary pituitary tumors. Arch Pathol Lab Med. 135(5):640-6, 2011
23. Nosé V: Familial thyroid cancer: a review. Mod Pathol. 24 Suppl 2:S19-33, 2011
24. Ozawa A et al: [Molecular pathophysiology and clinical phenotype of multiple endocrine neoplasia types 1 and 2.] Nihon Rinsho. 69 Suppl 2:681-5, 2011
25. Tonelli F et al: Pancreatic endocrine tumors in multiple endocrine neoplasia type 1 syndrome: review of literature. Endocr Pract. 17 Suppl 3:33-40, 2011
26. Vasilev V et al: Familial pituitary tumor syndromes. Endocr Pract. 17 Suppl 3:41-6, 2011
27. Wu T et al: Menin represses tumorigenesis via repressing cell proliferation. Am J Cancer Res. 1(6):726-39, 2011
28. Zada G et al: Atypical pituitary adenomas: incidence, clinical characteristics, and implications. J Neurosurg. 114(2):336-44, 2011
29. Zhang Y et al: Endocrine tumors as part of inherited tumor syndromes. Adv Anat Pathol. 18(3):206-18, 2011
30. Burgess J: How should the patient with multiple endocrine neoplasia type 1 (MEN 1) be followed? Clin Endocrinol (Oxf). 72(1):13-6, 2010
31. Nosé V: Thyroid cancer of follicular cell origin in inherited tumor syndromes. Adv Anat Pathol. 17(6):428-36, 2010
32. Powell AC et al: Multiple endocrine neoplasia type 1: clinical manifestations and management. Cancer Treat Res. 153:287-302, 2010
33. Rubinstein WS: Endocrine cancer predisposition syndromes: hereditary paraganglioma, multiple endocrine neoplasia type 1, multiple endocrine neoplasia type 2, and hereditary thyroid cancer. Hematol Oncol Clin North Am. 24(5):907-37, 2010
34. Sharretts JM et al: Clinical and molecular genetics of parathyroid neoplasms. Best Pract Res Clin Endocrinol Metab. 24(3):491-502, 2010
35. Shen HC et al: Multiple endocrine neoplasia type 1 deletion in pancreatic alpha-cells leads to development of insulinomas in mice. Endocrinology. 151(8):4024-30, 2010
36. Thakker RV: Multiple endocrine neoplasia type 1 (MEN1). Best Pract Res Clin Endocrinol Metab. 24(3):355-70, 2010
37. Vandeva S et al: The genetics of pituitary adenomas. Best Pract Res Clin Endocrinol Metab. 24(3):461-76, 2010

Frequency and Clinical Features of Various Organ Changes in Multiple Endocrine Neoplasia Type 1

Organ Changes	Frequency	Clinical Features
Parathyroid Gland ≥ 90%		
Microadenomatosis		Primary hyperparathyroidism
Multiglandular parathyroid disease: Multiple multiglandular microadenomas		Usually 1st manifestation of MEN1 patients
Endocrine Pancreas 30-75%		
Multiple microadenomas		
Diffuse microadenomatosis		Distinct feature of pancreas in MEN1
Nonfunctioning macrotumors		Distinctive trabecular/pseudoglandular pattern
Functioning macrotumors		
Insulinoma	10-30%	Hypoglycemia syndrome
Glucagon		Monoclonal glucagon cell proliferations
Duodenum		
Multiple gastrinomas	50-80%	ZES
Multicentric NETs in mucosa and submucosa of the duodenum		MEN1-associated ZES accounts for 20-30% of all ZES cases
Pituitary Gland		
Adenoma	70%	Clinically silent, local symptoms, pituitary insufficiency
Lactotroph adenoma	Frequent	Amenorrhea, galactorrhea
Somatotroph adenoma	9%	Acromegaly
Corticotroph adenoma	4%	Cushing syndrome
Others	Rare	
Other Lesions		
Neuroendocrine tumors (thymus, stomach, lung, intestinal)	5–10%	
Skin (facial angiofibromas, collagenoma, pigment lesions)	40–80%	
Adrenal cortical hyperplasia/ tumor	20–45%	
Lipoma	10%	
Spinal ependymoma	Rare	
Soft tissue tumors	Rare	

ZES = Zollinger–Ellison syndrome; NETs = Neuroendocrine tumors; MEN1 = Multiple endocrine neoplasia type 1.

Modified from: Komminoth P. et al. Multiple endocrine neoplasia type 1. In: WHO, 2017. p.243

38. Agarwal SK et al: The MEN1 gene and pituitary tumours. Horm Res. 71 Suppl 2:131-8, 2009

39. Daly AF et al: Update on familial pituitary tumors: from multiple endocrine neoplasia type 1 to familial isolated pituitary adenoma. Horm Res. 2009 Jan;71 Suppl 1:105-11. Epub 2009 Jan 21. Review. Erratum in: Horm Res. 71(5):297, 2009

40. Davenport C et al: The role of menin in parathyroid tumorigenesis. Adv Exp Med Biol. 668:79-86, 2009

41. Falchetti A et al: Multiple endocrine neoplasia type 1 (MEN1): not only inherited endocrine tumors. Genet Med. 11(12):825-35, 2009

42. Hofer MD et al: Immunohistochemical and clinicopathological correlation of the metastasis-associated gene 1 (MTA1) expression in benign and malignant pancreatic endocrine tumors. Mod Pathol. 22(7):933-9, 2009

43. Scheithauer BW et al: Multiple endocrine neoplasia type 1-associated thyrotropin-producing pituitary carcinoma: report of a probable de novo example. Hum Pathol. 40(2):270-8, 2009

44. Tsukada T et al: MEN1 gene and its mutations: basic and clinical implications. Cancer Sci. 100(2):209-15, 2009

45. Jensen RT et al: Inherited pancreatic endocrine tumor syndromes: advances in molecular pathogenesis, diagnosis, management, and controversies. Cancer. 113(7 Suppl):1807-43, 2008

46. Busygina V et al: Multiple endocrine neoplasia type 1 (MEN1) as a cancer predisposition syndrome: clues into the mechanisms of MEN1-related carcinogenesis. Yale J Biol Med. 79(3-4):105-14, 2006

47. Schnepp RW et al: Mutation of tumor suppressor gene Men1 acutely enhances proliferation of pancreatic islet cells. Cancer Res. 66(11):5707-15, 2006

48. Larsson C et al: Multiple endocrine neoplasia. Cancer Surv. 9(4):703-23, 1990

49. Oberg K et al: Multiple endocrine neoplasia type 1 (MEN-1). Clinical, biochemical and genetical investigations. Acta Oncol. 28(3):383-7, 1989

50. Yamaguchi K et al: Multiple endocrine neoplasia type 1. Clin Endocrinol Metab. 9(2):261-84, 1980

51. Neuroendocrine Tumors: NCCN Clinical Practice Guidelines in Oncology, Version I.2015 (I.2015) 2015

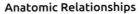

Anatomic Relationships

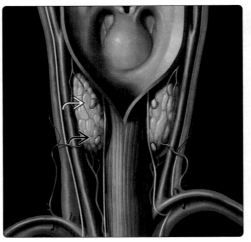

Parathyroid Adenoma

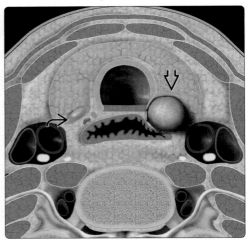

(Left) Coronal graphic displays the esophagus, parathyroid glands, and thyroid gland from behind. The drawing depicts the typical anatomic relationships of the paired superior ➡ and inferior ➡ parathyroid glands in the visceral space. (Right) Axial graphic at the level of the thyroid depicts a superior parathyroid adenoma ➡ in the visceral space just posterior to the thyroid gland. The parathyroid gland ➡ on the other side is of normal size.

Parathyroid Multiglandular Disease

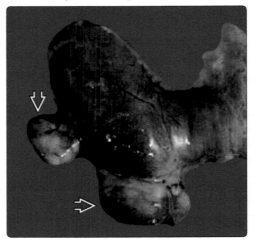

Multiglandular Parathyroid Disease

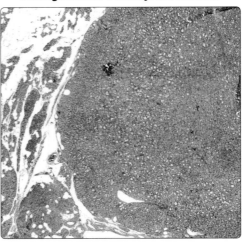

(Left) The usual finding in specimens from patients with MEN1 and multiglandular parathyroid disease is an uneven enlargement of the parathyroid glands. In this thyroid specimen, 2 attached parathyroid glands show multiglandular parathyroid enlargement ➡. (Right) Microscopic findings of nodular parathyroid gland shows a variable hypercellularity and variably sized nodules. The micronodular adenomatosis of parathyroid gland is usually seen in patients with MEN1.

Chief Cell Proliferation

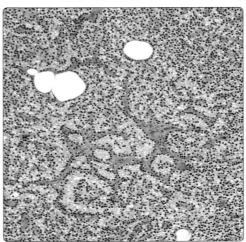

Parathyroid Clear Cell Area

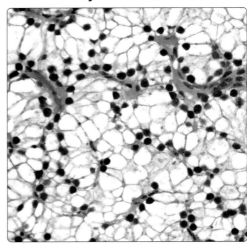

(Left) Microscopic image of a parathyroid in a patient with MEN1 is shown. This example shows chief cell predominant with focal clear cells. There are only scattered residual adipocytes present. (Right) MEN1-associated multiglandular parathyroid lesions are composed of multiple monoclonal cell proliferations consisting of multiglandular adenomas. Some may have abundant clear cell cytoplasm.

Pituitary Microadenoma

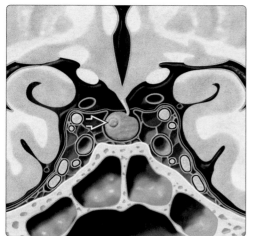

Pituitary Macroadenoma

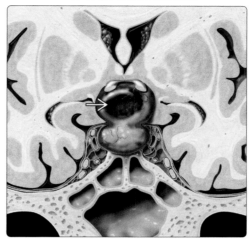

(Left) *Coronal graphic shows a small microadenoma* ⮞ *that slightly enlarges the right side of the pituitary gland and deviates the infundibulum toward the left.* (Right) *Coronal graphic shows a pituitary macroadenoma with suprasellar extension and acute hemorrhage* ⮞ *causing pituitary apoplexy.*

Touch Preparation of Pituitary Adenoma

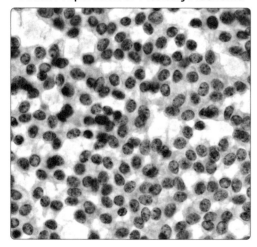

Microscopic View of Pituitary Adenoma

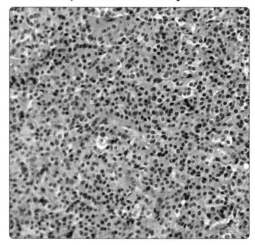

(Left) *Touch preparation of pituitary adenoma shows a monotonous population of cells with poorly defined pale cytoplasm and round to oval nuclei with typical salt and pepper chromatin.* (Right) *Pituitary adenomas are usually arranged in a solid pattern, which is formed by a homogeneous population of cells with no nuclear pleomorphism. The nuclei exhibit neuroendocrine cell features with finely dispersed chromatin and small distinct nucleoli.*

Prolactin-Producing Pituitary Adenoma

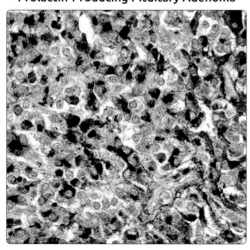

Prolactin-Producing Pituitary Adenoma

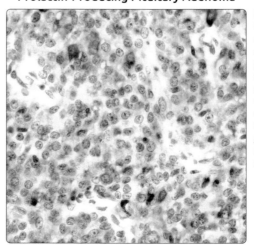

(Left) *Diffuse cytoplasmic as well as Golgi pattern immunoreactivity for PRL is usually present in densely granulated pituitary adenomas.* (Right) *Sparsely granulated lactotroph adenomas are composed of cells with typical Golgi-type staining for PRL. There is only focal and faint immunopositivity for prolactin in these tumors.*

Tumor in Pancreas

Tumor in Pancreatic Head

(Left) Graphic shows a small hypervascular lesion in the pancreatic body with regional lymph node metastases. Note the absence of pancreatic ductal dilatation. (Right) Axial CECT in the arterial phase shows an 8-mm hypervascular insulinoma ➡ in the pancreatic head; it was not detected on portal venous phase CT. Note the opacified superior mesenteric artery and unopacified superior mesenteric vein ➡.

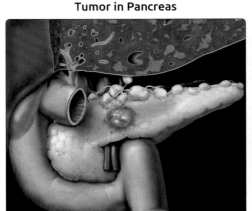

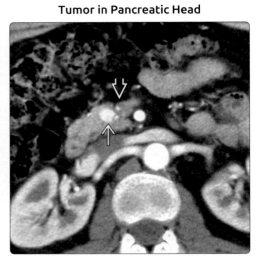

Pancreatic Microadenoma

Trabecular Arrangement

(Left) Microscopic image shows a well-demarcated endocrine tumor ➡ with pseudoglandular pattern surrounded by normal pancreatic parenchyma ➡ in a patient with known MEN1. The pseudoglandular arrangement is usually seen in these patients. (Right) At higher magnification, the tumor shows a distinct trabecular pattern with conspicuous connective tissue stroma. The nuclei of the cells show the typical salt and pepper pattern.

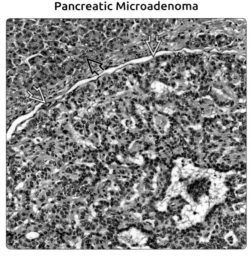

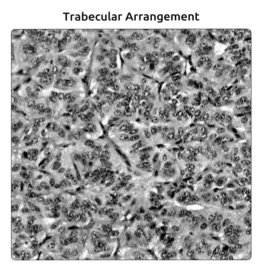

Amyloid in Pancreatic Endocrine Tumor

Pancreatic Endocrine Tumor

(Left) Pancreatic endocrine tumors may have abnormal amyloid deposition ➡, as seen in this insulin-producing tumor. (Right) Pancreatic endocrine tumors may be hormonally active or nonfunctional. The tumor cells in this example show cytoplasmic reactivity for glucagon.

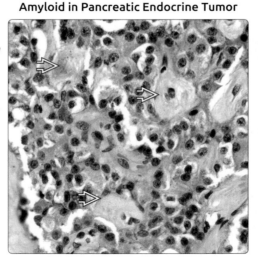

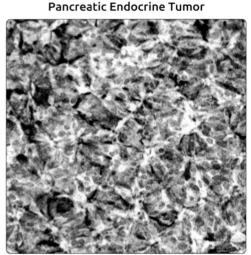

Pancreatic Endocrine Cells

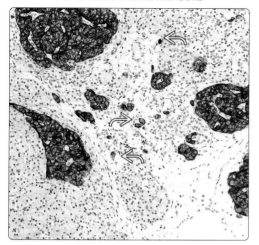

Pancreatic Microadenoma

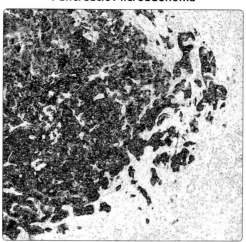

(Left) *Immunohistochemistry stain for synaptophysin in pancreas from a patient with MEN1 highlights the diffuse microadenomatosis. Both the increased number of pancreatic islets and the presence of numerous isolated endocrine cells* ➡ *within the exocrine pancreas are demonstrated in this picture.* **(Right)** *Immunohistochemistry stain for chromogranin A in pancreas from a patient with MEN1 highlights the small proliferation of endocrine cells with focal invasion into adjacent parenchyma.*

Irregularly Shaped Pancreatic Islet

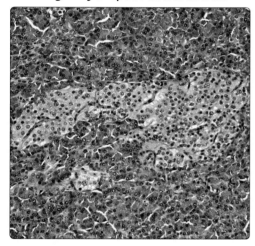

Enlarged Pancreatic Endocrine Islet

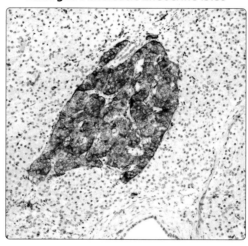

(Left) *Microscopic image of pancreas from a MEN1 patient shows an irregularly shaped pancreatic islet, with increase in the endocrine cell population. Immunohistochemistry for the pancreatic hormones in this pancreas shows multiple nonfunctioning microadenomas.* **(Right)** *An enlarged and irregularly shaped pancreatic islet in a patient with MEN1 is highlighted by diffuse synaptophysin reactivity in the cytoplasm.*

Endocrine Microadenoma and Hyperplasia

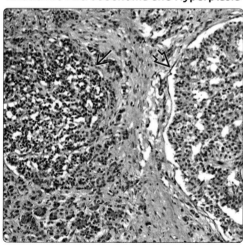

Microadenoma and Islet Cell Hyperplasia

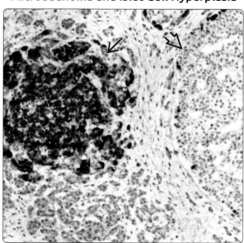

(Left) *Two distinct pancreatic endocrine cell proliferations are shown side by side. The lesion on the left* ➡ *has irregular borders, and the lesion on the right* ➡ *is well demarcated and larger. This is the characteristic microscopic appearance of a patient with MEN1 syndrome.* **(Right)** *The smaller pancreatic endocrine lesion present in this field* ➡ *is uniformly positive for glucagon (microadenoma), while the larger lesion* ➡ *shows a pattern of immunostaining similar to that of a normal island, indicating hyperplasia.*

Multiple Endocrine Neoplasia Type 2 (MEN2)

TERMINOLOGY

- Multiple endocrine neoplasia type 2 (MEN2): Inherited autosomal dominant tumor syndrome caused by activating germline mutations of *RET* gene

CLINICAL ISSUES

- MEN2A comprises ~ 35-40% of cases of MEN2
  - \> 90% of individuals with MEN2A develop medullary thyroid carcinoma (MTC)
  - ~ 35-50% develop pheochromocytoma (PCC)
  - 15-30% develop hyperparathyroidism (HPT)
- Familial medullary thyroid carcinoma subtype comprises 50-60% of cases of MEN2
  - MTC is only clinical manifestation of FMTC
- MEN2B subtype comprises ~ 5-10% of cases of MEN2
  - Characterized by early development of aggressive form of MTC associated with CCH
  - ~ 50% develop PCC
  - ~ 98-100% have neuromas
    - Presence of mucosal neuromas identified early in life
  - ~ 98-100% have asthenic marfanoid body habitus

MICROSCOPIC

- MTC diagnosed histologically when nests of C cells appear to extend beyond basement membrane and to infiltrate and destroy thyroid follicles
- Pheochromocytomas vary in morphology and may have variety of growth patterns
- Parathyroid hyperplasia: Intraparenchymal fat content reduced with great variation in this finding

DIAGNOSTIC CHECKLIST

- With advances of *RET* testing, genotype-specific risks, and management, molecular genetic testing is mandatory
- ATA Guidelines Task Force has classified mutations based on risk for aggressive MTC
  - Used to predict phenotype and recommendations of age to perform prophylactic thyroidectomy and to begin biochemical screening for PCC and HPT

Pheochromocytoma: Gross Cut Surface

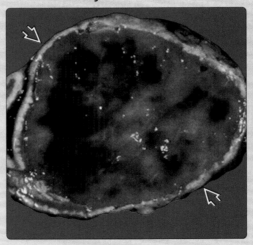

Bilateral Thyroid Tumors in MEN2

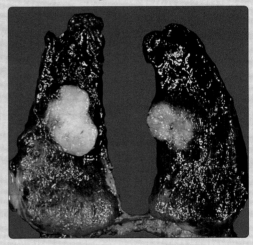

(Left) *The cut surface of a typical pheochromocytoma (PCC) has a gray-pink appearance with areas of hemorrhage. The tumor is distinct from the surrounding bright yellow adrenal cortex* ➡. (Right) *Bilateral medullary thyroid carcinoma (MTC) from a patient with multiple endocrine neoplasia type 2A (MEN2A) shows the characteristic well-circumscribed, tan-pink cut surface.*

C-Cell Hyperplasia in MEN2

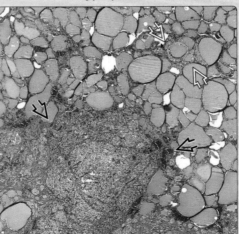

C-Cell Hyperplasia in MEN2

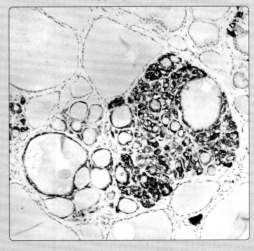

(Left) *C-cell hyperplasia (CCH) is usually present adjacent to MTC in MEN2 patients. This low-power view of the thyroid shows an area of CCH* ➡ *in close proximity to a medullary carcinoma* ➡. (Right) *In MEN2 thyroid, there are multiple foci of CCH. These areas are present in the vicinity of the tumor as well as in the contralateral lobe. This calcitonin stain highlights CCH adjacent to MTC.*

TERMINOLOGY

Abbreviations

- Multiple endocrine neoplasia type 2 (MEN2)

Synonyms

- MEN2A
  - Sipple syndrome
- MEN2B
  - Wagenmann-Froboese syndrome
  - Mucosal neuroma syndrome
  - Multiple endocrine neoplasia type 3

Definitions

- Autosomal dominant tumor syndrome caused by activating germline mutations in *RET* gene
- Characterized by coexistence of various endocrine tumors and lesions in nonendocrine organs and tissues
- 3 subtypes depending on clinical features and manifestations of different penetrances of *RET* mutations
  - **MEN2A**
    - ~ 70-80% of cases of MEN2
    - 70-95% of individuals with MEN2A develop medullary thyroid carcinoma (MTC), ~ 50% develop pheochromocytoma (PCC), and ~ 15-30% develop hyperparathyroidism (HPT)
    - Variants include
      - □ MEN2A with cutaneous lichen amyloidosis
      - □ MEN2A with Hirschsprung disease (HSCR)
      - □ Familial MTC
  - **Familial medullary thyroid carcinoma (FMTC)**
    - ~ 10-20% of cases of MEN2
    - Cases with MTC as their only feature were previously classified as FMTC
      - □ However, recent recommendations suggest including these cases as variant forms within spectrum of MEN2A
  - **MEN2B**
    - ~ 5% of cases of MEN2
    - Develop early-onset MTC
    - High risk of PCC
    - Pathognomonic physical appearance
      - □ Marfanoid body habitus
      - □ Oral mucosal neuromas
      - □ Intestinal ganglioneuromatosis
      - □ Medullated corneal nerve fibers

ETIOLOGY/PATHOGENESIS

RET Protooncogene

- Maps to 10q11.2 and encodes receptor tyrosine kinase rearranged during transfection protein
  - Tyrosine kinase plays integral role in transducing signals for growth and differentiation in tissues derived from neural crest
- Gain-of-function mutations that produce constitutively active protein or decreased specificity for its substrate cause MEN2
- In contrast, loss-of-function mutations associated with subset of HSCR

- **Pathologic allelic variants**: Major disease-causing mutations are nonconservative gain-of-function substitutions located in 1 of 6 cysteine codons in extracellular domain of encoded protein
  - Include codons 609, 611, 618, and 620 in exon 10 and codons 630 and 634 in exon 11
  - All these variants have been identified in families with MEN2A, and some have been identified in families with FMTC
    - Mutations in these sites have been detected in 98% of families with MEN2A
  - ~ 95% of all individuals with MEN2B have single point mutation at codon 918 in exon 16
  - 2nd point mutation at codon 883 has been found in 2-3% of individuals with MEN2B
- For families in which MEN2A and HSCR cosegregate, models to explain how same mutation can cause gain of function and loss of function have been proposed

CLINICAL ISSUES

Epidemiology

- Incidence
  - Unknown; estimated 1.25-7.5/10 million per year
    - MEN2A: 1 case per ~ 2 million per year
    - MEN2B: 1 case per ~ 40 million per year
    - Hereditary MTC accounts for 25% of all MTC
- Age
  - Mean age at clinical presentation
    - MEN2A: 25-35 years
    - MEN2B: 10-20 years
    - FMTC: 45-55 years
- Sex
  - F:M = 1:1
- Prevalence
  - ~ 1/30,000 population
- Relative frequency
  - MEN2A: 35-40%
  - MEN2B: 5-10%
  - FMTC: 50-60%

Presentation

- **MEN2A**
  - **MTC** generally 1st manifestation
    - Probands with MTC typically present with neck mass or neck pain, usually before age 35
      - □ Age-related progression of malignant disease, starting with C-cell hyperplasia (CCH)
      - □ Often associated with late onset when compared to MEN2B
    - Clinical disease: Palpable thyroid nodule &/or palpable lymphadenopathy
    - Subclinical disease: Identified only after clinical testing or early thyroidectomy performed on patient with pathogenic RET mutation
    - Diarrhea (most frequent systemic manifestation) occurs in affected individuals with plasma calcitonin concentration of > 10 ng/mL and implies poor prognosis
    - Rarely develop ectopic Cushing syndrome due to ACTH or CRH secretion

- Metastatic disease: Cervical lymph nodes, lungs, liver, and bone are most common sites
  - □ Up to 70% of such individuals already have cervical lymph node metastases when diagnosed
  - □ Usually occur years after onset of MTC
- All individuals with MTC-predisposing mutation who have not undergone prophylactic thyroidectomy demonstrate biochemical evidence of MTC by age 35
  - o **PCC** usually present after MTC or concomitantly; however, 1st symptom in 13-27% of individuals with PCCs and MEN2A
    - Adrenal involvement often diagnosed in patients aged 30-40 years
    - 40-60% of patients with MEN2 develop PCC with age-related and mutation-specific penetrance
    - Diagnosis of PCC warrants further investigation for MEN2A and other syndromes
      - □ Diagnosed at earlier age, subtler symptoms, and more likely to be bilateral than sporadic tumors
    - Malignant transformation occurs in ~ 4% of cases
    - Stroke and myocardial infarction with multiple microinfarcts can also occur
  - o **HPT** in MEN2A typically mild and may range from single adenoma to marked hyperplasia
    - Present in ~ 15-30% of patients with MEN2A
    - Affects adults (usually > 30 years) many years after diagnosis of MTC; average age of onset: 38 years
    - Most individuals with HPT have no symptoms; however, hypercalciuria and renal calculi may occur
    - If HPT longstanding and unrecognized, symptoms may become severe
  - o **Pruritic cutaneous lichen amyloidosis (CLA)** occurs in small number of families with MEN2A
    - Skin disorder associated with intense pruritus and secondary skin changes and dermal amyloid deposition that arises as consequence of repeated scratching
    - Typically located in interscapular region of back
    - Primarily associated with codon 634 mutations
  - o **Hirschsprung Disease (HSCR)**
    - Complete absence of neuronal ganglion cells (aganglionosis) in myenteric (Auerbach) and submucosal (Meissner) plexuses in variable lengths of gastrointestinal tract, primarily rectosigmoid colon
- **FMTC**
  - o By operational definition, MTC is only clinical manifestation of FMTC
  - o Age of onset of MTC later in FMTC, and penetrance of MTC lower than observed in MEN2A and MEN2B
  - o FMTC typically viewed as variant of MEN2A with decreased penetrance of PCC and HPT, rather than distinct subtype
    - Strict criteria should be met before family classified as having FMTC to avoid assumption of PCC risk
- **MEN2B**
  - o **MTC**: MEN2B is characterized by early development of aggressive form of MTC in all affected individuals
    - Individuals with MEN2B who do not undergo thyroidectomy at early age (< 1 year) are likely to develop metastatic MTC at early age

- Before intervention with early prophylactic thyroidectomy, average age of death in individuals with MEN2B 21 years
- Metastatic disease may already be present at time of diagnosis
- In patients with de novo MEN2B, MTC is usually diagnosed at more advanced stages, because there is often failure to recognize MEN2B phenotype in young patients
  - o **PCCs** occur in 50% of individuals with MEN2B; ~ 1/2 multiple and often bilateral
  - o **Parathyroid disease** is not related to MEN2B
  - o **Mucosal neuromas**: Individuals with MEN2B may be identified in infancy or early childhood
    - Mucosal neuromas on anterior dorsal surface of tongue, palate, or pharynx and distinctive facial appearance
    - Lips become prominent (or "blubbery") over time
    - Neuromas of eyelids may cause thickening and eversion of upper eyelid margins
    - Prominent thickened corneal nerves may be seen by slit lamp examination
  - o **Ganglioneuromatosis**: ~ 98-100% of MEN2B-affected individuals have neuroma and diffuse ganglioneuromatosis of GI tract
    - Associated symptoms include abdominal distension, megacolon, constipation, or diarrhea
    - Most individuals with MEN2B have gastrointestinal symptoms beginning in infancy or early childhood
  - o ~ 98-100% of affected individuals have **marfanoid habitus**, often with kyphoscoliosis or lordosis, joint laxity, and decreased subcutaneous fat

Laboratory Tests

- **MTC**: Calcitonin and CEA are excellent tumor markers
  - o Patients with clinical MTC show elevated calcitonin and CEA levels, but basal calcitonin levels can be normal with microscopic MTC
  - o In provocative testing, plasma calcitonin concentration is measured before (basal level) and 2 and 5 minutes after intravenous administration of calcium (stimulated level)
  - o Other calcitonin secretagogues also used, such as pentagastrin
  - o Reference levels for basal calcitonin vary across laboratories: < 10 pg/mL for adult men and < 5 pg/mL for adult women are typically considered normal
  - o Basal or stimulated calcitonin level of ≥ 100 pg/mL is indication for surgery
    - Caution should be used when interpreting calcitonin levels in children < 5 years
- **PCC** suspected when biochemical screening reveals elevated excretion of catecholamines and catecholamine metabolites
  - o At-risk individuals should undergo yearly screening via measurement of either plasma free metanephrines or urinary fractionated metanephrines
  - o In MEN2, PCCs consistently produce epinephrine or both epinephrine and norepinephrine
- Diagnosis of **parathyroid abnormalities** made when biochemical screening reveals simultaneously elevated serum concentrations of calcium and elevated or high-normal parathyroid hormone

Treatment

- **MTC**
  - Surgical removal of thyroid with regional lymph node dissection is standard
  - Small molecule kinase inhibitors of *RET* (vandetanib and cabozantinib) and other receptors now complementing classic surgical approaches
- **PCC**
  - When detected by biochemical testing and radionuclide imaging, removed by adrenalectomy
  - Strong probability that contralateral adrenal gland will develop tumor
    - Therefore, bilateral adrenalectomy indicated at time of demonstration of tumor within gland
- **Parathyroid lesions**
  - Parathyroid adenoma or hyperplasia diagnosed at time of thyroidectomy is treated with resection of visibly enlarged parathyroid glands, subtotal or total parathyroidectomy
- **Prevention of primary manifestations**
  - Prophylactic thyroidectomy
    - Primary preventive measure for individuals with identified germline *RET* mutation
    - Performed before age of 5 years for patients with MEN2A associated with high-risk (*RET* codon 634) mutations and before age of 1 year for patients with MEN2B
    - According to consensus statement from American Thyroid Association Guidelines Task Force, age at which prophylactic thyroidectomy is performed can be guided by codon position of *RET* mutation
  - Neck dissection
    - Central neck dissection
      - □ In early thyroidectomy, usually reserved for patients with basal calcitonin > 40 pg/mL, but recommended for cases with clinical suspicion of lymph node metastasis
      - □ Recommended for MTC because small lymph nodes may harbor metastatic tumor
    - Lateral neck lymph node compartments should be dissected only if radiologically or clinically suspicious for metastasis
  - Thyroidectomy for CCH, before progression to invasive MTC, may allow surgery to be limited to thyroidectomy with sparing of lymph nodes
  - Serum calcitonin screening
    - For children with MEN2B: Annual, beginning at age 6 months
    - For children with MEN2A or FMTC: Annual, beginning at age 3-5 years
    - Postoperative, if only precursor lesion found and no MTC: Every 3-6 months for 1st 2 years, then every 6 months until 5 years after surgery, and annually thereafter
- **Prevention of secondary manifestations**
  - Before any surgery, presence of functioning PCC should be excluded in any individual with MTC, MEN2A, or MEN2B
    - If PCC detected, adrenalectomy should be performed before thyroidectomy to avoid intraoperative catecholamine crisis and life-threatening hypertensive crisis

Prognosis

- 10-year survival rate
  - 75.5% for patients with MEN2B
  - 97.4% for patients with MEN2A
- **MTC**
  - Patients with hereditary MTC have better prognosis than patients with sporadic MTC
    - 10-year survival rates for patients with MTC of stages I, II, III, and IV, respectively, are 100%, 93%, 71%, and 21%
  - Worse survival rate directly related to
    - Older patient age at diagnosis
    - Larger tumor size
    - Lymph node disease
    - Distant metastases
  - Major preventive measure for MTC is prophylactic thyroidectomy
  - Calcitonin and CEA
    - Biochemical cure post surgery (i.e., undetectable basal calcitonin level) predicts 10-year survival rate of 97.7%
    - Short doubling times of calcitonin and CEA associated with more aggressive clinical course
    - MTC can rarely dedifferentiate and no longer produce calcitonin and CEA, which is harbinger of poor prognosis
- **PCC**
  - PCCs occurring as part of MEN2 almost always benign, with < 1-2% reported to be malignant
  - High risk of developing hypertensive crisis and stroke or myocardial infarction; must be treated before surgery
- **HPT**
  - MEN2A-related primary hyperparathyroidism generally mild; however, severe forms have been observed in rare cases

Genotype/Phenotype Correlations

- 1st clear genotype/phenotype associations to be found in inherited neoplasia syndromes: *RET* genotype-MEN2 phenotype correlations
- Most striking observation: Gain-of-function mutations affected several hotspot codons, with great majority mutating cysteine residues in exons 10 and 11
- Notably, mutations of codon 634 in exon 11 were highly associated with full-blown phenotype of MEN2A, i.e., with high prevalence of pheochromocytoma and hyperparathyroidism
  - Associated fulminant course with p.C634R, which is associated with higher probability of having metastases at diagnosis of MTC than other codon 634 mutations
  - Although 25% of FMTC kindreds harbor mutation in codon 634, most commonly p.C634Y, p.C634R mutations are virtually absent in this subtype
  - Codon 634 mutations also associated with development of CLA
- *RET* germline p.M918T mutations are associated with MEN2B

○ Somatic mutations at this codon frequently observed in MTC in individuals with no known family history of MTC
- Overrepresented in individuals with sporadic MTC who have particular germline *RET* variant, c.2439C>T
- Genotype/phenotype correlations suggest that exon 10 codon mutations, in particular at codons 609 and 611, have incidence of MTC in 77%, PCC in 17%, and HPT in 3%
- Mutations involving cysteine codons 609, 618, and 620 in exon 10 of *RET* associated with MEN2A or FMTC cosegregating with HSCR
- Mutations at codons 768, 804, and 891 associated with FMTC and in rare families with MEN2A
- Mutations in codons 790 or 804 may be associated with PTC as well as MTC
  ○ 40% of family members with p.V804M mutation had concomitant medullary and PTC
- American Thyroid Association Guidelines Task Force has classified mutations based on risk for aggressive MTC
  ○ May be used in predicting phenotype and recommendations for age at which to perform prophylactic thyroidectomy and to begin biochemical screening for PCC and hyperparathyroidism

Diagnostic Criteria

- MEN2A, FMTC, and MEN2B can all be diagnosed based on clinical features
- With advances of *RET* testing, genotype-specific risks, and management, molecular genetic testing is mandatory
  ○ Identify index patients (probands)
    - Most often used to distinguish sporadic from hereditary MTC
  ○ Facilitate timely diagnosis and therapy for at-risk relatives
- MEN2 should be highly suspected in any patient with
  ○ At least 2 tumors associated with MEN2
  ○ Diagnosis of MTC and ≥ 1 close relatives with MTC or another MEN2-defining tumor
  ○ Diagnosis of MTC with clinical features of MEN2B
- **MEN2A**
  ○ Diagnosed clinically by occurrence of ≥ 2 specific endocrine tumors (MTC, PCC, or parathyroid adenoma/hyperplasia) in single individual or in close relatives
- **FMTC**
  ○ Historically operationally diagnosed in families with ≥ 4 cases of MTC in absence of PCC or parathyroid adenoma/hyperplasia
  ○ Because *RET* mutation accounts for all clinical subtypes of MEN2, FMTC may be viewed as MEN2A with reduced organ-specific penetrance
- **MEN2B**
  ○ Diagnosed clinically by presence of mucosal neuromas of lips and tongue, as well as medullated corneal nerve fibers, distinctive facies with enlarged lips, asthenic marfanoid body habitus, and MTC

IMAGING

General Features

- Abdominal magnetic resonance (MR) imaging and computed tomography (CT) performed whenever PCC suspected clinically
  ○ MR more sensitive than CT in detection of PCC

- F-18 fluorodopamine positron emission tomography (PET) best overall imaging modality in localization of PCCs
- Postoperative parathyroid localizing studies with Tc-99m sestamibi scintigraphy may be helpful if HPT recurs
- For preoperative adenoma localization, 3D single-photon emission CT may also be used

MACROSCOPIC

MTC

- MTCs in MEN2 typically bilateral and multicentric
- Tumors well circumscribed but unencapsulated
- Smaller tumors located at junction of upper and middle 1/3 of thyroid lobes
- Larger tumors can occupy entire lobe

PCC

- Adrenal medullary hyperplasia-to-neoplasia progression sequence leading to bilateral and multifocal PCCs
- Associated with bilateral adrenal medullary hyperplasia, nodular and diffuse (gray to tan) in majority of patients with MEN2A and MEN2B
  ○ Normal medulla located in apex and corpus of adrenal gland and accounts for < 1/3 of gland's thickness
  ○ Adrenal medullary hyperplasia: When adrenal medulla exceeds 1/3 of gland's thickness in absence of cortical atrophy &/or when medulla noted in tail of gland
- Tumors tend to be bilateral and multicentric, gray, usually confined to adrenal medulla

Parathyroid Lesions

- All 4 glands enlarged with considerable variation in size of each gland
- Multiple enlarged cellular parathyroid glands
  ○ Individual gland measuring > 6-8 mm and weighing > 40-60 mg considered abnormal parathyroid gland

MICROSCOPIC

MTC and CCH

- Tumors from patients with heritable forms of MTC are virtually indistinguishable from those occurring sporadically, except for their bilaterality, multicentricity, and association with primary CCH
  ○ Primary CCH
    - Diagnosis suggested when > 6-8 C cells per cluster in several foci with > 50 C cells per low-power field are identified
    - Usually obvious on H&E-stained slides (counting often unnecessary)
    - Recognized on basis of expansile intrafollicular C-cell proliferation with varying degrees of dysplasia
  ○ Primary CCH in MEN2 and in some sporadic microcarcinomas constitutes thyroid intraepithelial neoplasia of C cells
- CCH-to-neoplasia progression is hallmark of inherited forms of MTC
  ○ In MEN2, age of transformation from CCH to MTC varies with different germline *RET* mutations

- o Earliest manifestation of invasive carcinoma characterized by extension of C cells through basement membrane of expanded C-cell-filled follicles into surrounding thyroid interstitium (confirmed on collagen IV stain)
- MTC diagnosed histologically when nests of C cells appear to extend beyond basement membrane and to infiltrate and destroy thyroid follicles
- MTC has variable histological appearance
  - o Morphology includes sheets, nests, trabeculae, or insular patterns
  - o Cells round, polygonal, or spindle-shaped
  - o ~ 80% show amyloid in stroma
- MTC and CCH suspected in presence of elevated plasma calcitonin concentration
  - o Specific and sensitive marker

PCC and Adrenomedullary Hyperplasia

- Mixed pattern of diffuse hyperplasia expanding into tail of gland
  - o May be intermingling of medullary and adrenocortical cells
  - o Cellular, architectural, and immunohistochemical features of hyperplastic lesions are similar to those of pheochromocytoma
- Classic pattern is small nests ("zellballen") of neuroendocrine cells with interspersed capillaries
- Sustentacular cells variably present
- PCCs vary in morphology and may have variety of growth patterns
  - o Most common are diffuse, large zellballen, cell cords, and cells may be round, oval, or spindled
  - o Extreme pleomorphism may be seen in benign tumors
- Hyaline globules usually present in PCCs of MEN2
- At molecular level, such lesions do not represent hyperplasia in MEN2 (microphaeochromocytoma)

Parathyroid Hyperplasia

- Intraparenchymal fat content reduced with great variation in this finding
- Predominant cell type chief cells arranged in cords and nests or in glandular or follicular pattern
- Corresponds to multiglandular adenomas in background of underlying genetic predisposition

ANCILLARY TESTS

Immunohistochemistry

- MTC: Calcitonin, calcitonin gene-related peptide (CGRP), chromogranin, and CEA
- PCC: Neuroendocrine markers; RET staining not helpful to distinguish MEN2-associated PCC from sporadic counterpart

Genetic Testing

- *RET* only gene known to be associated with MEN2
- *RET* molecular genetic testing indicated in all individuals with diagnosis of MTC, clinical diagnosis of MEN2, or primary CCH
- Algorithm for testing summarized in most recent American Thyroid Association MTC Practice Guidelines
  - o Young age of onset, significant CCH, &/or multifocal disease suggest inherited disorder

- o All individuals with MTC, regardless of other features or family history, and those with clinical features suspicious for MEN2 &/or with family history suspicious of MEN2 should be offered germline *RET* testing for exons 10, 11, and 13-16
- Knowledge of specific *RET* mutation present can help to predict patient age at onset of clinical disease, especially for MTC
  - o MEN2A: 98% of families have *RET* mutation in exon 10 or 11
  - o Most common mutation in MEN2A is in codon 634, followed by mutations in codons 609, 611, 618, 620, and 634, whereas M918T mutation is found in > 95% of patients with MEN2B
  - o De novo gene mutations occur rarely in patients with MEN2A, whereas de novo mutations account for vast majority (≥ 90%) of index cases of MEN2B
  - o Families with FMTC: *RET* mutation in ~ 95%
- Individuals with features suggestive of MEN2B: Mutation analysis or sequencing of exons 16 and 15 to detect p.M918T and p.A883F mutations
  - o If mutation negative, testing for p.V804M in exon 14 followed by sequencing of entire RET coding region should be performed
  - o Although isolated p.V804M mutation associated with FMTC, p.V804M co-occurring with 2nd *RET* variant seems to result in MEN2B
  - o This strategy will detect > 98% of mutations in individuals with MEN2B
- *RET* molecular genetic testing may be warranted in subsets of individuals presenting with apparently isolated adrenal pheochromocytoma
  - o Other differential diagnoses such as VHL and succinate dehydrogenase-associated pheochromocytoma should also be considered
  - o Testing algorithms for genes associated with paraganglioma and PCC have been proposed based on age of onset, location, laterality, malignancy, and family history
  - o Unexpected germline *RET* mutations are rarely (if ever) found in head and neck paraganglioma in absence of other features of MEN2 or family history of MEN2 phenotype
- Other clinical presentations may prompt consideration of genetic testing
  - o Exon 10 sequencing should be considered in individuals with HSCR
- Differential diagnosis in persons with intestinal ganglioneuromatosis should include MEN2B, and *RET* testing may be considered
- Rarely, germline *RET* mutation may not be detected in family with clinical diagnosis of MEN2A, MEN2B, or FMTC

Testing of Relatives at Risk

- At-risk relatives should be periodically screened for
  - o MTC with neck ultrasound examination, and basal &/or stimulated calcitonin measurements
  - o HPT with albumin-corrected calcium or ionized calcium
  - o PCC with measurement of plasma or 24-hour urine metanephrine and normetanephrine

- *RET* molecular genetic testing should be offered to probands with any MEN2 subtype and to all at-risk kindreds in which germline *RET* mutation has been identified in affected family member
- American Society of Clinical Oncologists identifies MEN2 as group 1 disorder, i.e., well-defined hereditary cancer syndrome for which genetic testing is considered part of standard management for at-risk family members
- *RET* molecular genetic testing should be performed as soon as possible after birth in all children known to be at risk for MEN2B
- In families with MEN2A or FMTC, molecular genetic testing should be offered to at-risk children by age 5 years, as MTC has been documented in childhood

DIFFERENTIAL DIAGNOSIS

Apparently Sporadic MTC

- Only 1 genetic differential diagnosis for MTC and that is MEN2
- Important for medical management of individual and his/her family to distinguish MTC + MEN2 from truly sporadic MTC
- Germline mutations in *RET* gene in individuals with simplex MTC: 6-9.5% (i.e., no known family history of MTC or personal history of other endocrine disease)

Physiological CCH

- Characterized by presence of ≥ 50 C cells per low-power field
- Unlike primary CCH, does not appear to be precursor of MTC
- C cells (identified by immunoperoxidase staining) identified beyond their normal geographical distribution or typically clustered in upper 2/3 of lateral lobes
- Observed in association with sporadic MTCs and other thyroid tumor types, Hashimoto thyroiditis, hypothyroidism, hypergastrinaemic and hypercalcemic states, and PTEN hamartoma tumor syndrome

Reactive CCH

- Not detected on H&E, unilateral, no cytological atypia

PCC

- Probability that PCC hereditary estimated to be 84% for multifocal (including bilateral) tumors and 59% for tumors with onset ≤ 18 years
- ~ 25% of individuals with PCC and no known family history of PCC may have inherited disease caused by mutation in 1 of following 4 genes
  - *RET*
    - ~ 5% of individuals with nonsyndromic PCC and no family history of PCC demonstrate *RET* mutation
    - Recent analysis of individuals with *RET* exon 10 mutations found that 25% of those with PCC were diagnosed at least 1 year before MTC
  - *VHL*
    - Any individual presenting with PCC should be evaluated for VHL disease
    - Germline *VHL* mutations was found in 11% of individuals with nonsyndromic PCC and no family history of PCC

- VHL disease characterized by PCC, renal cell carcinoma, cerebellar and spinal hemangioblastoma, and retinal angioma
- Some families with apparent autosomal dominant PCC have *VHL* gene mutations in absence of other clinical manifestations of VHL
  - *SDHx*
    - ~ 8.5% of individuals with apparently sporadic nonsyndromic PCC have mutation in 1 of the succinate dehydrogenase subunit genes *SDHD* or *SDHB*, or *SDHA*
    - *SDHC* germline mutations are rare in apparently sporadic PCC
    - These genes are associated with familial paragangliomas, a.k.a. extraadrenal pheochromocytomas or glomus tumors
    - When head and neck paraganglioma are associated with MEN2 or VHL, individuals almost always have other syndromic features or suggestive family history
  - *NF1*
    - Although *NF1* always included in genetic differential diagnosis of PCC, virtually all such presentations accompanied by clinical features of NF1
    - Similarly, PCC and paraganglioma considered rare components of MEN1
    - Personal or family history of MEN1 features should be evident
  - Metastatic medullary carcinoma
    - No single parameter predicts malignant behavior; malignancy is defined when metastasis occurs
    - PCCs can sometimes express calcitonin or calcitonin gene-related peptide
      - Positivity for tyrosine hydroxylase and negativity for cytokeratin and CEA can be used to distinguish PCC from metastatic medullary carcinoma

HPT

- Almost never initial presentation of MEN2, so formal differential diagnosis unnecessary
  - In contrast, HPT commonly (> 80%) initial manifestation of MEN1
- Role of surgical pathologist during intraoperative consultation for MEN2-related HPT is to identify tissue as parathyroid and to define an abnormal gland
- MEN2-related HPT associated with benign parathyroid proliferations; however, a few cases of parathyroid carcinoma have also been reported in this syndrome

Intestinal Ganglioneuromatosis

- Germline analysis for *RET* p.M918T and p.A883F mutations should be offered for infants and children presenting with intestinal ganglioneuromatosis
- Other than MEN2, only other genetic differential diagnoses to consider are Cowden syndrome and neurofibromatosis type 1
- Individuals with Cowden syndrome (*PTEN*-hamartoma tumor syndrome) more likely to exhibit ganglioneuromatous polyps than those with MEN2B or NF1

Genetically Related Disorder

- HSCR

o Complex genetic disorder characterized by aganglionosis of gut, likely due to absent gut ganglia from premature apoptosis of ganglia anlage

o Typically results in enlargement of bowel and constipation or even obstipation in neonates

o Because of seemingly similar clinical presentation, clinician should be careful differentiating diagnosis of HSCR from constipation/obstipation resulting from ganglioneuromatosis of MEN2B

o MEN2A and FMTC families segregate HSCR, seemingly unrelated neurocristopathy and developmental disorder

– Up to 50% of familial cases and up to 35% of simplex cases (i.e., single occurrence in family) of HSCR are caused by germline loss-of-function mutations in *RET* protooncogene

o Germline mutations causing HSCR occur throughout coding sequence of *RET*

o Subsets of families and individuals harboring germline *RET* mutations in exon 10, especially affecting codons 618 and 620, cosegregate MEN2A/FMTC and HSCR

- **PTC**

o ~ 20-40% of PTC associated with somatic gene rearrangements that cause juxtaposition of tyrosine kinase domain of *RET* to various gene partners (*RET/PTC*)

SELECTED REFERENCES

1. Accardo G et al: Genetics of medullary thyroid cancer: an overview. Int J Surg. 41 Suppl 1:S2-S6, 2017

2. Mathiesen JS et al: Distribution of RET mutations in multiple endocrine neoplasia 2 in Denmark 1994-2014: a nationwide study. Thyroid. 27(2):215-223, 2017

3. Mucha L et al: Phaeochromocytoma in multiple endocrine neoplasia type 2: RET codon-specific penetrance and changes in management during the last four decades. Clin Endocrinol (Oxf). 87(4):320-326, 2017

4. Reagh J et al: NRASQ61R Mutation-specific Immunohistochemistry also identifies the HRASQ61R mutation in medullary thyroid cancer and may have a role in triaging genetic testing for MEN2. Am J Surg Pathol. 41(1):75-81, 2017

5. Voss RK et al: Medullary thyroid carcinoma in MEN2A: ATA moderate or high-risk RET mutations do not predict disease aggressiveness J Clin Endocrinol Metab. 102(8):2807-2813, 2017

6. Essig GF Jr et al: Multifocality in sporadic medullary thyroid carcinoma: an international multicenter study. Thyroid. 26(11):1563-1572, 2016

7. Opsahl EM et al: A nationwide study of multiple endocrine neoplasia type 2A in Norway: predictive and prognostic factors for the clinical course of medullary thyroid carcinoma. Thyroid. 26(9):1225-38, 2016

8. Pacheco MC: Multiple endocrine neoplasia: a genetically diverse group of familial tumor syndromes. J Pediatr Genet. 5(2):89-97, 2016

9. Pappa T et al: Management of hereditary medullary thyroid carcinoma. Endocrine. 53(1):7-17, 2016

10. Frank-Raue K et al: Hereditary medullary thyroid cancer genotype-phenotype correlation. Recent Results Cancer Res. 204:139-56, 2015

11. Li Y et al: Endocrine neoplasms in familial syndromes of hyperparathyroidism. Endocr Relat Cancer. 23(6):R229-47, 2015

12. Romei C et al: 20 Years of lesson learning: how does the ret genetic screening test impact the clinical management of medullary thyroid cancer ? Clin Endocrinol (Oxf). 82(6):892-9, 2015

13. Coyle D et al: The association between Hirschsprung's disease and multiple endocrine neoplasia type 2a: a systematic review. Pediatr Surg Int. 30(8):751-6, 2014

14. Korpershoek E et al: Adrenal medullary hyperplasia is a precursor lesion for pheochromocytoma in MEN2 syndrome. Neoplasia. 16(10):868-73, 2014

15. Krampitz GW et al: RET gene mutations (genotype and phenotype) of multiple endocrine neoplasia type 2 and familial medullary thyroid carcinoma. Cancer. 120(13):1920-31, 2014

16. Posada-González M et al: Nonfunctional metastatic parathyroid carcinoma in the setting of multiple endocrine neoplasia type 2A syndrome. Surg Res Pract. 2014:731481, 2014

17. Yamazaki M et al: A newly identified missense mutation in RET codon 666 is associated with the development of medullary thyroid carcinoma [Rapid Communication]. Endocr J. 61(11):1141-4, 2014

18. Castro MR et al: Multiple endocrine neoplasia type 2A due to an exon 8 (G533C) mutation in a large North American kindred. Thyroid. 23(12):1547-52, 2013

19. Salehian B et al: RET gene abnormalities and thyroid disease: who should be screened and when. J Clin Res Pediatr Endocrinol. 5 Suppl 1:70-8, 2013

20. Laury AR et al: Thyroid pathology in PTEN-hamartoma tumor syndrome: characteristic findings of a distinct entity. Thyroid. 21(2):135-44, 2011

21. Nakao KT et al: Novel tandem germline RET proto-oncogene mutations in a patient with multiple endocrine neoplasia type 2B: report of a case and a literature review of tandem RET mutations with in silico analysis. Head Neck. 35(12):E363-8, 2013

22. Thosani S et al: The characterization of pheochromocytoma and its impact on overall survival in multiple endocrine neoplasia type 2. J Clin Endocrinol Metab. 98(11):E1813-9, 2013

23. Nosé V: Familial thyroid cancer: a review. Mod Pathol. 24 Suppl 2:S19-33, 2011

24. Raygada M et al: Hereditary paragangliomas. Adv Otorhinolaryngol. 70:99-106, 2011

25. Waguespack SG et al: Management of medullary thyroid carcinoma and MEN2 syndromes in childhood. Nat Rev Endocrinol. 7(10):596-607, 2011

26. Welander J et al: Genetics and clinical characteristics of hereditary pheochromocytomas and paragangliomas. Endocr Relat Cancer. Epub ahead of print, 2011

27. Zhang Y et al: Endocrine tumors as part of inherited tumor syndromes. Adv Anat Pathol. 18(3):206-18, 2011

28. Almeida MQ et al: Solid tumors associated with multiple endocrine neoplasias. Cancer Genet Cytogenet. 203(1):30-6, 2010

29. Grubbs EG et al: Do the recent American Thyroid Association (ATA) Guidelines accurately guide the timing of prophylactic thyroidectomy in MEN2A? Surgery. 148(6):1302-9; discussion 1309-10, 2010

30. Nosé V: Thyroid cancer of follicular cell origin in inherited tumor syndromes. Adv Anat Pathol. 17(6):428-36, 2010

31. Rubinstein WS: Endocrine cancer predisposition syndromes: hereditary paraganglioma, multiple endocrine neoplasia type 1, multiple endocrine neoplasia type 2, and hereditary thyroid cancer. Hematol Oncol Clin North Am. 24(5):907-37, 2010

32. American Thyroid Association Guidelines Task Force et al: Medullary thyroid cancer: management guidelines of the American Thyroid Association. Thyroid. 2009 Jun;19(6):565-612. Review. Erratum in: Thyroid. 19(11):1295, 2009

33. Boedeker CC et al: Head and neck paragangliomas in von Hippel-Lindau disease and multiple endocrine neoplasia type 2. J Clin Endocrinol Metab. 94(6):1938-44, 2009

34. Erlic Z et al: Familial pheochromocytoma. Hormones (Athens). 8(1):29-38, 2009

35. Hofer MD et al: Immunohistochemical and clinicopathological correlation of the metastasis-associated gene 1 (MTA1) expression in benign and malignant pancreatic endocrine tumors. Mod Pathol. 22(7):933-9, 2009

36. Margraf RL et al: Multiple endocrine neoplasia type 2 RET protooncogene database: repository of MEN2-associated RET sequence variation and reference for genotype/phenotype correlations. Hum Mutat. 30(4):548-56, 2009

37. Moore SW et al: Clinical and genetic differences in total colonic aganglionosis in Hirschsprung's disease. J Pediatr Surg. 44(10):1899-903, 2009

38. Pacak K et al: Diagnosis of pheochromocytoma with special emphasis on MEN2 syndrome. Hormones (Athens). 8(2):111-6, 2009

39. Waldmann J et al: Mutations and polymorphisms in the SDHB, SDHD, VHL, and RET genes in sporadic and familial pheochromocytomas. Endocrine. 35(3):347-55, 2009

40. Wu D et al: Observer variation in the application of the pheochromocytoma of the adrenal gland scaled score. Am J Surg Pathol. 33(4):599-608, 2009

41. Etit D et al: Histopathologic and clinical features of medullary microcarcinoma and C-cell hyperplasia in prophylactic thyroidectomies for medullary carcinoma: a study of 42 cases. Arch Pathol Lab Med. 132(11):1767-73, 2008

42. Frank-Raue K et al: Difference in development of medullary thyroid carcinoma among carriers of RET mutations in codons 790 and 791. Clin Endocrinol (Oxf). 69(2):259-63, 2008

43. Lodish MB et al: RET oncogene in MEN2, MEN2B, MTC and other forms of thyroid cancer. Expert Rev Anticancer Ther. 8(4):625-32, 2008

44. Machens A et al: Familial prevalence and age of RET germline mutations: implications for screening. Clin Endocrinol (Oxf). 69(1):81-7, 2008

45. Korpershoek E et al: Genetic analyses of apparently sporadic pheochromocytomas: the Rotterdam experience. Ann N Y Acad Sci. 1073:138-48, 2006

46. Gagel RF et al: The clinical outcome of prospective screening for multiple endocrine neoplasia type 2a. An 18-year experience. N Engl J Med. 318(8):478-84, 1988

Components of Multiple Endocrine Neoplasia Syndromes Type 2

Pathology	FMTC	MEN2A	MEN2B
Medullary thyroid carcinoma	> 90%	> 90%	> 90%
C-cell hyperplasia	100%	100%	100%
Pheochromocytoma	0%	30-50%	50%
Hyperparathyroidism	0%	15-30%	0%
Marfanoid habitus	0%	0%	98-100%
Mucosal neuromas	0%	0%	98-100%
Intestinal ganglioneuromatosis	0%	0%	60-90%
Thick corneal nerves	0%	Rare	60-90%
Cutaneous lichen amyloidosis	0%	10-15%	0%

FMTC = familial medullary thyroid carcinoma; MEN2A = multiple endocrine neoplasia type 2A; MEN2B = multiple endocrine neoplasia type 2B.

Differential Diagnosis of Micromedullary Thyroid Carcinoma

Characteristics	Sporadic	Familial
Multifocality	Rare (~ 10%)	Frequent (~ 90%)
Bilaterality	Rare (~ 10%)	Common (~ 70%)
Physiologic CCH	Common (~ 55%)	Rare (~ 10%)
Neoplastic CCH	Rare (~ 15%)	Frequent (90%)

RET Receptor Mutations Associated With MEN2 Phenotypes and Risk for Thyroidectomy

Codon/Mutations	MTC	+PCC	+PHPT	+CLA	+HSCR	MEN2B	ATA Risk[i]
Exon 10							
C609R/G/F/S/Y	✓	✓	✓		✓		M
C611R/G/F/S/W/Y	✓	✓	✓		✓		M
C618R/G/F/S/Y	✓	✓	✓				M
C620R/G/F/S/W/Y	✓	✓	✓				M
Exon 11							
C630R/F/S/Y C634R/G/F/S/W/Y	✓	✓	✓ ✓	✓			M
	✓						H
Exon 13							
E768D	✓	✓					M
L790F	✓						M
Exon 14							
V804L/M	✓	✓	✓	✓			M
Exon 15							
A883F	✓	✓	✓			✓	H
S891A	✓	✓					M
Exon 16							
M918T	✓	✓				✓	HST

Risk for thyroidectomy as defined by the American Thyroid Association (ATA) risk categories: Moderate (M), high (H), and highest (HST).
CLA = cutaneous lichen amyloidosis; HSCR = Hirschsprung disease; MTC = medullary thyroid carcinoma; PCC = pheochromocytoma; PHPT = primary hyperparathyroidism.
[i]Thyroidectomy is recommended before the age of 1 year for patients in the HST category (M918T) and before the age of 5 years for those in the H category; for patients in the M category, the timing of thyroidectomy is determined by calcitonin levels and parent/patient preference.

Modified from ATA: American Thyroid Association. Grubbs et al: WHO 2017.

47. Wolfe HJ et al: Familial medullary thyroid carcinoma and C cell hyperplasia. Clin Endocrinol Metab. 10(2):351-65, 1981

Ganglioneuromatosis

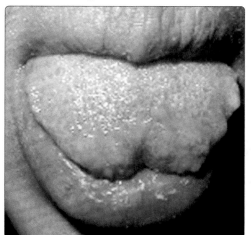

Ganglioneuromas

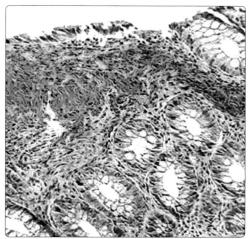

(Left) *Young patient with multiple endocrine neoplasia type 2B (MEN2B) displays marked thickening of the lips and tongue due to ganglioneuromatosis. This patient also had a MTC at a young age.* (Right) *S100 immunohistochemistry staining highlights ganglioneuromatosis of the intestine from a patient with MEN2.*

Cystic Pheochromocytoma

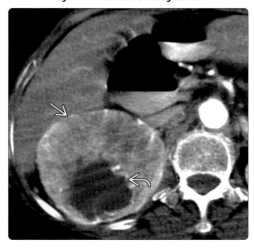

Adrenal Medullary Hyperplasia and Tumor

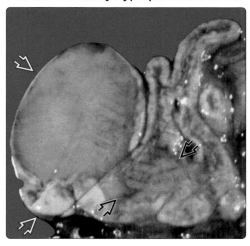

(Left) *Axial CECT shows a large, well-circumscribed, moderately enhancing right adrenal pheochromocytoma (PCC) ➡ with a hypodense area of cystic necrosis ➡.* (Right) *This adrenal gland shows both MEN2-associated PCC and adrenal medullary hyperplasia ➡, which is characteristic of MEN2. The cut surface is gray-pink, which distinguishes it from the yellow of adrenal cortex ➡ or adrenal cortical tumors.*

Hyaline Globules

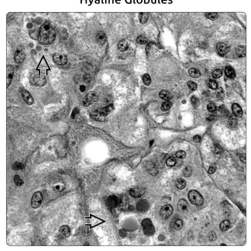

SDHB Maintained in MEN2

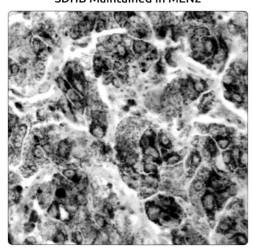

(Left) *Hyaline globules ➡ are present in some PCCs but also may be seen in some adrenal cortical neoplasms. They tend to be particularly conspicuous in PCCs from patients with MEN2.* (Right) *SDHB immunostaining reveals maintenance of immunoreactivity in a PCC associated with MEN2. SDHx mutations are seen in patients with hereditary PCC/paraganglioma syndromes.*

Normal C-Cell Distribution

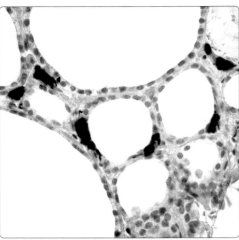

Prophylactic Thyroidectomy

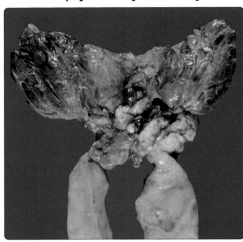

(Left) *Calcitonin stain highlights the normal C-cell distribution within the junction of the upper and middle 1/3 of the thyroid lobes. Normal C-cell population is characterized by < 50 calcitonin-positive cells/LPF.* (Right) *Total prophylactic thyroidectomy from a patient with family history of MEN2 and with mutation of the RET gene shows a grossly normal thyroid. However, on histological examination, CCH and a small medullary carcinoma were present.*

C-Cell Hyperplasia

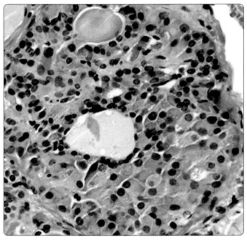

C-Cell Hyperplasia

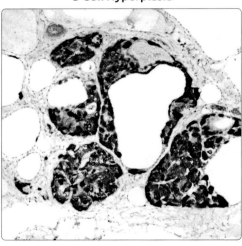

(Left) *Unlike sporadic MTC, MEN2 is frequently accompanied by CCH. C cells are usually highlighted by calcitonin stain; however, in many cases of MEN2, C cells are easily identified by H&E.* (Right) *Calcitonin stain highlights CCH, defined as nodular (> 6 cells forming nodules) or diffuse (> 50 calcitonin-positive cells/LPF) in a patient with MEN2A.*

Medullary Microcarcinoma

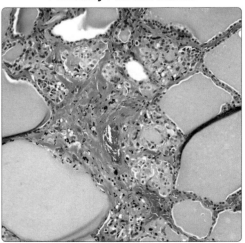

Medullary Thyroid Microcarcinoma

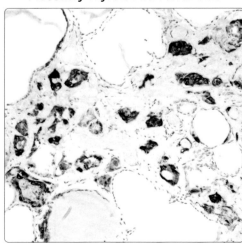

(Left) *Thyroid section from a patient with family history of MEN2 and mutation of the RET gene shows multiple medullary thyroid microcarcinoma. Note the infiltration by individual cells within the dense stromal fibrosis.* (Right) *Multiple medullary thyroid microcarcinomas are usually seen in thyroidectomy of MEN2 patients. This tumor is < 0.5 cm and has an infiltrative pattern showing desmoplasia and individual cells infiltrating the stroma.*

Thyroid Tumor and Metastases

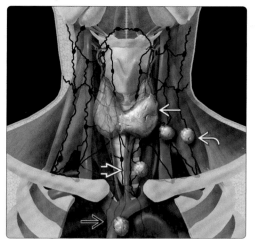

MTC Cytological Features

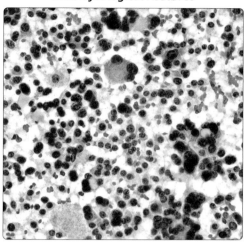

(Left) *Coronal graphic shows a left lobe thyroid carcinoma ➡ with multiple paratracheal ⇉, low jugular ⬈, and superior mediastinal ⇒ lymph node metastases. This presentation is usually seen in ~ 50% of patients with MTC in MEN2.* (Right) *FNA from MTC shows the characteristic cellular specimen with clusters of loosely cohesive cells and single cells in the background with salt and pepper quality of the nuclear chromatin. Many cells have a plasmacytoid appearance.*

TTF1 and Calcitonin Positivity

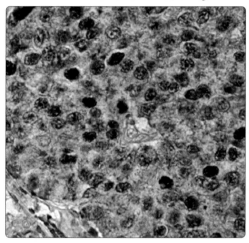

Cut Surface of Parathyroid

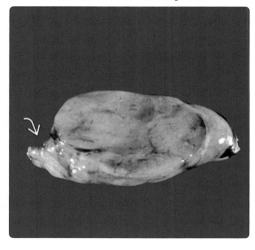

(Left) *Dual immunohistochemistry staining for TTF-1 and calcitonin in MTC shows variable immunopositivity for both TTF-1 (nuclear) and calcitonin (cytoplasmic) in the tumor cells. The endothelial cells are negative.* (Right) *This gross cut surface of an enlarged parathyroid shows a pink-yellow, slightly nodular surface with areas of hemorrhage. There is a small area of normal parathyroid ⬈, compressed by this micronodular adenomatosis.*

Parathyroid Micronodular Adenomatosis

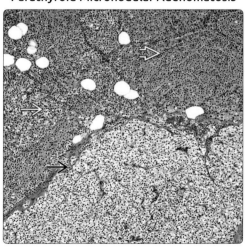

Oxyphilic Cells in Micronodular Adenomatosis

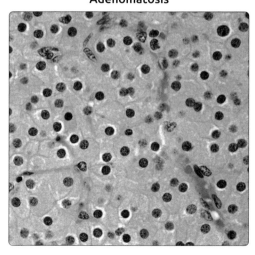

(Left) *Parathyroid has a nodular growth pattern in primary parathyroid hyperplasia with clear (water clear) cells ⇒, chief cells ➡, oxyphil cells ⇉, and a few scattered fat cells. The quantity of fat cells is highly variable both within a single gland and among glands.* (Right) *This enlarged parathyroid shows prominent parathyroid oxyphil cell composition. Oxyphil cells are not usually present in normal parathyroid in children; rather, they occur with increased age and can form small nodules in normal parathyroid in adults.*

DICER1 Syndrome

TERMINOLOGY

- Autosomal dominant pleiotropic tumor syndrome caused by germline *DICER1* mutations

ETIOLOGY/PATHOGENESIS

- DICER1 is multidomain protein with several known functions
- Mutations in *DICER1* expression &/or resultant protein activity initiate pathological processes
  - Germline mutations: Leading to premature truncation of protein, resulting in loss of RNAse III function
  - 2nd somatic missense mutations: Combination of neomorphic missense mutation within RNase IIIb domain and complete loss of function in other allele
  - Mosaicism for RNase IIIb domain hotspot mutations: More severe phenotypes

CLINICAL ISSUES

- Features number of highly characteristic tumor and tumor-like conditions that generally arise in childhood or young adulthood
- Some tumors are either so rare or so characteristic that any affected individual is likely to carry germline *DICER1* mutation
  - Pleuropulmonary blastoma
  - Cystic nephroma
  - Nasal chondromesenchymal hamartoma
  - Ciliary body medulloepithelioma
  - Pituitary blastoma
  - Embryonal rhabdomyosarcoma of cervix
  - Ovarian stromal tumors
  - Pineoblastoma
- Most often treatment involves surgical resection ± chemotherapy

Pineoblastoma

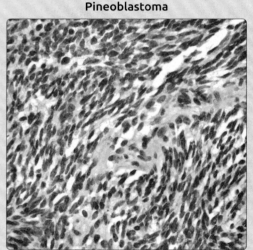

Intermediate SLCT

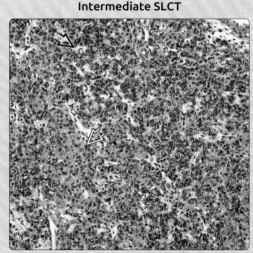

(Left) *Pineoblastoma is the most primitive of parenchymal tumors. These tumors are highly cellular and composed of patternless sheets of densely packed small cells with elongated nuclei and scant cytoplasm.* (Right) *This ovarian tumor is composed by cords of blue Sertoli cells ⊟ intermixed with Leydig cells. These cells are seen in clusters on bottom left ⊟ of this figure. DICER1-related Sertoli-Leydig cell tumors are typically intermediate to poorly differentiated. (Courtesy E. Oliva, MD.)*

Cystic Nephroma

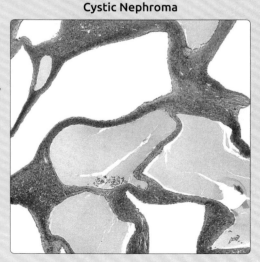

Pleuropulmonary Blastoma

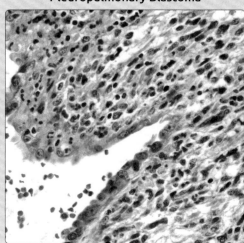

(Left) *Cystic nephromas are tumors that could occur in a patient with DICER1 syndrome. This low-power view of an epithelial and stromal tumor shows multiple, variably sized cysts.* (Right) *Pleuropulmonary blastoma (PPB) is multiloculated with interconnecting septa of variable thicknesses dividing the mass into multiple cysts. The septa are lined by predominantly flattened or cuboidal alveolar-type epithelium with nuclear pleomorphism.*

TERMINOLOGY

Synonyms

- Pleuropulmonary blastoma familial tumor and dysplasia syndrome

Definitions

- Autosomal dominant pleiotropic tumor syndrome caused by germline *DICER1* mutations
  - Tumors and dysplasias with onset in childhood, adolescence, or early adulthood
- Include pleuropulmonary blastoma (PPB), cystic nephroma, and endocrine-related lesions such as multinodular goiter, ovarian Sertoli-Leydig cell tumor (SLCT), gynandroblastoma, juvenile granulosa cell tumor, and pituitary blastoma (associated with infantile-onset Cushing disease)

ETIOLOGY/PATHOGENESIS

Genetics: *DICER1*

- Chromosomal location: 14q32.13
- DICER1 is multidomain protein
  - Encodes protein of 1922 amino acids
  - Comprises several structurally distinct domains (from N-terminus to C-terminus)
    - DExD/Hbox helicase
    - Transactivation response RNA-binding protein-binding
    - Helicase conserved C-terminal
    - DUF283 (unknown function)
    - Platform and PAZ
    - Connector helix
    - RNase IIIa and IIIb
    - Double-stranded RNA-binding
- *DICER1* has several known functions
  - Maturation of microRNAs from precursor molecules
    - Acts as molecular ruler, measuring and then cutting hairpin precursors into mature 5p and 3p forms
  - Chromatin structure remodeling
  - Inflammation and apoptotic DNA degradation
- Mutations may alter *DICER1* expression &/or resultant protein activity and consequently initiate pathological processes
- *DICER1* mutations
  - Germline mutations
    - Typically result in protein truncation and likely affect global processing
    - In majority of cases, germ-line mutations are nonsense, frameshift or splice-site mutations leading to premature truncation of protein, resulting in loss of RNAse III function
  - 2nd somatic missense mutations
    - Occur in most tumors studied to date
    - Occur in metal ion-binding RNase IIIa and IIIb domains, result in reduced 3p and 5p microRNAs, respectively
    - Commonly result of combination of neomorphic missense mutation at 1 of 5 specific "hotspot" codons within RNase IIIb domain and complete loss of function (LOF) in other allele
  - Mosaicism for RNase IIIb domain hotspot mutations
    - Rare individuals carry germline or mosaic mutations of critical metal ion-binding domains

- More severe phenotypes in terms of both patient age at onset and number of organs involved
- Likely that these RNase III mutations have oncogenic properties
  - ~ 10% of predisposing *DICER1* mutations are mosaic rather than germline
- Pathomechanism of Dicer-mutation-mediated diseases still poorly understood
- No clear correlation among *DICER1* expression, cancer type, and disease progression
  - Significant changes in *DICER1* expression have been detected during different stages of lung adenocarcinoma
    - Early stages: Transient upregulation in expression
    - More advanced stages: Downregulation in expression
  - Controversial whether *DICER1* acts as tumor suppressor or oncogene
    - Reduced expression may be associated with poor prognosis in some types of lung cancers
    - Increased expression associated to prostate adenocarcinoma cancer and Burkitt lymphoma

CLINICAL ISSUES

Epidemiology

- Incidence
  - Rare (~ 9:100,000 live births)
- Age
  - Childhood or young adulthood
    - PPBs: Nearly all present by age of 6 years
    - Cystic nephroma: > 90% of cases occur by age of 4 years
    - Ovarian sex cord-stromal tumors: 2-45 years, but most occur in patients aged 10-25 years
    - Pituitary blastoma (very rare): Occurs by age of 24 months
- Prevalence
  - Must be substantially higher
    - Many carriers go unidentified and most associated conditions are nonlethal

Presentation

- Features number of highly characteristic tumor and tumor-like conditions that generally arise in childhood or young adulthood
- Some tumors either so rare or so characteristic that any affected individual is likely to carry germline *DICER1* mutation
- **Pleuropulmonary blastoma**
  - Most common neoplasm in DICER1 syndrome
  - Clinical presentation of PPB varies by age and tumor type
    - Children < 2 years: Shortness of breath ± pneumothorax secondary to PPB cyst rupture
    - Older children: Advanced disease often present with shortness of breath, weight loss, and fever
  - Classically 3 types of PPB based on gross pathology, highly correlated with age at diagnosis and outcome, thought to represent natural history of disease
    - Type I PPB: Purely cystic
      - □ Present in youngest age group (median 9 months)
      - □ Has best prognosis

- – Type II PPB: Cystic and solid
  - □ Typically occur in children between ages of 18 months and 6 years (median: 36 months)
  - □ Retains grossly visible cystic component, also presents solid components
- – Type III PPB: Purely solid
  - □ Typically occur in children between ages of 18 months and 6 years (median: 43 months)
- **Cystic nephroma**
  - ○ 2nd most common neoplasm in DICER1 syndrome
  - ○ Most commonly presents in first 4 years of life as painless, enlarging abdominal or flank mass
  - ○ Finding of bilateral tumors rare event highly suggestive of germline *DICER1* pathogenic variant
- **Nasal chondromesenchymal hamartoma**
  - ○ Presents in nasal cavity or sinuses, commonly as unilateral polyp or mass, or rarely as bilateral
  - ○ Symptoms vary depending on size and location
    - – Persistent nasal drainage/rhinorrhea, nasal obstruction/swelling and respiratory or feeding difficulties
    - – Bony destruction can be seen
- **Ciliary body medulloepithelioma**
  - ○ Primitive neuroepithelial neoplasm, arises in anterior chamber of eye
  - ○ Present around 7 years of age with decreased visual acuity and pain
  - ○ Although viewed as malignant neoplasms, distant metastases are rare
- **Pituitary blastoma**
  - ○ Rare primitive malignant neoplasm of pituitary gland presenting in first 2 years of life
  - ○ Can present with ophthalmoplegia, proptosis, visual disturbance, &/or clinical endocrinopathy, typically Cushing disease
  - ○ Appears to be pathognomonic of *DICER1* mutation
- **Embryonal rhabdomyosarcoma of cervix**
  - ○ Older children and young adults
  - ○ Can present with vaginal spotting or passage of myxoid, hemorrhagic solid tissue
- **Ovarian stromal tumors**
  - ○ SLCT, juvenile granulosa cell tumor, and gynandroblastoma
  - ○ Seen in children and young adults
  - ○ Very highly suggestive of germline mutation
  - ○ Typically unilateral but can occur bilaterally, often large (≥ 10 cm) and predominantly solid
  - ○ May present as isolated adnexal mass ± clinical signs or laboratory findings of hormone production
  - ○ Signs of hormone production can include precocious puberty, menstrual irregularities, or signs of virilization such as hirsutism, acne, or voice changes
- **Pineoblastoma**
  - ○ Moderately suggestive of mutation
  - ○ Malignant primitive neuroectodermal tumor in region of pineal gland
  - ○ Typically presents with findings of increased intracranial pressure stemming from obstructive hydrocephalus due to compression of cerebral aqueduct by tumor mass
  - ○ Neuroophthalmologic abnormalities including upgaze paralysis and nystagmus may be seen

- ○ Focal neurologic deficits found in 25% of affected individuals
- **Most important endocrine manifestations**
  - ○ Nodular thyroid hyperplasia
    - – Can result in multinodular goiter
  - ○ More rarely differentiated thyroid carcinoma
  - ○ Ovarian sex cord-stromal tumors
    - – SLCT in particular
- **Other tumors reported**
  - ○ Anaplastic sarcoma of kidney
  - ○ Gynandroblastoma
  - ○ Primitive neuroectodermal tumors at other sites
  - ○ Cerebral sarcoma
  - ○ More common pediatric tumors, such as Wilms tumor
  - ○ Seminoma
  - ○ Rare forms of T-cell Hodgkin lymphoma
- Co-occurrence of ovarian SLCT with thyroid carcinoma highly suggestive of DICER1 syndrome
- Macrocephaly reported as common finding in DICER1 syndrome

Treatment

- Identification of tumor type and stage
- Most often treatment involves surgical resection ± chemotherapy
- Treatment of PPB may also include use of radiation to treat recurrence or metastases

Prognosis

- Favorable outcome
  - ○ Ovarian sex cord-stromal tumor, cystic nephroma, embryonal rhabdomyosarcoma of cervix, multinodular goiter, differentiated thyroid carcinoma, nasal chondromesenchymal hamartoma, or ciliary body medulloepithelioma
- Low survival rates (50%)
  - ○ PPB type II and III, pituitary blastoma, and anaplastic sarcoma of kidney
- Screening *DICER1* mutation carriers for cystic PPB at young age may permit early detection of PPB type I
  - ○ Subsequent surgical resection may prevent progression to types II and III with their higher morbidity and mortality

MACROSCOPIC

General Features

- **Pleuropulmonary blastoma**
  - ○ Type I PPB: Purely cystic
    - – Cysts can be unilocular, but more often multilocular, and located in periphery of lung
  - ○ Type II PPB: Cystic and solid
    - – Tumor cells within cyst wall have proliferated, creating grossly visible thickening of septa or formation of solid mass
  - ○ Type III PPB: Purely solid

MICROSCOPIC

Histologic Features

- **Pleuropulmonary blastoma**
  - ○ Type I PPB: Purely cystic

- Multilocular, thin-walled cyst lined by epithelium
- Cyst septa contain variably present primitive mesenchymal tumor cells beneath epithelium
  ○ Type II PPB: Cystic and solid
  ○ Type III PPB: Purely solid
    - Solid components best characterized as high-grade, multipatterned sarcoma that includes ≥ 2 of following patterns
      □ Embryonal rhabdomyosarcomatous pattern with ovoid, stellate, and spindled cells arranged in myxoid, pale blue background
      □ Blastemal pattern with cohesive clusters of primitive rounded cells with minimal cytoplasm
      □ Cartilaginous differentiation with fetal type or high-grade malignant cartilage nodules
      □ Spindle cell sarcoma
- **Cystic nephroma**
  ○ Cysts can sometimes be simpler in architecture compared with type I PPB and can resemble dilated tubules with plump, hobnail epithelium
  ○ In well-developed cystic tumors, delicate septa divide lesion into variably sized locules much like type I PPB
  ○ Cyst septa typically contain bland mesenchymal cells in pale, myxoid matrix with variable amount of inflammatory cells
- **Nasal chondromesenchymal hamartoma**
  ○ Composed of epithelial cysts lined by respiratory epithelium and nodules of immature or mature cartilage surrounded by spindle cell mesenchyme
  ○ Rest of polyp contains mucoid ground substance containing inflammatory cells, small vessels, and fibrosis
    - Occasional cases without cartilage nodules have been seen in individuals with *DICER1* mutations
- **Ovarian stromal tumors**
  ○ May be cystic and solid or solid and often contain heterologous epithelial glandular elements
  ○ Sertoli-cell component staining with inhibin staining invariably present in primary tumors
  ○ Tumors may also contain sarcomatous components
- **Embryonal rhabdomyosarcoma**
  ○ Subepithelial layer of primitive cells beneath intact epithelium (cambium layer), very similar to type I PPB
  ○ Deeper in polyp, stroma cells better differentiated, often showing tails of eosinophilic cytoplasm with striations
  ○ Background pale and mucoid and contains variable number of inflammatory cells
  ○ Cartilaginous nodules present in 35-40% of cervical ERMS
  ○ These polyps can be deceptively bland and confused with nonneoplastic polypoid lesions
- **Ciliary body medulloepithelioma**
  ○ Neuroblastic or embryonic-like neural tubules and Homer Wright rosettes accompanied by hyaluronic acid-rich stroma expanding region of ciliary body
  ○ Teratoid variant may have cartilage or immature skeletal muscle
- **Pineoblastoma**
  ○ Tumor cells are primitive with high nuclear:cytoplasmic ratio and hyperchromatic nuclei
  ○ Homer Wright and Flexner-Winsteiner type rosettes may be seen

- **Pituitary blastoma**
  ○ Combination of Rathke type epithelial rosettes/glands intermixed with small primitive appearing cells with blastemal features and larger secretory cells

ANCILLARY TESTS

Immunohistochemistry

- **Pleuropulmonary blastoma**
  ○ Typically shows diffuse vimentin positivity
  ○ Desmin positive in rhabdomyosarcomatous and blastemal elements
  ○ Myogenin and MyoD1 positive in proportion of tumor cells analogous to ERMS
  ○ Epithelial markers typically absent
- **Ovarian stromal tumors**
  ○ Positivity of hormonal markers such as inhibin A &/or B or estradiol (generally produced by granulosa cell elements) or testosterone (generally produced by Sertoli-Leydig cell elements)
- **Pituitary blastoma**
  ○ Synaptophysin and chromogranin immunoreactive
  ○ ACTH secreting
  ○ Some cases also include GH secreting subset

DIFFERENTIAL DIAGNOSIS

Cowden Disease and Bannayan-Ruvalcaba-Riley Syndrome (*PTEN*-Hamartoma Tumor Syndrome)

- Share clinical characteristics, such as mucocutaneous lesions, hamartomatous polyps of gastrointestinal tract, and increased risk of developing neoplasms
- Both conditions caused by mutations in *PTEN* gene
  ○ *PTEN* located on 10q23.31 and encodes phosphatidylinositol-3,4,5-triphosphate 3-phosphatase
  ○ Tumor suppressor gene that has been found mutated in number of tumors
- Thyroid usually affected by numerous adenomatous nodules, follicular adenomas, and follicular carcinoma
- Findings similar to those familial syndromes characterized by predominance of nonthyroidal tumors
  ○ PTEN-hamartoma tumor syndrome, Carney complex, Werner syndrome, and Pendred syndrome

Carney Complex

- Autosomal dominant syndrome
  ○ Caused by PRKA-R1A mutations
- Multiple neoplasia syndrome featuring endocrine overactivity, involving diverse endocrine organs as adrenal cortex, pituitary, thyroid, ovary and testes
- Presents spotty skin pigmentation, schwannomas, myxomatosis, neural tumors, and rarely tumors in liver and pancreas

Congenital Cystic Adenomatoid Malformation

- Type I PPB cannot be distinguished radiographically from benign congenital cystic lung malformations
  ○ Pneumothoraces and presence of multifocal or bilateral cysts more common in PPB than in other conditions
  ○ Difficulties in distinguishing from PPB have led some pediatric surgeons to advocate excision of all congenital cystic adenomatoid malformations

Lung Cysts and Pneumothoraces

- Multiple inherited and noninherited disorders can present with lung cysts &/or pneumothorax
- Many of these can be distinguished from PPB on basis of medical history and physical examination

Wilms Tumor (Nephroblastoma)

- Most common renal tumor of childhood
- Usually presents as abdominal mass in otherwise apparently healthy child
- Most commonly reported germline variants include WT1 and 11p15.5 locus
- Abdominal pain, fever, anemia, hematuria, and hypertension seen in 25-30% of affected children

Mixed Epithelial and Stromal Tumor (Adult CN)

- Cysts resemble those in *DICER1*-related CN but often contain cellular stroma resembling ovarian stroma
- Presents most commonly in adults

SELECTED REFERENCES

1. Bueno MT et al: Pediatric imaging in DICER1 syndrome. Pediatr Radiol. ePub, 2017
2. Cai S et al: Multimorbidity and genetic characteristics of DICER1 syndrome based on systematic review. J Pediatr Hematol Oncol. 39(5):355-361, 2017
3. Fernández-Martínez L et al: Identification of somatic and germ-line DICER1 mutations in pleuropulmonary blastoma, cystic nephroma and rhabdomyosarcoma tumors within a DICER1 syndrome pedigree. BMC Cancer. 17(1):146, 2017
4. Khan NE et al: Macrocephaly associated with the DICER1 syndrome. Genet Med. 19(2):244-248, 2017
5. Khan NE et al: Quantification of thyroid cancer and multinodular goiter risk in the DICER1 syndrome: A family-based cohort study. J Clin Endocrinol Metab. 102(5):1614-1622, 2017
6. de Kock L et al: High-sensitivity sequencing reveals multi-organ somatic mosaicism causing DICER1 syndrome. J Med Genet. 53(1):43-52, 2016
7. Durieux E et al: The co-occurrence of an ovarian Sertoli-Leydig cell tumor with a thyroid carcinoma is highly suggestive of a DICER1 syndrome. Virchows Arch. 468(5):631-6, 2016
8. Kuhlen M et al: Hodgkin lymphoma as a novel presentation of familial DICER1 syndrome. Eur J Pediatr. 175(4):593-7, 2016
9. Stewart CJ et al: Gynecologic manifestations of the DICER1 syndrome. Surg Pathol Clin. 9(2):227-41, 2016
10. Brenneman M et al: Temporal order of RNase IIIb and loss-of-function mutations during development determines phenotype in DICER1 syndrome: a unique variant of the two-hit tumor suppression model. F1000Res. 4:214, 2015
11. de Sousa GR et al: Low DICER1 expression is associated with poor clinical outcome in adrenocortical carcinoma. Oncotarget. 6(26):22724-33, 2015
12. Kurzynska-Kokorniak A et al: The many faces of Dicer: the complexity of the mechanisms regulating Dicer gene expression and enzyme activities. Nucleic Acids Res. 43(9):4365-80, 2015
13. Messinger YH et al: Pleuropulmonary blastoma: a report on 350 central pathology-confirmed pleuropulmonary blastoma cases by the International Pleuropulmonary Blastoma Registry. Cancer. 121(2):276-85, 2015
14. de Kock L et al: Pituitary blastoma: a pathognomonic feature of germ-line DICER1 mutations. Acta Neuropathol. 128(1):111-22, 2014
15. Foulkes WD et al: DICER1: mutations, microRNAs and mechanisms. Nat Rev Cancer. 14(10):662-72, 2014
16. Klein S et al: Expanding the phenotype of mutations in DICER1: mosaic missense mutations in the RNase IIIb domain of DICER1 cause GLOW syndrome. J Med Genet. 51(5):294-302, 2014
17. Pugh TJ et al: Exome sequencing of pleuropulmonary blastoma reveals frequent biallelic loss of TP53 and two hits in DICER1 resulting in retention of 5p-derived miRNA hairpin loop sequences. Oncogene. 33(45):5295-302, 2014
18. Rath SR et al: Multinodular goiter in children: an important pointer to a germline DICER1 mutation. J Clin Endocrinol Metab. 99(6):1947-8, 2014
19. Schultz KA et al: Judicious DICER1 testing and surveillance imaging facilitates early diagnosis and cure of pleuropulmonary blastoma. Pediatr Blood Cancer. 61(9):1695-7, 2014
20. Schultz KA et al: DICER1-pleuropulmonary blastoma familial tumor predisposition syndrome: a unique constellation of neoplastic conditions. Pathol Case Rev. 19(2):90-100, 2014
21. Stewart DR et al: Nasal chondromesenchymal hamartomas arise secondary to germline and somatic mutations of DICER1 in the pleuropulmonary blastoma tumor predisposition disorder. Hum Genet. 133(11):1443-50, 2014
22. Schultze-Florey RE et al: DICER1 syndrome: a new cancer syndrome. Klin Padiatr. 225(3):177-8, 2013
23. Heravi-Moussavi A et al: Recurrent somatic DICER1 mutations in nonepithelial ovarian cancers. N Engl J Med. 366(3):234-42, 2012
24. Foulkes WD et al: Extending the phenotypes associated with DICER1 mutations. Hum Mutat. 32(12):1381-4, 2011
25. Rio Frio T et al: DICER1 mutations in familial multinodular goiter with and without ovarian Sertoli-Leydig cell tumors. JAMA. 305(1):68-77, 2011
26. Slade I et al: DICER1 syndrome: clarifying the diagnosis, clinical features and management implications of a pleiotropic tumour predisposition syndrome. J Med Genet. 48(4):273-8, 2011
27. Hill DA et al: DICER1 mutations in familial pleuropulmonary blastoma. Science. 325(5943):965, 2009
28. Chiosea S et al: Overexpression of Dicer in precursor lesions of lung adenocarcinoma. Cancer Res. 67(5):2345-50, 2007
29. Bernstein E et al: Role for a bidentate ribonuclease in the initiation step of RNA interference. Nature. 409(6818):363-6, 2001
30. Priest JR et al: Pleuropulmonary blastoma: a marker for familial disease. J Pediatr. 128(2):220-4, 1996
31. Doros L et al: DICER1-Related Disorders 1993

Pleuropulmonary Blastoma

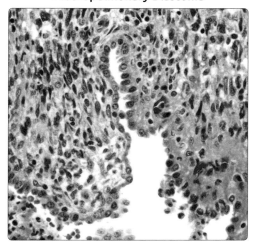

Pleuropulmonary Blastoma

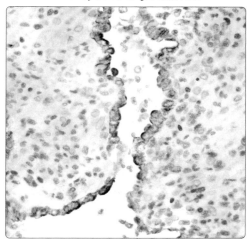

(Left) *Microscopically, the majority of PPBs are characterized as multilocular cysts containing primitive small mesenchymal cells within the cyst walls. Three pathologic types or stages in the evolution of PPB have been defined: Type I or purely cystic PPB, type II or cystic/solid PPB, and type III or purely solid PPB.* (Right) *The cystic spaces in type II PPB are lined by keratin-positive cells, whereas the solid component are negative. The solid areas consist of a collage of primitive sarcomatous patterns.*

Pleuropulmonary Blastoma

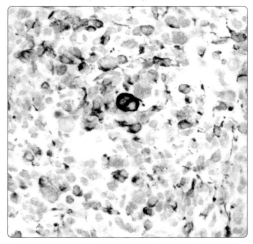

Cyst Lining Cells

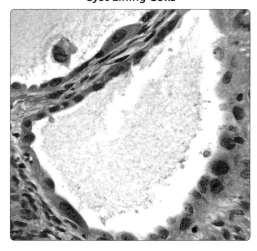

(Left) *The tumor cells in PPB usually show patchy immunopositivity for desmin. Definitive skeletal muscle differentiation characterized by cells with long tails of eosinophilic cytoplasm ± cross-striations may be identified. Myogenin and MyoD1 stains may show scattered positive cells.* (Right) *Cystic nephroma shows large epithelial cells with large, irregular nuclei with nucleoli. The cytoplasm is ample and eosinophilic.*

Patternless Pineoblastoma

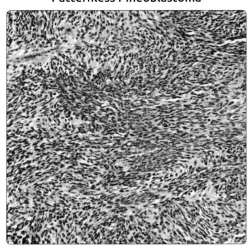

Synaptophysin in Pineoblastoma

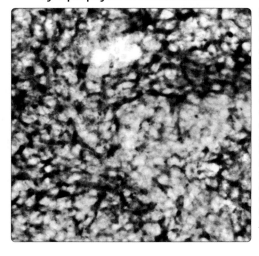

(Left) *Pineoblastomas are highly cellular with undifferentiated small cell histology and composed of patternless sheets of densely packed small cells and scant cytoplasm with high nuclear:cytoplasmic ratio. The cell borders are indistinct. The diffuse growth pattern is only interrupted by rare rosettes.* (Right) *The tumor cells in pineoblastoma show strong immunopositivity for synaptophysin. The tumor cells are also positive for NSE and chromogranin A but negative for GFAP and neurofilaments.*

KEY FACTS

TERMINOLOGY

- Autosomal dominant disease caused by germline mutations of *CDKN1B*
  - Resulting in phenotype similar to that of MEN1
  - Characterized by neuroendocrine neoplasms, particularly in parathyroid glands, pituitary, and pancreas

ETIOLOGY/PATHOGENESIS

- *CDKN1B* gene encodes p27
- p27: Cyclin-dependent kinase inhibitor whose main function is to control progression from G1 phase to S phase

CLINICAL ISSUES

- Wide variety of tumors have been reported in MEN4
- Most common neuroendocrine neoplasms
  - Parathyroid
    - Primary hyperparathyroidism seems to have fairly higher penetrance in MEN4 (75%) than in MEN1
    - Appears to occur later than in MEN1; average reported patient age: 56 years (vs. 20-25 years in MEN1)
  - Pituitary
    - Pituitary adenomas (37.5%): Corticotropinomas, somatotropinomas, and nonfunctioning PAs
- Patients presenting phenotype suggestive of MEN1 but with no MEN1 mutations should be tested for *CDKN1B* mutations
- No specific guidelines for diagnosis
- *CDKN1B*-associated tumors have no distinctive features from tumors with other genetic backgrounds
- Patients presenting phenotype suggestive of MEN1 but with no MEN1 mutations should be tested for *CDKN1B* mutations

Enlarged Parathyroid Gland

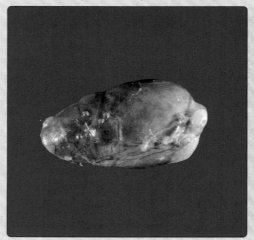

Pancreatic Neuroendocrine Tumor

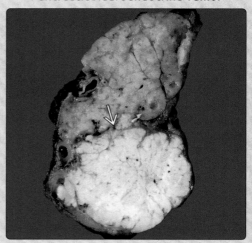

(Left) *Multiglandular parathyroid disease is a characteristic finding in patients with MEN4, as seen on this gross photo of an enlarged gland. These lesions are monoclonal proliferations of parathyroid cells, consisting of multiple microadenomas.* (Right) *Patients with MEN4 may have diffuse microadenomas associated with one or more macroadenomas. This gross cut surface of the pancreas shows the typical pancreatic neuroendocrine tumor, characterized by firm, pale-tan surface* ➡.

Pituitary Adenoma

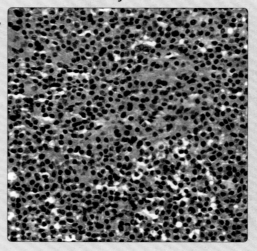

Glucagon-Producing Pancreatic NET

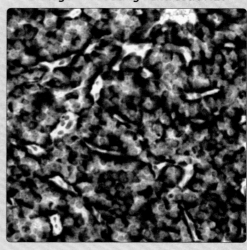

(Left) *MEN4-associated pituitary adenomas are usually functioning adenomas, and, as in MEN1 patients, they may be multiple and most frequently producing prolactin and growth hormone.* (Right) *As with MEN1 patients, MEN4 patients may have multiple pancreatic microadenomas and adenomas, as illustrated here. Glucagon-producing adenomas usually have a trabecular arrangement.*

TERMINOLOGY

Abbreviations

- Multiple endocrine neoplasia type 4 (MEN4)

Synonyms

- MEN1-like syndrome

Definitions

- Autosomal dominant disease, caused by germline mutations of *CDKN1B*, resulting in phenotype similar to that of MEN1
  - Characterized by neuroendocrine neoplasms, particularly in parathyroid glands, pituitary, and pancreas

ETIOLOGY/PATHOGENESIS

Etiology

- Caused by mutations in *CDKN1B* gene at 12p13

Pathogenesis

- *CDKN1B* gene encodes p27
  - p27: Cyclin-dependent kinase inhibitor whose main function is to control progression from G1 phase to S phase

CLINICAL ISSUES

Epidemiology

- Incidence
  - Extremely low
    - ~ 1.5-3.7% of MEN1 phenotype
- Age
  - Primary hyperparathyroidism (most frequent manifestation in patients with MEN4) appears to occur later than in MEN1
    - Average reported patient age: 56 years (vs. 20-25 years in MEN1)
- Penetrance
  - Has not been reliably calculated (limited data suggesting incomplete penetrance of CDKN1B mutations)

Presentation

- Clinical and histological manifestations seem to be more variable than in MEN1
  - Small number of patients so far reported; comprehensive phenotype has not been yet established
- Wide variety of tumors have been reported in MEN4
- Most common neuroendocrine neoplasms
  - Parathyroid
    - Primary hyperparathyroidism seems to have fairly higher penetrance in MEN4 (75%) than in MEN1
    - Appears to occur later than in MEN1
  - Pituitary
    - Pituitary adenomas (37.5%): Corticotropinomas, somatotropinomas, and nonfunctioning PAs
      - Growth hormone-secreting adenoma: Features of acromegaly
      - Adrenocorticotropic hormone-secreting tumors: Cushing disease
      - Lactotroph adenoma (suspected): High prolactin blood levels
      - Nonfunctioning adenoma
  - Pancreas
- Other sites
  - Cervix
  - Bronchus
  - Stomach
  - Thyroid
  - Breast
  - Duodenum

Treatment

- Hyperparathyroidism
  - Total parathyroidectomy with autotransplantation or subtotal resection of 3.5 parathyroid glands
- Pituitary adenoma
  - Surgery
- Other sites tumors
  - Surgery

Prognosis

- Depends on tumors with which they present or later develop
  - Currently not possible to predict which tumors patients with *CDKN1B* mutations will develop
- Poor prognostic factors
  - Functioning hormonal syndromes
  - Local or distant tumor spread
  - Aggressive &/or large tumors
  - Need for multiple surgical resections

Diagnostic Criteria

- No specific guidelines for diagnosis
  - *CDKN1B*-associated tumors have no distinctive features from tumors with other genetic backgrounds
  - Patients presenting phenotype suggestive of MEN1 but with no MEN1 mutations should be tested for *CDKN1B* mutations

MACROSCOPIC

General Features

- Clinical and histological manifestations seem to be more variable than in MEN1, and due to small number of patients so far reported, comprehensive phenotype has not been yet established

MICROSCOPIC

Histologic Features

- Neuroendocrine tumors with histological features similar to sporadic and other inherited tumors

Cytologic Features

- Neuroendocrine-type cells

ANCILLARY TESTS

Immunohistochemistry

- Pituitary adenoma can express 1 or several hormones
  - Prolactin
  - ACTH
  - GH
  - LH
  - FSH

  o TSH
- Pancreatic endocrine tumor can express 1 or several hormones
  o Pancreatic polypeptide
  o Glucagon
  o Insulin
  o Gastrin
  o Vasointestinal polypeptide
  o Somatostatin
  o Serotonin
  o Calcitonin

Genetic Testing

- *CDKN1B* gene
  o Located on chromosome 12p13
  o 2 coding exons resulting in 2.4 kb coding region
  o 16 germline base substitutions in *CDKN1B* have been identified in association with development of various endocrine tumors
    – Mutations reduce amount of protein, inhibit its binding to protein partners, or mislocalized p27 to cytoplasm, ultimately impairing protein's ability to regulate cell division
  o Encodes p27
    – Cyclin-dependent kinase inhibitor whose main function is to control progression from G1 phase to S phase
    – Activity tightly regulated at transcriptional, translational, and posttranslational levels
    – Multifunctional protein involved in control of various processes
      □ Migration and invasion, apoptosis, autophagy, progenitor/stem cell fate and specification, cytokinesis, and transcriptional regulation

DIFFERENTIAL DIAGNOSIS

Multiple Endocrine Neoplasia Type 1

- Autosomal dominant disease caused by mutations in *MEN1* gene at 11q13
- Characterized by proliferative lesions of multiple endocrine organs involving mainly parathyroid, endocrine pancreas/duodenum, and pituitary glands
- Phenotype similar to that of MEN4; appears to occur earlier than in MEN4

Multiple Endocrine Neoplasia Type 2

- Autosomal dominant tumor syndrome pattern caused by mutations of *RET* gene|
- Characterized by various endocrine tumors involving thyroid, adrenals, and parathyroids
- Additional abnormalities affecting nonendocrine tissues may be present
- Subdivided into 3 groups
  o Familial medullary thyroid carcinoma, MEN2A, and MEN2B

Hyperparathyroidism-Jaw Tumor Syndrome

- Autosomal dominant disorder caused by mutation in *CDC73* (previously known as *HRPT2*) gene
- Known as familial cystic parathyroid adenomatosis
- Parathyroid tumors usually single but may be multiple

- Often caused by parathyroid adenoma or carcinoma and follows much more aggressive behavior
- Parathyroid carcinoma cause of hypercalcemia in 15-37% of cases
  o Although diagnosis of carcinoma not made until recurrence
- Patients with apparently sporadic parathyroid carcinoma; up to 30% in fact have germline mutations in *CDC73*
  o Indicating occult syndrome

Carney Complex

- Autosomal dominant syndrome
  o Caused by *PRKA-R1A* mutations
- Multiple neoplasia syndrome featuring endocrine overactivity, involving diverse endocrine organs, such as adrenal cortex, pituitary, thyroid, ovary, and testes, as well as
  o Spotty skin pigmentation, schwannomas, myxomatosis, neural tumors, and rarely tumors in liver and pancreas

DIAGNOSTIC CHECKLIST

Clinically Relevant Pathologic Features

- Most common tumors are neuroendocrine tumors of diverse sites

Pathologic Interpretation Pearls

- *CDKN1B*-associated tumors have no distinctive features to distinguish them from tumors of other genetic backgrounds

SELECTED REFERENCES

1. Pellegata NS et al: Multiple endocrine neoplasia type 4. In: WHO; 253-254, 2017
2. Caimari F et al: Novel genetic causes of pituitary adenomas. Clin Cancer Res. 22(20):5030-5042, 2016
3. Schernthaner-Reiter MH et al: MEN1, MEN4, and Carney complex: Pathology and molecular genetics. Neuroendocrinology. 103(1):18-31, 2016
4. Elston MS et al: Early onset primary hyperparathyroidism associated with a novel germline mutation in CDKN1B. Case Rep Endocrinol. 2015:510985, 2015
5. Longuini VC et al: Association between the p27 rs2066827 variant and tumor multiplicity in patients harboring MEN1 germline mutations. Eur J Endocrinol. 171(3):335-42, 2014
6. Thakker RV: Multiple endocrine neoplasia type 1 (MEN1) and type 4 (MEN4). Mol Cell Endocrinol. Epub ahead of print, 2013
7. Tonelli F et al: A heterozygous frameshift mutation in exon 1 of CDKN1B gene in a patient affected by MEN4 syndrome. Eur J Endocrinol. 171(2):K7-K17, 2014
8. Lee M et al: Multiple endocrine neoplasia type 4. Front Horm Res. 41:63-78, 2013
9. Occhi G et al: A novel mutation in the upstream open reading frame of the CDKN1B gene causes a MEN4 phenotype. PLoS Genet. 9(3):e1003350, 2013
10. Malanga D et al: Functional characterization of a rare germline mutation in the gene encoding the cyclin-dependent kinase inhibitor p27Kip1 (CDKN1B) in a Spanish patient with multiple endocrine neoplasia-like phenotype. Eur J Endocrinol. 166(3):551-60, 2012
11. Pellegata NS: MENX and MEN4. Clinics (Sao Paulo). 67 Suppl 1:13-8, 2012
12. Tichomirowa MA et al: Cyclin-dependent kinase inhibitor 1B (CDKN1B) gene variants in AIP mutation-negative familial isolated pituitary adenoma kindreds. Endocr Relat Cancer. 19(3):233-41, 2012
13. Costa-Guda J et al: Somatic mutation and germline sequence abnormalities in CDKN1B, encoding p27Kip1, in sporadic parathyroid adenomas. J Clin Endocrinol Metab. 96(4):E701-6, 2011
14. Marinoni I et al: p27kip1: a new multiple endocrine neoplasia gene? Neuroendocrinology. 93(1):19-28, 2011
15. Wander SA et al: p27: a barometer of signaling deregulation and potential predictor of response to targeted therapies. Clin Cancer Res. 17(1):12-8, 2011
16. Molatore S et al: Characterization of a naturally-occurring p27 mutation predisposing to multiple endocrine tumors. Mol Cancer. 9:116, 2010

Germline *CDKN1B* Mutation in MEN4 and Phenotype

CDKN1B Germline Mutation	Parathyroid Disease	Pituitary Tumors	Other Manifestations
In 5 Untranslated Region			
-7G>C	PHPT		Bilateral adrenal mass (nonfunctioning)
-456_-453del(cctt)		GH-secreting (acromegaly)	Nonfunctioning pancreatic neuroendocrine tumor
-29_-26del(agag)		GH-secreting (young age)	
-32_-29del(gaga)	PHPT		Gastric carcinoid tumor
In Coding Sequence			
G9R	PHPT		
K25fs	PHPT	ACTH-secreting (Cushing disease)	
A55T	PHPT		Zollinger-Ellison syndrome, gastrinoma
P69L	PHPT	Nonfunctioning	Bronchial carcinoids, papillary thyroid carcinoma, bilateral multiple lung metastases
W76X	PHPT	GH-secreting (acromegaly)	
P95S	PHPT (2 parathyroid tumors)		Zollinger-Ellison syndrome, mass in duodenum and tail of pancreas
S125X	PHPT (2 parathyroid tumors)		Multiple gastroenteropancreatic tumors
K96Q		PRL-secreting (suspected lactotroph adenoma)	Breast tumor
I119T		GH-secreting (acromegaly)	
E126D	PHPT (young age)		
P133T	PHPT		
Stop>Q	PHPT (3 parathyroid tumors)		

ACTH = adrenocorticotropic hormone; GH = growth hormone; PHPT = primary hyperparathyroidism; PRL = prolactin

With modifications from Pellegata NS et al: Multiple endocrine neoplasia type 4. In: WHO; 253-254, 2017.

17. Molatore S et al: A novel germline CDKN1B mutation causing multiple endocrine tumors: clinical, genetic and functional characterization. Hum Mutat. 31(11):E1825-35, 2010
18. Molatore S et al: The MENX syndrome and p27: relationships with multiple endocrine neoplasia. Prog Brain Res. 182:295-320, 2010
19. Agarwal SK et al: Rare germline mutations in cyclin-dependent kinase inhibitor genes in multiple endocrine neoplasia type 1 and related states. J Clin Endocrinol Metab. 94(5):1826-34, 2009
20. Chu IM et al: The Cdk inhibitor p27 in human cancer: prognostic potential and relevance to anticancer therapy. Nat Rev Cancer. 8(4):253-67, 2008
21. Besson A et al: Discovery of an oncogenic activity in p27Kip1 that causes stem cell expansion and a multiple tumor phenotype. Genes Dev. 21(14):1731-46, 2007
22. Georgitsi M et al: Germline CDKN1B/p27Kip1 mutation in multiple endocrine neoplasia. J Clin Endocrinol Metab. 92(8):3321-5, 2007
23. Ozawa A et al: The parathyroid/pituitary variant of multiple endocrine neoplasia type 1 usually has causes other than p27Kip1 mutations. J Clin Endocrinol Metab. 92(5):1948-51, 2007
24. Pellegata NS et al: Germ-line mutations in p27Kip1 cause a multiple endocrine neoplasia syndrome in rats and humans. Proc Natl Acad Sci U S A. 103(42):15558-63, 2006
25. Philipp-Staheli J et al: p27(Kip1): regulation and function of a haploinsufficient tumor suppressor and its misregulation in cancer. Exp Cell Res. 264(1):148-68, 2001
26. Servant MJ et al: Differential regulation of p27(Kip1) expression by mitogenic and hypertrophic factors: Involvement of transcriptional and posttranscriptional mechanisms. J Cell Biol. 148(3):543-56, 2000
27. Slingerland J et al: Regulation of the cdk inhibitor p27 and its deregulation in cancer. J Cell Physiol. 183(1):10-7, 2000
28. Tomoda K et al: Degradation of the cyclin-dependent-kinase inhibitor p27Kip1 is instigated by Jab1. Nature. 398(6723):160-5, 1999
29. Fero ML et al: The murine gene p27Kip1 is haplo-insufficient for tumour suppression. Nature. 396(6707):177-80, 1998
30. Pagano M et al: Role of the ubiquitin-proteasome pathway in regulating abundance of the cyclin-dependent kinase inhibitor p27. Science. 269(5224):682-5, 1995

TERMINOLOGY

- Autosomal dominant genetic disease resulting from mutation in *VHL* tumor suppressor gene on chromosome 3p25.3
- Characterized by retinal and CNS hemangioblastomas, pheochromocytomas, pancreatic serous cystadenoma and cysts, and renal cell carcinoma of kidney

ETIOLOGY/PATHOGENESIS

- Type 1 is caused by deletions or truncation mutation of *VHL* gene
- Types 2A, AB, AC are caused by missense point mutations

MACROSCOPIC

- Multiple and bilateral renal cysts and renal cell carcinomas
- Multiple and bilateral pheochromocytomas
- Multiple pancreatic cysts and endocrine pancreatic tumors

MICROSCOPIC

- Multifocal and bilateral clear cell RCC are common in VHL patients
- Patients with type 2 disease have multiple and bilateral pheochromocytomas and paragangliomas
- Distinct pathological features from multiple endocrine neoplasia type 2 pheochromocytomas
  - Thick fibrous capsule, hyalinized stroma, and absence of cytoplasmic hyaline globules and adrenomedullary hyperplasia
- Pancreatic endocrine tumors are usually multiple and well circumscribed, characterized by solid, trabecular, &/or glandular architecture

DIAGNOSTIC CHECKLIST

- Bilateral renal cysts and liver cysts: Think ADPKD
- Bilateral renal cysts and pancreatic cysts: Think VHL

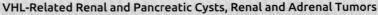

VHL-Related Renal and Pancreatic Cysts, Renal and Adrenal Tumors

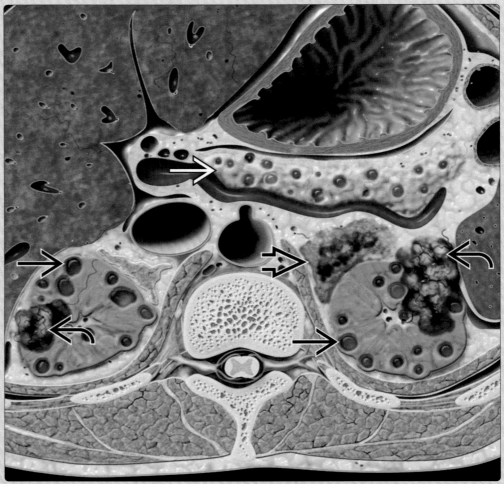

Graphic representation of abdominal lesions in von Hippel-Lindau (VHL) syndrome shows multiple bilateral renal cysts ➡, renal tumors ➡, pancreatic cysts ➡, and adrenal pheochromocytoma ➡.

TERMINOLOGY

Abbreviations

- von Hippel-Lindau disease (VHL)

Synonyms

- von Hippel-Lindau syndrome
- Familial cerebelloretinal angiomatosis

Definitions

- Rare autosomal dominant genetic disease resulting from mutation in *VHL* tumor suppressor gene on chromosome 3p25.3
- Characterized by development of multiple vascular tumors: Retinal and central nervous system (CNS) hemangioblastomas, pheochromocytomas, and paragangliomas, renal cell carcinomas (RCCs) and renal cysts, pancreatic serous cystadenomas and neuroendocrine tumors, endolymphatic sac tumors, and café au lait spots
  o If no family history, diagnosis requires 2 cardinal manifestations
    – Including retinal and CNS involvement (hemangioblastomas)
    – Excluding cysts
  o With positive family history
    – 1 cardinal manifestation, excluding cysts
- Member of phacomatosis familial cancer syndromes

ETIOLOGY/PATHOGENESIS

Tumorigenesis

- *VHL* gene encodes VHL protein, which is E3 ubiquitin ligase
  o Major regulator of hypoxic response by targeting transcription factor hypoxia inducible factor (HIF) for degradation
- VHL disease demonstrates marked phenotypic variability and age-dependent penetrance
  o Genotype-phenotype associations in VHL disease form basis of clinical classification
- Presumed that clinical presentation reflects quantitative or qualitative altered VHL protein function

Molecular Genetics

- Autosomal dominant
- Germline mutation of *VHL* gene (3p25-26)
  o *VHL* mutation in 50% of sporadic RCC
  o 2nd inactivating event predisposes to neoplasms
- VHL protein
  o Promotes destruction of HIF-1α via ubiquitin pathway
    – Loss of function leads to increased levels of vascular endothelial growth factor (VEGF), platelet-derived growth factor (PDGF), and transforming growth factor (TGF-α)
  o HIF-independent regulation of primary cilium and apoptosis via factors NF-κB
    – Loss of function promotes renal cysts
  o HIF contributes to overproduction of tyrosine hydroxylase and cathecolamines in pheochromocytomas

Subtypes

- **Classification**
  o Type 1 is caused by deletions or truncation mutation of VHL gene

  o Types 2A, AB, AC are caused by missense point mutations
- **Genotype/phenotype correlations**
  o Type 1 VHL (truncating and exon deletions)
    – Low risk of pheochromocytoma, high risk for RCC, high risk for CNS hemangioblastomas
  o Type 2 VHL (missense mutations)
    – High risk of pheochromocytoma
    – Type 2A: Low risk of RCC, high risk for CNS hemangioblastomas and pheochromocytoma
    – Type 2B: High risk of RCC, high risk for CNS hemangioblastomas and pheochromocytoma
    – Type 2C: Familial pheochromocytoma without hemangioblastoma or RCC

CLINICAL ISSUES

Epidemiology

- Incidence
  o 1 case per 36,000 live births
- Age
  o Age at diagnosis varies from infancy to age 60-70 years
  o Penetrance of up to 90% in patients aged ≥ 65 years
- Sex
  o No predilection is noted

Presentation

- CNS hemangioblastoma
  o Most common lesion associated with VHL disease (80% of patients)
  o Cerebellum, main stem and spinal cord tumors are major central nervous system manifestations
  o Benign vascular tumor, but may cause neurological deficits associated with significant mortality rate
  o Patients can present with headaches, numbness, dizziness, weakness or pain in arms and legs, incontinence, and spinal ataxia
- Retinal hemangioblastoma
  o Retinal capillary angiomas are typical ocular lesions of VHL disease and it earliest presentation
  o As many as 85% of patients develop retinal hemangioblastoma
  o Usually multifocal and bilateral
  o Patients present with painless loss of visual acuity or visual field
  o In advanced cases, can present with hemorrhage, leading to secondary glaucoma, and loss of vision
- RCC
  o Patients with VHL disease are at high risk of developing multiple renal cysts and RCC, affecting 2/3 of VHL patients
  o RCC is clear cell type, often multicentric &/or bilateral
- Pheochromocytoma
  o Catecholamine-producing neuroendocrine tumor derived from chromaffin cells that arise from adrenal medulla or extraadrenal chromaffin tissue (paraganglia)
  o Pheochromocytoma associated with VHL is usually asymptomatic, and patients are often young (< 40 years)
  o Hallmark of type 2 VHL disease

- o Tumor is usually bilateral, multiple, or extraadrenal, and hypertension with headache and sweating is most common presentation
- Pancreatic endocrine tumor and pancreatic cysts
  - o Tumors are usually nonsecretory and observed in 11-17% of patients with VHL
  - o Cystic lesions are present in as many as 91% of patients with VHL
- Other associated lesions
  - o Papillary cystadenoma of epididymis
  - o Endolymphatic sac tumor
  - o Papillary cystadenoma of broad ligament and mesosalpinx
  - o Cysts of pancreas, kidney, adrenal, testis, and ovary

Treatment

- Surgical approaches
  - o Nephron-sparing surgery
  - o Tumor resection when other organs affected
  - o Surgery for > 3 cm endocrine pancreatic tumor
  - o Adrenalectomy for pheochromocytoma

Prognosis

- Death due to RCC in 50%
  - o Metastases to liver, lung, and bone
- Pheochromocytoma is cured after surgery
  - o 5% of tumors present with metastasis, usually associated with large pheochromocytoma (> 5-6 cm in size) or paraganglioma

MACROSCOPIC

General Features

- Multiple and bilateral renal cysts
- Multiple and bilateral RCCs
  - o Solid and cystic clear cell RCCs
- Multiple and bilateral pheochromocytomas
- Multiple pancreatic cysts
- Well-circumscribed endocrine-type pancreatic tumors
- Microcystic adenoma and benign serous cysts of pancreas

MICROSCOPIC

Histologic Features

- Renal disease
  - o Cysts
    - – Lined by large cells with cleared-out cytoplasm
    - – Benign cyst lined by single cell layer
    - – Atypical cysts lined by piled up or stratified cells
  - o Clear cell RCC
    - – Sporadic and VHL-associated clear cell tumors are often indistinguishable
    - – Multifocal and bilateral tumors are more common and typically have microcystic growth pattern
    - – Microscopic to macroscopic lesions; early lesion: Intratubular proliferation of clear cells
    - – Tumors in VHL patients are usually multicystic &/or solid, surrounded by thick fibrous capsule
    - – Composed of cells with cleared-out cytoplasm and small nuclei
- Pheochromocytoma

- o Patients with type 2 disease have multiple and bilateral pheochromocytomas and paragangliomas
- o VHL pheochromocytoma have distinct pathological features from multiple endocrine neoplasia type 2 pheochromocytomas
  - – Presence of thick fibrous and vascular capsule
  - – Myxoid and hyalinized stroma
  - – Small- to medium-sized tumor cells with lack of nuclear atypia and mitosis
  - – Absence of cytoplasmic hyaline globules and adrenomedullary hyperplasia
- Pancreatic endocrine tumor and pancreatic cysts
  - o Tumors are usually multiple and well circumscribed
  - o Cystic lesions are usually multiple and benign
  - o Endocrine pancreatic tumors are characterized by solid, trabecular, &/or glandular architecture
  - o Stomal collagen is usually present and mitoses are rare
  - o Most tumors have clear cells, are hypervascularity, and marked nuclear atypia may be present
  - o Cystic lesions usually show histopathological features of serous cystic neoplasms (microcystic and macrocystic serous cystadenomas)
- CNS hemangioblastomas
  - o Histological features vary dependent on tumor size
  - o Nodules well circumscribed and high vascularized, often in wall of large cyst
  - o Non neoplastic component of abundant mature vascular structures with rich papillary network
  - o Neoplastic component of large vacuolated (called clear) lipid-containing stromal cells that harbor VHL gene deletion
  - o Stromal cells are immunonegative for vascular markers (CD31, cytokeratins, and EMA); important in differential diagnosis with metastatic RCC
  - o Strongly positive for vimentin
- Non-CNS hemangioblastomas
  - o Often multiple and bilateral, and histologically identical to CNS hemangioblastomas
  - o Tumors lack endothelial cells and some show glial cell proliferation
  - o Vacuolated or foamy stromal cells are interposed between variously sized vascular channels

DIFFERENTIAL DIAGNOSIS

Cystic Renal Diseases Associated With Renal Neoplasms

- Acquired cystic kidney disease
  - o Cyst frequency proportional to duration of ESRD
  - o Diverse array of RCCs
- Tuberous sclerosis complex/autosomal dominant polycystic kidney disease (ADPKD) contiguous gene syndrome
  - o Diffusely cystic kidneys identical to ADPKD
  - o Multiple and bilateral angiomyolipomas
  - o Rarely, clear cell RCC
- ADPKD
  - o Risk of renal carcinoma may be increased but controversial
  - o Far more numerous cysts than in VHL

Main Manifestations of von Hippel-Lindau Syndrome in Affected Organs

Affected Organ(s)	Tumors or Lesions
CNS	Hemangioblastomas
Retinas	Hemangioblastomas
Adrenal glands and paraganglia	Pheochromocytomas, paragangliomas, and hemangioblastomas*
Kidneys	Renal cell carcinomas, renal cysts, and hemangioblastomas*
Pancreas	Neuroendocrine tumors, serous cystadenomas, and simple cysts
Endolymphatic sac	Endolymphatic sac tumors
Epididymis	Epididymal papillary cystadenomas
Broad ligament and mesosalpinx	Cystadenomas of broad ligament and mesosalpinx
Others * (lungs, liver, gallbladder, ampulla, common bile duct, peripheral nerves)	Hemangioblastomas, cysts, and neuroendocrine tumors

*Very rarely described cases.

Couvelard A et al: Von Hippel-Lindau syndrome. In: WHO, 257-261, 2017.

Genotype-Phenotype Correlations in von Hippel-Lindau Syndrome

VHL Subtype	Hemangioblastomas	Renal Cell Carcinoma	Pheochromocytoma
Type 1	(+)	(+)	(-)
Type 2A	(+)	(-)	(+)
Type 2B	(+)	(+)	(+)
Type 2C	(-)	(-)	(+)

von Hippel-Lindau syndrome = VHL.

Couvelard A et al: Von Hippel-Lindau syndrome. In: WHO, 257-261, 2017.

Tuberous Sclerosis Complex

- Angiomyolipomas common
- Renal cancer and renal cysts rare
- Rare pancreatic lesions
- Cranial lesions are calcification and subependymal giant cell astrocytoma

DIAGNOSTIC CHECKLIST

Pathologic Interpretation Pearls

- Bilateral renal cysts and liver cysts: Think ADPKD
- Bilateral renal cysts and pancreatic cysts: Think VHL

SELECTED REFERENCES

1. Couvelard A. et al; Hammel P.; Komminoth P.; Mete O.; Pacak K.; Perren A.; Stratakis C. A. Von Hippel-Lindau syndrome. In: WHO, 257-261, 2017.
2. Okumura F et al: Hypoxia-inducible factor-2α stabilizes the von Hippel-Lindau (VHL) disease suppressor, Myb-related protein 2. PLoS One. 12(4):e0175593, 2017
3. O'Toole SM et al: Response to somatostatin analog therapy in a patient with von Hippel-Lindau disease and multiple pancreatic neuroendocrine tumors. Pancreas. 46(7):e57, 2017
4. Rednam SP et al: Von Hippel-Lindau and hereditary pheochromocytoma/paraganglioma syndromes: clinical features, genetics, and surveillance recommendations in childhood. Clin Cancer Res. 23(12):e68-e75, 2017
5. Sharma A et al: Clinical profile of pancreatic cystic lesions in von Hippel-Lindau disease: a series of 48 patients seen at a tertiary institution. Pancreas. 46(7):948-952, 2017
6. Ben-Skowronek I et al: Von Hippel-Lindau syndrome. Horm Res Paediatr. 84(3):145-52, 2015
7. Ashouri, L et al: Implications of von Hippel-Lindau syndrome and renal cell carcinoma. Journal of Kidney Cancer and VHL, 2(4), 163–173, 2015
8. Maher ER et al: von Hippel-Lindau disease: a clinical and scientific review. Eur J Hum Genet. 19(6):617-23, 2011
9. Rechsteiner MP et al: VHL gene mutations and their effects on hypoxia inducible factor HIFα: identification of potential driver and passenger mutations. Cancer Res. 71(16):5500-11, 2011
10. Salazar R et al: Retinal capillary hemangioma and von Hippel-Lindau disease: diagnostic and therapeutic implications. Arch Soc Esp Oftalmol. 86(7):218-221, 2011
11. Traen S et al: Central nervous system lesions in Von Hippel-Lindau syndrome. JBR-BTR. 94(3):140-1, 2011
12. Zhang Y et al: Endocrine tumors as part of inherited tumor syndromes. Adv Anat Pathol. 18(3):206-18, 2011
13. Barontini M et al: VHL disease. Best Pract Res Clin Endocrinol Metab. 24(3):401-13, 2010
14. Ellison J: Novel human pathological mutations. Gene symbol: VHL. Disease: Von Hippel-Lindau syndrome. Hum Genet. 127(4):477, 2010
15. Kaelin WG Jr: New cancer targets emerging from studies of the Von Hippel-Lindau tumor suppressor protein. Ann N Y Acad Sci. 1210:1-7, 2010
16. Safo AO et al: Pancreatic manifestations of von Hippel-Lindau disease. Arch Pathol Lab Med. 134(7):1080-3, 2010
17. Tamura K et al: Diagnosis and management of pancreatic neuroendocrine tumor in von Hippel-Lindau disease. World J Gastroenterol. 16(36):4515-8, 2010
18. Wu D et al: Observer variation in the application of the pheochromocytoma of the adrenal gland scaled score. Am J Surg Pathol. 33(4):599-608, 2009
19. Shehata BM et al: Von Hippel-Lindau (VHL) disease: an update on the clinico-pathologic and genetic aspects. Adv Anat Pathol. 15(3):165-71, 2008
20. Kaelin WG: Von Hippel-Lindau disease. Annu Rev Pathol. 2:145-73, 2007
21. Nakamura E et al: Clusterin is a secreted marker for a hypoxia-inducible factor-independent function of the von Hippel-Lindau tumor suppressor protein. Am J Pathol. 168(2):574-84, 2006

Cerebellar Hemangioblastomas

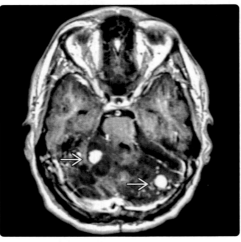

Pancreatic and Renal Cysts

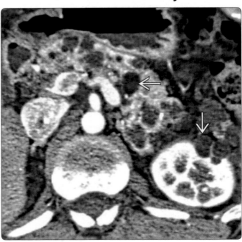

(Left) *Axial T1WI C+ MR shows 2 of several cerebellar hemangioblastomas ➡, a finding that is so characteristic as to be diagnostic of VHL by itself. The presence of multiple cysts and tumors in other organs is also characteristic of this disorder.* (Right) *Axial CECT shows innumerable pancreatic and renal cysts ➡. Either the CNS or abdominal findings would be considered diagnostic of this disorder. A patient's family history of VHL is also useful for corroboration.*

Multiple Cysts in Kidney and Pancreas

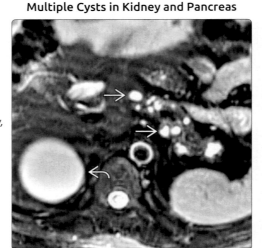

Renal Cysts and Renal Cell Carcinoma

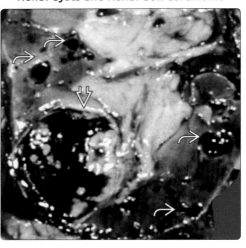

(Left) *Axial T2WI MR in a young man with multiorgan manifestations of VHL shows multiple pancreatic ➡ and renal ➡ cysts.* (Right) *Kidney from a patient with VHL disease shows multiple renal cysts ➡ within the renal parenchyma. There is a yellow, well-circumscribed renal cell carcinoma ➡ with extensive hemorrhage.*

VHL-Related Pancreatic Cysts

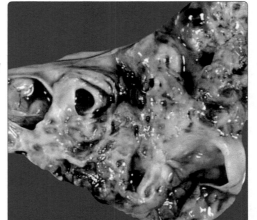

Pancreatic Cystadenoma

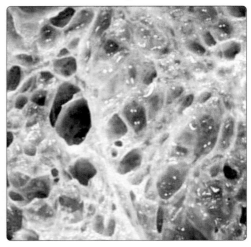

(Left) *This cut surface of a pancreas from a patient with VHL disease shows diffuse replacement of the normal architecture by variably sized cysts. The cysts are thin walled and have clear contents.* (Right) *Pancreas from a VHL patient shows a multicystic lesion with thin-walled cysts containing clear fluid. The cysts are derived from the pancreatic duct system, with different sizes, and have a thin, fibrovascular wall.*

Hemangioblastoma Sites

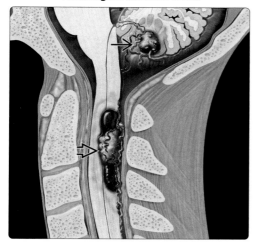

Retinal Hemangioblastoma

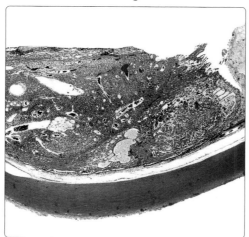

(Left) *Hemangioblastoma is the most frequently occurring tumor in VHL syndrome patients. The presence of multiple tumors is essentially pathognomonic of the disorder. The main locations involved are the cerebellum ⊡ and spinal cord ⊡. (From DP: Familial Cancer.)* (Right) *Although named hemangiomas in the past, given their rich vascular supply, retinal tumors afflicting VHL syndrome patients are hemangioblastomas, identical to tumors involving the CNS. (From DP: Familial Cancer.)*

Hematopoiesis in Hemangioblastoma

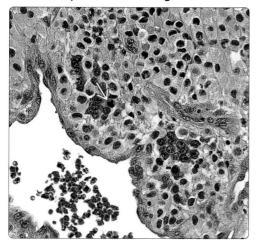

Cytoplasmic Vacuolization

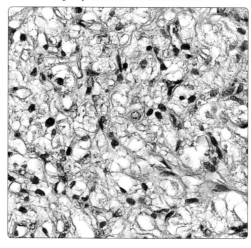

(Left) *An interesting histologic finding in a minority of hemangioblastomas is the presence of extramedullary hematopoiesis. This is characterized by variable clusters of large cells with prominent nucleoli and frequent mitotic figures ⊡. (From DP: Familial Cancer.)* (Right) *The reticular variant of hemangioblastoma is characterized by variable numbers of stromal cells containing prominent cytoplasmic microvacuoles. (From DP: Familial Cancer.)*

Reticulin Pattern in Hemangioblastomas

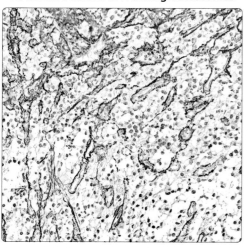

Intracellular Fat

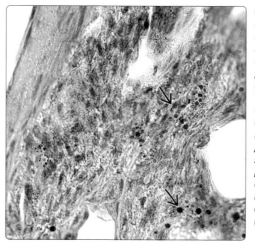

(Left) *Reticulin stain is useful in the evaluation of hemangioblastomas, since it highlights small lobules and even individual cells. This pattern is particularly characteristic of the reticular variant. (From DP: Familial Cancer.)* (Right) *Stromal cells contain variable amounts of intracytoplasmic lipid ⊡. In frozen section, an oil red O special stain may be particularly useful, since the characteristic microvacuolation of stromal cells may not be evident. (From DP: Familial Cancer.)*

(Left) *Hemangioblastomas contain a rich vascular supply and are not uncommonly grossly mistaken for vascular malformations. This particular example demonstrates congestion as well as a multinucleated megakaryocyte ⇾. (From DP: Familial Cancer.)* **(Right)** *A positive immunohistochemical reaction for inhibin is one of the most useful diagnostic features of hemangioblastoma, since most entities in the differential diagnosis are almost always negative. (From DP: Familial Cancer.)*

Multinucleated Cell

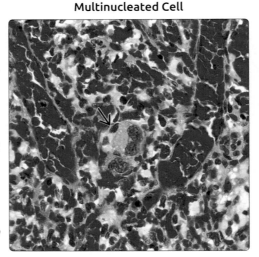

Immunopositivity for Inhibin

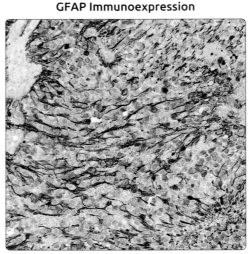

(Left) *A subset of hemangioblastomas may contain areas of glial differentiation and demonstrate overt immunoreactivity in neoplastic cells for glial markers such as GFAP. (From DP: Familial Cancer.)* **(Right)** *Gross cut surface of a kidney from a patient with VHL shows 2 encapsulated, yellow, solid and cystic renal cell carcinoma nodules ⇉ with focal hemorrhage.*

GFAP Immunoexpression

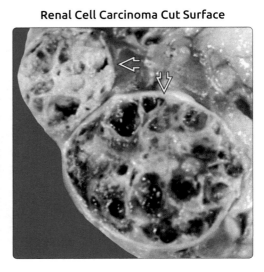

Renal Cell Carcinoma Cut Surface

(Left) *Renal cell carcinoma in a patient with VHL shows a solid component of the tumor. The tumor cells are round to oval, with irregular nuclei.* **(Right)** *This photomicrograph demonstrates a renal cell carcinoma in a patient with VHL with a predominant solid component of the tumor. The tumor in VHL is composed of clear cells and is morphologically indistinguishable from sporadic renal cell carcinoma.*

Renal Cell Carcinoma With Clear Cells

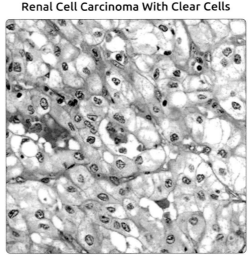

Clear Cell Renal Cell Carcinoma

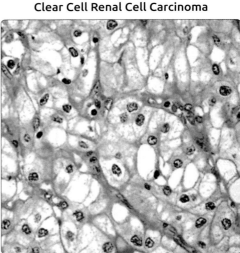

Cysts in Renal Cell Carcinoma

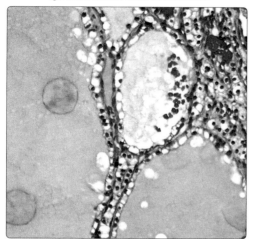

VHL-Associated Renal Carcinoma

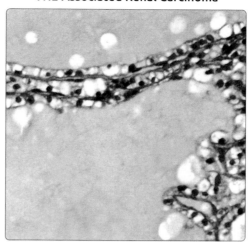

(Left) *Renal cell carcinoma with a cystic component is usually present in patients with VHL. The tumor is predominantly cystic, and the cysts are lined by cells with clear cytoplasm and low-grade nuclei.* (Right) *Grossly and microscopically, VHL-associated RCC resembles the classic clear cell type. This high-power figure of the renal tumor shows a predominantly cystic tumor, with cysts lined by cells with well-defined cytoplasmic membrane, clear cytoplasm, and low-grade nuclei.*

High Power of Clear Cells

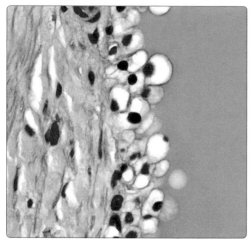

Solid and Cystic Renal Cell Carcinomas

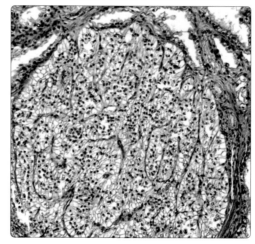

(Left) *The cyst lining from a renal cyst in a patient with VHL is composed of clear cells with ample cytoplasm and irregular grade 2 nuclei. The cyst is surrounded by a thick fibrous capsule.* (Right) *Most of the renal cell carcinomas in VHL patients are solid and cystic. The solid component is composed of cells with similar appearance to the cells lining the cystic spaces.*

Cell Morphology

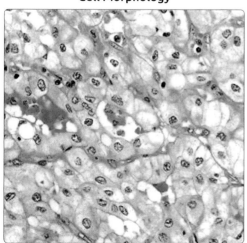

Clusterin Immunopositivity

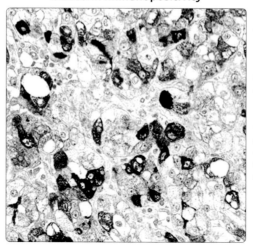

(Left) *Renal cell carcinoma in a patient with VHL shows a solid component of the tumor. The tumor cells are arranged in cords or trabeculae and are separated by thin fibrovascular stroma. The tumor cells are round to oval with irregular nuclei.* (Right) *Renal cell carcinoma in patients with VHL disease shows decreased clusterin staining in comparison with renal cell carcinoma in non-VHL patients.*

(Left) *Pancreas from a patient with VHL disease shows multiple thin-walled cysts of variable sizes. The cysts are filled with clear fluid, and there is extensive fibrosis of the pancreas.* **(Right)** *This photomicrograph of a pancreas from a patient with VHL disease shows multiple cysts lined by a single layer of cuboidal clear cells, surrounded by thick fibrous bands. There is residual pancreatic parenchyma ➡.*

Cut Surface of Pancreatic Cysts

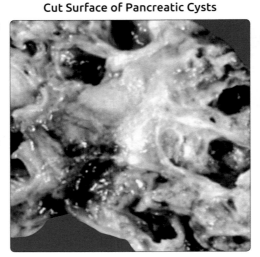

Pancreatic Cysts

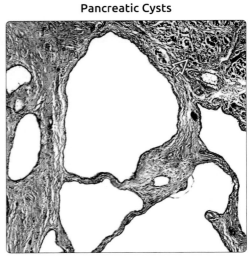

(Left) *The cut surface of this pancreas in a patient with VHL reveals numerous thin-walled cysts of variable sizes. The cysts have a thin fibrous wall and are filled with clear fluid.* **(Right)** *Pancreatic serous cystic neoplasms occur in as many as 90% of patients. The cells lining the numerous cyst wall are composed by small cells with indistinguishable cytoplasm and with bland nuclei.*

Cut Surface of Pancreatic Cystadenoma

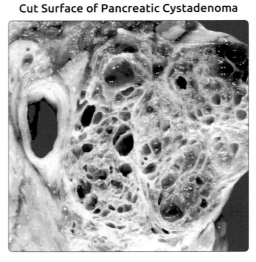

Cytological Features in Cystadenoma

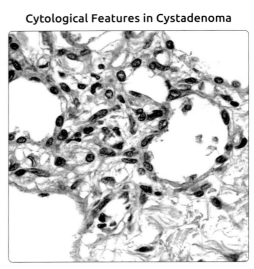

(Left) *This pancreatic gross photograph shows a solid adjacent to a cystic lesion in a VHL patient. Microscopically, there was a pancreatic neuroendocrine tumor and a serous cystadenoma. (Courtesy F. Fedeli, MD.)* **(Right)** *This neuroendocrine tumor in the pancreas in a patient with VHL shows a tumor with nested architecture with prominent, enlarged, irregular nuclei.*

Solid and Cystic Lesions in VHL in Pancreas

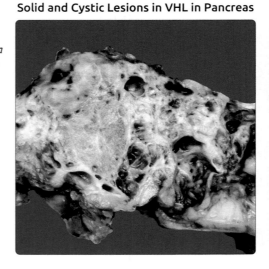

Pancreatic Endocrine Tumor in VHL Patient

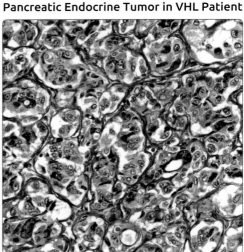

Pancreatic Endocrine Tumor and Cyst

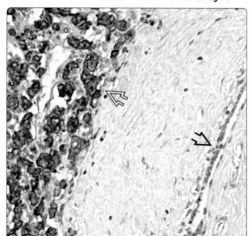

PET Adjacent to Cystadenoma

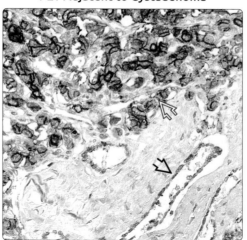

(Left) The immunohistochemistry stain for synaptophysin highlights the immunopositivity in the pancreatic neuroendocrine tumor ⇒, while the adjacent cystadenoma cells ⇒ lining one cyst wall are negative. (Right) The immunohistochemistry stain for CD56 highlights the pancreatic neuroendocrine tumor cells ⇒ in this pancreas of a patient with VHL. The adjacent cystadenoma cells ⇒ lining are negative for the neuroendocrine marker.

Pheochromocytoma

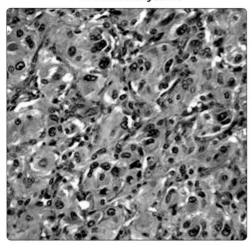

Clusterin in Pheochromocytoma

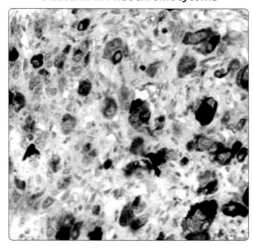

(Left) Pheochromocytoma in association with VHL disease shows tumor nests arranged in a nested and trabecular arrangement, composed of cells with ample cytoplasm and irregular nuclei. Note the absence of intracytoplasmic eosinophilic granules. (Right) Decreased clusterin staining in VHL pheochromocytoma is similar to the findings of decreased expression seen in VHL-associated renal cell carcinomas.

Immunopositivity for SDHA

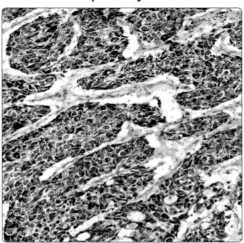

No SDHB in VHL Pheochromocytoma

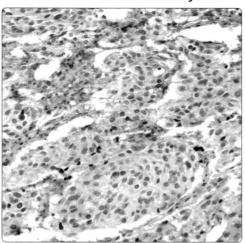

(Left) SDHA immunostain reveals preservation of the staining of the pheochromocytoma cells in VHL-associated tumors. (Right) SDHB staining in a VHL-associated pheochromocytoma may show loss of immunostaining, which is accompanied by preservation of SDHA. This finding is similar to the immunoexpression of these antigens in familial paraganglioma-pheochromocytoma syndromes (SDH-associated paraganglioma/pheochromocytoma syndrome).

KEY FACTS

TERMINOLOGY

- Autosomal dominant tumor disorder, which results from mutation in *NF1* gene
- Characterized by pigmentary or neoplastic involvement of neural crest and bony dysplasia

CLINICAL ISSUES

- Café au lait patches
- Neurofibromas
- Malignant peripheral nerve sheath tumor
- Freckling in axillary or inguinal region
- Optic nerve glioma
- Lisch nodules
- Duodenal carcinoid
- Pheochromocytoma
- Bone lesions
- Neurobehavioral abnormalities

MICROSCOPIC

- Plexiform neurofibroma
- Tortuous proliferation of peripheral nerves including
  - Axons, Schwann cells, fibroblasts, and perineurial cells
- Malignant peripheral nerve sheath tumor
  - Tortuous proliferation of peripheral nerves including axons, Schwann cells, fibroblasts, and perineurial cells
  - Often high grade, poorly differentiated, and aneuploid
- Optic nerve glioma
  - Fibrovascular septa within optic nerve are separated by tumor cells
- Duodenal carcinoid
  - Typically exhibit tubuloglandular structures

ANCILLARY TESTS

- NF1 gene was mapped to 17q11.2
- Genetic counseling; 50% of patients with NF1 are familial while other 50% arise from de novo mutation

---

Graphic Representation of Asymmetric Deformities Occurring in NF1 Patients

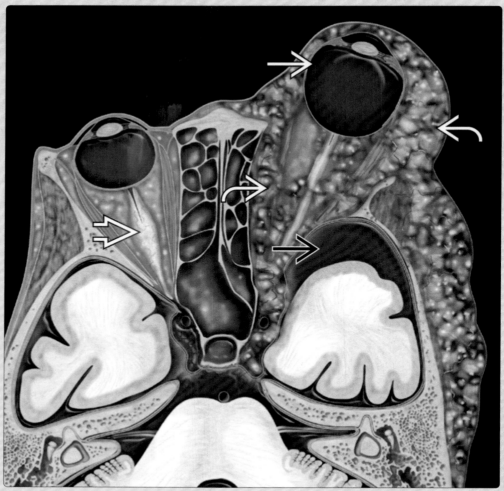

Axial graphic depicts sphenoid dysplasia with arachnoid cyst ⇨, optic nerve glioma ⇨, buphthalmos ⇨, and multiple plexiform neurofibromas ⇨.

TERMINOLOGY

Abbreviations

- Neurofibromatosis type 1 (NF1)

Synonyms

- von Recklinghausen disease
- Peripheral neurofibromatosis

Definitions

- Autosomal dominant tumor syndrome caused by mutations in *NF1* gene on chromosome 17q11.2, leading to multiple neurofibromas, café au lait spots, freckling of axila &/or groin, bone dysplasia, brain stem gliomas, malignant peripheral sheath tumors (MPNST), pheochromocytomas, duodenal neuroendocrine tumors, and gastrointestinal stromal tumors (WHO 2017)
- NF1 is most common inherited disease associated with neurofibromas

ETIOLOGY/PATHOGENESIS

Etiology

- Genetic syndrome resulting from germline mutations in *NF1* gene
- Inherited as autosomal dominant trait
- Result from mutation in or deletion of *NF1* gene encoding neurofibromin
- Neurofibromin is tumor suppressor, which downregulates p21-RAS oncoprotein
- Little genotype–phenotype correlation among patients with classic NF1 and NF1 mutations (other than chromosomal deletions)

CLINICAL ISSUES

Epidemiology

- Incidence
  - 1:2,500-3,000
- Age
  - Diagnosis of NF1 is often made in childhood

Presentation

- **Skin lesions**
  - **Café au lait patches**
    - Can be present at birth, and nearly every affected child has ≥ 6 by age 5 or 6
    - Often 1st feature of NF1; occur in > 95% of patients
    - Patches are usually round to ovoid, light brown in color with smooth borders, located over nerve trunks
    - Borders of patches are smooth, so-called "coast of California"
  - **Neurofibromas**
    - Pathognomonic for NF1; affect only 40–60% of patients
    - Cutaneous neurofibromas are soft, sessile, or pedunculated lesions that vary in number
    - Subcutaneous neurofibromas are often firm, round masses that are often painful
    - Plexiform neurofibromas contain numerous tortuous thickened nerves
      - Occur in about 30% of patients with NF1
  - **MPNST**

- Most common frequent malignant neoplasms associated with NF1 (8-13%)
- Often large, irregular, painful mass with rapid expansion
- Hematogenous metastasis to lung can occur
- 50% of MPNSTs are associated with NF1
- All deep-seated sarcomas with clear association to nerve and without clear line of differentiation should be considered MPNSTs
  - **Freckling in axillary or inguinal region**
    - Affects > 90% of NF1 patients by age of 7 years
    - Freckling occurs in non-sun-exposed skin
    - Appears later than café au lait spots
- **CNS lesions**
  - **Optic nerve glioma**
    - Occurs in around 15-20% of NF1 patients
    - Presents between birth and 7 years of age
    - Pilocytic astrocytoma is most common glioma affecting optic nerve
    - Can cause loss of vision and various visual abnormalities (e.g., strabismus, color vision changes, and proptosis)
  - **Macrocephaly**
  - **Unidentified bright objects**
    - Multiple, bilateral foci on MR, often affecting brainstem as well as cerebellum and deep cerebral gray matter
- **Lisch nodules**
  - Pigmented hamartomatous nevus of iris
  - Present in > 94% of patients > 6 years of age
  - Clear, yellow-brown, oval to round, dome-shaped papules that project from surface of iris
- **Endocrine lesions**
  - **Duodenal carcinoid**
    - Occurs in 1% of NF1 patients
    - Most patients presenting with NF1-related duodenal NETs are aged 40–50 years
    - Duodenal somatostatin-producing NETs usually occur at or in ampulla of Vater
    - Duodenal gangliocytic paragangliomas may coexist
    - Signs and symptoms are usually related to localization of tumor, including abdominal pain, anaemia, melaena, jaundice, and weight loss
  - **Pheochromocytoma**
    - Occurs in < 1% of NF1 patients; usually during 4th or 5th decade of life
    - Headache is most common presentation, usually frontal or occipital, starts suddenly and lasts about 15 minutes
    - Present with classic symptoms and signs related to excess release of epinephrine and metanephrine
      - Paroxysmal hypertension, palpitations, sweating, nervousness, anxiety, and pallor
    - Typically located in adrenal glands
      - Extraadrenal localization is rare
      - About 10% of patients have multiple tumors
      - Metastases develop in < 5% of cases
- **Bone lesions**
  - Most common lesions are skeletal dysplasias: Sphenoid wing, orbital bone, long bone dysplasias

- o Rare lesions: Ciliary bone cysts and giant cell granulomas
- o Very rare lesions (but can lead to metastatic disease): Fibrosarcomas, malignant fibrous histiocytomas, and primary neurogenic sarcomas
- **Neurobehavioral abnormalities**
  - o Headaches
  - o Seizures
  - o Learning disabilities occur in 50-75%

Treatment

- Genetic counseling; 50% of patients with NF1 are familial while other 50% arise from de novo mutation
- Cutaneous or subcutaneous neurofibromas can be removed surgically or by laser electrocautery
- Surgical or radiofrequency therapy for diffuse plexiform neurofibromas or café au lait spots
- Chemotherapy is treatment of choice for optic gliomas
- Bracing for progressive dystrophic scoliosis

Prognosis

- Average life expectancy of individuals with NF1 is reduced by 15 years
- Wide variability of outcomes, depending on tumor burden

Diagnostic Criteria

- Developed by National Institutes of Health (NIH) Consensus Conference in 1987
  - o Presence of 2 or more of following
    - ≥ 6 café au lait macules, greatest diameter of which is > 5 mm in prepubertal patients and > 15 mm in postpubertal patients
    - ≥ 2 neurofibromas of any type or 1 plexiform neurofibroma
    - Axillary or inguinal freckling (Crowe sign)
    - Optic glioma
    - ≥ 2 Lisch nodules
    - Distinctive osseous lesion such as sphenoid dysplasia or pseudoarthrosis
    - 1st-degree relative with NF1 according to these criteria
- By 8 years of age, 97% of children with NF1 clinically fulfill diagnostic criteria; by 20 years rate is 100%
- Diagnostic Criteria NIH 1991
  - o 2 or more of following
    - Café au lait macules (≥ 6) with diameter of 0.5 cm in children or 1.5 cm after puberty
    - Cutaneous or subcutaneous neurofibromas (≥ 2) or plexiform neurofibroma
    - Freckling of axillary or groin region
    - Glioma of optic pathways
    - Lisch nodules identified by slit-lamp examination (≥ 2)
    - Dysplasias of skeletal system (sphenoid wing, long bone bowing, pseudoarthrosis)
    - Diagnosis of NF1 in 1st-degree relative

MACROSCOPIC

Neurofibroma

- Benign tumor arising from Schwann cells that surround peripheral nerves of all sizes

Plexiform Neurofibroma

- Tortuous proliferation of all components of peripheral nerves including axons, Schwann cells, fibroblasts, and perineurial cells

Café au Lait Spot

- Vary in size, flat with smooth border

Malignant Peripheral Nerve Sheath Tumor

- Huge fusiform mass

Optic Nerve Glioma

- Grows within neural sheath to produce fusiform enlargement

Duodenal Carcinoid

- Neuroendocrine tumors of duodenum in NF1 are usually solitary and often polypoid, with mean diameter of 2 cm
- Typically affect major papilla &/or ampulla
- Advanced lesions infiltrate sphincter of Oddi, duodenal wall, &/or pancreatic head and are then associated with lymph node metastases

MICROSCOPIC

Café au Lait Spot

- Feature basilar hyperpigmentation ± suprabasilar melanosis
- Giant melanosomes within melanocytes are characteristic

Neurofibroma

- Neurofibromas reveal proliferation of all elements in peripheral nerve, including neuritides, Schwann cells, and fibroblasts in loose, myxoid stroma
- Consists mainly of uniform, spindle-shaped Schwann cells with barely discernible processes and delicate elongate or sinuous nuclei
- Diffuse cutaneous and subcutaneous neurofibroma is much less common and is characterized by plaque-like tumor, usually in head and neck region
- Pseudomeissnerian corpuscles are frequent

Plexiform Neurofibroma

- S100 positivity in Schwann cells
- Trichrome stains highlight proliferating fibroblasts
- Plexiform tumors may undergo malignant transformation to MPNST (risk of progression is 2-5%)
- Consists of tumor mass with multinodular and plexiform architecture that imparts bag of worms appearance

Malignant Peripheral Nerve Sheath Tumor

- Tumor may show glandular differentiation, skeletal muscle (triton tumor), or epithelioid elements
- Cells are pleomorphic with frequent mitotic figures
- About 50% of MPNSTs express S100 weakly, focal in majority of cases, and minority show perineurial differentiation
- Often high grade, poorly differentiated, and aneuploid

Optic Nerve Glioma

- In children almost all are pilocytic astrocytomas
- Fibrovascular septa within optic nerve are separated by tumor cells
- Minimal pleomorphism, lack of mitotic activity, and necrosis
- Tumor cells are reactive for glial fibrillary acidic protein

- 3 major patterns are recognized
  - Reticulated pattern
  - Microcystic pattern
  - Fibrillated; spindle-shaped cells form bundle pattern

Duodenal Carcinoid

- Typically exhibit tubuloglandular and pseudoglandular structures
- PAS(+) psammoma bodies composed of calcium apatite crystals

Pheochromocytomas

- NF1-associated pheochromocytomas do not differ from sporadic pheochromocytomas, except that they are more frequently of composite type

ANCILLARY TESTS

Genetic Testing

- *NF1* gene was mapped to 17q11.2
  - Massive gene containing > 300 kilobases of DNA divided into > 50 exons
- Most mutations are protein truncating, consisting of nonsense, frameshift, and splicing
- Large gene deletion can be detected by FISH
- *NF1* gene abnormalities are currently found in > 90% of patients with clinical diagnosis of NF1

DIFFERENTIAL DIAGNOSIS

McCune-Albright Syndrome

- Consists of polyostotic fibrous dysplasia, café au lait spots, and endocrinopathies caused by *GNAS* mutation
- Café au lait spots are larger than in NF1 and have "coast of Maine" border

Neurofibromatosis Type 2

- Autosomal dominant disorder caused by mutation of *NF2* gene, located on chromosome 22q12; encodes merlin
- Bilateral vestibular schwannomas, cutaneous schwannomas, meningiomas, and juvenile posterior subcapsular cataracts

Hereditary Nonpolyposis Colon Cancer

- Multiple café au lait spots, axillary freckling, and cutaneous neurofibromas are similar to NF1
- Colonic cancer at unusually young age

Multiple Endocrine Neoplasia Type 2B

- Autosomal dominant tumor syndrome pattern caused by mutations of *RET* gene
- High risk of pheochromocytoma but can be differentiated based on other clinical features

DIAGNOSTIC CHECKLIST

Pathologic Interpretation Pearls

- Diagnosis of NF1 is often made in children
- Plexiform neurofibromas, which contain numerous tortuous thickened nerves, are pathognomonic for NF1
- 50% of MPNST is associated with NF1

SELECTED REFERENCES

1. Blakeley JO et al: The path forward: 2015 International Children's Tumor Foundation conference on neurofibromatosis type 1, type 2, and schwannomatosis. Am J Med Genet A. 173(6):1714-1721, 2017
2. Sites ER et al: Analysis of copy number variants in 11 pairs of monozygotic twins with neurofibromatosis type 1. Am J Med Genet A. 173(3):647-653, 2017
3. Friedrich RE et al: Optic pathway glioma and cerebral focal abnormal signal intensity in patients with neurofibromatosis type 1: characteristics, treatment choices and follow-up in 134 affected individuals and a brief review of the literature. Anticancer Res. 36(8):4095-121, 2016
4. Hernández-Martín A et al: An update on neurofibromatosis type 1: not just Café-au-Lait spots, freckling, and neurofibromas. An update. Part I. Dermatological Clinical Criteria Diagnostic of the Disease. Actas Dermosifiliogr. 107(6):454-64, 2016
5. Karajannis MA et al: Neurofibromatosis-related tumors: emerging biology and therapies. Curr Opin Pediatr. 27(1):26-33, 2015
6. Okumura A et al: Development of a practical NF1 genetic testing method through the pilot analysis of five Japanese families with neurofibromatosis type 1. Brain Dev. 37(7):677-89, 2015
7. Abramowicz A et al: Neurofibromin in neurofibromatosis type 1 - mutations in NF1gene as a cause of disease. Dev Period Med. 18(3):297-306, 2014
8. Cai SP et al: A novel NF1 frame-shift mutation (c.702_703delGT) in a Chinese family with neurofibromatosis type 1. Genet Mol Res. 13(3):5395-404, 2014
9. Hirbe AC et al: Neurofibromatosis type 1: a multidisciplinary approach to care. Lancet Neurol. 13(8):834-43, 2014
10. Javed F et al: Oral manifestations in patients with neurofibromatosis type-1: a comprehensive literature review. Crit Rev Oncol Hematol. 91(2):123-9, 2014
11. Maruoka R et al: The use of next-generation sequencing in molecular diagnosis of neurofibromatosis type 1: a validation study. Genet Test Mol Biomarkers. 18(11):722-35, 2014
12. Pasmant E et al: Neurofibromatosis type 1 molecular diagnosis: what can NGS do for you when you have a large gene with loss of function mutations? Eur J Hum Genet. ePub, 2014
13. Jouhilahti EM et al: The pathoetiology of neurofibromatosis 1. Am J Pathol. 178(5):1932-9, 2011
14. Yap YS et al: The NF1 gene revisited - from bench to bedside. Oncotarget. 5(15):5873-92, 2014
15. Takenouchi T et al: Multiple café au lait spots in familial patients with MAP2K2 mutation. Am J Med Genet A. 164A(2):392-6, 2014
16. Bikowska-Opalach B et al: [Neurofibromatosis type 1 - description of clinical features and molecular mechanism of the disease.] Med Wieku Rozwoj. 17(4):334-40, 2013
17. Salvi PF et al: Gastrointestinal stromal tumors associated with neurofibromatosis 1: a single centre experience and systematic review of the literature including 252 cases. Int J Surg Oncol. 2013:398570, 2013
18. Raygada M et al: Hereditary paragangliomas. Adv Otorhinolaryngol. 70:99-106, 2011
19. Upadhyaya M: Genetic basis of tumorigenesis in NF1 malignant peripheral nerve sheath tumors. Front Biosci. 16:937-51, 2011
20. Welander J et al: Genetics and clinical characteristics of hereditary pheochromocytomas and paragangliomas. Endocr Relat Cancer. 18(6):R253-76, 2011
21. Zhang Y et al: Endocrine tumors as part of inherited tumor syndromes. Adv Anat Pathol. 18(3):206-18, 2011
22. Ferner RE: The neurofibromatoses. Pract Neurol. 10(2):82-93, 2010
23. Gilboa Y et al: Application of the international classification of functioning, disability and health in children with neurofibromatosis type 1: a review. Dev Med Child Neurol. 52(7):612-9, 2010
24. Jett K et al: Clinical and genetic aspects of neurofibromatosis 1. Genet Med. 12(1):1-11, 2010
25. Lodish MB et al: Endocrine tumours in neurofibromatosis type 1, tuberous sclerosis and related syndromes. Best Pract Res Clin Endocrinol Metab. 24(3):439-49, 2010
26. Katz D et al: Malignant peripheral nerve sheath tumour (MPNST): the clinical implications of cellular signalling pathways. Expert Rev Mol Med. 11:e30, 2009
27. Petri BJ et al: Phaeochromocytomas and sympathetic paragangliomas. Br J Surg. 96(12):1381-92, 2009
28. Ferner RE: Neurofibromatosis 1 and neurofibromatosis 2: a twenty first century perspective. Lancet Neurol. 6(4):340-51, 2007
29. Lee MJ et al: Recent developments in neurofibromatosis type 1. Curr Opin Neurol. 20(2):135-41, 2007
30. Pinson S et al: [Neurofibromatosis type 1 or Von Recklinghausen's disease.] Rev Med Interne. 26(3):196-215, 2005
31. Friedman JM. Neurofibromatosis 1. 1993-, 1998

Imaging Features of NF1 Glioma

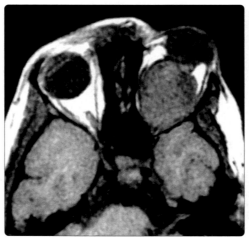

Optic Nerve and Chiasm Glioma

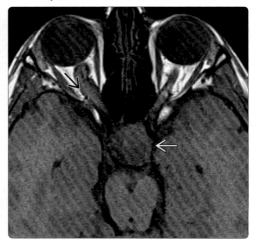

(Left) *Axial T1WI MR in a young girl with neurofibromatosis type 1 (NF1) reveals a massive optic nerve glioma that nearly fills the orbit. Notice the resultant proptosis and remodeling of the posterior orbit.* **(Right)** *The central nervous system hallmark of NF1 is multiple involvement of the optic pathways by low-grade gliomas. These may affect the optic nerve proper ⮕ as well as the chiasm ⮕. (From DP: Familial Cancer.)*

Graphic Features of Neurofibromas

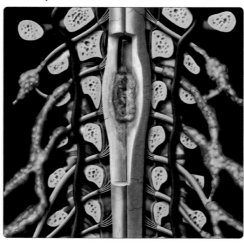

Graphic Features of Plexiform Neurofibromas

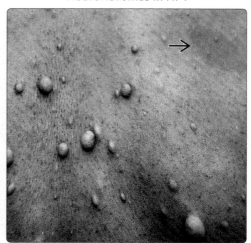

(Left) *Coronal graphic shows bilateral spinal nerve root and brachial plexus neurofibromas. Intramedullary cervical glial tumor produces focal cord expansion and cystic central canal dilatation.* **(Right)** *Graphic depicts plexiform neurofibromas in NF1 with multilevel, lobulated, tortuous expansion of cervical nerve roots and brachial plexus, with widening of the neural foramina.*

Café au lait Spots in NF1

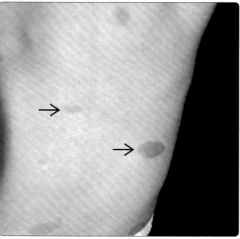

Neurofibromas in NF1

(Left) *Multiple café au lait spots represent an important cutaneous manifestation of NF1 ⮕. (Courtesy K. Yohay, MD.) (From DP: Familial Cancer.)* **(Right)** *Numerous cutaneous neurofibromas afflict a significant proportion of patients with NF1. They are characterized by sessile or pedunculated growths. An associated café au lait spot ⮕ is also present in this NF1 patient. (Courtesy K. Yohay, MD.) (From DP: Familial Cancer.)*

Gross Cut Surface of NF1-Related Tumor

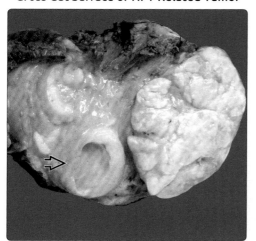

Neurofibromin Pathway

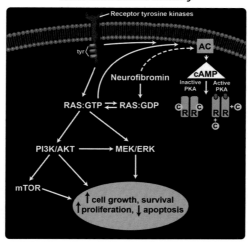

(Left) *Gross cut surface of a large MPNST arising from neurofibroma shows extensive areas of necrosis ⇨.* (Right) *NF1 syndrome is caused by germline mutations in the gene encoding for neurofibromin, a tumor suppressor protein that works by activating RAS GTPase function. Neurofibromin loss leads to constitutive RAS signaling and altered cAMP levels, resulting in a variety of neoplasms and other manifestations, particularly affecting the nervous system. (From DP: Familial Cancer.)*

Neurofibroma in NF1

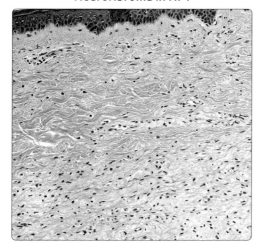

Plexiform Neurofibroma in NF1

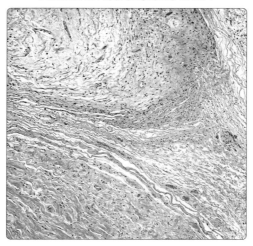

(Left) *Microscopically, neurofibromas reveal proliferation of all of the elements in the peripheral nerve, including neuritides, Schwann cells, and fibroblasts in a loose, myxoid stroma.* (Right) *Plexiform neurofibroma consists of multiple huge nerve bundles formed by proliferation of all components of peripheral nerves including axons, Schwann cells, fibroblasts, and perineurial cells.*

Iris Lynch Nodules in NF1

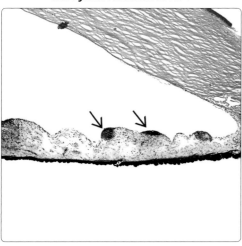

Lynch Nodules in NF1

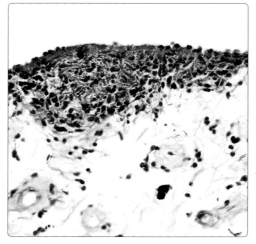

(Left) *Lisch nodules are asymptomatic nodular proliferations of pigmented cells involving the anterior surface of the iris in NF1 patients ⇨. They represent an important diagnostic criterion that is relatively easy to identify by ophthalmologic examination. (From DP: Familial Cancer.)* (Right) *Lisch nodules are composed of melanin-containing cells that form superficial aggregates in the iris. They usually do not affect vision and have no malignant potential. (From DP: Familial Cancer.)*

(Left) *Axial CECT in a patient with neurofibromatosis type 1 shows a right adrenal mass ➡ that proved to be a ganglioneuroma, although distinction from a pheochromocytoma is difficult and somewhat semantic.* **(Right)** *Both sporadic or NF1-associated pheochromocytomas have similar gross findings as well as histopathological findings. The cut surface of pheochromocytomas are grey-pink, which distinguishes it from the yellow adrenal cortex ➡. This tumor shows also areas of hemorrhage ➡.*

Adrenal Mass in NF1 Patient

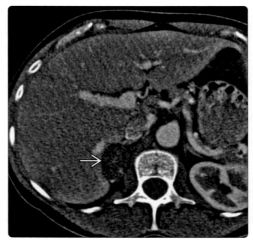

Adrenal Pheochromocytoma

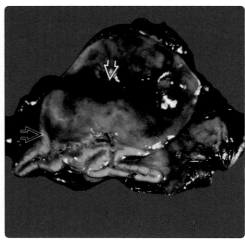

(Left) *Most neurofibromas are paucicellular tumors characterized by wavy, delicate eosinophilic collagen bundles colorfully referred to as "shredded carrots." A variable myxoid stroma may be identified in almost all neurofibromas. (From DP: Familial Cancer.)* **(Right)** *The majority of optic pathway gliomas are pilocytic astrocytomas. In this NF1-associated case, areas of tissue compaction, degenerative atypia ➡, and Rosenthal fibers ➡ are evident. (From DP: Familial Cancer.)*

Paucicellular Area

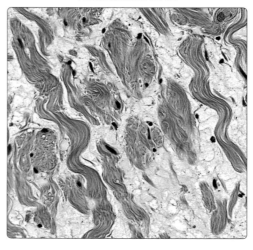

NF1-Associated Astrocytoma

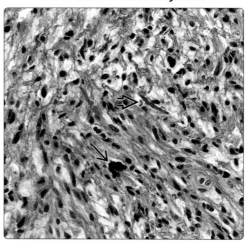

(Left) *The main diagnostic attributes of plexiform neurofibroma are evident on gross examination and low magnification, particularly a nodular or worm-like pattern of growth imparted by expansion of multiple peripheral nerve fascicles.* **(Right)** *Neurofibromas, including the plexiform variant, contain a myxoid stroma stained by Alcian blue. Such tumors also demonstrate cellular complexity, including Schwann cells, perineurial cells, fibroblasts, mast cells, and peripheral nerve axons. (From DP: Familial Cancer.)*

Plexiform Neurofibroma

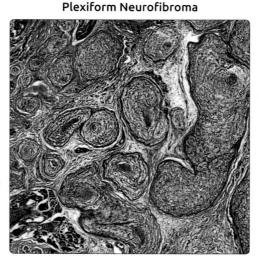

Plexiform Neurofibroma

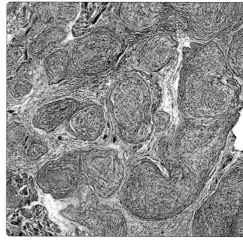

NF1-Associated MPNST

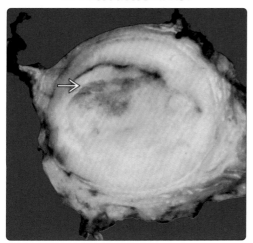

Large Epithelioid Cells in MPNST

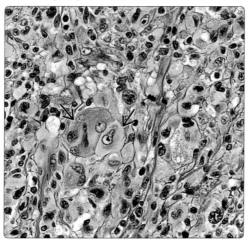

(Left) *Malignant peripheral nerve sheath tumor (MPNST) is the prototypical malignancy afflicting patients with NF1 syndrome. A suspicious finding on gross examination is the presence of necrosis ➡. MPNST may arise de novo or from a preexisting, usually plexiform neurofibroma.* **(Right)** *The morphologic variability of MPNST is wide, and pleomorphism may be marked in some NF1-associated and sporadic examples. Some tumors may contain epithelioid cells with well-defined borders ➡. (From DP: Familial Cancer.)*

Spindle Cells in MPNST

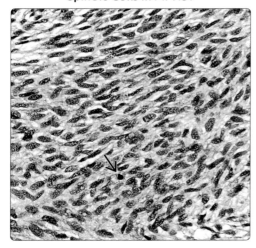

P53 Immunoexpression in MPNST

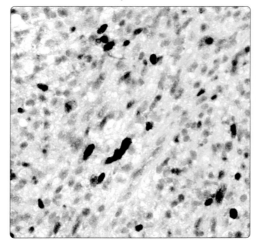

(Left) *MPNSTs are usually high-grade spindle cell malignancies. The neoplastic cells may be arranged in fascicles and resemble fibrosarcoma. Mitotic activity is variable but usually evident ➡. (From DP: Familial Cancer.)* **(Right)** *Strong nuclear immunoreactivity for p53 in a variable number of neoplastic cell nuclei is frequent in MPNST in contrast with benign neurofibromas. (From DP: Familial Cancer.)*

Loss of p16 in MPNST

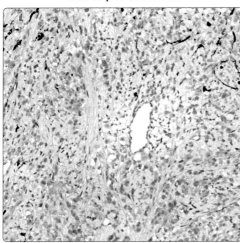

S100 in MPNST

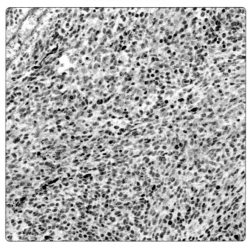

(Left) *p16 immunoreactivity is frequently lost in MPNST. p16 represents an important tumor suppressor that is frequently inactivated by gene mutations/deletions in MPNST. p16 loss at the gene or protein level may suggest malignant degeneration of neurofibromas in NF1 patients.* **(Right)** *S100, a ubiquitous Schwann cell marker, is characteristically weaker in areas of MPNST, or altogether negative. This is a useful distinguishing feature from cellular schwannoma. However, the latter is not typically NF1 associated.*

KEY FACTS

TERMINOLOGY

- Autosomal dominant tumor syndrome leading to spotty skin pigmentation, myxomatosis, endocrine overactivity, and schwannomas
- Associated endocrine disorders include functioning endocrine tumors of adrenal and pituitary glands and nonfunctioning tumors of thyroid, testes, and ovaries

ETIOLOGY/PATHOGENESIS

- Inactivating mutations in *PRKAR1A*/CNC1 gene (17q24)
- Activating mutation or increased copy number of one of protein kinase A (PKA) catalytic subunit genes (*PRKACA* or *PRKACB*)

CLINICAL ISSUES

- > 750 patients have been identified as having CNC
- Female predominance: F:M ~ 2:1
- Most tumors associated with CNC are slow growing with no malignant potential

- Sudden death due to cardiac myxoma may occur
- Complications of Cushing syndrome or acromegaly

DIAGNOSTIC CHECKLIST

- **Major diagnostic criteria for CNC**
  - Spotty skin pigmentation with typical distribution (lips, conjunctiva, and inner or outer canthi, vaginal and penile mucosa)
  - Cardiac, mucosal, and breast myxomas
  - Primary pigmented nodular adrenocortical disease with Cushing syndrome
  - Psammomatous melanotic schwannoma
  - Acromegaly due to GH-producing adenoma
  - Large cell calcifying Sertoli cell tumor
  - Thyroid carcinoma or multiple nodules in young patient
  - Blue nevus, epithelioid blue nevus
  - Breast ductal adenoma
  - Osteochondromyxoma

Cardiac Myxoma

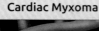
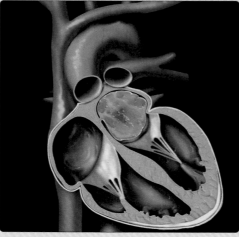

Adrenal Involvement in Carney Complex

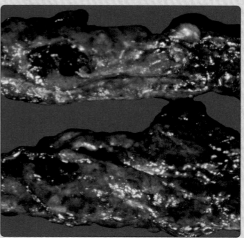

(Left) *Myxoid lesions associated with Carney complex are located in different sites, including skin, heart, and breast. The cardiac myxomas may occur in any chamber and at any age.* (Right) *The gross findings of primary pigmented nodular adrenocortical disease (PPNAD) include decreased, normal, or slightly increased weight, presence of small black-brown and yellow nodules, atrophy of the cortex, and loss of normal zonation.*

Skin and Mucosal Pigmentation in Carney Complex

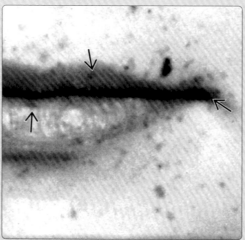

Eccentric Nuclei in Somatotroph Adenoma

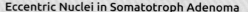
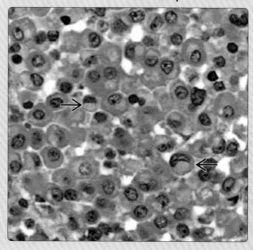

(Left) *Spotty skin pigmentation is characteristic of Carney complex, with typical distribution in lips ⇨, conjunctiva, inner or outer canthi, and vaginal and penile mucosa. (Courtesy of Aidan Carney, MD.)* (Right) *Photomicrograph shows sparsely granulated somatotroph adenoma composed of chromophobic cells. The nuclei tend to be eccentric, pushed to the cell periphery ⇨, and indented by the fibrous bodies.*

TERMINOLOGY

Abbreviations

- Carney complex (CNC)

Synonyms

- LAMB syndrome (lentigines, atrial myxomas, mucocutaneous myxomas, and blue nevi)
- NAME syndrome (nevi, atrial myxoma, myxoid neurofibroma, and ephelides)

Definitions

- Autosomal dominant tumor syndrome caused by *PRKAR1A* mutations leading to
  - Spotty skin pigmentation with typical distribution (lips, conjunctiva and canthi, and vaginal and penile mucosa)
  - Myxomatosis: Cutaneous, mucosal, and cardiac myxomas
  - Primary pigmented nodular adrenocortical disease (PPNAD)
  - Acromegaly due to growth hormone-producing adenoma
  - Schwannomas
  - Multiple other endocrine and nonendocrine neoplasms
    - Nonfunctioning tumors of thyroid, testes, ovary
  - Rarely tumors in liver and pancreas
- CNC may simultaneously involve multiple endocrine glands, as in classic multiple endocrine neoplasia syndromes 1 and 2
- CNC is in essence multiple endocrine neoplasia syndrome, but one that affects number of other tissues
  - This unique condition has similarities to other syndromes/diseases
    - Such as McCune-Albright
    - Peutz-Jeghers
    - Cowden, Bannayan-Zonana, and Birt-Hogg-Dube syndrome
    - Neurofibromatosis
    - Other phacomatoses and hamartomatoses

ETIOLOGY/PATHOGENESIS

Etiology

- Autosomal dominant disorder characterized by complex of myxomas, spotty pigmentation, and endocrine overactivity
  - Several patients described in earlier years under acronyms NAME and LAMB probably had CNC
  - CNC is not only multiple neoplasia syndrome but also causes variety of pigmented lesions of skin and mucosae
- Inactivating mutations in *PRKAR1A* gene (17q22-24)
  - *PRKAR1A* encodes regulatory R1 α-subunit of protein kinase A (PKA)
  - PKA heterotetramer consists of 2 regulatory (R) and 2 catalytic (C) subunits
  - Stimulation of adenyl cyclases through G protein subunit (Gs) activation leads to cAMP synthesis
  - cAMP, binds to regulatory subunits and leads to their dissociation from catalytic subunits
  - Catalytic subunits after their dissociation from PKA complex phosphorylate many downstream factors such as CREB

- *PRKAR1A* defects associated with CNC lead to PRKAR1A haploinsufficiency and, thus, to loss of this regulatory subunit's function
- Activating mutation or increased copy number of *PRKACA* or *PRKACB*

Criteria for Diagnosis

- Clinical characteristics of CNC have been recently reviewed
- **Definite diagnosis of CNC is given if**
  - 2 or more major manifestations are present
  - 1 major manifestation + 1 supplementary criteria
- **Major diagnostic criteria for CNC**
  - Spotty skin pigmentation with typical distribution (lips, conjunctiva, and inner or outer canthi, vaginal and penile mucosa)
  - Myxomas (cardiac, cutaneous, mucosal or breast) or fat-suppressed MR imaging findings suggestive of this diagnosis
  - PPNAD or paradoxical positive response of urinary glucocorticosteroid excretion to dexamethasone administration during Liddle test
  - Acromegaly due to GH-producing adenoma
  - Large cell calcifying Sertoli cell tumor or characteristic calcification on testicular ultrasound
  - Thyroid carcinoma or multiple hypoechoic nodules on thyroid ultrasound in young patient
  - Psammomatous melanotic schwannomas
  - Blue nevus, epithelioid blue nevus
  - Breast ductal adenomas
  - Osteochondromyxoma
- **Supplementary criteria**
  - Affected 1st-degree relative
  - Inactivating mutation of *PRKAR1A* gene
  - Activating mutation or increased copy number of *PRKACA* or *PRKACB*
- **Findings suggestive of, or possibly associated with, CNC but not diagnostic for disease**
  - Intense freckling (without darkly pigmented spots or typical distribution), blue nevus, common type (if multiple)
  - Café au lait spots or other "birthmarks"
  - Elevated IGF-I levels, abnormal GTT, or paradoxical GH response to TRH testing in absence of clinical acromegaly
  - Cardiomyopathy
  - Pilonidal sinus
  - History of Cushing syndrome, acromegaly, or sudden death in extended family
  - Multiple skin tags or other skin lesions
  - Lipomas
  - Colonic polyps (usually in association with acromegaly)
  - Hyperprolactinemia (usually mild and almost always combined with clinical or subclinical acromegaly)
  - Single, benign thyroid nodule in young patient; multiple thyroid nodules in older patient (detected on ultrasound)
  - Family history of carcinoma, in particular of thyroid, colon, pancreas, and ovary; other multiple benign or malignant tumors
- Cutaneous manifestations constitute 3 of major disease manifestations

- Spotty skin pigmentation with typical distribution (lips, conjunctiva, and inner or outer canthi, genital mucosa)
- Cutaneous or mucosal myxoma
- Blue nevi (multiple) or epithelioid blue nevus
- Findings that are suggestive of or associated with CNC findings but not diagnostic
  - Intense freckling (without darkly pigmented spots or typical distribution)
  - Multiple blue nevi of common type
  - Café au lait spots or other "birthmarks"
  - Multiple skin tags or other skin lesions, including lipomas and angiofibromas
- Relationship between cutaneous and noncutaneous manifestations of CNC appears to be essential clue to molecular etiology of disease
- > 1/2 of CNC patients present with both characteristic dermatological and endocrine signs
  - Significant number of patients present with skin lesions that are only "suggestive" and not characteristic of CNC
- Recent classification based on both dermatological and endocrine markers has subgrouped CNC patients as
  - Multisymptomatic (with extensive endocrine and skin signs)
  - Intermediate (with few dermatological and endocrine manifestations)
  - Paucisymptomatic (with isolated PPNAD alone and no cutaneous signs)

Similar Clinical and Pathological Features

- CNC shares skin abnormalities and some nonendocrine tumors with lentiginoses and certain hamartomatoses
  - Peutz-Jeghers syndrome, with which it shares mucosal lentiginosis and unusual gonadal tumor, and large cell calcifying Sertoli cell tumor
  - McCune-Albright syndrome, sporadic condition also characterized by multiple endocrine and nonendocrine tumors

CLINICAL ISSUES

Epidemiology

- Incidence
  - > 750 patients have been identified as having CNC
  - Cardiac myxomas are most common primary cardiac tumor and occur in 7 per 10,000 individuals
- Age
  - Mean patient age at diagnosis is 20 years
- Sex
  - F:M ~ 2:1

Presentation

- Skin
  - Multiple facial lentigines and mucosal labial pigmentation
  - Subcutaneous myxoid neurofibromas
- Atrial myxoma
  - Myxomas are most common primary tumor of heart
  - Majority of tumors arise from left atrial septum near fossa ovalis
  - Lesions arising from right atrium or in young adults are more likely to be associated with familial syndrome
  - May present with tumor emboli

- Endocrine organs
  - Thyroid
    - 75% of patients have multiple thyroid nodules
  - Adrenal gland
    - PPNAD with Cushing syndrome
- Testis
  - Large cell calcifying Sertoli cell tumor, often bilateral
- Gastrointestinal tract
  - Psammomatous melanotic schwannoma in esophagus and stomach
- There are groups of CNC patients who show specific genotype-phenotype correlation, and this also explains CNC heterogeneity
- Mutations in c.709–7del6 is present in most patients with isolated PPNAD, and most of remaining were c.1AOG carriers

Treatment

- Depends on main pathology
- Bilateral adrenalectomy, removal of cardiac myxomas, or removal of testicular tumor or other tumors

Prognosis

- Historic adjusted average life span for patients with CNC is 50-55 years
  - With careful surveillance, life expectancy may be normal
- Most tumors associated with CNC are slow growing with no malignant potential
- Sudden death due to cardiac myxoma may occur
  - Complications: Emboli (strokes), postoperative cardiomyopathy, and cardiac arrhythmias
  - Decreased lifespan expected
- Complications of Cushing syndrome or acromegaly

MACROSCOPIC

Cardiac Myxoma

- Mobile, pedunculated ball-shaped mass, 0.3-5.0 cm

Primary Pigmented Nodular Adrenocortical Disease

- Small to normal-sized adrenal glands
- Multiple bilateral, small cortical nodules, 0.1-0.4 cm
- Nodules may be pigmented, brown, or black
  - Some nodules may be pale to bright yellow

Large Cell Calcifying Sertoli Cell Tumor

- Ranges in size from microscopic to large tumor replacing entire testis
- Usually multicentric, bilateral, and calcified

Psammomatous Melanotic Schwannoma

- Black, multiple nodules that occur simultaneously or asynchronously at different sites

MICROSCOPIC

Histologic Features

- Pigmented nevi
  - Poorly circumscribed, located in dermis
  - 2 types of melanocytes: 1 heavily pigmented, globular, and fusiform, and other is lightly pigmented, polygonal, and spindled
- Cardiac myxoma

- o Composed of plump, stellate, or spindled cells arranged in cords and primitive-appearing vessels in loose, myxoid stroma
  - – Stroma often contains hemorrhage or hemosiderin with variable numbers of inflammatory cells
- o Heterologous elements such as glands or extramedullary hematopoiesis can be found in small minority of cases (2%)
- PPNAD
  - o Nodules composed of cells with compact eosinophilic cytoplasm, with abundant brown granular pigment (lipofuscin)
  - o Cell nuclei are vesicular and may contain prominent nucleoli
  - o Intervening cortical tissue is atrophic, and may present myelolipomatous changes
- Large cell calcifying Sertoli cell tumor
  - o Tumor has ill-defined periphery
  - o Multiple cellular arrangements patterns of distribution: Usually solid or trabecular
  - o Large tumor cells with abundant granular and eosinophilic cytoplasm
  - o Laminated calcospherites are characteristic
    - – May be only few or multiple, and often with confluence
  - o Mitoses are rare
  - o Neutrophilic infiltration is usually present
- Pituitary adenoma
  - o Adenoma with solid growth pattern
  - o Round and polygonal cells with granular eosinophilic cytoplasm with round to oval nuclei
  - o Usually GH- &/or prolactin-producing tumors
  - o Ultrastructural examination: Large, tightly packed cells with complex interdigitations, abundant rough endoplasmic reticulum and conspicuous Golgi complexes
- Psammomatous melanotic schwannoma
  - o Peripheral nerve sheath tumor affecting posterior spinal nerve roots, alimentary tract, bone, and skin
  - o Spindle and epithelioid cells intermixed with melanin, psammoma bodies, and adipose tissue
  - o Spindle cells are arranged in interlacing fascicles and show whorling and occasionally nuclear palisading
  - o ~ 10% are malignant and metastasize
  - o Ultrastructural examination: Cells with elongated processes, continuous basal lamina, and melanosomes, as well as premelanosomes and intercellular long spacing collagen
- Osteochondromyxomas
  - o Polymorphic histology, including areas of polygonal, stellate, or bipolar cells
  - o Immature osteoid, with increased numbers of osteoclasts, indicating rapid bone remodeling

ANCILLARY TESTS

Immunohistochemistry
- Atrial myxoma
  - o Cells stain positive for CD34, CD31, and S100
  - o Calretinin is positive in 74-100% of cases and can be useful to distinguish this lesion from myxoid thrombus
- PPNAD

- o Increased expression of glucocorticoid receptor
- o Positive for inhibin-α, Melan-A, and synaptophysin
- Large cell calcifying Sertoli cell tumor
  - o Positive for vimentin, inhibin-α, NSE, S100, desmin, and smooth muscle actin
  - o Negative for α-fetoprotein, HCG, PLAP, podoplanin, OCT3/4, and cytokeratin (may be focally positive)
- Psammomatous melanotic schwannoma
  - o Positive for S100 protein and vimentin, whereas staining for GFAP, actin, and keratin are negative

Genetic Testing
- Genetic heterogeneity, with at least 2 main loci for candidate genes
  - o Mutations of *PRKAR1A* gene on chromosome 17 (17q24)
  - o CNC2 on Chromosome 2 locus 2p16
  - o And 2 other rare genetic changes
    - – *PRKACA* copy number gain and *PRKACB*

DIFFERENTIAL DIAGNOSIS

Other Syndromes
- Shares clinical features and molecular pathways with other familial lentiginosis syndromes
  - o In all of these conditions, skin lesions accompany underlying endocrine &/or other abnormalities, and, similarly to CNC, are considered important diagnostic sign

McCune-Albright Syndrome
- Probably closest to CNC in terms of molecular pathway link
- Patients with this condition have characteristic lesions that affect predominantly 3 systems: Skin, endocrine system, and skeleton
- Café au lait spots in McCune-Albright syndrome patients are similar to those observed in CNC
  - o Tend to be more intensely pigmented
- Caused by postzygotic activating mutations of gene encoding adenylate cyclase stimulating G α protein (*GNAS1*) of heterotrimeric G protein

Peutz-Jeghers Syndrome
- Autosomal dominant familial lentiginosis syndrome characterized by melanocytic macules of lips, buccal mucosa, and digits, multiple gastrointestinal hamartomatous polyps, and increased risk of various neoplasms
- Lentigines observed in patients with Peutz-Jeghers syndrome (PJS) show similar density and distribution to those in CNC
- PJS was 1st mapped to chromosome 19p13.3, and gene encoding serine threonine kinase 11 (*STK11* a.k.a. LKB1) was found to be mutated in most patients

Cowden Disease and Bannayan-Ruvalcaba-Riley Syndrome (*PTEN*-Hamartoma Tumor Syndrome)
- Cowden disease and Bannayan-Ruvalcaba-Riley syndrome share clinical characteristics such as mucocutaneous lesions, hamartomatous polyps of gastrointestinal tract, and increased risk of developing neoplasms
- Both conditions are caused by mutations in *PTEN* gene
  - o *PTEN* is located on 10q23.31 and encodes phosphatidylinositol (3,4,5)-triphosphate 3-phosphatase

Genomic Locus and Genes Associated With CNC

Locus/Gene	Chromosomal Locus	Mutation Type	Expression/Protein
PRKAR1A (CNC1)	17q24	Missense, nonsense, Frameshift (Over 125 pathogenic mutations)	Altered protein, elongated protein, and shorter protein
CNC2	2p16	NA	NA
PRKACA	19p13.1	Large gene amplification	Overexpression
PRKACB	1p31.1	Large gene amplification	Overexpression

- – Tumor suppressor gene that has been found mutated in number of tumors
- Thyroid is usually affected by numerous adenomatous nodules, follicular adenomas, and follicular carcinoma
  - o Findings are similar to those familial syndromes characterized by predominance of nonthyroidal tumors
    - – PTEN-hamartoma tumor syndrome, CNC, Werner syndrome, and Pendred syndrome

LEOPARD

- Multiple **l**entigines, **e**lectrocardiographic conduction abnormalities, **o**cular hypertelorism, **p**ulmonic stenosis, **a**bnormal genitalia, **r**etardation of growth, and sensorineural **d**eafness
- Allelic to Noonan syndrome: Both diseases are linked to mutations in *PTPN11* (12q24), gene encoding nonreceptor tyrosine phosphatase Shp-2
- Protein encoded by this gene is member of protein tyrosine phosphatase family, proteins that are known to regulate variety of cellular processes including cell growth, differentiation, mitotic cycle, and oncogenic transformation

SELECTED REFERENCES

1. Idrees MT et al: The World Health Organization 2016 classification of testicular non-germ cell tumours: a review and update from the International Society of Urological Pathology Testis Consultation Panel. Histopathology. 70(4):513-521, 2017
2. Lowe KM et al: Cushing syndrome in Carney complex: clinical, pathologic, and molecular genetic findings in the 17 affected mayo clinic patients. Am J Surg Pathol. 41(2):171-181, 2017
3. Hannah-Shmouni F et al: Genetics of gigantism and acromegaly. Growth Horm IGF Res. 30-31:37-41, 2016
4. Schernthaner-Reiter MH et al: MEN1, MEN4, and Carney complex: pathology and molecular genetics. Neuroendocrinology. 103(1):18-31, 2016
5. Stratakis CA: Hereditary syndromes predisposing to endocrine tumors and their skin manifestations. Rev Endocr Metab Disord. 17(3):381-388, 2016
6. Stratakis CA: Carney complex: a familial lentiginosis predisposing to a variety of tumors. Rev Endocr Metab Disord. 17(3):367-371, 2016
7. Berthon AS et al: PRKACA: the catalytic subunit of protein kinase A and adrenocortical tumors. Front Cell Dev Biol. 3:26, 2015
8. Correa R et al: Carney complex: an update. Eur J Endocrinol. 173(4):M85-97, 2015
9. Salpea P et al: Carney complex and McCune Albright syndrome: an overview of clinical manifestations and human molecular genetics. Mol Cell Endocrinol. 386(1-2):85-91, 2014
10. Gaal J et al: SDHB immunohistochemistry: a useful tool in the diagnosis of Carney-Stratakis and Carney triad gastrointestinal stromal tumors. Mod Pathol. 24(1):147-51, 2011
11. Janeway KA et al: Defects in succinate dehydrogenase in gastrointestinal stromal tumors lacking KIT and PDGFRA mutations. Proc Natl Acad Sci U S A. 108(1):314-8, 2011
12. Laury AR et al: Thyroid pathology in PTEN-hamartoma tumor syndrome: characteristic findings of a distinct entity. Thyroid. 21(2):135-44, 2011
13. Lodish MB et al: The differential diagnosis of familial lentiginosis syndromes. Fam Cancer. 10(3):481-90, 2011
14. Nosé V: Familial thyroid cancer: a review. Mod Pathol. 24 Suppl 2:S19-33, 2011
15. Saggini A et al: Skin lesions in hereditary endocrine tumor syndromes. Endocr Pract. 17 Suppl 3:47-57, 2011
16. Smith JR et al: Thyroid nodules and cancer in children with PTEN hamartoma tumor syndrome. J Clin Endocrinol Metab. 96(1):34-7, 2011
17. Zhang Y et al: Endocrine tumors as part of inherited tumor syndromes. Adv Anat Pathol. 18(3):206-18, 2011
18. Almeida MQ et al: Solid tumors associated with multiple endocrine neoplasias. Cancer Genet Cytogenet. 203(1):30-6, 2010
19. Horvath A et al: Mutations and polymorphisms in the gene encoding regulatory subunit type 1-alpha of protein kinase A (PRKAR1A): an update. Hum Mutat. 31(4):369-79, 2010
20. Kirschner LS: PRKAR1A and the evolution of pituitary tumors. Mol Cell Endocrinol. 326(1-2):3-7, 2010
21. Nosé V: Familial follicular cell tumors: classification and morphological characteristics. Endocr Pathol. 21(4):219-26, 2010
22. Nosé V: Thyroid cancer of follicular cell origin in inherited tumor syndromes. Adv Anat Pathol. 17(6):428-36, 2010
23. Pan L et al: Novel PRKAR1A gene mutations in Carney complex. Int J Clin Exp Pathol. 3(5):545-8, 2010
24. Storr HL et al: Familial isolated primary pigmented nodular adrenocortical disease associated with a novel low penetrance PRKAR1A gene splice site mutation. Horm Res Paediatr. 73(2):115-9, 2010
25. Vezzosi D et al: Carney complex: Clinical and genetic 2010 update. Ann Endocrinol (Paris). 71(6):486-93, 2010
26. Zhang L et al: Gastric stromal tumors in Carney triad are different clinically, pathologically, and behaviorally from sporadic gastric gastrointestinal stromal tumors: findings in 104 cases. Am J Surg Pathol. 34(1):53-64, 2010
27. Horvath A et al: Carney complex and lentiginosis. Pigment Cell Melanoma Res. 22(5):580-7, 2009
28. Stratakis CA et al: The triad of paragangliomas, gastric stromal tumours and pulmonary chondromas (Carney triad), and the dyad of paragangliomas and gastric stromal sarcomas (Carney-Stratakis syndrome): molecular genetics and clinical implications. J Intern Med. 266(1):43-52, 2009
29. Stratakis CA: New genes and/or molecular pathways associated with adrenal hyperplasias and related adrenocortical tumors. Mol Cell Endocrinol. 300(1-2):152-7, 2009
30. Horvath A et al: Clinical and molecular genetics of acromegaly: MEN1, Carney complex, McCune-Albright syndrome, familial acromegaly and genetic defects in sporadic tumors. Rev Endocr Metab Disord. 9(1):1-11, 2008
31. Mateus C et al: Heterogeneity of skin manifestations in patients with Carney complex. J Am Acad Dermatol. 59(5):801-10, 2008
32. Nose' V: Familial non-medullary thyroid carcinoma: an update. Endocr Pathol. 19(4):226-40, 2008
33. Boikos SA et al: Pituitary pathology in patients with Carney complex: growth-hormone producing hyperplasia or tumors and their association with other abnormalities. Pituitary. 9(3):203-9, 2006
34. Horvath A et al: Serial analysis of gene expression in adrenocortical hyperplasia caused by a germline PRKAR1A mutation. J Clin Endocrinol Metab. 91(2):584-96, 2006
35. Lacroix A et al: Bilateral adrenal Cushing's syndrome: macronodular adrenal hyperplasia and primary pigmented nodular adrenocortical disease. Endocrinol Metab Clin North Am. 34(2):441-58, x, 2005
36. Libé R et al: Mutational analysis of PRKAR1A and Gs(alpha) in sporadic adrenocortical tumors. Exp Clin Endocrinol Diabetes. 113(5):248-51, 2005
37. Stratakis CA, Horvath A. Carney complex. 1993-, 2003
38. Kirschner L. S.; Lloyd R. V.; Stratakis C. A. Carney Complex. In: WHO, 2017. p.269-271

Inner and Outer Eye Canthi Pigmentation

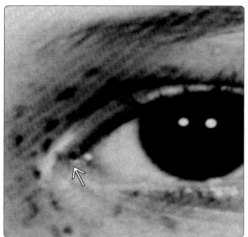

Large Atrial Myxoma

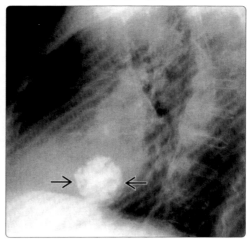

(Left) *There is conjunctival and inner* ➡ *and outer canthi pigmentation in Carney complex, usually associated with sooty skin pigmentation with typical distribution in lips and vaginal and penile mucosa. (Courtesy of A. Carney, MD.)* (Right) *Lateral radiograph shows densely calcified left atrial myxoma* ➡. *This patient had multiple transient ischemic attacks, a clinical feature associated with cardiac myxoma.*

Atrial Myxoma

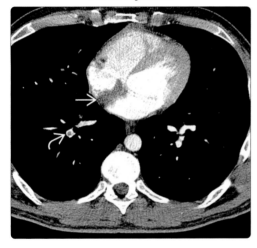

Calcification Seen in LCCSCT

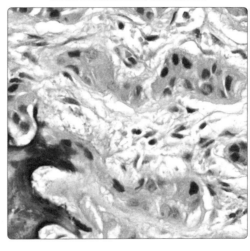

(Left) *Axial CECT shows myxoma involving the interarterial septum and extending into the right atrium* ➡. *A tumor embolism is seen in a right lower lobe pulmonary artery branch* ➡. *Tumor is of decreased density compared to contrasted heart chambers and has a different density than adipose tissue.* (Right) *Large cell calcifying Sertoli cell tumor (LCCSCT) is shown with nests of large epithelioid cells with abundant eosinophilic cytoplasm. A large area of calcification is seen in the loose fibromyxoid stroma.*

Epithelioid Cells and Neutrophils

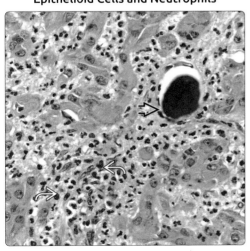

Calcifications

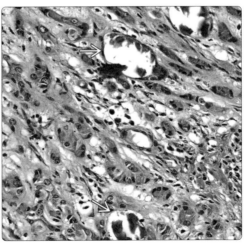

(Left) *LCCSCT shows cords and small nests of large epithelioid cells embedded in a fibrous background with dense neutrophilic infiltrate. A psammoma body* ➡ *is also seen. The neutrophilic background is an important diagnostic feature* ➡. (Right) *A LCCSCT is shown with cords of large epithelioid cells containing abundant eosinophilic cytoplasm. The hallmark of this tumor is the presence of scattered calcifications* ➡.

Subtle Changes in PPNAD

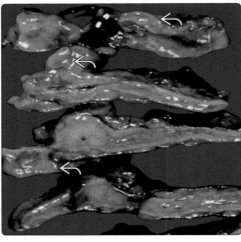

Variable-Sized Pigmented Nodules

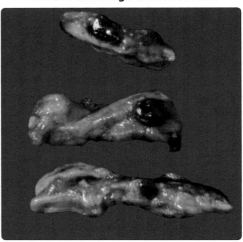

(Left) *Gross cross section of an adrenal gland from a patient with Cushing syndrome, Carney complex, and PPNAD shows the presence of small, yellow, nonpigmented nodules* 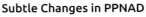*, most of which cannot be appreciated at gross examination.* (Right) *Gross cross section of an adrenal gland from a child with Cushing syndrome. There are multiple dark pigmented nodules from minute to large nodules. These gross findings are characteristic of Carney complex and PPNAD.*

Nodular Adrenal Cortex

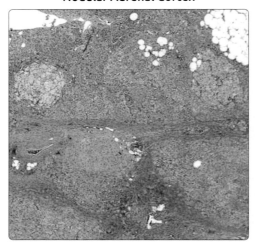

Pigment Deposition on PPNAD

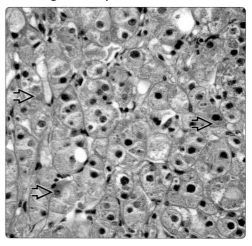

(Left) *On low-power magnification, the normal adrenal gland architecture is replaced by multiple nodules, most unencapsulated but some with a thin fibrous capsule. There is lipomatous metaplasia and the adjacent adrenal is atrophic.* (Right) *In PPNAD, there is loss of zonation of the adrenal cortex, which has multiple small cortical nodules, composed of enlarged globular cortical cells with granular and eosinophilic cytoplasm. Note variable amount of lipochrome pigment deposition* ➨.

Prominent Patchy Lipochrome Pigment

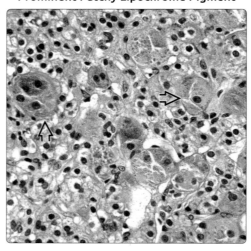

Diffuse Lipochrome Deposition

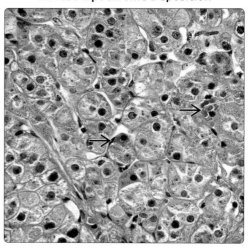

(Left) *The adrenal cortex show show numerous nodules in PPNAD. The nodules are composed by enlarged globular cortical cells with granular eosinophilic cytoplasm and with large amounts of lipochrome pigment* ➨. (Right) *In this field of an adrenal cortical nodule, there is a more uniform distribution of the lipochrome pigment with scattered areas* ➨ *of heavy pigment deposition.*

Graphic of Pituitary Adenoma

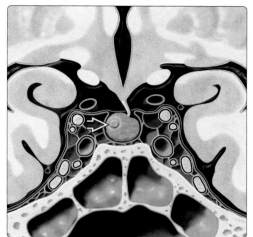

Cellular Morphology of Pituitary Adenoma

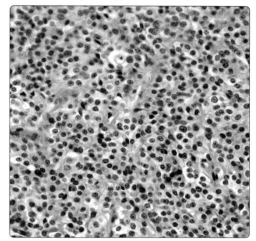

(Left) *Pituitary adenomas, microadenomas* ➡, *or macroadenomas, which are usually GH-producing adenomas, are typical findings in Carney complex.* **(Right)** *Photomicrograph shows a sparsely granulated, somatotroph adenoma composed of chromophobic cells. The nuclei can be centrally located but also tend to be eccentric, pushed to the cell periphery, and indented by the fibrous bodies.*

Keratin in Fibrous Bodies

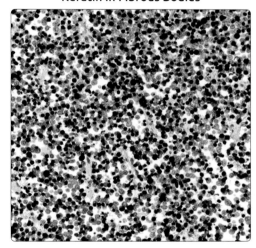

Keratin in Sparsely Granulated GH-Adenoma

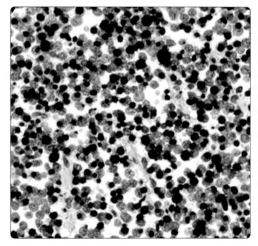

(Left) *CAM5.2 reveals diffuse paranuclear keratin aggresomes, "fibrous bodies", in sparsely granulated GH-adenomas. Occasional fibrous bodies can be seen in aggressive acidophil stem cell adenomas and other rare GH-adenomas.* **(Right)** *CAM5.2 reveals diffuse paranuclear keratin aggresomes ("fibrous bodies") in sparsely granulated somatotroph adenomas. Occasional fibrous bodies can be seen in aggressive acidophil stem cell adenomas, as well as in intermediate-type somatotroph adenomas.*

Growth Hormone Immunoexpression

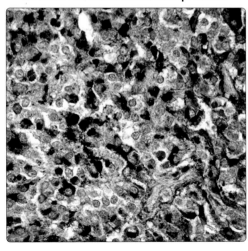

Variably GH Immunoexpression

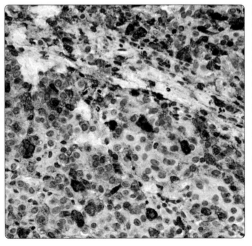

(Left) *GH in a densely granulated somatotroph adenoma shows numerous GH-containing cytoplasmic secretory granules that correlate with the cytoplasmic eosinophilic appearance on H&E.* **(Right)** *GH shows somatotroph adenomas harboring numerous GH-containing secretory granules with variable staining within the adenomatous cells.*

TERMINOLOGY

- Autosomal dominant disorder resulting from inactivating mutations in *CDC73* (HRPT2) gene

CLINICAL ISSUES

- Parathyroid hyperplasia or adenoma, increased risk of parathyroid carcinoma
  - Hyperparathyroidism: Severe hypercalcemia and higher incidence of parathyroid carcinoma
  - 80% of patients with hyperparathyroidism-jaw tumor syndrome (HPT-JT) present with hyperparathyroidism
  - Hyperparathyroidism usually develops late adolescence
  - 15% of patients with HPT-JT develop parathyroid carcinoma
- Tumor expansion of jaw bone
  - Ossifying fibroma
- Other features reported include: Renal cysts, Wilms tumor, hamartomas, and papillary thyroid carcinoma

IMAGING

- Ossifying fibroma: Well-demarcated, expansile mass with mixed soft tissue density central area surrounded by ossified rim
- Parathyroid adenoma or carcinoma: Tc-99m sestamibi scintigraphy or sonography identifies location but does not separate adenoma from carcinoma; mass on CT or MR with no specific features

MICROSCOPIC

- Ossifying fibroma: Densely cellular, well-defined fibrous tumor that ossifies beginning at periphery
- Parathyroid pathology: Parathyroid hyperplasia, adenoma, or parathyroid carcinoma
  - Caution: Complete loss of parafibromin (CDC73) protein expression helpful in separating parathyroid carcinoma from adenoma, but parafibromin expression may be lost in parathyroid adenomas associated with germline *CDC73* mutations such as with HPT-JT syndrome

Parathyroid Carcinoma Invading Skeletal Muscle

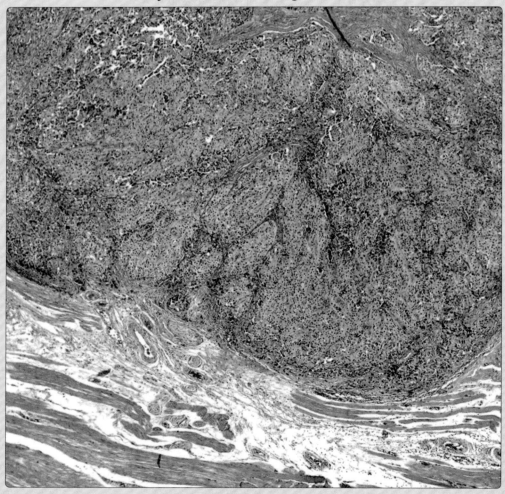

Approximately 15% of patients with hyperparathyroidism-jaw tumor syndrome develop parathyroid carcinoma. This parathyroid carcinoma is invading into the skeletal muscle.

TERMINOLOGY

Abbreviations

- Hyperparathyroidism-jaw tumor syndrome (HPT-JT)

Synonyms

- Familial cystic parathyroid adenomatosis

Definitions

- Autosomal dominant disorder characterized by parathyroid adenoma or carcinoma, ossifying fibromas of jaw bones, renal cysts and tumors, and hamartomas resulting from inactivating mutations in *CDC73* (HRPT2) gene

ETIOLOGY/PATHOGENESIS

Mutation of *CDC73* Gene on 1q25-q31

- Autosomal dominant
- Inactivating mutation of tumor suppressor gene *CDC73*
- 80% of mutations are truncating (frameshift and nonsense), most involve exon 1
- Strong association *CDC73* with mutation in familial and sporadic parathyroid carcinoma
- *CDC73* mutation uncommon in sporadic adenomas but identified in 20% of sporadic cystic adenomas
- HPT-JT associated with parathyroid adenoma or carcinoma, ossifying fibromas of jaw bones, renal cysts and tumors, and hamartoma
- *CDC73* encodes protein known as parafibromin (CDC73)
  - Germline *CDC73* mutations identified in subset of patients with mutation-positive carcinomas thought to be sporadic
- *CDC73*-related disorders
  - *CDC73* transcript spans 2.7 kb
  - CDC73 protein binds RNA polymerase II as part of PAF1 transcriptional regulatory complex, mediates H3K9 methylation that silences expression of cyclin-D1
  - *CDC73* mutation present in familial predisposition to parathyroid carcinoma (as with HPT-JT and familial isolated hyperparathyroidism)
  - CDC73 protein regulates gene expression and inhibits cell proliferation
  - Somatic inactivating *CDC73* mutations in some sporadic parathyroid carcinomas
    - Up to 75% *CDC73* inactivation, but may be higher as mutations may be outside of coding region sequenced in clinical testing and some research studies
    - Germline *CDC73* mutations present in substantial minority (20%) of clinically sporadic-appearing parathyroid carcinoma
    - Additional genes may be involved for malignant behavior
      - CCND1 overexpressed in many parathyroid carcinomas

CLINICAL ISSUES

Epidemiology

- Incidence
  - Yet unknown
  - First described in 1990; to date, < 40 families have been reported
  - Autosomal dominant

Presentation

- **Hyperparathyroidism**
  - 80% of HPT-JT patients present with hyperparathyroidism
  - Hyperparathyroidism usually develops in late adolescence
  - More aggressive course with severe hypercalcemia and higher incidence of parathyroid carcinoma
  - Penetrance of hyperparathyroidism is 80%
  - Parathyroid adenoma or carcinoma
  - 15% of patients with HPT-JT develop parathyroid carcinoma
  - Germline *CDC73* mutations identified in subset of patients with *CDC73* mutation-positive carcinomas
- **Jaw tumors**
  - Well-demarcated osseous lesion (ossifying fibroma) of mandible or maxilla
- Other features reported include renal cysts, hamartomas, Wilms tumor, and papillary thyroid carcinoma

Treatment

- Surgery

Prognosis

- Majority of patients with adenoma can be cured by surgery
- Guarded once parathyroid carcinoma confirmed
  - 15% of patients with HPT-JT develop parathyroid carcinoma

IMAGING

General Features

- Ossifying fibroma
  - Radiography: Well-demarcated, expansile mass with mixed soft tissue density central area surrounded by ossified rim
  - Bone scan: Increased uptake of affected bones
- Parathyroid
  - Tc-99m sestamibi scintigraphy or sonography identifies location but does not separate adenoma from carcinoma
  - Mass noted on CT and MR, often no specific features

MACROSCOPIC

General Features

- Ossifying fibroma gross pathology shows classic appearance of tumor with central pink-yellow area of fibrous tissue surrounded by pale yellow, dense, peripheral ossified tissue
- Parathyroid adenoma or carcinoma usually presents as single enlarged parathyroid gland
  - Parathyroid adenoma is single enlarged gland, tan to pink-tan, encapsulated, ± rim of normal tissue
    - Vary in size: < 1 cm to > 10 cm; weight: 0.2 to > 1 g
    - Cystic change may occur in adenomas, particularly larger adenomas and in those with HPT-JT syndrome
    - Larger adenomas may show fibrosis, hemosiderin, cystic degeneration, and calcification
  - Parathyroid carcinomas may be large, firm, and variably encapsulated, poorly circumscribed

- Large tumors (mean: 6.7 g, range: 1.5 to > 50 g); generally larger than adenomas, but overlap in size
- Lobulated appearance due to thick fibrous bands
- May be grossly encapsulated and resemble adenoma
- Firm tumors may be adherent to or invasive into adjacent structures
- Caution as large parathyroid adenomas, especially with cystic change, can become fibrotic and adhere to adjacent structures

MICROSCOPIC

Histologic Features

- **Hyperparathyroidism**
  o Caused by adenoma or carcinoma
  o Cystic changes
  o Both parathyroid adenoma and carcinoma are hypercellular
    - Mitoses may be seen in both adenoma and carcinoma but more mitoses in carcinoma than adenoma
    - Atypical mitoses generally seen only in carcinoma
    - Fibrous bands can be seen in both adenoma and carcinoma
    - Diagnosis of parathyroid carcinoma requires invasion (capsular, vascular, perineural, into adjacent structures) or metastases
- **Ossifying fibroma of jaw**
  o Microscopically, densely cellular, well-defined fibrous tumor that ossifies beginning at periphery
  o Tumor composed of dense, relatively avascular fibroblast-rich stroma and irregular spicules of woven bone with osteoblastic rimming

ANCILLARY TESTS

Genetic Testing

- DNA-based sequencing on *CDC73* gene
- *CDC73* mutation (tumor suppressor gene, 1q21-q31), encodes CDC73/parafibromin protein)
  o Strong association with *CDC73* mutation in familial and sporadic parathyroid cancer
    - 15% of patients with HPT-JT (caused by germine *CDC73* inactivating mutation) develop parathyroid carcinoma
    - Germline *CDC73* mutations identified in subset of patients with mutation-positive carcinomas
      □ Consider genetic testing in patients with parathyroid carcinoma
      □ Substantial minority of clinically sporadic parathyroid carcinomas may have germline mutation
      □ Up to 75% of parathyroid carcinomas have *CDC73* inactivation
      □ Clinical testing may not identify all mutations; inactivating *CDC73* mutations may be located outside coding region evaluated
  o *CDC73* mutation uncommon in sporadic adenomas but identified in 20% of sporadic cystic parathyroid adenoma (possibly HPT-JT related)

- Somatic *CDC73* mutations are common in sporadic parathyroid carcinomas and rare in sporadic adenomas but can be seen in adenomas in setting of HPT-JT syndrome
  o Complete loss of parafibromin (CDC73) protein expression helpful in separating parathyroid carcinoma from adenoma; however, parafibromin expression may be lost in parathyroid adenomas associated with germline *CDC73* mutations

Serologic Testing

- Blood test measuring ionized calcium and iPTH

DIFFERENTIAL DIAGNOSIS

Fibrous Dysplasia

- Caused by activating missense mutations of *GNAS* gene, which is benign bone tumor composed of woven bone and fibrous tissue in background
- In contrast to ossifying fibroma, fibrous dysplasia lacks osteoblastic rimming of woven bone

Multiple Endocrine Neoplasia Type 1

- Multiple endocrine neoplasia type 1 (MEN1) is characterized with hyperparathyroidism, pituitary adenoma, and pancreatic endocrine tumors caused by inactivation of *MEN1* gene
- Hyperparathyroidism in MEN1 is caused by multiglandular parathyroid hyperplasia in contrast to solitary adenoma or carcinoma in HPT-JT syndrome

SELECTED REFERENCES

1. Iacobone M et al: Surgical approaches in hereditary endocrine tumors. Updates Surg. 69(2):181-191, 2017
2. Pandya C et al: Genomic profiling reveals mutational landscape in parathyroid carcinomas. JCI Insight. 2(6):e92061, 2017
3. Simonds WF: Genetics of hyperparathyroidism, including parathyroid cancer. Endocrinol Metab Clin North Am. 46(2):405-418, 2017
4. Cetani F et al: Update on parathyroid carcinoma. J Endocrinol Invest. 39(6):595-606, 2016
5. Chen Y et al: CDC73 gene mutations in sporadic ossifying fibroma of the jaws. Diagn Pathol. 11(1):91, 2016
6. Thakker RV: Genetics of parathyroid tumours. J Intern Med. 280(6):574-583, 2016
7. DeLellis RA: Parathyroid tumors and related disorders. Mod Pathol. 24 Suppl 2:S78-93, 2011
8. Juhlin CC et al: Parafibromin as a diagnostic instrument for parathyroid carcinoma-lone ranger or part of the posse? Int J Endocrinol. 2010:324964, 2010
9. Wang P et al: Parafibromin, a component of the human PAF complex, regulates growth factors and is required for embryonic development and survival in adult mice. Mol Cell Biol. 28(9):2930-40, 2008
10. Carpten JD et al: HRPT2, encoding parafibromin, is mutated in hyperparathyroidism-jaw tumor syndrome. Nat Genet. 32(4):676-80, 2002
11. Szabó J et al: Hereditary hyperparathyroidism-jaw tumor syndrome: the endocrine tumor gene HRPT2 maps to chromosome 1q21-q31. Am J Hum Genet. 56(4):944-50, 1995
12. Jackson CE et al: Hereditary hyperparathyroidism and multiple ossifying jaw fibromas: a clinically and genetically distinct syndrome. Surgery. 108(6):1006-12; discussion 1012-3, 1990
13. Dinnen JS et al: Parathyroid carcinoma in familial hyperparathyroidism. J Clin Pathol. 30(10):966-75, 1977
14. Castleman B et al: The pathology of the parathyroid gland in hyperparathyroidism: a study of 25 cases. Am J Pathol. 11(1):1-72, 1935

Ossifying Fibroma

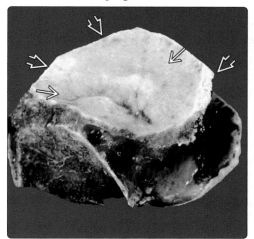

Axial Bone CT of Ossifying Fibroma

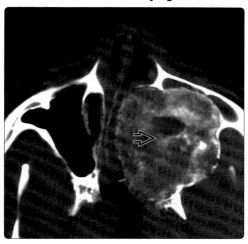

(Left) *Gross image shows the classic appearance of ossifying fibroma with central pink-yellow area of fibrous tissue* ➡ *surrounded by pale yellow, dense, peripheral ossified tissue* ➡. (Right) *Axial bone CT shows a large, well-demarcated left maxillary ossifying fibroma* ➡ *with mixed calcific and soft tissue density components. Note that the mass obstructs both sides of the nose.*

Ossifying Fibroma

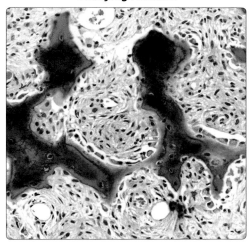

Parathyroid Adenoma With Rim

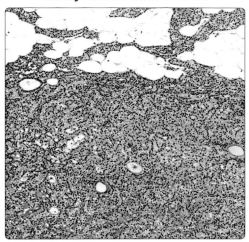

(Left) *Typical ossifying fibroma exhibits a dense, avascular, fibroblast-rich stroma and irregular spicules of woven bone with osteoblastic rimming.* (Right) *Approximately 80% of patients with hyperparathyroidism-jaw tumor syndrome develop hyperparathyroidism. Most occur by late adolescence. The hyperparathyroidism may be caused by parathyroid adenoma. However, 15% of patients develop parathyroid carcinoma.*

Parathyroid Adenoma

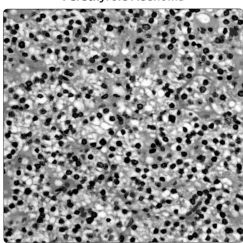

Chief Cells and Oxyphilic Cells in Parathyroid Adenoma

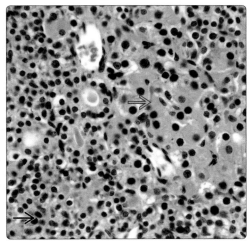

(Left) *Hypercellular parathyroid tissue is composed predominantly of parathyroid chief cells in this parathyroid adenoma.* (Right) *Parathyroid adenoma with chief cells* ➡ *and oxyphilic (oncocytic)* ➡ *cells is shown.*

TERMINOLOGY

- Paraganglioma syndromes 1-5 (PGL 1-5): Hereditary tumor syndromes caused by germline mutations of genes encoding subunits of succinate dehydrogenase (collectively *SDHx* genes)
- Carney triad: Nonhereditary combination of PGL, GIST, and pulmonary chondroma
- Carney-Stratakis dyad or syndrome: Not distinct entity, encompasses any combination of PGL and GIST

CLINICAL ISSUES

- *SDHx* mutations account for > 80% of familial groupings of PGLs, 15-25% of all patients, almost 30% of pediatric patients, > 40% of tumors that metastasize, almost 10% of apparently sporadic tumors,
- *SDHB* mutations most common (~ 6-8%), *SDHD* (~ 5-6%), *SDHC* (~ 1-2%), *SDHA* (~ 1%); *SDHAF2* mutations very rare
- Specific mutated gene determines number and distribution of tumors and risk of metastasis

- Penetrance very variable, no predetermined patterns of tumor development in individuals or families
- High risk of metastasis (> 30%) and poor long-term survival are associated with *SDHB* mutations

MICROSCOPIC

- Often small amphophilic to clear cells, can mimic primary or metastatic carcinomas

ANCILLARY TESTS

- Any *SDHx* mutation causes loss of enzyme activity, destabilization of enzyme complex, and loss of SDHB protein
- IHC for SDHB serves to triage for genetic testing or as surrogate where testing not available; also to validate genetic sequence variants of unknown significance and to assess whether any particular tumor is syndromic or coincidental in patient with known or suspected *SDHx* mutation

Metastatic Paraganglioma

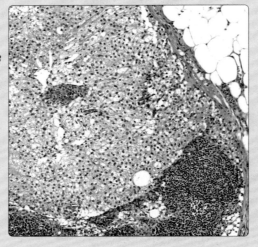

Negative IHC for SDHB in Metastatic Paraganglioma

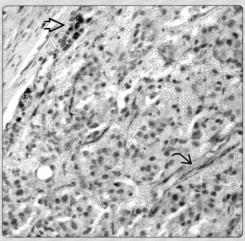

(Left) This lymph node shows metastatic paraganglioma (PGL) with SDHB mutation. (Right) IHC stain for SDHB in this metastatic PGL with SDHB mutation shows absent staining in tumor cells and strong granular staining in endothelial cells ⟹, which are a mandatory intrinsic control, and in a few peripheral histiocytes ⟹. A typical nested (zellballen) tumor architecture is also seen.

SDH-Deficient Renal Cell Carcinoma

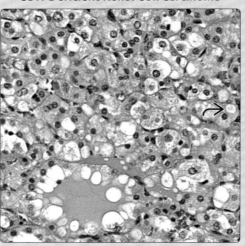

Negative IHC for SDHB in SDH-Deficient RCC

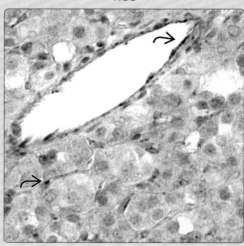

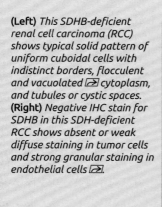

(Left) This SDHB-deficient renal cell carcinoma (RCC) shows typical solid pattern of uniform cuboidal cells with indistinct borders, flocculent and vacuolated ⟹ cytoplasm, and tubules or cystic spaces. (Right) Negative IHC stain for SDHB in this SDH-deficient RCC shows absent or weak diffuse staining in tumor cells and strong granular staining in endothelial cells ⟹.

TERMINOLOGY

Definitions

- Paraganglioma syndromes 1-5 (PGL 1-5): Hereditary tumor syndromes caused by germline mutations of genes encoding subunits of succinate dehydrogenase (*SDHA*, *SDHB*, *SDHC*, *SDHD*) or *SDHAF2*, collectively *SDHx* genes
- Carney triad: Nonhereditary combination of paraganglioma (PGL), gastrointestinal stromal tumor (GIST), and pulmonary chondroma
- Carney-Stratakis dyad or syndrome: Not distinct entity, encompasses any combination of PGL and GIST

ETIOLOGY/PATHOGENESIS

Genetics

- PGL 1-5: Autosomal dominant loss-of-function germline mutation followed by somatic 2nd hit, often large deletion that may involve tumor suppressor genes in addition to specific *SDHx* allele
  - PGL 1 and PGL 2 show parent-of-origin effect: Germline mutation transmissible by either parent, disease usually occurs only with paternal transmission
    - Resultant skipping of generations can obscure family histories
- Carney triad: Epigenetic silencing, predominantly by promoter methylation of *SDHC*

Postulated Mechanisms of Tumorigenesis

- Pseudohypoxic signaling, genomic hypermethylation, reactive oxygen species (ROS)
  - Normal SDH converts succinate to fumarate in Krebs cycle and functions in mitochondrial electron transport chain as complex ll
  - Loss of activity causes succinate buildup, interruption of oxidative phosphorylation, accumulation of ROS
    - Succinate inhibits α-ketoglutarate-dependent histone/DNA demethylases and prolyl hydroxylases that control levels of hypoxia-inducible transcription factors

CLINICAL ISSUES

Epidemiology

- *SDHx* mutations account for > 80% of familial groupings of PGLs, 15-25% of all patients, almost 30% of pediatric patients, > 40% of tumors that metastasize, and almost 10% of apparently sporadic tumors
  - *SDHB* mutations most common (~ 6-8%), *SDHD* (~ 5-6%), *SDHC* (~ 1-2%), *SDHA* (~ 1%); *SDHAF2* mutations extremely rare

Presentation

- Specific mutated gene determines number and distribution of tumors and risk of metastasis
- Penetrance very variable, no predetermined patterns of tumor development in individuals or families
  - Syndromically associated tumors [SDH-deficient GIST, renal cell carcinoma (RCC), or pituitary adenoma] can develop in some patients ± PGL
    - SDH-deficient GIST: Usually in children or young adults

- ~ 30% of all SDH-deficient GISTs occur in patients with *SDHA* mutations; ~ 50% in patients with Carney triad
- 5.0-7.5% of all gastric GISTs in adults; overwhelming majority in children
  - SDH-deficient RCC: Age range: 14-76 years; mean: 37 years with slight male predominance (M:F = 1.7:1.0); bilateral in 26% of patients
    - Occur in up to 14% of patients with *SDHB* and 8% with *SDHD* mutations
  - SDH-deficient pituitary adenomas appear very rare but possibly are under diagnosed

Treatment

- Only surgical excision is curative; no highly effective treatments available for metastases
  - Some benefit of temozolomide for tumors with hypermethylation of O6-methylguanine-DNA methyltransferase (*MGMT*) promoter and deficient expression of MGMT
  - **Peptide receptor radionuclide therapy (PRRT)**: Radiolabeled somatostatin analogs show efficacy in small series; most PGL strongly express somatostatin receptor SSTR2A
  - Potential new modalities target metabolic vulnerabilities caused by loss of SDH

Prognosis

- High risk of metastasis (> 30%) and poor long-term survival with *SDHB* mutations
  - Risk might reflect large size and extraadrenal locations of *SDHB* mutated tumors, both independent predictors of metastasis
  - Metastases may occur years after primary or be present at initial Dx
- Staging system introduced in 8th edition of AJCC staging manual
  - Size > 5 cm **or** extraadrenal abdominal location is automatically staged as T2
  - System does not account for *SDHB* mutation, which is most significant prognostic factor

IMAGING

General Features

- Somatostatin receptor imaging by PET/CT using recently developed "DOTA": Conjugated somatostatin analogs is most sensitive modality
  - DOTA peptides can be labeled with PET tracer (68Ga) for diagnosis or with therapeutic b-emitters (177Lu) or (90Y) for follow-up PRRT

MICROSCOPIC

Histologic Features

- SDH-related PC and PGL have no specific features distinguishing them from other hereditary or sporadic counterparts
  - Often small amphophilic to clear cells
  - Varied histologic patterns; classic zellballen architecture not always apparent, especially in small metastatic foci
  - Sustentacular cells rare in metastases and in some abdominal primaries

Familial Paraganglioma Syndromes

Syndrome	Gene	Chromosome	PC or PGL Distribution
PGL1	SDHD	11q23.1	H&N (~ 85%) , Adr (~ 10-25%), Abd, thorax ~ 60% multifocal
PGL2	SDHAF2	11q12.2	H&N (Adr, Abd & thorax very rare)
PGL3	SDHC	1q23.3	H&N, Thorax (Adr & Abd very rare) ~ 15-20% multifocal
PGL4	SDHB	1p36.13	Abd (~ 50%), H&N (~20-30%), Adr (~20-25%), thorax ~ 20-25% multifocal
PGL5	SDHA	5p15.33	Abd, Adr, H&N, (thorax very rare)

PC = pheochromocytoma; PGL = paraganglioma; H&N = head & neck; Adr = adrenal; Abd = abdomen; PC is intraadrenal PGL.

- Distinctive features exist for syndromically associated tumors
  - SDH-deficient GIST
    - Gastric location, predominantly epithelioid, often plexiform and multinodular architecture
  - SDH-deficient RCC
    - Typically uniform cuboidal cells with indistinct borders, flocculent and vacuolated cytoplasm, solid pattern surrounding tubules or cystic spaces
    - Historically misdiagnosed as clear cell or other RCC types
- SDH-deficient GIST or RCC can be poorly differentiated; IHC for SDHB advisable to rule out SDH deficiency for any morphologically or clinically unusual unusual examples of these tumors

ANCILLARY TESTS

Immunohistochemistry

- Any *SDHx* mutation causes loss of enzyme activity, destabilization of enzyme complex and loss of SDHB protein
- IHC for SDHB important for multiple purposes
  - Triage for genetic testing or surrogate where testing not available
  - Validate genetic sequence variants of unknown significance
  - Assess whether any particular tumor is part of syndrome or coincidental in patient with known or suspected *SDHx* mutation
- SDHA staining is preserved except when *SDHA* gene is mutated, can serve as adjunct to SDHB stain

DIFFERENTIAL DIAGNOSIS

Primary or Metastatic Carcinomas, Especially Those With Small Clear Cells

- Differential depends on anatomic location; includes squamous cell carcinoma, prostatic adenocarcinoma, RCC
  - PGLs positive for synaptophysin and chromogranin A, usually negative for keratins
    - Tyrosine hydroxylase shows excellent specificity but often negative in H&N PGLs

Paraganglioma Metastasis vs. 2nd Primary

- Metastases must be to site where normal paraganglionic tissue not present

- Very rare primary PGLs occur in lung and near hilum of liver; especially solitary lesions in these sites must be interpreted with caution
- Only sites that unequivocally qualify are bone and histologically confirmed lymph node

SELECTED REFERENCES

1. Kim E et al: Utility of the succinate: fumarate ratio for assessing SDH dysfunction in different tumor types. Mol Genet Metab Rep. 10:45-49, 2017
2. Jochmanova I et al: Pheochromocytoma: the first metabolic endocrine cancer. Clin Cancer Res. 22(20):5001-5011, 2016
3. Laukka T et al: Fumarate and succinate regulate expression of hypoxia-inducible genes via TET enzymes. J Biol Chem. 291(8):4256-65, 2016
4. Pinato DJ et al: Peptide receptor radionuclide therapy for metastatic paragangliomas. Med Oncol. 33(5):47, 2016
5. Benn DE et al: 15 years of paraganglioma: clinical manifestations of paraganglioma syndromes types 1-5. Endocr Relat Cancer. 22(4):T91-T103, 2015
6. Her YF et al: Oxygen concentration controls epigenetic effects in models of familial paraganglioma. PLoS One. 10(5):e0127471, 2015
7. Hoekstra AS et al: Models of parent-of-origin tumorigenesis in hereditary paraganglioma. Semin Cell Dev Biol. 43:117-24, 2015
8. Janssen I et al: Superiority of [68Ga]-DOTATATE PET/CT to other functional imaging modalities in the localization of SDHB-associated metastatic pheochromocytoma and paraganglioma. Clin Cancer Res. 21(17):3888-95, 2015
9. Kim E et al: Structural and functional consequences of succinate dehydrogenase subunit B mutations. Endocr Relat Cancer. 22(3):387-97, 2015
10. Papathomas TG et al: SDHB/SDHA immunohistochemistry in pheochromocytomas and paragangliomas: a multicenter interobserver variation analysis using virtual microscopy: a multinational study of the European Network for the Study of Adrenal Tumors (ENS@T). Mod Pathol. 28(6):807-21, 2015
11. Gill AJ et al: Succinate dehydrogenase (SDH)-deficient renal carcinoma: a morphologically distinct entity: a clinicopathologic series of 36 tumors from 27 patients. Am J Surg Pathol. 38(12):1588-602, 2014
12. Gill AJ et al: Succinate dehydrogenase deficiency is rare in pituitary adenomas. Am J Surg Pathol. 38(4):560-6, 2014
13. Hadoux J et al: SDHB mutations are associated with response to temozolomide in patients with metastatic pheochromocytoma or paraganglioma. Int J Cancer. 135(11):2711-20, 2014
14. Tischler AS et al: The adrenal medulla and extra-adrenal paraganglia: then and now. Endocr Pathol. 25(1):49-58, 2014
15. Letouzé E et al: SDH mutations establish a hypermethylator phenotype in paraganglioma. Cancer Cell. 23(6):739-52, 2013
16. Eisenhofer G et al: Plasma methoxytyramine: a novel biomarker of metastatic pheochromocytoma and paraganglioma in relation to established risk factors of tumour size, location and SDHB mutation status. Eur J Cancer. 48(11):1739-49, 2012
17. Xiao M et al: Inhibition of α-KG-dependent histone and DNA demethylases by fumarate and succinate that are accumulated in mutations of FH and SDH tumor suppressors. Genes Dev. 26(12):1326-38, 2012

Metastatic Paraganglioma

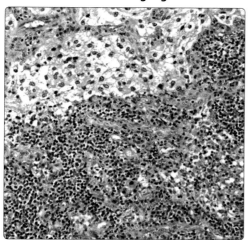

Sustentacular Cells in Metastatic Paraganglioma

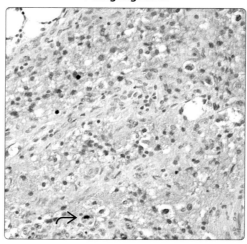

(Left) *The differential diagnosis for this focal lymph node metastasis includes squamous cell carcinoma and other tumors with clear cell features.* (Right) *Sustentacular cells are often absent or rare in PGL metastases, as shown in this IHC stain for S100 ⊠.*

Metastatic Paraganglioma

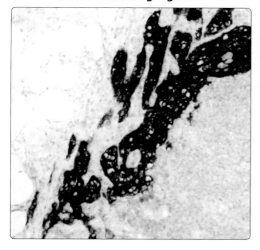

Somatostatin Receptor Expression

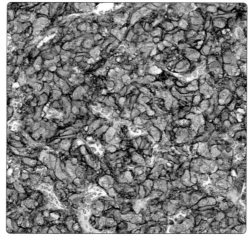

(Left) *IHC for synaptophysin discriminates this metastatic PGL from tumor types that are not neuroendocrine.* (Right) *SDHB-mutated PGL shows typical strong membrane staining for SSTR2A, consistent with the high sensitivity of somatostatin receptor imaging by PET/CT.*

Abdominal Paraganglioma With Intact SDHB

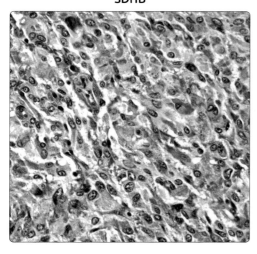

Positive IHC for SDHB in Sporadic Paraganglioma

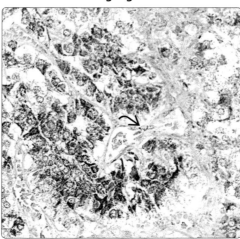

(Left) *Abdominal PGL with intact SDHB has somewhat basophilic cytoplasm and a poorly defined zellballen pattern.* (Right) *Tumor cells in this sporadic PGL show preserved granular cytoplasmic staining of the same intensity as in endothelial cells ⊠, consistent with intact SDHB. The granular staining reflects mitochondrial localization of SDHB protein.*

TERMINOLOGY

- Familial follicular cell tumors classified in 2 subgroups
  - Familial tumor syndrome with predominance of nonmedullary thyroid carcinoma (nonsyndromic)
  - Familial tumor syndromes characterized by predominance of nonmedullary thyroid carcinoma (syndromic)
    - PTEN-hamartoma tumor syndrome (PHTS)
    - Familial adenomatous polyposis (FAP)
    - Carney complex
    - Werner syndrome
    - Pendred syndrome
    - DICER1 syndrome
- Familial medullary thyroid carcinoma occurs in 3 distinct settings
  - Multiple endocrine neoplasia 2A
  - Multiple endocrine neoplasia 2B
  - Medullary thyroid carcinoma-only

ANCILLARY TESTS

- CMV-PTC has aberrant nuclear and cytoplasmic expression of β-catenin
- Immunostain for *PTEN* is lost in cases of PHTS/Cowden syndrome
- All other familial tumors have similar immunophenotype as their sporadic thyroid tumor counterparts
- Germline point mutation in *RET* gene responsible for hereditary MTC
- Patients with FAP-associated PTC have *APC* germline mutations
- Patients with PHTS have *PTEN* mutations

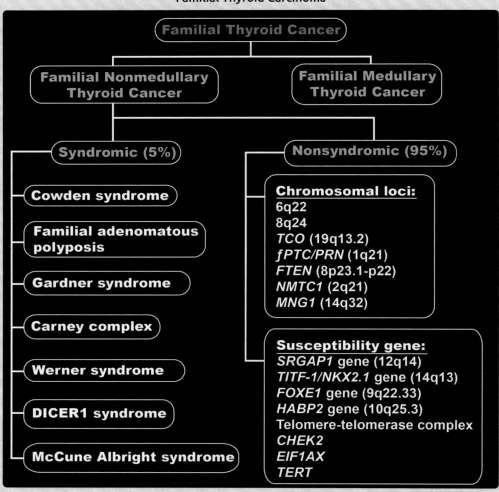

Familial Thyroid Carcinoma

Familial thyroid cancer are divided according to the cell of origin. Familial medullary thyroid carcinoma represents 25% of all medullary cancers. Familial nonmedullary thyroid carcinoma (FNMTC) constitutes ~ 10% of all thyroid cancers and only 5%, the syndromic forms, have known driver germline mutations. The susceptibility chromosomal loci and genes of the nonsyndromic FNMTC cases remain to be identified and characterized. Some of the genes on this chart still needs to be validated.

TERMINOLOGY

Abbreviations

- Familial nonmedullary thyroid carcinoma (FNMTC)
- Familial medullary thyroid carcinoma (FMTC)

Definitions

- Thyroid carcinoma occurring in familial setting
  - Can be syndrome-associated or nonsyndromic
- Familial thyroid carcinomas are divided into 2 subgroups: FNMTC and FMTC
- **FNMTC or familial follicular cell tumors**: Derived from thyroid follicular cells
  - Further subdivided into 2 subgroups
    - Familial tumor syndromes characterized by predominance of nonthyroidal tumors
    - Familial tumor syndromes characterized by predominance of nonmedullary thyroid carcinoma
- **FMTC**: Derived from thyroid calcitonin-producing C cells
  - Occurs in 3 distinct settings
    - FMTC (medullary thyroid carcinoma-only syndrome)
    - Multiple endocrine neoplasia 2A (MEN2A)
    - Multiple endocrine neoplasia 2B (MEN2B)

ETIOLOGY/PATHOGENESIS

Familial Nonmedullary Thyroid Cancer

- Constitutes 3-9% of all thyroid cancers
- Out of all FNMTC cases, only 5% in syndromic form have well-studied driver germline mutations
  - These associated syndromes include Cowden syndrome (CS), familial adenomatous polyposis (FAP), Gardner syndrome, Carney complex type 1, Werner syndrome, and DICER1 syndrome

Familial Follicular Cell Tumors or Familial Nonmedullary Thyroid Carcinoma

- Rare tumors encompassing heterogeneous group of diseases including both syndrome-associated and nonsyndromic tumors
- **Familial tumor syndromes characterized by predominance of nonmedullary thyroid carcinoma**
  - **PTEN-hamartoma tumor syndrome (PHTS)**: CS and Bannayan-Riley-Ruvalcaba syndrome are major entities composing PHTS
    - Characterized by multiple hamartomas involving multiple organs
    - Caused by germline mutations of *PTEN* gene and inherited in autosomal dominant fashion
    - *PTEN* (phosphatase and tensin homolog deleted on chromosome 10) is tumor suppressor gene located on 10q23.3
    - Can be caused by mutation of other genes: SDH genes, *PIK3CA*, *AKT1*, *KLLN*, *SEC23B*
  - **FAP**: Characterized by hundreds to thousands colorectal adenomas that develop during early adulthood
    - Inherited autosomal dominant syndrome caused by germline mutations in adenomatous polyposis coli (*APC*) gene on chromosome 5q21
  - **Carney complex**: Consists of myxomas, spotty pigmentation, and endocrine overactivity
    - Autosomal dominant disease

- Most cases classified as type 1 and associated with mutation of protein kinase A regulatory subunit type 1α (*PRKAR1A*) gene, probable tumor suppressor gene on chromosome 17q22-24
- Type 2 patients have mutation on chromosome 2p16, which may be regulator of genomic stability
  - **Werner syndrome**: Rare premature-aging syndrome that begins in 3rd decade
    - Autosomal recessive disease
    - Caused by mutations in *WRN* gene on chromosome 8p11-p12
  - **Pendred syndrome**: Most common hereditary syndrome associated with bilateral sensorineural deafness
    - Also called deaf-mutism and goiter
    - Autosomal recessive trait
    - Result of mutations in *SLC26A4* (*PDS*) gene, which encodes pendrin protein and is located on chromosome 7q21-34
    - 100 mutations identified in *PDS* gene, and most are family specific
  - **DICER1 syndrome**
    - Autosomal dominant pleiotropic syndrome caused by germline *DICER1* mutations
    - Tumors and dysplasias with early onset
      - Pleuropulmonary blastoma
      - Cystic nephroma
      - Multinodular thyroid hyperplasia
      - Ovarian tumors: Sertoli-Leydig cell tumor, juvenile granulosa cell tumor
      - Pituitary blastoma
- **Familial tumor syndromes characterized by predominance of nonmedullary thyroid carcinoma**
  - Characterized by ≥ 3 1st-degree relatives with follicular-derived nonmedullary thyroid carcinoma and occurs regardless of presence of another familial syndrome
  - Includes
    - **Pure familial papillary thyroid carcinoma (PTC) ± oxyphilia**: Mapped to chromosomal region 19q13
    - **Familial PTC (FPTC) with papillary renal cell carcinoma**: Mapped to chromosomal region 1q21
    - **FNMTC type 1**: Mapped to chromosome 2q21
    - **FPTC with multinodular goiter**: Mapped to chromosomal region 14q
  - Susceptibility chromosomal loci and genes of 95% of FNMTC cases remain to be characterized
    - To date, 4 susceptibility genes have been identified [*SRGAP1* gene (12q14), *TTF-1/NKX2.1* gene (14q13), *FOXE1* gene (9q22.33), and *HABP2* gene (10q25.3)]
      - Out of which only *FOXE1* and *HABP2* have been validated
    - Causal genes located at other 7 FNMTC-associated chromosomal loci [*TCO* (19q13.2), *fPTC/PRN* (1q21), *FTEN* (8p23.1-p22), *NMTC1* (2q21), *MNG1* (14q32), 6q22, 8q24] have yet to be identified
    - Increasingly, gene regulatory mechanisms (miRNA and enhancer elements) are recognized to affect gene expression and FNMTC tumorigenesis
    - Novel germline *SEC23B* variant, *SRGAP1* gene, *FOXE1* gene and *HABP2* genes in nonsyndromic FNMTC

Familial Medullary Thyroid Carcinoma

- Refers to those neoplasms arising from calcitonin-producing C cells derived from neural crest
- MTCs occur in sporadic or hereditary (25% of cases) forms, as part of MEN2 syndrome, or as MTC-only syndrome
  o MEN2 syndrome consists of 3 variants: MEN2A, MEN2B, and FMTC
  o MEN2A associated with pheochromocytoma and parathyroid hyperplasia
  o MEN2B associated with marfanoid habitus, mucosal neuromas, ganglioneuromatosis, and pheochromocytoma
- Germline gain-of-function mutations in *RET* protooncogene are major molecular drivers in pathogenesis of hereditary forms of MTC
  o ~ 85% of all *RET* mutations responsible for FMTC are known
  o In majority of MEN2A and FMTC patients, *RET* mutations clustered in 6 cysteine residues in *RET* cysteine-rich extracellular domain
  o Mutations detected in ~ 95% of MEN2A and ~ 85% of FMTC families
- Somatic *RET* point mutations identified in ~ 50% of patients with sporadic MTC

CLINICAL ISSUES

Epidemiology

- Incidence
  o Thyroid cancer accounts for only 1% of all malignant tumors
    – Advances in molecular genetics have confirmed presence of several familial cancer syndromes that have FNMTCs
  o 5% incidence of FNMTC in 95% of patients with well-differentiated thyroid cancer
  o Familial forms of follicular cell-derived tumors are rare and encompass heterogeneous group of diseases, including both syndrome-associated and nonsyndromic tumors
    – Thyroid neoplasms have been reported with increased frequency in familial syndromes, such as FAP, Cowden disease/PHTS, Carney complex type 1, Werner syndrome, Pendred syndrome, DICER1 syndrome
    – Among nonsyndromic tumors, predominant neoplasm is nonmedullary thyroid carcinoma, although other neoplasms may occur with increased frequency
  o Incidence of MTC in patients with familial disease is 25%
    – This group represents ~ 5% of all thyroid tumors and ~ 15% of all thyroid cancer-related deaths
- Age
  o **Familial follicular cell tumors or FMTC**
    – Age of diagnosis varies, but tumors generally occur in younger patients as compared to their sporadic counterparts
  o **Medullary thyroid carcinoma**
    – MEN2A syndrome or Sipple syndrome: In late adolescence or early adulthood; peak incidence of medullary thyroid carcinoma in these patients is in 3rd decade

– MEN2B patients usually develop medullary thyroid carcinoma early in life, diagnosed in infancy or early childhood; males and females are equally affected
– Inherited medullary thyroid carcinoma without associated endocrinopathies: Similar to other types of thyroid cancers, peak incidence ranges from 40-50 years

Presentation: FNMTC

- **Syndrome-associated group**
- Has increased prevalence of follicular cell-derived tumors within familial cancer syndrome, with preponderance of nonthyroidal tumors
  o **PHTS**
    – > 90% of individuals affected with CS manifest phenotype by age 20 years
    – By end of or during 3rd decade, almost all patients (99%) develop at least pathognomonic mucocutaneous lesions
    – Affected individuals with CS develop both benign and malignant tumors in variety of organs, such as breast, uterus, and thyroid gland
    – Individuals with germline *PTEN* mutation have 35% lifetime risk of thyroid cancer
    – Thyroid pathologic findings in this syndrome typically involves follicular cells
  o **FAP**
    – Extracolonic manifestations include osteomas, epidermal cysts, desmoid tumors, gastrointestinal tract polyps-hamartomas, congenital hypertrophy of retinal pigmented epithelium (CHRPE), hepatoblastomas
    – Papillary thyroid carcinoma in 2-12% of FAP patients
    – Young women with FAP at particular risk of developing thyroid cancer, ~ 160x that of normal individuals
    – PTC occurs with frequency of ~ 10x expected for sporadic PTC
  o **Carney complex**
    – Characterized by skin and mucosal pigmentation, diverse pigmented skin lesions, nonendocrine and variety of endocrine neoplasias: Pituitary adenoma, pigmented nodular adrenal disease, Sertoli and Leydig cell tumors, and thyroid tumors
    – Myxomas occur in heart, skin or soft tissue, external auditory canal, and breast
  o **Werner syndrome**
    – Elderly appearance with short stature, thin skin, wrinkles, alopecia, and muscle atrophy
    – Age-related disorders (e.g., osteoporosis, cataracts, diabetes, peripheral vascular disease, or malignancy) are present in these patients
    – Cardiac disease and cancer are most common causes of death in these patients
    – Mutations of *WRN* gene is specifically associated with malignancies such as melanoma, soft tissue sarcoma, osteosarcomas, and well-differentiated thyroid carcinoma
  o **Pendred syndrome**: Thyroid disease in these patients may range from minimal enlargement to large, multinodular goiter
    – Most patients are euthyroid

- ○ **DICER1 syndrome**: Multinodular goiter (MNG)
  - It has been associated with both familial MNG and MNG with ovarian Sertoli-Leydig cell tumors, independent of pleuropulmonary blastoma
  - Differentiated thyroid cancer (PTC and FTC) is infrequently observed in DICER syndrome
    - □ Papillary thyroid cancer had been reported in family with germline *DICER1* mutation
- **Familial tumor syndromes characterized by predominance of nonmedullary thyroid carcinoma (follicular cell-derived tumors)**
  - ○ **FNMTC** associated with multiple benign nodules, multifocality, bilateral disease, more aggressive clinical behavior, and worse prognosis than sporadic nonmedullary thyroid cancer
    - Diagnosed when ≥ 3 family members have nonmedullary thyroid cancer in absence of other known associated syndromes
    - Shorter disease-free survival than sporadic disease because of frequent locoregional recurrence
    - Increased risk of multifocal disease and more likely to have intraglandular dissemination, local invasion, local or regional recurrence, and lymph node metastases
  - ○ **Familial multinodular goiter syndrome** (mapped to 14q)
    - Some patients may develop associated PTC
  - ○ **Familial nonmedullary thyroid carcinoma type 1 syndrome** (chromosomal region 2q21)
    - Characterized by PTC without any distinguishing pathologic features
  - ○ **Familial PTC associated with papillary renal neoplasia syndrome** (mapped to chromosomal region 1q21)
    - Includes not only PTC and expected benign thyroid nodules but also papillary renal neoplasia
  - ○ **FPTC** (chromosomal region 19p13)
    - Characterized by multicentric tumors and multiple adenomatous nodules ± oxyphilia

Presentation: FMTC

- **MEN2A syndrome** or Sipple syndrome has bilateral medullary thyroid carcinoma or primary C-cell hyperplasia, pheochromocytoma, and hyperparathyroidism
  - ○ Inherited in autosomal dominant manner; males and females equally affected
- **MEN2B** associated with pheochromocytoma and alterations in nonendocrine tissue
  - ○ Syndrome also has medullary thyroid carcinoma and pheochromocytoma but only rarely hyperparathyroidism
  - ○ Patients have unusual appearance characterized by mucosal ganglioneuromas and marfanoid habitus
  - ○ Inheritance autosomal dominant, as in MEN2A
- **FMTC or inherited medullary thyroid carcinoma without associated endocrinopathies**
  - ○ Least aggressive form of medullary thyroid carcinoma
  - ○ MTC usually develops in patients with no other clinical manifestations

MACROSCOPIC

General Features

- Familial tumors have high incidence of multifocality, more likely to be bilateral

MICROSCOPIC

Histologic Features

- **Familial tumor syndromes characterized by predominance of nonmedullary thyroid carcinoma**
  - ○ Most tumors are PTC and have no distinct morphological findings to differentiate them from sporadic counterparts
  - ○ Mutations in patients with FNMTC syndromes have not been as well defined as in MTC
  - ○ Familial thyroid cancers more aggressive than sporadic thyroid cancer, with predisposition for lymph node metastasis, extrathyroidal invasion, and younger age of onset
- **PHTS**
  - ○ 2/3 of CS patients develop thyroid tumors; pathologic findings in this syndrome have been described as involving follicular cells
  - ○ Majority of thyroid lesions occurring in PHTS characteristically multicentric and bilateral; benign and malignant thyroid lesions observed in PHTS
  - ○ Multiple adenomatous nodules with multiple distinct well-circumscribed nodules, firm yellow-tan cut surface, diffusely involving thyroid gland
  - ○ Follicular adenomas are very common, occur at earlier age, and usually multicentric
  - ○ Follicular carcinoma is major criterion and important feature in PHTS; these tumors are more frequently multicentric
  - ○ PTC, follicular variant is associated with this syndrome
    - Cases with mutations of *SDH* or both *SDH* and *PTEN* show predominant classic PTC histology
  - ○ C-cell hyperplasia has been associated with this entity
- **FAP**
  - ○ Thyroid tumors in FAP occur almost exclusively in young females; tumors bilateral, multifocal, and well-differentiated
  - ○ Among patients with FAP who have synchronous PTC, > 90% exhibit histologic features of cribriform-morular variant (CMV), which focally shows typical nuclear features of PTC
  - ○ Characteristic cribriform pattern with solid areas and spindle cell component, associated with marked fibrosis and morular areas
  - ○ Characteristic PTC morphology associated with follicular, papillary, trabecular, solid, spindle cell, and squamoid areas
  - ○ Tumors with identical histology can occur as sporadic lesions without background of FAP
- **Carney complex**
  - ○ Thyroid is multinodular and has multifocal and bilateral thyroid disease
  - ○ Lymphocytic thyroiditis, multinodular hyperplasia, multiple follicular adenomas, characteristic multiple adenomatous nodules, follicular carcinoma, and PTC, usually present in ~ 15% of patients
- **Werner syndrome**
  - ○ Patients present at younger age and have ~ 3x ↑ risk for developing follicular carcinoma, 6x ↑ risk for anaplastic thyroid carcinoma, and slight ↑ risk for papillary thyroid carcinoma

Inherited Tumor Syndromes

- **Pendred syndrome**
  - Association of thyroid cancer and Pendred syndrome may be related to untreated congenital hypothyroidism and chronic stimulation by thyroid-stimulating hormone
  - Progression from thyroid goiter to cancer uncommon; risk likely related to longstanding untreated hypothyroidism
- **FMTC**
  - Morphologically indistinguishable form sporadic tumor counterpart
  - Associated with C-cell hyperplasia

ANCILLARY TESTS

Immunohistochemistry

- Immunostains of CMV-PTC show positivity for ER and PR, Bcl-2, E-cadherin, and galectin-3
- CMV-PTC is characterized by aberrant nuclear and cytoplasmic expression of β-catenin
- Immunostain for *PTEN* may be lost in cases of PHTS
- All other familial tumors have similar immunophenotype to sporadic thyroid tumor counterparts

Genetic Testing

- Germline point mutation in *RET* gene on chromosome 10q11.2 responsible for hereditary MTC
- Most patients with FAP-associated PTC have *APC* germline mutations
- Most patients with PHTS have germline mutations on gene *PTEN*
- Genetic inheritance of FNMTC remains unknown, believed to be autosomal dominant
  - To date, 4 susceptibility genes have been identified [*SRGAP1* gene (12q14), *TITF-1/NKX2.1* gene (14q13), *FOXE1* gene (9q22.33), and *HABP2* gene (10q25.3)]
  - Causal genes located at other 7 FNMTC-associated chromosomal loci [*TCO* (19q13.2), *fPTC/PRN* (1q21), *FTEN* (8p23.1-p22), *NMTC1* (2q21), *MNG1* (14q32), 6q22, 8q24] have yet to be identified

DIFFERENTIAL DIAGNOSIS

Follicular Cell Carcinoma

- **Sporadic follicular cell neoplasm**
  - Comprises ~ 95% of cases
  - Usually single and unilateral
  - Morphologically indistinguishable from tumor occurring in familial setting

Medullary Thyroid Carcinoma

- **Sporadic MTC**
  - Accounts for up to 75% of all cases of medullary thyroid cancer
  - Females outnumber males by 3:2
  - Peak of onset: 40-60 years of age; mean: 50 years
  - Typically unilateral
  - No associated endocrinopathies (not associated with disease in other endocrine glands)

DIAGNOSTIC CHECKLIST

Clinically Relevant Pathologic Features

- Familial thyroid carcinoma has been shown to occur at younger age, be associated with presence of multiple benign nodules, have high incidence of multifocality and bilateral disease, have more aggressive clinical behavior, and have worse prognosis than its sporadic counterparts

SELECTED REFERENCES

1. Marques IJ et al: Identification of somatic TERT promoter mutations in familial nonmedullary thyroid carcinomas. Clin Endocrinol (Oxf). ePub, 2017
2. Oh EJ et al: TERT promoter mutation in an aggressive cribriform morular variant of papillary thyroid carcinoma. Endocr Pathol. 28(1):49-53, 2017
3. Schultz KAP et al: PTEN, DICER1, FH, and their associated tumor susceptibility syndromes: Clinical features, genetics, and surveillance recommendations in childhood. Clin Cancer Res. 23(12):e76-e82, 2017
4. Scognamiglio T: C cell and follicular epithelial cell precursor lesions of the thyroid. Arch Pathol Lab Med. ePub, 2017
5. Vidinov K et al: Familial papillary thyroid carcinoma (FPTC): A retrospective analysis in a sample of the Bulgarian population for a 10-year period. Endocr Pathol. 28(1):54-59, 2017
6. Essig GF Jr et al: Multifocality in sporadic medullary thyroid carcinoma: An international multicenter study. Thyroid. 26(11):1563-1572, 2016
7. Nixon IJ et al: The impact of family history on non-medullary thyroid cancer. Eur J Surg Oncol. 42(10):1455-63, 2016
8. Valdes-Socin H et al: [A familial non medullary thyroid carcinoma (FNMTC): A clinical and genetic update.] Rev Med Liege. 71(12):557-561, 2016
9. Chernock RD et al: Molecular pathology of hereditary and sporadic medullary thyroid carcinomas. Am J Clin Pathol. 143(6):768-777, 2015
10. Dehner LP et al: Pleuropulmonary blastoma: Evolution of an entity as an entry into a familial tumor predisposition syndrome. Pediatr Dev Pathol. 18(6):504-11, 2015
11. Feng X et al: Characteristics of benign and malignant thyroid disease in familial adenomatous polyposis patients and recommendations for disease surveillance. Thyroid. 25(3):325-32, 2015
12. Gara SK et al: Germline HABP2 mutation causing familial nonmedullary thyroid cancer. N Engl J Med. 373(5):448-55, 2015
13. Sakorafas GH et al: Incidental thyroid C cell hyperplasia: clinical significance and implications in practice. Oncol Res Treat. 38(5):249-52, 2015
14. Sung TY et al: Surgical management of familial papillary thyroid microcarcinoma: A single institution study of 94 cases. World J Surg. 39(8):1930-5, 2015
15. Tomsic J et al: HABP2 Mutation and nonmedullary thyroid cancer. N Engl J Med. 373(21):2086, 2015
16. Laury AR et al: Thyroid pathology in PTEN-hamartoma tumor syndrome: characteristic findings of a distinct entity. Thyroid. 21(2):135-44, 2011
17. Mukherjee S et al: RET codon 804 mutations in multiple endocrine neoplasia 2: genotype-phenotype correlations and implications in clinical management. Clin Genet. 79(1):1-16, 2011
18. Nosé V: Familial thyroid cancer: a review. Mod Pathol. 24 Suppl 2:S19-33, 2011
19. Smith JR et al: Thyroid nodules and cancer in children with PTEN hamartoma tumor syndrome. J Clin Endocrinol Metab. 96(1):34-7, 2011
20. Zhang Y et al: Endocrine tumors as part of inherited tumor syndromes. Adv Anat Pathol. 18(3):206-18, 2011
21. Almeida MQ et al: Solid tumors associated with multiple endocrine neoplasias. Cancer Genet Cytogenet. 203(1):30-6, 2010
22. Cameselle-Teijeiro J: The pathologist's role in familial nonmedullary thyroid tumors. Int J Surg Pathol. 18(3 Suppl):194S-200S, 2010
23. Farooq A et al: Cowden syndrome. Cancer Treat Rev. 36(8):577-83, 2010
24. Frank-Raue K et al: Molecular genetics and phenomics of RET mutations: Impact on prognosis of MTC. Mol Cell Endocrinol. 322(1-2):2-7, 2010
25. Khan A et al: Familial nonmedullary thyroid cancer: a review of the genetics. Thyroid. 20(7):795-801, 2010
26. Nosé V: Familial follicular cell tumors: classification and morphological characteristics. Endocr Pathol. 21(4):219-26, 2010
27. Nosé V: Thyroid cancer of follicular cell origin in inherited tumor syndromes. Adv Anat Pathol. 17(6):428-36, 2010
28. Raue F et al: Update multiple endocrine neoplasia type 2. Fam Cancer. 9(3):449-57, 2010
29. Richards ML: Familial syndromes associated with thyroid cancer in the era of personalized medicine. Thyroid. 20(7):707-13, 2010

Familial Follicular Cell Carcinoma Classification

Disease	Histologic Subtype
Syndromic or Familial Tumor Syndrome With Preponderance of Nonthyroidal Tumors	
PTEN-hamartoma tumor syndrome (Cowden disease)	FTC or follicular variant of PTC, associated with follicular adenomas, multiple adenomatous nodules, and C-cell hyperplasia
Familial adenomatous polyposis (FAP)-hamartoma tumor syndrome	PTC with cribriform and morular pattern with sclerosis
Carney complex	FTC associated with follicular adenomas, multiple adenomatous nodules, and PTC
Werner syndrome	FTC, PTC, and ATC
Pendred syndrome	FTC
Nonsyndromic or Familial Tumor Syndrome With Preponderance of Nonmedullary Thyroid Carcinoma	
Familial papillary thyroid carcinoma	PTC, usual variant
Familial papillary thyroid carcinoma with papillary renal cell neoplasia	PTC, usual variant
Familial nonmedullary thyroid carcinoma type 1	PTC, usual variant
Familial papillary thyroid carcinoma and multinodular goiter	PTC and nodular hyperplasia

PTC = papillary thyroid carcinoma; FTC = follicular thyroid carcinoma; ATC = anaplastic thyroid carcinoma.

Familial Follicular Cell Cancer in Familial Cancer Syndromes

Syndrome	Inheritance	Gene	Gene Location	Thyroid Involvement (%)
PTEN-hamartoma tumor syndrome	Autosomal dominant	PTEN and other genes (SDH, PIK3CA, AKT1, KLLN, or SEC23B)	10q23.2	50 Thyroid cancer: 35%
Familial adenomatous polyposis	Autosomal dominant	APC	5q21	2-12
Carney complex	Autosomal dominant	PRKAR1-α	2p12-17q22-24	60; 4
Pendred syndrome	Autosomal recessive	SLC26A4 (pendrin)	7q21-24	1
Werner syndrome	Autosomal recessive	WRN	8p11-p12	18
DICER syndrome	Autosomal dominant	DICER1	14q32.13	

MEN2 Syndromes Associated With Heritable Medullary Thyroid Carcinoma

	MEN2A	MEN2B	Familial Medullary Thyroid Carcinoma
Frequency	35-30%	5-10%	50-60%
Mean age at presentation	25-35	10-20	45-55
Presence of C-cell hyperplasia	100%	100%	100%
Medullary thyroid carcinoma	> 90%	> 90%	> 90%

MEN2A = multiple endocrine neoplasia 2A; MEN2B = multiple endocrine neoplasia 2B.

30. Rubinstein WS: Endocrine cancer predisposition syndromes: hereditary paraganglioma, multiple endocrine neoplasia type 1, multiple endocrine neoplasia type 2, and hereditary thyroid cancer. Hematol Oncol Clin North Am. 24(5):907-37, 2010
31. Tran T et al: Familial thyroid neoplasia: impact of technological advances on detection and monitoring. Curr Opin Endocrinol Diabetes Obes. 17(5):425-31, 2010
32. Wohllk N et al: Multiple endocrine neoplasia type 2. Best Pract Res Clin Endocrinol Metab. 24(3):371-87, 2010
33. Alevizaki M et al: Multiple endocrine neoplasias: advances and challenges for the future. J Intern Med. 266(1):1-4, 2009
34. Dotto J et al: Familial thyroid carcinoma: a diagnostic algorithm. Adv Anat Pathol. 15(6):332-49, 2008
35. Etit D et al: Histopathologic and clinical features of medullary microcarcinoma and C-cell hyperplasia in prophylactic thyroidectomies for medullary carcinoma: a study of 42 cases. Arch Pathol Lab Med. 132(11):1767-73, 2008
36. Nosé V: Familial non-medullary thyroid carcinoma: an update. Endocr Pathol. 19(4):226-40, 2008
37. Yassa L et al: Long-term assessment of a multidisciplinary approach to thyroid nodule diagnostic evaluation. Cancer. 111(6):508-16, 2007
38. Zambrano E et al: Abnormal distribution and hyperplasia of thyroid C-cells in PTEN-associated tumor syndromes. Endocr Pathol. 15(1):55-64, 2004
39. DeLellis RA et al: C-cell hyperplasia and medullary thyroid carcinoma in the rat. An immunohistochemical and ultrastructural analysis. Lab Invest. 40(2):140-54, 1979
40. Wolfe HJ et al: Distribution of calcitonin-containing cells in the normal neonatal human thyroid gland: a correlation of morphology with peptide content. J Clin Endocrinol Metab. 41(06):1076-81, 1975

Inherited Tumor Syndromes

(Left) *Total prophylactic thyroidectomy and thymectomy from a patient with a family history of MEN2 with RET mutation shows a grossly normal thyroid. The entirely submitted specimen showed C-cell hyperplasia (CCH) and 2 foci of medullary thyroid carcinoma.* **(Right)** *Patient with family history of MEN2B with RET mutation had prophylactic thyroidectomy, which showed CCH and 2 foci of medullary thyroid carcinoma. Calcitonin stain highlights the focus of carcinoma.*

Grossly Normal Thyroid and Thymus

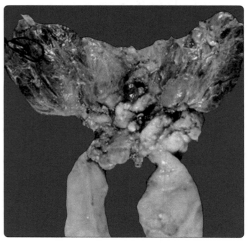

Medullary Thyroid Microcarcinoma

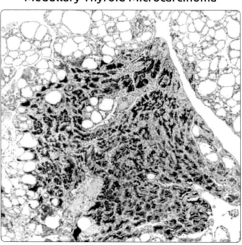

(Left) *CCH is present in a patient with MEN2 syndrome with C cells surrounding the entire thyroid follicle ➡ and replacing the follicular cells.* **(Right)** *Specimen from a patient with MEN2 syndrome who underwent prophylactic thyroidectomy shows CCH with calcitonin-positive C cells surrounding the thyroid follicle. Heritable medullary thyroid carcinoma is preceded by neoplastic CCH.*

C-Cell Hyperplasia

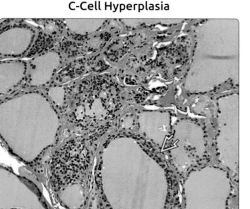

Calcitonin in C-Cell Hyperplasia

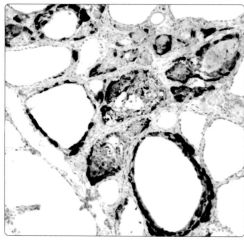

(Left) *Fused transaxial FDG PET/CT shows a focal hypermetabolic mass ➡ in the right thyroid lobe in a patient with medullary thyroid cancer.* **(Right)** *Gross cut surface of both thyroid lobes from a patient with MEN2A shows 2 well-circumscribed white-yellow thyroid tumor nodules. Medullary thyroid carcinomas are usually firm and gritty, and familial medullary thyroid carcinomas are usually bilateral and with associated CCH.*

PET/CT Imaging

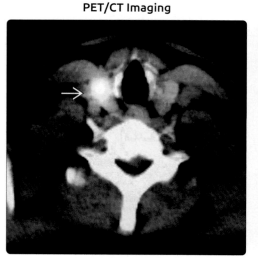

Bilateral Thyroid Tumors

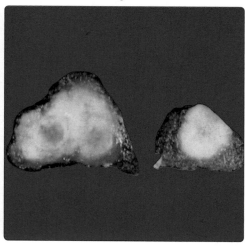

Amyloid Deposition

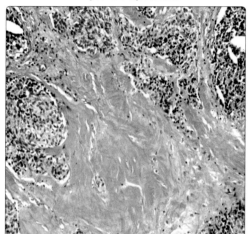

Calcitonin Staining

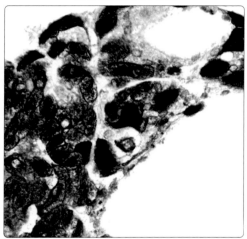

(Left) *H&E shows the characteristic histologic appearance of medullary thyroid carcinoma, a highly cellular tumor with a variable amount of fibrosis and amyloid deposition.* (Right) *Calcitonin immunostaining is usually strongly positive in the tumor cells, whereas the areas of fibrosis or amyloid deposition are characteristically negative.*

Histological Pattern

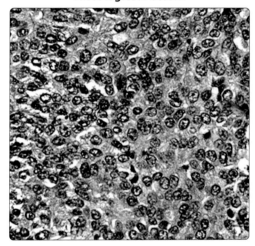

Variable Calcitonin Stain

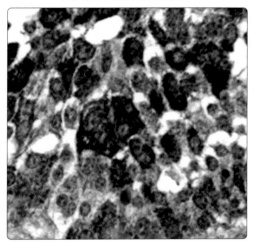

(Left) *The characteristic histopathological features of medullary thyroid carcinoma are solid sheets and groups of round to polygonal tumor cells separated by thin fibrovascular cores. There is a variable amount of cytoplasm, and the medium-sized nuclei have minimal nuclear pleomorphism. Mitoses are usually rare.* (Right) *Medullary thyroid carcinoma from a patient with familial medullary thyroid carcinoma syndrome shows variable cytoplasmic immunostaining for calcitonin.*

Congophilia

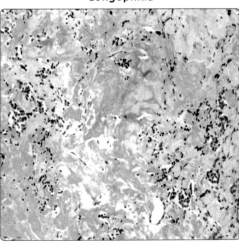

Amyloid Under Polarized Light

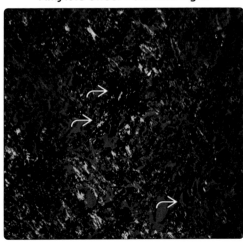

(Left) *Congo red-stained tumor shows extensive deposition of amyloid. Although amyloid is not essential for the diagnosis of medullary thyroid carcinoma, most of these tumors have at least some amyloid deposition.* (Right) *Congo red-stained medullary thyroid carcinoma under polarized light reveals the characteristic apple-green birefringence ➡, confirming amyloid deposition.*

Multinodular Cut Surface

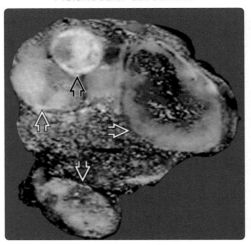

Multiple Pale Thyroid Nodules

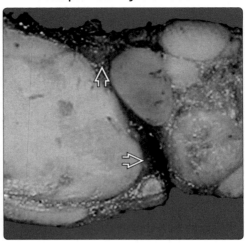

(Left) *Gross cut surface of a thyroid from a 12-year-old patient with Cowden syndrome/PTEN-hamartoma tumor syndrome (PHTS) shows multiple well-circumscribed nodules ⇒ and 1 encapsulated nodule ⇒.* (Right) *Gross cut surface of a thyroid from an 18-year-old woman with Cowden disease/PTEN hamartoma tumor syndrome shows multiple well-circumscribed nodules almost entirely replacing the thyroid parenchyma ⇒.*

Capsular Invasion

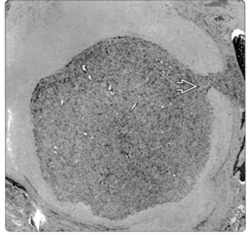

Multiple Adenomatous Nodules

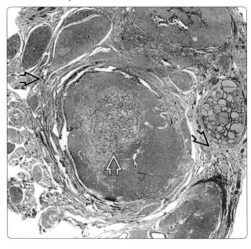

(Left) *An encapsulated follicular carcinoma from a 12-year-old girl with Cowden syndrome shows complete capsular invasion ⇒. Follicular carcinoma is a major criterion for diagnosis of this syndrome.* (Right) *H&E of the thyroid from a patient with Cowden disease shows diffuse involvement by diversely sized adenomatous nodules. The larger nodule shows focal central degenerative changes ⇒. Compressed intervening thyroid parenchyma ⇒ is observed.*

Adenomatous Nodules

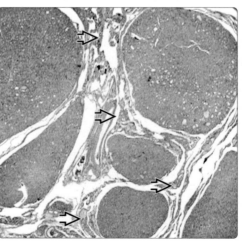

Numerous Adenomatous Nodules

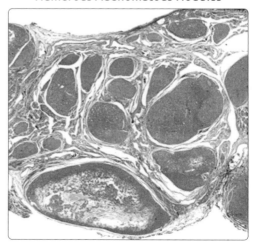

(Left) *H&E of the thyroid from an 18-year-old woman with Cowden disease shows multiple well-circumscribed adenomatous nodules with a small amount of compressed residual thyroid parenchyma ⇒.* (Right) *Multiple well-circumscribed adenomatous nodules distributed side by side with others are observed on low-power magnification. Residual compressed thyroid tissue can sometimes simulate a capsule.*

Follicular Adenoma

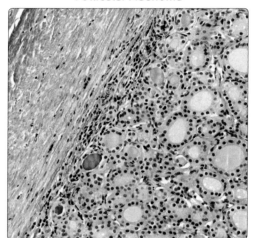

Microfollicles

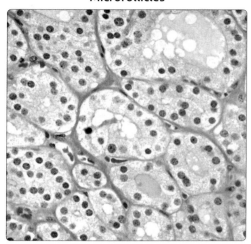

(Left) *Thyroid tissue from a patient with Cowden disease shows a well-encapsulated follicular adenoma. These lesions are usually present in association with multiple adenomatous nodules.* **(Right)** *High-power view of an adenomatous nodule in a patient with Cowden syndrome shows the characteristic homogeneous layer of follicular cells with uniform nuclei and no overlapping or nuclear changes of papillary thyroid carcinoma.*

Uniform Microfollicles

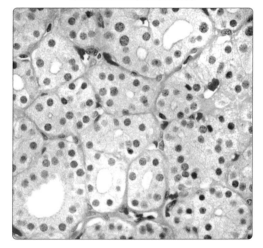

Loss of PTEN

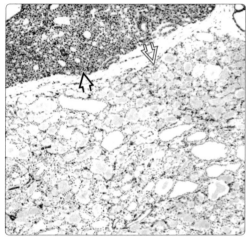

(Left) *High-power view of an adenomatous nodule in a patient with Cowden syndrome shows homogeneous microfollicles architecture, indistinguishable from their sporadic counterparts.* **(Right)** *Immunohistochemistry for PTEN shows loss of staining of the follicular cells with preservation of staining of the endothelial cells within one nodule ⇒ and preservation of PTEN immunostain in the adjacent nodule ⇒.*

Loss of PTEN Stain

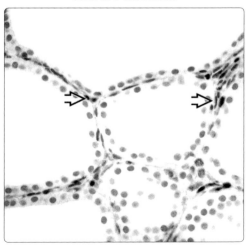

Loss of PTEN Stain

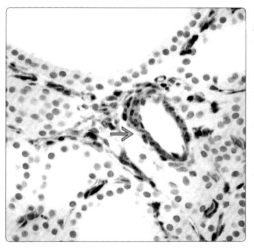

(Left) *Immunohistochemistry for PTEN in a thyroidectomy specimen from an 18-year-old woman with PHTS/Cowden disease shows loss of staining of the follicular cells with preservation of staining of the endothelial cells ⇒.* **(Right)** *High-power magnification shows loss of PTEN staining in the follicular cells. Preservation of PTEN staining of the endothelial cells and smooth muscle cells in a vessel wall ⇒ are well-illustrated in this image.*

Numerous Colonic Polyps

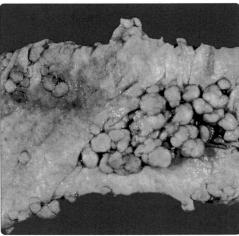

Eye Lesion in FAP

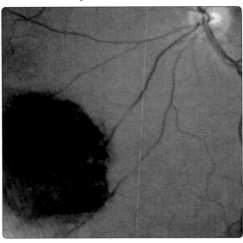

(Left) *Colectomy specimen from a 17-year-old girl with known thyroid tumor and familial adenomatous polyposis shows numerous polyps on the mucosal surface. This patient had multiple foci of cribriform-morular papillary thyroid carcinoma.* (Right) *Congenital hypertrophy of the pigmented retinal epithelium is shown. This condition is benign, and it is found in up to 2/3 of patients with FAP.*

Cut Surface of Large Tumor

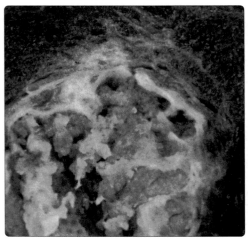

Cribriform Arrangement

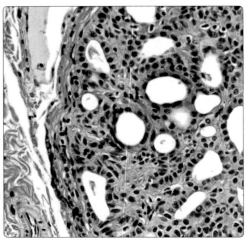

(Left) *Gross cut surface of a large PTC, cribriform-morular variant (CMV), shows irregular areas of fibrosis and a pale, soft, and friable tumor mass occupying most of the section. This variant usually has extensive fibrosis and a thick, fibrous capsule. They are usually multiple and bilateral.* (Right) *Cytologic features of tumor cells typically seen in PTC, CMV are shown. The cells are cuboidal with basophilic cytoplasm and hyperchromatic nuclei. Note the absence of classic PTC nuclei.*

Encapsulated Microcarcinoma

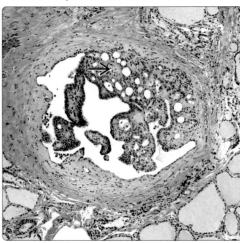

Solid Component

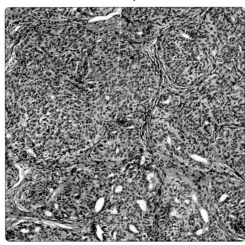

(Left) *Encapsulation is common in this variant of PTC. This example shows a thick, fibrous band encapsulating the tumor. Note the papillary and cribriform architecture. Also shown are eosinophilic foci of sclerosis/hyalinization ➡ within the stroma. This focus of tumor was < 1 cm.* (Right) *Solid pattern of PTC, CMV is shown. An area with the more common cribriform pattern is seen in the lower right corner of this field.*

Cribriform Arrangement

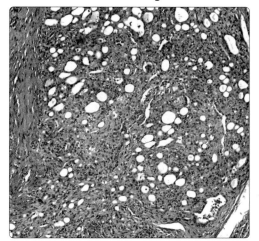

Squamous Morules

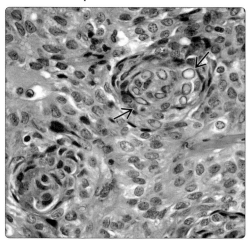

(Left) *PTC-CMV highlights the cribriform appearance of these types of tumors. This tumor shows areas of both cribriform pattern and solid pattern; however, this tumor has a predominantly cribriform architecture.* (Right) *Solid pattern of PTC, CMV is shown. In the center, there are squamous morules with the characteristic peculiar nuclear clearing* ⮕.

CD5(+) Squamous Morules

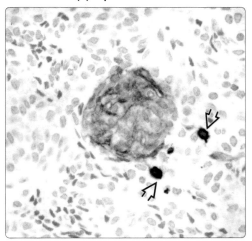

Keratin in Squamous Morule

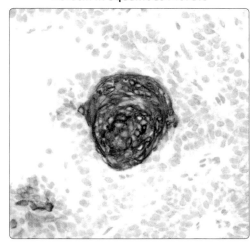

(Left) *The morules in CMV show immunopositivity for CD5 in the cell membranes and focally within cytoplasm. Note the adjacent T lymphocytes* ⮕ *demonstrates strong staining for CD5.* (Right) *Characteristically, the squamous morules are positive for cytokeratin 5/6 and also for CD5. The cribriform component is negative for these markers.*

Cribriform Pattern Lacking Colloid

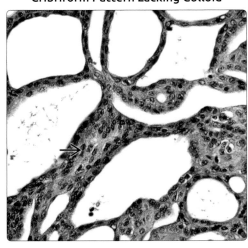

Nuclear β-Catenin

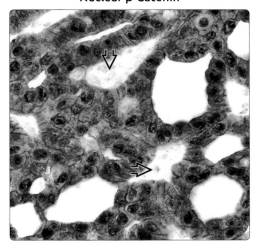

(Left) *A cribriform pattern tumor with focal solid areas and a spindle cell component* ⮕ *is shown at high magnification. The cells are spindled with basophilic cytoplasm and hyperchromatic nuclei with absence of typical PTC nuclei.* (Right) *High-power β-catenin immunostain of PTC, CMV demonstrates characteristic nuclear and cytoplasmic staining resulting from aberrant accumulation within the nucleus. Note the endothelial cells are negative* ⮕.

Familial PTC With Cell Oxyphilia

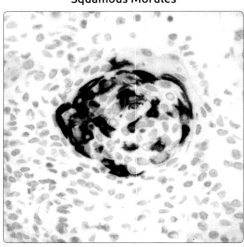

Squamous Morules

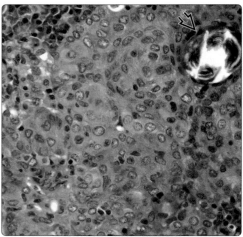

(Left) This figure shows one of the tumors in a patient with multifocal, bilateral tumors composed of follicles, papillae, trabeculae, and solid areas or an admixture formed by cells with pale to intense cytoplasmic eosinophilia. Psammoma body ⊟ is present. (Right) This familial papillary thyroid carcinoma with cell oxyphilia showed focal squamous morules. These are highlighted by cytokeratin 5/6 stain.

Lymphatic Involvement

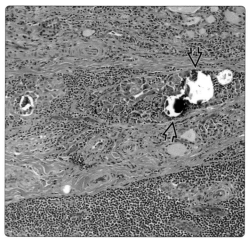

Lymphovascular Invasion

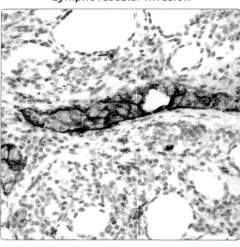

(Left) The thyroid of this patient with familial thyroid carcinoma with cell oxyphilia shows marked lymphocytic thyroiditis and numerous foci of tumor cells within intrathyroid vascular channels. Note the psammoma bodies ⊟ are present among the tumor cells. (Right) Immunohistochemistry for HBME1 highlights the tumor cells within intrathyroid vascular channels in this patient with familial thyroid carcinoma with cell oxyphilia.

Familial Papillary Thyroid Carcinoma

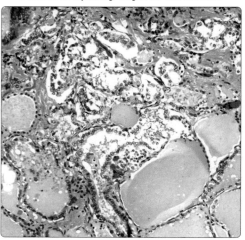

Multiple Tumors

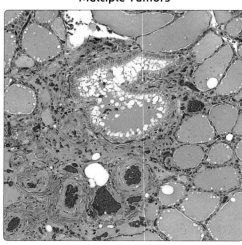

(Left) Classic features of PTC are shown in a patient with family history of brother and sister with numerous thyroid tumors. The morphological features of this tumor are indistinguishable from sporadic PTC. (Right) Papillary thyroid carcinoma is shown in a patient with numerous tumors measuring up to 1.3 cm and a family history of brother and sister with numerous thyroid tumors.

Hereditary Renal and Thyroid Carcinoma

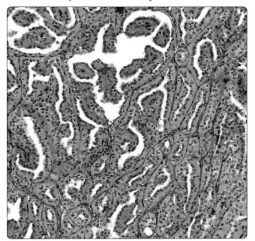

Papillary Arrangement

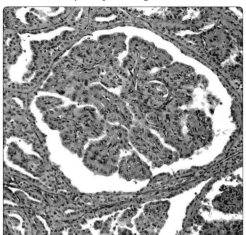

(Left) The familial papillary thyroid carcinoma associated with renal papillary neoplasia (fPTC/PRN) has been described as a familial association of PTC, thyroid nodules, and PRN. The thyroid of a 26-year-old woman with family history of hereditary papillary renal cell carcinoma and papillary thyroid carcinoma shows classic features of tumors. (Right) In hereditary papillary renal and papillary thyroid carcinoma, both tumors of the distinct sites are similar. However, only thyroid carcinoma is positive for TTF-1.

Papillae Formation

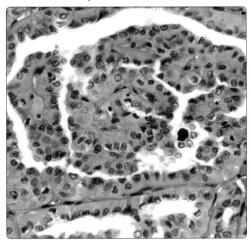

TTF1-Positive Papillary Tumor

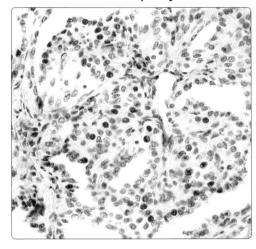

(Left) The high-magnification view shows the papillary arrangement of cells around a thin fibrovascular core. The cells have a pale-pink cytoplasm and irregular nuclear membranes. This picture shows papillary arrangement with a "glomeruloid" appearance. A psammoma body is present. (Right) The morphological features of both kidney and thyroid papillary carcinomas are similar. The immunostain for TTF-1 confirms the thyroid origin for thyroid tumor and not metastases from the kidney.

Hobnail Variant of PTC

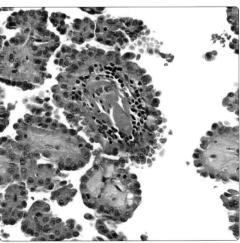

Hobnail Tumor Cells

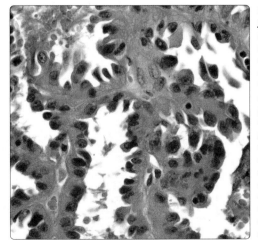

(Left) The thyroid tumor of a young female with CHEK2 mutation and with history of breast cancer and an ovarian tumor, shows a papillary carcinoma composed of cells with hobnail features. These tumors usually occur in older patients as nonsyndromic tumors. (Right) This high-power view highlights the cellular characteristics of the hobnail variant of papillary thyroid carcinoma. In this hereditary tumor, the morphological characteristics are similar. These tumors are know to be aggressive in a sporadic setting.

TERMINOLOGY

- **MAS consists of at least 2 features of triad**
  - Autonomous endocrine hyperfunction, such as precocious puberty, hyperthyroidism, and hypercortisolism
  - Polyostotic or monostotic fibrous dysplasia
  - Café au lait pigmented skin lesions
- **MAS caused by activating mutations in complex GNAS locus at 20q13**
  - Most common mutations are point mutations with Arg201 (most commonly R201H and R201C)

CLINICAL ISSUES

- Rare disease with estimated prevalence between 1:100,000 to 1 million
- Diagnosis of MAS often made within 1st decade of life

IMAGING

- Fibrous dysplasia: Ground-glass appearance on radiograph

MICROSCOPIC

- Endocrine organ hyperplasia or adenoma
  - Thyroid with multinodular hyperplasia
  - Adrenal gland with macronodular hyperplasia
  - Pituitary gland with pituitary adenoma
- Fibrous dysplasia
  - "Chinese writing" pattern, characterized by thin and disconnected bone trabeculae with interspersed fibrous tissue
  - Spicules of woven bone are surrounded by flat lining cells with retracted cell bodies, forming pseudolacunar spaces

TOP DIFFERENTIAL DIAGNOSES

- Neurofibromatosis
- Osteofibrous dysplasia
- Mazabraud syndrome
- Hyperparathyroidism-jaw tumor syndrome
- Carney complex

Variegated Cut Surface

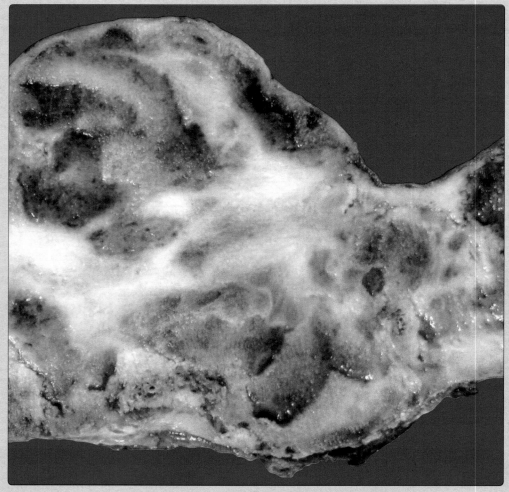

Gross photo of fibrous dysplasia of the rib shows an irregularly shaped bone lesion with a thinning of cortex and complete loss of marrow, which is occupied by a mass with a variegated appearance.

TERMINOLOGY

Abbreviations

- McCune-Albright syndrome (MAS)

Synonyms

- Albright syndrome
- Mazabraud syndrome
- Fibrous dysplasia (FD), polyostotic and monostotic

Definitions

- Mosaic disease with wide clinical variability and broad spectrum of lesions
- MAS consists of at least 2 features of triad of polyostotic or monostotic fibrous dysplasia, café au lait pigmented skin lesions, and autonomous endocrine hyperfunction
- Association of polyostotic fibrous dysplasia (POFD) and intramuscular myxomas categorized as Mazabraud syndrome

ETIOLOGY/PATHOGENESIS

Etiology

- MAS usually caused by early embryonic postzygotic somatic activating mutations in *GNAS1* gene (*GNAS* locus at 20q13.2-q13.3)
- Most common mutations are point mutations with Arg201 (most commonly R201H and R201C)
- Activating mutations lead to increased cAMP levels, which has multiple effects in different organs
- Significant variability observed in extent and severity of clinical presentation due to somatic mosaicism of *GNAS1* mutations
- Nonmosaic state of activating mutations presumably lethal to embryo
- Phenotype reflects distribution of GNAS mutations and role of Gs-alpha in mutation-bearing tissues
- Penetrance high and primarily determined by number and location of mutant cells

CLINICAL ISSUES

Epidemiology

- Incidence
  - Rare disease with estimated prevalence between 1:100,000 to 1 million
- Age
  - Diagnosis often made within 1st decade of life
- Sex
  - Occurs equally in both sexes

Presentation

- **Endocrine hyperfunction**
  - Precocious puberty
    - More frequent in girls, clinical presentation includes vaginal bleeding or spotting, development of breast tissue
    - Caused by gonadotropin-independent secretion of estrogen from large ovarian follicles
    - Ovarian cysts may be either present or absent due to episodic nature of their development
    - In boys, testicular and penile enlargement and precocious sexual behavior, ± excess testosterone production
    - Testicular enlargement often results from maturation and growth of seminiferous tubules
  - Thyroid
    - Hyperthyroidism due to multinodular hyperplasia
    - Clinical or subclinical hyperthyroidism, ± clinically detectable goiter or thyroiditis
    - Higher triiodothyronine:thyroxine ratio even in absence of hyperthyroidism (partially explained by cAMP-induced 5'-deiodinase activity)
    - Rare cases of inflammatory thyroiditis and thyroid carcinomas described
  - Adrenal gland
    - Hypercortisolism often due to macronodular cortical hyperplasia
    - Hypercortisolism in MAS always ACTH-independent and leads to Cushing syndrome, often mild and cyclical, but occasionally severe and with significant mortality
    - Weight gain and decreasing growth velocity: Cushing syndrome in childhood
    - Adrenal involvements manifests in 1st year of life (1.7-7.5% of patients affected)
    - Rare examples of bilateral adenomas have also been described in MAS
  - Pituitary gland
    - Acromegaly or gigantism due to pituitary adenoma
    - MAS-related acromegaly always associated with POFD of skull base
    - Synchronous hyperprolactinemia occurs in ~ 80% of patients
    - Acromegaly affects 20-30% of patients with MAS
  - Others
    - Chronic liver disease, tachycardia, and hypophosphatemia
    - Hyperphosphaturic hypophosphatemic rickets
      - Hypophosphatemia is FGF23-mediated (phosphaturic factor), which is released from FD tissue
      - Typically seen in patients with significant skeletal disease
    - Osteomalacia
- **POFD**
  - Benign fibroosseous bone lesion involving multiple bone sites
  - Clinical presentation includes
    - Abnormal gait
    - Visible bony deformities (leg length discrepancy, Shepherd's crook deformity, facial asymmetry, or bony enlargement)
    - Bone pain
    - Joint stiffness with pain
    - Pathological fractures
    - Nerve compression
    - Rarely undergoes sarcomatous degeneration
  - Location
    - Most commonly in femur, tibia, humerus, ribs, and craniofacial bones

- – Craniofacial FD, in particular, can vary widely in severity from asymptomatic to severe disfigurement and functional impairment
  - o POFD is thought to be secondary to increased proliferation and decreased osteoblastic differentiation of bone marrow stromal cells
- **Café au lait pigmented skin lesions**
  - o Likely result from increased intracellular cAMP in melanocytes, which leads to increased melanin production
  - o Flat macules that often follow segmental pattern of distribution of developmental lines of Blaschko
  - o Most common locations: Posterior neck, sacrum, head
  - o Skin pigmentation often covers large geographic area with irregular border
  - o May be present at birth or develop soon after; do not fade with age
  - o Often, lesions on same side affected by fibrous dysplasia
  - o Pigmentation becomes more obvious with age and may darken after sun exposure
- **Others**
  - o Oral pigmentation, gastrointestinal polyps, breast cancer
  - o Hepatobiliary and pancreatic neoplasms, hepatobiliary dysfunction, cardiac disease
  - o Platelet dysfunction, along with hyperplasia of thymus, spleen, and pancreatic islets

Treatment

- Endocrine hyperfunction
  - o Management depends on individual presentation
- Fibrous dysplasia
  - o Bony disease very difficult to treat and no specific treatments available
    - – Bisphosphonates often used to reduce bone pain, frequency of pathological fractures
- Café au lait skin lesions
  - o Totally benign and no treatment needed
- MAS-related pituitary disease
  - o Total hypophysectomy required for surgical cure

Prognosis

- MAS not associated with significantly increased mortality risk
- *GNAS* mutations in MAS/POFD weakly oncogenic
- Radiotherapy and uncontrolled GH excess may increase risk of malignant transformation
- Sudden cardiac death has been reported
- Endocrinopathies persist throughout childhood and adulthood
  - o Exception of FGF23-mediated hypophosphatemia, which may worsen during periods of rapid linear growth and ameliorate in adulthood (FD disease activity wanes)
  - o Hypophosphatemia increases fractures and bone pain

Complications

- Osteosarcoma in 1% of patients with POFD
- Females may have greater risk for breast cancer
- Secondary osteomyelitis
- Thyroid carcinoma
- Myositis
- Compressive neuropathy
- Sympathetic algodystrophy

IMAGING

General Features

- Fibrous dysplasia
  - o Radiograph: Ground-glass appearance
- Precocious puberty
  - o Ultrasonography: Ovarian cysts (may be present or absent)
    - – Testicular microlithiasis, hyperechoic and hypoechoic lesions, heterogeneity, and focal calcifications irrespective of precocity
- Hyperthyroidism
  - o Solitary or multiple functioning nodules that occur in MAS appear warm or hot on scan

MICROSCOPIC

Histologic Features

- Endocrine hyperfunction
  - o Ovary with enlarged follicles lined by granulosa cells
    - – Single case of borderline ovarian serous tumor and another of virilizing sclerosing stromal tumor have been reported in MAS
  - o Testicular enlargement results from maturation and growth of seminiferous tubules
    - – Leydig cell hyperplasia indistinguishable from Leydig cell tumors recently reported
    - – Sertoli cells proliferations (including Sertoli cell intraepithelial neoplasia), bilateral testicular cell tumors (including embryonal carcinoma), and testicular adrenal rests
  - o Thyroid with multinodular hyperplasia
    - – Multiple nodules with different size
      - □ Regardless of size, such nodules called follicular adenomas with papillary growth (or papillary adenomas)
      - □ Characterized by benign follicular epithelial proliferations with intrafollicular centripetal papillary projections
    - – Sanderson polsters (papillary-type projections into lumina of follicles)
    - – Varying degree of cellularity and colloid
  - o Adrenal gland with macronodular hyperplasia
    - – Shows multiple macronodules
    - – Macronodules composed of hypertrophied, globoid, lipid-depleted adrenocortical cells
    - – Residual normal gland often atrophic
    - – Bilateral nodular hyperplasia and bilateral primary bimorphic adrenocortical disease
      - □ Diffuse nodular hyperplasia juxtaposed with areas of atrophic cortex, resulting in bimorphic appearance
  - o Pituitary gland with pituitary adenoma
    - – Solid, diffuse, trabecular, sinusoidal, and papillary growth patterns common
    - – Tumor cells with typical neuroendocrine cell features
    - – Finely dispersed chromatin with distinct nucleoli
    - – Cytoplasmic granularity gives 3 morphologically distinct cell types: Chromophobic, eosinophilic, and basophilic

- – Evidence suggests hyperplasia-to-neoplasia progression sequence and multicentric microadenomas
- FD
  - ○ Composed of fibrous tissue and immature woven bone
    - – Spindle-shaped fibroblasts arranged in parallel arrays or in whorls
    - – Woven bone with "Chinese writing" pattern
    - – Spicules of woven bone surrounded by flat lining cells with retracted cell bodies, forming pseudolacunar spaces
- Café au lait skin lesions
  - ○ No change in number of melanocytes but increase in number of melanin-containing pigment melanosomes

ANCILLARY TESTS

Cytology

- Multinodular hyperplasia thyroid
  - ○ Abundant colloid
  - ○ Low cellularity
  - ○ Degenerative features
  - ○ Benign nuclear features
  - ○ Cellular atypia my be present
  - ○ Oncocytic changes
  - ○ Nuclear clearing
  - ○ Signet ring changes

Genetic Testing

- Activating mutation of GNAS1 at Arg201 codon
- Mutation spectrum
  - ○ Missense mutations on Arg201
    - – R201H
    - – R201C
    - – R201G
    - – R201L
    - – R201S
- Tests
  - ○ Sequencing

Serologic Testing

- Sexual precocity with increase of luteinizing hormone (LH) and follicle-stimulating hormone (FSH)
- Elevated serum alkaline phosphatase
- Elevated hormone level (thyroid hormone, cortisone, growth hormone, or estrogen)

DIFFERENTIAL DIAGNOSIS

Neurofibromatosis

- Café au lait spots also present (autosomal dominant)
- Multiple neurofibromas, Lisch nodules often present

Osteofibrous Dysplasia

- Rare, benign, nonneoplastic, self-limited intracortical fibroosseous lesion
- Most lesions of osteofibrous dysplasia affect cortex of tibiae and fibulae of children
- Radiograph shows that cortex often expanded and thinned with multiple radiolucencies

- Microscopically, lesion composed of spindle cell proliferation with production of woven bone trabeculae with prominent osteoblastic rimming

Mazabraud Syndrome

- Combination of polyostotic fibrous dysplasia and intramuscular myxomas
- Also caused by GNAS1 mutations

Hyperparathyroidism-Jaw Tumor Syndrome

- Caused by mutation of HRPT2 gene, which encodes parafibromin
- Hyperparathyroidism often caused by parathyroid adenoma or carcinoma with severe hypercalcemia
- Ossifying fibroma in jaw can be confused with fibrous dysplasia clinically, radiographically, and histologically

Carney Complex

- Autosomal dominant disease
- Shares some similarities with MAS
- Multiple endocrine neoplasia syndrome featuring cardiac, endocrine, cutaneous, and neural tumors
- Presence of variety of mucocutaneous pigmented lesions
- Involve several endocrine glands simultaneously
  - ○ Adrenal cortex
  - ○ Gonads
  - ○ Pituitary
  - ○ Thyroid

SELECTED REFERENCES

1. Mete O et al: WHO 2017. McCune-Albright Syndrome. 272-274, 2017
2. Angelousi A et al: McCune Albright syndrome and bilateral adrenal hyperplasia: the GNAS mutation may only be present in adrenal tissue. Hormones (Athens). 14(3):447-50, 2015
3. Pichard DC et al: Oral pigmentation in McCune-Albright syndrome. JAMA Dermatol. 150(7):760-3, 2014
4. Salenave S et al: Acromegaly and McCune-Albright syndrome. J Clin Endocrinol Metab. 99(6):1955-69, 2014
5. Elhaï M et al: McCune-Albright syndrome revealed by hyperthyroidism at advanced age. Ann Endocrinol (Paris). Epub ahead of print, 2011
6. Brown RJ et al: Cushing syndrome in the McCune-Albright syndrome. J Clin Endocrinol Metab. 95(4):1508-15, 2010
7. Moon S et al: Analysis of aberrantly spliced HRPT2 transcripts and the resulting proteins in HPT-JT syndrome. Mol Genet Metab. 100(4):365-71, 2010
8. Adegbite NS et al: Diagnostic and mutational spectrum of progressive osseous heteroplasia (POH) and other forms of GNAS-based heterotopic ossification. Am J Med Genet A. 146A(14):1788-96, 2008
9. Chapurlat RD et al: Fibrous dysplasia of bone and McCune-Albright syndrome. Best Pract Res Clin Rheumatol. 22(1):55-69, 2008
10. Dumitrescu CE et al: McCune-Albright syndrome. Orphanet J Rare Dis. 3:12, 2008
11. Keil MF et al: Pituitary tumors in childhood: update of diagnosis, treatment and molecular genetics. Expert Rev Neurother. 8(4):563-74, 2008
12. de Sanctis L et al: Genetics of McCune-Albright syndrome. J Pediatr Endocrinol Metab. 19 Suppl 2:577-82, 2006
13. Tinschert S et al: McCune-Albright syndrome: clinical and molecular evidence of mosaicism in an unusual giant patient. Am J Med Genet. 83(2):100-8, 1999
14. Riminucci M et al: Fibrous dysplasia of bone in the McCune-Albright syndrome: abnormalities in bone formation. Am J Pathol. 151(6):1587-600, 1997
15. Park YK et al: Osteofibrous dysplasia: clinicopathologic study of 80 cases. Hum Pathol. 24(12):1339-47, 1993

(Left) *Axial graphic shows expansion of the right lateral orbital rim, sphenoid wing, and temporal squamosa by fibrous dysplasia. Note the exophthalmos and stretching of the optic nerve on the ipsilateral side.* **(Right)** *Axial CT shows an expansion of the right anterior maxilla and right pterygoid plate with an internal ground-glass density* 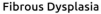.

Fibrous Dysplasia

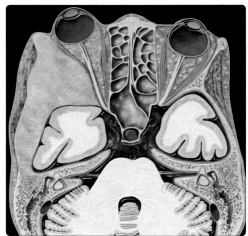

Maxillary Lesion

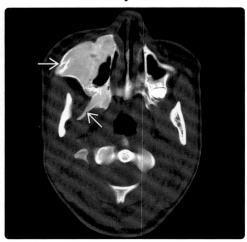

(Left) *Coronal graphic shows polyostotic fibrous dysplasia involving the proximal femur and acetabular roof. Cystic changes are shown in red, while the ground-glass appearance is shown in brown.* **(Right)** *Gross photo of a polyostotic fibrous dysplasia of the rib shows a bone lesion with a thinning of cortex occupying the entire bone marrow space.*

Polyostotic Fibrous Dysplasia

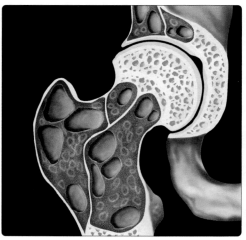

Mass in Rib

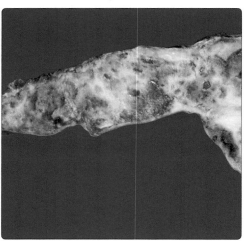

(Left) *Irregular, curvilinear trabeculae of woven bone are characteristic of fibrous dysplasia. The bone is surrounded by a fibrous-appearing stroma that contains scattered congested blood vessels. The amount of bone in an individual tumor can be very variable.* **(Right)** *High-power view of the neoplastic bone in fibrous dysplasia shows its composition of woven bone. Sharpey-like collagen fibers of the stroma can be seen extending into the matrix. The fibrous stroma is moderately cellular.*

Fibrous Dysplasia Trabeculae

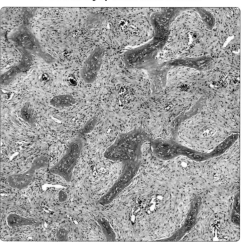

Woven Bone

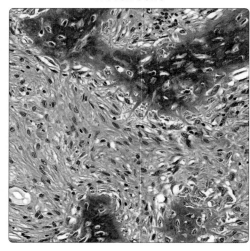

Large Adrenal Nodules

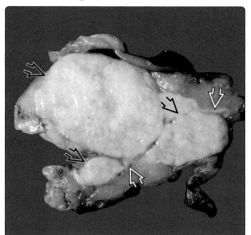

Adrenal Macronodules

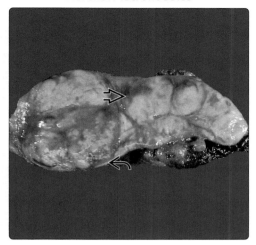

(Left) The cut surface of this adrenal gland shows multiple macronodules ⊡. The residual normal gland ⊡ is often atrophic, resulting in a bimorphic appearance. Hypercortisolism often is a result of macronodular cortical hyperplasia. (Right) ACTH-independent macronodular hyperplasia shows multiple adrenal cortical nodules > 1 cm ⊡. The residual overlying and intervening cortex appears atrophic or normal ⊡.

Adrenal Macronodular Hyperplasia

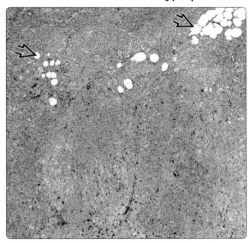

Touch Prep of Pituitary Adenoma

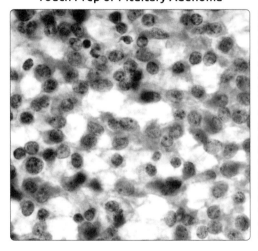

(Left) The macronodules are composed of hypertrophied, globoid, lipid-depleted adrenocortical cells. Lipomatous metaplasia ⊡ may be present in the areas of adrenal cortical hyperplasia. The residual normal gland is often atrophic. (Right) Touch prep of a pituitary adenoma shows uniform cells with round to oval nuclei with delicate chromatin. The pituitary tumors in these patients are usually GH-producing. Acromegaly affects 20-30% of patients with McCune-Albright syndrome (MAS).

Papillary Growth

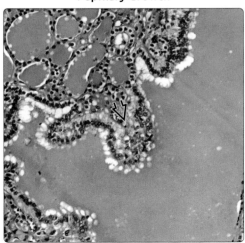

Hyperplastic Thyroid Changes

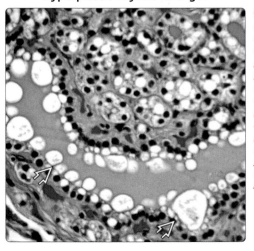

(Left) Hyperthyroidism is the 2nd most common endocrine manifestation in MAS, occurring in as many as 77% of patients with MAS-related goiter. The functioning thyroid nodules usually show intrafollicular centripetal papillary growth ⊡. (Right) Section from the thyroid in a patient with MAS shows multinodular hyperplasia with follicular hyperplasia and marked scalloping of colloid ⊡.

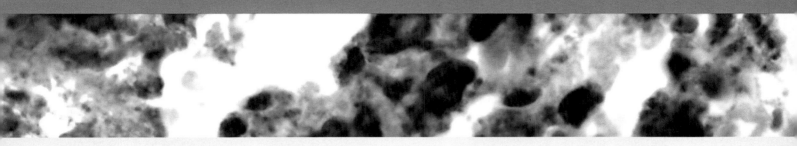

SECTION 8
Paraneoplastic Syndromes

ETIOLOGY/PATHOGENESIS

- Paraneoplastic (ectopic) syndromes are due to production of substances (hormones, growth factors, cytokines, or autoantibodies) by tumor cells, immunologic response to tumor cells, or blockade of hormone effects
  - Signs and symptoms are not due to invasion or mass effect of tumor itself
- Tumors may
  - Secrete hormones in greater quantities (quantitatively abnormal) than corresponding normal cells
  - Produce abnormal hormone product (i.e., precursor) or hormone or amine that corresponding normal tissue does not produce
- Many mechanisms have been suggested for ectopic or excess hormone production, but poorly understood

CLINICAL ISSUES

- Paraneoplastic syndromes may be presenting manifestation of neoplasm (and prompt search for underlying tumor) or may occur late in disease
- Ectopic hormones or substances may be used as markers for effectiveness of treatment and may herald recurrence
- Hypercalcemia is most common paraneoplastic endocrine syndrome
  - Markedly elevated calcium and often recent diagnosis of malignancy (lung, head and neck, skin, esophagus, breast, genitourinary, lymphoma, myeloma)
- Syndrome of inappropriate antidiuretic hormone is 2nd most common paraneoplastic endocrine syndrome
- Other ectopic (paraneoplastic) syndromes include carcinoid syndrome, virilization, Cushing syndrome (ectopic ACTH causes 10-20% of Cushing syndrome), tumor-induced hypoglycemia, among many others

Small Cell Lung Carcinoma

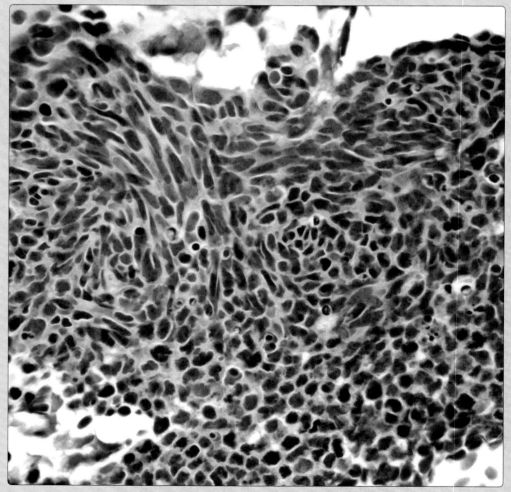

Small cell carcinoma of lung is often associated with paraneoplastic syndromes, such as hypercalcemia, which is the most common paraneoplastic endocrine syndrome.

TERMINOLOGY

Synonyms

- Paraneoplastic endocrine syndrome
- Ectopic hormone production
- Inappropriate hormone production

Definitions

- Paraneoplastic syndrome
  - Signs and symptoms caused by substances (e.g., hormone, growth factors, cytokine, autoantibody, biologically active amine, etc.) produced by tumor cells, immune response to tumor cells, or blockade hormone effects
    - Signs and symptoms are not due to direct invasion or mass effect of tumor

ETIOLOGY/PATHOGENESIS

Abnormal Hormone Production

- Hormone or hormone-like substance can be produced by nonendocrine tumors
- Most bioactive substances ectopically produced are peptides and hormones, but can also be biogenic amines, steroids, and thyroid hormones
- Endocrine tumors can excrete hormones not usually produced by corresponding benign endocrine cells
- Tumors can secrete hormones in greater quantities than corresponding normal cells or abnormal hormone product (i.e., precursor)
- Tumor can produce > 1 hormone
- Tumor can secrete hormones or substances it does not normally secrete (ectopic)
  - With newer testing, many substances thought to be "ectopic" have been identified in corresponding normal tissue
  - Term "ectopic" is now often used for types of hormone production or abnormal production of precursors
  - Symptoms of endocrine paraneoplastic syndromes cannot be attributed to presence of secreting neoplastic lesion related to tumor's anatomic site, and is thus regarded as ectopic
  - Neoplasms without endocrine differentiation may acquire ability to synthesize and secrete bioactive substances

Mechanisms of Ectopic or Excessive Hormone Production

- Many mechanisms suggested for ectopic or excess hormone production, but poorly understood
- Molecular and cytogenetic abnormalities
  - Somatic genetic rearrangements result in growth advantage or abnormal regulation
  - e.g., lung cancer bHLH transcription factor hASH-1 highly expressed, resulting in ectopic adrenocorticotrophic hormone (ACTH)
  - Alterations of gene function may occur under conditions such as neoplastic process that may activate genes regulating hormone synthesis and resulting in endocrine paraneoplastic syndrome
  - Inappropriate gene expression may occur, but mechanism initiating ectopic hormone synthesis and secretion in neoplasia remains unknown
- Cellular dedifferentiation
  - Poorly differentiated malignancies may express substances normally expressed early in development in corresponding tissues
  - Possible that cancer stem cells initiate tumors that express hormones or factors not normally produced by associated tissue type

CLINICAL ISSUES

Presentation

- Paraneoplastic syndromes may be presenting manifestation of neoplasm or may occur late in disease
- Production of hormone or substance significant in associated clinical manifestations and morbidity
- Ectopic hormones or substances may be markers for treatment effectiveness and can herald recurrence
- Prevalence of paraneoplastic syndrome ~ 8% among all malignant neoplasms
- Clinical manifestations may be clinically indistinguishable to those seen when tumor found in expected site of origin (eutopic hormonal secretion), which can cause diagnostic difficulties
- Majority of endocrine paraneoplastic syndromes produced from nonendocrine tumors occur in highly malignant tumors
  - Most commonly: Lung, breast, prostate, ovary, skin, colon, lymphoproliferative
    - However, almost any tumor type can be associated with paraneoplastic syndrome
- Benign and low-grade tumors can also be associated with paraneoplastic syndromes

Treatment

- Remove underlying tumor
- If tumor cannot be removed, treatment may be directed toward inhibiting hormone secretion
  - e.g., bisphosphonates and possibly denosumab may be useful in intractable hypercalcemia
  - Cinacalcet may be helpful in PTHrP-related hypercalcemia

Hypercalcemia

- Most common paraneoplastic endocrine syndrome
- Up to 25% of hospitalized patients with hypercalcemia have underlying malignancy
- Hypercalcemia poor prognostic factor; 30-day mortality up to 50%
- Often recent diagnosis of malignancy and markedly elevated serum calcium
- Tumors: Lung, head and neck, skin, esophagus, breast, genitourinary, lymphoma, myeloma
- Occurs without metastases or altered parathyroid gland function
- Symptomatic when calcium levels markedly elevated
  - Fatigue, dehydration, nephrolithiasis, bone pain, polyuria, nausea, vomiting, confusion, lethargy, coma, death

○ Symptom severity depends on degree of hypercalcemia, speed of onset, and patient's underling renal and neurologic function

- **Humoral hypercalcemia of malignancy**
  ○ Causes 80% of hypercalcemia in malignancy; occurs in 20% of patients with malignancy
  ○ Overproduction of parathyroid hormone-related protein (PTHrP), which acts as circulating humoral factor and also binds parathyroid hormone (PTH) receptor
    - Tissues producing PTHrP in development (skin, marrow, breast) may produce it in malignancy
    - PTHrP also produced by bone metastases
    - Most common with squamous cell carcinomas and squamous cell lung cancer, but can also occur with other tumors such as neuroendocrine tumors of gastrointestinal tract and nonneuroendocrine tumors
    - PTHrP-related hypercalcemia is most common mechanism of endocrine tumor-related hypercalcemia
    - In recent study, 29 colorectal carcinomas with PTHrP-mediated hypercalcemia were associated with advanced metastatic disease, severe hypercalcemia, and high mortality
    - Nonendocrine neoplasia-induced hypercalcemia can occur with breast cancers, testicular malignancies, multiple myeloma, and other lymphoproliferative disorders
  ○ Tumors can produce enzyme to convert 25-hydroxyvitamin D to active 1,25-dihydroxyvitamin D, which can also result in humoral hypercalcemia of malignancy
  ○ *RAS* oncogene mutation can be associated with PTHrP expression
  ○ Features favoring hypercalcemia of malignancy over primary hyperparathyroidism
    - History of malignancy
    - Recent onset hypercalcemia with markedly elevated serum calcium (> 14 mg/dL)
    - Elevated PTHrP (increased in 80% of hypercalcemic patients with malignancy)
    - PTH level suppressed in hypercalcemia of malignancy and elevated in primary hyperparathyroidism
    - Both hypercalcemia of malignancy and primary hyperparathyroidism associated with hypercalciuria and hypophosphatemia
  ○ Ectopic 1,25-dihydroxy(OH)2 vitamin D secretion or ectopic PTC secretion may be associated with hypercalcemia in some lymphomas and neuroendocrine tumors
    - Hypercalcemia from true ectopic PTH secretion is rare
  ○ Granulocyte colony stimulating factor may cause osteoclastic bone resorption or increase in osteoclast progenitors with long-term use and may be associated with hypercalcemia
- **Localized osteolytic hypercalcemia**
  ○ Causes 20% of hypercalcemia of malignancy
- Treatment: Saline, diuretics, bisphosphonates, dialysis or calcitonin in severe hypercalcemia
  ○ Hypercalcemia with hematolymphoid disorders may respond to glucocorticoids
- Prognosis: Median survival of hypercalcemic cancer patients is 1-3 months

Syndrome of Inappropriate Antidiuretic Hormone

- 2nd most common paraneoplastic endocrine syndrome
- 1-2% of patients with malignancies
- Most common with small cell lung cancer, but can occur in large cell lung cancer and prostate cancer, breast cancer, adrenal cancer, and lung carcinoids
- Hypo-osmotic, euvolemic hyponatremia in absence of hypotonicity
- Vasopressin: Antidiuretic hormone abnormally produced by tumor cells, resulting in hyponatremia
  ○ Vasopressin gene becomes activated as does adjacent oxytocin gene
  ○ Relationship between syndrome and ectopic ADH production by tumor cells
- Tumors: Small cell lung (15-50%), carcinoids, other lung cancers, head and neck, central nervous system tumors, gastrointestinal, genitourinary, ovarian tumors
- Most asymptomatic, identified by serum electrolyte
  ○ Symptoms depend on degree and speed of onset of hyponatremia
  ○ Hyponatremia and reduced serum osmolality occur in setting of inappropriately normal or increased urine osmolality
- Exclude other causes of hyponatremia (renal, adrenal, or thyroid insufficiency) and vasopressin stimulation (lung disease, CNS lesions), hypotension, cirrhosis, heart failure, medications
- Symptoms: Fatigue, mental status, weakness, nausea
- SIADH associated with increased central nervous system metastases, poor chemotherapy response and high tumor stage
- Treatment: Remove/treat underlying tumor; monitor fluid intake and correct electrolyte balance, medications to block effects of hormone (demeclocycline), etc.
  ○ ADH receptor agonist raised as possible symptom treatment

Pancreatic Endocrine Tumors

- In addition to histologic classification and stage, pancreatic endocrine tumors are classified by hormonal status
  ○ Insulin-producing (insulinoma), glucagon-producing (glucagonoma), somatostatin-producing (somatostatinoma), and nonfunctioning
  ○ Other ectopic hormones produced
    - ACTH and corticotrophin-releasing hormone (CRH) (Cushing syndrome)
    - Growth hormone (GH) and GHRH (acromegaly)
    - Luteinizing hormone (LH) (oligomenorrhea)
    - Vasoactive intestinal peptide (VIP) (VIPoma, pancreatic cholera)
    - Gastrin (gastrinoma)
- Functional status of pancreatic tumors is based on clinical symptoms caused by inappropriate hormonal secretion, not by immunohistochemical findings
  ○ Hormone causing clinical syndrome can usually be detected by immunohistochemistry
- Many tumors immunophenotypically multihormonal, but only 1 hormone usually associated with patient's symptoms
- Histologic patterns not specific for tumor type, except amyloid (insulinoma) and glandular structures with psammoma bodies (somatostatinoma)

- ○ **Glucagonoma**
  - − Necrolytic migratory erythema: Migratory erythematous maculopapular dermatosis with annular configuration on face, abdomen, thighs, and perianal area
  - − Stomatitis, angular cheilitis, glossitis, diabetes mellitus, weight loss, deep venous thrombosis, and anemia as well

Carcinoid Syndrome

- Well-differentiated neuroendocrine tumors, particularly those metastatic to liver, are associated with carcinoid syndrome
- Bronchospasm, right-sided cardiac fibrosis with tricuspid stenosis and regurgitation, and watery diarrhea
- Cutaneous features: Intense flushing of face, neck, chest, abdomen; telangiectasias
  - ○ Scleroderma-like skin changes and pellagra-type of dermatitis due to serotonin

Virilization (Androgens)

- Tumors: Adrenal carcinomas, ovarian tumors, polycystic ovaries, congenital adrenal hyperplasia
- Symptoms and signs: Virilization, acne, hirsutism, hyperpigmentation, androgenic alopecia

Gynecomastia or Precocious Puberty (Estrogens)

- Tumors: Ovarian & testicular tumors
- Gynecomastia in males; precocious puberty in females

Acromegaly (GH and GHRH)

- Tumors: Pituitary adenomas, lung cancer, pancreatic neuroendocrine tumors, lymphoma
  - ○ But acromegaly unrelated to pituitary growth hormone-secreting adenoma is very rare (< 1% of acromegaly)
  - ○ Most GHRH-secreting tumors are neuroendocrine tumors, usually well differentiated, and most often from pancreas or bronchus
- Symptoms and signs: Thick skin, coarse facial features, hypertrichosis, hyperpigmentation, macroglossia
- Tumors often large and easily localized with normal imaging of pituitary; plasma measurement of GHRH very helpful

Cushing Syndrome (ACTH and CRH)

- Ectopic ACTH causes 10-20% of Cushing syndrome
  - ○ Increased/abnormal expression of proopiomelanocortin (*POMC*) gene encodes ACTH and melanocyte-stimulating hormone, resulting in excess glucocorticoids and mineralocorticoids
- Tumors: Small cell lung cancer and bronchial carcinoids (> 50%), thymic carcinoid (15%), pancreatic neuroendocrine tumors, bronchial carcinoids, medullary thyroid carcinoma, pheochromocytoma, gastrointestinal, head and neck, ovary, prostate, among others
- ACTH-independent Cushing syndrome can be caused by ectopic G protein-coupled receptors
  - ○ Gastric inhibitory peptide → adrenal cortex → glucocorticoid
- Rarely, corticotropin-releasing hormone (CRH) is produced by pancreatic neuroendocrine tumors, lung cancer, medullary thyroid cancer, carcinoid, or prostate cancer
  - ○ Increased CRH → pituitary corticotrope hyperplasia → Cushing syndrome
- Clinical manifestations
  - ○ Most ectopic ACTH production asymptomatic
  - ○ Weight gain and fat redistribution (often less due to associated cachexia of malignancy)
  - ○ Increased pigmentation (due to MSH), skin fragility and easy bruisability
  - ○ Fluid retention, hypertension, hypokalemia, metabolic alkalosis, glucose intolerance, elevated urine free cortisol, and ectopic ACTH
- Treatment: Remove underlying malignancy, reduce cortisol levels

Tumor-Induced Hypoglycemia Caused by Excess Production of IGF2

- Rare
- Caused by insulin-producing non-islet cell tumors and tumors secreting substances that can cause hypoglycemia by means other than insulin
- Insulin-like growth factor 2 (IGF2) precursor binds IGF1 receptors and insulin receptors → insulin-like effect → hypoglycemia
  - ○ Methylation and loss of imprinting *IGF2* gene (11p15) suggested mechanism for induction *IGF2* gene expression
  - ○ Serum IGF2 levels may not be elevated as precursor may not be identified by IGF2 assays
    - − But increased protein identified in tumors
  - ○ Also, reduced IGF binding protein 3 and other substances that sequester IGF2 are decreased
- Clinical: Symptoms of hypoglycemia with fasting (low serum glucose, suppressed insulin levels)
- Tumors: Sarcomas (leiomyosarcoma, fibrosarcoma, etc.), hemangiopericytoma, hepatocellular, adrenal, mesothelioma, carcinoid, lymphoma/leukemia
- Treatment: Remove underlying malignancy; frequent meals and IV glucose or glucagon or glucocorticoids to increase glucose

Osteogenic Osteomalacia (Tumor-Induced Osteomalacia)

- Fibroblast growth factor 23 (FGF23, phosphatonin circulating phosphaturic factor) inhibits renal reabsorption of phosphate and conversion of 25-hydroxyvitamin D to 1,25-dihydroxyvitamin D
- Synonyms: Tumor-induced osteomalacia, hypophosphatemic oncogenic osteomalacia
- Laboratory: Decreased serum phosphorus, renal phosphate wasting, normal serum calcium, normal PTH, low 1,25-dihydroxyvitamin D
- Mesenchymal tumors (hemangiopericytomas, giant cell tumors, sarcomas), lung and prostate cancers
- Treatment: Remove tumor, supplement phosphate and vitamin D

Human Chorionic Gonadotropin

- Tumors: Lung, ovary, testicular, germ cell, prostate, breast, adrenal, bladder, liver, and pancreatic neuroendocrine; osteosarcoma, etc.
- Females often asymptomatic, males precocious puberty or gynecomastia

Calcitonin and Calcitonin Gene-Related Peptide

- Tumors: Medullary thyroid (eutopic), also ectopic expression in pancreatic endocrine tumors, adrenal cortical tumors, pheochromocytoma, small cell, breast, gastrointestinal, renal, and prostate cancer
- No well-defined clinical syndrome

Ectopic Renin

- Rare
- Paragangliomas, carcinoids, small cell lung cancer, and very rare reports of desmoplastic small round cell tumor, lung cancer
- May cause hypertensive paraneoplastic syndrome
- Treat underlying tumor; antihypertensives, spironolactone, etc.; may be symptomatically helpful

Ectopic Gonadotrophin

- Rare
- Follicle stimulating hormone: Ovarian hyperstimulation syndrome
- Luteinizing hormone: Resemble polycystic ovarian disease

Ectopic B-Human Chorionic Gonadotrophin

- Rare
- Gynecomastia in men; virilization and menstrual irregularity in women; precocious puberty in children
- Small cell lung cancer, lung carcinoids, extragonadal germ cell tumors

MICROSCOPIC

Histologic Features

- Individual tumors generally cannot predict if that individual tumor will be associated with paraneoplastic endocrine syndrome
- Some tumors (small cell carcinoma, squamous cell carcinoma, etc.) more commonly associated with paraneoplastic endocrine syndromes

SELECTED REFERENCES

1. Abubakar S et al: Source of ectopic ACTH secretion easily identified by 68 Ga DOTANOC PET/CT. Clin Nucl Med. 42(4):295-296, 2017
2. Dimitriadis GK et al: Paraneoplastic endocrine syndromes. Endocr Relat Cancer. 24(6):R173-R190, 2017
3. Elston M et al: Severe Cushing's syndrome due to small cell prostate carcinoma - a case and review of literature. Endocr Connect. ePub, 2017
4. Zhang HY et al: Ectopic Cushing syndrome in small cell lung cancer: A case report and literature review. Thorac Cancer. 8(2):114-117, 2017
5. Galindo RJ et al: Hypercalcemia of malignancy and colorectal cancer. World J Oncol. 7(1):5-12, 2016
6. Kamp K et al: Prevalence and clinical features of the ectopic ACTH syndrome in patients with gastroenteropancreatic and thoracic neuroendocrine tumors. Eur J Endocrinol. 174(3):271-80, 2016
7. Murakami K et al: Pancreatic solitary fibrous tumor causing ectopic adrenocorticotropic hormone syndrome. Mol Cell Endocrinol. 436:268-73, 2016
8. Owen CE: Cutaneous manifestations of lung cancer. Semin Oncol. 43(3):366-9, 2016
9. Kunc M et al: Paraneoplastic syndromes in olfactory neuroblastoma. Contemp Oncol (Pozn). 19(1):6-16, 2015
10. Maragliano R et al: ACTH-secreting pancreatic neoplasms associated with Cushing syndrome: clinicopathologic study of 11 cases and review of the literature. Am J Surg Pathol. 39(3):374-82, 2015
11. Santhanam P et al: PET imaging in ectopic Cushing syndrome: a systematic review. Endocrine. ePub, 2015
12. Sternlicht H et al: Hypercalcemia of malignancy and new treatment options. Ther Clin Risk Manag. 11:1779-88, 2015
13. van Raalte DH et al: Sarcoidosis-related hypercalcaemia due to production of parathyroid hormone-related peptide. BMJ Case Rep. 2015, 2015
14. Witek P et al: Ectopic Cushing's syndrome in light of modern diagnostic techniques and treatment options. Neuro Endocrinol Lett. 36(3):201-8, 2015
15. Ferone D et al: Ectopic Cushing and other paraneoplastic syndromes in thoracic neuroendocrine tumors. Thorac Surg Clin. 24(3):277-83, 2014
16. Iglesias P et al: Management of endocrine disease: a clinical update on tumor-induced hypoglycemia. Eur J Endocrinol. 170(4):R147-57, 2014
17. Johnston PC et al: Ectopic ACTH-secreting pituitary adenomas within the sphenoid sinus. Endocrine. 47(3):717-24, 2014
18. Borson-Chazot F et al: Acromegaly induced by ectopic secretion of GHRH: a review 30 years after GHRH discovery. Ann Endocrinol (Paris). 73(6):497-502, 2012
19. Neary NM et al: Neuroendocrine ACTH-producing tumor of the thymus—experience with 12 patients over 25 years. J Clin Endocrinol Metab. 97(7):2223-30, 2012
20. Pelosof LC et al: Paraneoplastic syndromes: an approach to diagnosis and treatment. Mayo Clin Proc. 2010 Sep;85(9):838-54. Review. Erratum in: Mayo Clin Proc. 86(4):364, 2011
21. Yeung SC et al: Lung cancer-induced paraneoplastic syndromes. Curr Opin Pulm Med. 17(4):260-8, 2011
22. Chapireau D et al: Paraneoplastic syndromes in patients with primary oral cancers: a systematic review. Br J Oral Maxillofac Surg. 48(5):338-44, 2010
23. Kaltsas G et al: Paraneoplastic syndromes secondary to neuroendocrine tumours. Endocr Relat Cancer. 17(3):R173-93, 2010
24. Oberg K: Pancreatic endocrine tumors. Semin Oncol. 37(6):594-618, 2010
25. Shanbhogue AK et al: Clinical syndromes associated with ovarian neoplasms: a comprehensive review. Radiographics. 30(4):903-19, 2010
26. Müssig K et al: Syndrome of inappropriate antidiuretic hormone secretion and ectopic ACTH production in small cell lung carcinoma. Lung Cancer. 57(1):120-2, 2007
27. DeLellis RA et al: Paraneoplastic endocrine syndromes: a review. Endocr Pathol. 14(4):303-17, 2003
28. Kaltsas G et al: Paraneoplastic syndromes related to Neuroendorine Tumours 2000
29. Wajchenberg BL et al: Ectopic ACTH syndrome. J Steroid Biochem Mol Biol. 53(1-6):139-51, 1995

Paraneoplastic Endocrine Syndromes

Syndrome	Hormone, Cytokine, or Substance	Tumors	Symptoms and Signs
Hypercalcemia	Parathyroid hormone releasing hormone, vitamin D, interleukins, parathyroid hormone	Squamous cell lung and head and neck, small cell lung, genitourinary, gastrointestinal, lymphoma, myeloma, etc.	Fatigue, mental status change, dehydration, nephrolithiasis, bone pain, polyuria, nausea, vomiting, confusion, lethargy, coma
Syndrome of inappropriate antidiuretic hormone (SIADH)	Vasopressin	Small cell lung, carcinoids, other lung cancers, head and neck cancers, central nervous system tumors, gastrointestinal, genitourinary, ovarian cancers	Usually asymptomatic, fatigue, mental status, weakness, nausea
Carcinoid syndrome	Serotonin	Pancreatic or gastrointestinal neuroendocrine tumors (particularly those metastatic to liver)	Bronchospasm, watery diarrhea, right-sided cardiac fibrosis, scleroderma, and pellagra-like skin
Virilization	Androgens	Adrenal carcinomas, ovarian tumors, polycystic ovaries, congenital adrenal hyperplasia	Virilization, acne, hirsutism, hyperpigmentation
Gynecomastia in males, precocious puberty in females	Estrogen	Ovarian and testicular tumors	Gynecomastia in males, precocious puberty in females
Acromegaly	GH, GHRH	Pituitary tumors, pancreatic endocrine tumors, gastrointestinal endocrine tumors, lung, lymphoma	Thick skin, coarse facial features, hypertrichosis, hyperpigmentation, macroglossia
Cushing syndrome	Corticotropin (ACTH), corticotropin-releasing hormone (CRH)	Small cell lung, lung and other carcinoids, pheochromocytomas, medullary thyroid carcinomas, rarely other nonneuroendocrine tumors	Weight gain, fat redistribution, fluid retention, hypertension, hypokalemia, metabolic alkalosis, glucose intolerance, increased pigmentation
Osteogenic osteomalacia	Fibroblast growth factor 23	Phosphaturic mesenchymal tumor, lung carcinoma, prostate carcinoma	Osteomalacia, fractures, muscle weakness
Hypoglycemia	Insulin-like growth factor 2 (IGF2) (precursor)	Sarcomas (leiomyosarcoma, fibrosarcoma, etc.), adrenocortical carcinomas, hepatocellular carcinomas, mesotheliomas, carcinoid tumors, lymphoma, and leukemia	Symptoms of hypoglycemia with fasting (faintness, dizziness, fatigue, etc.)
Necrolytic migratory erythema	Glucagon	Pancreatic glucagon-producing neuroendocrine tumor (rarely extrapancreatic)	Necrolytic migratory erythema, stomatitis, angular cheilitis, glossitis, diabetes mellitus, weight loss, deep venous thrombosis, and anemia
Pancreatic cholera syndrome	Vasoactive intestinal peptide (VIP)	Pancreatic endocrine tumors, small cell lung, neuroblastoma, ganglioneuroma, medullary thyroid	Marked diarrhea

ACTH = adrenocorticotrophic hormone; GH = growth hormone; GHRH = growth hormone receptor hormone.

(Left) *Small cell neuroendocrine carcinoma of the lung is often associated with paraneoplastic syndromes such hypercalcemia, and is the most common tumor associated with syndrome of inappropriate antidiuretic hormone secretion.* **(Right)** *Small cell carcinoma can be associated with hypercalcemia of malignancy, syndrome of inappropriate antidiuretic hormone, Cushing syndrome, acromegaly, gynecomastia, among other syndromes.*

Small Cell Lung Carcinoma

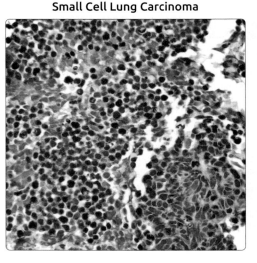

Small Cell Lung Carcinoma

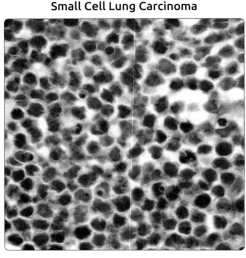

(Left) *Squamous cell carcinomas of the lung and head and neck may be associated hypercalcemia of malignancy due to overproduction of parathyroid hormone-related protein.* **(Right)** *Squamous cell carcinomas of the lung and head and neck often produce parathyroid hormone-related, protein-related hypercalcemia as well as syndrome of inappropriate antidiuretic hormone.*

Squamous Cell Carcinoma

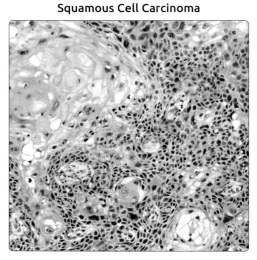

Squamous Cell Carcinoma

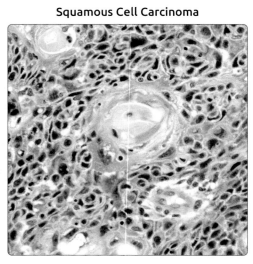

(Left) *Breast cancer can be associated with ectopic (paraneoplastic) syndromes such as hypercalcemia.* **(Right)** *Hypercalcemia associated with breast cancer is common.*

Breast Carcinoma

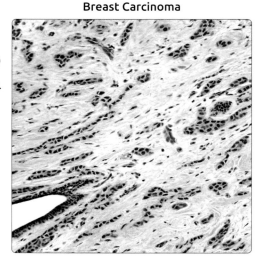

Breast Carcinoma

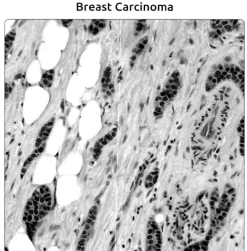

Well-Differentiated Neuroendocrine Carcinoma of Gastrointestinal Tract

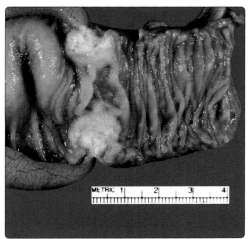

Well-Differentiated Neuroendocrine Carcinoma

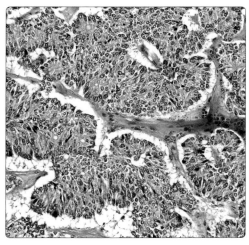

(Left) *Well-differentiated neuroendocrine (carcinoid) carcinoma is shown involving the gastrointestinal tract.* (Right) *Well-differentiated neuroendocrine (carcinoid) carcinoma shows nested and partially trabecular growth pattern of cells with neuroendocrine stippled chromatin.*

Metastatic Well-Differentiated Neuroendocrine Carcinoma to Liver

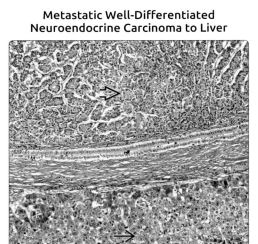

Neuroendocrine Carcinoma of Pancreas

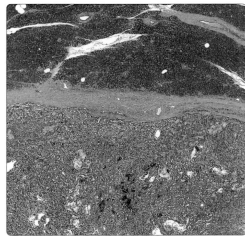

(Left) *Metastatic well-differentiated neuroendocrine carcinoma ⊡ to the liver ⊡ may be associated with carcinoid syndrome. Serotonin and other amines are responsible for the carcinoid syndrome in patients who develop extensive liver metastases, which inhibit the capacity of the liver to rapidly inactivate serotonin and tachykinins.* (Right) *Pancreatic neuroendocrine tumors may be classified by clinical hormonal status. These tumors can also produce ectopic hormones.*

Neuroendocrine Carcinoma of Pancreas

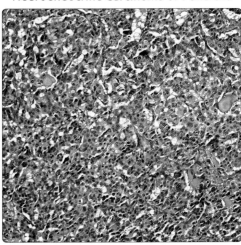

Neuroendocrine Carcinoma of Pancreas

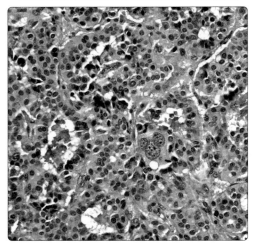

(Left) *Functional status of pancreatic neuroendocrine tumors is based on clinical symptoms caused by inappropriate hormonal secretion, not by immunohistochemical findings.* (Right) *Neuroendocrine carcinomas of the pancreas can produce excess hormones, such as insulin, glucagon, somatostatin, or be nonfunctioning. They can also produce ectopic hormones such as ACTH, growth hormone, luteinizing hormone, vasoactive intestinal peptide, and gastrin.*

(Left) *Pancreatic endocrine tumors can produce a variety of hormones, eutopic and ectopic. The functional classification of a pancreatic neuroendocrine tumor is based on the hormone being produced clinically and not on immunohistochemical identification.* **(Right)** *Malignant lymphoma can be associated with hypercalcemia of malignancy and with other paraneoplastic disorders such as hypoglycemia with insulin-like growth factor II and acromegaly with growth hormone production.*

Glucagon Immunostain in Glucagonoma

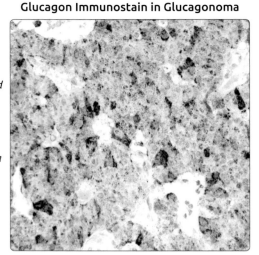

Malignant Lymphoma

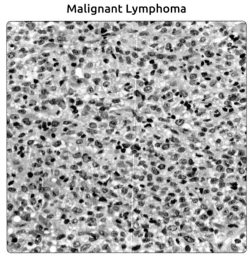

(Left) *Myeloma can be associated with hypercalcemia of malignancy. This is usually PTHrP-associated hypercalcemia.* **(Right)** *PTHrP-mediated hypercalcemia can occur in colorectal carcinoma and adenosquamous carcinoma of the colon and rectum. The syndrome of inappropriate antidiuretic secretion, gynecomastia (HPL) and ectopic calcitonin production have also been reported.*

Multiple Myeloma

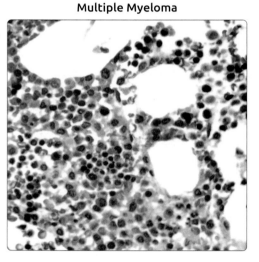

Colorectal Carcinoma

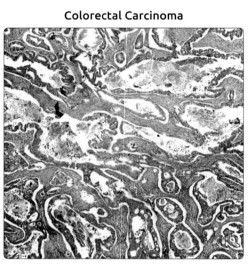

(Left) *Patients with PTHrP-mediated hypercalcemia in the setting of a colorectal malignancy were found to have advanced metastatic cancer, severe hypercalcemia, and high mortality.* **(Right)** *Thymoma can be associated with paraneoplastic syndromes associated with auto-antibodies and can be associated with hypercalcemia of malignancy.*

Colorectal Carcinoma

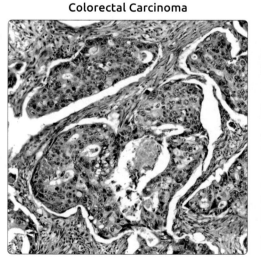

Thymoma

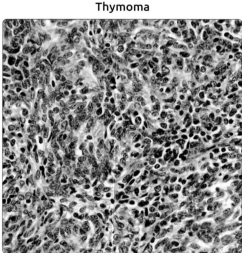

Adrenal Cortical Carcinoma

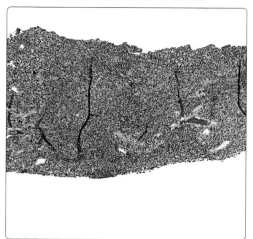

Adrenal Cortical Carcinoma

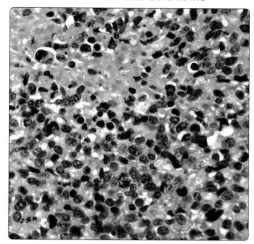

(Left) *Adrenocortical carcinoma is associated with hormonal secretion in ~ 45-49% of cases. Patients may experience hypercortisolism, virilization, adrenogenital syndrome, feminization, hyperaldosteronism, or precocious puberty.* (Right) *Patients with adrenal cortical carcinoma often experience symptoms caused by excess hormone secretion.*

Medullary Thyroid Carcinoma

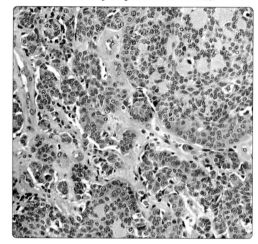

Medullary Thyroid Carcinoma

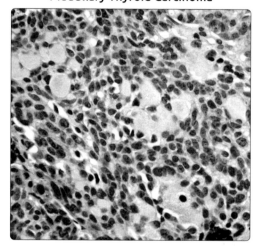

(Left) *Medullary thyroid carcinomas are associated with increased calcitonin, but it is not associated with specific paraneoplastic features. Medullary thyroid carcinomas can have ectopic production of other substances.* (Right) *Medullary thyroid carcinoma can be associated with ectopic production of ACTH and VIP.*

Non-Small Cell Lung Cancer

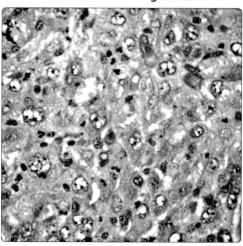

Pheochromocytoma

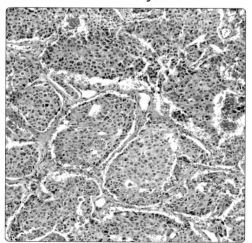

(Left) *Although small cell lung cancers are often associated with ectopic paraneoplastic syndromes, non-small cell lung cancer can be associated with hypertension (renin), gynecomastia (HPL or hCG), and acromegaly (GH). Squamous cell and small cell lung carcinomas are not infrequently associated with hypercalcemia.* (Right) *On rare occasion, pheochromocytoma can ectopically produce adrenocorticotropic hormone or corticotropin-releasing hormone and be associated with Cushing syndrome.*

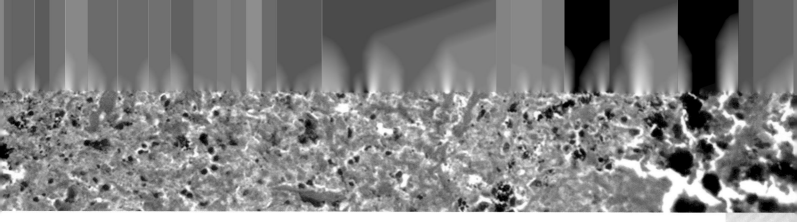

INDEX

D

I

L

N

R

U

V

W

X

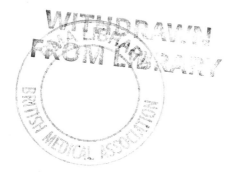

WITHDRAWN
FROM LIBRARY

BMA LIBRARY

BRITISH MEDICAL ASSOCIATION